Neuro-ophthalmology

Third Edition

Neuro-ophthalmology

Third Edition

Edited by

Joel S. Glaser, M.D.

Professor
Departments of Neurology and Ophthalmology
Bascom Palmer Eye Institute
University of Miami School of Medicine, Miami;
and
Consultant in Neuro-ophthalmology
Cleveland Clinic Florida
Ft. Lauderdale, Florida

with 20 contributors

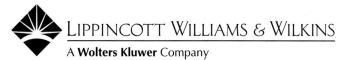

LIPPINCOTT WILLIAMS & WILKINS
A **Wolters Kluwer** Company
Philadelphia · Baltimore · New York · London
Buenos Aires · Hong Kong · Sydney · Tokyo

Acquisitions Editor: Paula Callaghan
Developmental Editor: Delois Patterson
Manufacturing Manager: Tim Reynolds
Production Manager: Liane Carita
Production Editor: Jeffrey Gruenglas
Cover Designer: Patty Gast
Indexer: Mary Kidd
Compositor: Bi-Comp Inc.
Printer: Edwards Brothers

Printed in the United States of America

9 8 7 6 5 4 3 2 1

Library of Congress Cataloging-in-Publication Data
Neuro-ophthalmology / edited by Joel S. Glaser ; with 20 contributors.
  — 3rd ed.
     p.   cm.
  Includes bibliographical references and index.
  ISBN 0-7817-1729-9
  1. Neuro-ophthalmology.   I. Glaser, Joel S., 1938–   .
  [DNLM: 1. Eye—innervation. 2. Eye Diseases.   WW 101 N494 1999]
  RE725.N4568 1999
  617.7—DC21
  DNLM/DLC   99-24157
  for Library of Congress   CIP

Neuro-ophthalmology is included (first section, Volume 2) in *Clinical Ophthalmology,* a six-
volume looseleaf series edited by William Tasman, M.D., and Edward Jaeger, M.D., published
by Lippincott Williams & Wilkins.

Contents

Contributors vii

Preface ix

Preface to the Second Edition xi

Preface to the First Edition xiii

1. The Neuro-ophthalmologic Case History: Elucidating the Symptoms 1
   Frederick E. Lepore

2. Neuro-ophthalmologic Examination: The Visual Sensory System 7
   Barry Skarf, Joel S. Glaser, Gary L. Trick, and Erkan Mutlukan

3. Neuro-ophthalmologic Examination: General Considerations and
   Special Techniques 51
   Joel S. Glaser

4. Anatomy of the Visual Sensory System 75
   Joel S. Glaser and Alfredo A. Sadun

5. Topical Diagnosis: Prechiasmal Visual Pathways
   Part I. The Retina 95
   Part II. The Optic Nerve 118
   Joel S. Glaser

6. Topical Diagnosis: The Optic Chiasm 199
   Joel S. Glaser

7. Retrochiasmal Visual Pathways and Higher Cortical Function 239
   Matthew Rizzo and Jason J. S. Barton

8. The Facial Nerve and Related Disorders of the Face 293
   Steven L. Galetta and Mark May

9. Eye Movement Characteristics and Recording Techniques 327
   Louis F. Dell'Osso and Robert B. Daroff

10. Supranuclear Disorders of Eye Movements 345
    R. John Leigh, Robert B. Daroff, and B. Todd Troost

11. Nystagmus and Saccadic Intrusions and Oscillations 369
    Louis F. Dell'Osso and Robert B. Daroff

    Glossary (Chapters 9 through 11) 402

12. Infranuclear Disorders of Eye Movement 405
    Joel S. Glaser and R. Michael Siatkowski

13. Pediatric Neuro-ophthalmology: General Considerations and Congenital Motor and Sensory Anomalies 461
R. Michael Siatkowski and Joel S. Glaser

14. Orbital Disease and Neuro-ophthalmology
Part I: An Overview 489
Joel S. Glaser

Part II: Surgery of the Orbit and Optic Nerve 509
David T. Tse and Warren J. Chang

15. The Pupils and Accommodation 527
Thomas L. Slamovits and Joel S. Glaser

16. Migraine and Other Headaches 553
B. Todd Troost

17. Aneurysms, Arteriovenous Communications, and Related Vascular Malformations 589
B. Todd Troost, Joel S. Glaser, and P. Pearse Morris

18. The Dizzy Patient: Disturbances of the Vestibular System 629
Ronald J. Tusa

Subject Index 647

Color Plates
5–1 between pages 146 and 147
5–2 between pages 146 and 147
5–3 between pages 146 and 147
5–4 between pages 146 and 147
7–1 between pages 274 and 275
7–2 between pages 274 and 275

Contributors

Jason J. S. Barton, M.D., Ph.D., F.R.C.P. *Assistant Professor, Departments of Neurology and Ophthalmology, Beth Israel Deaconess Medical Center; and Harvard Medical School, Boston, Massachusetts*

Warren J. Chang, M.D. *Professor, Bascom Palmer Eye Institute, University of Miami School of Medicine, Miami, Florida*

Robert B. Daroff, M.D. *Professor and Associate Dean, Department of Neurology, Case Western Reserve University; and Chief of Staff and Senior Vice-President for Medical Affairs, University Hospitals of Cleveland, Cleveland, Ohio*

Louis F. Dell'Osso, Ph.D. *Professor, Departments of Neurology and Biomedical Engineering, Schools of Medicine and Engineering, Case Western Reserve University; and Director, Ocular Motor Neurophysiology Laboratory, Veterans Administration Medical Center, Cleveland, Ohio*

Steven L. Galetta, M.D. *Van Meter Professor of Neurology, Department of Neurology; and Director, Division of Neuro-ophthalmology, University of Pennsylvania Medical Center, Philadelphia, Pennsylvania*

Joel S. Glaser, M.D. *Professor, Departments of Neurology and Ophthalmology, Bascom Palmer Eye Institute, University of Miami School of Medicine, Miami; and Consultant in Neuro-ophthalmology, Cleveland Clinic Florida, Ft. Lauderdale, Florida*

R. John Leigh, M.D. *Professor, Department of Neurology, Case Western Reserve University; and Neurology Service, Veterans Affairs Medical Center, Cleveland, Ohio*

Frederick E. Lepore, M.D. *Professor, Departments of Neurology and Ophthalmology; and Attending Physician, Department of Neurology, Robert Wood Johnson University Hospital, New Brunswick, New Jersey*

Mark May, M.D. *Clinical Professor (Emeritus), Department of Otolaryngology, Head, and Neck Surgery, University of Pittsburgh, Pittsburgh, Pennsylvania*

P. Pearse Morris, M.B., B.Ch., B.A.O. *Interventional Neuroradiologist, Department of Ophthalmology, Wake Forest University School of Medicine, Winston-Salem, North Carolina*

Erkan Mutlukan, M.D. *Fellow, Glaucoma Service, Wills Eye Hospital, Philadelphia, Pennsylvania*

Matthew Rizzo, M.D. *Professor, Departments of Neurology and Engineering; and Visual Function Laboratory, Division of Behavioral Neurology and Cognitive Neuroscience, University of Iowa College of Medicine, Iowa City, Iowa*

Alfredo A. Sadun, M.D., Ph.D. *Professor, Departments of Ophthalmology and Neurosurgery, University of Southern California; and Professor and Vice-Chairman for Education, Department of Ophthalmology, Doheny Eye Institute, Los Angeles, California*

R. Michael Siatkowski, M.D. *Assistant Professor, Department of Ophthalmology, Dean A. McGee Eye Institute, University of Oklahoma, Oklahoma City, Oklahoma*

Barry Skarf, M.D., Ph.D. *Adjunct Associate Professor, Department of Ophthalmology, University of Toronto; and Director, Neuro-ophthalmology Unit, Eye Care Services, Henry Ford Health Sciences Center, Detroit, Michigan*

Thomas L. Slamovits, M.D. *Professor and Vice Chairman, Departments of Ophthalmology, Neurology, and Neurosurgery, Albert Einstein College of Medicine/Montefiore Medical Center, Bronx, New York*

Gary L. Trick, M.D. *Associate Professor, Department of Ophthalmology, Case Western Reserve University, Cleveland, Ohio; and Senior Scientist, Department of Eye Care Services, Henry Ford Hospital, Detroit, Michigan*

B. Todd Troost, M.D. *Professor and Chair, Department of Neurology, Wake Forest University School of Medicine; and Chief, Department of Neurology, North Carolina Baptist Hospital, Winston-Salem, North Carolina*

David T. Tse, M.D. *Professor, Bascom Palmer Eye Institute, University of Miami School of Medicine, Miami, Florida*

Ronald J. Tusa, M.D., Ph.D. *Professor, Department of Neurology, Bascom Palmer Eye Institute; and Dizziness and Eye Movement Center, Department of Neuro-ophthalmology, Anne Bates Leach Hospital, Miami, Florida*

Preface

This third edition of *Neuro-ophthalmology* appears some two decades after publication of the first. As the page of the century turns we reflect that the discipline of neuro-ophthalmology continues to expand rather than retract, inarguably spurred by the spectacular newer techniques of neuroimaging, genetics, and immunology. And if these innovations of the passing century are viewed as entirely remarkable, how much more so will be the advent of radiologic, genetic, and immunologic interventions in the century to come.

This edition is enlarged by the considerable contributions of visual physiologists, interventional radiologists, and authorities on that unique character of Man: higher cortical functions. The sections concerned with the afferent visual pathways, the retina, and the optic nerve are enlarged, and pediatric neuro-ophthalmology is thoroughly renovated. A chapter dealing with vestibular disorders is a vital addition.

It is the intent that the contents of this single volume of work continue to provide a sound foundation for accurate diagnosis and proper management of the great majority of conditions and disorders, not only within the purview of neuro-ophthalmologists but also encompassed by broader categories of patients attended by ophthalmologists, neurologists, neurologic surgeons, and otologists—especially for young physicians training in these specialities. Again, the pragmatic is stressed over exoticisms, and newer references and subject reviews are cited in preference to ancient (if classic) but often inaccessible publications. As in the game of poker, it is often more important to know what to *discard*, and the volume's Editor takes responsibility for any flagrant errors of omission.

I take the liberty of dedicating this small work in remembrance of Irena, my wife and greatest teacher; and to Larah, Benjamin, and Jacob, from whom I will no longer steal time.

Joel S. Glaser, M.D.

Preface to the Second Edition

The eyes reflect a true picture of the measure of body strength, providing that vision and lid opening are normal.

Medical Aphorisms of Maimonides
Moshe ben Maimon (1135–1204)

The subject matter that compromises the discipline of neuro-ophthalmology continues to evolve in several directions, the most notable of which is surely the clinical impact of neuro-imaging procedures, specifically the advent of magnetic resonance imaging. And, though this is not a text of neuro-radiology, this second edition does bear the imprint of at least the salient features of current imaging techniques. We are interested here more in the rational and judicious application of such studies in clinical diagnosis rather than in the specifics of radiologic analysis.

As with the previous edition, an attempt is made to assimilate important and frequently encountered clinical problems, but not to ignore the rare or fascinating, in the comprehensive overview of our subject. Hopefully, the reader will excuse the absence of much discussion of experimental investigations and will pardon the inclusion of a modicum of visual and ocular motor physiology that has more or less direct pragmatic application.

This volume is enriched by the considerable efforts of fourteen knowledgeable contributing authors, including seven neurologists, five ophthalmologists, and an otorhinolaryngologist. This diverse assembly reflects the spectrum of disorders and ailments encountered under the aegis of neuro-ophthalmology and also attests to the extensive overlapping of these medical and surgical domains.

We recognize with genuine empathy our long-suffering patients, from whose unfortunate illnesses flow the science of art of our vocation. Also I should like to dedicate this small work to the memory of my father and teacher, Dr. Benjamin Glaser, who took exceptional care and concern for his patients throughout a lifetime of medical practice.

Joel S. Glaser, M.D.
1990

Preface to the First Edition

Knowledge is of two kinds. We know a subject ourselves, or we know where we can find information upon it.

SAMUEL JOHNSON (1775)

Among medical practitioners, the ophthalmologist should be most capable of evaluating the visual sensory and ocular motor systems. He has at his disposal specialized techniques and apparatus with which to make accurate observations and measurements, and this art is in no situation more critically relevant than in the diagnosis of neuro-ophthalmologic disorders. Certainly the ophthalmologist should be more expert in analyzing disorders of ocular motility than is the neurologist, and more adept in meaningful pronouncements on the appearance of optic discs than is the neurosurgeon. Basically, it is far more practical for the ophthalmologist to familiarize himself with a modicum of neuroanatomy and neurologic disorders, than for his colleagues in neurology and neurosurgery to become proficient in the use of ophthalmologic instruments. Yet the truly competent physicians in these related specialities have managed to bridge apparent clinical gaps and have come to appreciate the multitude of diseases that form the foundation for the discipline of neuro-ophthalmology.

There is ample historic precedent for the intimate rapport between ophthalmology and the neurologic specialities. In the United States, ophthalmology owes a debt to the renowned neurosurgeon Harvey Cushing for stimulating interest in investigation of the visual fields. Cushing emphasized the major role that perimetry should play in the localization of intracranial lesions involving the visual pathways. During that same decade in Germany, the ophthalmologist Wilbrand and the neurologist Saenger produced an epic 10-volume work in neuro-ophthalmology, *Die Neurologie des Auges* (1917).

During World War I, the British neurologist Gordon Holmes utilized cases of cerebral gunshot wounds to conceptualize the topographic representation of the retina on the cortex. A major contribution to visual field studies followed in 1927 when the Scots ophthalmologist Traquair published *An Introduction to Clinical Perimetry,* a classic work which helped transform perimetry from the realm of special studies to ordinary clinical practice. Von Graefe, decades before, had emphasized the practical value of visual field testing, and his publications on that subject appeared concurrently with the introduction of opthalmoscopy.

Neuro-ophthalmology is not a clinical discipline *sui generis*: It belongs to the greater body of ophthalmology. In fact, it is one of the oldest fields of specialized knowledge within the parent speciality. Neurologic diagnosis in ophthalmology requires a passing familiarity with neuroanatomy, an understanding of the disease processes that affect the ocular motor and visual sensory systems, the training to competently examine such patients, and the experience to effectively utilize additional laboratory and radiologic studies. For the trainee in ophthalmology, to set more myopic goals is a disadvantage to himself and an injustice to his patients.

It is beyond the scope of this present work to cover in minute detail the voluminous material pertaining to neuro-ophthalmology. I have endeavored instead to cover basic topics with reasonable completeness and in sufficient depth to enable the student to attain a substantial foundation and to provide for the practitioner an available source of reference. The subjects herein discussed have for the most part passed the tests of pragmatism and are applicable within the confines of office practice. Reference material reflects a bias toward clinically important current information or reviews, or classic publications in the English language. Certain topics have been discussed at length, in the absence of accessible and adequate coverage elsewhere in the neuro-ophthalmologic literature.

xiii

I would like to recognize the substantial contributions of Doctors Robert B. Daroff, B. Todd Troost, and Louis F. Dell'Osso in the preparation of those chapters related to the ocular motor system. Moreover, if this text has merit it reflects the influence of three men who are my patient teachers, generous colleagues, and warm friends: Edward Norton and Lawton Smith of the Bascom Palmer Eye Institute, Miami, and William Hoyt of the University of California, San Francisco.

Joel S. Glaser, M.D.
1977

Neuro-ophthalmology

Third Edition

CHAPTER 1

The Neuro-ophthalmologic Case History: Elucidating the Symptoms

Frederick E. Lepore

An Overview
Afferent Visual Symptoms
  Visual Loss Arising from Structures Anterior to the
    Optic Nerve

Visual Loss Arising from Optic Nerve Chiasm
Visual Loss Arising from Postgeniculate Structures
Symptoms of Disordered Motility
Pain

Once again he would go over the points in the history, elucidating, elaborating. His own examination would follow—full, detailed, but without the tedious slowness of some other neurologists. A clinical point, or any unusual symptom or sign would attract his attention. He would perhaps send for a copy of his manual to verify an observation. Often he would produce his pocket-book and make some shorthand memorandum which at home would be simplified and indexed for later reference.

The basis of his assessment of the problem was hence solid and substantial. Aided by an adequate knowledge of neuropathology as it stood in his day, and by a thorough grounding in neuroanatomy, he interpreted his observations scientifically. Hence he did not have to rely on clinical memory, or clinical "instinct"—useful though they were to him. There was nothing flashy or meretricious therefore in his bedside technique.

Hence it was that his diagnostic accuracy proved uncanny.

M. Critchley: *Sir William Gowers*

AN OVERVIEW

The case history remains one of the last strongholds of the clinician, besieged by dire predictions of its imminent replacement by continually refined neurologic imaging techniques. These computer-based procedures, and the thoroughness of the neuro-ophthalmologic examination, must raise doubts regarding the usefulness of the labor-intensive (supposedly anachronistic) elicitation of the detailed account of each patient's illness. Holmes,[1] one of the great students of the eye and nervous system, succinctly rebutted similar doubts by affirming that "the final diagnosis is often as dependent on an accurate history as on a clinical examination."

Holmes had a twofold approach to the medical his-

tory. First, he included a description of the illness in the patient's words, uninfluenced by the physicians leading questions. Second, the chronology or any ambiguous terminology was clarified by "a definite system of investigation . . . to determine: (a) the exact nature of each symptom; (b) its relations in space; (c) its relations in time; (d) the factors which influence it."[1]

Ideally, the history begins a process of diagnosis and directs the clinician to focus the examination on structures most likely to have caused particular neuroophthalmologic complaints. In addition to suggesting a tentative topographic localization, the patient's recollection of onset, progression, and recurrence of symptoms also may hint at etiology. Specific clinical paradigms (*e.g.,* the sudden onset of visual loss stemming from optic nerve ischemia or inflammation, the fluctuating diplopia of myasthenia, or the indolent visual decline of tumoral compression of the anterior visual pathways) are invaluable leads to precise diagnosis. Circumstantial aspects of visual dysfunction, such as an inability to adapt visually in a darkened theater (pigmentary retinopathy), blurred vision during a hot bath (demyelinating optic neuropathy), or image degradation in bright light (posterior subcapsular cataracts), provide important etiologic clues.

The past medical background often sheds light on the acute complaint. In a patient with a prior history of diabetes or thyroid disease, the evaluation of acquired diplopia may be streamlined. Similarly, neuroradiologic studies are superfluous when slit lamp detection of posterior subcapsular cataracts or ophthalmoscopic observation of pigmentary macular retinopathy confirms the cause of visual loss in the setting of chronic corticosteroid or thioridazine use, respectively. The details of personal and nutritional habits may prove critical: a puzzling progression of bilateral central visual loss is recognized as nutritional "amblyopia" with the revela-

F. E. Lepore: Departments of Neurology and Ophthalmology; and Department of Neurology, Robert Wood Johnson University Hospital, New Brunswick, New Jersey

tion of excessive alcohol intake and an especially poor diet; an immunodeficient basis of cytomegalovirus retinopathy may be brought forward in the self-confessed intravenous drug abuser or homosexual.

The transition from appropriate inquiries to diagnostic precision is most readily conveyed by specific instances of history-taking. In this chapter, the diagnostic choices prompted by frequently encountered historical paradigms and the symptom complexes of visual sensory or ocular motility disturbances, or of ocular/cephalic pain, will be examined.

AFFERENT VISUAL SYMPTOMS

As described by Traquair,[2] the field of vision is "a portion of an immense hollow sphere upon the inner surface of which is spread a panoramic picture of external objects showing the central feature depicted with minute detail and vivid colouring, while objects at increasing distance from the centre are indicated with correspondingly diminished clearness and duller hues." These external objects are not merely projected onto a static retina. James[3] likened peripheral areas to "sentinels, which when beams of light move over them, cry 'Who goes there?' and call the fovea to the spot." The clinician must know that the dynamic process of normal vision is heir to transient and benign vagaries of function, such as fleeting constriction and dimming of the visual field periphery with relative retinal hypoperfusion induced by rapid postural changes. Some phenomena such as suppression of vision[4] and visual masking during saccades occur constantly and do not intrude upon the observer's awareness. Other benign visual obscurations may be caused by the following:

Tear film opacities
Physiologic halos
Vitreous floaters
Retinal capillary circulation
Orthostatic visual field constriction
Phosphenes induced by
    Mechanical pressure
    Accommodation
    Saccadic eye movement
    Vitreous traction
    Cosmic particles
Afterimages
Visual suppression during saccades
Blankout associated with ganzfeld
Monocular patching

Stimuli as diverse as a flashbulb ignition or a video display terminal can affect vision with afterimages of retinal[5] or cerebral[6] origin.

Intermittent darkening of the visual field (blankout) can occur in patients undergoing bowl-type perimetry and is attributed to the effects of full-field illumination (ganzfeld).[7] Momentary loss of vision or "snowstorm" in the intact eye of patients wearing an eye patch may result from binocular rivalry suppression.[8] Visual interference can occur as a result of images (entoptic phenomena) caused by the inherent structure of the eye. Bright lights may be encircled by entoptic halos that are produced by a normal lens and cornea but have a smaller diameter than the pathologic halo of glaucomatous corneal edema.[9] When one observes a uniformly illuminated background, such as the sky, vitreous floaters consisting of a condensation of collagen fibrils are more readily perceived. The insidious or abrupt appearance of these *muscae volitantes* is usually a benign concomitant of aging, although the sudden onset of many floaters and phosphenes may signify intravitreal hemorrhage or retinal detachment. Pinpoint luminosities darting more rapidly than the gentle drift of vitreous floaters probably represent cells moving within the retinal capillary circulation.

Phosphenes are luminous sensations that may be perceived spontaneously on eye closure, especially in children,[10] or by astronauts exposed to high-energy, heavy cosmic particles.[11] They are also caused by mechanical distortion of the retina induced by pressure on the globe, accommodation, rapid (saccadic) eye movement, or forward separation of the vitreous from the retinal surface. The latter phenomenon triggers the entoptic "lightning streaks" described by Moore,[12] who emphasized their benign prognosis. These symptoms alarm the patient and may prove difficult to distinguish from similar symptoms of less benign origin.

Pathologic disturbances of vision may be transient or permanent, simple or complex, and negative or positive. Patients detect a startling positive complex visual obscuration, such as a scintillating scotoma, more readily than a simple negative peripheral field defect. The ability to ignore small scotomata, or even more extensive visual depressions, is exemplified by the subjective imperception of the physiologic blind spot or of angioscotomata during monocular viewing conditions. Similarly, Helmholtz[13] remarked on the deep inattention to visual defects occasionally encountered in "cases where one eye has gradually gone blind, and the patient lived for an indefinite time without knowing it, until through accidental closure of the healthy eye alone, the blindness of the other was brought to attention." Nonawareness of homonymous hemianopias may aid in cerebral localization, because such neglect may signify a large parietal lesion or lesions interrupting the associative pathways to the primary or secondary visual cortices. Partial or full awareness of hemianopia is more typical of purely occipital lesions.[14] Alternatively, patients may attribute visual loss to one eye when in reality an ipsilateral hemianopia is present.

Transient pathologic visual loss can occur from events at any level of the afferent visual system, from the cornea to the occipital poles.[15] The following lists give examples of these events.

Visual Loss Arising from Structures Anterior to the Optic Nerve

Amaurosis fugax
Retinal microembolization or hypoperfusion
Retinal migraine
Acute glaucoma (corneal edema)
Reversible cataract (*e.g.,* acute hyperglycemia)
Aphakic dyschromatopsia
Aphakic microhyphema (recurrent iris bleed)
G force–induced "red out"
Glycine urologic irrigating solution[16] (retinal inhibition)
Quinine, digitalis, clomiphene citrate[17] (retinal toxicity)

Visual Loss Arising from Optic Nerve and Chiasm

Obscurations preceding ischemic optic neuropathy
Photopsias with optic neuropathies
Synesthesiae—phosphenes induced by sound
Movement-induced phosphenes, with multiple sclerosis
Uhthoff's phenomenon
Optic disc swelling
Retrobulbar tumors
Intracranial hypotension[18]

Visual Loss Arising from Postgeniculate Structures

Carotid or vertebrobasilar ischemia
Contralateral diaschisis following occipital lobe cerebrovascular accident
Classic migraine and variants
Occipital lobe seizures
Occipital trauma
Release and irritative hallucinations
Dazzle
Osmotic disruption of occipital blood-brain barrier by angiographic contrast agents[19]

All too often, transient visual disturbances are attributed to extracranial carotid artery atheromatous disease, and further critical diagnostic analysis ceases when a normal study of the carotid bifurcation is obtained. The abrupt onset and transience (seconds to a few minutes) of a gray, monocular curtain or diaphragm-like constriction of the visual periphery, or positive visual phenomena in about one third of patients,[20] may herald embolism or momentarily decreased perfusion in the distribution of the internal carotid artery (see Chapter 5). These symptoms of amaurosis fugax ("fleeting blindness") can readily be distinguished from the migraineur's scintillating scotoma that expands into the visual periphery over a period of 15 to 25 minutes.[21]

Pain can reveal the origin of visual loss, as in angle-closure glaucoma that is characterized by attacks of nauseating ocular pain and by vision obscured by halos around light sources, or reduced to mere perception of light.[22] A several-day siege of central visual blurring and orbital ache aggravated by eye movement (possibly due to an inflamed dural sheath) is typical of demyelinating optic neuritis, and absence of pain is more typical of papillitis or ischemic optic neuropathy.[23] Eye or supraorbital pain on the side contralateral to homonymous hemianopia may indicate ischemia of the occipital lobe and surrounding dural structures, which are innervated by the ophthalmic division of the trigeminal nerve.[24] Temporal artery and scalp tenderness and jaw/lingual claudication point to giant-cell arteritis as the origin of permanent or (infrequently) transient monocular visual loss.

Other elucidating features of visual dysfunction include a worsening of central scotoma with exercise (Uhthoff's phenomenon) associated with demyelinating optic neuropathies. An enigmatic history of frequent, brief, painless visual obscurations with postural changes need not be elucidated by angiography, but can be explained by ophthalmoscopic detection of swollen optic discs.[25] These few examples should underscore the heterogeneity of "transient visual loss" and bolster the principle that meticulous history-taking may obviate the need for elaborate diagnostic devices or invasive neuroimaging procedures.

History-taking of complex visual disturbances may be hindered by a reluctance to disclose apparently bizarre symptoms or by a lack of insight (*e.g.,* a patient who seeks a new refraction because he "can't read" but who is found to be alexic). Other defective associative (suprastriate) visual processing includes visual agnosia, in which an object is clearly seen but cannot be recognized, and simultanagnosia, in which the details of a picture cannot be synthesized into an intelligible whole. The inability to recognize faces (prosopagnosia) and the inability to recognize colors, despite normal visual acuity and color matching, are further examples of selective "mind blindness" in which the clinical history merges into a battery of tests of higher cortical function. Visual perseveration in space and time may transform a moving light into a series of multiple discrete lights along its path (polyopia),[26] or it may cause a visual afterimage to loom before the patient after gaze is directed elsewhere (palinopsia) (see Chapter 7). It has been proposed that defects of object recognition,[27,28] such as visual agnosia, prosopagnosia, simultanagnosia, and cerebral achromatopsia, result from an interruption of occipital-temporal projections, whereas disordered spatial localization and motion perception (*e.g.,* polyopia) are produced by an impairment of occipital-parietal pathways.

Hallucinations encompass a spectrum of false sensory impressions, ranging from unformed light to complex cinematic visions. The content of the latter may be sufficiently distressing that the patient may be coaxed to answer whether there are ever "dreams with the eyes open." The clinical concept of equating calcarine cortex dysfunction with unformed positive visual phenomena, and more rostrally placed temporoparietal lesions with increasingly complex hallucinations, has been repeatedly criticized and supplanted by classifying hallucinations as irritative or release in origin. The former variety may allow tentative localization, but the latter can be formed or unformed in appearance regardless of the site of visual pathway lesions. Most hallucinations are release hallucinations, and they are typically continuous and nonstereotypic. Cogan[29] suggests that these originate when the "removal of normal visual impulses releases indigenous cerebral activity of the visual system."

SYMPTOMS OF DISORDERED MOTILITY

Stability and fusion of binocular images are among the most demanding exercises of the central nervous system and are liable to disruption, as anyone who has experienced vertigo after sudden cessation of spinning, or diplopia after alcoholic intoxication,[30] can attest. Momentary visual blurring or diplopia is a common complaint. Although causes such as decompensation of a pre-existent phoria or physiologic diplopia[31] are often invoked, other more precise explanations may not evolve. More persistent diplopia, or as the patient will term it, "seeing double," is the most distressing and constant symptom of an ocular palsy. "It is due to failure of the images of the objects towards which the eyes are directed to fall on corresponding parts of the two retinae; the images are consequently projected separately into space, and the patient perceives them separately."[1]

If the patient acknowledges that the diplopia disappears with closure of one eye, the origin of the symptom is a disturbance of motility. Double vision (subjectively perceived perhaps more accurately as "ghost images") that persists despite closure of one eye is termed monocular diplopia and is usually caused by optical aberrations of the refractive media of the eye, especially oil droplets in the tear film, excessive tearing, and corneal disease (e.g., keratoconus). Multirefractile cataracts are much more common causes of monocular diplopia than are retinal diseases, which physically distort or displace the fovea.[32] Anomalous retinal correspondence is an uncommon sensory adaptation that occurs after strabismus surgery; it may be a rare cause of nonparetic diplopia.

The use of a pinhole should eliminate monocular diplopia ("ghost images") caused by refractive errors of the ocular media. Persistence of monocular diplopia despite pinhole "refraction," and without evidence of posterior visual pathway disease, is very suggestive of a functional disorder. Similarly, binocular diplopia may have a functional origin, as in spasm of the near reflex,[33] which can resemble bilateral abduction palsies but is accompanied by telltale accommodative miosis (see Chapter 15, Fig. 17).

The process of identifying paretic extraocular muscles begins when the patient reports in which direction of gaze image separation is greatest or smallest; whether images are separated vertically, horizontally, or obliquely; and whether image separation is greater at near or far distances. For example, a report of image tilt or vertical diplopia that increases on down-gaze and is minimized by compensatory head tilt or tucking the chin down on the chest practically pinpoints a superior oblique palsy.

When an up-gaze attempt results in increasing vertical diplopia, then signs of lid retraction or proptosis should be sought. Restrictive myopathy of the inferior rectus due to Graves' ophthalmopathy is a likely cause of such spontaneously acquired vertical eye muscle imbalance. An acute onset of rather severe periorbital ache, horizontal diplopia with ptosis, dilated pupil, and exotropia may herald compression of the oculomotor nerve by distention or bleeding of a posterior communicating, internal carotid, or rostral basilar artery aneurysm.[34] Pupil-sparing oculomotor palsy of benign vascular origin is much more common in the aging population. Other diagnostic maxims of diplopia include the diurnal fluctuations and ubiquitous ptosis of myasthenia, the confusion and ataxia accompanying Wernicke's alcoholic ophthalmoplegia, and the subjective bruit with chronic red eye of a carotid-cavernous or dural fistula.

Vertigo, oscillopsia (apparent shimmering movement of the environment), and visual tilt are symptoms of dynamic disturbances of ocular motility. Vertigo is the memorable illusory rotation of self or environment, and the patient's recollection of the discomfort of vertigo, its induction by changes in head position, and its association with nausea or tinnitus can reliably localize disease of the semicircular canals or their central connections (see Chapter 11, Fig. 3). Oscillopsia, the false perception of back-and-forth movement of the environment created by the repeated transit of images of stationary objects across the retina, can be caused by impairment of the vestibulo-ocular reflex, by any acquired pathologic nystagmus, by ocular fixation instability, by superior oblique myokymia, or even by "pseudonystagmus" induced by eyelid myokymia.[35] The striking complaint of a 90° tilt, or complete inversion of the environment, is prompted by a distorted perception of gravity that arises from lateral medullary infarction damaging otolith connections.[36]

There may be inherent ambiguity in some patients' subjective descriptions of "blurry vision," which can cover a multitude of conditions ranging from a central scotoma, to subtle diplopia, to impaired accommodation. Some patients complain more bitterly about narrowly separated double images, whereas others can paradoxically ignore the widely parted images produced by a large-angle heterotropia. Similarly, a patient who "can't see" may not be the victim of disease of the afferent visual system, but rather of the involuntary lid closure found in blepharospasm or of immobile globes found in chronic progressive external ophthalmoplegia.

Although most of these symptom complexes can be easily elucidated by a few pertinent questions or even by "across-the-room" observations, a painstaking history may assign relative values to the causes of disability and suggest avenues of therapy. Consider such complicated visual scenarios as albinism: acuity is impaired by relative foveal hypoplasia, by refractive error, by photophobia, and by motor anomalies in the form of congenital pendular or jerk nystagmus and strabismus, probably related to misrouting of retinogeniculate projections.[37]

PAIN

Sherrington[38] believed that pain was an integral component of nervous activity and proclaimed it to be "the psychical adjunct of an imperative protective reflex." Pain potentially serves as a guide to localization of disease and as an indicator of response to therapy. Pain is the overwhelming symptom in cluster headaches and in tic douloureux, where suffering appears disproportionately excessive for the minor degree of tissue injury. Conversely, a mildly painful compressive oculomotor palsy may lack the symptomatic "drama" appropriate to the life-threatening impending rupture of a posterior communicating artery aneurysm. In addition to the relatively well-known tic douloureux, there are infrequently encountered entities such as glossopharyngeal neuralgia in which burning throat pain may be triggered by swallowing. Pain in the distribution of the ear, palate, or occiput may arise from neuralgias of the geniculate ganglion, sphenopalatine ganglion, and greater occipital nerve, respectively.[39] The somatic distribution and variations of neuralgias distinguish them from other sources of cephalic pain, such as temporomandibular joint syndrome, cranial arteritis, sinusitis, retrobulbar neuritis, and acute glaucoma.

A troublesome group of patients has facial pain lacking discernible origin, not conforming to any classic neuralgia or pain syndrome. Such atypical facial pain is characterized by the following:

1. It is not limited to the somatic area supplied by a single cranial or cervical nerve.
2. It is often bilateral.
3. It is constant rather than occurring in paroxysmal attacks.
4. External stimuli do not precipitate attacks.
5. It is deep rather than superficial.
6. The patient has a tendency for drug (or doctor) addiction.
7. The patient suffers from depression or has a neurotic personality.[40]

Eye discomfort may be simply an indication of local ocular disease, running the gamut from the chronic irritation of relative tear deficiency or the acute foreign-body sensation of corneal abrasion to the throbbing ache and photophobia of iritis or the nauseating agony of acute angle-closure glaucoma (see Chapter 3). Despite the common occurrence of these ocular disorders

in the general population, other occult sources of "ocular pain" must be sought beyond the globe and adnexa.

Migraine may consist of several hours of throbbing hemicranial and retro-orbital pain. This pain differs in degree from that of cluster headaches. The latter assail the patient with briefer but agonizing bouts of unilateral periocular pain accompanied by lacrimation and ipsilateral sympathetic paresis. Historical details such as a positive family history, "triggering" foodstuffs, a clocklike regularity of attacks, and visual scintillations lend credence to the diagnosis of vascular headache (see Chapter 16).

Physicians rarely encounter a disorder more distinctive than trigeminal neuralgia, with its lancinating pain affecting the mandibular, maxillary, or ophthalmic divisions (in decreasing order of frequency). During the crescendo agony, Wilson[41] observed that the patient's face is "often screwed up, voluntarily or half-consciously, or becomes the seat of flickers or twitches (tic douloureux) . . . As the paroxysm dies down it may leave behind it a nerve 'on edge' which seems loath to cease its troubling." Speaking, eating, or even the contact of a washcloth or breeze on the face may trigger a terrible spasm of facial pain. In addition to the demyelinative lesions or vascular compression that underlies some cases of tic douloureux, the trigeminal nerve is also prey to the neurotropism of herpes zoster. A complaint of steady, burning pain in a unilateral facial segment usually accompanies the appearance of herpetic vesicles emblazoning the cutaneous distribution of the affected trigeminal division. The further torturous course of postherpetic neuralgia, long after resolution of the cutaneous eruptions, is a common additional affliction.

Diplopia accompanied by pain should prompt a meticulous review of other symptoms, an assessment of nonocular cranial nerves, and a medical/surgical history. For example, the pain of self-limited ischemic oculomotor palsy can mimic an intracranial aneurysm, and diagnostic priorities may be assigned according to age-related general medical status (*e.g.*, hypertension, diabetes), absence of meningismus, and typical pupillary findings. Other "painful ophthalmoplegias" may involve one of the ocular motor, trigeminal, or sympathetic nerves (or combinations of these nerves) and indicate a locus in the continuum of anterior orbit, posterior orbit (apex), superior orbital fissure, and cavernous sinus. However, the steady, boring eye pain associated with these lesions is insufficiently distinctive to accurately predict a neoplastic, aneurysmal, or inflammatory source (see Chapter 12).

Lastly, pain may herald a precise cause of visual loss, as is well known to the physician who confidently begins steroid therapy when confronted by an elderly individual with severe monocular visual loss, head and neck pain, and tenderness of the scalp and temporal arteries, and then commences the workup of giant-cell arteritis. The severe pain accompanying visual loss in angle-closure glaucoma and the eye movement that induces orbital ache of optic neuritis are specific admonitions against a nonsensical diagnosis of "painful amaurosis fugax" or the vagaries of "brain tumor."

The linchpin of accurate diagnosis remains a detailed account of neuro-ophthalmologic disease as seen through the patient's eyes. Each individual's interpretation of visual experience is unique. As Carlyle[42] observed, "To Newton and to Newton's dog Diamond, what a different pair of universes; while the painting on the optical retina of both was, most likely, the same!" The clinician in general and the neuro-ophthalmologist in particular must listen carefully to the patient's visual experiences so that they can proceed with effective diagnosis.

REFERENCES

1. Holmes G: Introduction to Clinical Neurology. Edinburgh, E & S Livingston, 1946
2. Traquair HM: An Introduction to Clinical Perimetry, p 1. London, Henry Kimpton, 1949
3. James W: The Principles of Psychology, vol 2, p 175. Mineola, NY, Dover, 1950
4. Burr DC, Morrone MC, Ross J: Selective suppression of the magnocellular visual pathway during saccadic eye movements. Nature 371:511, 1994
5. Craik KJW: Origin of visual after-images. Nature 145:512, 1940
6. Rosner M, Belkin M: Video display units and visual function. Surv Ophthalmol 33:515, 1989
7. Fuhr PS, Hershner TA, Daum KM: Ganzfeld blankout occurs in bowl perimetry and is eliminated by translucent occlusion. Arch Ophthalmol 108:983, 1990
8. Ellingham RB, Waldock A, Harrad RA: Visual disturbance of the uncovered eye in patients wearing an eye patch. Eye 7:775, 1993
9. Cavender JC: Entoptic imagery and afterimages. In Duane TD, Jaeger EA (eds): Biomedical Foundations of Ophthalmology, Vol 2, Chap 20, pp 1–22. Hagerstown, MD, Harper & Row, 1982
10. Oster G: Phosphenes. Sci Am 222:82, 1970
11. Fugii MD, Patten BM: Neurology of microgravity and space travel. Neurol Clin 10:999, 1992
12. Moore RF: Subjective "lightning streaks." Br J Ophthalmol 31:46, 1947
13. Helmholtz H: Handbuch der Physiologischen Optik, p 431. Hamburg and Leipzig, Voss, 1910
14. Koehler PF, Endtz LJ, TeVelde J, Hekster REM: Aware or nonaware. J Neurol Sci 75:255, 1986
15. Lepore FE: Visual obscurations: evanescent and elementary. Semin Neurol 6:167, 1986
16. Barletta JP, Fanous MM, Hamed LM: Temporary blindness in TUR syndrome. J Clin Neuro Ophthalmol 14:6, 1994
17. Purvin VA: Visual disturbance secondary to clomiphene citrate. Arch Ophthalmol 113:482, 1995
18. Horton JC, Fishman RA: Neurovisual findings in the syndrome of spontaneous intracranial hypotension from dural cerebrospinal fluid leak. Ophthalmology 101:244, 1994
19. Lantos G: Cortical blindness due to osmotic disruption of the blood-brain barrier by angiographic contrast material: CT and MRI studies. Neurology 39:567, 1989
20. Goodwin JA, Gorelick P, Helgason C: Symptoms of amaurosis fugax in atherosclerotic carotid artery disease. Neurology 37:829, 1987
21. Hupp SL, Kline LB, Corbett JJ: Visual disturbances of migraine. Surv Ophthalmol 33:221, 1989
22. Ravits J, Seybold M: Transient monocular visual loss from narrow-angle glaucoma. Arch Neurol 41:991, 1984
23. Lepore FE: The origin of pain in optic neuritis. Determinants of pain in 101 eyes with optic neuritis. Arch Neurol 48:748, 1991
24. Knox DL, Cogan DG: Eye pain and homonymous hemianopsia. Am J Ophthalmol 54:1091, 1962
25. Sadun AA, Currie JN, Lessell S: Transient visual obscurations with elevated optic disks. Ann Neurol 16:489, 1984
26. Kampf D, Piper HF, Neundorfer B et al: Palinopsia (visual perseveration) and cerebral polyopia—Clinical analysis and computed tomographic findings. Fortschr Neurol Psychiatr 51:270, 1983
27. Tusa RJ: Neuro-ophthalmology of the Cerebral Cortex. New Orleans, American Academy of Neurology, April 1986
28. Mishkin M, Ungerleider LG, Macko KA: Object vision and spatial vision: two cortical pathways. Trends Neurosci 6:414, 1983
29. Cogan DG: Visual hallucinations as release phenomena. Graefes Arch Clin Exp Ophthalmol 188:139, 1973
30. Wilkinson IMS, Kime R: Alcohol and human eye movement. Trans Am Neurol Assoc 99:38, 1974
31. Trevor-Roper PD: The Eye and Its Disorders, p 176. Boston, Little, Brown & Co, 1974
32. Lepore FE, Yarian DL: Monocular diplopia of retinal origin. J Clin Neuro Ophthalmol 6:181, 1986
33. Griffin JF, Wray SH, Anderson DP: Misdiagnosis of spasm of the near reflex. Neurology 26:1018, 1976
34. Bartleson JD, Trautman JC, Sundt TM: Minimal oculomotor nerve paresis secondary to unruptured intracranial aneurysm. Arch Neurol 43:1015, 1986
35. Krohel GB, Rosenberg PN: Oscillopsia associated with eyelid myokymia. Am J Ophthalmol 102:662, 1986
36. Wertenbaker C, Gutman I: Unusual visual symptoms. Surv Ophthalmol 29:297, 1985
37. Kinnear PE, Jay B, Witkow CJ: Albinism. Surv Ophthalmol 30:75, 1985
38. Sherrington C: The Integrative Action of the Nervous System, p 229. New Haven, CT, Yale University Press, 1947
39. Ross GS, Chipman M: The neuralgias. In Baker AB, Baker LH (eds): Clinical Neurology, Vol 3, Chap 39, pp 1–28. Philadelphia, Harper & Row, 1984
40. White JC, Sweet WH: Pain and the Neurosurgeon, pp 408, 409. Springfield, IL, Charles C Thomas, 1969
41. Wilson SAK: Neuritis. In Bruce AN (ed): Neurology, p 279. Baltimore, Williams & Wilkins, 1940
42. Carlyle T: The French Revolution, p 5. New York, AL Burt, 1925

CHAPTER 2

Neuro-ophthalmologic Examination: The Visual Sensory System

Barry Skarf, Joel S. Glaser, Gary L. Trick, and Erkan Mutlukan

Anatomy and Physiology of the Sensory Visual Pathways
Retina
  Receptive Fields
  Ganglion Cells and On/Off Dichotomy
  Retino-Cortical Visual Pathway
  Parallel Visual Pathways
    Magnocellular and Parvocellular Parallel Pathways
  On and Off Pathways
Visual Cortex and Magnification Factor
Visual Acuity
Contrast Sensitivity
Color Vision
Neuro-ophthalmologic Evaluation of Visual Function
Symptoms
Tests of Macular and Foveal Function
  Visual Acuity
  Contrast Sensitivity
  Color Vision
Pupillary Light Response
Photostress Test
Steropsis and Binocular Fusion
Visual Fields and Perimetry
Anatomic Considerations

Physiologic Considerations
Clinical Testing of the Visual Field
  Confrontation Methods
    Visually Elicited Eye Movements
    Finger Mimicking
    Finger Counting
    Hand Comparison
    Color Comparison
  Tangent Screen
  Factitious (Functional) Fields
  Clinical Perimetry
    Goldmann Kinetic Perimetry
    Automated Static Threshold Perimetry
    Automated Visual Field Interpretation
Electrophysiology Tests of the Eye and Visual Pathway
Electroretinography
  Standard (Full-Field) Electroretinography
  Focal Electroretinography
  Pattern Electroretinography
Visual Evoked Potential
Other Tests of Visual Function
  Light and Dark Adaptation
  Motion Sensitivity
  Acuity at Reduced Illumination

We have instruments of precision in increasing numbers with which we and our hospital assistants at untold expense make tests and take observations, the vast majority of which are but supplementary to the careful study of the patient by a keen observer using his eyes and ears, and fingers and a few simple aids.
—Harvey Cushing

B. Skarf: Department of Ophthalmology, University of Toronto; and Neuro-ophthalmology Unit, Eye Care Services, Henry Ford Health Sciences Center, Detroit, Michigan
J. S. Glaser: Departments of Neurology and Ophthalmology, Bascom Palmer Eye Institute, University of Miami School of Medicine, Miami; and Neuro-ophthalmology, Cleveland Clinic Florida, Ft. Lauderdale, Florida
G. L. Trick: Department of Ophthalmology, Case Western Reserve University, Cleveland, Ohio; and Department of Eye Care Services, Henry Ford Hospital, Detroit, Michigan
E. Mutlukan: Glaucoma Service, Wills Eye Hospital, Philadelphia, Pennsylvania

The goal of the neuro-ophthalmologic examination of the visual sensory system is to discover and diagnose abnormalities of the neural projections from the retina to the visual centers in the brain, and of disturbances of higher visual integration. In order to succeed at this task, we must take into account the physical properties of light and, more importantly, the anatomic and physiologic properties of the retina and of the eye's optical system. Consequently, a review of relevant anatomy and physiology is essential.

ANATOMY AND PHYSIOLOGY OF THE SENSORY VISUAL PATHWAYS

Normal human vision is not a single unitary faculty, but rather a synthesis of multiple semiautonomous functional subsystems, segregated into sets of separate pathways or "channels" between the eye and the brain.[1,2] This functional division into multiple channels is evident for both subcortical visual processes and in the primary visual cortex. Although there is extensive interaction, these visual channels transmit particular classes of visual information.[1-4] Visual deficits that arise from diverse disease processes can selectively disturb these subsystems at various levels, giving rise to localizing subjective and objective signs.

Retina

There are an average of 57.4 million rods and 3.3 million cones in the human retina.[5] The cones each contain 1 of 3 photopigments with a maximum absorption at about 440 nm (S, short wavelength sensitive; blue) 535 nm (M, medium; green), and 577 nm (L, long; red), respectively. The fovea centralis contains approximately 200,000 cones/mm². Outside the fovea, the average density of cones is about 5000/mm², but the distribution of cones is not uniform. Cone density declines rapidly with distance from the fovea. In contrast, the density of rods is nil at the foveola, increasing rapidly with eccentricity to peak at 3 mm (20°) from the fovea, where there are 150,000 rods/mm². The concentration of rods then decreases more gradually than does cone density, to about 35,000 rods/mm² at the periphery of the retina.

The photoreceptor cells of the retina connect to the ganglion cells via bipolar cells that respond to either increments in light ("on-type") or to decrements ("off-type"). Rods connect only to "on-type" bipolar cells, whereas cones connect with both "on" and "off" types.[6] One "on-type" and one "off-type" bipolar cell innervate each ganglion cell, with the "on" bipolar exciting an "on" ganglion cell or inhibiting an "off" ganglion cell and vice versa. Bipolar cells also provide lateral connections to horizontal, amacrine, and interplexiform cells.[7]

The distribution of retinal ganglion cells is even more uneven than that of rods and cones. In the foveola, approximately 150,000 cones are connected to twice as many ganglion cells, because each cone connects via bipolar cells to 2 ganglion cells, 1 on and 1 off type.[8] With increasing eccentricity from the fovea, gradually more photoreceptors converge onto single bipolar and retinal ganglion cells, which decrease markedly in density toward the periphery.[8,9] In the far retinal periphery, there may be as many as 10,000 rods connected in clusters to a single ganglion cell, with considerable overlapping of clusters so that a point stimulus of light can trigger responses from several ganglion cells at once.

Patterns of neural interactions among various cell types in the retina have been studied and described. Rods and cones differ substantially in the patterns of their respective connections. These different patterns result in low spatial frequency (large size) contrast sensitivity for rod (scotopic) vision and high spatial frequency (fine detail) sensitivity for cone (photopic) vision.[10]

Receptive Fields

As a result of this architecture, it is possible to define the receptive field as the unit area of retinal function. The receptive field of a neuron is the retinal area for which a visual stimulus causes a change in the activity of that neuron. Receptive field sizes are smallest at the fovea and enlarge with retinal eccentricity as a consequence of the increase in the ratio of photoreceptors to ganglion cells.[11] Under photopic conditions, the size of the on-type receptive field center is 4.5' to 9' at the fovea, increasing to 60' to 90' at 10° to 15° beyond the fovea and to 120' to 200' at 60° to 70° from fovea. Similar to the inverse relationship between receptive field size and ganglion cell density, the number of overlapping receptive field centers at a given retinal point also decreases towards the periphery, from 32 centers at 10° of eccentricity to 13 at 70° eccentricity.[12] As a result, visual sensitivity decreases gradually with distance from the fovea.[13] The retinal ganglion cell population, like the number of photoreceptors, decreases with aging,[14] along with neuronal loss in the visual cortex of the brain. These phenomena are reflected in the decrease in overall visual sensitivity that occurs with aging.

Ganglion Cells and On/Off Dichotomy

One million retinal ganglion cells can be subdivided into at least 11 different classes. An average of 85% of these cells have concentrically organized "center-surround" receptive fields with 2 antagonistic regions. There are two types: "on-center" cells have a center that is activated by light, with a surround that is inhibitory, whereas "off-center" cells are excited by decrements in light falling inside their center and are inhibited by light decrements in their surround zone.[15] The remaining 15% of the ganglion cells have no antagonistic surround mechanism, and the receptive field is "non-concentric." Generally, the diameter of the ganglion cell excitatory receptive field center is equal to the field size of its dendritic distribution within the retina.[16]

Studies have shown that the surround area of a receptive field is formed by interactions among horizontal and amacrine cells and not by convergence of inputs from "on" and "off" ganglion cells.[17] Furthermore, the "on" and "off" retino-geniculo-striate pathways remain segregated up to the visual cortex, where they first converge onto single cortical neurons. The organization of cortical receptive fields is likely the product of intracortical circuitry, and not the result of convergence of the "on" and "off" pathways.[6,17]

Retino-Cortical Visual Pathway

Visual information originating from the retinal ganglion cells is transmitted through the optic nerve, which is formed at the optic disc by the retinal nerve fiber layer. The retinal nerve fiber layer can be divided into three topographic sectors: (1) the papillomacular bundle, which serves the macula and hence the central field of vision; (2) the relatively thick superior and inferior arcuate bundles, which roughly parallel their respective vascular arcades; and (3) the nasal radial bundles, which expand outward from the nasal aspect of the disc (see Fig. 4–2). Lesions affecting each of these topographic sectors of the retina or optic disc produce characteristic patterns of visual field loss. Disruption in the papillomacular bundle results in a central or centro-cecal scotoma; lesions of the arcuate bundles cause nasal depressions that form a "step" border at the horizontal meridian and arcuate scotomas in the superior and inferior hemifields (see Figs. 5–4 and 5–7). Lesions of the nasal bundles produce wedge-shaped, sectorial defects radiating from the temporal aspect of the blind spot.

The optic nerve leaves the eye at the lamina cribrosa of the optic disc and meets the fellow optic nerve intracranially at the optic chiasm, where the optic nerve fibers coming from the nasal hemiretina cross to join the temporal hemiretinal fibers from the fellow eye. Lesions of the optic chiasm characteristically lead to complete or incomplete bitemporal hemianopia that are morphologically limited by the vertical meridian, at least in part (see Chapter 6).

Behind the optic chiasm, the retinal ganglion cell axons form the optic tract and travel to synapse in the lateral geniculate nucleus (LGN) of the posterior thalamus. The LGN is a compact structure made up of six layers in which the projections from each eye remain segregated. Layers 1, 4, 6 receive inputs exclusively from the contralateral eye, and layers 2, 3, 5 are innervated only by the ipsilateral eye (see Chapter 4). LGN postsynaptic neurons project to the visual cortex via the optic radiations. Lesions affecting the optic tract, LGN, optic radiations and visual cortex produce hemifield defects (hemianopia) that are "homonymous," that is, they occupy the same side of the visual field in both eyes, respecting the vertical meridian (see Chapter 7).

Parallel Visual Pathways

Visual stimuli are processed via multiple neural channels, or "parallel pathways" (see Fig. 4–12), which are specialized to transmit specific visual information.[1,2,4] These neural channels become differentiated in the retina, where complex neural interactions and processing begin. They project from the retinal ganglion cells to the cortex, which is ultimately responsible for subjective visual perception.

Magnocellular and Parvocellular Parallel Pathways

Based on their morphology and response characteristics, retinal ganglion cells have been classified as P type, for those projecting to the parvocellular layers (layers 3 to 6) of the LGN; and M type, for those projecting to the magnocellular layers (layers 1 and 2) of LGN.[18] Parvocellular (P) retinal ganglion cells have small receptive field diameters, and small somal and axonal caliber, whereas magnocellular (M) retinal ganglion cells have large receptive fields (nearly six times larger), large cell bodies, and axons.[18] In accordance with their smaller receptive fields, P cells have higher spatial resolution.[19] The conduction velocity of the visual signal is higher in M cells, as expected from their large axons, but M-type ganglion cells are 3 to 10 times less numerous than the P-type cells.[20] The center-surround mechanism of M cells is more sensitive to achromatic luminance contrast as opposed to the dominant feature of color opponency in 80% of P-type cells. The sensitivity of M cells to achromatic contrast becomes most pronounced at short stimulus exposure durations as they respond to the visual stimuli transiently, at lower stimulus contrasts (below 15% contrast),[20] and at lower levels of adapting background luminance.[21]

Most cones providing input to the center and surround of M cells are red and green type, and only some appear to receive signals from blue cones. The signals from blue (short wavelength sensitive) cones are transmitted via P cells and almost exclusively via the on pathway.[22]

In monkey eyes, selective lesions of the parvocellular system impair visual acuity, color vision, high spatial frequency (i.e., small size) and low temporal frequency (i.e., slow flicker) contrast sensitivity, brightness discrimination, pattern (shape and texture) discrimination, and stereopsis, whereas magnocellular lesions distort low spatial frequency contrast sensitivity, fast flicker, and low-contrast fast motion perception.[2,23] In humans, the parvocellular system is affected by optic neuritis,[24] and the magnocellular system is damaged preferentially in glaucoma.[25]

On and Off Pathways

On and off pathways remain morphologically segregated in the LGN also. On-center ganglion cells are concentrated in layers 5 and 6, and off-center cells are concentrated in layers 3 and 4 of parvocellular LGN.[25] The magnocellular layers 1 and 2 have a mixture of both type cells.

On and off pathways provide equal sensitivity and rapid information transfer for both light increments and decrements and facilitate the transmission of high-contrast sensitivity information,[6] which is processed mainly by the magnocellular system. On and off pathways that subserve brightness are important contributors to color contrast perception, which is mediated mainly by the parvocellular pathway.[26]

Visual Cortex and Magnification Factor

The scale with which the visual field is mapped onto the striate cortex is dependent on eccentricity; the fovea is represented by a large area of visual cortex, and the periphery claims a relatively much smaller portion[27] (see Fig. 4–11). The recent advances in neuro-imaging have revealed that the central 10° of field is represented by at least 60% of the occipital cortex. The cortical magnification factor (M) indicates the surface area of cortex associated with each unit area of visual field and is determined by the following relationship: $M^2 = mm^2$ cortex/degree^2.[28]

Visual Acuity

"Visual acuity" refers to the overall sensitivity of the visual system to spatial detail and is typically measured by determining the threshold for detecting a spatial component of a visual stimulus. This concept was introduced by Helmholz,[29] who first coined the term "minimum separable" to indicate the minimum spatial interval between two points of light sufficient to permit the visual system to perceive their duality. He thought that a distance just greater than one cone diameter should allow stimulation of two cones in the foveola, each with its own ganglion cell and "private line" into the central nervous system. In actual testing, however, the frequency with which subjects correctly identify dual lines increases gradually as the actual separation is increased (a frequency-of-seeing curve is used to represent this phenomenon),[30] and the threshold separation is often specified as an arbitrary percentage, somewhat greater than 50%, of correct responses that an individual could theoretically achieve by random guessing. Clinically,

however, the term visual acuity has come to describe standard measures of "minimal angle of resolution," that is, the threshold or minimal separation between two distinct visual stimuli (measured in degree of visual angle) that can be perceived visually under certain controlled operative conditions.[31]

Visual acuity measures both the optical quality of the retinal image and the functionality of the neural structures carrying the foveal projections to the striate cortex. Therefore, reduced visual acuity can be produced either by degrading the optical quality of the eye or by a disruption of the fovea or of its neural projections to the brain. The optical system of the eye is adversely affected by refraction (focus), light scattering, and diffraction, and absorption by the pre-retinal media. Among optical factors, diffraction will cause spreading of light even in a perfectly focused system, and it varies inversely with pupil size.[31] With pupil diameter of less than about 2.5 mm, "spread" of an optimally focused single point becomes progressively larger and, thus, acuity decreases as pupil size is reduced below this diameter. For eyes with pupils between 2.5 mm and 6 mm in diameter, acuity remains relatively constant, whereas with pupils larger than 6 mm, *optical aberration* degrades acuity.[31] Optical aberration occurs when light rays entering a large pupil do not converge precisely to a point.

Campbell and Green[32] showed that the human visual system is capable of resolving a higher–spatial frequency (finer) grating if the optics of the eye are bypassed by producing the grating directly on the retina using laser-generated interference fringes. Diffraction in the eye lowers contrast of an optical image grating, but not the contrast of a laser-generated interference fringe grating. Improvement of performance (resolution of higher–spatial frequency gratings) with increased contrast indicates that, for the foveolar cones, contrast sensitivity is a key factor determining the minimal angle of resolution, that is, acuity. Another factor, the ultrastructure of the ocular media, can cause both backward and forward scattering of light that degrades the quality of the optical image. In addition, the ocular media are neither fully nor uniformly transparent to light, and some light is absorbed by these media. This absorption tends to be wavelength dependent such that the shorter the wavelength of light entering the eye (*i.e.,* toward the blue-violet), the greater the absorption.

Visual acuity also depends on the spatial arrangement and concentration of the photoreceptor mosaic in the foveolae, which set an upper limit of spatial resolution. As Helmholz first proposed, acuity is limited because of the finite size of the retinal receptors, but, in addition, the neural connections among retinal cells may converge to produce larger summation areas less sensitive to fine detail.

The physical properties of the visual stimulus used to

test acuity, and the situation in which it is presented, also influence discrimination. Most factors that affect light sensitivity influence visual acuity. Maximal acuity occurs in the range of photopic light levels at which the foveolar cones function optimally.[33] These cone pathways have the highest light thresholds and operate poorly in dim (scotopic) light. Visual acuity falls off abruptly as light levels are reduced, principally because parafoveal cones and rods, which have greater light sensitivity, also have poorer spatial resolution.[33] This is primarily due to neural factors such as the larger summation area of the parafoveal receptor fields (greater numbers of cones and rods converging onto the same single ganglion cell). Visual acuity, maximal at the center of the fovea, decreases with eccentricity; for example, there is a 60% decrease in acuity at 1° off the foveola. Of course, adequate illumination is critical to cone function, and at very low light levels, when vision is dependent exclusively on rod function, acuity falls off abruptly. Maximal rod acuity is about 8 minutes of arc (20/160).[33]

Acuity is also dependent on background adapting luminance and stimulus contrast. The sensitivity of the eye for the detection of a stimulus varies with the level of adaptation to ambient light levels. The light and dark adaptations have two mechanisms, namely, a neural process that is completed in about 0.5 seconds and a slower photochemical process involving molecular changes in visual pigment that occurs in about 1 minute for light adaptation and 45 minutes for dark adaptation.[34] Above the retinal illuminance level of 3.2×10^{-3} cd/m^2, cones begin to contribute to visual sensitivity along with the rods (mesopic light level). Traditionally, rods are taken to be saturated about 3 cd/m^2, but above this level, rods still contribute to color vision and pupil size.[35] Nonetheless, the conventional adapting luminance used with the Goldmann perimeter, which is 10 cd/m^2, is regarded as representative of the mesopic level.

The duration of stimulus presentation also influences measured acuity. For very brief presentations, acuity remains constant as long as the number of quanta absorbed remains constant (by increasing stimulus intensity in proportion to the decrease in the duration it is presented). For longer presentations, lasting 100 to 500 milliseconds, acuity improves with increased duration, even though summation is no longer a factor.[33]

Finally, interactions between the stimulus used to test acuity and objects adjacent to it can also adversely affect acuity measures. This phenomenon is often referred to as "crowding" because visual acuity suffers when neighboring contours are too close (i.e., within a few minutes of arc).[36]

In clinical practice, visual acuity is expressed as the threshold value for which some aspect of the spatial dimension of the visual stimulus is the relevant variable. Typically, visual acuity is specified in terms of the visual angle defined by a particular spatial detail. The visual angle depends on the physical size of the stimulus and its distance from the observer. Because visual acuity is a sensory threshold, it is important to recognize that different subjective criteria will produce different types of acuity. The three most common acuity criteria are detection, resolution, and identification (recognition).[31] Detection acuity is a measure of the smallest stimulus object or pattern of elements that can be discriminated from a uniform background or distinguished as a single feature. Consequently, detection acuity is typically specified as minimum angle of detection or minimum angle visible. Resolution acuity refers to the smallest amount of spatial detail necessary to distinguish a difference between patterns or to identify features in a visible target. When resolution acuity is measured, the size of the stimulus is increased or decreased to determine the threshold size that elicits a correct response. Resolution acuity is specified as minimum angle of resolution, or MAR. Identification (or recognition) acuity is a measure of the minimum spatial detail necessary to recognize an object (such as an optotype) or to identify the relative location of visible features in an object (e.g., the open segment of a ring). Identification acuity is also specified in terms of MAR.

Traditional Snellen charts and similar displays of letters, numbers, or symbols (optotypes) have been used to measure visual acuity clinically. These charts provide a high-contrast, clearly visible target and require that the patient identify or recognize the letters or symbols based on the spatial arrangement of their components. The size (minimum angle subtended by the components of the stimuli) varies, and, hence, the patient's MAR is determined. However, as indicated above, MAR can fluctuate depending on proximity or presence of adjacent stimuli. In order to control this effect, especially in clinical studies such as controlled trials, the standard types of acuity charts have been replaced by other types of charts, most notably the Bailey-Lovie logMAR acuity chart,[37] which was first widely used in the Early Treatment Diabetic Retinopathy Study (ETDRS).[38] This system of acuity measurement addresses several key deficiencies of the standard clinical (Snellen-type) chart. It uses (1) letters that are comparably difficulty to identify, (2) an equal number of letters on each line, (3) proportional spacing between letters, and (4) *logarithmic* progression of size from line to line. These innovations adjust for the fact that not all letters of the alphabet are equally recognizable, and they attempt to standardize the effects of crowding while allowing proportional reductions of acuity to represent equivalent (logarithmic) decrements in resolution.

Other methods of visual acuity testing use letters or symbols of different contrast. The Pelli-Robson chart[39] uses alphabet letters of constant size that vary in contrast and measures the minimum contrast necessary for letter recognition. On the other hand, the chart devised by Regan and Neima[40] resembles the Snellen and logMAR charts, with letters of decreasing size that are used as a measure of MAR. However, the Regan test provides a series of charts, each progressively decreasing in contrast (from black, to medium, to light gray optotypes on a white background) permitting measurement of low- as well as high-contrast acuity. Another sensitive index of visual-neural interactions is the measurement of *hyperacuity,* which refers to certain spatial distinctions that can be observed for which the thresholds are lower than even normal acuity.[33] Hyperacuity thresholds can even exceed the upper limit for discrimination that is implied by the spatial arrangement of the foveal cones, a finding indicating that such testing measures a different mechanism than resolution acuity. The best-known example of hyperacuity is *Vernier alignment,* in which the displacement of one linear element (line segment) relative to another element, within the same target, must be judged.[33]

Although many useful and sensitive tests of visual acuity have been developed, none has succeeded in displacing high-contrast character acuity as the standard. Because Snellen (optotype) acuity remains the most widely used measure of visual function in clinical practice, it is important to understand its nomenclature, value, and limitations. Snellen acuity is generally reported in a fractional notation (*e.g.,* 20/20) in which the numerator refers to the distance at which an individual can successfully read the letters, and the denominator refers to the distance at which "a normal eye" should distinguish the same letters. An eye with 20/40 vision therefore is able to read at a distance of 20 ft the letters a normal eye could read at 40 ft, but it is unable to read smaller letters.

The fractional notation used for character acuity must be interpreted with caution for several reasons. First, Snellen notation cannot be treated mathematically as a fraction. Instead, the Snellen notation must be converted to decimal form (20/20=1.0, 20/30=0.66, 20/40=0.5, etc.) for mathematical treatment. Even when this is done, however, it must be realized that Snellen acuity is a logarithmic measure and that equal increments in the decimal notation do not represent equivalent changes in acuity. For example, acuity of 20/50 (=0.40) represents twice the resolution of 20/100 (=0.2), and it is represented by an incremental change of 0.2, whereas the doubling of acuity represented by a change from 20/200 (=0.1) to 20/100 (=0.2) is represented by an incremental change of 0.1. Perhaps more importantly, nominal changes in acuity do not reflect comparable changes in the health of the optical or neural substrates. Abnormalities resulting in 20/80 vision are not necessarily twice as severe as those producing 20/40 vision. Another

limitation on the interpretation of character acuity is that 20/20 is an excessively lenient criterion for "normal" MAR. Depending on age, the typical normal eye is often able to see considerably better than 20/20.[41] Visual acuity testing in infants and children is addressed in Chapter 13.

Contrast Sensitivity

Standard tests of visual acuity, for example, Snellen optotypes, generally measure resolution of fine detail at high contrast (black on white). However, common everyday visual experience is not a high-contrast phenomenon. Most objects are seen against a diffuse background or with other objects at a moderate or intermediate level of contrast. The visual scene is typically made up of large and small objects with coarse outlines intermingled with fine detail and producing a mixture of stimuli that include gradual transitions between areas of light and dark, as well abrupt transitions and sharp edges. This means that visual acuity as measured clinically does not begin to assess the capacity of our visual system to distinguish and identify a wide variety of different images. Selective loss of intermediate and low spatial frequencies may produce disturbing visual symptoms in patients with nominally "normal" visual acuity as measured with standard high-contrast, sharp-edged optotypes.

In visual physiology, *contrast* is defined as change in brightness across space or time. The change, whether spatial or temporal, may be gradual or abrupt (Fig. 2–1), single (only one transition) or repetitive (steady-state). If the visual stimulus consists of a repetitive pattern of varying luminance (*e.g.,* a pattern of stripes or checks), then the pattern can be described in terms of spatial contrast. For most clinical and research purposes, the contrast of a visual stimulus is defined by the relationship between these intensities (I) such that contrast $=(I_{max}-I_{min})/(I_{max}+I_{min})$. Thus, contrast can vary from a minimum of 0 to maximum of 1.0. Using stimuli of decreasing contrast, visual function can be assessed by determining the minimum contrast, or contrast sensitivity, at which a specific test pattern can be detected. Visual resolution, on the other hand, is more directly related to the degree of spatial detail (*i.e.,* the spatial frequency) of the pattern. Thus, spatial contrast sensitivity is a measure of the ability to resolve diverse patterns with a more obvious relationship to the range of everyday visual experience of discrimination and identification than is provided by routine clinical tests of visual acuity.

The most common stimuli for clinical evaluation of spatial contrast sensitivity are repetitive patterns of alternating light and dark bars in which the luminance of the bars varies sinusoidally along a single axis. This

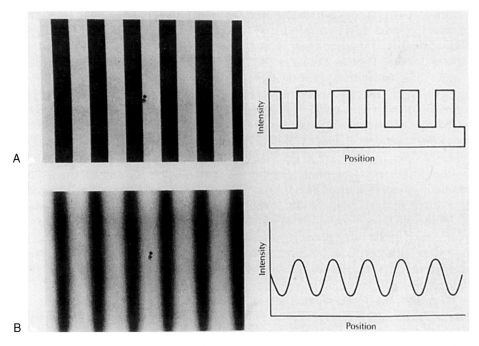

Fig. 2–1. Contrast sensitivity function. **A.** Sharp edge luminance change; square wave transition. **B.** Gradual luminance change; sine wave transition. (From Cornsweet TN: Visual Perception, p 313. New York, Academic Press, 1970)

pattern is known as a sine wave grating (see Fig. 2–1B). The periodicity of the pattern, is referred to as its spatial frequency and is generally specified in cycles (pairs of light and dark bars) per degree of visual angle. The spatial frequency is used to represent the degree of spatial detail in the stimulus. Thus, a relatively broad wave with cycles subtending 2° has a spatial frequency of 0.5 cycles per degree (cpd), whereas a narrower wave subtending 0.2° per cycle has a spatial frequency of 5 cpd. A true sinusoidal grating can be described by a single frequency and by the contrast between the brightest and dimmest parts of the wave. On the other hand, a square wave grating is a pattern with sharp edges such as a series of dark and light bars (see Fig. 2–1A). Square wave gratings are complex visual stimuli made up of mixed spatial frequency components (many different waves of low and high frequencies). Similarly, a complex visual image in the real world, characterized by abrupt transitions from bright to dark, is made of numerous high–spatial frequency components. In contrast, an image made up primarily of low–spatial frequency components should contain gradual transitions and little fine detail.

Human contrast sensitivity is usually tested using sine wave gratings of various frequencies. The contrast sensitivity for a particular spatial frequency grating is the inverse of the contrast threshold, that is, the minimum contrast necessary for the pattern to be "just detectable." The contrast sensitivity of the human visual sys-

tems varies with spatial frequency such that maximum sensitivity is normally for spatial frequencies of about 1 to 2 cpd; sensitivity falls off at both higher and lower spatial frequencies. However, many factors affect the shape of the human contrast sensitivity curve (function), including background adaptation level, stimulus field size, retinal eccentricity, pattern orientation, pupil size, and defocus. Abnormalities of contrast sensitivity are known to occur in numerous retinal and optic nerve disorders as well as in anterior segment disease. However, the utility of contrast sensitivity testing for differentiating particular disorders remains an unresolved issue.

Color Vision

Within the limits of the visible spectrum (approximately 400 to 700 nm), the human visual system has a remarkably good sensitivity to differences in color. Color is largely determined by the physical properties of light energy entering the eye. However, the eye and visual pathways also influence subjective color perception. The physical properties of light (and their corresponding perceptual attributes) that characterize color are (1) wavelength (hue), (2) intensity (luminance), and (3) colorometric purity (saturation).[42] Significantly, the color perceived also depends upon the chromatic properties of surrounding objects and background.

Normal human color vision is *trichromatic*, that is, an

individual with normal color vision can match the color appearance of any colored field by appropriately adjusting the relative intensity of three suitably chosen unique primary colors. Indeed, Thomas Young in 1802 speculated that only three individual color-sensitive mechanisms, each with broad spectral sensitivity, are necessary to account for all color perception. However, it was not until 1964 that color-matching experiments performed by the Nobel laureate George Wald[43] revealed that mixtures of three primary colors are sufficient to produce the entire spectrum of perceptible colors. The trichromatic nature of normal human color vision is based on three distinct types of photopigments, each found in the outer segments of the specific cone photoreceptors. Each of the three photopigments has a broad-band spectral absorption function with peak absorption in a distinct region of the visual spectrum, but with considerable overlap. This overlap provides for the fact that any given wavelength of light will stimulate all three photopigments, but the strength of the photoreceptor response will be at different levels for each wavelength. Based on the unique absorption peak of the pigment in a particular cone photoreceptor, the designation of long- (L or red), medium- (M or green), and short-wavelength (S or blue) photoreceptors has become widely adopted. The population of cones with peak absorption close to the wavelength of a given light stimulus will be activated most intensely, and the cones with peak sensitivity farthest from that wavelength will respond least. It is the ratio of the activity generated by the three mechanisms that is specific for each wavelength of light. In this way, the retina can provide for discrimination of all wavelengths at each retinal locus by way of only three differentially sensitive cones at each locus.

The neural processing of color information is known to involve transformation of the signals from the three cone types such that, at the level of the optic nerve, color coding is not based on individual cone-specific responses, but it reflects excitatory (facility) and inhibitory (opponent) interactions between the signals from the specific cone types. There are three color-opponent neural pathways that convey color information from the three classes of retinal cone photoreceptors: a red-green pathway that signals differences between L and M cone responses; a blue-yellow pathway that signals differences between S cone responses and a sum of L and M cone responses; and a luminance pathway that signals a sum of L and M cone responses. Functional magnetic resonance imaging suggests color-opponent encoding of cortical neurons with the strongest response to red-green stimuli in cortical areas V1 and V2.[44] These concepts have implications on the nature of color deficits associated with optic nerve disease in which the photoreceptor response may be normal, but the interactions among the neural signals may be defective.

One of the major hurdles in understanding color vision is the obscure terminology that has evolved and persisted as physiologic concepts developed. For example, the three major types of congenital color defects were termed protan, deutan, and tritan, respectively, but these words mean only the "first, second, and third" defects and have nothing whatsoever to do with the pathology of the underlying color vision mechanisms. Color vision deficits (dyschromatopsias) are best understood in relation to the trichromacy of normal color vision. Dyschromatopsias are either congenital or acquired as a function of disease of the eye or visual pathways. Almost 10% of males and approximately 0.5% to 1.0% of females in the general population have congenital defects of color vision that impair their ability to make normal color discriminations. The least severe form is *anomalous trichromacy,* characterized technically by the ability match the color appearance of any colored field by adjusting three suitably chosen unique primary colors (similar to normal trichromats), but requiring significantly different relative radiances of the primary colors to do so. Such refined color sense is assessed on an *anomaloscope,* which permits a combination of colored filters (usually red and green) that are adjusted subjectively to match a standardized yellow. Historically, anomalous trichromats are considered to have an abnormal photopigment in one of the three types of cone photoreceptors (L, M, or S). Consequently, anomalous trichromats are typically referred to as protanomalous, deuteranomalous, or tritanomalous depending on whether the abnormal photopigment is L, M, or S wavelength photoreceptors, respectively. Depending on the extent of the anomaly in the photopigment absorption and the severity of the resulting color discrimination deficit, anomalous trichromats may be classified as having mild, moderate, or even severe deficiencies. Dichromats exhibit more pronounced color vision deficits than anomalous trichromats. Dichromacy is characterized by the ability to match the color appearance of any colored field by adjusting two, rather than three, primary colors. This feature suggests the failure, or perhaps absence, of one of the underlying photoreceptors types. Dichromats are typically referred to as protanomalous, deuteranomalous, or tritanomalous depending on whether the defect is related to the response to L, M, or S wavelength photoreceptors, respectively. The smallest group of congenitally color-deficient individuals is that of the achromats. *Achromacy* is characterized by the ability to match the color appearance of any colored field by adjusting of the radiance of any single primary color. Simplistically, these individuals may possess only a single cone photopigment, or they may have no functioning cones at all. In the latter case, only rods are responsive, and central vision is also reduced.

Acquired color vision deficits due to pathologic changes of the eye, retina, or visual pathways are frequently referred to as protan, deutan, or tritan defects. However, the use of this terminology has, at least in part, evolved from the application of tests originally designed to detect congenital color defects. It is important to recognize that, with the possible exception of diseases specifically affecting the cone photoreceptors, it is unlikely that similar mechanisms underlie acquired "protan, deutan, or tritan" defects. Other factors aid in differentiating congenital from acquired color vision defects. In particular, congenital anomalies are bilateral and symmetric, whereas acquired defects are rarely symmetric. Furthermore, congenital defects are non-progressive, whereas acquired defects generally progress. Kollner[45] originally proposed that acquired dyschromatopsias due to optic nerve disease typically produce red-green deficits, whereas a loss of blue-yellow discrimination is more characteristic of retinal/macular disorders. There are numerous exceptions to this "rule," and it should be considered no more than a casual guide; indeed, some macular diseases may show red-green confusion deficits, whereas optic neuropathies have blue-yellow deficits early in their pathogenesis. In either instance, both red-green and blue-yellow deficits usually evolve as the disease progresses. Finally, in considering acquired color vision deficiencies, it is important to recognize that changes in the optical properties of the pre-retinal media, in particular, wavelength-specific changes in the absorption properties of the lens, can produce significant color discrimination defects. In addition, the normal aging process can contribute to a reduction in color discrimination that can confound the interpretation of color test results.

NEURO-OPHTHALMOLOGIC EVALUATION OF VISUAL FUNCTION

The neuro-ophthalmologic examination of the sensory visual system employs various strategies and examination techniques for the dual purpose of (1) determining the probable cause or at least the topographic localization of the lesions causing a visual disturbance or symptom and (2) documenting the character and extent of the visual disturbance. Frequently, these two objectives are so closely linked that they cannot be truly separated. By evaluating the character and extent of a visual deficit, the site of the lesion and the probable cause can often be deduced. A trivial example will suffice. If a patient's visual symptoms are found to be associated with a true bitemporal hemianopia, the disorder is certainly situated at the chiasm and the cause is most likely a tumor in or close to the sella turcica. The neuro-ophthalmic examination of patients with occult visual problems or with otherwise unexplained visual disturbances must use this goal-directed approach.

Frequently, the neuro-ophthalmologic approach involves considerable "detective work," namely, collecting evidence and assembling clues that can identify the origin and nature of the visual disturbance with increasing certainty. The more supporting evidence that can be accumulated, the stronger is the likelihood of a correct diagnosis. Information that does not "fit" must first be rechecked, reconfirmed, modified, or discarded. All genuine findings should be explained and, if possible, reconciled. Failure to account for observations that appear incompatible with a diagnosis can be perilous.

The principles, examination procedures, and techniques described here are not restricted to the patient with a suspected neuro-ophthalmic disorder. They are useful in localizing and diagnosing any disturbance of vision, and particularly those involving occult processes, because the systematic approach used in neuro-ophthalmology frequently results in the accurate diagnosis of optical, retinal, and anterior segment disorders. However, the emphasis here is on the basic maneuvers and techniques essential in the elucidation of neuro-ophthalmic problems. Consequently, measurements of foveal and optic nerve function, sensitivity to color and brightness, and the visual field examination are of major importance and receive special attention.

The technology available to assess visual function and to evaluate the sensory visual system is increasing dramatically from year to year. In addition to traditional Snellen and more recent logMAR optotype acuity, foveal function can also be scrutinized using various types of contrast sensitivity testing, suprathreshold contrast matching tests, spatial frequency–filtered acuity tests, and a variety of electrophysiologic tests, including focal and pattern electroretinography (ERG) and visual evoked potentials (VEPs). Visual fields can now be evaluated by a selection of computerized tests, performed using several different instruments, as well as by the more traditional methods. However, as always, the diagnostic process begins with history taking. The characteristics of visual symptoms, their evolution, and their associated neurologic and systemic problems provide important, often unique, clues to neurologic localization and etiology of visual pathway lesions, and they are arguably more critical for the accurate and timely diagnosis of lesions involving the sensory visual pathway than for diseases involving other parts of the visual apparatus.

Symptoms

Blurring is the most common complaint of patients with vision problems; unfortunately, it is also the most nonspecific. Blurring or indistinctness of boundaries and lines is produced by degradation of the optical image on the retina in refractive disorders and by opacities of the ocular media. These optical causes of blur must be distinguished from similar symptoms of neurologic lesions. Associated symptoms such as color loss or dyschromatopsia (hue desaturation) or dimness of vision should be sought to make this distinction.

The word "scotoma" implies a circumscribed area of darkness or dimness in the visual field. Some patients, however, refer to a scotomatous area as blurred rather than dark. Localized blur or otherwise degraded vision in the center of the visual field may indicate either macular changes or optic nerve disease with predominant involvement of the papillomacular nerve fiber bundle. Pronounced central field depression is not indicative of refractive errors or ocular media opacities, which rather produce diffuse or non-localized blurring of vision.

The sensory visual system seems to be organized into a series of neural channels having specific functions (see the discussion of parallel pathways, above). There are even separate channels for contrast perception of coarse versus fine detail, and there may be diminished sensitivity for one stimulus category and not for others. For instance, specific loss of sensitivity for medium spatial frequency visual information is a common residual dysfunction following recovery from optic neuritis. When viewed with the affected eye, objects appear faded or washed out, even though the contours still appear sharp. The latter aspect correlates with relatively normal function at high–spatial frequency channels that detect fine detail (see the discussion of contrast sensitivity below).

The term "ghost image" is used to describe a form of monocular diplopia in which an image appears to be edged or outlined by a secondary, usually dimmer, image; or it may appear as a line faintly duplicated in a second superimposed image. This type of symptom is almost always a result of irregularities in the optical media of the eye, often attributable to cataracts and even to uncorrected astigmatism. Ghost images are always visible monocularly, although they may be present for each eye, and they are almost always eliminated by the use of a pinhole aperture. Ghost images must be distinguished from small-angle diplopia, in which the second image will disappear on occlusion of either eye. In addition, in true binocular diplopia resulting from muscle imbalance or paresis, the two images have equal visual density or clarity if vision in the two eyes is good. However, it should be noted that the combination of diplopia and reduced contrast sensitivity in one eye may mimic the faded ghost image seen with monocular diplopia.

Curvilinear distortion of straight lines or patterns is called *metamorphopsia* and indicates the presence of macular edema, submacular fluid, epimacular membrane, retinochoroidal folds, or other retinal distortion that results in alteration of photoreceptor orientation. Objects may seem too large (*macropsia*) or too small (*micropsia*) as a result of abnormal compression or separation of photoreceptor elements in the fovea. Metamorphopsia is usually monocular or, at least, asymmetric and it cannot be a result of retro-bulbar optic neuropathy.

A sense of darkness or of dimmed lights often accompanies optic neuropathy, even when central vision is relatively preserved. It seems as if the visual pathway has separate channels encoding brightness information that may be altered selectively in optic nerve disease. A sense of darkness is more strongly associated with depression of the entire field, rather than with small central scotomas. In addition, persons with central scotomas note relatively better vision in dim lighting[46] because the paracentral and peripheral rod photoreceptors operate better at low light levels (scotopic conditions).

A dynamic sensation of continuous dimming or darkening of vision can more readily be attributed to retinal disease and can occur when retinal or choroidal perfusion is insufficient to meet the retina's metabolic demands. In such cases, an interval in darkness promotes temporary improvement, and an abnormal photostress test (see below) confirms the diagnosis. Dimness may also be the principal complaint with hemianopia, particularly when the lesion involves the chiasm or optic tract.

Acquired disorders of the afferent visual pathways commonly disrupt color perception. Patients may report a sense of reduced vividness of colors, or they may state that colors are "washed out" (desaturated) or dull when they are questioned. Although red seems disproportionally susceptible to this subjective alteration, patients usually agree that all colors are less vivid. Some patients characterize the altered shades of color as *darker,* that is, red is shifted toward amber or brown, whereas others say colors appear *faded* or lighter, that is, red is shifted toward orange or yellow. This subjective variability may result from the degree to which the associated brightness channels in the afferent visual system are involved. Central dyschromatopsia can occur rarely with lesions of the inferior occipital cortex. These lesions may produce color vision defects that are quite distinctive and bilateral (see Chapter 7). Patients complain that color sensation is absent and the world appears in "black-and-white." Inability to name colors, but with intact color discrimination, characterizes alexia without agraphia (see below). Color discrimination is within the purview of the right hemisphere, but naming requires transfer of visual information to the left hemisphere.

How a patient reads is a little like how a patient walks. For the physician, it provides a wealth of information on visual system function; reading requires coordinated participation of the sensory visual systems and of the ocular motor apparatus. Patients with simple hemianopias that split fixation (*i.e.,* that pass through the fovea) may complain of difficulty reading, particularly with the loss of the right hemifield, because they cannot scan forward adequately on the written page. Patients with left hemianopsia may read a line of text fluently, but they have difficulty finding the lefthand margin and the beginning of the next line. Hemifield loss may be evident when testing acuity as the patient may fail to see letters toward the side of the chart corresponding to the side of the hemianopsia (Fig. 2–2).

Reading difficulties resulting from hemianopic field loss occur when there is loss of the macular representation in the hemianopic field and usually are not present when the central portion of the hemianopic field is preserved, as occurs with *macular sparing* (see below). Conversely, patients with partial hemianopias involving only the paracentral region adjacent to fixation (*i.e.,* half the macula) often complain of difficulty reading, and they may read the eye chart in the selective manner described above, leaving out letters on the side of their hemianopic field defect. This type of limited central homonymous hemianopia can occur when the lesion is confined to the occipital pole of the visual cortex, or it can occur in one or both eyes in cases of chiasmal dysfunction. Patients who read the chart selectively in this way provide a strong clue to the nature of their field defect (see Fig. 2–2). This reading behavior may be critical in

suggesting the correct diagnosis in patients with normal peripheral fields and a small, occult, central hemianopic defect.

Migraine frequently affects reading because visual auras at or close to fixation, with shifting patches of mixed negative and bright positive scotomas, can obscure one or two letters at a time. This transient hemianopic scotoma must be distinguished from the common "running together" of print as occurs with insidious presbyopia and that is relieved with appropriate correction of refraction for near.

Alexia without agraphia (see Chapter 7) is an extreme and specific reading disorder in which the right occipital cortex is disconnected from the language mechanism in the left hemisphere because of a lesion involving the splenium of the corpus callosum, where an extensive bundle of commissural fibers links the right and left visual association cortices. A second lesion, most commonly involving the left calcarine cortex, produces a dense right homonymous hemianopsia, so that visual information enters only the right occipital cortex from the left hemifield. The written word is perceived accurately as a complex form in the right occiput, but linguistic analysis of the words, which requires participation of the left hemisphere in most individuals, is blocked by the callosal lesion. Auditory and tactile input to the language mechanism is intact, so the patient is not aphasic and can write spontaneously or in response to spoken dictation. This was one of the first disconnection syndromes to be demonstrated adequately in clinical neurology.

Tests of Macular and Foveal Function

Visual Acuity

Visual acuity must be recorded each time a patient is examined. Standard acuity measures can be extremely helpful in diagnosing lesions of the visual pathway, but, paradoxically, they may be *relatively* insensitive to pathologic processes involving the optic nerves, chiasm and the retro-chiasmal pathways. If acuity is reduced more than a few lines by a lesion of the optic nerve or chiasm, there is also accompanying diminished color sense, a relative afferent pupillary defect (RAPD), and a significant field defect. Ocular disease, on the other hand, including most occult processes involving the macula, can reduce acuity substantially, without necessarily producing dramatic deficits in color perception, pupillary response, or visual field.

Snellen letter visual acuity testing is firmly entrenched in clinical ophthalmology. It is measured using printed "eye charts" or facsimiles of these charts on projection slides, computer-generated displays, and light boxes. The individual characters (letters or numbers) on the

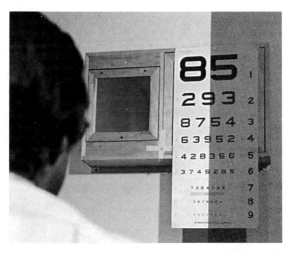

Fig. 2–2. A patient with hemianopia may ignore half the reading chart. Such defects can be asymptomatic.

acuity chart are called *optotypes.* Standards for the printing of charts and projection slides dictate that letters be high in contrast (usually greater than 85% to 90%). Block characters (*sans serif* or Gothic fonts) and overall letter width and height should be nearly equal. By definition, the 20/20 letter subtends 5 minutes of visual angle at the retina, and each component stroke of the letter is 1 minute wide. Thus, 20/20 vision could be interpreted as the ability to resolve images with details subtending as little as 1 minute of arc. However, as discussed below, this is a gross oversimplification. The usual fractional notation (20/20), although easily recognized, is not a particularly useful designation because it is awkward to manipulate arithmetically and statistically. Alternatively, the fraction is expressed as a decimal (20/20=1.0; 20/30=0.66; 20/40=0.5, and so on). However, it is not really a fraction in the mathematical sense. The numerator refers to the distance from which the patient reads the letters, and the denominator is the distance at which a "normal" eye could identify the same letters. An eye with 20/40 vision can make out letters of a certain size at 20 feet that a "normal" eye could discern even at 40 feet. As an observer moves from a viewing distance of 40 to one of 20 feet, the retinal image becomes twice as large. In a sense then, acuity of 20/40 is "half as good" as 20/20, and the decimal notation 0.5 expresses this concept. Similarly, 20/80 can be considered "half as good" again as 20/40, but what is not clear is whether a pathologic process producing 20/80 vision is twice as severe as that which results in 20/40 vision. Measured acuity depends greatly on the conditions under which the subject is tested, the criteria applied to subject performance on reading an eye chart, and the construction of the chart itself.

Frisén and Frisén,[41] in a normative study of 100 individuals at various ages, found that 20/20 is an excessively lax criterion for normal acuity. Using a 50% frequency-of-seeing criterion and a 10-letter Sloan chart, average performance was considerably better than 20/15, even for the elderly groups. An average normal subject had a 10% probability of discriminating letters just larger than 20/10 (decimal acuity 1.9) and a 90% probability of discriminating letters just larger than 20/15 (1.3). However, rather than using the usual office practice of requiring almost 100% performance on a line of letters, these authors chose the 50% probability-of-seeing (discriminating) criterion as most suitable. Whether one agrees with this choice or not, it is necessary to recognize that the criterion used in that study produces higher (better) acuities compared with the more stringent (90% to 100%) performance criterion used routinely in clinical practice.

Because acuity can vary with environment and exposure to light, it should be measured under controlled conditions. Abnormalities of the ocular media and macular disease may adversely affect visual acuity depending on current and recent exposure to light, if such

exposure can result in glare or prolonged recovery after bleaching of retinal photoreceptors (as occurs in macular edema, serous detachment, and photoreceptor degenerations). Thus, patients with vague visual complaints that may result from glare or dazzle may have normal acuity in a dim room or after resting their eyes. When the symptoms occur under certain specific environmental conditions, the astute clinician is advised to test acuity and visual function under lighting conditions mimicking those prevailing during the offending situations. In this way, the circumstances that induce or aggravate visual disturbances can be used advantageously to help localize the cause of the visual disturbance (*e.g.,* see Photostress Test below).

When testing acuity or other aspects of visual sensory function, there is a tendency to be limited by the equipment at hand. This is an artificial constraint. A patient who cannot read the Snellen or equivalent distance chart needs to be evaluated further, and quantitative measures of acuity should be still be sought. Some patients may be able to identify the large numbers or symbols on a reading card, especially at close range. Patients with central scotomas can often identify single letters presented within their paracentral field. Tests designed to evaluate acuity in children such as the Sheridan-Gardner, "HOTV" tests or a simple "E" card can be very useful. The most sensitive portion of the visual field can be identified at close range, and then the distance from the smallest symbol that can be reliably identified should be recorded. Thus, a patient who can see a 20/100 "E card" at 5 ft, fixing eccentrically with the superior nasal quadrant, should have acuity recorded as follows: "5/100 S(upra)N(asal) with single E card." When presenting this type of stimulus at close range, appropriate near correction must be used with patients older than 40 years, and it may even be helpful in younger patients. These cards are also useful with the occasional patient who has a central disorder (such as dyslexia, aphasia, or agnosia) that limits the ability to name characters, although these characters can be seen and recognized. Anyone who can "count fingers" should be able to identify large single letters, but those patients who cannot should have acuity recorded as "counts fingers," "hand movements," or "perceives light" in a particular quadrant, at a specified distance. Some patients who cannot see well enough to count fingers can see movement of just the fingers, so that "finger movement" can be used as an intermediate grade between count fingers and hand movements. When testing perception of movement or of light, care must be taken to interrupt the stimulation and to ask that the patient identify *when,* and not just *if,* he or she detects the stimulus. With hand movements, one can also ask the direction of movement. Many of these methods are also useful when testing acuity at the bedside and whenever a patient cannot be brought to an examining site.

Additional clues to the nature of a visual disturbance can be derived from the actual process of obtaining a patient's acuity. Most practitioners recognize that the failure to see characters on the right or left side of an acuity chart should arouse suspicion of a hemianopsia. However, patients frequently state that certain portions of a line of characters appear blurred, absent, distorted, doubled, or deviated. This information can be useful in determining the site of the disturbance. Diseases of the optic nerves, chiasm, and tracts, as well the posterior visual pathway, do not produce monocular *metamorphopsia,* whether it is described as distortion, doubling, or deviation of images. On the other hand, central lesions can occasionally generate distorted images and visual illusions that may mimic true metamorphopsia, but they are seen with either eye. Thus, unilateral metamorphopsia is certainly ocular in origin. Of course, ocular diseases include disturbances of the optic disc, such as papilledema, which can distort the retina and can produce metamorphopsia.

Depending on a patient's symptoms, it may be advisable to determine best corrected visual acuity at distance and near, and both monocularly and binocularly, because some symptoms may appear only under selected circumstances. Any unexplained discrepancy in visual function should arouse concern. For example, a patient with latent nystagmus may have substantially better acuity when using both eyes as compared to the monocular acuity of each eye when the other is covered. Moreover, there may be significant inconsistencies in the findings when the visual problem is factitious or "functional," thus providing a clue to its origin (see below).

Contrast Sensitivity

The measurement of contrast sensitivity in a clinical setting has been simplified by the appearance of a variety of new charts and electronic devices. The scientific method for determining contrast sensitivity is to measure sensitivity thresholds at a series of different spatial frequencies using sine wave gratings displayed on a video monitor. The gratings are displayed while the contrast is varied, and the patient signals when the pattern is first detected. The mean and standard deviation of this threshold are calculated for various spatial frequencies, typically ranging from 0.5 to 23 cpd, and the graphic representation of these data determines the contrast sensitivity function or curve. In humans, there is a contrast sensitivity peak around 4 cpd (Fig. 2–3). Although commercially designed equipment that simplifies this process is now available, determining contrast sensitivity functions is time-consuming and impractical in most clinical settings. However, research studies[39] using this method have led to the detection of four basic patterns of selective loss in pathologic states: (1) high-frequency loss; (2) broad or generalized loss at all frequencies; (3) mid-frequency

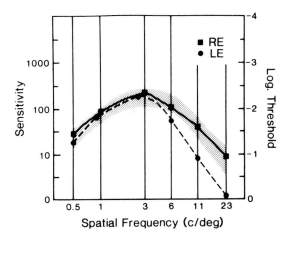

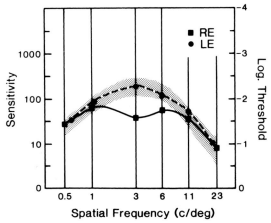

Fig. 2–3. Graphs of contrast sensitivity (*ordinate*) versus spatial frequency (*abscissa*). The normal range is shaded in gray. In the *upper plot,* there is gradual fall-off of sensitivity at high spatial frequencies resulting from optical blur. The *lower plot* illustrates selective loss of mid-spatial frequencies in a patient with optic neuritis of the right eye. (Courtesy of Nicollet Co., Chicago)

("notch") defects; and (4) low–mid-frequency loss. Thus, in practice, only two measurements are needed in order to detect all patterns of loss: (1) visual acuity, which is a measure of high-frequency contrast; and (2) an intermediate spatial frequency contrast threshold. Concentrating on developing a simplified test of contrast sensitivity in the intermediate-frequency range, Regan and Neima[40] and Pelli et al[39,47] developed charts using familiar optotypes, varying in contrast (black to light gray letters on a white background).

The *Pelli-Robson* chart was designed using optotypes of fixed size, but varying contrast (gray to black) to test for mid-range spatial-frequency loss.[47] This technique reliably discriminates normal from abnormal peak contrast sensitivity.[39] Regan and Neima[40] also developed a set of low-contrast optotype acuity charts aimed at testing discrimination that depends on mid-range spatial frequencies. The charts are at least equal to sine wave grating tests in detecting spatial frequency loss in the mid-range of the contrast sensitivity function in patients with diabetes, glaucoma, ocular hypertension, and Parkinson's disease. These tests offer the clinician a familiar, practical method of measuring contrast sensitivity at mid-spatial frequencies.

In contrast, the Vistech wall chart[48] differs from the Pelli-Robson and Regan charts because it uses sine wave gratings presented at different orientations and contrasts. In place of individual letters, each grating is presented as a small, circular spot on the chart, which consists of five rows, each with nine spots. The spatial frequency of the gratings in a particular row is constant, but it increases toward the bottom. The contrast of the individual grating decreases from left to right along each row. Subjects are asked to identify the orientation of the individual gratings. Rubin[49] compared the Pelli-Robson, Regan, and the Vistech charts and reported that the Pelli-Robson charts were the most sensitive in *detecting* loss of peak contrast sensitivity (at midrange spatial frequencies) and gave the most reproducible results. He found that measurement of peak contrast sensitivity alone was extremely effective in detecting pathologic states and concluded that, in clinical testing, it is not necessary to measure sensitivity to individual spatial frequencies using different sine wave gratings. In the Optic Neuritis Treatment Trial, it was found that Pelli-Robson contrast sensitivity testing was the most sensitive indicator of visual dysfunction in the setting of normal visual acuity (see Chapter 5, Part II).

Color Vision

The subjective appreciation of color saturation or brightness is one of the most useful clinical components of the sensory neuro-ophthalmologic examination. As indicated above, color sensitivity is typically reduced dramatically in inflammatory, infiltrative, and compressive optic and chiasmal neuropathies, even when acuity is relatively well preserved. Color sensitivity will be depressed in ischemic optic neuropathy if both superior and inferior portions of the central field are involved. The effect of optic neuropathies on color is in marked contrast to the relatively well preserved color sensitivity in most acquired macular and ocular disease, in which acuity is usually more disturbed than color vision.

Simple or complex tests are used to evaluate color vision clinically. Booklets of color plates such as the Hardy-Rand-Rittler (HRR) series or various versions of Ishihara's pseudo-isochromatic plates, as well as a number of imitators, are also used. The neuro-ophthalmic color evaluation is concerned primarily with topical diagnosis and semiqualitative assessment of color sense rather than the determination of congenital color vision deficiencies, and standardized lighting and viewing distances are less strictly enforced. The number of characters identified correctly is recorded ("7 of 9 plates"), rather than the specific identity of plates. It is important to note the ease and rapidity with which patients identify characters. Some patients may identify characters only after tracing them with a finger. (The patient preferably should point or use an artist's soft paintbrush, because actual contact eventually produces damage.)

Patients may be asked simply to describe the color of various objects (bottle caps or colored sheets of paper). If one eye has normal or substantially better vision, comparison of gross color saturation between the two eyes, and between paired quadrants of the visual field, can be assessed (see Visual Fields and Perimetry). During such comparison testing, care must be taken to keep constant the size of the colored stimulus, the distance from the eyes, eccentricity in the visual field, and incident illumination. Overhead fluorescent lighting usually is sufficient. The patient must understand, however, that the task is to compare the relative intensity, color saturation, or brightness (*e.g.*, "redness" of an object) when the stimulus is presented alternately to each eye, or at two positions in the visual field, usually to either side of the vertical meridian (see below). Inconsistent or uninterpretable responses include the subjective sensation of a darker, less saturated red, as seen with an impaired eye, but identified as "redder" than the brightly, saturated hue of the stimulus as seen with the normal, or less impaired, eye.

After bright light exposure (pupil light reactions or ophthalmoscopy), or any significant asymmetries in the ocular media, such as the presence of unilateral pseudophakia, aphakia, cataract, or other opacities, the subjective perception of hue and saturation of colors may be falsely enhanced. In these situations, objective tests, such as the pupillary responses, are more reliable indicators of anterior pathway dysfunction.

Special mention must be made of patients who have congenital color deficiencies. Red-green color confusion affects approximately 10% of the male population, and many mildly and moderately affected patients unaware of their deficiencies score poorly on the Ishihara series of plates. Therefore, patients should be asked about difficulty discriminating colors or whether color sense has previously been tested (*e.g.*, in the military service). If color vision in both eyes is symmetrically depressed, and there is no other reason to account for dyschromatopsia, a congenital deficit should be suspected. The HRR plates are very useful in these cases, because 6 of the 20 plates are designed to test non–red-green types of congenital color deficiency. The symbols on these 6 plates will be missed by patients with acquired anterior visual pathway disease affecting central vision, but they are easily identified by patients whose vision is otherwise normal and who have congenital red-green dyschromatopsia, who have much greater difficulty with some of the more brightly saturated characters on the remaining 14 plates.

Nichols et al[50] found that using a subset of the lengthy Farnsworth-Munsell 100-hue test (F-M 100), consisting of chips 22 to 42, had nearly the same sensitivity and specificity for detecting optic neuropathies. These workers found that the majority of the clinical value can be achieved in one-fourth of the time required for the standard F-M 100 test protocol.

Pupillary Light Response

The pupillary light response is an objective indicator of anterior visual pathway function, in general, but it is a particularly practical and sensitive measure of optic nerve dysfunction. The speed and amplitude of the pupillary light reaction generally depend on the overall intensity and speed with which the afferent neural signal is transmitted to the brain stem. Diseases of the retina, optic nerve, chiasm, and tract produce definite decreases in pupillary reactivity that last as long as the lesion persists. Moderate media opacities, such as cataract, do not have this effect (see Chapter 15).

In practice, a pupillary reaction diminished by a lesion of the anterior visual pathway is most easily uncovered using the *swinging flashlight test,* probably the single most useful diagnostic test in neuro-ophthalmology. In a darkened room, each eye is alternately stimulated with a bright light stimulus, which is moved rhythmically from one eye to the other. The pupillary reactions elicited during stimulation of one eye are compared with the reaction produced during identical stimulation of the other eye. A pathologic process of the anterior pathway disrupting function disproportionally on one side produces a "relative afferent pupillary defect" (RAPD), also known as a "Marcus Gunn" pupil. The characteristic observation is "release" or dilation of both pupils when the light is moved from the better to the affected eye.

Several principles apply: (1) to avoid pupillary constriction associated with accommodation (the near response), the subject should fixate a distant target; (2) each eye must be stimulated identically in an alternating fashion, with the brightness, incident angle, and duration of stimulus the same for both eyes; (3) the alternating swing interval from one eye to the other should be equally rapid in both directions; (4) the direct reaction of each pupil to the stimulus can only be identical if the efferent motor pathway is intact and if the irides are mechanically and structurally identical; (5) if there is marked anisocoria or other pathologic changes of the globe that could influence the pupil's reaction, the direct and consensual reactions of only one pupil (usually the one with the better reaction or more preserved structure) should be observed while performing the swinging flashlight test; (6) when in doubt, the test should be repeated using two alternation rates, "slow" and "fast," approximately 1 second per eye for fast rate and a 3-second stimulus for slow rate; (7) if an asymmetry in the response is noted, a grading system may be used to describe it (see Chapter 15 for detailed descriptions of qualitative and quantitative RAPD grading). For example, grades can be described as one plus (1+), two plus (2+), and so forth, with four plus (4+) corresponding to an amaurotic or non-reactive pupil in a blind eye. According to this scheme, a 3+ RAPD indicates that the pupils dilate readily or "release" when the affected eye is stimulated, and 2+ when the pupils fail to constrict or dilate slightly when the light swings to the weaker eye. A 1+ RAPD is a minimally detectable asymmetry. This grading system is subjective, and its reliability will depend on consistency of the technique applied. Every clinician should establish a clear sense of what each grade represents.

Neutral density filters may be used to quantify the asymmetry in the afferent input from each eye. A set of progressive neutral density filters (usually incorporated into a bar holder) is used over the normal eye while performing the swinging flashlight test. The density of the filter that just balances (neutralizes) the defect in the abnormal eye is determined and the RAPD is then specified as the *density* in log units of this filter (see Chapter 15).

If the patient has strabismus, care must be taken to direct the light stimulus in the identical position with respect to the visual axis of each eye. The key factor that cannot be overemphasized is to provide the exact same stimulus to each eye. Under rigidly identical stimulating conditions, any asymmetry in the pupillary reaction to light is significant and usually implies a pregeniculate lesion. Rarely, afferent pupillary defects can be attributed to mid-brain lesions, but in these cases, visual function is usually preserved on all other tests. With relatively symmetric bilateral neural visual loss, both eyes may show sluggish pupillary light reactions.

Photostress Test

A variety of choroidal and retinal diseases, particularly those affecting the macula, can cause subjective visual disturbances. At times, funduscopy and fluorescein angiography can fail to reveal structural changes in the tissues and vessels sufficient to account for these symptoms. In these situations, the disturbance is often erroneously attributed to an occult optic neuropathy. One of the most useful techniques available to help distinguish a maculopathy from optic nerve dysfunction is the photostress test.

The photostress test records visual recovery after a

retinal bleach, and as such it is a measure of photopigment regeneration. This, in turn, depends on the metabolic activity and general health of the retina, retinal pigment epithelium, and choroid. Recovery of vision after exposure to a bright light stimulus is not generally prolonged when visual dysfunction is due to diseases affecting the optic nerve. Consequently, prolonged recovery after photostress effectively localizes the dysfunction to the macula.

The photostress test is a rapid and uncomplicated maneuver.[51] A modified photostress test may be conducted as follows (Fig. 2–4):

1. Best corrected visual acuity is recorded in each eye.
2. With the defective eye covered, the normal or "better" eye is subjected to a strong light directed into the pupil for a specific time (*e.g.,* 10 to 15 seconds).
3. The light is removed, and the patient is instructed to begin reading the chart as soon as any letters can be identified. The end point is the interval until the "next largest" line (just above the one for best acuity) is read. This recovery period is timed and recorded.
4. Now the defective or "worse" eye is exposed to the same bright light directed into the pupil for the same length of time.
5. The light is removed, and the recovery period (*i.e.,* the interval until the patient can again begin to read the "next largest" line) is recorded.
6. The recovery period of the two eyes is compared.

Normal recovery depends on age, but in a young, healthy eye, it is usually 15 to 30 seconds. In older individuals, normal recovery can take 30 to 50 seconds. Markedly asymmetric recovery periods for each eye or periods longer than 60 seconds are definitely abnormal. For example, if decreased acuity is caused by retinal edema, central serous choroidopathy (retinopathy), or similar macular lesions, recovery time in the abnormal eye will be prolonged to between 90 and 150 seconds (see Fig. 2–4D). In contrast, if the deficit of central vision is, for example, due to retro-bulbar neuritis or compression of the optic nerve, visual recovery following light stress to the eye with decreased vision will occur over approximately the same period as recovery in the normal eye.

There are ample experimental and clinical data to support the concept of prolonged recovery time following light stimulation of the retina in the presence of defects in the choriocapillaris, retinal pigment epithelium, and outer retinal layers.[51,52] For example, in the case of a small serous detachment of retinal pigment epithelium or retina, a positive scotoma is induced following exposure of the fundus to bright light. The "afterimage" is prolonged until visual pigments are regenerated. Similarly, a primary maculopathy or inadequate macular perfusion can markedly prolong the recovery of a bleached retina producing symptoms of

"glare," visual "wash out" or "white out," or a perception of continual dimming of the environment.[52] With mild macular dysfunction, symptoms may only be present during or after exposure to bright surroundings. More advanced maculopathies may produce symptoms at normal indoor light levels, but in a dark or dim room, they can be virtually asymptomatic, and affected patients may continue to score well on standard eye tests performed under these idealized conditions. Photostress can also be used to elicit or enhance a central scotoma during visual field examination or when the patient is tested using the Amsler grid.

Stereopsis and Binocular Fusion

Binocular depth perception and fusion are not tested routinely in adults, but their determination can be useful in certain situations. Patients with mild to moderate reduction in visual acuity that cannot be explained and those complaining of intermittent diplopia, but with eyes that appear to be aligned, should be evaluated using standard clinical tests of binocular fusion, such as the Worth 4-dot test and the four diopter base-out prism test. Binocular depth perception and stereoacuity can be estimated with simple stereographic tests, such as the Titmus Fly and Randot tests. These tests may help to uncover mild occult amblyopia, microtropias, or intermittent, decompensated strabismus. Such testing can also be extremely instructive in situations of feigned or hysterical visual loss, when the measured stereoacuity or binocular perception is attainable, but the patient's subjective near and distant monocular acuity as determined using standard acuity charts is seemingly grossly abnormal.[53] Descriptions of these and other test of binocular function are beyond the scope of this chapter.

VISUAL FIELDS AND PERIMETRY

Traquair's classic definition of the visual field is: "that portion of space in which objects are visible at the same moment during steady fixation of the gaze in one direction."[54] Perimetry measures the visual field and involves recording of visual function of the eye at topographically defined loci in space. Understanding the visual field as it relates to neuro-ophthalmologic diagnosis is a complex subject requiring knowledge of the anatomy of the optic pathways and contiguous related structures, of the intrinsic organization of retinal projection through the pathways and in the cortex, and of the nature of various lesions and the mechanisms by which they produce field defects. The specific localizing characteristics of field defects are discussed subsequently in the chapters dealing with topical diagnosis in the visual sensory system.

The visual field is too often considered peripheral visual space, exclusive of central function, that is termed "acuity." That is, the field is defined as extrafoveal visual

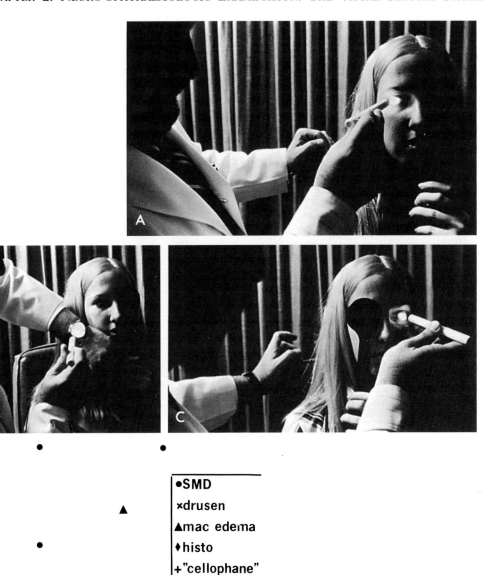

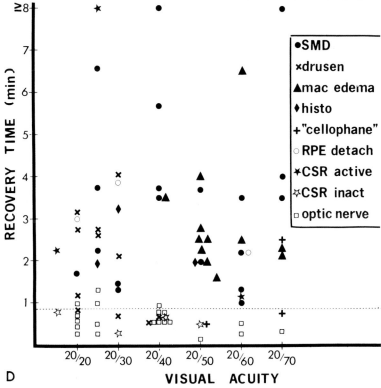

Fig. 2-4. Light stress test. **A.** The retina is bleached with bright light as the patient occludes the other eye. **B.** The recovery phase is timed. **C.** The second eye is exposed to light. **D.** Photostress recovery times in macular and optic nerve disease. The *dotted line* represents 50 seconds, the upper limit of normal for 99% of control eyes. *SMD,* senile macular degeneration; *histo,* histoplasmosis syndrome; *RPE,* retinal pigment epithelium; *CSR,* central serous retinopathy. (From ref. 51.)

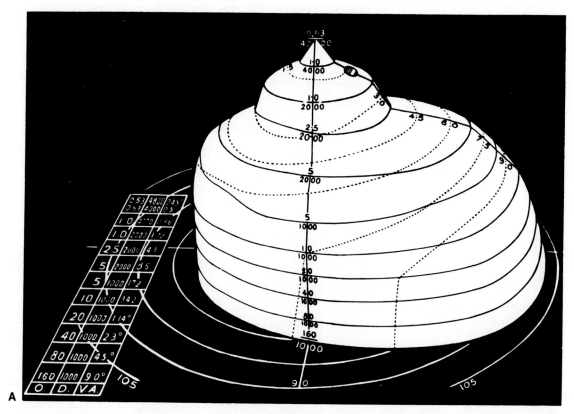

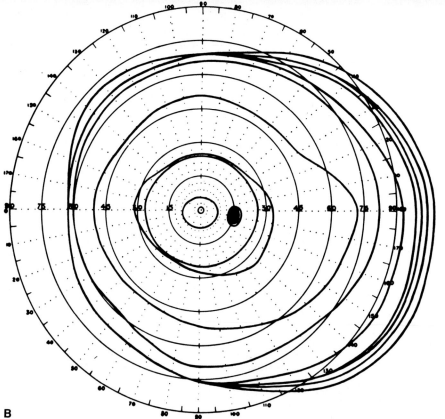

Fig. 2–5. A. Three-dimensional model of Traquair's "Island of Vision." The right visual field is shown. **B.** Standard flat plot of isopters, as if viewed from above.

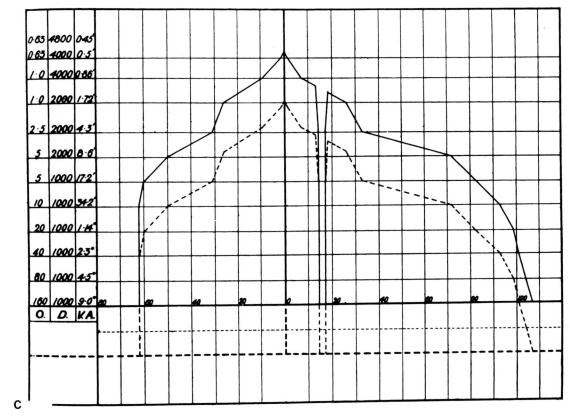

Fig. 2–5. (*continued*) **C.** Vertical (section along horizontal) meridian. *O,* target size in millimeters. **D.** Distance from the eye in millimeters. *VA,* visual angle. (From ref. 54.)

function. As is inherent in Traquair's definition, however, the visual field in more appropriately thought of as a three-dimensional "island of vision surrounded by a sea of blindness" crowned by a sharp pinnacle of central vision (Fig. 2–5). Certainly in the context of neurologic dysfunction, the central portion of the visual field is at least as important as the periphery.

There are many techniques and a variety of equipment available for evaluating visual fields. In essence, however, all methods depend on the patient's subjective response to a visual stimulus. The threshold of perception for a specific visual stimulus is determined either qualitatively or quantitatively by varying the size, brightness, color, or some other physical attribute of the stimulus and the point at which that stimulus is just perceived (*i.e.,* the threshold sensitivity) is determined. With Goldmann-type perimetry recording, a line is drawn connecting peripheral points of equal threshold sensitivity, thereby defining the *isopter* for that specified stimulus. This convention is roughly analogous to the isobar lines on weather maps, which define areas of equal atmospheric pressure. Complex manual and computerized perimeters have been developed to determine threshold sensitivity to a variety of stimuli and either to plot the position and shape of isopters or to graphically

represent the sensitivity thresholds otherwise. Before dealing with these devices, however, we consider some basic principles of visual field measurement and the relatively simple, yet sensitive, confrontation techniques that are easily available to any clinician, at any time, and in all clinical settings.

Anatomic Considerations

In general, field defects due to lesions of the retina optic nerve, chiasm, and visual pathways conform to a limited set of patterns. The variations in these patterns are elaborated elsewhere in discussions of topical diagnosis (see Chapters 5, 6, and 7), but several anatomic concepts necessary for understanding the basic principles of perimetry are considered here.

Pathologic processes involving the retina may produce general or geographically focal field defects or areas of diminished sensitivity (*i.e.,* scotomas); these deficits frequently correspond to lesions visible on funduscopy. Macular lesions produce *central* (at fixation) scotomas, sparing the periphery, whereas widespread tapeto-retinal degenerations result in generalized field constriction, often sparing central fixation (see Chapter 5, Part I).

Lesions of the optic nerve head or immediate peripapillary region, as well as some vascular diseases, tend to produce retinal "nerve fiber bundle defects," which are segmental defects extending radially outward from the blind spot. The configurations of these scotoma patterns are as follows: temporal wedge-shaped when the lesion is at the nasal aspect of the disc; or arcuate curves toward the nasal periphery with damage to axonal bundles at the superior or inferior poles of the optic disc. Superior or inferior arcuate scotomas point to, or originate at, the blind spot and terminate at the nasal horizontal meridian, which represents the anatomic temporal raphe that extends from the fovea to the temporal retinal periphery. These defects frequently spare central vision, leaving acuity intact. Lesions at the temporal aspect of the optic disc result in centrocecal scotomas that encompass the blind spot and the central (macular) region, resulting in decreased visual acuity. Large lesions on or near the optic disc may result in areas of visual field loss that combine two or more of these segmental patterns.

Typically, and rather consistently, retro-bulbar disorders of the optic nerves (*e.g.*, optic neuritis, toxic neuropathies) have a predilection for especially depressing function in the central core of the nerve. This central core is occupied predominantly by small caliber myelinated fibers subserving the cone system of the fovea and macular area of the retina (the papillomacular nerve fiber bundle). Defects in this system cause diminished visual acuity, depression of central field, and alterations in color vision. A central scotoma occurring in the absence of macular disease is the classic, but not exclusive, hallmark of a lesion involving the optic nerve (see Chapter 5, Part II).

At the chiasm, all afferent nerve fibers from both eyes are segregated into crossed and uncrossed systems (Fig. 2–6). It is at the chiasm that the visual system becomes functionally divided by a vertical demarcation through the fixation point, the retino-cortical projections representing the left hemifields of both eyes blending and coursing toward the right cerebral hemisphere and the projections representing the right homonymous halves of the field joining and coursing to the left. In the optic nerve (*i.e.*, anterior to the chiasm), there is no functional vertical demarcation of right and left fields. At the chiasm, and in the pathways posterior to it, there is an *inviolate* lateralizing separation of homonymous hemifields. It is thus that the vertical meridian that divides the hemifields assumes critical importance in the elucidation and exploration of field defects due to lesions of the chiasm, optic radiations, and occipital cortex.

The optic tract forms a compact fascicle of fibers that passes to the LGN of the thalamus. Lesions of this tract or of the LGN are relatively infrequent, and when they occur, they typically produce fairly incongruent (unequally sized) homonymous hemianopic field defects,

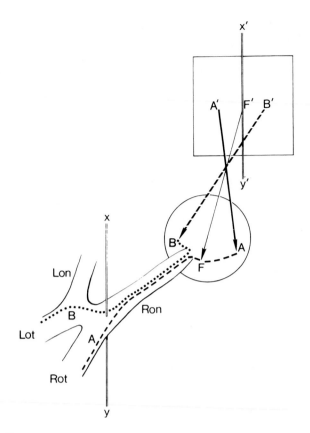

Fig. 2–6. Visual field of the right eye divided into a temporal (*B′*) and nasal (*A′*) hemifield, by a vertical line (*X′, Y′*) through the point of fixation (*F′*). There is no anatomic or functional segregation of crossed (nasal retinal) and uncrossed (temporal retinal) fibers before the junction of the optic nerve with the chiasm. Therefore, lesions anterior to the chiasm produce defects that extend across the vertical, whereas chiasmal and retro-chiasmal lesions produce defects confined to one hemifield. *Lon,* left optic nerve; *Ron,* right optic nerve; *Lot,* left optic tract; *Rot,* right optic tract.

unless, of course, the hemianopia is complete and total. Lesions of the retro-geniculate pathways also can produce partial or complete homonymous hemianopias. Partial hemianopias tend to be more congruent because the lesions responsible are situated more posteriorly toward the occipital lobe. Lesions involving the temporal lobe are associated with somewhat incongruent defects in the superior portion of the contralateral hemifields, whereas disturbances of the pathway in the parietal lobe characteristically cause slightly incongruent homonymous defects in the inferior part of the hemifield. Lesions of the visual cortex in the occipital lobe have three localizing characteristics: (1) they are exquisitely congruent; (2) they can give rise to true homonymous quadrantanopsias that respect both horizontal and vertical meridians because anatomically the geniculocortical projections representing the upper and lower visual field quadrants become segregated to the lower and upper gyri of the calcarine cortex, respectively; and

(3) macular sparing is frequently a characteristic feature when occipital homonymous hemianopsia is otherwise complete, and this is a result of the differential blood supply to the anterior and posterior portions of the visual cortex.

Physiologic Considerations

The utility of Traquair's concept of an island or a hill of vision (see Fig. 2–5) has proven consistent throughout the 50-year period during which Goldmann-type kinetic perimetry dominated clinical testing. Remarkably, Traquair's analogy remains current as an excellent way of conceptualizing automated static perimetry that has now largely superseded formal kinetic perimetry in clinical and investigational protocols.

Traquair's three-dimensional representation (see Fig. 2–5A) sits on a base plane, represented as a circular grid identical to that for plotting Goldmann isopters. This plane represents the horizontal and vertical dimensions of visual space. The third dimension, rising upward from the base plane is *differential light sensitivity* (DLS), which is the degree to which the visual system, at each point, is capable of detecting a circular spot of light that is brighter than the background. The foveal pinnacle is the most sensitive point in the field where the dimmest target (least different from background) can be detected. Traquair's various slopes and rises are zones within the visual field where DLS varies from point to point. In a gently sloping region (*e.g.*, the temporal side of fixation), sensitivity changes gradually along the horizontal meridian, whereas in a steeply sloped region (*e.g.*, the nasal periphery), there is a precipitous drop of sensitivity across a short lateral distance.

Traquair likened the process of perimetry to a geographic survey of an elevated surface wherein the lines encircling the island at various levels indicate a certain elevation above sea level. In perimetry, the lines encompass zones within the field that have achieved a certain elevation of DLS above the base plane, that is, at "sea level." These isopters lines refer to points or zones of equal visual sensitivity. In dynamic perimetry of the Goldmann type, isopters are determined by moving projected light points across the inner surface of a bowl-shaped hemisphere; the light stimulus is moved from a non-seeing to a seeing region, at various locations around the "island," and the patient signals when the moving light is first detected. This corresponds to mapping the isopter by choosing a DLS level and moving horizontally at this fixed DLS "altitude" above the base plane toward the island, noting where contact would occur with the rising slope of land.

Figure 2–5B shows the aerial view Traquair's hypothetic observer would have just above the foveal pinnacle, with the isopters now projected upon the base plane. The series of concentric circles indicate discrete levels of DLS, each elevation (sensitivity) determined by a specific stimulus size and brightness. Although several stimulus levels are required to adequately map the surface of Traquair's island generally no more than three isopters are plotted. A vertical slice (see Fig. 2–5C) through the island along the horizontal midline shows a steep nasal side (left) and the more gently sloping temporal field (right). On the temporal side of fixation is the physiologic blind spot, a dark shaft ("bottomless pit") extending to the base plane.

One category of visual field loss, generalized depression, implies that all points on the DLS surface are displaced downward by an equal proportion, that is, sensitivity is depressed equally at all points. This is represented as a concentric contraction of all isopters as Traquair Island sinks in the sea (see Fig. 2–5C, dotted profile). With depression of the entire field, a stimulus target would have to move further inward to be detected.

Traquair used the geologic term "erosion" to describe the consequences on the visual field of disease of the afferent pathways. For example, a dense inferior altitudinal field defect resulting from anterior ischemic optic neuropathy is illustrated in Figure 2–7, showing Traquair's island with a steeply excavated "cliff face" along the nasal horizontal mid-line, where the field undergoes transition to nearly zero DLS as a result of the nerve infarction. Small localized depressions ("pits") on the surface could be missed if flanked by two isopters that are too widely spaced. For this reason, it is common practice in Goldmann perimetry to present blinking but static light targets positioned well within the peripheral isopters in order to search small focal depressions or scotomas. Because the target used to determine a particular isopter should be brighter than threshold for field zones *within* the isopter, any missed points can be considered as within a field defect. This technique of presenting target lights statically within their isopter is referred to as *suprathreshold static perimetry*. The concept of slope may be applied to the DLS contour of field defects in the same way as it is applied to the slope of normal field regions.

Imagine a temporal lobe infarction in which a central zone is necrotic and even the brightest stimulus is not perceived in the corresponding field; surrounding the necrotic zone are edematous, partially compressed visual fibers that are not functioning at peak efficiency but permit some visual function. This translates into a region of reduced DLS (a relative scotoma) surrounding the absolute visual field defect (an absolute scotoma). The area of non-seeing field in the upper right quadrant (Fig. 2–8A) is considerably enlarged with reduced stimulus intensity. This is a gently sloped area of field defect that is consistent with an acute lesion surrounded by a zone of relative dysfunction. When the pathologic changes have stabilized and the secondary edema has

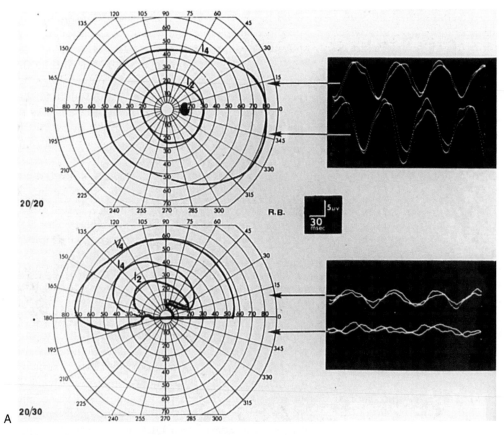

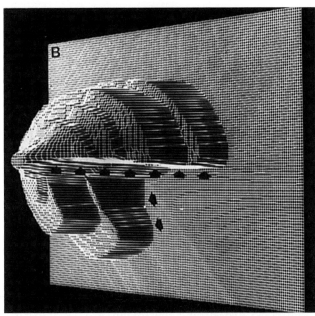

Fig. 2–7. Dense inferior altitudinal field defect resulting from anterior ischemic optic neuropathy of the left eye. **A.** Goldmann perimetric plots for the right eye (*R*), which is normal, and the left eye (*L*), which shows complete loss of the lower half-field. Tracings show results of steady-state (8-Hz reversals) evoked potentials: normal in both half-fields of the right eye and with diminished amplitudes, especially from inferior field, of the left eye. **B.** Three-dimensional computer reconstruction of same field defect; *furrows* define the sharp edge of the absolute defect. (Courtesy of H. Stanley Thompson, MD)

cleared, the absolute scotoma persists, corresponding to the necrotic zone (see Fig. 2–8B). The visual field defect mapped with the two weaker stimuli is now the same size as the absolute defect (*i.e.*, the relative scotoma has cleared). This produces a steeply sloped defect along the horizontal meridian, which is characteristic of a stable established lesion.

Clinical Testing of the Visual Field

Confrontation Methods

Innumerable and ingenious methods can be employed to screen patients for field defects. Screening generally involves rapid testing, which is usually done without special equipment, but at some sacrifice of sensitivity.

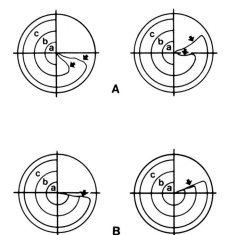

Fig. 2–8. Right homonymous upper quadrant visual field defect resulting from a left temporal lobe infarction. **A.** In the acute stage, the field defect is moderately incongruous (greater in left eye) and shows a relative slope along the horizontal edge (*arrows*). **B.** In the chronic stage, the defect is steep along the horizontal edge (*arrows*).

Using confrontation screening, examiners compare patients' fields with their own while in a face-to-face position and without using the tangent screen or perimeter.

Confrontation screening of fields provides a rapid, practical, and readily available technique that can be used at the bedside or in the office, with either children or adults (Table 2–1). When used knowledgeably, it is both sensitive and accurate. It is critical to realize, however, that confrontational methods are most useful in uncovering field defects such as central scotomas, altitudinal defects, and bitemporal and homonymous hemianopsias, but they are generally not sensitive enough to reveal subtle defects due to glaucoma or minor peripheral retinal lesions. Fortunately, most neurologic field defects do not fall into that category and can frequently be detected using confrontational methods. It is also obvious that these techniques may uncover

TABLE 2–1. Confrontation Field Techniques

Visually elicited eye movements	Infants
	Obtunded, dysphasic adults
Finger mimicking	Toddlers (3–5 yr)
	Dysphasic adults
Finger counting	Young children (5–8 yr)
	Adults
Hand comparison*	Children (8–12 yr)
	Adults
Color comparison*	Children (8–12 yr)
	Adults
Threat	Infants
	Obtunded adults

* Although it is highly subjective, comparison testing is very sensitive.

retinal detachments, choroidal tumors, and dense glaucomatous defects. However, our discussion is confined to lesions involving the optic nerves, chiasm, and posterior pathways.

Determining the best corrected visual acuity is usually a prerequisite for proceeding with the visual field examination. However, in infants, toddlers, and bedridden, semiobtunded, and confused patients, the inability to determine acuity neither invalidates nor excuses the performance of confrontation fields. Table 2–1 indicates the approximate age at which reasonable cooperation for various types of confrontation testing may be expected.

Visually Elicited Eye Movements

The "foveation reflex," wherein reflex eye movements are made to bring a stimulus presented in the peripheral field onto the central area (fovea) of the retina, develops at a very young age. The eye movement that accomplishes refixation is objective evidence that the stimulus was perceived in the periphery. Therefore, such involuntary visually provoked fixational movements provide a mechanism to test gross function of the peripheral retina (field) (Fig. 2–9). Clearly, this technique can be used to test infants, but it is also valuable with semiobtunded patients who may have homonymous or bitemporal hemianopic field defects.

Finger Mimicking

Even before the "E game" can be learned, a young child can be shown how to mimic finger patterns by playing "Do this!" (Fig. 2–10), first with both eyes opened, then with each alternately occluded. This technique does not require the ability either to count or to conceptualize spatial orientation and provides good approximations of field function. Because a young child has great difficulty in controlling ocular fixation, finger targets should be "flashed" (*i.e.*, briefly exposed before the child looks toward the hand). In the temporal field, fixation can be further controlled by turning the child's face toward the opposite side, carrying the eye into abduction, and rendering further movement toward the temporal field anatomically impossible. For the nasal field, this maneuver is more difficult because the nose and the object occluding the other eye may obscure the examiner's fingers. Finger patterns should be limited to the presentation of one, two, or five fingers, or the fist, because other combinations are difficult to distinguish.

Finger Counting

Most children and adults are able to identify accurately the number of fingers presented in each quadrant of the monocular field. Visual acuity 10° from fixation

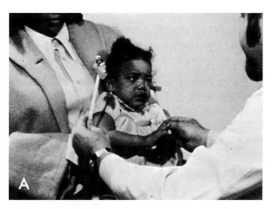
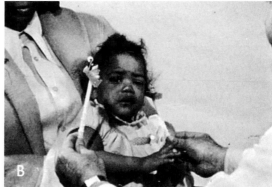

Fig. 2–9. Visually elicited eye movements provide gross estimate of field function and are demonstrated here in an 11-month-old infant. **A.** The infant watches the face of a cooing examiner while a brightly colored object is moved into her peripheral field. **B.** The head and eyes perform a fixation reflex, which is objective evidence of field function.

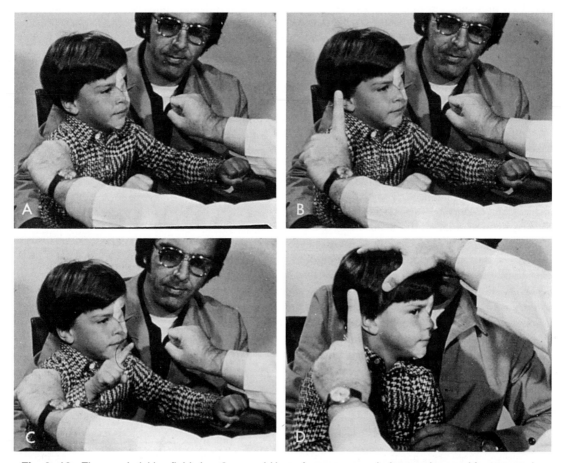

Fig. 2–10. Finger-mimicking fields in a 3-year-old boy. A press-on occluder may be used for monocular testing. **A.** The child and examiner face each other with both hands poised. **B.** With the child fixating on the examiner's face, a number of fingers (1, 2, or 5) is "flashed." **C.** The child responds. **D.** When fixation is a problem, the face may be turned such that the abducted eye can move no farther toward the right.

is roughly 20/200; at 30°, it falls to 20/400. Therefore, because the fingers represent an approximation of the 20/200 "E" optotype, finger counting at an eccentric point between 10° and 20° from fixation should be accomplished easily at confrontation distances (approximately 0.5 m).

If a patient seems to have some difficulty counting fingers in a quadrant or hemifield, simultaneous testing (Fig. 2–11) may help confirm a field defect. Simultaneous presentation of visual stimuli may also elicit a response similar to other sensory extinction phenomena. When the defective hemifield is tested alone, it may appear intact, but simultaneous presentation of stimuli to both hemifields may suppress the perception on one side, revealing the deficit.

Hand Comparison

The simultaneous presentation of targets to either side of the vertical meridian provides a sensitive subjective comparison of visual function in the two hemifields. In a similar way, the hands can be placed in the superior and inferior nasal quadrant to determine whether there is an altitudinal defect or nasal step, which will usually respect the horizontal nasal meridian (see below).

In performing hand comparisons, the examiner's hands or matched targets should provide large, light-colored paired stimuli about which the patient can be asked to make critical judgments in brightness perception (Fig. 2–12). The physician must determine that both hands or targets are illuminated equally, preferably by a light source directed toward the hands from behind the patient's head. Overhead lighting may be uniform, but positioning of the hands will be critical as a slight tilting will alter the reflected luminance. The following are typical questions asked during the comparison: "Do my hands appear the same? Is one hand lighter or darker than the other? Is one hand blurred or less distinct? Does one appear in shadow?"

It is obvious that for such confrontational screening methods to succeed, the physician must gain experience testing persons with normal vision as well as patients with known field defects. As with practically all other forms of field testing, hand comparison is totally dependent on the patient's subjective response and the ability of the physician to interpret that response. However, a consistent and reproducible response by the patient must be construed as an indication of a field defect and is a definite indication for formal perimetry.

Color Comparison

Functionally, the optic nerves and chiasm may be considered macular structures (*i.e.*, they predominantly subserve the central field) because more than 90% of the nerve fibers that comprise the anterior visual pathways arise from the small ganglion cells associated with cone receptors that populate the macula (Fig. 2–13). These fibers occupy the central core of the optic nerves and the median bar (decussating fibers) of the chiasm, which are especially vulnerable to compression by tumors or to intrinsic demyelinating or toxic processes. Therefore, depression of central field function, including loss of sensitivity to color, is a feature of both optic nerve and chiasmal disease. In fact, color desaturation may occur disproportionally with relative preservation of acuity and form perception.

In optic nerve disease, central depression (scotoma) of the field can be easily detected by asking the patient to describe changes in the saturation of the color of a large test object moved away from or toward central fixation (Fig. 2–14). Alternately, two similar targets may be used, one placed centrally and the other eccentrically, and the patient is asked to describe differences in color

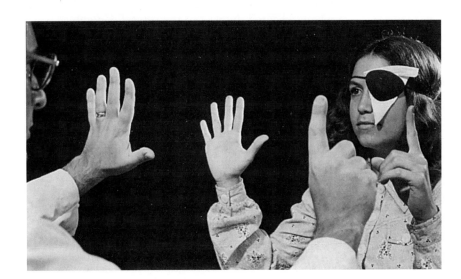

Fig. 2–11. Finger-counting fields in adults. Four quadrants of each eye should be tested. The patient may name or hold up the same number of fingers. Simultaneous finger counting may bring out a subtle hemianoptic defect.

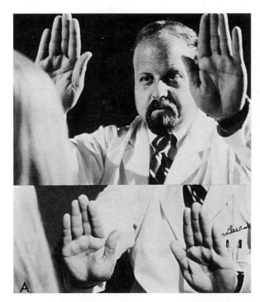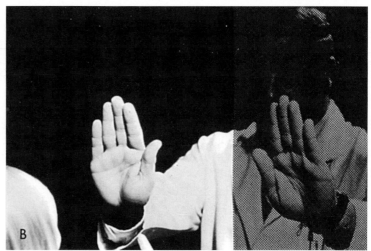

Fig. 2–12. The use of simultaneous hand comparison for detecting subtle hemianoptic depressions. **A.** Hands are first compared above the horizontal (superior quadrants), then below. **B.** The hand in hemianoptic depression appears "darker," "in shadow," or "blurred."

intensity or saturation. Normally, color is brighter or more saturated the closer one comes to fixation.

In suspected chiasmal syndromes, color perception should be compared on either side of the central fixation point. Moving a single large stimulus from one side to the other, or simultaneously presenting two targets, one on either side of fixation, provides the patient with a large visual stimulus about which he or she may make

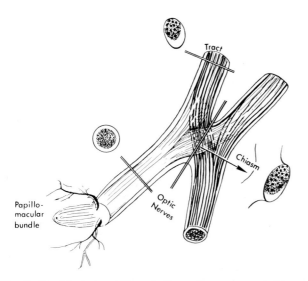

Fig. 2–13. Most visual fibers in the optic nerves and chiasm subserve macular function and, therefore, the central visual field. Anatomically and functionally, the nerves and chiasm may be considered macular projection structures. Note that the section through the median bar of the chiasm demonstrates distribution of macular crossing fibers (after Hoyt) and that macular projection is not limited to a small decussation at posterior chiasmal notch.

subjective yet sensitive judgments concerning color saturation (Fig. 2–15). To substantiate an apparent temporal field defect further, the test target should demonstrably "brighten" or take on color as it passes across the vertical meridian into the nasal hemifield (Fig. 2–16). Similar color comparison can be used to detect altitudinal visual field defects, which typically border on the horizontal nasal meridian. In those cases, the comparison is made between the upper and lower nasal quadrants. This is extremely useful because visual field defects that align at the horizontal nasal meridian *must* be caused by lesions at the optic nerve head or adjacent to it, that is, their origin is anterior. The most common causes are glaucoma, anterior ischemic optic neuropathy, branch artery occlusion, and retro-bulbar neuritis. Chiasmal compressive lesions do not produce this pattern, and so imaging studies can be avoided or at least, when indicated, limited to the orbital contents.

Tangent Screen

Although largely superseded by automated static threshold and Goldmann-type perimetry, the tangent screen still offers a valuable, sensitive, and readily available method for formally evaluating visual fields or for screening visual field defects. One of the major advantages of the tangent screen is the relative magnification of the surface area at 1 or 2 m when compared to perimeters that are viewed from 33 cm or less. This allows detailed exploration of small central scotomas and certain suspected nerve fiber layer defects. The relationship of central anatomic areas of the retina and their geometric enlarged projection in space (field) are shown in

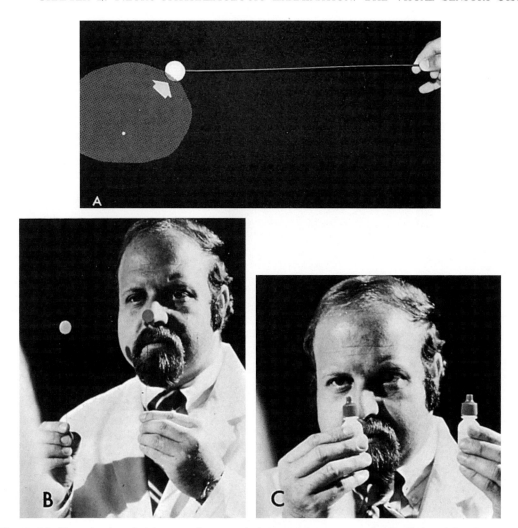

Fig. 2–14. Use of colored objects to detect and plot central scotomas. **A.** The limits of the detect are most easily defined when the target subjectively increases in color intensity as it is moved out of scotoma. **B.** Two targets of same color used for simultaneous comparison, one centrally (on nose), the other at approximately 10°. Normally, the central fixation target is brighter. **C.** Use of brightly colored bottle tops (mydriatic red) for color comparison.

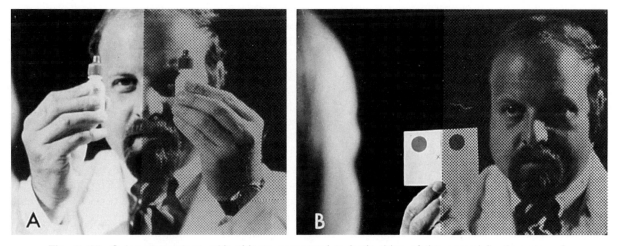

Fig. 2–15. Color comparison with objects presented to both sides of the central fixation area. **A.** Mydriatic red bottle tops. **B.** A card with two large red patches.

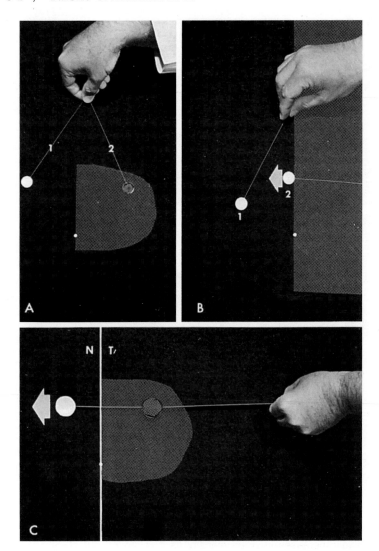

Fig. 2–16. Central exploration of the vertical meridian. **A.** Simultaneous color comparison for subtle central depression of the temporal hemifield, especially helpful in early chiasmal syndromes. Target 2 is desaturated. **B.** The vertical border of the defect is corroborated by the patient's objective perception of increased color intensity (now equal to the color of target 1) as target 2 passes into intact hemifield. **C.** Single large colored target brightens as it is moved across the vertical from the temporal field (*T*) into the nasal field (*N*).

Figure 2–17. The tangent screen examination, generally carried out by a physician and not a technician, also provides an opportunity for a goal-directed examination of the visual fields, depending on the site or nature of the suspected lesion. Compared with automated perimetry, it is rapid and convenient, even if less quantitative or standardized.

For tangent screen examination, the patient is seated comfortably 1 or 2 m from the center of the screen, which should be evenly illuminated, and each eye is alternately tested. The patient is instructed to gaze steadily at a central fixation point. With central scotomas, a large X may be taped across the fixation point and the patient instructed to look at the center of the X mark even if the line intersection is inapparent. The patient's fixation should be observed while the field stimulus is presented, and the examiner must be particularly vigilant for eccentric refixation eye movements, especially at the start of testing. A suprathreshold stimulus is first used, such as a 3- or 5-mm white target at 1 m. As with all field testing, the stimulus is moved from non-seeing areas to seeing areas. A flat disc stimulus is preferred, white or red on one side, black on the obverse, that can be flipped over and thus "hidden." Patients are instructed to indicate verbally or by gesture when they first see the target, and not the wand, hand, or vague movement. Occasional sham presentations of the wand with the black obverse side of the disc stimulus will ensure that the patient is responding correctly. If the chosen target is above threshold everywhere on the screen except for the blind spot, a smaller stimulus is then selected. On the other hand, the depth and size of scotomas or other field defects can be explored with larger stimuli. Shallow central field defects can be defined more easily with a red target, particularly when a small white target is seen in the area of the presumed scotoma. The blind spot should be initially explored and mapped to demonstrate the concept of target detection and disappearance; this is best accomplished with a relatively large (*e.g.,* 5 mm) suprathreshold stimulus. If the blind spot is enlarged, further testing with larger stimuli is required. The points at which a particular target is

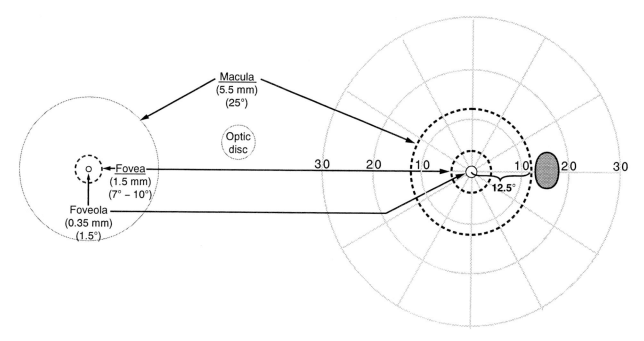

Fig. 2–17. Anatomic dimensions in millimeters (mm) of macular areas and the optic disc of the right eye and corresponding circular zones in degrees (°) of the right visual field. (From Gray LG, Galetta SL, Siegal T et al: The central visual field in homonymous hemianopsia. Arch Neurol 54:312, 1997)

detected can be marked with pins, and these points can then be transcribed to a standard visual field chart. With tangent screen field plots, the stimulus is specified by notations such as 5/1000/W, which defines a white (W) stimulus, 5 mm in diameter, presented at a viewing distance of 1 m (1000 mm) (see Fig. 2–5C).

The importance of the central field (especially the fixational area) in the diagnosis of optic nerve disease and the significance of the vertical meridian in the diagnosis of chiasmal and homonymous hemianopic defects have been emphasized previously. Therefore, the examiner's attention and time should be directed to exploring these areas (Fig. 2–18).

Although the peripheral field may be defective, there is almost always depression of central field in optic nerve disease. Therefore, special emphasis should be given to exploring for scotomas in the central region of fixation and the area between the blind spot. As indicated above, this area is best explored with relatively large colored targets while the patient is asked to indicate when the color appears or brightens (see Fig. 2–14A).

Ischemic optic neuropathy and occasionally optic neuritis tend to produce altitudinal and arcuate visual field defects and nasal steps, which usually are limited by the horizontal nasal meridian (see Fig. 2–7). Responses to targets presented in the superior and inferior hemifields and specifically the upper and lower nasal quadrants can be compared across the horizontal meridian. Field defects with sharp borders and steep gradients across the horizontal nasal meridian, if not also present as a homonymous defect in the other eye (i.e., involving

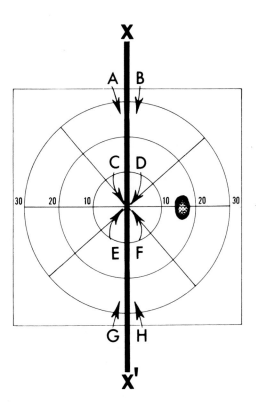

Fig. 2–18. Importance of the vertical meridian (*X, X'*) in neurologic diagnosis. Testing of visual function, whether form (standard targets) or color, should consist of comparisons along *X, X'*, at *A-B* and *G-H* for detection of "hemianoptic step" in periphery, and at *C-D* and *E-F* centrally.

the homonymous temporal quadrant), always implicate the optic nerve head or peripapillary retina as the site of the lesion producing the field defect.

Chiasmal syndromes tend to produce bitemporal depression. Characteristically, the field defect is hemianopic, extending toward the periphery, but occasionally the scotoma can be limited to the temporal paracentral region (see Fig. 2–16). For these field defects, testing to either side of the vertical meridian is critical because visual function in the temporal and nasal hemifields must be compared. The same holds true in homonymous hemianopic defects resulting from retro-chiasmal lesions. Hemianopic field defects have sharp borders at the vertical meridian, which neither optic nerve nor chorioretinal lesions manifest. A vertical step or discontinuity in the isopter should be sought along the vertical at the upper and lower extremes of the tangent screen. Within the central few degrees of field, it is often useful to employ colored targets, for here the patient can comment on relative color intensity and note when the target enters or emerges from a zone of color desaturation.

Homonymous hemianopsia results most frequently from infarction of the calcarine cortex, with occlusion of the posterior cerebral artery or its branches (see Chapter 7). The occipital pole receives collateral blood supply from the middle cerebral artery and may be spared when an infarction occurs in the more anterior portions of the visual cortex supplied by the posterior cerebral artery. This mechanism produces a field feature referred to as "macular or fixation sparing," for the area around the fixation point that represents the large cortical projection of the macula. Testing for spared remnants near fixation is practically accomplished at the tangent screen or by confrontation.

During field testing, patients may shift their gaze a few degrees to either side of fixation and the hemianopic midline will shift with gaze angle. Therefore, the patient with a complete hemianopsia will seemingly detect test objects into the presumed hemianopic field, a form of pseudo-sparing. With face-to-face confrontation testing, the examiner can maintain direct eye contact while bringing a target from the periphery across the hemianopic field toward fixation and thus can detect even slight refixation movements. In the absence of refixation movements, the patient without macular sparing will not see a target until it crosses the vertical midline passing through the visual axis shared by patient and examiner. When macular sparing is present, the target will be seen by the patient in the "blind" hemifield well before it reaches the visual axis.

Factitious (Functional) Fields

The visual field defects of hysteria and malingering typically result in an alleged claim of marked peripheral or "tubular" constriction. Unlike the organic causes of

generalized field constriction (see Chapter 5, Part I), a tubular field maintains the same diameter, that is, it does not expand geometrically with increasing test distances. Thus, assessment of peripheral field constriction involves testing at least two viewing distances (Fig. 2–19); this maneuver is easily accomplished at the tangent screen or by confrontation field testing. The average person is not aware that the eye, like a camera, encompasses a certain linear diameter at a 1-m viewing distance, and that this field size will measure roughly twice the linear diameter at 2 m. In an attempt at consistency, patients with non-physiologic field constriction will dissemble and respond as if the field diameter at a 2-m distance remains the same or smaller, rather than showing physiologic conical expansion. Of course, genuine pathologic causes of constricted fields, similar to a camera, will show enlarged diameters at increasing distances.

Clinical Perimetry

Routine field testing at the classic 1-m distance from a black tangent screen has been more or less replaced by the modern bowl perimeter, with a reduced viewing distance of about 0.33 m, but with the great advantage of standardized and reproduceable target and background luminance (i.e., contrast). The goal of conventional clinical perimetry remains to measure subjective detection

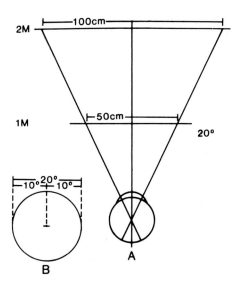

Fig. 2–19. A. Diagram of tangent screens placed at 1-m and 2-m viewing distances. **B.** A 20° diameter of central field is used as an example. Measured at the screens, the circle has a diameter of 50 cm at 1 m and a diameter of 100 cm when viewed from a distance of 2 m. The physiologic field of vision is actually a cone with the base outward. Visual field constrictions of functional origin show a "tubular" pattern with the patients failing to understand the effect of testing at variable distances, so the field diameter is usually the same (or worse) at the more remote viewing distance.

sensitivity to the onset of a white light stimulus in different locations of the field, at low photopic background luminance levels, in order to identify normal areas and regions showing retinal sensitivity loss (scotomas). Two general techniques for visual field assessment are widespread: Goldmann-type manual kinetic perimetry and computer automated static perimetry.

Goldmann Kinetic Perimetry

In manual kinetic perimetry, a stimulus of fixed size, luminance, and contrast on a defined background is moved from non-seeing to seeing areas until the appearance of the stimulus is detected by the patient. This procedure is repeated along several radial meridians. The contour line connecting all the detection loci defines the isopter and *field abnormalities for that particular stimulus-background combination.* Certain of isopters may be determined, and the visual field defect may be quantified by altering the stimulus intensity or size.

A Goldmann visual field examination typically involves determining three isopters (Fig. 2–20), and this is usually sufficient to characterize the surface of Traquair's island adequately (see Fig. 2–5). More isopters may be required to define certain defects, tailored to explore the region of the defect and to avoid unnecessary patient fatigue. If a scotoma is discovered during

suprathreshold static screening in the central field, the stimulus is moved radially outward from the center of the defect in a series of presentations to explore borders of the defect. Progressively larger or brighter stimuli are then presented within the scotoma to define the density of the defect. (Conceptually, this is plotting the shape and depth of local erosions in Traquair's island.)

Kinetic perimetry allows fairly rapid field examination, but sometimes it lacks reliability because of its dependence on the patient's reaction time, the speed of target movement and variability introduced by different perimetrists. In kinetic perimetry, the very motion of the stimulus also contributes to its detection (Riddoch phenomenon).[55]

Egge[56] carried out a useful study of normal Goldmann visual fields on 374 persons ranging in age from 15 to 69 years, categorized by decades. Isopter size declined steadily by decade throughout the sample, with regression greatest for the temporal quadrants and more marked for central rather than peripheral isopters. Variation over time fluctuated most for the I-1 isopter, especially in the temporal quadrants. The isopters were uniformly oval with a long horizontal diameter. Variation from this shape was most common for the I-1 isopter, with the temporal margin falling either outside (52%) or inside (11%) the physiologic blind spot. With increasing age, a greater proportion of subjects' I-1 isopters passed

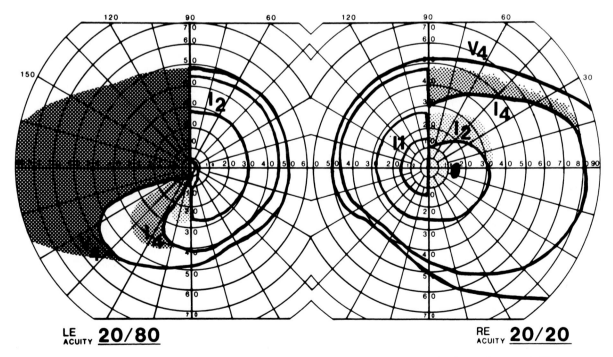

Fig. 2–20. Goldmann-type visual field plot. Four isopters (*V-4, I-4, I-2,* and *I-1*) are illustrated. There is a bitemporal defect that is more severe in the left eye than the right. This illustrates how multiple isopters give a complete quantitative representation of the defect in various areas of the visual field from the far periphery (*V-4*) to the paracentral field (*I-1*).

inside the blind spot; 76% of subjects in the 60- to 69-year age group demonstrated this pattern.

Automated Static Threshold Perimetry

At present, automated static perimetry has largely supplanted manual kinetic perimetry for routine field examinations, although Goldmann type kinetic perimeters are still especially useful in certain clinical settings. The following review emphasizes the appropriate use of automated perimetry in clinical practice.

Static Perimetry. Static perimetry refers to the technique of visual field testing performed with non-moving stimuli. Purely static examination with manual perimetry of the Goldmann-type is time-consuming and has been used in the past only on a limited scale to spot-check selected locations, such as the Bjerrum arcuate bundles, or otherwise within the isopters initially defined with manual kinetic perimetry. Computerized static perimetry has gained rapid acceptance by providing systematically controlled presentation of brief, non-moving stimuli at selected locations. It is therefore more objective and mathematically more exacting than possible with the most rigorous manual kinetic techniques. Furthermore, the random ordering of stimuli presentations across the field of vision and the accurate registry of patient responses without the need for a perimetrist facilitated visual field examination substantially by decreasing the test time and eliminating operator variability. The latest of a series of different types of computerized static perimeters are the Humphrey and Octopus visual field analyzers (VFAs), which are now the most widely used automated perimeters.

In automated static perimetry, the stimulus is constant in size and is presented at programmed loci in the visual field for a controlled exposure time. The most commonly employed threshold determination is a staircase method in which true threshold is bracketed by presentations at luminance levels *brighter than and dimmer than* ("bracketing") threshold. Typically, between three and five presentations are needed at each test locus. It should be recalled that the stimuli are randomly presented at successive and subjectively unpredictable locations; the bracketing presentations at a given locus may take place minutes apart. A special strength of computer-assisted perimetry is the capacity of the computer to keep track of stimulus-response relationships at all test locations and to place subsequent stimuli randomly at the proper brightness to approach threshold as determined by the patient's response to earlier presentations at that locus. The staircase procedure used for threshold determination proceeds as follows. The intensity of the stimulus at a given locus is either increased (ascending) or decreased (descending) by the computer until the stimulus is, respectively, detected or missed by the observer. After this initial threshold estimate is deter-

mined, the stimulus intensity may be altered in the opposite direction using smaller steps. The staircase procedure in current practice terminates after crossing the threshold once or twice, and that design is considered closest to ideal.[57]

Computerized automatic projection perimeters are capable of producing the standard-size Goldmann test stimuli across the range of stimulus brightness levels. It is customary to define the intensity of the stimuli used by computerized perimeters and the thresholds measured in decibel (dB) units. The dB notation indicates attenuation in stimulus brightness. The brightest stimuli produced by the perimeter have the intensity of 0 dB, which may represent an intensity of 10,000 apostilb. Increasing sensitivity (the ability to see dimmer stimuli) is denoted by higher dB values, so that 10 dB and 20 dB indicate attenuation of the stimulus brightness by 10 and 100 times, respectively (*i.e.,* down to 1000 and 100 apostilb). The stimulus intensity may be changed by as little as 1 dB (*i.e.,* 0.1 log-unit steps) with each presentation after the initial estimate of threshold sensitivity at a particular locus.

With a normative database that is age specific, computer-driven perimetry begins at a stimulus luminance close to the expected threshold for each test point. However, threshold sensitivity may vary from the normal at many test locations, making the normal threshold a poor starting point. Another strategy selects a starting brightness based on thresholds at adjacent points tested.[58] This approach is efficient because there is a high degree of correlation between thresholds at adjacent points, even within visual field defects.

The Humphrey VFA starts the full-threshold examination and the various screening protocols by testing four points, one in each quadrant. For threshold determination, starting levels at adjacent points are based on the threshold levels determined for these first four points, and as testing proceeds, starting levels at subsequent loci are based on thresholds that have been determined for adjacent or other nearby points.

For screening tests on the Humphrey VFA, threshold values at the same four original test locations are determined and the expected threshold at each other point is calculated from the normal shape of the "hill of vision," which is adjusted up or down according to the thresholds at the four original test locations. The basic Humphrey screening strategy tests each point twice, with stimulus brightness set 6 dB above expected threshold for each location. If the first stimulus presented at a given location is detected, no further presentations are made at this location. Thus, any defect deeper than 6 dB should be detected. This method, known as the "threshold related screening strategy," is used to screen for abnormalities without any quantification, thus saving time at the cost of reduced information. Additional data can be collected on points missed. Using the "three zone strategy," each missed location is retested with a maximally bright stimulus to determine whether the loss of sensitivity is relative or absolute, whereas when the "quantify defects strategy" is used, missed points undergo full-threshold determination. These alternate screening strategies take more time than simple screening, but they provide more information.

The main purposes of screening visual field examination programs are to establish the presence or absence of a visual field defect and to indicate the boundaries of any scotomas. Screening is particularly useful for those patients who have not had previous visual field examinations. The tests are not suitable for quantification of field defects or for careful follow-up of patients to determine the progression of the disease or the effectiveness of the treatment.

Most computerized perimeters have various programs designed to increase the grid density in areas of field known to be involved in specific conditions. For example, extra test points are added above and below the nasal horizontal midline and in the arcuate regions in examinations designed to detect early glaucomatous field loss, whereas tests to screen for neurologic disease commonly emphasize straddling the vertical midline and the central 10°, to detect hemianopic defects and central scotomas.

Among a number of full-threshold test grids available, a rectangular grid of points at 6° intervals in the central 30° has become the most standardized and frequently used array. The Humphrey VFA 30-1 and 30-2 full-threshold examinations use 6° test grids to evaluate the central 30° field, whereas the Humphrey 24-1 and 24-2 programs test only the most central 24° by dropping most of the peripheral test points on the same 6° grids. The Humphrey 30-2 (Fig. 2–21) and 24-2 programs, which test 76 or 54 test locations, respectively, have become the most frequently used and standardized programs because their test loci straddle the vertical and horizontal meridians, providing the optimal strategy for determining whether neurologic or glaucomatous field defects respect these boundaries. Various screening strategies, such as those described above, may be applied to any of these specialized or standard test grids. The Humphrey central 76-point screening grid is identical to that of central 30-2 threshold program.

Some studies have compared automated static threshold perimetry with kinetic Goldmann perimetry in different clinical settings.[59,60] For example, Trope and Britton[59] compared findings using the Humphrey VFA and the Goldmann perimeter on 25 patients with glaucoma, whereas Beck and colleagues[60] compared the 2 perimeters in 171 eyes: 69 with glaucoma or intraocular hypertension, 69 with neurologic vision disorders, and 33 with normal vision. Overall, these studies have demonstrated that both the Humphrey VFA and the Octopus perimeter are excellent at detecting glaucomatous and neuro-

ophthalmic field defects with high degree of sensitivity and specificity. However, it is important to note that, in contrast to Goldmann perimetry, a significant percentage of the results with automated perimetry were inadequate or unreliable, mostly because of fixation problems, and patients much preferred the manually administered Goldmann fields.[59] Improving patient reliability and convenience by shortening the time and effort required to obtain full-threshold tests has been a major challenge that is being addressed by increasingly sophisticated systems and protocols.

Representation of Results (Cartography).

Graphic display. In manual kinetic perimetry, loci where a particular stimulus is detected are marked and are later connected with lines (like isobars on a weather map) to form isopters (see Figs. 2–5B and 2–20), as has been described. Scotomas are outlined in a similar manner. With automated static perimetry, the test data are not usually converted to isopter lines, *per se.* Instead, one or more of several different displays may be used, depending on the program (screening or threshold) chosen. Usually, graphic and numeric representations of the measurements made at each tested point in the visual field are presented topographically on a chart of the particular test grid used. Figure 2–21 demonstrates key portions of the graphic display generated by the central 30-2 threshold test produced by the Humphrey VFA, which we describe below. Other automated perimeters provide similar displays.

Gray-scale (symbols) display. The most common visual graphic representation of automated visual field test results is the gray-scale plot (see Fig. 2–21, upper right). The sensitivity values obtained from the examination are assigned different sized or shaded symbols on the computer printout of the test result. Generally, the larger or darker the symbol, the lower is the sensitivity (the denser the defect). The symbols may appear only at the discrete test locations or the spaces between test loci can be assigned interpolated values such that the entire visual field projection appears in various shades of gray. Because the peripheral visual field has lower sensitivity than the center, the gray scale plot will normally become darker toward the periphery of the field.

Numeric display. A numeric display of the actual threshold values in decibels for each test location on automated perimeters such as Humphrey VFA (see Fig. 2–21, upper left) can be charted to provide a topographic printout of the "raw data." Decreased sensitivity at any point can be derived by comparing numeric threshold value at that point to the following: (1) the values at surrounding locations; (2) the threshold values at mirror image test locations in both eyes of the same individual; or (3) to mirrored points across the horizontal and vertical meridians of each field. A few test points with significantly reduced sensitivity may occasionally occur by chance alone. However, falsely abnor-

Numeric (dB) Results   **Grayscale Results**

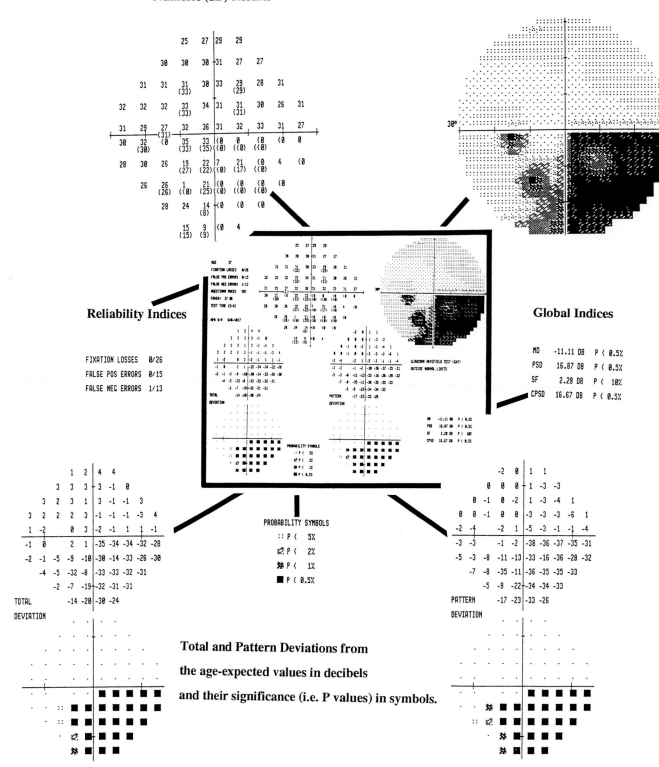

Reliability Indices

FIXATION LOSSES   0/26
FALSE POS ERRORS 0/15
FALSE NEG ERRORS 1/13

Global Indices

MD   -11.11 DB   P < 0.5%
PSD   16.87 DB   P < 0.5%
SF   2.28 DB   P < 10%
CPSD   16.67 DB   P < 0.5%

PROBABILITY SYMBOLS

:: P < 5%
⬚ P < 2%
✳ P < 1%
■ P < 0.5%

Total and Pattern Deviations from the age-expected values in decibels and their significance (i.e. P values) in symbols.

Fig. 2–21. Graphic display produced by the Humphrey Visual Field Analyzer, central 30-2 threshold test. *Center:* Actual display arranged as dot-matrix printout; enlarged key components are shown surrounding the central display. *Top right: GS,* gray-scale graph. *Top left: Num,* numeric threshold values in decibels. *Center left: RI,* reliability indices. *Lower left:* Plot of total deviation, representing differences between patients' measures and age-matched persons with normal vision. *Bottom left: PP,* probability plot showing the probability deviation from normal values. *Lower center: PS,* legend for probability symbols used in PP showing significance levels. *Lower right: PD,* plot of pattern deviation values at each tested point (see text). *Bottom right: PP,* equivalent probability plot for pattern deviation values. *Right center: GI,* global indices (see text).

mal points arising by chance should be scattered randomly in the field. Clusters of two or more depressed points must be regarded as true defects.

The detection sensitivity at each locus in the visual field decreases with age. This decline with increasing age requires that the limits of normal for all test locations be defined to enable comparisons among the results from same or different individuals. The statistical software packages, OCTOSOFT and STATPAC/FASTPAC incorporated in Octopus and Humphrey VFAs, respectively, perform comparisons between the each patient's test results and age-expected normal visual field threshold values. For the Humphrey VFA, the difference between STATPAC and FASTPAC is simply the method of threshold determination at the test locations.[62] The differences between the measured and age-expected threshold values at each test location are shown in the total deviation map (see Fig. 2–21, lower left). In addition, for each tested point, these programs calculate the statistical significance of the deviation in sensitivity and compile empiric *probability maps*[61] (see Fig. 2–21, bottom left and right). Such maps are easier and more accurate to interpret than the numeric and gray-scale maps. These statistical packages further facilitate the recognition and analysis of the defects on a single visual field test by calculating *global visual field indices* (see Fig. 2–21, right middle), which are interpreted below. In addition, these programs compile and print out a longitudinal series of repeat fields obtained on the same eye, facilitating the evaluation of field changes that occur over time.

Automated Visual Field Interpretation

Reliability Indices (Catch-Trials).

Fixation losses. The frequency of fixation losses is used to assess the patient's cooperation with the requirement of steady fixation during the test (see Fig. 2–21, left center). In the Humphrey VFA, the ratio of the number of fixation losses to the total number of stimulus presentations in the physiologic blind spot is recorded. Fixation losses exceeding 20% are regarded as a sign of low patient cooperation. Although lack of accurate fixation does not cause false field defects in normal eyes, this leads to underestimation of the existing defects in glaucomatous eyes.[63]

False-positive responses. The number of occasions when the response button is pressed without a stimulus being presented represents the patient's overwillingness to see in the field of vision. If the number of false-positive responses is greater than 33% of sham stimulus presentations, the patient is considered unreliable. A high number of false-positive responses is an indication that existing field defects will be underestimated.

False-negative responses. Occasionally, an easily detectable suprathreshold (too bright) stimulus is pre-

sented, and the patient is expected to press the button indicating the target was seen. False-negative responses are recorded when the patient misses these suprathreshold stimuli; the percentage of false-negative responses should be less than 33% for the patient to qualify as reliable. Abnormally high numbers of false-negative responses indicate the patient's lack of attention to stimulus presentations during the test and may lead to apparently abnormal fields in healthy persons and may overestimate the existing glaucomatous field defects.[63]

During their first threshold test, 30% to 45% of patients produce unreliable results because of difficulty in maintaining a fixation or because of too many false-negative responses.[64] Subject reliability improves to 25% with experience;[65] however, even with repeat testing, 4% to 9% of patients consistently fail to generate reliable results, and the poor reliability is due almost exclusively to fixation losses. Factors such as age, pupil diameter, and visual acuity do not influence the reliability parameters.[64]

Global Visual Field Indices. Global visual field indices (see Fig. 2–21, right center) are intended to summarize clinically important features in the visual field by using conventional statistical methods such as the mean and standard deviation.[66] The calculation of the global field indices is possible only when the age-expected normal threshold values are known for each of the individual test locations in different age groups. Global field indices on the Humphrey VFA are calculated and are presented in the same way by STATPAC and FASTPAC programs (see Fig. 2–21).

Mean sensitivity. The mean sensitivity reflects the mean of the decibel threshold values measured at all test locations in a given field. That index is sensitive to a diffuse change in the visual field and insensitive to small localized changes. It is also affected by media opacities, refractive errors, and small pupil size. Because it is not corrected for age, the mean sensitivity should decrease with age in all individuals.

Mean defect. The mean of the differences between the measured and age-expected threshold values at all points represents the total deficit and is termed "mean defect." The concept was introduced by Flammer[66] and is mostly influenced by diffuse damage and also by preretinal factors such as pupil size, refractive error, and media opacity. It is not sensitive to small localized areas of field loss. Unlike mean sensitivity, mean defect should not increase with age in a normal individual. "Mean deviation" on the Humphrey VFA is the reciprocal of mean defect.

Loss variance. The loss variance is an index of irregularity in the shape of the hill of vision and is intended to reflect localized depressions in the visual field.[67] The square root of the loss variance is used in the Humphrey VFA and is named "pattern standard deviation."

Short-term fluctuation. This index reflects the variability in the individual threshold values with repeated testing during the test (*i.e.,* intratest and intra-individual variability). Thresholds for at least 10 randomly selected stimulus locations are measured twice during the test session, and the average variability in the repeat threshold values obtained from both measurements is calculated. The square root of the mean variance of all tested locations is taken as the short-term fluctuation (STF). The STF for a patient's first threshold test may be 3 dB, but it should decrease to less than 2 dB with repeat testing (STF less than 2 dB is normal). When the STF is higher, it may represent a low level of patient cooperation and vigilance, especially if there are other abnormal reliability indices. When the other reliability indices are within normal limits, a high STF may be the first sign of a visual field disturbance. Patient fatigue may also increase the STF.

The variability of the threshold results from the same individual on different test occasions (intertest variability) is termed "long-term fluctuation" (LTF). LTF (not shown in the single field analysis shown in Fig. 2–21) seems to be dependent on the presence of visual field abnormalities and is greater in patients with deteriorating fields, although it is unrelated to age or eccentricity.[68] LTF remains one of the major challenges in automated threshold visual field testing.

Corrected loss variance. Corrected loss variance (CLV) is the "loss variance" adjusted for STF. CLV is analogous to the "corrected pattern standard deviation" (CPSD) index on the Humphrey VFA. CLV provides a more accurate estimate of localized damage because both STF and localized damage can cause an elevated loss variance. The CLV filters out the intratest variability component and provides a more accurate index of the true localized defects in the visual field. CLV and CPSD must be interpreted cautiously in patients with advanced visual field loss, in whom the decrease in these values results from an overall reduction in visual sensitivity.

Deviation and Empiric Probability Maps. STAT-PAC/FASTPAC on the Humphrey VFA calculates and prints out graphic displays of "total deviation" and "pattern deviation" and empiric probability maps to assist in interpretation of the threshold field results. Because the normal sensitivity threshold at each test point varies, it is impossible to define a minimum normal value for all test points. Consequently, the deviation from the age-related normal threshold at each individual test location must be determined. Deviations of 4 dB of more are presented topographically in a map labeled "total deviation." Using normative data, the "significance limits" for the deviations at each test point are calculated so that statistical significance can be attached to deviations from the normal age-related values shown at specific test locations on the map. The statistical significance of the deviation at each test location is also presented in a graphic display called the "total deviation probability map" on the Humphrey VFA (see Fig. 2–21, lower left). Using defined probability symbols (see Fig. 2–21, bottom center), the highest p value ($p<5\%$, $p<2\%$, $p<1\%$, and $p<0.5\%$), reached at each location is plotted at the corresponding point on the map.

The total deviation at an individual test point is the sum of the deviation caused by diffuse (generalized, homogenous) reduction in sensitivity plus localized reduction in sensitivity. The total deviation plot therefore reflects the global depression introduced by media opacities, small pupils, and uncorrected refractive errors (preretinal sensitivity loss), in addition to localized decreases in field sensitivity due to retinal and neurologic disease. The "pattern deviation map" (see Fig. 2–21, lower right) is designed to filter out the diffuse or global component of field depression and to highlight the localized "pattern" loss only. To accomplish this, it is assumed that the most sensitive points in the field are outside any existing localized defects. An estimate of the diffuse component of field depression is based on the deviations from normal measured at 51 most sensitive locations within the central portion of the field. The value estimated for the diffuse component is subtracted from each of the individual total deviations to derive the final numeric value of the pattern deviation at each test point. A pattern deviation probability map (using the same symbols for p values described above) is then generated to display the significance (p value) of the pattern deviation reached at each measured point.

Thus, the empiric probability maps (see Fig. 2–21, bottom left and right corners) indicate even the most shallow significant deviation from normal and also help to categorize the abnormal points according to the depth and statistical significance of the defects. However, it is important to realize that test point significance on an empiric probability map indicates only how often a particular threshold value can be expected to occur in the normal population. The significance level does not indicate the chance that a given deviation is normal.

Color Perimetry and Blue-on-Yellow Stimulus. Some retinal diseases influence rod or cone function differentially and selectively. Such specific rod or cone anomalies may be missed with white luminous stimuli because the rods continue to operate at the modest photopic background levels of conventional perimeters. However, it is possible to measure the threshold to a positive contrast (incremental) stimulus of one particular wavelength while the background is illuminated using a different wavelength composition, thus increasing the sensitivity of the test for cone disease. For instance, a strong yellow adapting background selectively reduces the sensitivity of the red and green cones, but it only minimally influences blue cone sensitivity. When a blue test target is presented on a yellow background, the visibility of the stimulus reflects the functionality of the blue cone system.

Blue-on-yellow (short-wavelength) automated perimetry has been reemphasized as a "more sensitive" method of detecting field loss in glaucoma[69] and has become an optional testing mode on the Humphrey VFA. In that mode, static blue stimuli of Goldmann size V are presented against a high-luminance (200 cd/m^2) yellow adapting background that saturates the red- and green-sensitive cones and isolates the blue- (short-wave-) sensitive cones. A prospective 5-year follow-up study of patients with glaucoma and ocular hypertension indicated that visual field defects mapped using this short wavelength technique could appear larger and seem to increase in size more rapidly than those mapped with conventional white stimuli.[70] In addition, early defects picked up only with blue-yellow testing converted to visual field defects with conventional testing with progression of disease.[71] Although short wavelength automated perimetry remains promising and has been shown to improve the discrimination of abnormal fields from normal fields, the increase in variability that occurs with this technique is a problem, and it has not yet replaced conventional automated perimetry in the detection of early field loss.[70]

ELECTROPHYSIOLOGY TESTS OF THE EYE AND VISUAL PATHWAY

Electroretinography

The ERG is a retinal biopotential that can be evoked by either flash or pattern stimuli. For more than 100 years, it has been known that this potential could be recorded from the cornea of the human eye, and clinical ERG has now become a relatively standard and routine technique available in most clinical centers as well as in some private practices. Standards and recommended protocols have been published for many ERG procedures, and attempts are being made to standardize the technique so that results can be easily shared among different clinics throughout the world. Nevertheless, new ERG techniques continue to emerge, our understanding of the neural basis of the response continues to evolve, and new components of the response are being recognized. Consequently, this overview primarily deals with the most widely accepted and routinely used aspects of ERG.

Standard (Full-Field) Electroretinography

The traditional full-field flash ERG (FERG) is recorded using either discrete single flashes of short duration (less than 0.2 per second) that elicit a transient response or to a series of rapidly flickering flashes (30 to 40 Hz) that generate a steady-state sinusoidal waveform. The FERG can be recorded as a response to a single flash, although off-line averaging may be used to improve signal-to-noise characteristics. The steady-state or flicker FERG is typically averaged on line with 10 to 100 repetitions included in each average. Because both single-flash and flicker ERGs are elicited by diffuse light sources that stimulate the full visual field, they represent the mass response of retinal generators distributed across virtually the entire retina. However, the generators of the FERG are located in the distal (outer) two-thirds of the retina. Retinal ganglion cells do not contribute appreciably to this response. Because most photoreceptors are located outside the fovea, the full-field FERG originates primarily from the electrical activity generated by extramacular rods and cones.

The full-field flash ERG is a complex waveform that results from the interaction of electrical potentials arising from multiple generators. In the dark-adapted human eye, the flash ERG waveform typically includes an initial negative component (a-wave), followed by a larger positive component (b-wave), and then a slower biphasic (negative followed by positive) component (c-wave). The ascending limb b-wave may contain a set of higher-frequency oscillations known as the oscillatory potentials. In addition, both the a-wave and the b-wave may exhibit notches that result from differences in timing between the rod and cone components of the response. The a-wave of the flash ERG is believed to be generated by the photoreceptors, whereas the b-wave that occurs later is generated by the Müller cells, whose electrical potentials result from ionic fluxes driven largely by the bipolar cells. Exclusive rod responses can be produced by using low-intensity white or blue light, whereas cone responses can be isolated with bright backgrounds (to suppress the rods) or by using the flicker ERG, which drives only the cones. Amplitude and latency measures as shown in Figure 2–22 are used to quantify the responses.

The most important use of the FERG is to diagnose and evaluate apparent and occult retinal dystrophies and diseases (See Figs. 13–2 and 13–3), such as retinitis pigmentosa and cancer associated retinopathy. However, as noted above, the FERG reflects the integrity of only the more distal retinal layers, and it is not altered by atrophy of the ganglion cells, the axons of which make up the optic nerve. Thus, the FERG cannot be used as an indicator of neurologic visual dysfunction beyond the photoreceptors and bipolar cells of the retina, because it remains completely unaffected by lesions affecting the inner retina and the retro-bulbar visual pathway. This characteristic can also be useful, however, because the presence of a normal FERG can eliminate the outer retina as a possible source of widespread visual dysfunction of the type that would produce severe visual field constriction, for example.

FERG can also be helpful in certain settings by providing evidence of retinal disease when the distinction from optic nerve disease is not certain. A common ex-

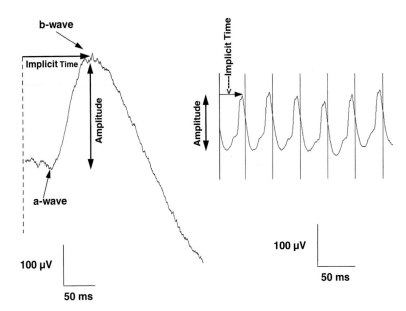

Fig. 2–22. Transient and steady-state electro-retinographic response to a bright single flash (*right*) and to a 30-Hz flicker (*left*), respectively. The amplitude and latency measures are indicated.

ample is the problem of diagnosing slowly progressive, bilaterally symmetric visual loss in a young person. The differential diagnosis may be between a heredofamilial optic atrophy in which the optic nerve head may demonstrate only minimal pallor, and a photoreceptor degeneration such as a progressive cone dystrophy, in which the appearance of the retina may be equally benign. An abnormal FERG definitely implicates retinal disease. However, because the FERG reflects primarily extramacular retinal function, the converse is not valid. A normal FERG does not rule out a macular dystrophy or degeneration or the early stages of a more widespread process, such as Stargardt's disease.

Focal Electroretinography

Localized retinal disturbances can be evaluated using a technique that has become known as focal ERG. The focal ERG represents the retinal electrical activity generated while simultaneously stimulating and visualizing a small spot on the retina. A specially constructed, hand-held or mounted stimulator-ophthalmoscope that produces a rapidly flickering spot stimulus is required, and the stimulus is positioned under direct visualization on the retinal area of interest (usually the macula). The stimulus is designed to activate only the cone component of the ERG by virtue of its high frequency (30 to 40 Hz) and bright intensity, which is above the rod saturation level. In addition, the flickering stimulus is surrounded by a bright, steady ring of light that minimizes the possible effects of stray light.

The focal ERG is thought to be derived from the same retinal elements that generate the full-field ERG, but the area of retina that is stimulated (approximately 4°) and the resultant response amplitude are extremely small (a fraction of a microvolt versus 250 mV for

the normal full-field ERG). However, this tiny signal can be measured using advanced signal-averaging and frequency-filtering techniques. These techniques were first introduced to enhance and isolate sensory evoked cortical potentials from background electrical activity generated intrinsically in the brain and externally by the environment. They are essential in recording the VEP and the pattern ERG, as well as the focal ERG, and are now frequently used to enhance the full-field ERG, which is the only visually derived electrical signal that does not routinely *require* the use of these methods.

Instrumentation used to extract and isolate small, repetitive electrical responses from undesirable background "noise" largely depends on digital computers to provide dynamic frequency filtering and signal averaging. Signal averaging combines and averages multiple short segments of the electrical potential, most often about 0.25 second (250 milliseconds) long, which are synchronized to follow each repetitive presentation of the visual stimulus. After a succession of identical stimuli are presented, the computer sums and averages all synchronized waveforms. All the electrical potential shifts generated by the stimulus should occur at the same interval after each stimulus and are additive. Electrical potentials unrelated to the presentation of the stimulus and those that occur at random intervals may be positive or negative and are expected to cancel each other out, averaging to near zero after many stimulus repetitions.

For the focal ERG, the amplitude of the response and its phase relationships to the stimulus are the parameters usually measured. The focal ERG has proven useful in distinguishing occult macular from optic nerve disease, especially in patients with unexplained decreased acuity, shallow central scotomas, or complaints of blurred vision with normal or near-objective visual function. Patients with optic neuropathies unassociated with macular pathology have normal focal ERGs. Macular disease, in contrast, can be associated with abnormal focal ERG responses, even when the fluorescein angiogram is normal. This objective finding can help to support the diagnosis of a degenerative or dystrophic macular process, resolving uncertainty and conflict concerning possible causes, prognosis, and management decisions.

Pattern Electroretinography

Retinal biopotentials can also be recorded in response to counterphasing (reversing) checkerboard or grating patterns. Although the pattern evoked ERG (PERG) was originally recorded by Riggs and co-workers in the early 1960s, it was Maffei and Fiorentini[72] who first reported that, under appropriate conditions, the pattern ERG may reflect the neural activity of the retinal ganglion cells. In their original work, they found that following transection of the cat optic nerve, flash or flicker ERGs remained stable, whereas the PERG progressively disappeared over 4 months, an interval that closely followed the time course of ganglion cell degeneration.[72] This and subsequent studies have supported the belief that the generators of this response lie in the proximal 30% to 50% of the retina.

Therefore, changes in the waveform of the pattern ERG are believed to reflect abnormalities in retinal ganglion cell function from either dysfunction of the retinal ganglion cells themselves or disruption of input to the ganglion cells resulting from pathology in the distal (inner) retina. The PERG can be recorded in response to the same slow or fast counterphase reversing stimuli that are used routinely in visual electrodiagnostic facilities to generate VEPs. However, unlike the VEPs, but in common with all ERGs, the PERG records electrical potentials directly from the eye. This fact and the small retinal potentials generated by pattern stimuli make this technique extremely sensitive to variation in electrode type and placement, thus limiting its utility to those few facilities with the requisite technical expertise. However, when coupled with measurement of the FERG and the VEP, the value of the PERG is its facility for further electrophysiologic dissection of the sensory visual pathway. Consequently, disease of the inner retina can be localized. If, for example, the full-field and focal ERGs are normal and the pattern ERG and VEP are abnormal, a lesion involving the inner retina can be postulated. Although any form of optic atrophy producing degeneration of retinal ganglion cells could produce these findings, certain retro-bulbar processes such as compression and demyelination, which impede conduction but do not destroy cells, can leave the PERG unaffected. Furthermore, the PERG can assist in the diagnosis of diffuse cerebral degenerative or ischemic processes that can mimic the visual dysfunction of generalized anterior pathway disease. The PERG has been used to evaluate clinical cases of optic nerve damage in glaucoma,[73,74] in multiple sclerosis,[73] and in Alzheimer's disease.[75] Other studies have found, however, that the PERG is not a consistently strong indicator of demyelinating damage.[76]

Visual Evoked Potential

Electrical activity generated by visual stimuli can be recorded from the scalp overlying the occipital cortex and other areas of the brain using surface electrodes. These cortical potentials are similar to the spontaneous activity that makes up the electroencephalogram, except they are specifically elicited by visual stimulation, to which they are linked temporally. Unlike the full-field ERG but in common with both focal and pattern ERGs, visually evoked electrical signals recorded from the scalp are of relatively small amplitude when compared with the background random electrical activity of the brain and the ambient electrical noise. The visual component of this activity must be extracted from the background electrical activity using the signal averaging and filtering techniques described above. When isolated from the diffuse cortical activity not directly linked to the visual input, the visually elicited component forms a characteristic waveform, the VEP. These electrical waves, also known as visual evoked responses (VERs) or visual evoked cortical potentials (VECPs), may be produced by either diffuse light flashes (flash VEP or FVEP) or by counterphase-reversing gratings or checkerboard patterns (pattern VEP or PVEP). The waveform morphology of the FVEPs and PVEPs, although similar, is not identical. It is customary to plot the amplitude of the electrical potential on the ordinate and time after stimulus presentation on the abscissa. Depending on the convention used, positive potentials may be either upward or downward (Fig. 2–23).

Generally, the VEP can be considered to reflect almost exclusively macular function. This is because of two factors: (1) the cortical magnification factor, which represents the relatively disproportionate and expansive cortical area dedicated to processing foveal and macular input; and (2) the physical fact that this representation of the macula is closer to the surface of skull than the deeper portions of calcarine cortex that subserve peripheral vision. Change in a pattern stimulus centered on the fovea constitutes a powerful activator of receptive fields in the foveal and perifoveal region. Even if the stimulus is large enough, there is little contribution to the PVEP from areas outside the central 5°. Although the diffuse FVEP stimulus activates receptive fields that extend to the periphery of the retina, for the reasons given, the FVEP also has a predominant macular com-

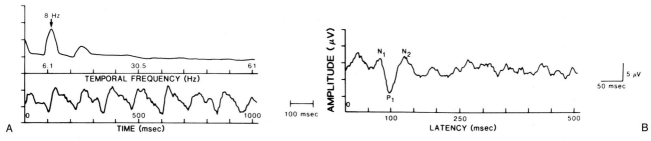

Fig. 2–23. Pattern visual evoked potentials (*PVEP*). **A.** Steady-state: the *lower trace* is a steady-state sinusoidal waveform resulting from 4-Hz (eight pattern reversals per second) stimulation. The *upper trace* is a Fourier transform indicating peak power at the second harmonic of the stimulus frequency (8 Hz). **B.** Transient PVEP waveform resulting from 1-Hz stimulation. The major positive deflection (*P1*) occurs normally at about 100 milliseconds after each stimulus.

ponent. However, in certain instances, when the peripheral field is primarily affected, the FVEP will reflect the abnormality more adequately than the PVEP. However, some disorders that typically show peripheral field abnormality, such as glaucoma, have significantly abnormal PVEPs,[73] and evidence of early involvement of foveal function in glaucoma is evident if the proper measurement techniques are applied.[77]

The main parameters measured with the VEP are its amplitude and latency, the latter being more informative. VEP amplitude is quite variable in persons with normal vision. Latency of the transient VEP is most commonly assessed using the time delay from the stimulus presentation to the P1 (or P100) peak of the VEP waveform, a large positive potential that, in persons with normal vision, occurs around 100 milliseconds after stimulus presentation (see Fig. 2–23, bottom).

The VEP may be employed to detect or analyze various disorders of the anterior afferent visual pathway. By understanding the mechanisms of damage, some of the abnormalities in the VEP can be predicted. In anterior ischemic optic neuropathy (see Fig. 2–7), for example, the VEP is frequently low in amplitude but normal in latency.[78] On the other hand, delayed VEP responses are characteristic in demyelination of the optic nerve secondary to optic neuritis[73] or compression.[73] The lack of specificity in VEP abnormalities, however, is a major drawback in clinical assessment. Latency delays occur not only in demyelination, but also in neurotransmitter disorders,[80] glaucoma,[73,77] with uncorrected refractive error,[81] with media opacities and in normal human aging. Amplitude reduction occurs regularly in all causes of optic atrophy, but also in amblyopia[82] and with uncorrected refractive errors.[81] As a matter of course, therefore, proper testing technique mandates that refractive correction be optimized for the testing distance and that ocular causes of blurring be noted whenever recording the pattern VEP.

VEPs have also been used to evaluate disease affecting the chiasm, the optic tract, and the posterior visual pathway. In general, hemifield stimulation (that is, presentation of the stimulus to one hemifield of one eye at a time) is required for proper topographic localization of chiasmal and retro-chiasmal lesions. Although this procedure has been shown to be helpful, the hemifield technique requires that the patient maintain steady fixation. Patients who are able to perform this test usually can be tested at a perimeter, which provides more specific and useful information. Therefore, the technique of obtaining hemifield VEPs is of limited clinical value, especially when neuroimaging is by far more productive.

One of the most useful applications of pattern VEPs is to evaluate the visual function of young children and infants using a series of pattern stimuli with different component (*e.g.,* check or stripe) sizes. Various investigators have demonstrated methods of estimating visual acuity, color vision, stereopsis, and other parameters in pre-verbal children. Amblyopia may be diagnosed, and other developmental conditions of childhood that compromise vision can be followed and effects of therapy monitored. The interested reader is directed to the appropriate bibliographic references for description of techniques and protocols.[83,84]

More relevant to neuro-ophthalmology, VEPs can be used to document normal activity in patients with feigned or hysterical visual loss. Although it is possible to avoid looking or focusing on the pattern stimulus, many patients fail to realize that responses to a pattern consisting of small checks or stripes are evidence of good visual acuity. Normal VEPs to pattern stimuli are not an absolute guarantee of good central visual function, but there are very few instances when normal VEPs to small and medium-size checks are associated with markedly decreased visual acuity, and these must always be central, usually involving higher-order cognitive processing or disconnection syndromes. Thus, a normal VEP should support or generate suspicion of non-physiologic visual loss. Of course, an abnormal VEP does not necessarily imply physiologic visual impairment because a variety of technical problems and patient avoidance can degrade the VEP waveform.

Other Tests of Visual Function

Light and Dark Adaptation

The rod and the cone systems adjust sensitivity thresholds across an enormous variation in overall light levels. This regulation is *dark and light adaptation,* and it occurs when going from a higher to a lower light level, and vice versa. Retinal adaptation to light occurs much more quickly than dark adaptation, requiring less than 5 minutes for the process to stabilize. During the first minute of this process, sensitivity changes rapidly and may include both a desensitization and a resensitization process. Following the first minute, a slower and less pronounced desensitization occurs. The first of these periods appears to be associated with a neural adaptation, whereas the second sensitivity change is primarily a photochemical effect.

At the onset of *dark adaptation,* both the rods and cones instantaneously begin to modify. During the first 10 to 12 minutes, the sensitivity of the cone system continues to exceed the the rod system, because of both a higher initial sensitivity and a faster recovery. After 10 to 12 minutes, however, the sensitivity of the rods surpasses the cone sensitivity, which approaches its maximum scotopic adaptation. Rod sensitivity continues to increase for approximately 30 to 60 minutes toward its ultimate plateau. Consequently, after the first 10 to 12 minutes of dark adaptation, vision is primarily governed by rod function.

Clinically, the full course of dark adaptation can be measured with standard dark adaptometers, or testing can be limited to the determination of final thresholds after prolonged adaptation. Dark adaptometry applies exclusively to retinal diseases that do not touch on neuro-ophthalmologic subjects, and it is beyond the scope of this discussion.

Motion Sensitivity

Motion perception refers to the visual inference that objects have changed relative position, and it is a fundamental visual capability involved in many aspects of visually guided behavior. Motion perception provides information about our movements in space, the motion of objects relative to our position in space, the three-dimensional structure of objects and depth perception. Impaired motion perception can adversely affect activities as simple as pouring a glass of water and as complex as flying an airplane.

Although motion perception is an important visual capacity with obvious survival value, there has been limited consideration of the clinical utility of assessing motion perception. Most studies on motion blindness in humans have dealt with individual cases reports of specific patients in which reductions in motion sensitivity occurred following cortical lesions. However, more recent studies have shown that motion sensitivity deficits are not limited to brain injury but also occur with retinal damage that limits neural input to higher-order motion detection centers. Disordered motion sensitivity has been reported in patients with retinitis pigmentosa,[85] diabetic retinopathy, and glaucoma.[86] Furthermore, there is evidence that the motion perception deficits of patients with Alzheimer-type dementia[87] and Parkinson's disease[88] are at least partially attributable to retinal dysfunction. Comparisons of the perceptual and ocular motor response to motion also demonstrate a dissociation between motion sensitivity deficits and ocular motor abnormalities in patients with Alzheimer's dementia.[89]

Acuity at Reduced Illumination

A practical technique to determine whether reduced acuity is due to long-standing functional amblyopia or to an organic lesion (macular or optic nerve disease) is to use a neutral density filter.[90] If a 2-log unit filter (Kodak No. 96, ND 2.00) is placed before a normal eye, vision will be reduced approximately two lines (*e.g.,* from 20/20 to 20/40). With an optic nerve conduction defect such as retro-bulbar neuritis, vision is usually drastically reduced when a neutral density filter is used, for example, from 20/60 to 20/200 or 20/400. The effect of such reduced contrast testing on functional amblyopia is of great interest because vision in such eyes decreases minimally or not at all. Thus, the use of neutral density filters can distinguish between functional amblyopia and an acquired retro-bulbar lesion. However, if amblyopia is severe, this test is difficult to interpret.

REFERENCES

1. Livingstone MS, Hubel DH: Psychophysical evidence for separate channels for the perception of form, color, movement and depth. J Neurosci 7:3416, 1987
2. Schiller PH, Logothetis NK, Charles ER: Role of the color-opponent and broad-band channels in vision. Vis Neurosci 5:321, 1990
3. Van Essen DC, Anderson CH, Fellman DJ: Information processing in the primate visual system: an integrated systems perspective. Science 255:419, 1992
4. Merigan WH, Maunsell JHR: How parallel are the primate visual pathways? Annu Rev Neurosci 16:369, 1993
5. Panda-Jonas S, Jonas JB, Jacobczyk M, Schneider U: Retinal photoreceptor count, retinal surface area, and optic disc size in normal human eyes. Ophthalmology 101:519, 1994
6. Schiller PH, Sandell JH, Maunsell JH: Functions of the ON and OFF channels of the visual system. Nature 322:824, 1986
7. Masland RH: The functional architecture of the retina. Sci Am 254:102, 1986
8. Drasdo N: Receptive field densities of the ganglion cells of the human retina. Vision Res 29:985, 1989
9. Curcio CA, Allen KA: Topography of ganglion cells in human retina. J Comp Neurol 300:5, 1990
10. D'Zmura M, Lennie P: Shared pathways for rod and cone vision. Vision Res 26:1273, 1986
11. Rovamo J, Raninen A: Cortical acuity and the luminous flux collected by retinal ganglion cells at various eccentricities in human rod and cone vision. Vision Res 30:11, 1990
12. Ransom-Hogg A, Spillmann L: Perceptive field size in fovea and

periphery of the light and dark adapted retina. Vision Res 20:221, 1980

13. Crook JM, Lange-Malecki B, Lee BB, Valberg A: Visual resolution of macaque retinal ganglion cells. J Physiol 396:205, 1988
14. Gao H, Hollyfield JG: Aging of human retina. Invest Ophthalmol Vis Sci 33:1, 1992
15. Bishop PO: Processing of visual information within the retinostriate system, p 357. In Darian-Smith I (ed): Handbook of Physiology. Bethesda, MD, American Physiological Society, 1984
16. Silveira LC, Perry VH: The topography of magnocellular projecting ganglion cells (M-ganglion cells) in the primate retina. Neuroscience 40:217, 1991
17. Schiller PH: The on and off channels of the visual system. In Cohen B, Bodis-Wollner I (eds): Vision and the Brain: The Organisation of the Central Visual System, p 35. New York, Raven Press, 1990
18. Shapley R, Perry VH: Cat and monkey retinal ganglion cells and their visual functional roles. Trends in Neurosci May:229, 1986
19. Derrington AM, Lennie P: Spatial and temporal contrast sensitivities of neurones in lateral geniculate nucleus of macaque. J Physiol (Lond) 357:219, 1984
20. Brannan JR, Bodis-Wollner I: Evidence for two systems mediating perceived contrast. Vis Neurosci 6:587, 1991
21. Purpura K, Kaplan E, Shapley RM: Background light and the contrast gain of primate P and M retinal ganglion cells. Proc Natl Acad Sci USA 85:4534, 1988
22. Evers HU, Gouras P: Three cone mechanisms in the primate electroretinogram: two with, one without off-center bipolar responses. Vision Res 2:245, 1986
23. Merigan W, Katz LM, Maunsell JHR: The effects of parvocellular lateral geniculate lesions on the acuity and contrast sensitivity of macaque monkeys. J Neurosci 11:994, 1991
24. Wall M: Loss of P retinal ganglion cell function in resolved optic neuritis. Neurology 40:649, 1990
25. Chaturvedi N, Hedley-Whyte ED, Dreyer EB: Lateral geniculate nucleus in glaucoma. Am J Ophthalmol 116:182, 1993
26. Kolb H: Anatomical pathways for color vision in the human retina. Vis Neurosci 7:61, 1991
27. Horton JC, Hoyt WF: The representation of the visual field in human striate cortex: a revision of classical Holmes map. Arch Ophthalmol 109:816, 1991
28. Wood JM, Wild JM, Drasdo N, Crews SJ: Perimetric profiles and cortical representation. Ophthalmic Res 18:301, 1986
29. Helmholtz H: Handbuch der Physiologischen Optik. Leipzig, Leopold Voss, 1867
30. Frisén L: Visual acuity and visual field tests: psychophysical versus pathophysical objectives. In Kennard C, Clifford Rose F (eds): Physiological Aspects of Clinical Neuro-Ophthalmology, p 3. Chicago, Year Book, 1988
31. Johnson CA: Evaluation of visual function. In Tasman W, Jeager EA (eds): Foundations of Clinical Ophthalmology. Philadelphia, Lippincott-Raven, 1995
32. Campbell FW, Green DG: Optical and retinal factors affecting visual resolution. J Physiol (Lond) 181:576, 1965
33. Westheimer G: Visual acuity. In Hart WM (ed): Adler's Physiology of the Eye, p 502. St. Louis, Mosby–Year Book, 1992
34. Hart WMJ: Visual adaptation. In Hart WM (ed): Adler's Physiology of the Eye, p 502. St. Louis, Mosby–Year Book, 1992
35. Rea MS: Some basic concepts and field applications for lighting, color and vision. In Nadler PM, Miller D, Nadler DJ (eds): Glare and Contrast Sensitivity for Clinicians, p 120. New York, Springer-Verlag, 1990
36. Flom MC, Weymouth FW, Kahneman D: Visual resolution and contour interaction. J Optom Soc Am 1026, 1963
37. Bailey IV, Lovie JE: New design principles for visual acuity letter charts. Am J Optom Physiol Opt 53:740, 1976
38. Ferris FL, Kassof A, Bresnick GH, Bailey IL: New visual acuity charts for clinical research. Am J Ophthalmol 94:91, 1982
39. Pelli DG, Robson JG, Wilkins AJ: The design of a new letter chart for measuring contrast sensitivity. Clin Vision Sci 2:187, 1988
40. Regan D, Neima D: Low contrast letter charts as a test of visual function. Ophthalmology 90:1192, 1983
41. Frisén L, Frisén M: How good is normal visual acuity? Graefes Arch Clin Exp Ophthalmol 215:149, 1981

42. Adams AJ, Verdon WA, Spivey BE: Color vision. In Tasman W, Jeager EA (eds): Duane's Foundations of Clinical Ophthalmology, p 1. Philadelphia, Lippincott–Raven, 1995
43. Wald G: The receptors of human color vision. Science 145:1007, 1964
44. Engel S, Zhang X, Wandell B: Colour tuning in human visual cortex measured with functional magnetic resonance imaging. Nature 388:68, 1997
45. Kollner H: Die Stoungen des Farbensinnes. Ihre Klinische Bedeutung und ihre Diagnose. Berlin, Karger, 1912
46. Safran AB, Kline LB, Glaser JS: Positive visual phenomena in optic nerve and chiasm disease: photopsia and photophobia. In Glaser JS (ed): Neuro-Ophthalmology, p 225. St. Louis, CV Mosby, 1980
47. Pelli DG, Robson JG: Are letters better than gratings? Clin Vision Sci 6:409, 1991
48. Ginsberg AP: A new contrast sensitivity vision test chart. Am J Optom Physiol Opt 61:403, 1984
49. Rubin GS: Reliability and sensitivity of clinical contrast sensitivity tests. Clin Vision Sci 2:169, 1988
50. Nichols BE, Thompson HS, Stone EM: Evaluation of a significantly shorter version of the Farnsworth-Munsell 100-hue tests in patients with three different optic neuropathies. J Neuro-ophthalmol 17:1, 1997
51. Glaser JS, Savino PJ, Sumers KD: The photostress recovery test: a practical adjunct in the clinical assessment of visual function. Am J Ophthalmol 83:255, 1977
52. Wu G, Weiter JJ, Santos S et al: The macular photostress test in diabetic retinopathy and age-related macular degeneration. Arch Ophthalmol 108:1556, 1990
53. Johnson LN: The relative afferent pupillary defect and a novel method of fusion recovery with the Worth 4-dot test. Arch Ophthalmol 114:171, 1996
54. Scott GI: Traquair's Clinical Perimetry, 7th ed. London, Henry Kimpton, 1957
55. Safran AB, Glaser JS: Stato-kinetic dissociation in lesions of the anterior visual pathways: a reappraisal of the Riddoch phenomenon. Arch Ophthalmol 98:291, 1980
56. Egge K: The visual field in normal subjects. Acta Ophthalmol Suppl 169:1, 1984
57. Johnson CA, Chauhan B, Shapiro LR: Properties of staircase procedures for estimating thresholds in automated perimetry. Invest Ophthalmol Vis Sci 33:2966, 1992
58. Heijl A, Drance SM: A clinical comparison of three computerised automatic perimeters in the detection of glaucoma defects. Arch Ophthalmol 99:832, 1981
59. Trope GE, Britton R: A comparison of Goldmann and Humphrey automated perimetry in patients with glaucoma. Br J Ophthalmol 71:489, 1987
60. Beck RW, Bergstrom TJ, Lichter PR: A clinical comparison of visual field testing with a new automated perimeter, the Humphrey Field Analyzer, and the Goldmann perimeter. Ophthalmology 92:77, 1985
61. Heijl A, Lindgren G, Olsson J, Asman P: Visual field interpretation with empiric probability maps. Arch Ophthalmol 107:204, 1989
62. Mills RP, Barnebey HS, Migliazzo CV, Li Y: Does saving time using FASTPAC or suprathreshold testing reduce quality of visual fields? Ophthalmology 101:1596, 1994
63. Katz J, Sommer A: Screening for glaucomatous visual field loss: the effect of patient reliability. Ophthalmology 97:1032, 1990
64. Katz J, Sommer A: Reliability indexes of automated perimetric tests. Arch Ophthalmol 106:1252, 1988
65. Bickler-Bluth M, Trick GL, Kolker AE, Cooper DG: Assessing the utility of reliability indices for automated visual fields: testing ocular hypertensives (see comments). Ophthalmology 96:616, 1989
66. Flammer J: The concept of visual field indices. Graefes Arch Clin Exp Ophthalmol 1986; 224:389, 1986
67. Flammer J, Drance SM, Fankhauser F, Augustiny L: Differential light threshold in automated static perimetry: factors influencing short-term fluctuation. Arch Ophthalmol 102:876, 1984

68. Boeglin RJ, Caprioli J, Zulauf M: Long-term fluctuation of the visual field in glaucoma. Am J Ophthalmol 113:396, 1992

69. Johnson CA: Modern developments in clinical perimetry. Curr Opin Ophthalmol 4:7, 1993

70. Johnson CA, Adams AJ, Casson EJ, Brandt JD: Progression of early glaucomatous visual field loss as detected by blue-on-yellow and standard white-on-white automated perimetry. Arch Ophthalmol 111:651, 1993

71. Johnson CA, Adams AJ, Casson EJ, Brandt JD: Blue-on-yellow perimetry can predict the development of glaucomatous visual field loss. Arch Ophthalmol 111:645, 1993

72. Maffei L, Fiorentini A: Electroretinographic responses to alternating gratings before and after transection of the optic nerve. Science 211:953, 1981

73. Bobak P, Bodis-Wollner I, Harnois C et al: Pattern electroretinograms and visual evoked potentials in glaucoma and multiple sclerosis. Am J Ophthalmol 96:72, 1983

74. Ringens PJ, Vijfvinkel-Bruinenga S, Van Lith GHM: The pattern-elicited electroretinogram. 1. A tool in the early detection of glaucoma? Ophthalmologica 192:171, 1986

75. Barris M, Trick G, Bickler-Bluth M: Abnormal visual function in patients with early senile dementia of the Alzheimer's type (SDAT) revealed by retinal evoked potentials. Invest Ophthalmol Vis Sci 28(Suppl):432, 1988

76. Plant GT, Hess RF, Thomas SJ: The pattern evoked electroretinogram in optic neuritis: a combined psychophysical and electrophysiological study. Brain 109:469, 1986

77. Atkin A, Podos SM, Bodis-Wollner I: Abnormalities of the visual system in ocular hypertension and glaucoma: seeing beyond routine perimetry. In Krieglstein GK, Leydhecker W (eds): Glaucoma Update 11. Berlin, Springer-Verlag, 1983

78. Cox TA, Thompson HS, Hayreh SS et al: Visual evoked potential and pupillary signs: a comparison in optic nerve disease. Arch Ophthalmol 100:1603, 1982

79. Halliday AM, Halliday E, Kriss A et al: The pattern evoked potential in compression of the anterior visual pathways. Brain 99:357, 1976

80. Bodis-Wollner I, Yahr MD, Mylin L et al: Dopamine deficiency and delayed visual evoked potentials in humans. Ann Neurol 11:478, 1982

81. Bobak P, Bodis-Wollner I, Guillory S: The effect of blur and contrast on VEP latency: comparison between checks and sinusoidal grating patterns. Electroencephalogr Clin Neurophysiol 68:247, 1987

82. Sokol S, Bloom B: Visually evoked cortical responses of amblyopes to a spatially alternating stimulus. Invest Ophthalmol Vis Sci 12:936, 1973

83. Taylor MJ, McCulloch DL: Visual evoked potentials in infants and children. J Clin Neurophysiol 9:357, 1992

84. Fulton AB, Hartmann EE, Hansen RM: Electrophysiologic testing techniques for children. Doc Ophthalmol 71:341, 1989

85. Turano K, Wong X. Motion thresholds in retinitis pigmentosa. Invest Ophthalmol Vis Sci 33:2411, 1992

86. Trick GL, Steinman SB, Amyot M: Motion perception deficits in glaucomatous optic neuropathy. Vision Res 35:2225, 1995

87. Trick GL, Silverman SE: Motion perception deficits in aging and senile dementia of the Alzheimer's type (SDAT). Neurology 41:1437, 1991

88. Trick GL, Kaskie B, Steinman SB: Visual dysfunction in Parkinson's disease: deficits in orientation and motion perception. Optom Vis Sci 71:242, 1994

89. Silverman SE, Tran DB, Zimmerman KM, Feldon SE: Dissociation between the detection and perception of motion in Alzheimer's disease. Neurology 44:1814, 1994

90. von Noorden GK, Burian HM: Visual acuity in normal and amblyopic patients under reduced illumination. 1. Behavior of visual acuity with and without neutral density filter. Arch Ophthalmol 65:533, 1959

CHAPTER 3

Neuro-ophthalmologic Examination: General Considerations and Special Techniques

Joel S. Glaser

Ocular Motility
  Range and Character of Eye Movements
    Fixation and Ocular Stabilization
    Conjugate Gaze: Versions
    Convergence
  Special Techniques
    Examination of Infants
    Optokinetic Nystagmus
    Diplopia
    Bell's Phenomenon and Spasticity of Conjugate
      Gaze
Eyelids
  Neuroanatomy and Physiology
  Position and Movements

  Lid Retraction
  Ptosis
  Lid Nystagmus
Ocular Sensation and Pain
  Functional Anatomy
    Peripheral Trigeminal Afferents
    Trigeminal Sensory Nuclei
    Trigeminal Ascending Pathways
  Clinical Evaluation of Trigeminal Function
  Abnormal Corneal Reflexes
  Pain in and about the Eye
  Defective Tearing
  Neuralgia and Atypical Facial Pain
The Comatose Patient

Since neuro-ophthalmologic examination makes use of ophthalmologic means and devices but aims at a neurologic diagnosis, it occupies a kind of intermediate position and suffers neglect from both sides. Many neurologists are not familiar enough with the detailed technique of the ophthalmologic methods; ophthalmologists are often not concerned with the details of neurologic localization.

Alfred Kestenbaum, 1946
Clinical Methods of Neuro-
ophthalmologic Examination

OCULAR MOTILITY

In the examination of ocular motility, it is helpful for the physician to follow an orderly protocol that logically subdivides the different types of eye movement. There is sufficient clinical and experimental evidence to substantiate the existence of several subsystems for the control of eye movement and position. The pragmatic clinical analysis of defective eye movements must take into account these newer concepts of ocular motor mechanisms. A complete discussion of the anatomy and physiology of eye movements is found in Chapter 10.

  J. S. Glaser: Departments of Neurology and Ophthalmology, Bascom Palmer Eye Institute, University of Miami School of Medicine, Miami; and Neuro-ophthalmology, Cleveland Clinic Florida, Ft. Lauderdale, Florida

Range and Character of Eye Movements

It is through familiarity with the normal that we may distinguish the abnormal. Therefore, this discussion begins with a brief description of typical and normal eye movement. As with the determination of visual function, observation of ocular motility begins as the patient enters the examination room and continues during history taking. The physician should note normal or abnormal spontaneous gaze and eye position. It is especially rewarding to observe the spontaneous eye movements of infants and young children, before the "threat" of actual physical examination.

Fixation and Ocular Stabilization

In the human, eye movements occur so that a focused image is projected onto the central fixational area of the retina, the fovea. Here visual function is greatest because of the concentration of receptor cells. A stimulus that falls on the peripheral retina provokes an eye movement that realigns the visual axis of the eye so that the fovea "acquires" the visual direction of that stimulus; that is, the eye "fixates" the stimulus that now becomes the object of regard. The eye movement that acquires the target is the "fixational reflex," and the steady "lock on" of the fovea is "fixation."

It is obvious that ocular fixation, in acquiring and

holding a target, requires reasonably good visual acuity, although more peripheral parts of retina have some fixational capacity. Therefore, the afferent visual pathways from retina to cortex play a major role in fixation, but there must be a counterpart motor efferent that precisely guides the fixational eye movement to target and then maintains punctilious gaze. The ability of one or both eyes accurately and steadily to fixate a target (muscle light, finger, or pencil) is a prerequisite for evaluating other types of eye movement. For example, if one eye fixates poorly due to dense central scotoma, the cover-uncover or alternate-cover test has limited value.

Fixational movements may be *voluntary* (the quick eye movements as one looks about a room) or *involuntary* (when a bright light suddenly appears in the far peripheral field). The involuntary fixational reflex may alternately be called a "visually elicited eye movement"; that such eye movements may be provoked, is used as evidence of peripheral field function in infants (see below). In either case, when the object of regard is acquired by the fovea, fixation is steady, and the eye continues smoothly to track (a pursuit movement) a target that is slowly moved, much as a radar system acquires a target, locks on, and smoothly tracks.

The stability of fixation is quickly determined simply by having a patient (even a baby) gaze at a target (light, pencil, small cartoon character, or hand puppet). Fixation should be steady and unwavering. If the target is slowly moved from side to side, the eyes move smoothly to maintain fixation without "slippage" off the target. These ocular pursuit movements are discussed below. Fixation should be tested binocularly as well as with each eye separately.

Conjugate Gaze: Versions

The ability of the eyes to move symmetrically and synchronously in the same direction, horizontally or vertically, is termed "conjugate" (yoked together) gaze. These versional movements may be rapid (a *saccade*), as in the command to "look left", or during the reflex to take up fixation (see above), or may be slow as in the smooth tracking (*pursuit*) of a slowly moving target. Saccadic and pursuit sub-systems are discussed in some detail in Chapters 9 through 11.

Conjugate gaze is tested by asking the patient to "look right . . . left." The patient is then asked to "follow" ("let your eyes follow") some target such as the examiner's hand-held light (Fig. 3–1). Command horizontal eye movements should be rapid and symmetric in the two eyes. Binocular excursions (both eyes open) are generally smaller than monocular (one eye covered), and the eyes move through approximately 45° to either side of the straight forward position (*i.e.*, primary gaze). Abduction is difficult to sustain beyond 35° of eccentricity, and a physiologic *end-gaze nystagmus* is quite com-

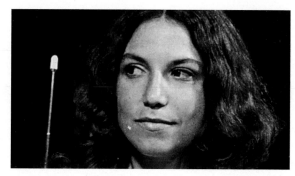

Fig. 3–1. Examination of ocular versions. Horizontal pursuit is toward the right.

mon (see Chapter 11). In the abducting eye, the temporal aspect of the corneal margin should almost approximate the outer angle (lateral canthus) of the lids, with little sclera visible. In elderly patients with lax facial tissues, the external lid angle may be displaced so that a minimal rim of sclera is still visible in the abducted position. The adducting eye is positioned such that 1 mm to 2 mm of the nasal aspect of the cornea may be buried in the folds of conjunctiva and caruncle at the inner canthal angle.

Vertical conjugate gaze is somewhat more difficult to assess. Downward gaze should be at least 45°, but since the lower lid is indented by the cornea, there is no constant landmark. Upward gaze is even more difficult to assess. Chamberlain[1] reported a progressive restriction in upward ocular versions with advancing age: 95 patients aged 5 to 34 years had 36° to 40° of elevation; 125 patients aged 65 to 94 years had 16° to 22° of elevation.

Conjugate versions may also be tested without the patient's active cooperation, by directing attention to a distant target (*e.g.*, a wall-mounted light, or even while an acuity chart is being read), and passively rotating the patient's face to the right, left, up, and down.

Convergence

Convergence is an associated, but disjugate, movement, in that the eyes move toward each other, rather than turning toward the same side (*i.e.*, conjugate). It is usually accomplished by synchronous action of both medial recti muscles as in reading or other near-visual tasks, but convergence may be blended with a conjugate gaze, for example, fixating a near object directly in front of one eye. The neural mechanisms responsible for adduction during lateral conjugate gaze, and during convergence, are separate and may be dissociated in pathologic states, for example, in patients with internuclear ophthalmoplegia.

It is helpful to test convergence capability in the following neuro-ophthalmologic situations: (1) if pupillary light reactions are absent or sluggish, the pupils are observed during convergence (more precisely, during the near-effort reflex); (2) if there is lag of the adducting eye on lateral conjugate gaze suggesting an internuclear ophthalmoplegia; (3) any bilateral external ophthalmoplegia; and (4) in acquired exotropia, in which monocular ductions are full, suggesting convergence paralysis.

Convergence strength varies considerably and depends principally on the cooperation of the patient. A sure sign that the patient is indeed attempting to converge is simultaneous pupillary constriction. Of course, there are pathologic states that involve both convergence and pupillary constriction (*e.g.*, Parinaud's dorsal midbrain syndrome). It is helpful if the patient's own finger is used as a convergence target. Thus, even in a blind patient, convergence may be examined using proprioceptive clues to the nearness of one's finger or hand. Reticence to attempt to gaze at one's finger, or histrionic avoidance, may signal a functional disorder or dissembling.

Special Techniques

Examination of Infants

In order to determine the extent of conjugate eye movements in infants, it is often necessary to resort to special clinical techniques and manipulations. However, initial observation of spontaneous versions and fixation may suffice, and such observations should begin before the infant or young child is startled or anxious. Otherwise, visually elicited eye movements are provoked by objects that attract an infant's attention (see Chapter 2, Fig. 2–9) and therefore also provide a gross estimation of visual function. Similarly, a child turns head and eyes toward a sound (jingling keys). This is an *acoustically elicited* eye movement that does not require sight, however, and so no conclusions may be drawn regarding vision. If the child accurately fixates and follows any silent object, that is good evidence of reasonably intact vision.

If the examiner holds a neonate upright, face to face, and turns, the neonate's eyes undergo a tonic deviation in the direction of the turn (Fig. 3–2). This tonic, conjugate eye deviation is a result of labyrinthine stimulation and does not depend on vision. The fast phase (jerk) of such rotation induced nystagmus may be absent in the premature neonate, but it is usually present before 1 week of age. Rotational maneuvers are helpful in determining the state of brain stem systems for conjugate horizontal gaze. Failure to elicit eye movement on rotational testing infers a major pontine or extraocular muscle abnormality. Brisk rotation of the head, vertically and horizontally, on the long axis of the body ("doll's head" phenomenon), produces tonic contralateral horizontal deviation of the eyes in the neonate.

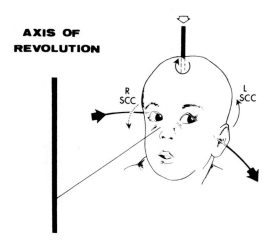

Fig. 3–2. Rotational testing for eye movement function in infants. As the infant is spun toward its left (toward the examiner's right), the eyes will tonically deviate in the direction of the movement, with the jerk phase of nystagmus toward the opposite side. The *open arrow* indicates the induced axis of rotation of the infant's head. Note the influence of head rotation on the right and left semicircular canals (*SCC*).

Optokinetic nystagmus (OKN; see below) may be used to determine ocular motility, but induced OKN movements are less extensive than with rotational stimulation. Disparity between vertical and horizontal response or between optokinetic and rotational responses may indicate a disorder of supranuclear gaze mechanisms, such as in congenital ocular motor apraxia or congenital nystagmus (see Chapter 13).

Optokinetic Nystagmus

If a series of vertical bars or other such patterned contours is passed before the eyes (Fig. 3–3), a visually induced nystagmus occurs. This nystagmus was apparently first adequately described by Helmholtz, who observed the eyes of passengers gazing out of train windows at the passing countryside. This phenomenon is easily noted in riders of subway trains, buses, and so forth. There is a slow following phase toward the side of target movement (or at the passing scene) and a rapid jerk return in the opposite direction. The character of OKN is partially dependent on the speed of target movement, the pattern density, and the subject's visual function and state of attentiveness. Because the slow phase is initiated by vision, OKN may be used as a rough parameter of visual function. As noted by Linksz,[2] OKN is more closely related to movement perception or contour recognition than to visual acuity. Actually, suppression of OKN response by interposition of a fixation target of variable size is best correlated with "acuity." It should be recognized that OKN represents an innate and highly complex ocular motor reflex evoked by perception of moving contours, which is only distantly related to visual

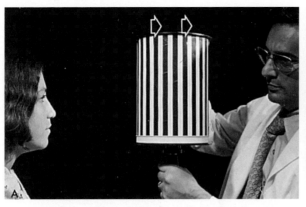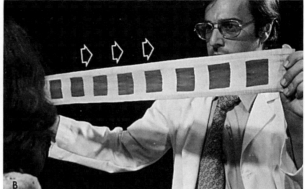

Fig. 3–3. Optokinetic nystagmus. The movement of a striped drum **(A)** or squares on a cloth **(B)** evokes a nystagmus that beats opposite the direction of target movement.

acuity. In clinical practice, only a rough estimate of visual "acuity" is obtained with the usual optokinetic devices. Examples of the *minimum* visual requirement with a stimulus at *2 to 4 feet* (see Fig. 3–3) are presented below:

1. Striped drum: finger count 3 to 5 feet.
2. Squares on flag: finger count 3 to 5 feet.
3. Tailor's tape: 20/400 to 3/200.

OKN is an especially useful technique in infants as a test of gross visual function, and it should be demonstrable to some degree even in newborns. It is positive evidence of sight in malingerers and hysteric patients, and it is similarly productive in evaluating uncooperative, semiobtunded, or dysphasic patients. Central vision need not be good to have intact OKN response if gross pattern stimuli are used (see Fig. 3–3).

It is evident that visual impulses trigger a cerebral mechanism that more or less regulates the rhythmicity of the nystagmus. OKN is affected by non-visual factors and may even be observed in hypnotic states, although the character of the OKN is not strictly parallel to that induced by actual visual stimuli. An optokinetic after-nystagmus may be demonstrated on cessation of target rotation, especially if fixation is inhibited by dark environment or lid closure. Further evidence of non-linearity of visual input and optokinetic response was demonstrated in the rabbit by Collewijn,[3] but it is also true in the human patient who meets the criteria for conducting the demonstration; if a gross OKN stimulus is presented monocularly before a seeing but immobile eye, optokinetic response is observed in the occluded or blind, but mobile, fellow eye.

Optokinetic response as a useful clinical tool was first popularized by Kestenbaum,[4] and later by Cogan and Smith,[5] and others. Cerebral lesions deep in the parietal lobe cause homonymous hemianopias and also interrupt the descending occipitomesencephalic system for slow (pursuit) eye movements.

The occipital optomotor fibers descend in the internal sagittal stratum and are medial to the geniculocalcarine radiations in their posterior course through the parietal lobe. Lesions here consistently produce a homonymous hemianopia (contralateral) and a defective OKN when targets are moved toward the side of the lesion. The defective OKN (a "positive OKN sign") is not due to targets coming out of the hemianopia, as originally thought by Barany, because strictly occipital or temporal lobe lesions producing profound hemianopias are not associated with a positive (*i.e.*, asymmetric) OKN response. Therefore, in the presence of a homonymous hemianopia, a defective OKN response indicates deep parietal involvement. This sign is considerably more helpful when the non-dominant (right) parietal lobe is involved (left hemianopia). When the dominant (usually left) parietal lobe is involved, there are consistently other localizing signs and symptoms, such as motor and sensory dysphasias.

OKN may be helpful in elucidating volitional (saccadic) gaze palsies, with intact pursuit movement. For example, a patient with a right frontal lesion may show an inability to make command eye movements to the left, but slow-moving targets will produce smooth pursuit toward the left. Because pursuit to the left is intact and saccades to the right are normal, with targets rotated toward the left a normal OKN response is seen. However, with targets toward the right, the fast phase leftward cannot be generated, and a tonic deviation toward the right will result, as though the eyes are drawn in that direction by the rotating drum or tape.

OKN is a useful mechanism to amplify muscle pareses by inducing an asymmetric response of yoke muscles, best observed in the fast (saccadic) phase. For example, a subtle weakness of adduction (as seen in internuclear ophthalmoplegia) may be uncovered by observing a grossly dissociated OKN response when the paretic muscle is challenged to make a saccade (*i.e.*, with targets rotated opposite the field of action of the paretic muscle). Thus, the adduction lag of the left eye with left internuclear ophthalmoplegia is enhanced by target rotation toward the left that induces fast phase to the (defective) right. Similarly, a command saccade from left to right also enhances the adduction lag; that is, a grossly slowed rightward saccade of the left eye is observed.[6] Despite the complexities of the neurophysiologic basis for OKN, it is a simple and practical clinical maneuver with multiple applications in elucidating defects in the ocular motor system (see Chapter 10).

Diplopia

Double vision is a disturbing symptom that most patients cannot ignore, but many are unable to describe adequately. Diplopia may be intermittent at first, as the patient's fusional mechanism is not overtaxed, or it may first be noticed only for distant vision (suggesting lateral rectus paresis) or principally during near-vision tasks (suggesting medial rectus or superior oblique paresis). The issue may be clarified by the following questions:

1. When and how was the double vision first noticed?
2. Were there other symptoms when the double vision began: light-headedness, dizziness, or spinning; weakness or tingling in face, arm, or leg; difficulty with speech or swallowing (or other signs and symptoms of vertebrobasilar ischemic episode); facial or ocular pain?
3. Did one or both lids droop? Before or since?
4. Are the images side by side, one above the other, or a combination?
5. Is one image tilted (suggests superior oblique palsy)?
6. Is it worse in the distance or while reading?
7. Is the double vision the same throughout the day?
8. Since first noticed, has it gotten worse, better, or stayed about the same?
9. Can the head and face be turned or tilted to avoid the double vision?
10. Is there a medical history of trauma, diabetes, hypertension, or dysthyroidism?

General inspection of the patient should include observation for spontaneous head tilt or face turn. While taking the history, the physician notes the position of the lids and looks for partial or total ptosis (myasthenia, third nerve palsy, Horner's syndrome) or unilateral or bilateral lid retraction (dysthyroidism). Signs of local orbital disease should be sought: proptosis, lid edema, and inflamed or hypervascular conjunctiva (see Chapters 12 and 14).

Almost all diplopia occurs as the result of an acquired paresis or palsy of one or more extraocular muscles. However, a child who insidiously develops a non-paralytic comitant squint may rarely complain of diplopia.

In addition, in instances of fusional disturbances, such as convergence insufficiency, double vision may be a major symptom (see Chapter 13). These conditions are defined by appropriate examination techniques that demonstrate their non-paralytic characteristics; that is, monocular ductions are full, and angle of deviation remains the same regardless of which eye is made to fixate a target. In other words, in non-paralytic strabismus, the angle of muscle imbalance (squint) is essentially constant, and each eye has a full range of motion if tested separately.

Monocular diplopia (or perhaps more accurately, a "ghost image") is an uncommon complaint and is usually the result of opacities of the cornea or lens, a high degree of astigmatism, or a partially dislocated lens. The use of a pinhole should solve this diagnostic dilemma (see Chapter 1). Kommerell[7] described monocular diplopia caused by pressure of the upper lid that deforms the regular curvature of the cornea. The diagnosis is confirmed by an abnormal retinoscopic reflex, the "Venetian blind phenomenon."

Bender[8] reported instances of polyopia and monocular diplopia of cerebral origin (cerebral polyopia) accompanied by major field defects and other signs of parietal dysfunction, including: spatial disorientation, fluctuating extinction of images, extinction of cutaneous sensation, and disturbances of ocular fixation, which he attributed to occipital lobe disease (see Chapter 7).

In general, the complaint of diplopia indicates an acquired cranial nerve or extraocular muscle disorder that must be confirmed and investigated in an orderly, step-by-step analysis of ocular motility. It is beyond the scope of this work to present a detailed discussion of the anatomy and physiology of the extraocular muscles. However, a brief outline of basic ocular motility follows, primarily for the convenience of readers not formally trained in ophthalmology.

Each eye is maneuvered by six extraocular muscles, each of which has a partner in the contralateral orbit for coordinated simultaneous movement of the fellow eye. Muscles working in pairs for conjugate gaze are called "yoke" muscles. If we consider six cardinal positions of gaze, there are six pairs of yoke muscles that act as the prime movers in those six positions of gaze. Thus, on gaze rightward, the right lateral rectus and left medial rectus are yoke muscles. Each extraocular muscle has an ipsilateral antagonist that must relax if the globe is to move. Therefore, as the lateral rectus contracts to abduct the globe, its antagonist, the medial rectus, is simultaneously inhibited.

The six muscles of each eye may functionally be grouped in three pairs: the two horizontal recti (lateral and medial); the two vertical recti (superior and inferior); and the two obliques (superior and inferior). Each of these pairs represents an agonist-antagonist combination.

Numerous procedures have been devised to assess the function of the extraocular muscles, but if weakness is recent and moderate to marked, a simple test of versions (conjugate gaze) will usually suffice. It is also helpful to note the relative positions of the binocular corneal light reflections, as well as the gross positions of the globes. Mild limitations of movement often can more readily be detected during observation of binocular movements, as the eyes are turned into the "field of action" of the paretic muscle.

According to Hering's law, yoke muscles receive equal and simultaneous innervation. This phenomenon provides a sensitive mechanism for the detection of subtle muscle pareses. For example, the right lateral rectus and left medial rectus are yoke muscles for right horizontal gaze. If the right lateral rectus is paretic and fusion is consequently broken, the patient must elect to fixate an object with one eye or the other. If the non-paretic left eye fixates, there is an inward deviation (esotropia) of the right eye resulting from paresis of right lateral rectus, as well as relatively unopposed contraction of the medial rectus. This is called the *primary deviation* (Fig. 3–4). If, however, the paretic eye fixates, or is forced to fixate (by occluding the intact eye), then additional innervation is required in an attempt to activate the paretic lateral rectus. This excessive innervation determined by the effort of the paretic eye to fixate, according to Hering's law, will also be equally transmitted to the intact left medial rectus, which now "overacts" and excessively adducts the sound eye. This overaction of the non-paretic eye, when the paretic eye is forced to fixate, is termed *secondary deviation* and is greater than primary deviation.

The difference in size of primary and secondary deviation is evident when the *alternate cover test* is used. This is an excellent objective and reproducible method to analyze paretic ocular muscles, but it requires sufficient visual function for adequate central fixation with each eye. The previous discussion (and see Fig. 3–4) showed that the occluded eye deviates; for example, the right eye with a lateral rectus paresis deviates inward behind the occluder. If the occluder is now quickly switched to the other eye, the right eye will make an outward movement to "take up fixation," and this movement is easily observed. Rapid alternation of occluder from one eye to the other (approximately 1 to 2 seconds) provokes an easily discernible and reproducible pattern of fixational eye movements. The alternate cover test may be performed in the six cardinal positions of gaze to discover (1) the field of gaze in which deviation is greatest and (2) in *that* field of gaze, which eye fixation produces the greater deviation. The difference in the angle of deviation from one field of gaze to the other, and with each eye fixating, may be roughly estimated or accurately measured by prism neutralization.

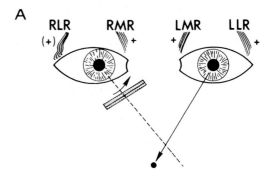

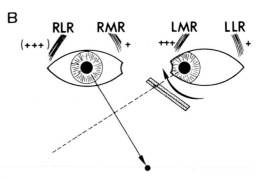

Fig. 3–4. Alternate cover test used, for example, with palsy of the right lateral rectus muscle (*RLR*). **A.** With a cover over the right eye, the left (nonparetic) eye fixates and the right eye is moderately deviated inward (primary deviation). **B.** If the paretic right eye is forced to fixate, increased innervation (+++) is delivered to both the paretic RLR and its normal yoke muscle, the left medial rectus (*LMR*). Subsequent overaction of the LMR markedly deviates the non-paretic eye (secondary deviation).

Diplopia "fields" may be performed by placing a red glass over one eye (by convention, the right) and having the patient indicate the field of gaze of greatest subjective separation of images. This test demonstrates the relative position of the two eyes with respect to one another. With an esotropic deviation (inward turn) the images are uncrossed, that is, the red (right eye) image is toward the right; with an exotropic deviation, the images are crossed, the red image toward the left. The more peripheral-appearing image belongs to the paretic eye. It is helpful if the patient holds up two fingers to demonstrate the relative position of the two images, which should change as the eyes are moved into different gaze directions (Fig. 3–5).

The Maddox rod is a series of parallel cylindrical bars that transform a point source of light into a line perpendicular to the cylinder axes (see Fig. 3–5). If a red Maddox rod is used, the right eye sees a straight vertical or horizontal red line, which may be compared with the position of a white point source of light seen

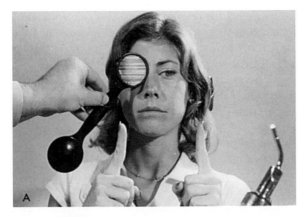

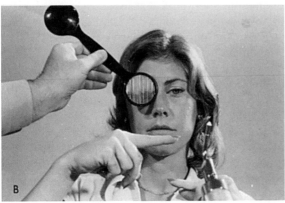

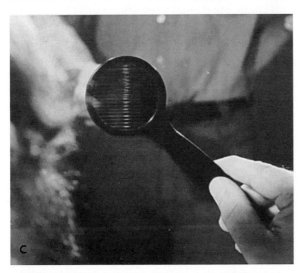

Fig. 3–5. Subjective diplopia examination using a Maddox rod. With the cylinders held horizontally **(A)** or vertically **(B)**, the patient indicates position of images. **C.** Demonstration of the effect of the Maddox rod on the point light source, that is, formation of a line perpendicular to the axes of the series of cylinders.

with the left eye. Torsional deviations, such as those that occur with superior oblique palsies, may be uncovered by subjective appearance of tilting of the Maddox rod image. Special techniques for testing function of the superior oblique are discussed in the section related to fourth nerve palsy (see Chapter 12).

Every patient with diplopia, the cause of which is not obvious, and that is not accompanied by pain or involvement of the pupil, should raise the possibility of myasthenia, for which an intravenous edrophonium (Tensilon) test should be considered. Myasthenia gravis can affect the extraocular muscles singly or in any combination, with or without ptosis, and it is most assuredly a commonly missed diagnosis unless the physician keeps the disease in mind and a syringe at hand (see Chapter 12).

The local orbital inflammatory reaction that consistently accompanies dysthyroid states is a common cause of extraocular muscle restriction. The situation of a middle-aged woman with isolated vertical diplopia represents a monotonous clinical picture with which neurologists and ophthalmologists alike should be thoroughly familiar. If, for good measure, there is unilateral or bilateral lid retraction, the diagnosis is made regardless of the absence of other clinical or chemical signs of dysthyroidism (see Chapters 12 and 14).

In order to establish the presence of a restrictive local orbital myopathy, the *forced duction test* is used. This test determines the presence of mechanical resistance by actually taking hold of the globe and attempting to move it in the direction that the patient cannot (Fig. 3–6; see Chapter 14). It should be pointed out that in any long-standing ocular deviation, whether due to sixth nerve palsy, ocular myasthenia, or congenital esotropia, there may be secondary changes in muscles with contractures and therefore a "positive forced duction test." The conclusions of Kommerell and Oliver[9] are apparently valid: any paresis of an extraocular muscle ultimately results in a contracture of the ipsilateral antagonist; and secondary changes in the non-paretic eye (contracture of yoke muscle) occur only if the paretic eye fixates continuously.

The characteristics of paralytic strabismus, that is, differences in primary and secondary deviation and variation of squint angle with different fields of gaze, are most marked when the paresis is recent. These differences become less marked with time, and the strabismus becomes more symmetric, that is, less incomitant. This phenomenon is the so-called *spread of comitance*. A sequence of events takes place such that comitance emerges; for example, if the right lateral rectus muscle is paretic, the following occur in some degree: (1) overaction (secondary deviation) of the contralateral yoke, the left medial rectus; (2) contracture of the ipsilateral antagonist, the right medial rectus, such that the angle of the inward turn increases; (3) in the presence of hypoactivity of the antagonist, the right medial rectus, its contralateral yoke muscle, the left lateral rectus, will become apparently paretic, especially if the paretic eye is used for fixation (inhibitional palsy of Chavasse); and (4) therefore, the esotropic deviation increases in the

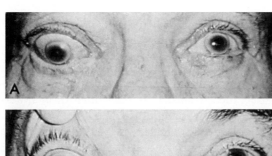
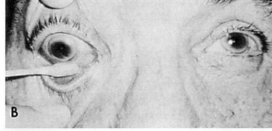
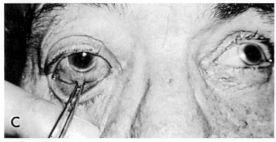
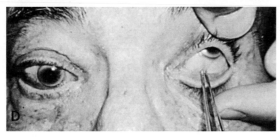

Fig. 3–6. Forced duction test. **A.** Inability of the patient to elevate the right eye on upward gaze. **B.** Using cocaine 10%, the insertion of the right inferior rectus muscle is anesthetized. **C.** The insertion of the inferior rectus is grasped with toothed forceps (Elschnig), and, with the patient looking upward, an attempt is made manually to rotate the right globe upward. **D.** For comparison, the left globe is manually rotated upward following instillation of cocaine.

the eyelids against resistance (Fig. 3–7). The exact neural mechanism for this integrated movement is unknown, but it involves brain stem pathways between the seventh nerve nucleus in the pons and the third nerve nuclear complex in the rostral midbrain. In patients who cannot volitionally elevate the eyes, intact Bell's phenomenon (like doll's head deviation upward) indicates that brain stem pathways, the nuclear cell complex for upward gaze, the associated motor neurons, and the extraocular muscles related to eye elevation are functioning, and that the upward-gaze palsy is due to a supranuclear defect.

Cogan[11] studied the occurrence of abnormal Bell's phenomenon and found that in a series of 156 persons with no known neurologic disease, 132 showed upward or upward and outward deviation of the eyes, that is, the anticipated ocular deviation with forced lid closure. In that presumed normal control group, no deviation from the primary position was observed in 11, convergence occurred in 5, downward deviation was noted in 3, wandering movements occurred in 2, and conjugate lateral deviation was seen in 3. A second group of patients in Cogan's study was composed of 78 patients with unilateral cerebral or infratentorial lesions, with reasonably definite localizing signs. Of the 54 patients with presumed unilateral cerebral disease, 34 showed a lateral conjugate deviation of the eyes to the side *opposite* the lesion, 5 to the same side, and 15 showed no deviation, with forced lid closure. Twenty-four patients with unilateral lesions of the cerebellum, brain stem, or labyrinth demonstrated no consistent deviation. Eye movements related to simple blinking are rapid, and the eyes actually deviate and return to their original position even before the blink is completed.[12]

The pathologic reflex of conjugate deviation of the eyes to the side opposite a cerebral lesion, was called "spasticity of the conjugate oculomotor mechanism" by Cogan. The spastic deviation is not dependent on conjugate-gaze paralysis and, in fact, occurs toward the side opposite that which would be anticipated with a

field of gaze of the left lateral rectus, as well as in the field of gaze of the originally paretic right lateral rectus.

Bell's Phenomenon and Spasticity of Conjugate Gaze

In 1823, Sir Charles Bell reported on the oculogyric phenomenon that accompanies forceful closure of the eyelids, which Bell first noted as an upward deviation of the globe during attempted eyelid closure in the presence of the peripheral facial palsy that now bears his name.[10] Bell's phenomenon is an associated movement of eyes and orbicularis oculi, such that the eyes typically roll upward and outward when efforts are made to close

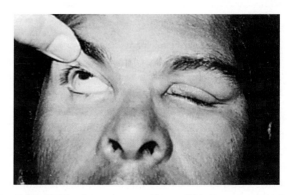

Fig. 3–7. Bell's phenomenon. Forced lid closure against resistance produces upward and outward deviation of the eye.

cerebral gaze palsy. Smith et al[13] emphasized that spasticity of conjugate gaze has lateralizing rather than localizing significance; this phenomenon has its highest correlation with temporo-parietal lesions, is less frequent with occipital disorders, and is not seen with frontal lobe disease. There is apparently no consistent association of spasticity of conjugate gaze with homonymous hemianopia, long-tract signs, or abnormal optokinetic response. As an isolated finding, spasticity of conjugate gaze should bear no diagnostic weight.

EYELIDS

Careful observations of the resting position of the eyelids, rate and extent of blinking, synkinetic movement with the eyes and facial muscles, and spontaneous movement abnormalities all provide useful information for neuro-ophthalmologic diagnosis. "Lid watching" is a lost art, and errors of omission in the physical examination have cost more than one dysthyroid patient the price of inappropriate diagnostic procedures.

Neuroanatomy and Physiology

The neural control of eyelid function is well reviewed by Schmidtke and Buttner-Ennever.[14] The eyelid is elevated and its resting position is maintained primarily by the levator palpebrae superioris. This muscle is innervated by the superior division of the oculomotor nerve, with motoneurons that originate in a midline dorsocaudal nucleus of the oculomotor nuclear complex in the midbrain. Because of its dorsal position, the levator nucleus may be spared or preferentially involved exclusive of other oculomotor nerve functions. Damage to the levator nucleus results in *bilateral* ptosis.

Pre-motor neurons that influence lid movements are located in the brain stem reticular formation and receive input from multiple suprasegmental sources that execute bilateral lid widening (via oculomotor nerve branches to the levator palpebrae superioris) or aperture narrowing (orbicularis oculi). There is a direct relationship of tonic activity of the levators and level of alertness; the lids widen with attentiveness and arousal, they lower involuntarily with increasing fatigue, and eventually, it is impossible to keep them from closing. During sleep, levator activity ceases completely.

Blink reflexes occur in response to touch or other corneal stimulation and to sudden bright illumination (perhaps via a direct pre-tectal–facial projection that bypasses the occipital cortex), or they are induced by sound or general startle reflex.[15] During a simple blink, the levator palpebrae is abruptly inhibited and the palpebral portion of the orbicularis oculi contracts; thus, there is a coordinated synkinesis involving the oculomotor nerve (levator) and facial nerve (orbicularis) during both spontaneous and voluntary blinking.

Motor cortex, extrapyramidal system, and rostral midbrain structures are involved with levator palpebrae control, and coordination with vertical gaze is integrated by the rostral interstitial nucleus of the medial longitudinal fasciculus. For example, on downward gaze, the levators are progressively inhibited, but the orbicularis oculi does not contract.

The ventral periaqueductal gray is assumed to control generation of tonic levator neuronal activity, and caudal supraocular neurons mediate converging inhibitory inputs to the levator motor neurons. Cerebral localization for voluntary lid widening, or reflex elevation in coordination with eye and head movements, is not precisely understood. Experimental cortical lesions of the frontal motor area, angular gyrus, and temporal lobe can all produce ptosis, and electrode stimulation of the frontal, temporal, and occipital cortices results in lid opening. Unilateral or bilateral ptosis, *cerebral ptosis,* may occur from unilateral temporal and temporo-parietal or bilateral frontal lobe disease.[16,17] Lesions in frontal, temporal, and occipital areas have been associated with ptosis or dysfunction of voluntary lid control.[14] Extrapyramidal system disorders such as parkinsonism and progressive supranuclear palsy are associated with blepharospasm and supranuclear apraxias of lid opening; these are discussed in Chapter 8.

In the upper lid, Müller's muscle consists of a thin sheet of smooth muscle fibers that connects the upper tarsus to the undersurface of the levator. The superior tarsal muscle is innervated by the cervical sympathetics, damage to which results in ptosis as part of Horner's syndrome. A small inferior tarsal muscle also regulates the height of the lower lid. Sympathetic tone appears to modulate static lid position.

The two upper lids are "yoked," and their synkinetic movements with the eyes in vertical gaze positions are synchronous and symmetric,[18] but with horizontal gaze one eye may widen more than the other.[19] That Hering's law of equivalent innervation may be applicable to the two levators, even in the primary gaze position, is debatable.[20] In some patients with partial unilateral ptosis, such as in myasthenia, retraction of the contralateral upper lid may be attributable to increased innervation in an attempt to widen the abnormally narrowed palpebral fissure (see Fig. 3–10). If the ptotic side is occluded, the opposite "retracted" lid assumes a normal position.

Compensatory unilateral lid retraction is uncommon, and factors other than Hering's law may play an important role. For example, if the eye with ptosis is also preferred for visual fixation, as opposed to fixation preference for the non-ptotic eye, compensatory retraction is more likely.[21] Other examples of compensatory lid retraction include deficits of supraduction of a downward deviated eye, such as in Graves' disease, that disproportionately raise the contralateral lid.[22]

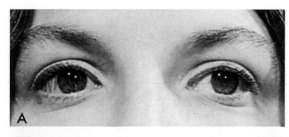

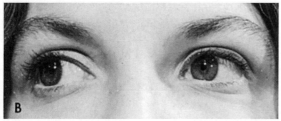

Fig. 3–8. Normal lid positions. **A.** With the eyes in primary position, palpebral fissures are equal. Note the position of the lid margins with respect to the corneas. **B.** In conjugate lateral gaze, the lid fissure of the abducting eye may widen.

Position and Movements

In neuro-ophthalmologic context, the eyelid examination should include the following observations:

1. Position at rest with eyes straight ahead: the palpebral fissures should be equal (from lower to upper lid margin measures 9 mm to 12 mm); the prevalence of physiologic fissure asymmetry (1 mm or more) is reckoned at about 6%;[19] the upper lids drape over the corneal limbus covering the superior 1 mm to 2 mm of cornea; the lower lid edge touches at or just above the lower corneal limbus (Fig. 3–8). (Lid position obviously varies with individual physiognomy, laxity of facial tissues, and the position of the globe with respect to the orbital rim).

2. The shape of the lid may be altered by local inflammations of the lid margins or conjunctiva, or after trauma, including surgical manipulations; on occasion, the configuration of the lid margin takes on special significance, such as the S-shaped lid in neurofibromatosis (Fig. 3–9)

3. Synkinetic coordination with eye movements; in conjugate lateral gaze (see Fig. 3–8), Lam et al[19] found that palpebral fissure asymmetry increased by a tendency of the adducting eye to widen slightly; levator tone increases on upward gaze and diminishes on downward gaze, such that the lids smoothly follow vertical ocular versions; when testing for lid lag, the patient should be made to follow a moving target from above downward; any consistent lag, especially if unilateral, is *prima facie* evidence of Graves' ophthalmopathy.

Lid Retraction

Abnormal elevation of the upper lid is seen in a variety of conditions, but it is most commonly associated

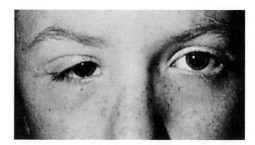

Fig. 3–9. S-shaped configuration of the right upper lid margin in neurofibromatosis, usually resulting from diffuse neurofibroma of the lid.

with Graves' disease (Fig. 3–11). In this disorder, the exact mechanism of lid retraction is obscure, but it is probably not due simply to sympathetic overaction. In fact, if the upper lid margin or lashes are gently grasped, there is mechanical resistance to drawing the lid downward.

Lid retraction is well documented in lesions involving the posterior third ventricle or rostral midbrian (Collier's sign of the posterior commissure). Fissure widening is increased on attempted upward gaze, which is also usually defective (Parinaud's syndrome), but lid position on downward gaze typically is normal (Fig. 3–12). Galetta et al[23] documented eyelid retraction and lid lag, with minimal impairment in vertical gaze, in patients with rostral midbrain lesions. Hydrocephalus in infancy is also thought to produce lid retraction via involvement of the periaqueductal area of the rostral midbrain.

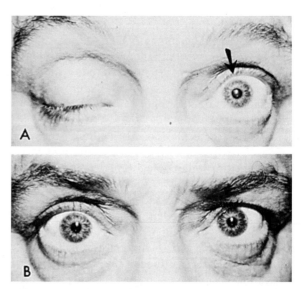

Fig. 3–10. Demonstration of the law of equivalent innervation (Hering's law) applicable to lid levators. **A.** A patient with myasthenia attempts to overcome right ptosis. Increased levator innervation results in contralateral lid retraction (*arrow*). Note also elevated brows resulting from frontalis effort. **B.** After administration of edrophonium chloride (Tensilon), right ptosis is relieved and the left fissure narrows. Note frontalis relaxation with descent of the brows.

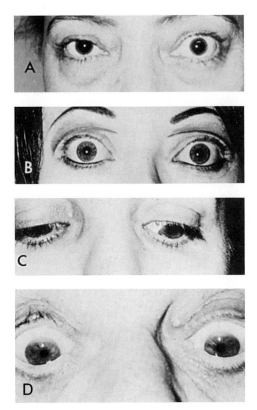

Fig. 3–11. Spectrum of lid retraction in dysthyroidism. **A.** Mild unilateral lid retraction. **B.** Moderate bilateral "stare." **C.** Modest unilateral lid lag on downward gaze. **D.** Marked lid retraction in downward gaze.

Whereas topical instillation of sympathomimetic drugs is a well-recognized cause of lid retraction, only in rare instance do systemically administered agents result in lid position changes. Prolonged high doses of corticosteroids apparently cause lid retraction (in patients with normal thyroid function studies) in some cases[24] (Fig. 3–13). Lid retraction has also been documented in cirrhotic patients without dysthyroidism.[25]

Lid retraction may be seen with congenital anomalous synkineses, of which the Marcus Gunn jaw-winking phenomenon (Fig. 3–14A) is most widely known (see Chapter 13). Other congenital anomalous patterns are occasionally seen, such as lid retraction on downward gaze (Fig. 3–14B,C). The relationship of such anomalous synkineses with aberrant regeneration (misdirection) in the third cranial nerve is tenuous, because preceding oculomotor palsies have not been documented, and embryopathic miswiring is a more likely mechanism.

Bartley[26] has suggested that lid retraction may be roughly classified as "neurogenic, myogenic and mechanistic"; this author also includes an extensive catalog of miscellaneous disorders purported to be associated with eyelid retraction.

Ptosis

The causes of lid ptosis are numerous, as outlined below, and the most common are discussed in sections

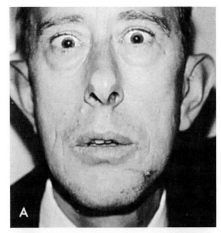

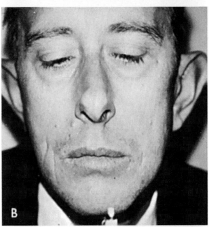

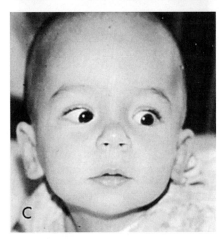

Fig. 3–12. Pathologic lid retraction (Collier's sign) in rostral mesencephalic disorders. **A.** A patient with pinealoma. Note the position of the lids in forward gaze. The pupils are mid-dilated and light fixed. **B.** On downward gaze, the lids follow the eyes smoothly without retraction. **C.** A "setting sun" sign with lid retraction associated with infantile hydrocephalus.

dealing with the primary disorder (*e.g.,* myasthenia, Horner's syndrome, oculomotor nerve palsies):

I. Congenital ptosis
    A. Isolated
    B. With double-elevator palsy

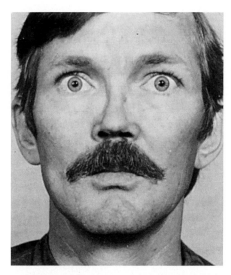

Fig. 3–13. Lid retraction in a patient taking long-term high doses of steroids for renal disease. All thyroid function studies are repeatedly normal.

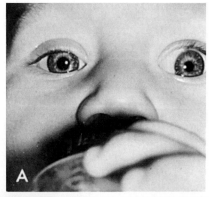
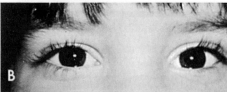
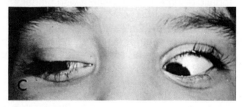

Fig. 3–14. Congenital lid retraction. **A.** Overaction of the levator (*left*) during the non-ptotic phase of Marcus Gunn jaw-winking. **B.** Normal lid position in the forward eye position. **C.** Overaction of levator in downward gaze. (There is no history of birth trauma or other signs of third nerve misdirection.)

C. Anomalous synkineses (including Gunn jaw-winking)
D. Lid or orbital tumor (hemangioma, dermoid)
E. Neurofibromatosis (neurofibroma, neurilemmoma)
F. Blepharophimosis syndromes
G. First branchial arch syndromes (*e.g.,* Hallermann-Streiff, Treacher Collins)
H. Transient neonatal myasthenia (myasthenic mother)
II. Myopathic ptosis
A. Myasthenia
B. Myotonic dystrophy
C. Progressive external ophthalmoplegia ("ocular myopathy")
D. Familial variants of external ophthalmoplegias
E. Graves' disease (rare; rule out myasthenia)
III. Sympathetic oculoparesis (Horner's syndrome)
IV. Oculomotor nerve palsies
A. Peripheral
B. Central
V. Miscellaneous
A. Age-related levator dehiscence
B. Allergic blepharochalasis; other recurrent lid edema
C. Manipulation of levator complex: cataract, retina, corneal surgery
D. Contact lenses, prolonged and long-term usage
E. Orbito-facial trauma
F. Lid and conjunctival infections/inflammations
G. Obtundation, lethargy, drowsiness, intoxication
H. Cortical (cerebral) "ptosis"
I. Blepharospasm, hemifacial spasm, spastic contracture, facial nerve misdirection
J. Apraxia of lid opening
K. Hysteria or malingering

In the neonate, unilateral partial ptosis is only rarely due to birth trauma and is not likely to resolve on its own. Although occult tumors of the lid or orbit may be the hidden cause, nonetheless observation is usually the most prudent initial course in the neonate. Neurofibromatosis, for example, may present as ptosis without exophthalmos (see Fig. 3–9). Certainly before performing lid surgery in a young child, neuroimaging of the orbit and Tensilon testing should be accomplished. At any age, unexplained ptosis may eventually require a Tensilon test (Fig. 3–15A,B), but there are other observations and diagnostic maneuvers to uncover myasthenia. For example, levator fatigue may be demonstrated by observing slow lid curtaining during sustained upward gaze (usually, the lids become fatigued well before 1 minute). Cogan[27] has described a useful "twitch" sign, which is elicited by having the patient rapidly redirect gaze from the downward to the primary position. The lid is seen initially to overshoot (twitch) upward and then slowly to resettle to the customary

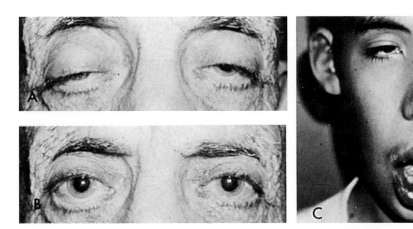

Fig. 3–15. Myopathic ptosis. **A** and **B.** An elderly patient with "afternoon ptosis" and dramatic response to edrophonium chloride (Tensilon). **C.** A young boy with ptosis and the "hatchet face" of myotonic dystrophy.

ptotic position. Occasionally, fine fluttering vibrations of the lash margins are observed in myasthenic lids. After brief eye closure, the relaxed myasthenic lid may momentarily recover before again drooping. A form of "pseudomyasthenia," composed of fatigable ptosis with lid twitch that mimics myasthenia, even with improvement with acetylcholinesterase inhibitors, has been described in patients with skull base tumors and intrinsic brain stem tumors.[28]

Ptosis may be familial, or it may occur as a symmetric, slowly progressive disorder of senescence. Before contemplating surgical repair of ptotic lids, it is critical to establish the state of upward deviation of the globes. With defective upward gaze, as occurs in progressive external ophthalmoplegia (see Chapter 12, Figs. 12–31 and 12–32), serious corneal complications due to exposure may follow ptosis surgery.

In cases of newly acquired unilateral ptosis, the size and reactivity of the ipsilateral pupil usually establish whether sympathetic or oculomotor paresis is present. Abrupt or progressive ptosis occurring without pain or pupillary abnormality, or alternating sides, is likely to be myasthenic in origin. The levator muscle–aponeurosis complex seems especially sensitive to mechanical processes that may take the form of trauma, including manipulation during common ophthalmic surgical procedures (for cataract, retinal detachment, or any procedure that includes the placement of a lid speculum or other disturbance of the superior rectus muscle, the latter being intimately attached to the levator). Traumatic (including the foregoing) weakening of the levator complex may follow even mild injury, and age alone takes its toll on the lids. Involutional, otherwise *idiopathic*, ptosis is related to the following: sagging and redundancy of lid and brow tissues; weakening and dehiscences of levator fascial attachments to the tarsus; medial dehiscence of Whitnall's ligament; focal levator atrophy (primary myopathy ?); and prolapse of retroseptal fat.[29]

Of special note in younger patients, prolonged wearing of hard contact lenses distinctly may cause ptosis, usually asymmetric, which may be due to levator disinsertion.[30] However, in my experience, the lid slowly recovers after several weeks of lens discontinuance, a finding that suggests a reversible mechanism such as reactive edema. Ptosis and *lagophthalmos* suggest infiltration of the lids by tumor such as breast carcinoma,[31] which may also be accompanied by *enophthalmos* (see Fig. 14–9A–C).

Confused with genuine ptosis is *apraxia of lid opening,* an inability volitionally to open the eyes that is not due to infranuclear paralysis or myopathy. The syndrome variably keeps company with extrapyramidal system disorders such as parkinsonism, progressive supranuclear palsy, and multiple system atrophy.[32] At times, this disabling condition may be associated with blepharospasm, although simple involuntary levator inhibition without hyperactive facial movement permits sudden release of apparently immobile lids; thus, the somewhat inaccurate term "apraxia" is applied. The precise nature of the central defect is unclear, and specific therapies are not yet clarified (see Chapter 8).

Lid Nystagmus

Upper lid nystagmus is a pathologic condition when *not* part of synchronous vertical beating ocular nystagmus, that is, when the lid jerking does not simply reflect movement secondary to eye displacement. It is a rare observation, usually evoked by convergence (Pick's sign) or by horizontal conjugate gaze. It has been reported in patients with multiple sclerosis, cerebellar diseases, cranial polyneuropathy (Miller Fisher syndrome), and midbrain astrocytoma.[33] Lid nystagmus is usually accompanied by other neuro-ophthalmologic findings such as ptosis, ophthalmoparesis, gaze-evoked nystagmus, and dorsal midbrain or cerebellar signs.

OCULAR SENSATION AND PAIN

Pain in and about the eye is a compelling symptom that the patient cannot ignore and the physician cannot dismiss. Most eye pain is indeed due to ocular disease, most of which is diagnosed by ophthalmologic evaluation. Diminished sensation, on the other hand, is a relatively rare finding and an even less frequent complaint. However, the symptoms of pain or numbness in the trigeminal distribution deserve careful consideration as a neuro-ophthalmologic signal.

Functional Anatomy

The sensory innervation of the globe is mediated through the ophthalmic division (V_1) of the fifth cranial nerve (trigeminal) (Fig. 3–16). The anterior ocular segment, including the cornea, iris, trabecular meshwork, and ciliary body, transmits pain, temperature, and touch sensations via the ciliary nerves, which join the nasociliary nerve directly (long ciliary nerve) or by traversing the ciliary ganglion (short ciliary nerves). Nerve endings contain neuropeptide vesicles, and antidromic stimula-

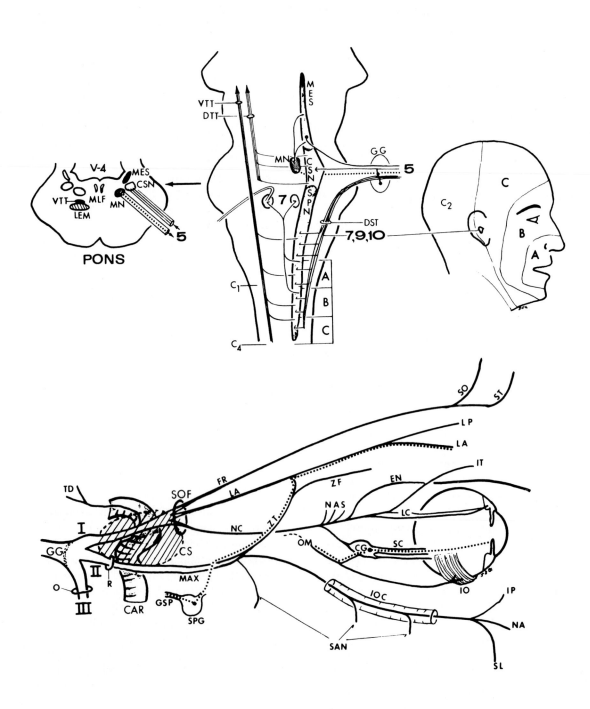

tion of the trigeminal nerve causes release of neuropeptide into the aqueous that provokes uveal vasodilation and an inflammatory response;[34] that is, the sensory trigeminal exerts an "ocular injury response" by modulating parasympathetic neurons in the pterygopalatine ganglion.[35] The role of minute sympathetic innervation to the cornea is obscure. Other branches of the nasociliary nerve supply sensation to the upper lid skin and conjunctiva, caruncle, medial canthus, lacrimal sac, bridge of the nose, nasal mucosa, and tip of the nose.

The upper lid and its conjunctiva, as well as the brow, forehead, and scalp, are supplied by the supratrochlear and supraorbital branches of the frontal nerve. The temporal aspect of the upper lid and outer canthus is supplied by the lateral palpebral branch of the lacrimal nerve, and the lower lid is in the sensory distribution of the infraorbital nerve of the maxillary division (V_2) of the trigeminal nerve (Fig. 3–17).

The non-ocular distribution of the ophthalmic division is of major clinical importance because disturbances

Fig. 3–16. Top. Trigeminal-sensory complex. Ocular and facial sensation is mediated by the trigeminal nuclear complex, which extends from the midbrain downward into the upper cervical segments (*C1* through *C4*). The rostral nucleus (*MES*encephalic) serves proprioception and deep sensation from the tendons and muscles of mastication. Axons of afferent cells also terminate in the motor nucleus (*MN*) of the trigeminal, which innervates the masticatory muscles (*dotted line*) via the mandibular division. The midportion of the trigeminal complex contains the chief sensory nucleus (*CSN*) located in the pons. This nucleus serves light touch from the skin and mucous membranes. Without a distinct transition, the nuclear complex continues caudally as the spinal nucleus (*SPN*), which receives pain and temperature afferents via the descending spinal tract (*DST*); cutaneous sensory components of *7, 9,* and *10* also join the spinal tract, conducting sensation from the ear and external auditory meatus. Concentric areas of the face (*A, B,* and *C*) are projected on corresponding portions of the caudal aspect of the spinal nucleus. The corneal reflex is mediated via internuclear fibers to the facial nuclei. The fibers ascend to the thalamus via the ventral (*VTT*) and dorsal trigeminothalamic (*DTT*) tracts; an ipsilateral ascending DTT tract is not shown. The gasserian ganglion (*GG*) contains cell bodies of neurons mediating touch, pain, and temperature from three trigeminal divisions; cell bodies for proprioception and deep pain are contained in the MES. Cross-section of the pons at the level of the trigeminal roots includes the fourth ventricle (*V-4*), the median longitudinal fascicule (*MLF*), and the medial lemniscus (*LEM*). **Bottom.** Peripheral trigeminal distribution. Three major divisions arise from the gasserian ganglion (*GG*). The ophthalmic (*I*) enters the cavernous sinus (*shaded area CS*) lateral to the internal carotid artery (*CAR*), passes into the orbit via the superior orbital fissure (*SOF*), and divides into the frontal (*FR*), lacrimal (*LA*), and nasociliary (*NC*) branches. The supraorbital (*SO*) nerve supplies the medial upper lid and the conjunctiva, forehead, scalp, and frontal sinuses; the supratrochlear nerve (*ST*) supplies the conjunctiva, medial upper lid, forehead, and side of the nose. The lacrimal nerve (*LA*) serves the conjunctiva and skin in the area of the lacrimal gland (lateral palpebral branch, *LP*) and carries post-ganglionic parasympathetic fibers (*dotted line*) for reflex lacrimation. Pre-ganglionic fibers traverse the vidian canal with the greater superficial petrosal nerve (*GSP*) and enter the sphenopalatine ganglion (*SPG*), thence to the maxillary nerve, which transmits post-ganglionic fibers to the lacrimal nerve via an anastomosis, the zygomaticotemporal nerve (*ZT*). The nasociliary (*NC*) branch of the ophthalmic nerve supplies sensation to the globe. A series of nasal nerves (*NAS*) serves the mucosa of nasal septum, middle and inferior turbinates, and lateral nasal wall. An external nasal (*EN*) branch innervates skin of nose tip. The infratrochlear (*IT*) branch supplies the canaliculi, caruncle, lacrimal sac, conjunctiva, and skin of the medial canthus. Two long ciliary (*LC*) nerves carry sensory fibers from the ciliary body, iris, and cornea, and sympathetic innervation to the pupil dilator. Multiple short ciliary (*SC*) nerves transmit sensory fibers from the globe that pass through the ciliary ganglion (*CG*) and join the nasociliary nerve via its sensory root; short ciliaries also carry post-ganglionic parasympathetic fibers (*dotted line*) from the ciliary ganglion to the pupil constrictor and ciliary muscle. These fibers reach the ciliary ganglion via the inferior division of the oculomotor nerve (*OM*) destined to innervate the inferior oblique (*IO*) muscle. The maxillary division (*MAX, II*) does not usually traverse the cavernous sinus, but exits the skull through the foramen rotundum (*R*) into a variable "trigeminal" sinus, thence into the pterygopalatine fossa in relation to the sphenopalatine ganglion, thence into the inferior orbital fissure, continuing along the orbital floor into the infraorbital canal (*IOC*). The posterior, middle, and anterior superior alveolar nerves (*SAN*) supply the upper teeth, maxillary sinus, nasopharynx, tonsils, soft palate, and roof of the mouth. The infraorbital nerve exits onto face through infraorbital foramen, supplying the lower lid via the inferior palpebral (*IP*), side of the nose via the nasal (*NA*), and upper lid via the superior labial (*SL*) nerves. A zygomaticofacial (ZF) innervates side of cheek. The mandibular (*III*) is the only mixed motor-sensory division of the trigeminal. Both roots pass through the foramen ovale (*O*) into the infratemporal fossa; the motor branches supply the pterygoid, masseter, and temporalis muscles; the sensory branches supply the mucosa and skin of the mandible and lower lip, tongue sensation, external ear, and tympanum. A tentorial-dural branch (*TD*) arises from the intracavernous portion of the opthalmic, to supply sensation to the dura of the cavernous sinus, anterior fossa, sphenoid wing, petrous ridge, trigeminal cave (Meckel's), tentorium cerebelli, posterior aspect of falx cerebri, and dural venous sinuses. Sensation from cerebral veins and arteries, as well as nerves III, IV, and VI, may be mediated by these dural nerves.

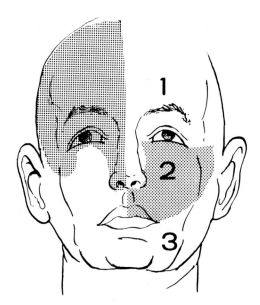

Fig. 3–17. Cutaneous sensory distribution of the trigeminal nerve: *1*, ophthalmic; *2*, maxillary; *3*, mandibular divisions.

of intracranial structures, including dura, dural venous sinuses, cerebral arteries and veins, all typically refer pain to the eye, orbit, or brow. Referral of pain from dural stimulation was reviewed by Wirth and van Buren,[36] who found that pain patterns secondary to intracranial disease were not sufficiently specific to provide precise clinical localization.

Peripheral Trigeminal Afferents

The trigeminal nerve conveys pain and mechanoreceptor afferents from the intracranial dura, except the infratentorial dura of the posterior fossa, from which afferents are carried by the vagus. There are vagal somatosensory afferent fibers that run in the spinal tract of the trigeminal and synapse with cells in the spinal nucleus; although the vagus is the *peripheral* nerve, the central connections are essentially trigeminal. Cell bodies for the peripheral trigeminal fibers and for the primary nociceptive and other afferents are situated in the gasserian ganglion in Meckel's cave at the base of the sphenoid bone (see Chapter 12, Figs. 12–5 and 12–20). Cells here vary in size; the smaller (C-nociceptors) synapse in the caudal end of the spinal nucleus, which is consonant with clinical evidence that pain results mainly from lesions in the caudalmost part of the spinal nucleus and tract. In addition, there is layering of the inputs in the spinal tract: the ophthalmic fibers that terminate caudally are ventral; the maxillary division fibers end in a more dorsal and rostral layer; and the mandibular division fibers insert above the maxillary layer. Dorsal to three trigeminal layers in the spinal nucleus are path-

ways served peripherally by cranial nerves IX, X, and the facial intermedius (VIIi).

Trigeminal Sensory Nuclei

The spinal nucleus is an area of sensory integration, as evidenced by the presence of ascending spinal cord afferents[37] and descending fibers primarily from contralateral somatosensory cortex, but also with inputs from the red nucleus, the reticular formation, and of course the primary trigeminal afferents. The spinal tract and nucleus descend to the level of C2 to C4 and merge with the dorsal horn of the spinal gray matter. In fact, the histologic organization of the trigeminal spinal tract *pars caudalis* is strikingly similar to that of the dorsal horn. There are three layers: an outer marginal zone occupied by large Waldeyer-type cells; a gelatinous layer; and a deeper *subnucleus magnocellularis.* In the more rostral parts of the spinal nucleus (the *interpolaris* and the *rostralis subnuclei*), the histologic organization differs from the caudalis portion. This suggests functional specialization even within the spinal tract, in which the caudalis part is homologous to the dorsal horn pain-carrying system, and the oralis subnucleus is homologous with the nuclei of the dorsal columns, carrying non-nociceptive touch and mechanoreceptor sensation.

Trigeminal Ascending Pathways

Afferents from the main sensory nucleus travel in the contralateral medial-dorsal portion of the *medial lemniscus (trigeminal lemniscus)* to the ventral posteromedian nucleus of the thalamus. A smaller uncrossed output from the dorsal part of the main sensory nucleus ascends to the dorsomedial part of the ipsilateral ventral postero-median nucleus. Outflow from the pars caudalis of the spinal nucleus probably runs or originates in the reticular formation. Horseradish peroxidase injections into the thalamus have revealed labeled cells in the reticular formation adjacent to the pars caudalis, as well as labeled units in the marginal zone of the spinal nucleus itself.[38] This situation suggests a certain similarity with the dorsal horn output, some of which goes directly to the thalamus in the spinothalamic tract, and some goes indirectly via spinoreticular and spinomesencephalic tracts. The caudal spinal trigeminal nucleus input to the thalamus is scanty, according to many of the anatomic studies. Perhaps available methods underestimate these afferents, there being possibly a greater number of polysynaptic neural chains rather than direct monosynaptic inputs from the caudal spinal nucleus. Moreover, physiologic studies indicate that units in the main sensory nucleus, in addition to caudalis spinal nucleus units, respond to tooth-pulp stimulation. Thus, there appears to be duality of nociceptive input, with ascending and descending collaterals from fibers entering via the trigeminal sensory root innervating both the main sensory and the spinal nuclei.

Clinical Evaluation of Trigeminal Function

Sensory testing of the globe and face may be accomplished rapidly and without need for special equipment. Corneal sensation obviously cannot be adequately evaluated after instillation of topical anesthetics for intraocular tension measurements. In clinical practice, pain sensation is routinely assessed rather than other sensory modalities. In the otherwise intact patient, both subjective and objective responses may be evaluated. In the lethargic or obtunded patient, blink reflex and head withdrawal are gross objective signs of corneal sensitivity.

In office practice, an applicator with a cotton tip drawn to a point (Fig. 3–18) may be lightly touched to, or drawn across, the inferior aspect of the cornea. In ocular inflammatory disease, the same cotton probably should not be used in both eyes (*e.g.,* with herpes simplex keratitis). The applicator cotton wisp may also be used to test light touch sensation of the brow and face, looking for differences from one side of the midline to the other. Such cutaneous sensory testing is best accomplished with the patient's eyes closed, the response indicating which side of the face has been touched. Subjective and objective responses to eye drop instillation are useful indications of relative corneal sensation.

The motor function of the mandibular division is conveniently tested by palpating masseter mass (over the rami of the madibles) and temporalis muscle bulk during the command, "Grit your teeth." Pterygoid function

may be assessed by having the patient attempt to deviate the jaw laterally against the palm of the examiner's hand (weakness toward the right indicates palsy of left pterygoid group).

Abnormal Corneal Reflexes

The causes of diminished sensation in the trigeminal distribution are outlined below:

I. Cornea
   A. Herpes simplex
   B. Ocular surgery
   C. Cerebellopontine angle tumors
   D. Dysautonomia
   E. Congenital
II. Ophthalmic division
   A. Neoplasm, orbital apex
   B. Neoplasm, superior orbital fissure
   C. Neoplasm, cavernous sinus
   D. Neoplasm, middle fossa
   E. Aneurysm, cavernous sinus
III. Maxillary division
   A. Orbit floor fracture
   B. Maxillary antrum carcinoma
   C. Perineural spread of skin carcinoma
   D. Neoplasm, foramen rotundum, sphenopterygoid fossa
IV. Mandibular division
   A. Nasopharyngeal tumor
   B. Middle fossa tumor
V. All divisions
   A. Nasopharyngeal carcinoma
   B. Cerebellopontine angle tumors
   C. Brain stem lesions (dissociated sensory loss)
   D. Intracavernous aneurysm
   E. Demyelinative
   F. Middle fossa or Meckel's cave tumor
   G. Benign sensory neuropathy
   H. Tentorial meningioma
   I. Toxins (*e.g.,* trichlorethylene)
   J. Trigeminal neurofibroma

In addition to hypesthesia, corneal sensory testing may uncover other abnormal reflexes. For example, the motor arc (facial nerve) of the corneal reflex may be absent or diminished. Both the afferent (pain) and efferent (blink) portions of the reflex may be diminished, as in patients with cerebellopontine angle tumors.

A corneo-mandibular reflex may be seen in patients with bilateral corticobulbar tract lesions, either hemispheral or at the midbrain level, or in parkinsonism. When the cornea is stimulated, the jaw momentarily deviates to the opposite side, concurrent with eye closure. As pointed out by Paulson and Bird,[39] the corneo-mandibular reflex is quite common in normal infants,

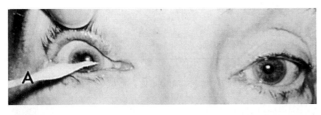
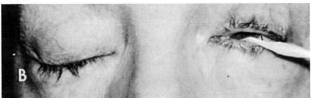

Fig. 3–18. Examination of corneal sensation. **A.** The patient has a right intracavernous aneurysm and an insensitive right cornea that "permits parking" of a cotton-tipped applicator. **B.** When the cotton wisp is gently placed on the left cornea, a blink occurs, and the patient subjectively indicates discomfort.

contrary to Wartenberg's opinion. Therefore, this infantile reflex may "return" in cerebral and extrapyramidal diseases of senescence.

Pain in and about the Eye

The causes of eye pain are numerous and consist, for the most part, of diseases of the globe and ocular adnexa. However, discomfort in the ocular segment or orbit may be a harbinger of neurologic disease ranging from innocent vascular cranial mononeuropathies (*e.g.,* diabetic ophthalmoplegia) to bleeding aneurysm, sinus inflammation, or atypical migraine (see Chapter 16). An outline of relatively common entities associated with ocular and facial pain is presented below. Painful ophthalmoplegia syndromes are discussed in Chapter 12.

I. Ocular
   A. Local lid, conjunctival, and anterior segment disease
   B. Ocular inflammation
   C. Dry eye and tear deficiency syndromes
   D. Chronic ocular hypoxia, carotid occlusive disease
   E. Angle-closure glaucoma
II. Ophthalmic division
   A. Migraine, cluster headaches
   B. Raeder's paratrigeminal neuralgia
   C. Painful ophthalmoplegia syndromes
   D. Herpes zoster
   E. Referred (dural) pain, including occipital infarction
   F. Tic douloureux (infrequent in V_1)
   G. Sinusitis
III. Maxillary division
   A. Tic douloureux
   B. Nasopharyngeal carcinoma
   C. Temporo-mandibular joint syndrome
   D. Dental disease
   E. Sinusitis
IV. Mandibular division
   A. Tic douloureux
   B. Dental disease
V. Miscellaneous
   A. Atypical facial neuralgias
   B. Pain with medullary lesions
   C. Cranial arteritis
   D. Trigeminal tumors

Many patients, especially middle-aged and elderly women, complain of vague aches, "stabs," and other discomfort in and about the eyes. Neither ocular nor neurologic disease is demonstrable, although the patient often anticipates that a grave cause will be uncovered. Often, nonspecific symptoms are considered due to "eyestrain," the need for new spectacle lenses, or exposure to lights (especially fluorescent) or to the elements.

Having examined the patient and determined that no substantial disease is present, the *quantity and quality of the tear film* must be suspect. Dry eye syndrome (keratoconjunctivitis sicca) consists of the following: foreign body sensation with "gritty" feeling, itching, burning, redness, and excessive tearing (epiphora); photophobia; reduced tear meniscus, abundant mucous threads, debris in the pre-corneal tear film, and hyperemic palpebral and conjunctival conjunctiva; rapid (less than 10 seconds) breakup of the fluorescein-stained tear film over the cornea and rose-bengal staining of the interpalpebral conjunctiva; Schirmer strip test typically showing minimal wetting.[40,41] In women especially, there is an age-related progressive loss of tear film constituents that ordinarily keep the eyes lubricated and comfortable, and dry mouth is also common.

Patients with secretory dysfunction of the lacrimal gland develop pathologic changes of the corneal epithelium, squamous metaplasia. Epithelial cells reflect inflammation, fail to mature, and no longer produce the mucus that normally coats and lubricates the ocular surfaces. Thus, some patients with "dry eye" experience both ocular irritation and, occasionally, visual disturbance that may be mistaken for occult neurologic disease.

Many patients with vague ocular discomfort and nonspecific findings are made comfortable by the following regimen: (1) eye and facial cosmetics are cut to the minimum; (2) hair "stiffeners" with shellac bases must be discontinued; (3) on arising, at midday, and before retiring, a basin of warm water with a few drops of baby shampoo is used with a washcloth to cleanse the brows, lids, and lashes thoroughly; and (4) as needed for comfort, but at least four times per day, a tear substitute is instilled.

Defective Tearing

In general, defective lacrimation is an uncommon problem in neuro-ophthalmology. This finding is usually encountered in the context of diminished corneal sensation subsequent to local corneal disease (including herpes zoster, keratitis), to neurosurgical lesions of the ophthalmic division (ganglion or sensory root), or to medullary infarction. Reflex tearing is diminished in the presence of a hypesthetic cornea, and severe complicated keratitis may develop (neuroparalytic keratitis). If facial nerve function is also defective such that some degree of corneal exposure occurs, the keratitis is usually even more severe.

Reflex tearing, that is, that evoked by trigeminal sensory stimulation, is mediated by pre-ganglionic parasympathetic fibers that arise near the facial nucleus in the pontine tegmentum. These fibers exit the brain stem and travel with the sensory root (nervus intermedius) of the facial nerve (see Chapter 8), traverse the geniculate ganglion, and enter the greater superficial petrosal nerve, which lies in the floor of the middle fossa in a position lateral to the trigeminal ganglion (gasserian). After joining the deep petrosal nerve to form the vidian nerve, the pre-synaptic fibers enter the sphenopalatine ganglion, where they synapse with post-ganglionic fibers. These latter fibers gain the lacrimal gland by joining the zygomatic branch of the maxillary division of the trigeminal (see Fig. 3–16).

The efferent limb of reflex tearing may be interrupted by lesions involving the facial nerve in the cerebellopontine angle or petrous bone, the greater superficial petrosal nerve in the floor of the middle fossa, or the sphenopalatine ganglion in the retro-antral space. The onset of facial pain or numbness associated with a sixth nerve palsy (medial aspect of middle fossa) and deficient tearing, or numbness in the maxillary division with diminished tearing, are syndromes typical of malignant nasopharyngeal tumor. Defective reflex tear secretion is assessed semiquantitatively by Schirmer filter paper technique, without application of topical anesthetics.

Paradoxical tearing may occur months following facial palsies, wherein the anticipation or taste of food provokes excessive tearing. This gustatory-lacrimal reflex ("crocodile tears") is caused by misdirection of regenerating salivary axons in the proximal portion of the facial nerve that then aggrandize the peripheral pathways to the lacrimal gland. On rare occasions, this autonomic dyskinesis is congenital and has been reported in Duane's retraction syndrome (see Chapter 8).

Neuralgia and Atypical Facial Pain

Most ocular pain is caused by actual pathologic changes observable in or on the globe, or with evidence of adnexal or orbital disease. Gritty or sandy sensations, made worse with blinking or eye movement, usually accompanied by copious tearing, surely point to foreign body of the cornea or hidden under the lid. Fluorescein staining of the cornea with slit-lamp examination is indicated. Most, but not all, "red eyes" are caused by local infections or inflammations. Iritis (anterior uveitis) is usually accompanied by photophobia and evidence of anterior chamber cells and protein flare. The "dry eye" and its symptoms, and the vagaries of "eyestrain" (asthenopia), are considered above. With regard to the question of "eyestrain" and ocular neuroses, in 1930, Derby[42] quipped: "I wish we could banish the term eyestrain from our vocabulary. If the general public could learn that the eyes are seldom strained, this would be a much happier world to live in. . . . Eyestrain is a terrible and serious bugbear to the public; would that the word had never been coined." At any rate, these conditions are all strictly the business of the ophthalmologist.

The subject of painful ophthalmoplegia is covered at length in Chapter 12, and orbitopathies are discussed

TABLE 3–1. Pain In and About the Eye

Ocular
 Cornea and conjunctival inflammations, foreign body, "dry eye"
 Blepharitis, chalazion, scleritis, episcleritis
 Anterior uveitis, angle-closure glaucoma, chronic ocular ischemia
 Accommodative spasm, convergence insufficient; ? refractive errors
 Graves' disease, inflammatory pseudotumor, other congestive orbitopathies
Neuralgias
 Herpes zoster ophthalmicus
 Trigeminal neuralgia
 Infiltrative (perineural) neuralgias
Atypical facial pain
 Temporo-mandibular joint syndrome
 Dental malocclusion
 Cluster headaches
 Sinus disease
 Giant cell (cranial) arteritis
 Carotid dissection
 Occult perineural infiltration

in Chapter 14. Table 3–1 is a brief outline emphasizing neuralgias and atypical facial pain syndromes, which are not to be confused with standard headache syndromes or the variants of migraine.

Herpes zoster (from the Greek *herpein*, to spread, and *zoster*, girdle or zone) ophthalmicus is a common cause of first trigeminal division acute pain and more-or-less simultaneous or slightly delayed cutaneous vesiculation (Fig. 3–19), followed by pustule formation. The

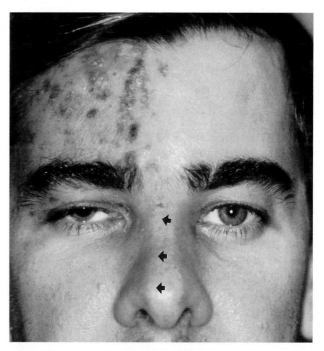

Fig. 3–19. Herpes zoster ophthalmicus involving the first (ophthalmic) division of right trigeminal nerve distribution. Note ptosis and lid edema; the pupil is dilated to relieve iritis pain. Note involvement of the nose (*arrows*).

infection occurs in otherwise healthy persons, but with increasing frequency in immunocompromised patients, including those with malignancies and especially in acquired immunodeficiency syndrome.[43] After primary varicella infection (chickenpox), the virus lies dormant in the sensory trigeminal ganglion, until the virus is reactivated as zoster. An inflamed eye with dendritiform keratopathy and iritis is frequent, but it is the disabling post-herpetic neuralgia that constitutes the major challenge in pain control. The risk of post-herpetic neuralgia increases with age.

Corticosteroids by systemic administration and antiviral agents such as oral or intravenous acyclovir or famciclovir are reported to ameliorate acute pain significantly and arguably to reduce the likelihood of neuralgia.[44] Zoster of the geniculate ganglion, the Ramsay Hunt syndrome, results in ear and facial vesiculation, pain, and facial palsy (see Fig. 8–10), as discussed in Chapter 8. Abducens, trochlear, and oculomotor nerve palsies are reported, as well as Horner's syndrome and optic neuritis.[45]

Trigeminal neuralgia is characterized by episodic, recurring electric shock–like or lancinating (knife-like) pain of severe magnitude, often triggered by stimulation of facial cutaneous areas or mucous membranes of the oral cavity. Usually of idiopathic origin, trigeminal neuralgia also occurs in patients with tumors or vascular compression at the trigeminal root exit zone,[46] and infrequently in patients with multiple sclerosis.[47] Trigeminal *neuropathy* implies prominent sensory loss, in which case an infiltrative, inflammatory, or compressive cause must be explored.[48]

Cutaneous carcinomas of the face, and some nasopharyngeal carcinomas, may present with facial dysesthesias ("ants crawling," formication), pain, or numbness, at times associated with facial nerve palsies or unilateral ophthalmoplegia. Centripetal perineural spread may eventually carry the disease to the cavernous sinus. Magnetic resonance imaging can disclose involved peripheral trigeminal nerve branches, for example, the infraorbital nerve, that may be biopsied.[49] A past history of treatment for facial carcinoma, especially squamous cell, is highly suggestive of this diagnosis.

THE COMATOSE PATIENT

Although the diagnosis and treatment of coma are the purview primarily of the neurologist and neurosurgeon, the ophthalmologist may at times be of great help in the analysis of eye-movement patterns, state of the pupils, and condition of the fundus. Indeed, the neurologist or neurosurgeon also must be conversant with the neuro-ophthalmologic assessment of the patient who cannot respond. Local disorders of the globe and the ocular adnexa must first be excluded. These possibilities include the following: pre-existing pupillary abnormalities such as surgical aphakia (we have seen arteriography performed on a comatose patient because of a "dilated pupil," which actually was unilateral aphakia with a sector iridectomy); miosis due to glaucoma medication; and anterior segment inflammation with iris adhesions. In patients with trauma, orbital fractures may limit eye movement, and mydriasis may be due to direct blunt injury to the globe and may not signify oculomotor palsy.

The "swinging flashlight test" may be used to evaluate the afferent and motor pathways of the anterior visual system. It should be re-emphasized that anisocoria cannot be due to a strictly afferent defect (*e.g.*, optic nerve contusion) (see Chapter 15). Eyelid blink to sudden bright illumination may be mediated through subcortical reflexes[50] and may not be taken to indicate intact cerebral pathways.

In general, in patients with metabolic coma or drug overdose, the pupils are small but reactive, in keeping with depression of the reticular activating system and removal of its inhibition of the pre-tectal center for pupillary constriction. Such miotic pupils ("pontine miosis") may dilate momentarily with pain or other psychosensory stimuli. In the terminal (anoxic) stage of metabolic encephalopathies, pupillary dilation occurs and is considered a grave prognostic sign. Paulson and Kapp[51] suggested that such pupillary widening in cerebral ischemia is due to massive sympathetic discharge.

A dilated and fixed pupil may herald progressive third nerve palsy due to temporal lobe herniation (Hutchinson's pupil) occurring with hemispheral mass lesions (*e.g.*, subdural hematoma). Injury of the third nerve sustained at the time of head trauma is usually complete and nonprogressive, as is oculomotor palsy due to bleeding intracranial aneurysm, although instances of isolated pupillary paresis are reported (see Chapter 12).

Examination of ocular motility in the comatose patient requires special maneuvers. It is first necessary to note spontaneous eye movement, more specifically, the range of movement of each eye, the degree of coordinated movement of the two eyes, and any intermittent or continuous pattern of eye movement. Various degrees of non-conjugate eye movements are to be expected in patients in a coma. In cases of drug intoxication or simple concussion, surprisingly incoordinate and erratic slow wandering of the eyes may be observed. These movements themselves neither signify major brain stem damage nor portend a lasting or disastrous neurologic deficit. Note should be made of persistent tonic deviation or lack of spontaneous movement in a particular direction. Further details of specific eye movements in coma (*e.g.*, ocular bobbing) are discussed in Chapter 11.

In the comatose, obtunded, or lethargic patient, voluntary or visually evoked eye movements cannot be

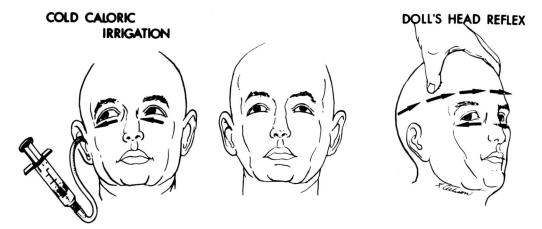

COLD CALORIC
IRRIGATION

DOLL'S HEAD REFLEX

Fig. 3–20. Examination of ocular motor function in a comatose patient.

evaluated. Other than spontaneous movements, the ocular motor system may be analyzed by reflex ocular deviations: rotational, oculocephalic, and caloric stimulation.Rotational testing is of no practical value in the comatose patient (other than perhaps an infant). The oculocephalic (doll's head, Roth-Bielschowsky deviation) reflex is dependent on stimulation of the vestibular system by rapid passive head turning, with an anticipated contraversive conjugate eye movement. For example, if the examiner suddenly rotates the head of a comatose patient toward the left (Fig. 3–20), the eyes will move contraversively to the right, if pontine gaze mechanisms are intact. These oculocephalic versions may be of relatively short duration, but they provide a rapid approximation of brain stem function. Vertical movements may similarly be tested by rapid extension and flexion of the head.

In patients with cerebral and brain stem hemorrhages or increased intracranial pressure, one may argue against the advisability of maneuvers entailing rapid displacement of the head, and certainly such abrupt rotations are contraindicated in cervical injuries. By contrast, as Rodriguez-Barrios[52] pointed out, caloric stimulation of the labyrinth is a harmless, simple procedure that may be repeated at will. Caloric irrigation of the ear canal cannot be carried out on the side of an otorrhagia from basal skull fracture, and this complication should first be excluded by otologic examination.

The technique of caloric testing may be simplified for bedside diagnosis by using available sources, either cool tap water or ice water. The external canal and tympanum should first be inspected, and wax or other debris

should be removed. With the patient's head on a pillow, that is, at an angle of 30° with the horizontal (for maximum stimulation of the horizontal semicircular canals), 10 ml to 20 ml of cold water is flushed into the ear canal using a small rubber tube fitted onto a syringe (see Fig. 3–20; Fig. 3–21B). One of several responses may be observed: (1) a slow tonic ocular deviation toward the side of cold irrigation (a bilateral positive response indicates integrity of pontine oculogyric mechanisms); (2) nystagmus, with the jerk phase directed *away from* the side of cold irrigation (usually the eyes drift toward the side of irrigation, but the nystagmus beats toward the *opposite* side); (3) no deviation elicited (total abolition of responses to caloric labyrinthine stimulation usually corresponds to an extensive pontine lesion); (4) vertical responses preserved in the absence of horizontal movement, indicating relative sparing of the midbrain (upward deviation is tested by *bilateral irrigation with warm water,* and downward tonic deviation attempted by *bilateral cold water* instillation); and (5) an ocular motor nerve palsy (III or VI) further elucidated by observing one eye responding while the other does not, an internuclear ophthalmoplegia may be uncovered.

In barbiturate intoxication with coma, all oculocephalic and vestibulo-ocular reflexes may be temporarily lost (see Fig 3–21). Similar cases with phenytoin alone or in combination with primidone have been reported.[53]

Table 3–2 provides an overview of ocular signs in the comatose patient. A complete discussion of neurologic signs in coma is available in the text by Plum and Posner.[54]

TABLE 3–2. Ocular Signs in Coma

Level of impairment	Extraocular movements				Pupils	
	Rest position	Doll's head	Cold calorics	Defective system	Size	Reactivity
Unilateral hemispheral	Tonic deviation toward lesion	Intact*	Intact*	Frontomesencephalic (saccadic)	In hemispheral disease pupillary signs inconstant and usually of little help; in coma, pupil usually small but reactive	
Bilateral or diffuse hemispheral	Straight†/divergent; slow disconjugate wandering	Intact*	Tonic phase only	Bilateral frontomesencephalic		
Metabolic, including drugs						
Light	Straight†/divergent	Intact*/diminished	Intact*/diminished	(Above)	Small	Reactive
Deep	Slow disconjugate wandering or fixed	Absent	Absent	Brain stem reticular		
Midbrain	Straight† or skew; ±III	Horizontal only; adduction lag	Horizontal only; adduction lag; ±skew	Rostral mesencephalic vertical gaze	Mid-dilated; ±III	Fixed
Pons	Straight† or deviated opposite lesion; ±skew; ±bobbing	May fail to one/both sides; ±internuclear; ±VI	May fail to one/both sides; ±internuclear; ±VI	Pontine paramedian reticular	Pinpoint	Reactive
Cerebellum‡						
Early	Deviated opposite lesion; gaze palsy toward lesion	Normal or diminished toward side of gaze palsy	Normal or diminished toward side of gaze palsy	?	(Normal)	
Late	±Skew	Diminished/absent toward side of gaze palsy	Diminished/absent toward side of gaze palsy		Pinpoint	Reactive

* Bilaterally intact doll's head or caloric deviations preclude the possibility of severe pontine lesions. (The onset of reflex paralysis of eye movements in the course of coma is considered a sign of secondary brain stem hemorrhages.)

† In coma, eyes directed straight have no localizing value.

‡ The syndrome of acute cerebellar hemorrhage consists of occipital headache, ataxia, vertigo, conjugate gaze palsy, and progressive lethargy.

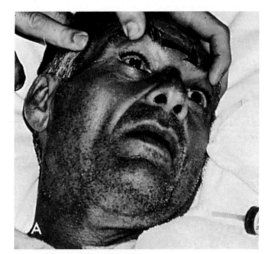
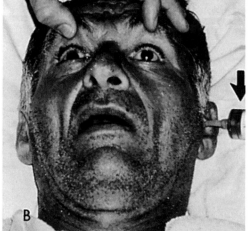

Fig. 3–21. Ocular signs in coma. A patient with barbiturate overdose shows no ocular motor response to doll's head maneuver **(A)** or cold caloric irrigation **(B)**.

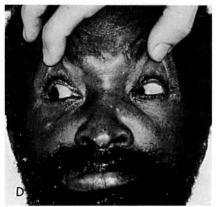

Fig. 3–21. (*continued*) **C.** Pupils are small but reactive, and the eyes are slightly divergent. **D.** A patient with a right frontoparietal infarct demonstrates tonic deviation of the eyes to the right.

REFERENCES

1. Chamberlain W: Restriction in upward gaze with advancing age. Am J Ophthalmol 71:341, 1971
2. Linksz A: Visual acuity in the newborn, with notes on some objective methods to determine visual acuity. Doc Ophthalmol 34:259, 1973
3. Collewijn H, Kleinschmidt HJ: Vestibulo-ocular and optokinetic reactions in the rabbit: changes during 24 hours of normal and abnormal interaction. In Lennerstrand G, Bach-y-Rita R (eds): Basic Mechanisms of Ocular Motility and Their Clinical Implications. Oxford, Pergamon Press, 1975
4. Kestenbaum A: Clinical Methods of Neuro-Ophthalmologic Examination, p 344. New York, Grune & Stratton, 1961
5. Smith JL, Cogan DG: Optokinetic nystagmus: a test for parietal lobe lesions. Am J Ophthalmol 48:187, 1959
6. Smith JL, David NJ: Internuclear ophthalmoplegia: two new clinical signs. Neurology 14:307, 1984
7. Kommerell G: Monocular diplopia caused by pressure of the upper lid on the cornea: diagnosis on the basis of the retinoscopic "Venetian blind phenomenon." Klin Monatsbl Augenheilkd 203:384, 1993
8. Bender MD: Polyopia and monucular diplopia of cerebral origin. Arch Neurol Psychiatry 54:323, 1945
9. Kommerell G, Oliver D: Contractures following paresis of ocular muscles. Albrecht von Graefes Arch Klin Ophthalmol 183:169, 1971
10. Wilkins RH, Brody IA: Bell's palsy and Bell's phenomenon. Arch Neurol 21:661, 1969
11. Cogan DG: Neurologic significance of lateral conjugate gaze phenomenon. Arch Neurol 21:661, 1969
12. Riggs L, Kelley JP, Manning A et al: Blink related eye movements. Invest Ophthalmol Vis Sci 28:334, 1987
13. Smith JL, Gay AJ, Cogan DG: The spasticity of conjugate gaze phenomenon. Arch Ophthalmol 62:694, 1959
14. Schmidtke K, Buttner-Ennever JA: Nervous control of eyelid function: a review of clinical, experimental and pathologic data. Brain 115:227, 1992
15. Wilkins DE, Hallett M, Wess MM: Audiogenic startle reflex of man and its relationship to startle syndromes. Brain 109:561, 1986
16. Lepore FE: Bilateral cerebral ptosis. Neurology 37:1043, 1987
17. Lowenstein DH, Koch TK, Edwards MS: Cerebral ptosis with contralateral arteriovenous malformation: a report of two cases. Ann Neurol 21:404, 1987
18. Becker W, Fuchs AF: Lid-eye coordination during vertical gaze changes in man and monkey. J Neurophysiol 60:1, 1988
19. Lam BL, Lam S, Walls RC: Prevalence of palpebral fissure asymmetry in white persons. Am J Ophthalmol 120:518, 1995
20. Lepore FE: Unilateral ptosis and Hering's law. Neurology 38:319, 1988
21. Komiyama A, Hirayama K: Paradoxical reversal of ptosis in myasthenia gravis by edrophonium administration. J Neurol Neurosurg Psychiatry 51:315, 1988
22. Wesely RE, Bond JB: Upper eyelid retraction from inferior rectus restriction in dysthyroid orbit disease. Ann Ophthalmol 19:34, 1987
23. Galetta SL, Gray LG, Raps E et al: Pretectal eyelid retraction and lag. Ann Neurol 33:554, 1993
24. Slansky HH, Kolbert G, Gartner S: Exophthalmos induced by steroids. Arch Ophthalmol 77:579, 1967
25. Summerskill WHJ, Molnar GD: Eye signs in herpetic cirrhosis. N Engl J Med 266:1244, 1962
26. Bartley GB: The differential diagnosis of eyelid retraction. Ophthalmol 103:168, 1996
27. Cogan DG: Myasthenia gravis: a review of the disease and a description of lid twitch as a characteristic sign. Arch Ophthalmol 74:217, 1965
28. Ragge NK, Hoyt WF: Midbrain myasthenia: fatigable ptosis, "lid twitch" sign and ophthalmoparesis from a dorsal midbrain glioma. Neurology 42:917, 1992
29. Shore JW, McCord CD: Anatomic changes in involutional blepharoptosis. Am J Ophthalmol 98:21, 1984
30. van den Bosch WA, Lemij HG: Blepharoptosis induced by hard contact lens wear. Ophthalmology 99:1759, 1992
31. Po SM, Custer PL, Smith ME: Bilateral lagophthalmos: an unusual presentation of metastatic breast carcinoma. Arch Ophthalmol 114:1139, 1996
32. Boghen D: Apraxia of lid opening: a review. Neurology 48:1491, 1997
33. Brodsky MC, Boop FA: Lid nystagmus as a sign of intrinsic midbrain disease. J Neuro-ophthalmol 15:236, 1995
34. Burton H: Somatosensory sensations from the eye. In Hart WM (ed): Adler's Physiology of the Eye, 9th ed, p 71. St. Louis, CV Mosby, 1992
35. ten Tusscher MPM: The trigeminal nerve supply to the eye. Orbit 12:183, 1993
36. Wirth FP, van Buren JM: Referral of pain from dural stimulation in man. J Neurosurg 34:630, 1971
37. Kerr FWL: The divisional organization of afferent fibers of the trigeminal nerve. Brain 86:721, 1963
38. Albe-Fessard D, Boivie J, Grant G et al: Labelling of cells in the medulla oblongata and the spinal cord of the monkey after injections of horseradish peroxidase in the thalamus. Neurosci Lett 1:75, 1975
39. Paulson GW, Bird MT: The corneomandibular reflex. Confin Neurol 33:116, 1971
40. Whitcher JP: Clinical diagnosis of the dry eye. Int Ophthalmol Clin 27:7, 1987
41. Schein OD, Tielsch JM, Munoz B et al: Relation between signs and symptoms of dry eye in the elderly: a population-based study. Ophthalmol 104:1395, 1997
42. Derby GS: Ocular neuroses: an important cause of so-called eyestrain. JAMA 95:13, 1930
43. Sellitti TP, Huang AJW, Schiffman J et al: Association of herpes zoster ophthalmicus with acquired immunodeficiency syndrome and acute retinal necrosis. Am J Ophthalmol 116:297, 1993

44. Kost RG, Straus SE: Postherpetic neuralgia: pathogenesis, treatment, and prevention. N Engl J Med 335:32, 1996
45. Mansour AM, Bailey BJ: Ocular findings in Ramsey Hunt syndrome. J Neuro-ophthalmol 17:199, 1997
46. Meaney JFM, Eldridge PR, Dunn LT et al: Demonstration of neurovascular compression in trigeminal neuralgia with magnetic presonance imaging: comparison with surgical findings in 52 operative cases. J Neurosurg 83:799, 1995
47. Temser RB: Trigeminal neuralgia: mechanisms of treatment. Neurology 51:17, 1998
48. Rovick MB, Chardar K, Colombi BJ: Inflammatory trigeminal sensory neuropathy mimicking trigeminal neurinoma. Neurol 46:1455, 1996
49. ten Hove MW, Glaser JS, Schatz NJ: Occult perineural tumor infiltration of the trigeminal nerve: diagnostic considerations. J Neuro-ophthalmol 17:170–177, 1997
50. Tavy DL, van Woerkom TC, Bots GT, Endtz LJ et al: Persistence of the blink reflex to sudden illumination in a comatose patient. Arch Neurol 41:323, 1984
51. Paulson GW, Kapp JP: Dilatation of the pupil in the cat via the oculomotor nerve. Arch Ophthalmol 77:536, 1967
52. Rodriguez Barrios R, Botinelli MD, Medoc J: The study of ocular motility in the comatose patient. J Neurol Sci 3:183, 1966
53. Orth DN, Almeida H, Walsh FB, Honda M: Ophthalmoplegia resulting from diphenylhydantoin and primadone intoxication. JAMA 201:225, 1962
54. Plum F, Posner JB: The Diagnosis of Stupor and Coma, 3rd ed. Philadelphia, FA Davis, 1982

CHAPTER 4

Anatomy of the Visual Sensory System

Joel S. Glaser and Alfredo A. Sadun

Functional Anatomy
  Retina
  Optic Disc
  Optic Nerve
  Optic Chiasm
  Optic Tracts
  Lateral Geniculate Nucleus

Visual Radiations
Occipital Cortex
Visual Association Areas and
    Interhemispheric Connections
Extrageniculate Visual Systems
Retinotopic Organization
Vascular Supply

> Those who have dissected or inspected many, have at least learned to doubt when the others, who are ignorant of anatomy, and do not take the trouble to attend to it, are in no doubt at all.
>
> Morgagni GB
> *The Seeds and Causes of Diseases Investigated by Anatomy, 1761*

The retina, optic nerves, optic chiasm, optic tracts, lateral geniculate nuclei, other brainstem primary visual nuclei (superior colliculus, pretectum), hypothalamic nuclei, pulvinar, and accessory optic system, geniculostriate radiations, striate cortex, visual association areas, and related interhemispheric connections constitute the primary visual sensory system in man.[1] Most of this specialized afferent system lies in a horizontal plane that crosses at right angles the major ascending sensory and descending motor systems of the cerebral hemispheres (Fig. 4–1). The anterior portion of the visual system is intimately related to the vascular and bony structures at the skull base and undersurface of the brain. The posterior portions are intimately applied to the lateral aspects of the ventricular system that extends throughout the cerebral hemispheres. Thus, defects of the visual pathways, as revealed by visual field assessment or other methods, have great localizing value in neurologic diagnosis. The dominant role of vision in man may be expressed numerically by considering, for example, the number of axons in the human optic nerve

(greater than 1.2 million), as compared with the axons in the acoustic nerve (approximately 31,000).[2,3] Thus, the ratio of afferent neurons in the peripheral visual apparatus to the afferent neurons in the aural system is roughly 40:1. It has been estimated that the optic nerves comprise about 40% of all fibers that enter or exit the brain.[4]

The first distinct evidence of the human eye is found in the eight-somite stage of embryologic development, at about the third to fourth week. The two primordial optic bulbs extend to either side of the anterior end of the neural tube, the prosencephalon. A slight thickening between the two represents the *torus opticus* (*i.e.,* the primitive chiasmal anlage). The optic primordia evaginate to form the laterally placed cuplike vesicles, which contact overlying surface ectoderm and induce lens growth. The optic stalk and cups are notched ventrally (the "fetal" fissure), which permits entry of blood vessels, and primitive retina develops by about 5 weeks' gestation. Retinal ganglion cells differentiate, and optic nerve fibers begin to fill the optic stalk, now surrounded by a cellular sheath. The retinal precursor cells are multipotential (each has the ability to produce all retinal neuron types up to the final cell division).[5] These afferent visual neurons reach the area of the optic chiasm at about the seventh week as the ventral fissure closes.

At about 50 days of gestational age, the optic nerve contains a full complement of retinal ganglion cell axons, the optic disc and scleral opening are well defined, and endochondral ossification of the sphenoid begins.[6] The ultimate number of axons in the mature human optic nerve is the result of an initial overproduction of axons during the first half of gestation, followed by a 70% reduction ("die-back") between 16 and 30 weeks' gestation.[7] The optic nerve, as a part of the central

J. S. Glaser: Departments of Neurology and Ophthalmology, Bascom Palmer Eye Institute, University of Miami School of Medicine, Miami; and Neuro-ophthalmology, Cleveland Clinic Florida, Ft. Lauderdale, Florida

A. A. Sadun: Departments of Ophthalmology and Neurosurgery, University of Southern California; and Department of Ophthalmology, Doheny Eye Institute, Los Angeles, California

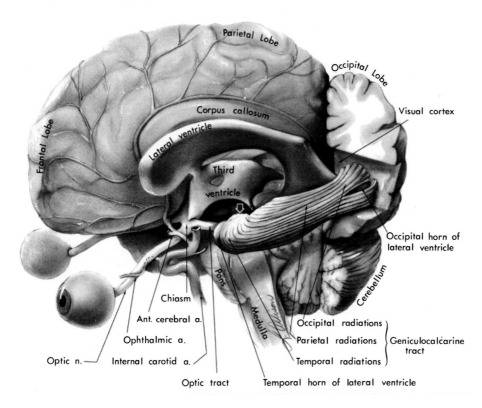

Fig. 4–1. The visual sensory system. The left cerebral hemisphere has been removed, with the exception of the occipital lobe and the ventricular system. The left lateral geniculate body is hidden (*arrow*). Note the following relationships: optic nerve with internal carotid and anterior communicating arteries; chiasm in floor of third ventricle; forward sweep of temporal radiations around lateral ventricle; course of occipital radiations toward interhemispheral surface of occipital lobe. The cerebral falx and cerebellar tentorium are not illustrated.

nervous system (CNS), is incapable of further axonal growth or regeneration, although there is interesting new work on what inhibits this regeneration.[8,9] Myelination begins centrally at the optic chiasm early in the seventh fetal month and progresses toward the eye, reaching (but not passing) the lamina cribrosa of the optic disc at about the first postpartum month.[10]

FUNCTIONAL ANATOMY

Retina

The functional organization of the visual sensory system begins at the retina. It is beyond the scope of this chapter to describe the complex vertical and horizontal organization of retinal elements, synaptic patterns, receptive field physiology, and other details of visual signal propagation. However, it is important to emphasize that there is a considerable degree of retinal processing that modifies neural signals before transmission to central structures, such as the lateral geniculate nuclei and cortical areas. It would be incorrect to describe the retina as "film in the back of the camera." There is a great deal of temporal and spatial modulation of the signal between the percipient elements, the middle retina (bipolar cells, horizontal cells, and amacrine cells), and the retinal ganglion cells. Ganglion cell subsets selectively encode specific aspects of visual information, such as acuity (resolution), color, image velocity and movement direction, and contrast; thus, visual signal processing takes place in parallel and simultaneously, through separate "channels."[11-14]

The distribution of visual function across the retina is not uniform but rather is a pattern of concentric zones that increase in sensitivity toward the central retinal area, the fovea, which subserves the highest sensitivity. At progressively eccentric retinal locations, there is a nonlinear decrease in sensitivity (conversely, an elevation of thresholds). Ultimately, retinal sensitivity is a manifestation of the underlying cytoarchitecture and the distribution of the percipient elements, the cones and rods. The fovea itself is essentially without rods but is composed of about 100,000 compactly arranged slender cones. The entire posterior pole of the retina is dominated by the foveal and parafoveal cone system, which occupies an area about 1.5 mm in diameter. Small ganglion cells subserving this central cone cell system send their axons directly to the temporal aspect of the optic disc, forming the papillomacular nerve fiber bundle. This discrete bundle of nerve fibers is relatively isolated from other retinal nerve fibers that reach the optic disc by an arcuate course above and below the papillomacular bundle, forming dense superior and inferior bands (Fig. 4–2).

Østerberg[15] quantitatively examined the arrangement of photoreceptors in the human retina and found a skewed distribution; rod and cone populations are denser in the superonasal retina and less dense in the inferotemporal retina. Van Buren[16] performed retinal ganglion cell counts and demonstrated the same eccentric pattern of a denser packing of ganglion cells that reached nearly twice as far on the nasal side of the fovea as on the temporal side. This asymmetric distribution

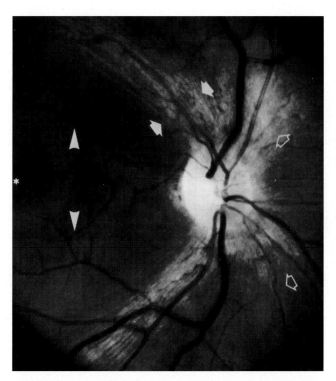

Fig. 4–2. Retinal nerve fiber layer pattern. The dense temporal arcuate fiber bundles (*solid arrows*) are most easily seen. Nasal fibers (*open arrows*) take a more direct radial course. The papillomacular bundle (*arrowheads*) is most difficult to visualize.

of retinal elements about the fovea is reflected in the asymmetry of the nasal visual field versus the temporal visual field, and it may in part account for the relative foreshortening of the nasal field.[17] Curcio et al[18,19] quantitated the number of percipient elements and retinal ganglion cells in the human retina, noted these and other asymmetries, and found moderate attrition in both aging and disease.

In advanced primates, the fovea occupies the central 3° of retina and is a roughly circular pit devoid of ganglion cells, surrounded by a multilayered annulus of densely packed small ganglion cells. Central projections, traced by horseradish peroxidase, indicate that ipsilaterally projecting ganglion cells in the temporal foveal rim can generate 2° to 3° of *bilateral* representation in the geniculocortical pathways because of an intermingling with contralaterally projecting cells on the nasal side of the foveal pit.[20] These findings provide a potential retinal neural basis for foveal (fixational) "sparing" or "splitting," which is demonstrated by perimetry in the presence of lesions of the posterior visual pathways.

Ogden[21] has extensively studied horizontal and vertical retinotopy in the geographic bundles of ganglion cell axons as they traverse the retina to the optic disc. Despite previous reports that the nerve fiber layer is well organized, Ogden has demonstrated that horizontal retinotopic organization is present within nasal but not temporal nerve fiber bundles, and that vertical retinotopic

stratification is orderly within temporal, but not nasal, retinal bundles. Also, temporal axons in the nerve fiber layer intermingle freely along the intraretinal course of the arcuate bundles. Therefore, the segregation of fibers into a retinotopic distribution occurs at the level of the optic disc or more posteriorly in the optic nerve. Species differences do occur; the macaque retina most resembles the human nerve fiber layer.[22]

Optic Disc

The optic nerve head can be seen funduscopically end-on and appears as a flat disc with a central depression of variable width and depth, the optic cup. *Papilla*, a term that implies a nipple-like eminence, is used less often. The optic disc is the collective exit site of all retinal ganglion cell axons, via the nerve fiber layer. The optic disc is located about 3 mm nasal and 1 mm superior to the fovea and represents a 1.5×2 mm hiatus in the sclera, choroid, retinal pigment epithelium, and retina proper. The mean horizontal disc diameter is 1.76 ± 0.3 mm, the mean vertical diameter is 1.92 ± 0.3 mm, the mean horizontal cup/disc ratio is 0.39, and the mean vertical cup/disc ratio is 0.34 mm.[23] There are no percipient or other retinal elements on the disc, which is represented in visual space as an absolute scotoma, the blind spot of Mariotte.

The retinal axons bend posteriorly 90° over the scleral disc margin and pass through the perforations of the collagen plates of the lamina cribrosa.[24] This fenestrated connective tissue is lined by astrocytes and other specialized glial elements to form a "seal." The lamina cribrosa is continuous with the surrounding sclera and partitions the nerve head into prelaminar, laminar, and retrolaminar compartments (Fig. 4–3). The extracellular matrix of the human lamina cribrosa contains collagen macromolecules resembling CNS basement membrane and is distinct from the collagen of the surrounding sclera.[25] Axonal bundles are compartmentalized by glial-collagen pial septae as they traverse the lamina cribrosa into the posterior portion of the optic nerve. These well-defined septae and the myelination of axons cause the optic disc to increase in diameter from about 1.8 mm in the disc to about 3.5 mm in the retrobulbar optic nerve. The interaxonal glial tissue and connective tissue septae, in addition to the lamina cribrosa and scleral canal, constrain the propagation of edema in the optic disc that occurs with ischemic optic neuropathies or when intraocular pressure is raised.[26]

Optic Nerve

The optic nerve consists of four segments: intraocular (1 mm in length), intraorbital (about 25 to 30 mm), intracanalicular (about 9 to 10 mm), and intracranial (about 16 mm). Thus, the entire length of the optic nerve from the globe to the optic chiasm is about 5 to

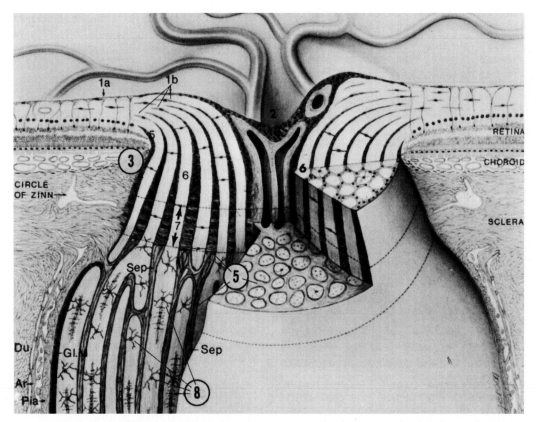

Fig. 4–3. Schematic structure of optic disc and nerve. *1a,* internal limiting membrane of retina; *1b,* nerve fiber layer; *2,* optic cup, lined by astroglial cells, and central retinal vessels; *3,* ophthalmoscopically visible disc edge; *5,* glial and connective tissue columns; *6,* nerve fiber fascicles; *7,* major portion of lamina cribrosa; *8,* oligodendrocytes; *Du,* dura; *Ar,* arachnoid. *Pia,* pia; *Gl. M,* glial mantle; *Sep,* pial septum. (Modified from Anderson DR, Hoyt WF: Ultrastructure of intraorbital portion of human and monkey optic nerve. Arch Ophthalmol 82:506, 1969)

6 cm. The intraocular portion (optic disc) can be further divided into retinal, choroidal, and scleral levels as the retinal ganglion cell axons from the nerve fiber layer turn sharply in a posterior direction to exit the globe (see Fig. 4–3). Anderson and Hoyt[27,28] and Minckler[26] have extensively described the microanatomic structure of the nerve as consisting of a neuroectodermal (nervous tissue proper) and a mesodermal (providing support and nourishment) component. Mesodermal connective tissue includes the sclera, fibroblasts, meningothelial cells, and blood vessels. The collagenous component of the perforated lamina (also termed the lamina cribrosa scleralis) can be considered continuous with, but distinct from, both the sclera and the perioptic meninges. The more anterior aspects of the optic nerve head contain less connective tissue, and there is a correspondingly greater glial presence. The anterior optic nerve head consists of unmyelinated axons and astrocytes. It is unusual for oligodendrocytes or myelinated axons to be anterior to the laminar scleralis; funduscopically visible myelinated nerve fibers are associated with anomalous rests of retinal oli-

godendrocytes. Patches of myelination are observed in the retina in about 1% of the general population.[29]

Behind the laminar cribrosa, the optic nerve abruptly increases in diameter from 3 mm to 4 mm in midorbit and to 5 mm intracranially. At this point, oligodendrocytes (responsible for the formation of myelin, which ensheathes the axons) constitute about two thirds of the interstitial cells. Because the optic nerve contains oligodendrocytes rather than Schwann cells to produce myelin, the optic nerve must be considered analogous to the white-matter tracts of the brain rather than to peripheral nerves; this composition makes the optic nerve susceptible to diseases of CNS tracts, such as multiple sclerosis. The orbital and intracanalicular portions of the optic nerve contain a well-developed septal system continuous with the pia mater. The septae form porous cylindrical walls aligned along the long axis of the nerves and may permit strength and support in the context of flexible movement.[30] The septae divide the nerve fibers into parallel columns of variable shape and size. Astrocytes are intimately related to the pial septae and play a role in the support and nutrition of axons; they are also a component of the blood-brain barrier.

Fibers, grouped into fascicles maintain retinopy at all locations along the nerve, except intracranially, close to the chiasm where this pattern is lost. Relatively large fascicular numbers are found directly behind the eye and in the region of the optic canal, but decline in the mid-orbital segment of the nerve. Connective tissue is present in the extra-fascicular matrix throughout the fasciculated segment, but in many cases it does not fully encircle axon fascicles.[31]

About 1 cm posterior to the globe, the major branch of the ophthalmic artery pierces the inferior aspect of the meninges of the optic nerve, passes through the cerebrospinal fluid–filled subarachnoid space, and gains a central axial position, emerging in the middle of the optic disc as the central retinal artery. The central retinal artery does not contribute directly to the blood supply of the laminar and prelaminar portions of the optic nerve head. These areas of the optic nerve are supplied by an anastomotic arterial complex, the circle of Zinn-Haller, which is usually fed by about four short posterior ciliary arteries.[32] This perioptic nerve arteriolar anastomosis also receives a much smaller contribution from the pial arterial network and the peripapillary choroid (Fig. 4–4).[33] Autoregulated radial branches from the circle of Zinn-Haller supply the laminar optic disc.[34] Thus, the blood supply of the optic nerve head itself is derived primarily from choroidal and posterior ciliary vessels, as opposed to the inner retina, whose blood supply is provided by the central retinal artery.[35,36]

The intraorbital segment of the optic nerve (about 25 mm) exceeds in length the distance from the back of the globe to the orbital apex (less than 20 mm). Therefore, within the orbit, the optic nerve has redundancy in length and a sinuous course. This permits the nerve to move freely in its cushion of fat behind the globe during eye movements, and also allows up to 6 or 8 mm of proptosis before the nerve begins to tether and distort the back of the globe. At the orbital apex, the optic nerve enters the bony optic canal, and is surrounded by the connective tissue origins of the superior, medial, and inferior recti muscles, which collectively constitute the so-called annulus of Zinn.

The optic canal runs posteromedially in the sphenoid bone at an angle of about 35° with the midsagittal plane (Fig. 4–5). The optic canal is 4 to 10 mm in length and contains not only the optic nerve but the ophthalmic artery, branches of the carotid sympathetic plexus, and extensions of the intracranial meninges that form the sheaths of the optic nerve. Many fine blood vessels must cross from the dura affixed to the periosteum, through the subarachnoid space to feed the pial plexus covering the optic nerve.[37] Usually, the ophthalmic artery gives off three main branches that pierce the dura.[37] Hence, inertial and shearing forces can rupture these vessels,

leading to optic nerve damage in the optic canal with or without canal fracture after blunt trauma to the head (especially the lateral forehead).[38] The medial wall of the optic canal is the thinnest and is the most likely to fracture in blunt trauma.[38] The dural covering of the nerve and the periosteum of the canal are fused, but the arachnoid is continuous, permitting the subarachnoid space of the optic nerves to communicate freely with the intracranial subarachnoid space, both of which contain cerebrospinal fluid.

The mesial surface of the optic canal protrudes into the superolateral aspect of the sphenoid sinus. According to Rhoton et al,[39] the optic nerves are separated from the sinus cavity by only the nerve sheath and mucosa in about 4% of specimens; in 78%, less than a 0.5-mm thickness of bone separates the optic nerves from the sinus cavity. Therefore, manipulations at the lateral sphenoid sinus wall during transsphenoidal surgical procedures may damage the optic nerves.

The optic nerves are fixed at the intracranial opening of the optic canals, the upper margins of which are formed by an unyielding falciform fold of dura. This constriction may notch the superior surface of the optic nerve when sellar-based adenomas or internal carotid artery aneurysms elevate the chiasm, or even in cases of generalized severe brain edema. From the internal (posterior) foramina of the canals, the optic nerves converge toward the chiasm in the anteroinferior floor of the third ventricle. The two nerves ascend toward the chiasm at an angle of about 45° with the nasotuberculum line (Fig. 4–6). The intracranial nerve segment averages 17 ± 2.4 mm in length, and the optic chiasm itself sits 10.7 ± 2.4 mm above the dorsum of the sella turcica.[40] Occasionally, the intracranial optic nerves are shorter, and the chiasm may lie directly above the sella in a position that is called "prefixed." More commonly, the optic chiasm is positioned 10 to 12 mm above the insertion of the diaphragma sellae onto the dorsum.[41] Hence, it should be recognized that pituitary tumors must extend well above the sella before the optic chiasm is encroached upon. The neurosurgical correlate is as follows: By the time that chiasmal field defects evolve, pituitary tumors are already large and have major suprasellar extensions. On average, a pituitary adenoma will have a diameter of 22 to 24 mm before any visual field defect is detectable.[42] Smaller tumors are detected clinically when signs of unilateral optic nerve compression evolve.

The inferior surfaces of the frontal lobes (gyri recti) of the cerebral hemispheres are above the optic nerves. The anterior cerebral and anterior communicating arteries lie between the frontal lobes and the optic nerves (see Fig. 4–1 and also Fig. 12–17). Medial to the anterior clinoid process (see Fig. 4–5B and also Fig. 12–17), the optic nerve lies just above the siphon of the intracavernous portion of the internal carotid artery and is sepa-

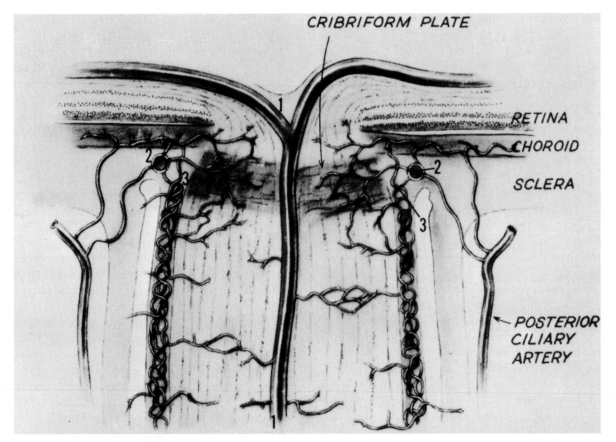

Fig. 4–4. Blood supply of the optic nerve head. *1,* central retinal artery; *2,* arterial circle of Zinn-Haller; *3,* pial arterial network. Contribution to Zinn-Haller circle from posterior ciliary arteries, pial plexus, and peripapillary choroid; the latter also sends branches directly to prelaminar disc substance. (Modified from Kolker AE, Hetherington J Jr: Becker-Shaffer's Diagnosis and Therapy of the Glaucomas, ed 3. St. Louis, Mosby, 1970)

rated from the cavernous sinus by the optic strut. Thus, expanding lesions of the cavernous sinus, such as an aneurysm or meningioma, can also impinge on the optic nerve. At the origin of the ophthalmic artery, aneurysms can compress the nerve from a medial and ventral direction. An ophthalmic artery aneurysm can also expand across the midline to compress the contralateral optic nerve nasally.[43]

Optic Chiasm

The anatomy of the optic chiasm has been an intriguing subject since the time of Galen, who, in the 2nd century, likened the structure to the Greek letter *chi,* with subsequent additions and emendations by Leonardo da Vinci (1504), William Briggs (1676), Thomas Willis (1681), Descartes (1686), Isaac Newton (1704), and Santiago Ramon y Cajal (1898), among others.[44] Both Descartes and Newton, on theoretic grounds, defined the essential character of the organization of the central visual pathways in animals that have overlapping binocular vision. By the end of the 19th century, the

partial decussation of retinal axons in most mammalian chiasms was histologically ascertained. Moreover, Ramon y Cajal saw the chiasm as a structure that corrected the inversion of sensory space imposed by the optical system of the eye. These considerations of physiologic optics led Ramon y Cajal to elaborate a general theory of cerebral crossings that provides the basis for contralateral motor and sensory projections.

The optic chiasm derives from the merging of the two optic nerves. The superior and posterior aspects of the optic chiasm are contiguous with the anteroinferior floor of the third ventricle (see Fig. 4–6). The optic chiasm measures about 8 mm from the anterior to the posterior notch, 12 to 18 mm across, and 4 mm in height.[45] The regional vascular relationships of the intracranial optic nerves and optic chiasm are critical, because aneurysms commonly involve the internal carotid arteries and the basal arterial circle. As the internal carotid arteries curve posteriorly and upward out of the cavernous sinuses, they lie immediately below the optic nerves. The carotid arteries then ascend vertically along the lateral aspects of the chiasm (see Fig. 4–1 and also Figs. 12–5

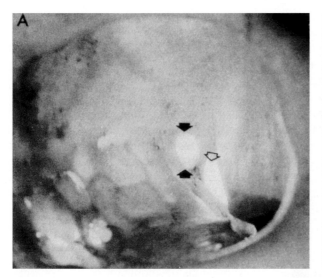

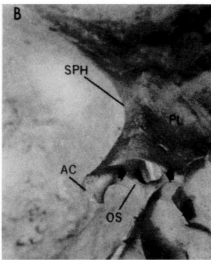

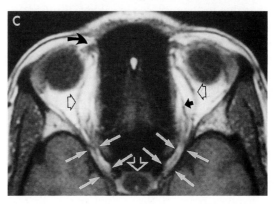

Fig. 4–5. The optic canal. **A.** Anterior view of left orbital apex. Orbital end of optic canal is vertically oval (*black arrows*) and separated from superior orbital fissure (*open arrow*) by optic strut. Note transilluminated ethmoidal and sphenoidal air cells, which form medial orbital wall and medial wall of optic canal. **B.** Posterior view of intracranial aspect of left optic canal demonstrating horizontally oval contour. The optic strut (OS) forms the ventrolateral margin of the canal and separates it from the carotid artery. In this preparation the ethmoidal and sphenoidal air cells have been opened. AC, anterior clinoid; PL, planum; SPH, sphenoidal wing. **C.** MRI axial section. Optic canals (*white arrows*) converge toward sella at base of skull. Venous sinus (*open white arrow*) indicates location of tuberculum of planum sphenoidale. Superior ophthalmic veins (*open black arrows*), ophthalmic artery (*black arrow*) on right, and trochlea (*curved black arrow*) on left.

and 12–17). The precommunicating portions of the anterior cerebral arteries are closely related to the superior surface of the chiasm and optic nerves. Dolichoectasias of the internal carotid arteries can produce visual field

defects.[46] Because the entire Circle of Willis is less than an inch in diameter, even aneurysms of the posterior circle can impinge on the optic chiasm.

According to Barber et al,[47] the human optic chiasm anlage is visible in the floor of the forebrain between the optic vesicles at the 3-mm stage of embryogenesis. Between 4 and 8 weeks' gestation, axons and retinal ganglion cells grow toward the brain into the floor of the third ventricle and partially decussate to form a true hiasm (30-mm stage). Kupfer et al[48] calculated in the adult human that the ratio of crossed to uncrossed fibers in the optic chiasm was about 53 to 47, respectively; the uncrossed portion was greater than that seen in other primates. After the 8-week stage of development, retinofugal axons swing laterally around the diencephalon to reach a collection of cells that differentiate from the dorsolateral portion of the thalamus to form the dorsal nucleus of the lateral geniculate body. During the second month, the eyes assume a frontal position, such that the optic nerves must pass upward and medially to gain the optic canals. At about the 10th week, uncrossed

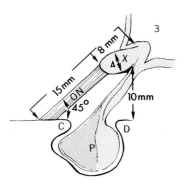

Fig. 4–6. Relationships of the optic nerves (*ON*) and chiasm (*X*) to the sellar structures and third ventricle (*3*). *C,* anterior clinoid; *D,* dorsum sellae; *P,* pituitary gland in sella. Lateral view.

retinal fibers begin to appear. They are prohibited from crossing a central chiasmal zone by trophic factors, such as stage-specific embryonic antigen 1 (SSEA-1).[49] The primitive optic recess forms at the anterior aspect of the third ventricle; the recess extends variably a short distance into the proximal ends of the optic nerves but is eventually obliterated as more retinofugal axons reach the optic chiasm. Ultimately, the small optic recess represents the remnant of the proximal ends of the optic vesicles.

As the thalamic nuclear masses increase in size, the third ventricle becomes a vertical slit (at about 12 weeks' gestation or the 60-mm stage). At the beginning of the fourth month, the optic tracts continue to form by decussating fibers that pass around the hypothalamic nuclei. During the last few months of gestation, the development of the optic chiasm consists mainly of an increase in size, which is due to the increase in caliber of retinal axons. Its ultimate topographic configuration is dictated by the growth of contiguous structures and modification of the shape of the third ventricle. Myelination of these axons commences only after the visual pathways are otherwise complete. Sometime during the fifth month, myelination begins at the brainstem visual nuclei. Myelination reaches the chiasm during the sixth month and progresses from a proximal to a distal direction along the optic nerves during the eighth and ninth months of gestation. It stops abruptly at the lamina cribrosa. About 1% of the time, myelination "escapes" anterior to the lamina and involves parts of the retinal nerve fiber layer.[30]

There is evidence suggesting that each neuroretina has contributions from *both* sides of the prospective forebrain. By cell-labeling techniques (induced chromosomal mosaicism or horseradish peroxidase) it has been demonstrated in the frog embryo[50] that there is reciprocal movement (translocation) of cells from each side of the primitive forebrain into the contralateral retinal anlage. This migration begins before neural tube closure and results in the formation of a primitive optic chiasm into which grow axons from each retina. These axons are destined for synaptic sites on the *opposite* side of the brain, from which the precursor cells originated. Thus, translocated cells establish a pattern for chiasmal crossing even before ganglion cell axonal outgrowth from the retina occurs. Pioneer neurons, perhaps exquisitely sensitive to trophic cues, lead the way and are later followed by the general optic nerve axonal population.[51–53]

Melanin may play a role in axonal guidance during development of the primitive optic nerves and chiasm.[54] In rodents, parts of the distal eye stalk are transiently pigmented during the migration of pioneer visual axons, which avoid the area of melanosomes. Hence, melanin-producing stalk cells may play a role in controlling the topographic pattern of optic nerve fibers by inhibiting axonal growth within their territory. Indeed, in the albino there is an anomalous topographic arrangement of retinal axons such that most temporal retinal ganglion cells decussate at the optic chiasm and project to the wrong lateral geniculate nucleus. This results in abnormal field representations of the geniculate and visual cortex. Hypomelanosis syndromes such as oculocutaneous or ocular albinism regularly show an intermediate abnormality of misrouted retinal axons, with retinal fibers from 20° or more temporal to the fovea anomalously crossing at the chiasm. Hence, each hemisphere receives predominantly monocular input from the contralateral eye, with only the peripheral nasal field represented ipsilaterally.[55] Strabismus and nystagmus are likely results.

Anomalous development of the optic chiasm otherwise occurs from faulty development of one or both optic vesicles, or with forebrain malformations (see Chapter 5). In bilateral anophthalmia, the optic nerves, chiasm, and optic tracts do not develop.[56] In unilateral anophthalmia, an asymmetric and small optic chiasm is found composed of nerve fibers from the intact eye.[57]

Most of the retinofugal fibers exit the optic chiasm posteriorly to form the primary optic tracts. However, a few fibers have been shown to exit from the dorsal surface of the optic chiasm and enter directly into the hypothalamus to terminate in the suprachiasmatic nucleus or the supraoptic nucleus of the hypothalamus.[58,59] These two fiber pathways probably represent the neuroanatomic basis for light/dark entrainment of the neuroendocrine circadian rhythm. Bilateral transection of the optic nerve in the rat results in a loss of synchronized endogenous circadian rhythms, whereas bilateral transection of the optic tract (distal to these fibers from the chiasm to the hypothalamus) does not.[60] Conversely, although in humans complete blindness generally results in the loss of diurnal rhythms (and insomnia), if patients maintain minimal integrity of the retinal-hypothalamic pathway, circadian rhythms can be maintained.[61]

Optic Tracts

As the retinofugal fibers pass through the chiasm, they form the optic tracts immediately posterior to the optic chiasm. Each tract begins at the posterior notch of the chiasm and is separated from the other optic tract by the pituitary stalk inferiorly and the third ventricle more superiorly. Across the basal arachnoidal cistern, the inferolateral aspect of the tract faces the uncal gyrus of the temporal lobe. As the tracts proceed posteriorly, they diverge in the interpeduncular cistern and embrace the ventral aspect of the rostral midbrain contiguous with the cerebral peduncles (see Fig. 7–6).

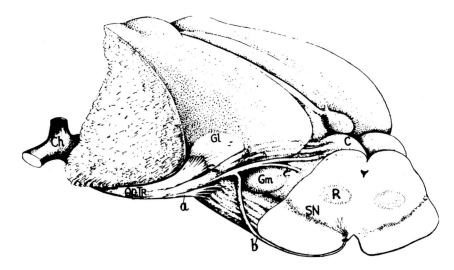

Fig. 4–7. Terminal relations of optic tract in mammalian brain. *Ch,* chiasm; *Op Tr,* optic tract; *Gl,* lateral geniculate body; *Gm,* medial geniculate body; *C,* superior colliculus; *R,* red nucleus; *SN,* substantia nigra; *a,* anterior accessory optic tract; *b,* posterior accessory optic tract; *c,* fibers to large-cell nucleus of optic tract. (LeGros Clark WE: The structure and connections of the thalamus. Brain 55:442, 1932)

At the level of the mamillary bodies, the optic tracts are located more laterally in the choroidal fissures, with the uncus below, the internal capsule above, and the amygdala lateral to them. Most of the fibers in the optic tract terminate in the ipsilateral lateral geniculate nucleus; however, just posterior to the optic chiasm a small fascicle of fibers emanates from the optic tract, travels between the two lobes of the ipsilateral supraoptic nuclei, and ascends to terminate in the paraventricular nucleus of the hypothalamus.[62] The paraventricular nucleus also mediates visual input to control diurnal rhythms.[60] Further posteriorly, a larger fascicle of axons leaves the optic tract and turns medial just ventral to the medial geniculate nucleus. These axons then proceed, via the brachium of the superior colliculus, to terminate in the tectal and pretectal nuclei of the rostral mesencephalon (Fig. 4–7).[63] These latter fibers represent the afferent limb of the pupillomotor reflex.

Lateral Geniculate Nucleus

The bulk of the optic tract terminates in the lateral geniculate nucleus (LGN) or "body." The LGN is the largest, and the most important, primary visual nucleus in man. Here, crossed and uncrossed retinal fibers are ultimately organized into homonymous pairs. Neurons of the LGN contribute axons that form the geniculocalcarine radiations. The LGN is part of the thalamus and is folded deep in the lateral recess of the choroidal fissure, obscured from direct view by the hippocampal gyrus of the temporal lobe (see Fig. 7–6). The lateral relationship of the LGN is the so-called temporal isthmus, the white matter structure lying between the auditory cortex above and the temporal horn of the lateral ventricle below.

Polyak and other anatomists have traditionally di-

vided the LGN into a large dorsal and a small ventral (pregeniculate) nucleus. However, there is little evidence that the ancient ventral portion functions in the visual system of primates. Hence, the LGN described in man always refers to the dorsal LGN of other mammals. In man there are six nuclear layers of neurons discernible in the dorsal LGN. These can be best appreciated in coronal section through the middle of the LGN (Fig. 4–8). In other planes and at the poles, the LGN may appear to have fewer than six layers. Since the early studies of Minkowski, it is evident that crossing visual axons from the contralateral eye terminate in laminae 1, 4, and 6, and uncrossed ipsilateral axons end in laminae 2, 3, and 5.[64,65] Each lamina receives input from one eye only.

The LGN is shaped like a three-cornered hat. Degeneration studies[66] reveal that there is a rather sharply defined dorsal central wedge that extends through all laminae and represents the macular projection. The macular fibers are also relatively confined to the dorsal section of the optic tract (Fig. 4–9). Upper retinal quadrants are represented medially, and lower retinal projections terminate laterally. This situation is the exception to the useful generalization that upper retinal fibers continue dorsally and lower fibers continue ventrally, throughout the visual pathways. Thus, the retinotopic organization of the posterior optic tract appears to rotate 90° (intorted) as it enters the LGN.

There is a retinotopic organization within the LGN, as demonstrated by degeneration and electrophysiology techniques.[67] Any point in the visual field is projected to a vertical column of cells whose long axis is approximately perpendicular to the LGN laminae. These "projection lines" have been established in all mammals thus far studied.[67,68] Even the physiologic blindspot is represented in the contralateral LGN as a cell-free verti-

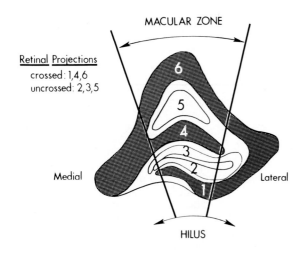

Fig. 4–8. Coronal section of lateral geniculate nucleus. Note extensive macular representation.

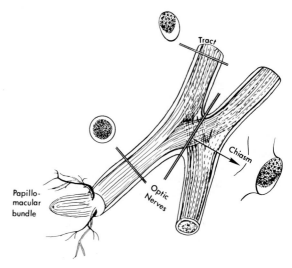

Fig. 4–9. Representation of the macular (central field) projection in the anterior visual pathways. Most afferent visual fibers are related to the papillomacular bundle, which subserves the central visual field and constitutes the central core of the optic nerve. Note that the crossing macular projection occupies an extensive area of the median bar of the chiasm.

cal column, suggesting a preset and extremely accurate alignment of projection columns through adjacent laminae.[68] Autoradiographic tracing methods[69] in owl monkeys have confirmed the nature of projection fibers from cortical visual area 17; the striate cortex projects to all laminae and interlaminar zones of the LGN.

By comparing the locations of cortical injection sites (^{3}H-proline) with positions of subsequent labels in the LGN, it is clear that the corresponding loci in the paired representations of the visual field are interconnected. Also, vertical columns of labels are noted to be roughly perpendicular to the LGN laminae and in line with projection lines. Input to the LGN from cortical area 18 is relatively sparse and is found predominantly in the ventral magnocellular layer. The functional significance of these cortical inputs to the LGN is not clear, but differences in laminar location and density patterns or projections from each cortical area further suggest different functions for each set of connections. Layers 1 (receiving contralateral retinal projections) and 2 (receiving ipsilateral retinal projections) contain larger neurons and are therefore termed the *magnocellular* LGN layers. Conversely, layers 3 through 6 are termed *parvocellular* layers. There is considerable evidence that there are at least two types of retinal ganglion cells that project in a segregated fashion to either magnocellular (M cells) or parvocellular (P cells) LGN. Indeed, the retinal ganglion cells that project to magnocellular LGN are themselves larger and associated with larger dendritic fields; they have a faster conducted transient response compared with the smaller P cell–bound retinal ganglion cells.[70] Thereafter, this segregation remains true insofar as the magnocellular LGN projects to cortex

area 4C alpha, which eventually projects to middle temporal cortical area MT.[71–73] Conversely, the parvocellular LGN projects to cortical area 4C beta, and from there to layers 2 and 3 of area 17, to the "pale stripe" region of area 18, and finally to areas V3 and V4. Thus, at the LGN a major division between lines of information is already established.

The processing of visual signals occurs in part by means of a highly complex synaptic organization of relay cells within the LGN. Cortical and subcortical (including pontine reticular formation, pulvinar and superior colliculus) centers also have neural input to the LGN. For example, electrode stimulation of the optic radiation evokes LGN inhibition, and the LGN layer 2 response to electrical stimulation of the ipsilateral optic nerve is depressed by stimulation of the contralateral optic nerve. Therefore, there is ample evidence of corticofugal inhibition by descending projections (such as those described above) from visual cortex areas 17, 18, 19 (also termed V1, V2, and V3) and the middle temporal cortex. There is also evidence of retinogeniculate inhibition from the indirect input of the optic nerve. A detailed analysis of geniculate cytoarchitecture, synaptology, and neurophysiology is available elsewhere.[74,75]

The LGN has often been considered as a model system for the phenomenon of transsynaptic degeneration. Following lesions to retinal ganglion cell axons (in the optic nerve or elsewhere), changes are noted in the neurons and cytoarchitecture of the LGN that have been described as evidence of cell death consequent to presynaptic deafferentation.[76] Indeed, this has also been described as occurring in the reverse direction; optic atrophy can be seen following destruction of the geniculocortical radiations.[77] However, this phenomenon occurs primarily in children and is seen in adults only after very long-term intervals following lesions of the radiations or occipital cortex.[78] Anterograde transsynaptic degeneration probably does not occur; instead, atrophy (not cell death) of LGN neurons is the transsynaptic event that follows the loss of retinal ganglion cell axons.[79]

Visual Radiations

The geniculocalcarine fiber tract begins in the LGN and constitutes the "posterior" visual pathway that projects to the primary visual cortex. The primary visual cortex goes by many names, such as striate cortex, area 17, or as used in experimental research, V1. These myelinated fibers exit from the dorsal aspect of the LGN and then fan laterally and inferiorly through the temporal isthmus to sweep around in the anterior extension of the temporal (inferior) horn of the lateral ventricle (see Fig. 4–1). The most anteroinferior fiber fascicle forms a bend (Meyer's loop) containing fibers that represent the homonymous inferior retinal quadrants, which mediate information from the contralateral superior visual field. This loop is located approximately 4 to 5 cm caudal to the anterior tip of the temporal lobe. This configuration of the anterior portion of the visual radiations is the anatomic substrate that explains the tendency for superior quadrantanopic field defects ("pie in the sky") encountered in some temporal lobe lesions (see Chapter 7).

Both the superior and inferior fascicles of the visual radiations pass posteriorly as a vertically narrow fillet in the external sagittal striatum. This striatum lies just lateral to the tapetum of the corpus callosum, which separates the radiations from the cavities of the lateral ventricle. In the deep parietal lobe, the radiations pass just external to the trigone and occipital horn of the lateral ventricle. These visual fibers then turn medially above and below the occipital horn to terminate in the mesial surface of the occipital lobe, the striate (calcarine) cortex.

Occipital Cortex

The primary visual cortex (Brodmann area 17, or V1) lies in the interhemispheric fissure in relationship to the falx cerebri (Figs. 4–10 and 4–11). However, the large macular projection area extends 1 to 2 cm laterally onto

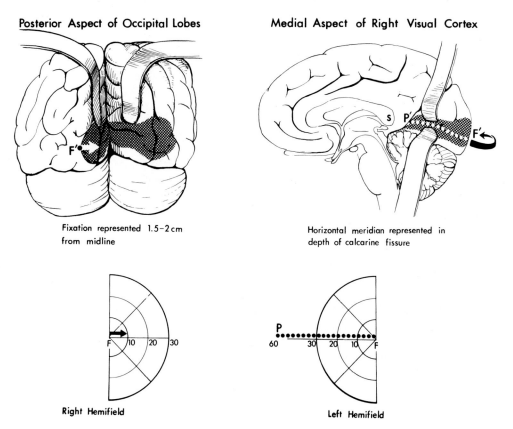

Fig. 4–10. Location of visual cortex primarily in interhemispherical fissure. Lateral extension as illustrated is variable. Point F′ corresponds to central fixation point F in contralateral field. Peripheral field point P is represented in rostral portion of cortex, P′. S, splenium of corpus callosum.

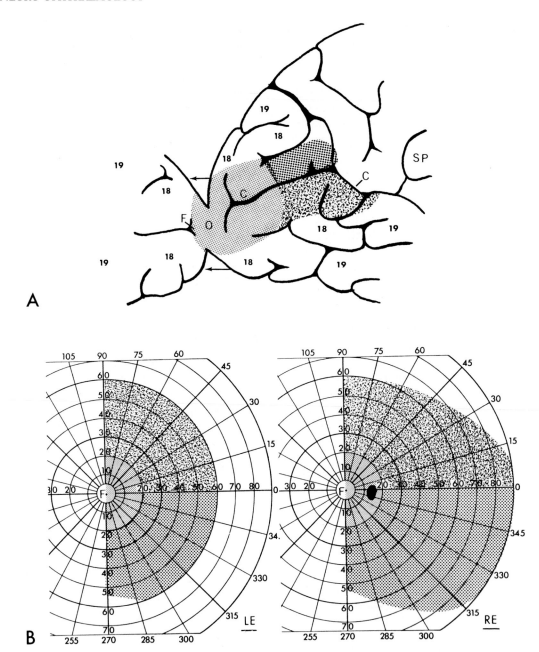

Fig. 4–11. Occipital lobe and the corresponding projection of the visual field. **A.** Mesial aspect of left occipital lobe. The posterior pole (*O*) is flattened to illustrate the lateral surface (*arrows*), which is composed primarily of areas 18 and 19. The extension of striate cortex onto the lateral surface of the occipital pole is variable. The calcarine fissure (*C*) separates the striate or calcarine cortex into an upper and a larger lower strip, which also extends further forward toward the splenium (*SP*) of the corpus callosum. The visual cortex is about 5 cm in horizontal diameter, and the macular projection (*fine stipple*) may occupy as much as the posterior 2.5 cm. The border zone between macular and peripheral retinal cortical projections is arbitrarily illustrated. **B.** The right hemifields. Note that the upper field is represented in the inferior calcarine strip and the lower field in the superior calcarine strip. The central field has a disproportionately large cortical representation. *F,* point of fixation. The temporal field of the right eye extends to 90° as compared with the nasal 60° limit of the left eye. This 30° monocular temporal crescent is represented only in the contralateral hemisphere at the rostral extreme of the striate cortex.

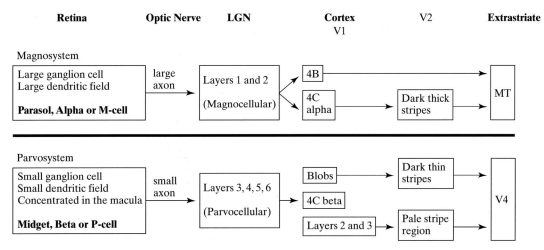

Fig. 4–12. Parallel processing in the primate visual system. *LGN,* lateral geniculate nucleus; *Magnosystem:* high contrast sensitivity, low spatial frequency, motion stereopsis. *MT,* middle temporal cortex; *Parvosystem:* low contrast sensitivity, high spatial frequency, color. V1, striate cortex (area 17); V2, parastriate cortex (area 18); V3 and V4, extrastriate cortex.

the posterior surface of the occipital cortex. The visual cortex extends anteriorly toward the splenium of the corpus callosum and is separated into a superior and an inferior portion by the calcarine fissure, which runs horizontally. This area about the calcarine fissure is termed the calcarine cortex (see Figs. 4–11 and 4–15). The macular projection area is disproportionately large, and the anterior extent of the calcarine fissure represents most of the contralateral visual field.[80] These anatomic features are relatively constant, even in patients with developmental defects of the anterior pathways, such as congenital anophthalmia.[81,82]

The visual cortex is further identified by specialized histologic features. Although the arrangement of cell nuclei and myelinated fibers is much the same as in other regions of the cortex, the visual cortex is characterized by a pronounced lamination oriented parallel to the cortical surface that produces more than the usual six cortical layers. Although the cellular population is greater here, the V1 visual cortex is thinner (about 1.5 mm) than most other cortical areas because the neuropil (intercellular spaces) is reduced. This homogeneous cellular composition suggested the appearance of dust to von Economo, for which reason he employed the term koniocortex. However, the most dramatic feature that distinguishes the visual cortex is the presence of a conspicuous, relatively acellular, myelinated fiber layer that is visible without magnification in sections perpendicular to the cortex. This is the white stria or stripe of Gennari or Vicq d'Azyr, which gives us the term striate cortex. An excellent description of the visual cortex and its cellular types and fiber connections is found in *The Vertebrate Visual System,* by Polyak.[83]

The anatomy and cytoarchitecture of the striate cortex have been well elucidated by electrophysiologic studies in the cat and monkey and by special staining techniques in the monkey and human. With microelectrodes placed in the cortex, visual stimuli are projected onto a tangent screen placed before the animal, such that the visual image is focused on the retina. The spatial and temporal properties of cortical cells are thus explored. Most cells in V1 respond only to stimuli in very restricted locations in the visual field and with very specific psychophysical properties. The position and diameter of a stimulus in the visual field by which a single cortical cell can be excited or inhibited in a specific manner is the "receptive field" of that cell. Hubel and Wiesel have been pioneers in the elucidation of cortical visual physiology.[84] Their description of visual cascade specification has been recognized with a Nobel prize.

A more precise understanding of the neurophysiology of the central visual pathways in the cortex has been obtained with the use of horseradish peroxidase, cytochrome oxidase, and other histologic techniques. The functional architecture of the striate cortex can be best appreciated by analysis of its input from the LGN (Fig. 4–12). Axons originating from magnocellular cells of the LGN project to area 4C alpha of V1, which projects to area 4B alpha of V1, which in turn projects both directly and indirectly to the middle temporal cortical area (MT). Conversely, parvocellular cells of the LGN project to 4C beta of V1, which projects to interblobs (identified by cytochrome oxidase) and interblob areas also in V1. Cells in these areas then project to the pale stripe zone of V2, and from there to other higher visual centers. Thus, there exists a magnocellular system that probably mediates low spatial resolution with high contrast sensitivity orientation, and movement sensitivity, directionality, and stereopsis. In contradistinction, the parvocellular system mediates primarily color and low contrast sensitivity at high spatial resolutions (visual acuity), without directionality or stereopsis.

Additionally, a third system termed the "blob" system has been described. The blobs (stained by cytochrome oxidase) probably receive both magnocellular and parvocellular input, analyze color, and convey information on brightness. In actuality, the segregation is neither quite so simple nor complete. Authoritative review of this rather complex functional anatomy and histoarchitecture is available elsewhere.[13,14,70,85,86]

Visual Association Areas and Interhemispheric Connections

For the visual environment to be analyzed, recognized, and interpreted, afferent visual information must be transferred from the striate cortex to higher visual association areas 18 (V2 or parastriate cortex), area 19, and to other analytic locations termed V3, V4, and MT.[70] In a simplified schematic, area 18 integrates the two halves of the visual fields by means of a major interhemispheric commissural pathway that traverses the splenium (most posterior portion) of the corpus callosum. Thus, areas V1, V2, and V3 in one hemisphere are interconnected to the same areas in the other hemisphere. Visual cortex area V2 probably participates in sensorimotor eye movement coordination through frontooccipital pathways and perhaps is a site of origin of corticomesencephalic optomotor pathways concerned with the smooth pursuit of visual targets. Cortical area V3 (peristriate cortex) accounts for the major lateral expanse of the occipital lobe and extends into the posterior parietal as well as the temporal lobes.

Visual information must be ultimately analyzed in the dominant parietal lobe, which is usually in the left hemisphere (Fig. 4–13). Objects in the right homonymous field of vision are "seen" by the left calcarine cortex; these stimuli are then transmitted to higher cortical centers (including the area of the angular gyrus) for processing. Visual stimuli arriving at the right visual cortex (coming from the left homonymous hemifields) must be passed through the splenium of the corpus callosum to the left parietal area to be recognized and, for reading or verbal description, interpreted. Therefore, lesions of the left angular gyrus will result in faulty verbal description of the visual target despite intact primary visual pathways. Patients with these lesions may experience any or all of the following as part of the subsequent communicative deficit: alexia, the inability to read despite normal vision; object agnosia, the inability to recognize objects

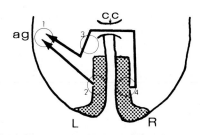

Fig. 4–13. Higher integration of vision. Diagram of primary visual cortices (*stippled*) and their projection to area of angular gyrus (*ag*) of left parietal lobe for analysis of visual stimuli. Note that right calcarine cortex is connected to left parietal area via pathway through splenium of corpus callosum (*cc*). Lesion 1 produces alexia and agraphia; lesion 2 produces only right homonymous hemianopia; combination of 2 and 3 produces right hemianopia and alexia despite intact left hemifields (*i.e.*, the right visual cortex is disconnected from visual analytic areas in the left parietal lobe); lesion 4 produces only left homonymous hemianopia.

by sight but maintain the ability to recognize them by touch; symbolic agnosia, the inability to recognize words, numbers, musical notes, actions, and gestures; and agraphia, the inability to write.

Lesions of the left visual cortex and splenium of the corpus callosum result in a remarkable clinical syndrome of visual disconnection called Geshwind's syndrome. In addition to the expected right homonymous hemianopsia, there is an inability to verbally interpret visual stimuli in the otherwise intact left hemifields. That is, only the right visual cortex remains intact, but it is "disconnected" from the angular gyrus (because of the callosal lesion) that deciphers written language for the perisylvian area of the left hemisphere. Thus, the patient is not able to read, but the capacity to write accurately is not disturbed (*i.e.*, alexia without agraphia). Patients with nondominant (right) parietal lobe lesions may demonstrate peculiar visual spatial anomalies. These include neglect or ignorance of left visual space (even without a left homonymous hemianopia) and spatial disorientation, including the inability to make skilled, purposeful movements (apraxia) in copying diagrams, dressing, and so forth. However, in apraxia there is no motor paralysis, ataxia, or sensory disturbance. Such patients make wrong turns on familiar routes, become confused in their own homes, misplace objects, and find routine and simple activities such as toothbrushing or hair combing exceedingly difficult (see Chapter 7).

Extrageniculate Visual Systems

It has long been known that subcortical visual systems exist in animals, as demonstrated by a variety of sophisticated tracing techniques.[83] However, until recently, these pathways were not demonstrated in man.[87] Retinotopic organization of the visual system in the superior colliculus has been established in many animals, including the monkey.[88] The superior colliculus (optic tectum) is critical in providing orientation and visually guided eye movements. Cells of the monkey superior colliculus respond to moving stimuli within specific receptor fields, and stimulation of these collicular cells results in predictable, reciprocal saccadic eye movements toward the specific visual field area. Recent studies in human brains[89] suggest that, as in simians, the human superior colliculus plays a role in the control of saccadic eye movements, visual orientation, tracking, and binocular vision. Additionally, a direct retinal projection to the human pulvinar nucleus has been demonstrated.[72] It is likely that the pulvinar contributes, along with the superior colliculus, to the visual processing that expedites the recognition of the position of objects in space, which in turn helps guide eye movements. Lesions of the pulvinar have been described in Alzheimer's disease, perhaps explaining the deficits of visual attention and eye movement control.[90]

The inter-relationship between the visual cortex, the superior colliculus, and the pulvinar is not fully understood. However, the visual acquisition of a target with accurate saccadic eye movements is probably dependent on both superior colliculus and pulvinar function, as well as on cortical input. Additionally, cells in the ventral superior colliculus have been shown to respond to auditory and tactile stimuli. Thus, it appears that the superior colliculus has more generic responsibilities regarding multimodal stimulus location and the integration of eye movement.

The accessory optic system (AOS) has also been extensively studied in vertebrates, including primates, and it has recently been identified in man.[91] In mammals, the AOS consists of two sets of retinofugal optic fibers that project to three target nuclei in the midbrain (dorsal, lateral, and medial terminal nuclei [DTN, LTN, and MTN, respectively]). On the basis of known inputs and outputs of the AOS, as well as on physiologic data, it is possible to postulate the functional importance of this set of nuclei. In man, the main function of the AOS nuclei is probably to correct for the "retinal slip" that results during head and eye movements. Thus, the AOS connections, in coordination with other brainstem nuclei, can be considered as "visual proprioception" and assist in providing dynamic stabilization of the eyes, neck, trunk, and limbs during body movement.[91]

Subjective visual phenomena have been recorded during subcortical (optic radiations and posterior hippocampus)[92] and brainstem[93] stimulation in humans. In some patients who are cortically blind for all other visual stimuli, there remains a recognition of movement or of sudden changes in illumination.[94] Other clinical visual

dissociations include the retention of movement perception in areas of field blind to formed targets, the so-called Riddoch phenomenon (see Chapter 7), and "blindsight," which consists of a retained capacity to localize objects in otherwise blind hemifields even as the subject denies any conscious visual sense.[95]

Although clinicians rarely consider any visual input other than the "primary" pathway to the LGN and striate cortex, and the luminance system of the pretectum that drives pupil constriction, it is clear that there are at least eight different retinofugal projections to visual sensory nuclei in the human brain. It is implied that each of these eight projections mediates a different visual function. It is also likely that classes of retinal ganglion cells with separate physiologic and psychophysical properties project to these distinctive visual nuclei. The schematic demonstrated in Figure 7 is a provisional neuroanatomic outline for parallel processing of vision in the human brain.

RETINOTOPIC ORGANIZATION

Visual space is represented on the retina in a direct point-to-point relationship. Because of the optical system of the eye, the superior visual field is projected onto the inferior retina, and the nasal field is projected onto the temporal retina. In general, this relationship holds true throughout the visual system, including the optic nerves, the optic chiasm, the radiations, and the visual cortex. Thus, the inferior visual field is transduced in the superior retina, and this information is mediated by the most superior axons throughout the visual pathways (except as the fibers approach the lateral geniculate nucleus).

The "retinotopic" projection of visual fibers through the anterior visual pathways has been carefully mapped in primates by Hoyt et al,[96-98] who used retinal photocoagulation and axonal degeneration staining techniques. Much of the following discussion is derived from that work.

Most visual fibers in the optic nerves and optic chiasm are derived from the large population of cells described as "midget" ganglion cells by Polyak.[83] These cells are now termed "P cells" because they project to the parvocellular LGN. The P cells largely subserve macular vision where they outnumber M cells by about 60 to 1. Potts et al[99] have analyzed the axonal population in the primate optic nerve with special reference to foveal outflow. They concluded that the total number of retinal ganglion cell axons in man was 1.1 to 1.3 million fibers per optic nerve. They confirmed the high density of small axons in the area of the optic nerve known to carry macular fibers and noted a loss of these small-caliber fibers after foveal photocoagulation in the monkey. Therefore, both anatomically and functionally, the optic nerves and optic chiasm can be considered as largely macular projection structures (see Fig. 4–9). The larger caliber peripheral retina axons subserving extramacular visual space tend to be distributed toward the periphery of the optic nerve. However, intermingling of fibers without strict boundaries is the rule. Generally, fibers that originate in the inferior retina remain inferior in the nerve and optic chiasm. The probable retinotopic organization of visual fibers in the optic nerves, optic chiasm, and optic tracts is demonstrated in Figure 4–14. Curiously, the retinotopic order is tighter in the orbital optic nerve and becomes less accurate as the fibers approach the chiasm.[51]

The arrangement of the retinal ganglion cell axons becomes considerably more complex as they approach the lateral geniculate body. In the LGN, a pattern of cellular layers is found (see Fig. 4–8). The extent of macular representation in humans has been well documented by Kupfer.[66] Focal vascular lesions of the LGN are only rarely recognized; this is most likely due to the dual blood supply through the anterior choroidal branch

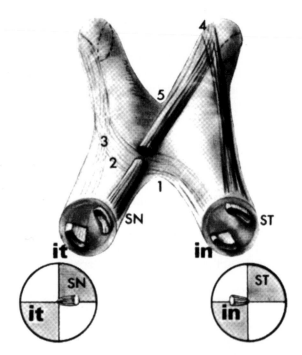

Fig. 4–14. Retinotopic organization of visual fibers in the anterior visual pathways (after Hoyt). Diagram of homonymous retinal quadrants and their fiber projections, anterior aspect. *it,* inferior temporal; *in,* inferior nasal; *SN,* superior nasal; *ST,* superior temporal. Note the following: the superior fibers retain a superior course, and the inferior fibers retain an inferior position; the anterior notch (*1*) is occupied by inferonasal (superior temporal field) fibers; the inferonasal fibers bend slightly into the contralateral nerve (*2*), Wilbrand's knee; inferior homonymous fibers converge in the chiasm (*3*) but superior homonymous fibers converge beyond the chiasm in the tract (*4*); the posterior notch (*5*) is occupied by superior nasal (inferior temporal field) fibers, as well as macular fibers (cf. Fig. 4–9).

of the middle cerebral artery (anterior circulation) and the thalamogeniculate branches that derive from the posterior cerebral and lateral choroidal arteries (posterior circulation).

As the geniculocalcarine radiations begin, the inferior retinal fiber projection (representing the superior visual field) takes an indirect and variable course for a short distance anteriorly around the tip of the temporal horn of the lateral ventricle, forming Meyer's loop. In the parietal mid-radiations, superior peripheral fibers are seemingly separated from inferior peripheral fibers by the mass of macular projection fibers. Further details of the distribution of fibers in the visual radiations are found in the works of Spalding[100] and of van Buren and Baldwin.[101]

The currently accepted conceptualization of the projection of the visual field on the occipital cortex in man is attributed primarily to the British neurologist Holmes,[102] who studied visual field defects that occurred after head injuries in World War I. Spalding also took advantage of material that accrued during World War II by examining visual field defects occurring after high-velocity penetrating head injuries.[103] With the use of modern imaging technique, Horton and Hoyt have modified this map of representation of the visual field in the human striate cortex.[104] The representation of the field of vision in the visual cortex as modified from the work of Holmes and Spalding is outlined in Figure 4–11.

The topographic anatomy of the human primary visual cortex has been studied with regard to the area, distribution, and variability of the striate cortex on the surface and also within the fissures of the occipital lobe.[105] The following conclusions may be drawn:

1. Only about one third of the striate cortex is on the surface of the occipital lobe, the major portion lying buried in the calcarine fissure, its branches, and accessory sulci.
2. As a rule, only a small portion (about 3% of the total area) of the striate cortex is exposed on the posterolateral aspect of the occipital poles.
3. There is more striate cortex above the calcarine fissure (about 60%) than below, and the inferior gyrus extends 1 to 2 cm more anteriorly than the superior gyrus.
4. The horizontal extent of the visual cortex is variable but usually measures about 5 cm from the occipital pole to the anterior extreme (in the lower calcarine lip).
5. There is variation in both area and general configuration when paired visual cortices from the same brain are compared.

Because of these anatomic variations in visual cortices, no finite point-to-point retinotopic representation, such as that based on surface landmarks, can be consistently applied at the occipital lobe. Brindley[106] has reported the effects of electrode stimulation in the human visual cortex (during attempts at designing a visual prosthesis device) in terms of evoked phosphenes in the visual field. His results were generally consistent with the established visual map of Holmes-Spalding.

Several other points deserve emphasis in regard to the retinotopic organization of the visual cortex.

1. The macular field (including the foveal fixation area) is predominantly represented unilaterally (see also Leventhal et al[20] above)
2. The central portion of the visual field is represented in the caudal cortex, but the correspondence of visual field position (*e.g.,* 10°) with the cortex locus (*e.g.,* 1 cm anterior to the occipital pole) is variable and thus uncertain.
3. The horizontal meridian of the visual field is represented in the depth of the calcarine fissure, but the middle of the calcarine fissure probably corresponds to a meridian 5° below fixation.
4. The vertical meridian of the visual field is represented in the perimeter of the striate cortex.
5. The unpaired monocular temporal crescent of field is represented in the most anterior aspect of the contralateral calcarine cortex.
6. The central 15° of field occupies about 40% of the surface area of the medial occipital lobe.[107]

VASCULAR SUPPLY

The microvasculature of the human optic nerve was well portrayed by Onda et al, who showed a stunning array of micrographs of methacrylate casts made from 18 normal eyes.[32] They confirmed that the vascular supply of the optic disc is derived mainly from the arteriole anastomotic circle of Zinn-Haller (see Fig. 4–4), which receives contributions primarily from the short posterior ciliary arteries. Additional contributions come from the pial arteriole plexus and the peripapillary choroid. The latter may also send small arterioles directly to the prelaminar disc substance. The central retinal artery nourishes the retina but probably contributes little or no blood to the optic nerve itself.

The intraorbital portion of the optic nerve is vascularized by perforating arteries derived from branches of

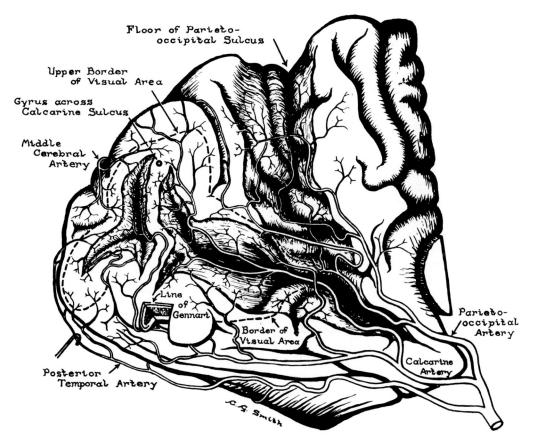

Fig. 4–15. Blood supply of striate cortex. Medial surface of left occipital lobe with visual cortex outlined by broken line. Calcarine and parieto-occipital fissures are opened to show course of cortical branches of posterior cerebral artery. Note potential triple supply to macular area, via the calcarine, posterior temporal, and middle cerebral arteries. (Smith CG, Richardson WFG: The course and distribution of the arteries supplying the visual (striate) cortex. Am J Ophthalmol 61:1391, 1966)

the ophthalmic artery. In the optic canal and suprasellar space, the optic nerve receives small pial branches from the internal carotid, anterior cerebral, and anterior communicating arteries. The ophthalmic artery is usually the first major intradural branch of the internal carotid artery. Rarely, the ophthalmic artery derives from the carotid artery while still within the cavernous sinus. Within the optic canal, the ophthalmic artery lies below the nerve and is enveloped within the dural sleeve of the optic nerve.

The arterial supply of the optic chiasm comes from a superior and an inferior group of vessels.[108] The superior group comprises multiple small branches from the pre-communicating portions of the anterior cerebral arteries. These vessels supply the upper surface of the optic nerves, the optic tracts, and the lateral portions of the optic chiasm. The inferior group of vessels is part of an extremely rich, anastomotic system described as the superior hypophyseal arteries. This system derives from the internal carotid, posterior communicating, and posterior cerebral arteries.

Anterior thalamic perforating branches of the posterior cerebral artery supply the optic tract; thalamogeniculate branches provide some of the blood supply to the LGN. A branch of the middle cerebral artery, the anterior choroidal artery, also supplies the optic tract, the LGN, and, variably, the initial portions of the visual radiation. Given the multiple blood supplies, it is not surprising that the posterior optic tract and LGN are rarely the site of a primary vascular lesion.

The anterior visual radiations may receive a branch of the middle cerebral artery, the deep optic artery, which passes through the putamen to the internal capsule. Branches of the middle cerebral artery in the sylvian fissure (*e.g.,* the inferior temporo-occipital artery) variably supply the temporal radiations. The superior temporo-occipital sylvian artery is the major blood supply of the posterior radiations and can anastomose with posterior cerebral vessels at the occipital pole, providing a dual blood supply to the visual cortical convexity. This arterial configuration forms the basis of one of the explanations for "macular sparing," which often characterizes cortical hemianopsias.

The posterior cerebral artery courses around the midbrain between the cerebral peduncle and the hippocampal gyrus of the temporal lobe, the inferior aspect of which is supplied by the anterior temporal artery, the first cortical branch of the posterior cerebral artery. The remaining three major cortical branches of the posterior cerebral artery—the posterior temporal, calcarine, and parieto-occipital arteries—may contribute to the visual cortex (Fig. 4–15). The blood supply of the striate cortex usually comes from the calcarine artery, but branches of the other two aforementioned vessels commonly share this responsibility and may account for the preserved portions of the visual field (including the macular

area), despite calcarine artery occlusion.[109] The terminal branches of the middle cerebral artery also supply the posterior aspect of the occipital pole.

REFERENCES

1. Sadun AA: Editorial prologue to the following three papers on parallel processing in the human visual system: a new perspective. J Clin Neuro Ophthalmol 6:351, 1986
2. Bruesch SR, Arey LB: The number of myelinated and unmyelinated fibers in the optic nerve of vertebrates. J Comp Neurol 77:631, 1942
3. Johnson BM, Miao M, Sadun AA: Age-related decline of human optic nerve axon populations. Age 10:5, 1987
4. Bruesch SR, Arey LB: The number of myelinated and unmyelinated fibers in the optic nerve of vertebrates. J Comp Neurol 77:631, 1942
5. Price J: The origins of neurons in the central nervous system. Eye 8:217, 1994
6. Lemire R, Loeser J, Leech R et al: Normal and Abnormal Development of the Human Nervous System. The Optic System, pp 196–205. New York, Harper & Row, 1975
7. Provis JM, van Driel D, Billson FA et al: Human fetal optic nerve overproduction and elimination of retinal axons during development. J Comp Neurol 238:92, 1985
8. Berry M, Hall S, Shewan D, Cohen J: Axonal growth and its inhibition. Eye 8:245, 1994
9. Targett MP, Blakemore WF: The use of xenografting to evaluate the remyelinating potential of glial cell cultures. Eye 8:238, 1994
10. Collelo RJ, Schwab ME: A role for oligodendrocytes in the stabilization of optic axon numbers. J Neurosci 14:6446, 1994
11. Livingstone M, Hubel D: Segregation of form, color, movement, and depth: anatomy, physiology, and perception. Science 240:740, 1988
12. Sadun AA: Vision: a multi-modal sense. Bull Clin Neurosci 50:61, 1985
13. Gegenfurtner KR, Kiper DC, Beusmans JM et al: Chromatic properties of neurons in macaque MT. Vis Neurosci 11:455, 1994
14. Beckers G, Zeki S: The consequences of inactivating areas V1 and V5 on visual motion perception. Vis Neurosci 11:455, 1994
15. Østerberg G: Topography of the layer of rods and cones in the human retina. Acta Ophthalmol (suppl 6), 1935
16. van Buren JM: The Retinal Ganglion Cell Layer, p 130. Springfield, IL, Charles C Thomas, 1963
17. Glaser JS: The nasal visual field. Arch Ophthalmol 77:358, 1967
18. Curcio CA, Sloan KR: Packing geometry of human cone photoreceptors: variation with eccentricity and evidence for local anisotropy. Vis Neurosci 9:169, 1992
19. Curcio CA, Millican CL, Allen KA, Kalina RE: Aging of the human photoreceptor mosaic: evidence for selective vulnerability of rods in central retina. Invest Ophthalmol Vis Sci 34(12):3278, 1993
20. Leventhal AG, Ault SJ, Vitek DJ: The nasotemporal division in primate retina: the neural bases of macular sparing and splitting. Science 240:66, 1988
21. Ogden TE: Nerve fiber layer of the owl monkey retina: retinotopic organization. Invest Ophthalmol Vis Sci 24:265, 1983
22. Hoyt WF, Luis O: Visual fiber anatomy in the infrageniculate pathway of the primate. Arch Ophthalmol 68:94, 1962
23. Jonas JB, Gusek GC, Naumann GOH: Optic disc, cup and neuroretinal rim size, configuration and correlations in normal eyes. Invest Ophthalmol Vis Sci 29:1151, 1988
24. Minckler DS: Histology of optic nerve damage in ocular hypertension and early glaucoma (summary). Surv Ophthalmol 33:401, 1989
25. Hernandez MR, Igoe F, Neufeld AH et al: Extracellular matrix of the human optic nerve head. Am J Ophthalmol 102:139, 1986
26. Minckler DS: Correlations between anatomic features and axonal transport in primate optic nerve head. Trans Am Ophthalmol Soc 84:429, 1986
27. Anderson DR, Hoyt WF: Ultrastructure of intraorbital portion of human and monkey optic nerve. Arch Ophthalmol 82:659, 1969

28. Anderson DR: Ultrastructure of the optic nerve head. Arch Ophthalmol 83:63, 1970
29. Ali BH, Logani S, Kozlov KL et al: Progression of retinal nerve fiber myelination in childhood. Am J Ophthalmol 118:515, 1994
30. Kurosawa H, Kurosawa A: Scanning electron microscopic study of pial septa of the optic nerve in humans. Am J Ophthalmol 99:490, 1985
31. Jeffery G, Evans A, Albon J et al: The human optic nerve. Fascicular organization and connective tissue types along the extra-fascicular matrix. Anat Embryol 191:491, 1995
32. Onda E, Cioffi GA, Bacon DR, van Buskirk EM: Microvasculature of the human optic nerve. Am J Ophthalmol 120:92, 1995
33. Olver JM, Spalton DJ, McCartney AC: Quantitative morphology of human retrolaminar optic nerve vasculature. Invest Ophthalmol Vis Sci 35:3858, 1994
34. Cioffi GA, van Buskirk EM: Microvasculature of the anterior optic nerve. Surv Ophthalmol 38:107, 1994
35. Anderson DR: Vascular supply of the optic nerve of primates. Am J Ophthalmol 70:341, 1970
36. Hayreh SS: Anatomy and physiology of the optic nerve head. Trans Am Acad Ophthalmol Otolaryngol 78:240, 1974
37. Chou PI, Sadun AA, Lee H: Vasculature and morphometry of the optic canal and intracanalicular optic nerve. J Neuroophthalmol 15:186, 1995
38. Chou PI, Sadun AA, Chen YC et al: Clinical experiences in the management of traumatic optic neuropathy. Neuro-Ophthalmology 16:325, 1996
39. Fujii K, Chambers SM, Rhoton AL: Neurovascular relationships of the sphenoid sinus. A microsurgical study. J Neurosurg 50:31, 1979
40. Walker AE: The neurosurgical evaluation of the chiasmal syndromes. Am J Ophthalmol 54:563, 1962
41. Bergland RM, Ray BS, Torack RM: Anatomical variations in the pituitary gland and adjacent structures in 225 human autopsy cases. J Neurosurg 28:93, 1968
42. Ikeda H, Yoshimoto T: Visual disturbances in patients with pituitary adenoma. Acta Neurol Scand 92:157, 1995
43. Sadun AA, Smythe BA, Schaechter JD: Optic neuritis or ophthalmic artery aneurysm? Case presentation with histopathologic documentation utilizing a new staining method. J Clin Neuro-Ophthalmol 4:265, 1984
44. Rucker CW: The concept of a semidecussation of the optic nerves. Arch Ophthalmol 59:159, 1958
45. Daniels DL, Haughton VM, Williams AC et al: Computed tomography of the optic chiasm. Radiology 137:123, 1980
46. Sadun AA: Commentary on optic nerve compression by a dolichoectatic internal carotid artery: case report by Colapinto EV, Cabeen MA, Johnson LN. Neurosurgery 39:606, 1996
47. Barber AN, Ronstrom GN, Mueeling RJ: Development of the visual pathway: optic chiasm. Arch Ophthalmol 52:447, 1954
48. Kupfer C, Chumbley L, Downer J, De CC: Quantitative histology of optic nerve, optic tract and lateral geniculate nucleus of man. J Anat 101:393, 1967
49. Marcus RC, Blazeski R, Godement P, Mason CA: Retinal axon divergence in the optic chiasm: uncrossed axons diverge from crossed axons within a midline glial specialization. J Neurosci 15:3716, 1995
50. Jacobson H, Hirose G: Origin of the retina from both sides of the embryonic brain: a contribution to the problem of crossing at the optic chiasma. Science 202:637, 1978
51. Guillery RW, Mason CA, Taylor JS: Developmental determinants at the mammalian optic chiasm. J Neurosci 15:4727, 1995
52. Marcus RC, Blazeski R, Godement P, Mason A: Retinal axon divergence in the optic chiasm: Uncrossed axons diverge from crossed axons within a midline glial specialization. J Neurosci 15:3716, 1995
53. Naito J: Retinogeniculate projection fibers in the monkey optic chiasm: a demonstration of the fiber arrangement by means of wheat germ agglutinin conjugated to horseradish peroxidase. J Comp Neurol 346:559, 1994
54. Silver J, Sapiro J: Axonal guidance during development of the optic nerve: the role of pigmented epithelia and other extrinsic factors. J Comp Neurol 202:521, 1981
55. Strongin AC, Guillery RW: The distribution of melanin in the developing optic cup and stalk and its relation to cellular degeneration. J Neurosci 1:1193, 1981
56. Recordon E, Griffith SG: A case of primary bilateral anophthalmia. Br J Ophthalmol 22:353, 1938
57. Rogalski T: The visual path in a case of unilateral ophthalmia with special reference to the problem of crossed and uncrossed visual fibers. J Anat 80:153, 1946
58. Sadun AA, Schaechter JD, Smith LEH: A retinohypothalamic pathway in man: light mediation of circadian rhythms. Brain Res 302:371, 1984
59. Sadun AA, Johnson BM, Schaechter JD: Neuroanatomy of the human visual system: Part III. Three retinal projections to the hypothalamus. Neuro-Ophthalmology 6(6):371, 1986
60. Stephan FK, Sucker I: Circadian rhythms in drinking behavior and locomotor activity are eliminated by hypothalamic lesions. Proc Natl Acad Sci USA 69:1583, 1982
61. Czissler CA, Shananhan TL, Klerman EB et al: Suppression of melatonin secretion in some blind patients by exposure to bright light. N Engl J Med 332:6, 1995
62. Schaechter JD, Sadun AA: A second hypothalamic nucleus receiving retinal input in man: the paraventricular nucleus. Brain Res 340:243, 1985
63. Sadun AA, Johnson BM, Smith LEH: Neuroanatomy of the human visual system: Part II. Retinal projections to the superior colliculus and pulvinar. Neuro-Ophthalmology 6:363, 1986
64. Chacko LW: The laminar pattern of the lateral geniculate body in primates. J Neurol Neurosurg Psychiatry 11:211, 1948
65. Hubel DH, Wiesel TN, LeVay S: Plasticity of ocular dominance columns in monkey striate cortex. Philos Trans R Soc Lond Biol Sci 278(961):377, 1977
66. Kupfer C: The projection of the macula in the lateral geniculate nucleus of man. Am J Ophthalmol 54:597, 1962
67. Bishop PO, Kozak W, Levick WR, Vakkur GJ: The determination of the projection of the visual field on the lateral geniculate nucleus in the cat. J Physiol (Lond) 163:503, 1962
68. Kaas JH, Guillery RW, Allman JM: Some principles of organization in the dorsal lateral geniculate nucleus. Brain Behav Evol 6:253, 1972
69. Lin CS, Kaas JH: Projections from cortical visual areas 17, 18 and MT onto the dorsal lateral geniculate nucleus in owl monkeys. J Comp Neurol 173:457, 1977
70. Livingstone MS, Hubel DH: Psychophysical evidence for separate channels for the perception of form, color movement, and depth. J Neurosci 7:3416, 1987
71. Leventhal AG, Rodieck RW, Dreher B: Retinal ganglion cells in the Old World monkey: morphology and central projections. Science 213:1139, 1981
72. Zeki SM: Representation of central visual fields in prestriate cortex of monkeys. Brain Res 14:271, 1969
73. Lund JS, Boothe RG: Intralaminar connections and pyramidal neuron organization in the visual cortex, area 17, of the macaque monkey. J Comp Neurol 159:305, 1975
74. Szentagothai J: Neuronal and synaptic architecture of the lateral geniculate nucleus. In Jung R (ed): Handbook of Sensory Physiology, Vol VII/3B, pp 141–176. Berlin, Springer-Verlag, 1973
75. Freund J-H: Neuronal mechanisms of the lateral geniculate body. In Jung R (ed): Handbook of Sensory Physiology, Vol VII/3B, pp 177–246. Berlin, Springer-Verlag, 1973
76. Matthews MR: Transneuronal cell degeneration in the lateral geniculate nucleus of the macaque monkey. J Anat 94:145, 1960
77. van Buren JM: Transsynaptic retrograde degeneration in the visual system of primates. J Neurol Neurosurg Psychiatry 26:402, 1963
78. Beatty B, Sadun A, Smith L, Richardson E: Direct demonstration of transsynaptic degeneration in the human visual system: a comparison of retrograde and anterograde changes. J Neurol Neurosurg Psychiatry 45(2):143, 1982
79. Sadun AA: The neuroanatomy of the human visual system: Part I. Retinal projections to the LGN and PT as demonstrated with a new stain. Neuro-Ophthalmology 6(6):353, 1986
80. Horton JC, Hoyt WF: The representation of the visual field in human striate cortex. Arch Ophthalmol 109:816, 1991
81. Kuljis RO: Development of the primary visual (striate) cortex in patients with congenital anophthalmia. Int Pediatr 10:133, 1995

82. Kuljis RO, Rakic P: Hypercolumns in primate visual cortex can develop in the absence of cues from photoreceptors. Proc Natl Acad Sci USA 87:5303, 1990

83. Polyak S: The Vertebrate Visual System. Chicago, University of Chicago Press, 1957

84. Holden AL: The central visual pathways. In Davson H (ed): The Eye: Visual Function in Man, Vol 2A, pp 357–474. New York, Academic Press, 1976

85. Lund JS: Anatomical organization of macaque monkey striate visual cortex. Annu Rev Neurosci 11:253, 1988

86. Kuljis RO, Rakic P: Neuropeptide Y–containing neurons are situated predominantly outside cytochrome oxidase puffs in macaque visual cortex. Vis Neurosci 2:57, 1989

87. Sadun AA: Parallel processing in the human visual system: a new perspective. Neuro-Ophthalmology 6:351, 1986

88. Schiller PH: The role of the monkey superior colliculus in eye movement and vision. Invest Ophthalmol Vis Sci 11:451, 1972

89. Sadun AA, Johnson BM, Smith LEH: Neuroanatomy of the human visual system: Part II. Retinal projections to the superior colliculus and pulvinar. Neuro-Ophthalmology 6:363, 1986

90. Kuljis RO: Lesions in the pulvinar in patients with Alzheimer's disease. J Neuropathol Exp Neurol 53:202, 1994

91. Fredericks CA, Giolli RA, Blanks RH, Sadun AA: The human accessory optic system. Brain Res 454:116, 1988

92. Adams JE, Rutkin BB: Visual responses to subcortical stimulation in the visual and limbic systems. Confin Neurol 32:158, 1970

93. Nashold BS: Phophenes resulting from stimulation of the midbrain in man. Arch Ophthalmol 84:433, 1970

94. Brindley GS, Gautier-Smith PC, Lewin W: Cortical blindness and the functions of the non-geniculate fibers of the optic tracts. J Neurol Neurosurg Psychiatry 32:259, 1969

95. Weiskrantz L: Blindsight: A Case Study and Implications. Oxford Psychological Series No. 10, New York, Oxford Press, 1986

96. Hoyt WF, Luis O: Visual fiber anatomy in the intrageniculate pathway of the primate: uncrossed and crossed retinal quadrant fiber projections studied with Nauta silver stain. Arch Ophthalmol 68:94, 1962

97. Hoyt WF, Luis O: The primate chiasm: details of visual fiber organization studied by silver impregnation techniques. Arch Ophthalmol 70:69, 1963

98. Hoyt WF, Tudor RC: The course of parapapillary temporal retinal axons through the anterior optic nerve: a Nauta degeneration study in the primate. Arch Ophthalmol 69:503, 1963

99. Potts AM, Hodges D, Shelman CB et al: Morphology of the primate optic nerve I-III. Invest Ophthalmol Vis Sci 11:980, 1972

100. Spalding JMK: Wounds of the visual pathway: I. The visual radiation. J Neurol Neurosurg Psychiatry 15:99, 1952

101. van Buren JM, Baldwin M: The architecture of the optic radiation in the temporal lobe of man. Brain 81:15, 1958

102. Holmes G: A contribution to the cortical representation of vision. Brain 54:470, 1931

103. Spalding JMK: Wound of the visual pathway: II. The striate cortex. J Neurol Neurosurg Psychiatry 15:169, 1952

104. Horton JC, Hoyt WF: The representation of the visual field in human striate cortex. A revision of the classic Holmes map. Arch Ophthalmol 109:816, 1991

105. Stensaas MA, Eddington DK, Dobelle WH: The topography and variability of the primary visual cortex in man. J Neurosurg 40:747, 1974

106. Brindley GS: Sensory effects of electrical stimulation of the visual and paravisual cortex in man. In June R (ed): Handbook of Sensory Physiology, Vol VII/3B, pp 583–594. Berlin, Springer-Verlag, 1973

107. Wong AMF, Sharpe JA: Representation of the visual field in the human occipital cortex. A magnetic resonance imaging and perimetric correlation. Arch Ophthalmol 117:208, 1999

108. Bergland RM, Ray BS: The arterial supply of the human optic chiasm. J Neurosurg 31:327, 1969

109. Smith CG, Richardson WFG: The course and distribution of the arteries supplying the visual (striate) cortex. Am J Ophthalmol 61:1391, 1966

CHAPTER 5

Topical Diagnosis: Prechiasmal Visual Pathways

Part I. The Retina

Joel S. Glaser

Symptomatology
Heredodegenerations and Abiotrophies
　Pigmentary Retinopathies
　Cone and Cone-Rod Dystrophies
Chorio-retinal Inflammations
Metabolic Storage Disorders
Retinal Arterial Occlusions
　Carotid Atheromatous Disease
　Other Retinal Arterial Occlusions
　Retinal Migraine

Retinal Vasculitis
Uveo-Meningeal Syndromes
Human Immunodeficiency Virus Infection and AIDS
Toxic Retinopathies
Congenital Hamartoma Syndromes
　Tuberous Sclerosis
　Neurofibromatosis

To suppose that the eye, with all its inimitable contrivances for adjusting the focus to different distances, for admitting different amounts of light, and for the correction of spherical and chromatic aberration, could have been formed by natural selection, seems, I freely confess, absurd in the highest possible degree.

Charles Darwin
"Organs of extreme perfection and complication"
In *The Origin of Species,* 1859

Accurate diagnosis of disorders of the visual sensory system is dependent on knowledgeable history taking and competent evaluation of visual function, including acuity, visual fields, and color perception, of pupillary light reactions and of the fundi. There are no valid diagnostic shortcuts; rather, there are guiding principles and axioms that should at least determine a provisional impression and course of investigation, if not provide a conclusive diagnosis. Part I of this chapter is intended to provide a reasonably detailed overview of those retinal disorders and diseases that may confound or otherwise touch on neuro-ophthalmologic diagnosis.

J. S. Glaser: Departments of Neurology and Ophthalmology, Bascom Palmer Eye Institute, University of Miami School of Medicine, Miami; and Neuro-ophthalmology, Cleveland Clinic Florida, Ft. Lauderdale, Florida

SYMPTOMATOLOGY

Diseases and pathologic alterations involving the retina provoke the least clinical dilemma in that, for the most part, the ophthalmoscope resolves the question of the *anatomic level* at which the visual pathways are involved. The problem of complicated neurodiagnostic studies should not arise, although fluorescein angiography, electroretinography (ERG), and other retinal function tests (see Chapter 2) may prove valuable. There are two major pitfalls to be avoided. First, minimal retinal changes may be misconstrued as the cause of disproportionately perturbed visual function, or a normal macula may be misinterpreted as abnormal. For example, a patient with relentless monocular visual loss, a central field depression, and afferent-defect pupil, with a few drusen or minimal derangement of retinal pigment epithelium at the fovea, must not be dismissed with an inappropriate diagnosis of "macular degeneration." In this instance, the afferent-defect pupil indicates a conductive lesion of the optic nerve and cannot be attributed to minimal retinochoroidal disease. Second, true macular disease, especially when bilateral and ophthalmoscopically subtle, should raise the question of macular dystrophies that masquerade as neurologic disease or for which no cause is apparent (Fig. 5–1). Indeed, there are increasing numbers of retinal disorders that

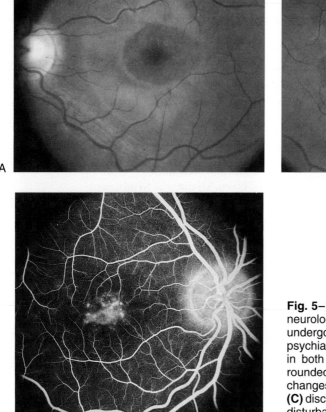

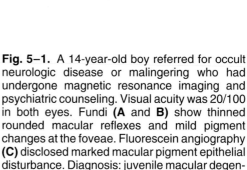

Fig. 5–1. A 14-year-old boy referred for occult neurologic disease or malingering who had undergone magnetic resonance imaging and psychiatric counseling. Visual acuity was 20/100 in both eyes. Fundi **(A** and **B)** show thinned rounded macular reflexes and mild pigment changes at the foveae. Fluorescein angiography **(C)** disclosed marked macular pigment epithelial disturbance. Diagnosis: juvenile macular degeneration (Stargardt's type).

produce subtle or even insignificant objective fundal changes that may escape conventional ophthalmoscopic detection.

These "hidden" retinal disorders include the following: congenital and hereditary photoreceptor or pigment epithelial abiotrophies and dystrophies; immune-mediated retinopathy associated with distant carcinoma; and an enlarging list of acute zonal occult outer retinopathies, conveniently labeled AZOOR by Gass and associates.[1,2] Previously lumped as the "big blind spot syndrome," AZOOR now encompasses a variety of heterogeneous, presumably inflammatory, retinopathies to be discussed below. Other lesions such as serous detachment of the macula (central serous choroidopathy) or cone dystrophies may be quite subtle on funduscopic examination alone, even during biomicroscopy with the use of a corneal contact lens or Hruby lens. It is in such situations that auxiliary tests of visual function, including color function, Amsler grid, photostress, ERG, and fluorescein angiography are critical in distinguishing modest lesions involving the choroid and retina from early optic nerve compression and demyelination.

In the assessment of visual function, the role of retinal aging alone is noteworthy. Even as macular photoreceptors are incompletely developed at birth and do not reach maturity until at least 4 years post partum, so virtually every parameter of visual function declines from midadulthood onward. Age-related degradations in reading acuity, color perception, and feature recognition (contrast sensitivity) are caused by senescent changes of neuronal elements, and, in fact, over a 70-year life span there is a loss of almost 50% of retinal ganglion cells, some half of which serve the macula.[3] After the age of 40 years, there is apparently a linear net loss of cone photoreceptors especially from the fovea, to which is added the nonneural factors of increasing pupillary miosis and decreasing lens transparency.[4] Other studies dispute an age-related reduction in rod and cone counts.[5]

The *temporal profile* of monocular visual deficit is often an important clue in differential diagnosis. Abrupt, non-transient visual symptoms usually indicate retinal artery or vein occlusion, infarction of the optic disc, retinal detachment, or hemorrhage into the vitreous. Age-related macular degeneration may suddenly cause hemorrhage beneath the fovea. In addition, on occasion, optic neuritis may run a course that is interpreted by the patient as abrupt, rather than subacute or rapidly progressive. Transient visual events are considered below (see Table 5–3).

HEREDODEGENERATIONS AND ABIOTROPHIES

Pigmentary Retinopathies

Heredodegenerative retinal disorders such as retinitis pigmentosa are almost always separable from "neurologic" causes of visual deficits on the basis of chronicity, bilaterality, and typical funduscopic appearance of pigmentary retinopathy, attenuated arteriolar tree, and waxy disc pallor. "Retinitis pigmentosa" is actually a misnomer twice over: the progressive photoreceptor degeneration is not inflammatory, as "-itis" would imply; and pigmentary changes evolve relatively late and may not be obvious. The term "retinitis pigmentosa sine pigmento" is not a separate entity, but it represents a stage of disorder when the retina appears relatively unaltered but photoreceptor function is defective.

A thorough account of retinal photoreceptor dystrophies is beyond the scope of neuro-ophthalmologic subjects, but A. C. Bird's Jackson Lecture[6] provides an overview of current concepts of clinical classification, molecular biology, and therapeutic advances. Hereditary transmission may follow autosomal dominant or recessive, or X-linked, patterns, with a spectrum of responsible gene mutations. Indeed, molecular geneticists have now identified numerous mutations in literally dozens of genes that are associated with or cause photoreceptor degeneration, findings suggesting an extraordinary vulnerability of these cells, possible stemming from their high-oxygen–requiring metabolism and physiologic population culling. These detailed genetic elaborations are replacing imprecise, if more classic, clinical descriptions.[6]

In the fully developed disorder, there is usually profound constriction of the fields with relative sparing of the central fixational area, resulting in so-called "gun-barrel" or "tubular" field constriction. End-stage retinitis pigmentosa is actually one of the few organic causes of markedly narrowed visual fields. The causes of such "gun-barrel" field constrictions are listed in Table 5–1. The retained field function actually mimics a *cone* (see Fig. 2–19), because the central remnant enlarges as the

TABLE 5–1. Constricted Field with Retained Acuity

Glaucoma, late
Retinitis pigmentosa
Post-papilledema optic atrophy
Hyaline bodies (drusen) of optic disc
Bilateral occipital infarcts with "macular sparing"
Malingering or hysteria

testing distance is increased between the patient and, for example, the tangent screen. The field diameter does *not* enlarge with increasing testing distances in hysteria or malingering, and, in fact, the diameter of the field may shrink further if this possibility is suggested to the naive patient.

Atypical cases of selective pigmentary degeneration of the nasal retinal sectors (Fig. 5–2) produce field defects that may mimic bitemporal hemianopias. Such preferential involvement of the fundus *nasal* to the optic disc occurs in at least one-third of patients with *sectoral* retinitis pigmentosa. Nerve fiber bundle scotomas, somewhat mimicking glaucoma, are also recorded.[7,8]

Acuity is reduced when cystic or wrinkling changes occur at the fovea or as the central aperture of field finally darkens. Disc pallor and retinal arteriolar attenuation are *not* simply the result of ganglion cell death because the ganglion cell and nerve fiber layer of the retina are affected only late in the disease. Unilateral or bilateral disc hyaline bodies (drusen), at times most marked in peripapillary and juxtapapillary locations, occur in some 10% of all genetic subtypes.[9]

Central field defects with acuity loss occur with photoreceptor degeneration that especially affects the macula, so-called retinitis pigmentosa *inversa*, but this disorder likely represents a separate nosologic class, the cone-rod dystrophies (see below) (Fig. 5–3). Severe visual defect in early infancy is frequently enough caused by a primary outer segment retinal abiotrophy, Leber's *congenital amaurosis,* although this is probably not a single clinical entity. This disorder is characterized by the following: severe impairment of vision, present at birth or becoming evident during early to late infancy; a fundus that may initially approach normal, but within years, optic atrophy, diffuse fine pigmentary degeneration, and attenuation of the arteriolar tree are evident; and either an absent or a markedly reduced ERG response. Other variable features include nystagmus, photophobia, digito-ocular maneuver (forceful eye rubbing with sunken globes; "blindisms"), strabismus, cataracts, hyperopia, mental retardation, deafness, renal anomalies, seizures, hydrocephalus, and focal neurologic deficits (*e.g.,* cerebral diplegia). Hereditary transmission is typically autosomal recessive[10] (see Chapter 13).

Cone and Cone-Rod Dystrophies

As noted above, the macular ("inversa") form of abiotrophic pigmentary retinopathy is actually a selective loss of cone function, but rod function also is defective. Indeed, retinal dystrophies accompanying many systemic disorders are typically, but not exclusively, this macular form. Of special neuro-ophthalmologic interest is the association of this and other geographic pigmentary patterns with hereditary cerebellar ataxias,[11,12] with olivopontocerebellar and spinocerebellar degener-

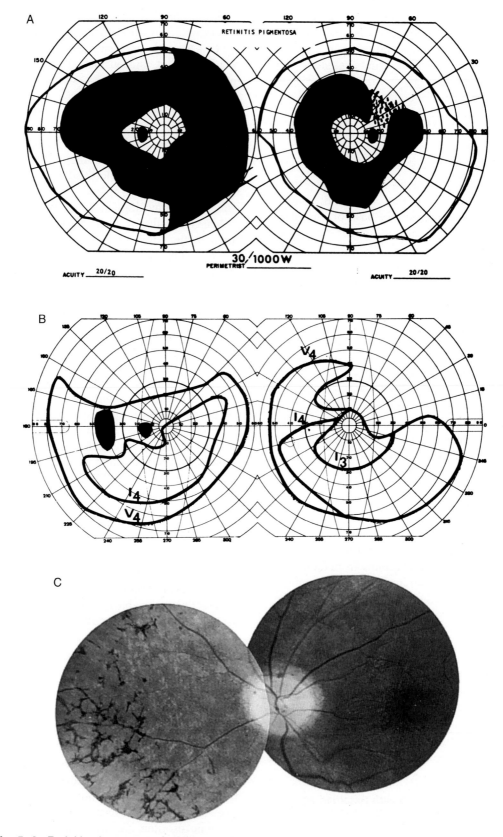

Fig. 5–2. Retinitis pigmentosa. **A.** Advanced field loss showing dense annular defects. Deficits start in the 20° to 30° middle zone (as compared with Bjerrum's zone defects in glaucoma) and proceed toward fixation and outward toward the periphery. Central fixation is relatively spared, producing "gun-barrel fields." **B.** The pseudobitemporal field defects of sector retinitis pigmentosa. Unlike chiasmal interference, the defects cross the vertical meridian. **C.** Left fundus of patient with nasal-sector retinitis pigmentosa.

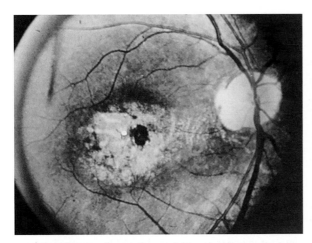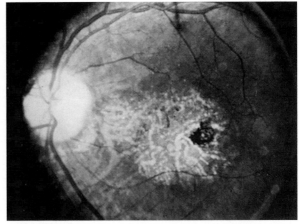

Fig. 5–3. Cone-rod dystrophy or so-called "retinitis pigmentosa inversa" in a young man with progressive spinocerebellar degeneration and 20/200 acuity in each eye.

ations,[12–14] and with Friedreich's ataxia.[15] These disorders are usually dominantly inherited, with variable expression of early life onset of progressive spasticity, ataxia, slowed saccades or supranuclear ophthalmoplegia, and chorioretinal macular dystrophy. Trinucleotide gene expansion (point mutation) is incriminated, but not exclusively. In Friedreich's ataxia, the most common inherited, if clinically inhomogeneous, spinocerebellar ataxia, a mitochondrial location of frataxin (Friedreich's ataxia protein) has been identified; this locus on chromosome 9 reflects the relationship with vitamin E deficiency ataxia and certain neuropathies with mutations in nuclear genes.[16]

Other subsets of pigmentary retinopathies are due to mitochondrial DNA mutations and are associated with migraine, ataxia, dementia, and Leigh's disease[17]; the sporadic or maternally inherited MELAS syndrome of mitochondrial myopathy, encephalopathy, lactic acidosis, and stroke-like episodes, usually presents in the teens as cognitive regression, headaches, and cerebral lesions causing field defects.[18–20] Even in family members, there is considerable variation of genotypic and phenotypic specificity in metabolic disorders mediated by mitochondrial DNA aberrations, including Kearns-Sayre progressive external ophthalmoplegia (see Chapter 12) and other conglomerations of pigmentary retinopathies. Further identification of gene point mutations will eventually provide a more precise classification.

Progressive cone degenerations present as bilaterally diminished acuity, defective color vision, and aversion to bright lights (photophobia) with "day blindness" (hemeralopia). Central field defects progress, at times showing a fenestrated central scotoma. This widespread loss of cone function usually begins in the first 2 decades of life, but severe cone disease may begin at any age. Heredity is autosomal dominant, but sporadic cases are common, and both severity and rate of progression are variable. The fundus may appear quite normal, a finding that, when coupled with photophobia, provokes an im-

pression of hysteria, but defective pigment epithelium in the form of a "bullseye," nonspecific mottling, and crystalline deposits are usually enhanced by fluorescein angiography (see also Fig. 5–1). Mild disc pallor is not unusual. Abnormal single-flash photopic and flicker (*i.e.,* cone-mediated) responses define the disorder by ERG[21]; fluorescein angiography and full-field ERG may be inconclusive, yet focal ERG is abnormal.[22] If considered sooner rather than later, full-field or focal ERG should obviate more exhaustive and inappropriate diagnostic studies for optic nerve disease.

Cones may be congenitally absent, as in the case of *rod monochromatism,* a rare form of "color blindness" with acuity of about 20/200 and reduced visual capacity under bright light situations; that is, these children show a preference for dim illumination. Pendular or mixed jerk-pendular nystagmus patterns are typical, and the fundus foveal reflex may be blunted. ERG shows absent or markedly subnormal photopic (cone) responses, but normal scotopic (rod) responses.

Pigmentary retinopathies, or more typically cone-rod dystrophies, keep company with a large number of other neurodegenerative and metabolic disorders, such as Bassen-Kornzweig syndrome, Refsum's disease, Kearns-Sayre progressive ophthalmoplegia (see Chapter 12), Laurence-Moon-Bardet-Biedl cerebellar ataxia, and sensorineural hearing loss. A complete description of the retinal abiotrophies, dystrophies and degenerations may be found in topical reviews, and pertinent texts. Age-related macular degenerations and other macular dystrophies and abiotrophies without neurologic implications are beyond the scope of this chapter.

CHORIO-RETINAL INFLAMMATIONS

As noted above, Gass[1] and others have elaborated a class of acute and subacute, diffuse or focal, presumed inflammatory zonal disorders of the outer retinal layers, now termed AZOOR. Roughly described as "enlarged blind spots" and thus confounding neurologic diagnosis, this somewhat heterogeneous rubric includes MEWDS (multiple evanescent white dot syndrome), multifocal choroiditis, acute macular neuroretinopathy, pseudo-presumed histoplasmosis, and idiopathic blind spot enlargement. These entities share a constellation of signs and symptoms and so raise the question of a spectrum of common origin involving geographic zones of retinal photoreceptors and pigment epithelium. Characteristics include the following: predilection for female patients; acute onset in one or both eyes, associated with photopsias; minimal fundus findings at onset, but eventual minor pigment epithelial disturbances; ERG abnormalities; fluorescein angiographic evidence of geographic thinned pigment epithelium; vitreous cells; and permanent field depressions often close to the physiologic blind spot. Taken as a group, Jacobson et al[2] investigated the nature of retinal dysfunction and found patchy but dense scotomas and ERG abnormalities, but no evidence of autoantibodies to specific retinal antigens. Recurrent central nervous system (CNS) inflammation in association with AZOOR is reported,[23] characterized by cerebrospinal fluid (CSF) lymphocytosis and multiple magnetic resonance imaging (MRI) signal abnormalities, followed in 6 years by an episode of cervical myelopathy.

Acute multifocal retinitis, another idiopathic inflammation in eyes of healthy young to middle-aged adults, may be associated with optic disc edema and may follow flu-like prodromes.[24] Mild vitrous reaction and macular exudative stars are characteristic, and a self-limited benign outcome is usual, with no evidence of specific infectious or autoimmune causes. Other relatively acute multifocal chorio-retinal inflammations include presumed ocular histoplasmosis, coccidioidomycosis, *Pneumocystis carinii* infection, cryptococcosis, mycobacterial or syphilitic choroiditis, birdshot (vitiliginous) retinochoroidopathy, punctate inner choroidopathy, and acute multifocal posterior placoid pigment epitheliopathy (AMPPPE). Although specific infectious agents may also be incriminated in meningeal reactions, such as cryptococcosis, AMPPPE is associated with CSF pleocytosis and protein elevation, findings suggesting possible viremia.[25] The foregoing discussion has focused on retinal pigmentary and macular disease in relation to neurologic disorders, not simple isolated macular dystrophies, which are considered at length elsewhere.[23,26]

METABOLIC STORAGE DISORDERS

Biochemical assays have considerably clarified the nosologic status of the group of storage diseases previously classified as the "cerebromacular degenerations," of which Tay-Sachs disease is the eponymous prototype. Although these disorders share a superficial resemblance, showing a progressive neurodegenerative course with variable fundus findings, they are now best classified by abnormal storage products (*e.g.,* sphingolipidoses, mucopolysaccharidoses, and mucolipidoses) and lysosomal enzyme deficiencies. Lysosomes contain hydrolytic enzymes that degrade proteins, polysaccharides, and nucleic acids; if undegraded, these materials accumulate in lysosomes and impair cell function. The complex lipids and saccharides indigenous to neural cells produce symptoms and signs related to eye and brain, including corneal clouding, macular "cherry-red spot," pigment epithelial degenerations, optic atrophy, mental deterioration, seizures, motor incoordination, myoclonus, and death.

The ganglion cell layer of the retina is a principal site of abnormal accumulation of anomalous storage products, such that ophthalmoscopic changes are observable either in the form of retinal "graying" or the well-known cherry-red spot. The ganglion cell layer densely surrounds the thin fovea, which transmits the normal red color of underlying choroid (Fig. 5–4). The storage disorders with cherry-red spot or macular graying are listed in Table 5–2.[27]

In addition to retinal changes, pallor of the optic disc occurs in numerous storage disorders, the nerve being affected by several mechanisms. Optic atrophy occurs when abnormal glycolipids are stored in retinal ganglion cells with subsequent neuronal death and nerve pallor, such as occurs in Tay-Sachs disease (Gm_2 gangliosidosis), but ophthalmoscopic evidence of optic atrophy is not invariable. Tay-Sachs is an autosomal recessive inherited disease, resulting from mutations of the hexosaminidase (Hex) A gene coding for the alpha-subunit of beta-D-*N*-acetyl-hexosaminodase. Juvenile and adult Hex A deficiencies are rare, less severe variants. Both

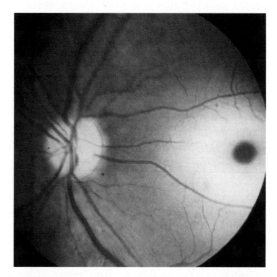

Fig. 5–4. "Cherry-red spot" of advanced Tay-Sachs disease (gangliosodosis). Note the central foveal window surrounded by a ring of densely opaque retinal ganglion cell layer; also, optic atrophy.

TABLE 5–2. Storage Diseases with Macular Changes

Sphingolipidoses
  Gm_1 gangliosidosis ("Generalized" gangliosidosis)
  Tay-Sachs disease (Gm_2 gangliosidosis type I)
  Sandhoff's disease (Gm_2 gangliosidosis type II)
  Niemann-Pick disease
  Lactosyl ceramidosis
  Childhood metachromatic leukodystrophy
Mucolipidoses
  Mucoliposaccharidosis (MLS) type I
    (lipomucopolysaccharidosis)
  Farber's disease
  Sea-blue histiocyte syndrome or chronic Niemann-Pick
    disease (yellow perifoveal granules)
  Mucolipidosis I (lipomucopolysaccharidosis) (Spranger)
Unclassified

infantile and late forms are most prevalent among Ashkenazi (roughly, Middle and Eastern European) Jews, but are reported in non-Jews, in whom clinically benign mutations may occur.[28,29] MRI findings include hyperintensities in basal ganglia and thalamus, with marked brain atrophy and diffuse white matter lesions; these findings likely reflect accumulation of Gm_2 ganglioside.[30] Similarly, in Gm_1 gangliosidosis (generalized gangliosidosis; "Tay-Sachs disease with visceral involvement"), there is also an abnormal deposition of ganglioside in the retina, with subsequent atrophy of the nerve, but it is a mucopolysaccharide that accumulates in the viscera.

Metachromatic leukodystrophy (sulfide lipidosis) is an autosomal recessive deficiency of arylsulfatase A, with ceramide-galactose sulfate in retinal ganglion and glial cells and macrophages in the optic nerve; a cherry-red spot occurs occasionally. The optic atrophy of Krabbe's disease (formerly considered one of the familial diffuse scleroses) is due to extensive demyelination associated with the accumulation of globoid bodies containing ceramide-galactose resulting from beta-galactosidase deficiency.

The *ceroid lipofuscinoses* are among the most commonly inherited childhood neurodegenerative disorders. These autosomal recessive syndromes are caused by accumulation of an insoluble, complex lipopigment that demonstrates autofluorescence and appears microscopically as characteristic curvilinear bodies. Histopathologic examination discloses degeneration of rods and cones beginning at the macula, narrowing of retinal vessels, atrophy of pigment epithelium with pigment migration, and curvilinear bodies in ganglion cells. These progressive disorders are not genetically homogeneous and are separable into infantile, late infantile, juvenile, and Finnish variants. These share seizures, motor disturbances, visual impairment, dementia, and autosomal inheritance.[31]

The late infantile type (Bielschowsky-Jansky) is a fatal recessively inherited disorder with genomic defect localized to chromosome 13q22, thus delineating this disease as a separate entity.[32] Presentation is with developmental arrest and seizures at 2 to 5 years of age, with motor and visual symptoms thereafter. There is massive tissue accumulation of lysosomal hydrophobic subunit-c protein of the mitochondrial adenosine triphosphate synthase. Ganglion cells are decreased in number, with thinning of the nerve fiber layer and optic atrophy. In addition, there is involvement of the outer segments with degeneration of the rods and cones and pigmentary clumping in the outer retinal layers. On MRI, hyperintense periventricular signals correlate with severe loss of myelin.[33]

Juvenile amaurotic idiocy (Batten-Mayou, Vogt-Spielmeyer) presents as visual loss in early adolescence and is characterized by retinal pigmentary changes predominantly at the macula, with late and minimal pallor of the disc. Apoptosis of photoreceptors and brain neurons has been confirmed as the mechanism of cell death.[34] At a later stage, motor and mental deficits evolve. The late or adult form of amaurotic idiocy ascribed to Kufs paradoxically is associated neither with amaurosis nor with retardation to the degree of idiocy, but rather, with dementia with cerebellar and extrapyramidal motor signs.

Optic nerve involvement may occur in the *mucopolysaccharidoses* (MPS), taking the form of optic atrophy or papilledema. Although true papilledema doubtlessly occurs in association with hydrocephalus seen in these disorders, there are other instances of "papilledema" in which fundus descriptions or photographs are not convincing. Goldberg and Duke[35] reported the ocular histopathologic findings in a patient with Hunter's syndrome (MPS II), in which pre-mortem examination included the observation of "bilateral chronic papilledema." On microscopic examination, the optic nerve was normal, despite marked retinal pigmentary degeneration, showing neither consecutive atrophy nor changes compatible with chronic papilledema. Similarly, Kenyon et al[36] reviewed the systemic mucopolysaccharidoses and included an instance of a 26-year-old man with Hunter's syndrome (MPS II), whose ophthalmoscopic examination revealed "blurred disc margins in both fundi (without venous congestion, hemorrhages or exudates) compatible with mild chronic papilledema," but no further comment was made in elucidation of this finding. Hunter's syndrome is an X-linked recessive disorder characterized by facial and skeletal dysmorphism, stiff joints, and mental slowing. Deafness and chronic disc edema occur, without raised intracranial pressure, and mucopolysaccharide deposition in the sclera and optic nerve septa, especially at the lamina cribrosa, is described.[37] MRI may disclose large multifocal cystic areas of hypointense or hyperintense signals in white matter, including the corpus callosum, likely reflecting deposition of mucopolysaccharide and increased fluid content.[38]

Mailer[39] reviewed 16 patients with optic atrophy in gargoylism and concluded that communicating hydrocephalus was the most frequent cause. Although hydrocephalus has long been recognized to occur in mucopolysaccharidosis, it is uncovered more frequently at autopsy than clinically. Goldberg et al[40] reported a case of Maroteaux-Lamy syndrome (MPS VI) with hydrocephalus and papilledema, treated with a ventriculojugular shunt. Those authors discussed the following possible pathogenetic mechanisms of visual dysfunction due to optic nerve involvement in mucopolysaccharidosis: optic atrophy secondary to glaucoma, retinal pigmentary degeneration, or mucopolysaccharide deposition in the retinal elements; infiltration of the nerve substance or meninges; narrowing of the optic canals; and hydrocephalus, with or without papilledema. Retinal pigmentary dystrophy occurs in MPS I-H (Hurler), MPS III (Sanfilippo), and MPS I-S (Scheie), all resulting from storage of heparan sulfate.

The *cherry-red spot myoclonus syndrome* is an autosomal recessive oligosaccharidosis due to deficiency of lysosomal acetylneuraminidase. The syndrome is comprised of typical cherry spot macula, resting and intention myoclonus, and preserved intellect. Sogg et al[41] also described flutter-like ocular oscillations attributed to possible cerebellar involvement.

RETINAL ARTERIAL OCCLUSIONS

Retinal arterial occlusions of neuro-ophthalmologic pertinence occur in patients with carotid athero-occlusive disease, heart disease, arteritis (giant cell, collagen vasculitides), and, rarely, migraine. Cranial arteritis is considered in a subsequent discussion of ischemic optic neuropathies (see Chapter 5, Part II).

The onset of retinal arterial occlusion rarely goes unnoticed by the patient, but unlike venous thrombosis, arterial occlusions of a minor degree may be difficult to discern ophthalmoscopically, especially if days or weeks pass before the fundus is examined. Muci-Mendoza et al[42] used fluorescein fundus angiography to demonstrate ophthalmoscopically occult emboli and post-embolic endothelial damage after episodes of *amaurosis fugax* (see below, Carotid Atheromatous Disease).

With acute infarction, the retina becomes opaque and takes on a creamy or gray appearance. Atheromatous material in the form of "bright plaques" of cholesterol or other microemboli may be seen, especially lodged at arterial bifurcations (Fig. 5–5). Segmental arteriolar mural opacification (see Fig. 5–5D) may follow retinal microembolization by weeks to months, and such sheathing may be as useful as the recognition of the cholesterol embolus itself.[43] ERG may show diminished B-wave amplitude, a finding indicating inner retinal ischemia. Weeks following retinal infarction, the optic disc becomes pale, and the arterial tree becomes narrowed in the sector corresponding to the arterial occlusion.

The visual field defects with arterial occlusion are variable, but they usually take the form of arcuate scotomas or "altitudinal hemianopias" of the superior or inferior half fields (Fig. 5–6). These altitudinal or pseudo-quadrantic defects are dense and are easily discovered by hand- or finger-counting confrontation techniques. The localizing value of the position of the "vertex" of quadrantic and wedge-shaped defects was pointed out by Alfred Kestenbaum. When the wedge originates at or points toward the blind spot, the defect is due to a retinal arterial occlusion or a lesion at the edge of the optic disc (including the arcuate defects seen in glaucoma). The differential diagnosis of arcuate scotomas, that is, with radial borders originating at the blind spot (see Fig. 5–6, right field), includes glaucoma, ischemic optic neuropathy, branch retinal artery occlusion, hyaline bodies of optic disc, congenital optic pit, juxtapapillary inflammation, and, rarely, chiasmal interference (see Fig. 6–1F).

Carotid Atheromatous Disease

The pathogenesis of embolic retinal arterial occlusions is diverse, but most are associated with atheromatous degeneration of the cervical carotid arteries. Since the observations by Fisher[44] of mobile intravascular material during episodes of transient retinal ischemic episodes (amaurosis fugax), an embolic source is commonly invoked, especially when any material is detected ophthalmoscopically within the retinal circulation. Such retinal emboli have been examined histopathologically and may consist of cholesterol crystals,[45] platelet aggregates,[46] fibrin and blood cells,[47] and neutral fat.[48] A study of the prevalence of *asymptomatic retinal emboli* among 3654 persons aged 49 years or older disclosed photographic evidence in 1.4%, the majority being judged as cholesterol; risk for subsequent stroke is not yet calculated.[49] On the other hand, the incidence of visible emboli in retinal arterial occlusion is estimated at about 20%.[50] Wilson et al[51] compared the incidence of carotid and cardiac disease in 103 patients with retinal artery occlusions and reported cardiac valve abnormalities in 28; of 62 carotid arteriograms, 35% were normal, 13% were occluded, and the remainder showed irregularity or significant stenosis. In a small group of 41 patients with transient monocular visual loss or retinal artery occlusion, no cardiac or carotid source was uncovered in two-thirds of subjects, ipsilateral carotid disease was seen in 11 (27%) cases, and a cardiac source was noted in a single patient.[52]

Even in those patients without ophthalmoscopically visible emboli, it is possible that the embolus either has lodged in the retro-laminar portion of the optic disc or has disintegrated and passed to the retinal periphery.

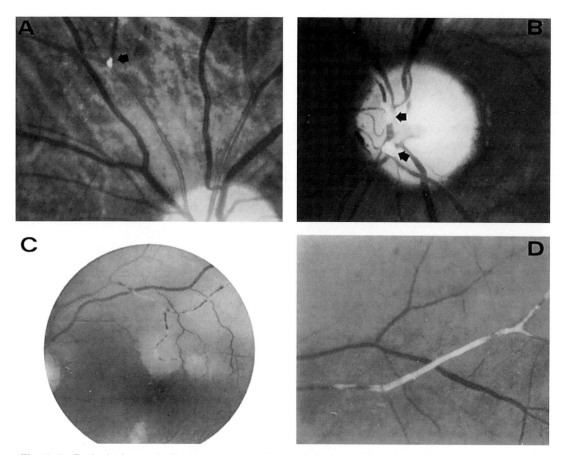

Fig. 5–5. Retinal microembolic phenomena. **A.** Bright cholesterol plaque (*arrow*) impacted at an arterial bifurcation. Thin crystal does not obstruct flow. **B.** Cholesterol crystals in disc vessels (*arrows*). Often, the plaque appears larger than the vessel diameter. **C.** Infarcted opaque retina. The artery contains emboli (? fibrin platelets) that have obstructed flow. **D.** Reactive opacification of the arterial wall. Fluorescein angiography demonstrated flow through this formerly occluded vessel.

Primary thrombosis in the retinal arterial circulation, beyond evidence of frank vasculitis or hypercoagulable states, is considered obsolete. Vasospasm, on the other hand, is an unlikely candidate to explain arterial occlusion, although rare instances of otherwise unexplained transient visual loss are reported.[53] Other non-carotid sources of emboli, including cardiogenic, are discussed below.

Transient ischemic episodes involving the retinal arterial tree produce the well-known symptom of *amaurosis fugax* ("fleeting darkness, or blindness"; ocular transient ischemic episode). This phenomenon may be defined as a painless unilateral, transient loss of vision that usually progresses from the periphery toward the center of the field. Often, the visual deficit takes the pattern of a dark curtain descending from above or ascending from below. Complete or subtotal blindness follows in seconds and lasts from 1 to 5 minutes (rarely longer). Vision returns to normal within 10 to 20 minutes, at times by reversal of the pattern of progression. Incomplete variations produce less distinctive sensations such as "looking through a fog . . . through raindrops . . .

through haze." By convention, the term amaurosis fugax is reserved for the ocular symptoms as described, which are usually distinguishable from other episodic visual disturbances (see Chapter 1), and it implies transient ischemia in retinal arterial circulation. Those conditions with principally monocular transient visual loss are listed in Table 5–3.[54]

It is likely that microembolic material in the form of fibrin-platelet aggregates momentarily occludes retinal vessels, then fragments and passes into the retinal periphery. If disaggregation with reconstitution of blood flow does not take place within several minutes, ischemic damage to inner retinal layers may be irreversible, and permanent visual defects may ensue. Most evidence indicates that the major source of retinal microemboli is the extracranial internal carotid artery, specifically an ulcerating atheromatous lesion at the level of the bifurcation.[55] The incidence of carotid atheromatous disease in patients with retinal strokes or amaurosis fugax, as noted above, ranges from a low of 27%[52] to an estimated high from 57 to 67%.[56] Moreover, retinal ischemic events may be more frequent when carotid stenosis is greater

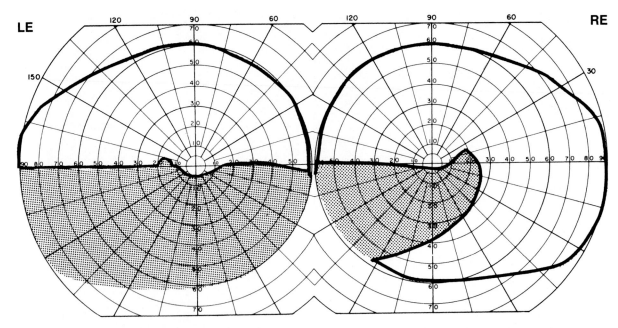

Fig. 5–6. Field defects of vascular origin. **RE.** Arcuate nerve fiber bundle defect of the right eye extending from the blind spot into the nasal quadrant. **LE.** Inferior altitudinal "hemianopia" of the left eye. These patterns are common to both retinal arterial occlusions and segmental infarction of nerve head (ischemic optic neuropathy).

than 50% to 70% or in the presence of ulcerative atheromatous plaques.[57,58] The diagnosis of amaurosis fugax and the implied underlying carotid atheromatous disease may usually be made on the basis of signs and symptoms (Table 5–4).

The presence of a carotid bruit is suggestive evidence of turbulent flow, but, however practical, auscultation and tender palpation of the carotid arteries and performance of ophthalmodynamometry or ocular plethysmography no longer suffice. At any rate, in the patient with amaurosis fugax, in whom carotid disease must be evaluated, further technical procedures are mandatory. Such tests of carotid morphology and hemodynamics assume two distinct forms: arteriographic, requiring in-

traluminal contrast opacification of arteries; and non-arteriographic ("noninvasive"), using ultrasound, Doppler imaging, and, most recently, MRI (magnetic resonance angiography or MRA). Noninvasive panels are commonly employed for preliminary assessment, with the advantages of risk-free, outpatient application. Carotid *duplex* scanning combines simultaneous real-

TABLE 5–3. Transient Obscurations of Vision

Amaurosis fugax (retinal microembolization or hypoperfusion)
Papilledema of raised cerebrospinal fluid pressure
Migraine: retinal, monocular; cortical, hemianopic
Hyaline bodies of optic nerve
Hypotension (orthostatic, arrhythmia)
Refractive errors (myopia)
Congenital dysplasias of optic disc
Anemia
Arteritis
Polycythemia/thrombocythemia
Coagulopathies
Angle-closure glaucoma
Spontaneous anterior chamber micro-hyphema, especially after lens implantation[54]

TABLE 5–4. Symptoms and Signs of Carotid Atheromatous Disease

Transient symptoms
  Amaurosis fugax
  Photopsias
  Orbital and ocular pain
Ophthalmoscopic signs
  Arteriosclerotic retinopathy
  Hypertensive retinopathy
  Bright plaques
  Occluded arteries
  Optic atrophy
Chronic ocular hypoxia
  Dilated episcleral veins
  Edematous cornea
  Anterior chamber reaction
  Rubeosis and iris atrophy
  Synechiae
  Cataract
  Glaucoma (or hypotony)
  Retinal venous dilation
  Microaneurysms, hemorrhages
  Neovascularization
  Arterial occlusions

time B-mode ultrasonography with gated, pulsed Doppler ultrasonography. These studies provide color-coded images of the degree of stenosis and plaque morphology, although not without limitations and artifactual data.[59] MRA imaging of carotid vessels is currently an evolving field, but preliminary drawbacks include overestimation of stenosis and perturbation by signal voids related to turbulent flow. MRA images are useful in combination with duplex ultrasonography, especially when the carotid bifurcation is involved.[58]

The general consensus[58] is that there is a sharp decline in the risk of stroke and in benefit from endarterectomy as the degree of angiographically defined stenosis diminishes from 99% to 70%, and this critical point underscores the importance of precise measurement of stenosis. Whereas modern techniques of angiography carry a 0.09% to 0.3% stroke rate risk, it is generally recognized that duplex ultrasonography be used as a screening tool to exclude patients with no detectable carotid disease from further testing, but patients suspected of harboring carotid disease, who are otherwise suitable candidates for endarterectomy, should undergo confirmatory contrast angiography. Ultrasonography may also be applied to monitor for progression of stenosis. Therefore, the elimination of conventional carotid angiography in favor of combined Doppler and MRA, to assess for stroke risk or determination of proper therapy, is premature, cost-containment strategies notwithstanding.

In contrast to transient symptoms and signs of retinal microembolic episodes, a condition of *chronic ocular hypoxia* (ocular ischemic syndrome) occurs less frequently, resulting from diffuse vascular occlusive disease of the aortic arch or common carotid artery. Acute or chronic occlusion with insufficient collateralization produces an ischemic pseudo-inflammatory uveitis, which variably includes an injected painful globe, corneal edema, aqueous flare and cells, a mid-dilated fixed pupil, rubeosis and iris atrophy, rapidly advancing cataract, either hypotony or elevated intraocular pressure ("neovascular glaucoma"), retinal microaneurysms and new vessel formation, posterior pole and mid-peripheral blot hemorrhages, macular edema, venous dilation and "sausaging," cytoid infarcts (cotton-wool spots) of the nerve fiber layer, and arterial occlusions (Fig. 5–7; see Table 5–4). The hypoxemic fundus changes constitute a picture of *venous stasis* (low-pressure) *retinopathy*, perhaps the commonest ocular sign of chronic carotid obstruction.

Ischemic photoreceptor metabolism accounts for subjective afterimages following exposure to bright light, including a positive photostress test[60] (see Chapter 2). Low retinal arterial pressure may be detected by observing pulsation or collapse of the disc arterioles with even slight fingertip pressure exerted on the globe. Such borderline perfusion associated with carotid stenosis and retinopathy may be heralded by postprandial visual loss.[61] In the situation of chronic, subacute, or rapidly progressive ischemic oculopathy, giant cell arteritis must be considered in the differential diagnosis, and chronic venous obstruction or diabetic retinopathy may produce similar fundus appearance.

From a series of 32 patients[62] with ocular ischemic syndrome manifested by anterior segment neovascularization, the following data were accrued: mean age 68 ± 8 years; visual symptoms presented as amaurosis fugax,

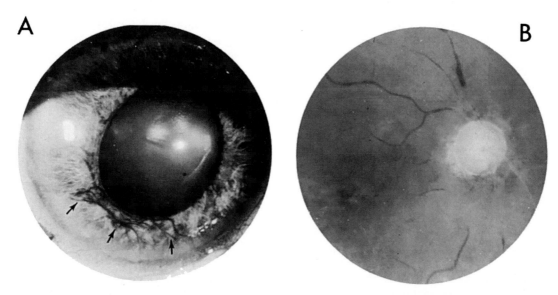

Fig. 5–7. Ocular hypoxia with subacute carotid occlusion. The patient complained of a painful red eye. **A.** Anterior segment shows an irregular, fixed pupil and iris rubeosis (*arrows*). **B.** Fundus demonstrates combined retinochoroidal infarction with acute excavation of the optic disc. Arteriography revealed right internal carotid occlusion.

15%, gradual, 28%, or sudden, 41% loss; initial visual acuity less than or equal to 20/400 in 64%, and in 77% at final follow-up; iris neovascularization, 87%; iridocorneal angle neovascularization, 59%; disc pallor, 40%, or cupped, 19%, or edematous, 8%; retinal circulatory stasis, 21%; retinal hemorrhages, 24%. Intraocular pressures ranged widely from 4 mmHg to 60 mmHg. Ipsilateral carotid occlusion or severe stenosis (80% to 99%) was found in 74%, but endarterectomy in 7 patients did not influence visual outcome, which was poor at onset. Other significantly associated systemic diseases included diabetes (56%), arterial hypertension (50%), coronary artery disease (38%), and previous stroke or transient ischemic attack (TIA) (30%).

Visual outcome in such ischemic globes is guarded, but endarterectomy may prevent progressive infarction of ocular tissues and may alleviate pain (ocular "angina"). Improvement or stabilization of vision and some resolution of retinopathy are reported, especially if carotid reconstruction is performed before irreversible neovascular glaucoma.[63] A vasospastic form of ocular ischemia is reported, with improvement with the calcium channel blocker verapamil.[64]

It is exceedingly difficult to predict which patients with amaurosis fugax will develop permanent visual loss or suffer a hemispheral vascular accident, and it is not yet clear that patients with asymptomatic carotid stenosis benefit from arterial surgery. From the exacting North American Symptomatic Carotid Endarterectomy Trial (NASCET),[65] in patients with 70% or greater stenosis and cerebral TIAs within the past 4 months, stroke risk is estimated at up to 25% per year; with first-time amaurosis fugax and high-grade stenosis, the risk is 8.5% per year, but apparently with less severe stoke deficits.[66] These risks are compared with surgical complication rate of carotid endarterectomy, with a perioperative stroke or death rate of 5.8% in the NASCET study, but as much as 8.5% even in academic centers,[67] and the surgical morbidity/mortality figures may be greater outside major vascular surgery facilities.

Regarding the Asymptomatic Carotid Atherosclerosis Study (ACAS),[68] in 1662 patients with greater than 60% stenosis but no symptoms, after 4465 cumulative patient-years, aggregate risk of stroke or death was 4.8% among surgical patients and 10.6% among patients who did not have surgery; both groups received aspirin and attempts at reduction of risk factors; perioperative morbidity/mortality risk was 3%, but patients were selected to avoid those with confounding factors to avoid excessive surgical risk. Interestingly, patients with 80% stenosis or greater had a lower subsequent events rate than those with less stenosis.

To reiterate, carotid endarterectomy may be recommended for properly selected asymptomatic patients with stenosis of 80% to 90% by modern contrast angiography and when angiography and surgery can be performed with a combined stroke or death rate of less than 3%. In patients with asymptomatic carotid stenosis who are prepared to undergo coronary artery bypass grafting for symptomatic coronary artery disease, there are no data suggesting benefit from prophylactic endarterectomy.[69]

In a British study,[70] retinal infarction was believed to have some prognostic value, the presence of retinal emboli being associated with increased mortality rate of 8% per year. It was emphasized that the most deaths in such patients were related to cardiac infarctions.

In recent years, aspirin, in daily low doses of 75 mg to 325 mg, has been used as a platelet antiaggregant. A collaborative overview[71] summarizing data from 173 randomized trials of antiplatelet therapy in patients at high risk for occlusive vascular disease showed a definite protective value for myocardial infarction, nonfatal stroke, and vascular death, with respective risk reductions of one-third, one-third, and one-sixth. Other previous analyses showed stroke reduction rates as high as 42% in both men and women; dipyridamole (Persantine) has no established role in stroke prophylaxis.[72] Most interestingly, an analysis of published randomized studies of the medical treatment (chronic anticoagulation or platelet inhibitors, versus no treatment or placebo) of TIAs showed that *neither treatment modality significantly reduced mortality rates.*[73] Failure to prevent cardiac complications appears independent of therapeutic effectiveness in reducing the incidence of cerebral strokes in patients with TIAs.

Not without controversy, there is general agreement with the following management recommendations regarding indications for endarterectomy, as modified from Trobe.[74] Patients *for whom carotid endarterectomy is indicated:* cerebral hemispheric ischemic symptoms within the carotid artery distribution occurring within the past 6 months; ipsilateral stenosis of 70% or greater, without intraluminal thrombosis or substantial syphon stenosis (*i.e.,* distal intracranial segment stenosis does not exceed cervical segment stenosis); age less than 75 years; no evidence of significant disease (organ failure) of kidney, liver, lung; no severe disabling stroke or progressing neurologic dysfunction; no recent myocardial infarct, unstable angina pectoris, or a cardiac valvular or rhythm disorder that could be a source of embolic symptoms; no uncontrolled hypertension; life expectancy of at least 2 years and adequate quality of life. Patients with acute ocular ischemia (amaurosis fugax, recent retinal infarction, ischemic optic neuropathy) *do not qualify.* Again, it is imperative that a proficient vascular surgical team with a perioperative stroke and death rate less than 2% to 4% should be available. It also must be reiterarated that atherosclerotic disease is multifocal, and most patients succumb to myocardial infarcts, not stroke.

Other non-atheromatous carotid diseases may manifest as transient visual obscurations. *Fibromuscular dysplasia,* most common in younger women, is also a likely source of recurrent microembolization, requiring angiography for confirmation, and surgical intraluminal dilation may be required.[75] Spontaneous *dissection* of the cervical segment of the internal carotid artery is increasingly recognized as a cause of stroke, with a mean age of 45 years (range, 16 to 76 years), and an estimated annual incidence of 2.5 to 3.5 per 100,000.[76] Symptoms of dissection frequently include headache, neck and jaw pain, dysphagia, metallic dysgeusia, Horner's syndrome, and amaurosis fugax. According to Biousse et al.,[76a] nearly two-thirds of patients have ocular signs or symptoms, 5,270 at presentation; almost half have a painful Horner's syndrome, one-third with transient monocular vision loss, and rarely ischemic optic neuropathy occurs. Trivial trauma or exertion such as weight-lifting may be inapparent contributing factors, but predisposing conditions include fibromuscular dysplasia, Marfan's or Ehler-Danlos syndrome, and cystic medial necrosis.[77] Diagnosis is made on angiography, which shows irregular narrowing, and MRI discloses hyperintense signal of mural hematoma. Duplex echography demonstrates arterial enlargement due to mural hematoma and stenosis distal to the point of dissection. Recanalization is the anticipated outcome, but antithrombotic therapy such as heparin is usually used to prevent subsequent embolization.

Pulseless disease (Takayasu's arteritis), suggested by the inability to obtain peripheral pulses in the arms and confirmed by aortic arch angiography,[78] is also associated with transient obscurations of vision and chronic retinal ischemic changes. This disorder is an idiopathic chronic inflammation of the aorta and proximal segments of its major branches, producing progressive stenosis and end-organ hypoperfusion. Although there is a predilection for Asians and for women, pulseless disease has been described in all racial groups. Ophthalmologic signs and symptoms are considered late manifestations, and visual loss may be noted when the patient assumes an erect posture. Ischemic retinopathy, iris neovascularization, cataract, vitreous hemorrhage, and anterior segment ischemia are chief ophthalmic findings.

Color Doppler ultrasound imaging is a relatively recent noninvasive technique to assess blood flow dynamics in the eye and orbit, although the accuracy and applicabilities are not yet fully explored. Nonetheless, preliminary investigations suggest effective application in retinal arterial occlusions, cranial arteritis, ischemic neuropathies, and carotid artery disease.[79] In a study of 24 persons with greater than 75% carotid stenosis,[80] all patients showed lower mean peak systolic velocities in the central retinal, posterior ciliary, and ophthalmic arteries, with improvement after endarterectomy.

Other Retinal Arterial Occlusions

Although atherosclerotic disease of the extracranial carotid system is by far the most common source of emboli to the retina and brain, other sites should be considered. Embolic material may originate from damaged endocardium following myocardial infarction, a significant difference being noted between observed and expected probabilities of stroke at 1 and 2 months.[81] Rheumatic or atherosclerotic aortic and mitral valvular disease may serve as a nidus for recurrent embolus formation. Patent foramen ovale is found in one-third of normal hearts at autopsy, as well as other septal defects (right-to-left shunts), and atrial fibrillation, are all potential sources of retinal and cerebral microemboli. In recent years, mucoid degeneration of the mitral valve and chordae tendineae ("prolapsing mitral valve"; Barlow's syndrome) has been recognized as a source for ocular and cerebral stroke and transient ischemic events.[82,83] In 59 patients with mitral prolapse, Lesser et al[83] found an incidence of 22% with amaurosis fugax. This syndrome should come to mind especially in non-hypertensive patients younger than the sixth decade; both men and women may be affected, and most patients with native valve endocarditis have mitral valve prolapse.[84] This condition is suggested by chest pain, dyspnea and cardiac arrhythmias, and midsystolic click or murmur. The diagnosis is confirmed by echocardiography and angiocardiography. Otherwise, endocarditis of native or prosthetic valves is rarely unaccompanied by systemic manifestations of malaise, fever, petechiae, and heart murmur. Other ocular manifestations include conjunctival petechiae, Roth's spots, choroidal septic emboli with subretinal vascularization, embolic retinitis, and endophthalmitis.[85]

Retinal arterial obstructions in children and young adults are only rarely the result of embolization in the absence of detectable cardiac disease. Of 27 patients with retinal artery occlusions occurring before the age of 30 years, Brown et al[86] found a history of migraine headaches in 8 patients, but no instance of a previous history of "retinal migraine" attacks (see below), and emboli were detected in only 7%. In a similar series of retinal arterial occlusions in 27 eyes of 21 persons aged 22 to 33 years, 67% of whom were women, Greven et al[87] found identifiable emboli in 7 (33%) patients and cardiac valvular disease (atrial myxoma, bacterial endocarditis, mitral valve lesions) in only 4; hypercoagulable or embolic factors included various admixtures of oral contraceptives, cigarette use, pregnancy, obesity, and migraine; 2 patients with either anticardiolipin antibody elevation or protein S deficiency were both pregnant, and no patient in the series had typical migrainous symptoms at the time of retinal arterial occlusion. The role of transesophageal echocardiography is stressed, especially in young patients with unaccountable arterial occlusions, with or without visible emboli.[88] In a retrospective review[89] of 16 patients with idiopathic *recurrent* branch arterial occlusions and no particular common risk factor, the long-term visual, neurologic, and systemic prognosis remained favorable after a mean follow-up of 9 years, with no systemic thromboembolic events.

Coagulation studies (*e.g.*, prothrombin and partial thromboplastin times, total platelet count) are generally unrevealing unless specific thrombophilic (coagulants and fibrinolytics) factors are evaluated, such as lupus anticoagulants, other immunoglobulins against phospholipids, proteins C and S (inhibit clotting cascade), antithrombin III, and homocysteine.[90,91] The antiphospholipid antibody syndrome accounts for both venous and arterial occlusions. Antibodies to negatively charged phospholipid include anticardiolipin antibodies, lupus anticoagulant, and those responsible for biologic false-positive Venereal Disease Research Laboratory tests. Antiphospholipid antibodies are detectable in 2% of healthy persons, but in 35% to 50% of patients with lupus erythematosus and in 25% to 50% of young patients with stroke.[92] However, in a prospective study[93] of 75 patients with retinal vascular occlusions, mostly venous, no increased prevalence of antiphospholipid antibodies was found. With regard to homocysteine, there is unequivocal evidence that hyperhomocysteinemia is a risk factor in carotid artery stenosis,[94] likely related to impaired production of endothelium-derived relaxing factor, to stimulated proliferation of smooth muscle cells that play a key role in atherogenesis and affecting the expression of thrombomodulin and activation of protein C.

Among young patients with stroke, 17% exhibit a deficiency of natural anticoagulants, with protein S deficiency in 12%, protein C deficiency in 2%, and antithrombin III deficiency in 2%. However, 5 to 10 times more common than these conditions is functional resistance to activated protein C (APC), especially in youthful patients with venous thrombosis, and it is prevalent in the general population in 2% to 5% of individuals. APC, also known as *factor V Leiden,* is due to a single point mutation altering coding for residue 506 from arginine to glycine and is dominantly inherited.[92]

Branch arterial occlusion is documented in association with Lyme disease,[95] and arterial and venous retinal vascular disease is rarely associated with Crohn's ulcerative colitis.[96] Other systemic ("collagen") vasculitides such as lupus erythematosus, polyarteritis nodosa,[97] and dermatomyositis are also infrequent causes of retinal arterial occlusions, but they must be suspected especially in young women. Serum complement (C3, C4) and antinuclear antibody (ANA) levels, erythrocyte sedimentation rate (ESR), and other rheumatologic evaluations are mandatory.

The *single and multiple influences of some risk factors remain speculative.* For example, the previously described mitral valve prolapse syndrome, with or without "sticky platelets," occurs in some 20% of otherwise healthy women, migraine affects *at least* 10% (other estimates run as high a prevalence as 20% in men and 30% in women) of the population, and millions of women regularly use oral anovulatory agents.

It bears emphasizing that the origin of transient, monotonously stereotyped *visual obscurations in healthy young persons* often proves elusive, but fortunately most of these attacks are self-limited and benign, with neither identifiable risk factors nor need for therapy. Of course, echocardiography should be considered. Extrapolating from general stroke data,[98] there is no consensus that low-dose oral contraceptives increase the risk of retinal vascular occlusions. However, other reviews[99] suggest that the presence of complex or prolonged migraine aura, or of additional stroke risk factors (increased age, smoking, hypertension), likely increases the ischemic stroke risk further in patients with migraine when oral contraceptives are added. Otherwise, intraocular pressure, occult vasculitis, and hemoglobinopathies should be considered in patients with retinal arterial occlusions, as well as the multiple causes considered here, and judiciously selective laboratory assessments should be applied. That is not to say that definitive diagnosis is forthcoming, nor do abnormal laboratory data necessarily imply cause and effect; for example, antiphospholipid antibodies are found in healthy persons. Optimal, or even minimal, therapy remains controversial, and only basic regimens currently suffice: systemic corticosteroids to suppress antibody production; anticoagulants to block thrombosis; and antiplatelet agents. In the acute period, perhaps hours after occlusion, ocular massage may lower intraocular tension, and microcatheter infusion of urokinase or tissue plasminogen activator is advocated,[100] but there is little evidence to support anterior chamber paracentesis or other medical therapies.[85]

Retinal vein occlusion has far fewer neuro-ophthalmologic implications than do arterial retinal infarctions. Significant associations are found with hypertension, diabetes, glaucoma, cardiovascular disease, and increased ESR in women, but not with estrogen use, alcohol consumption, or physical activity.[101] Vein occlusion is reported in association with hyperhomocysteinemia,[102] and with antiphospholipid antibody syndrome,[103] although in larger series[94] no direct relationship with anticardiolipin antibodies or lupus anticoagulant is found. However, in patients younger than 45 years, dominantly inherited APC resistance (see above) is a distinct risk factor.[104] Venous stasis retinopathy may be found in instances of arteriovenous shunts or fistulas, as discussed in Chapter 17. The general problem of venous occlusions is reviewed elsewhere.[105]

Retinal Migraine

Retinal migraine implies stereotypical transient monocular loss of vision of rapid onset, usually followed by ipsilateral headache, in persons usually with other migrainous symptoms, including typical common migraine headaches. The following case history is exemplary:

A 22 year-old male medical student complained of "blackouts" in the left eye, lasting between 10 and 20 minutes, often followed by mild diffuse headache local-

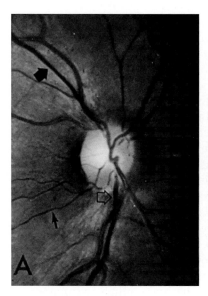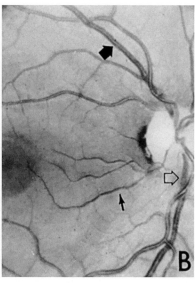

Fig. 5–8. Retinal migraine. **A.** During amaurotic episode. Note the dusky appearance of the fundus, increased retinal sheen (? edema), and dark narrowed veins (*arrows*). The disc is also hyperemic. **B.** Fundus after episode. Compare *paired arrows.* (Courtesy of Dr. J. Reimer Wolter)

ized to the left side of the head. Cephalgia usually began as the visual deficit was clearing. These episodes began at age 16, at first occurring once or twice per year, but currently every 4 weeks for the past 6 months, especially at "exam time." The patient had no other particular headache pattern, and the family history was negative. Standard cardiac echography was unremarkable.

The retinal variety may be admixed in a person who suffers the more conventional attacks of migraine. It is presumed that vasospasm in the retinal circulation determines transient hypoxia, perhaps somewhat similar to the visual cortical event. On rare occasions, the fundus has been examined during typical retinal migraine episodes, and arterial constriction has been described.

Wolter and Burchfield[106] photographically documented such an episode and demonstrated mild "retinal edema"; vessel narrowing is also evident (Fig. 5–8).

Fortunately, permanent complications of retinal migraine are rare. These may take the form of central retinal artery occlusion or ischemic papillopathy (see Chapter 16); nerve fiber bundle visual field defects may be demonstrated (Fig. 5–9).

RETINAL VASCULITIS

Mild monocular visual blurring and a fundus picture of disc swelling with dilated veins and multiple small

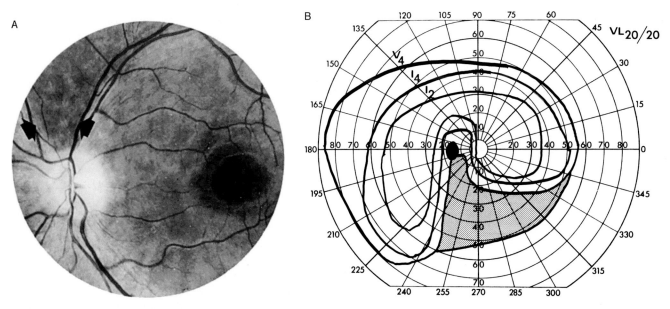

Fig. 5–9. An 18-year-old student with recurrent episodes of left retinal migraine. After a typical attack, he noted an inferior field defect. **A.** Fundus shows a defect in the superior arcuate nerve fiber bundle (between *arrows:* compare fiber layer below disc). **B.** Visual field defect corresponds to a retinal nerve fiber layer defect.

nerve fiber layer hemorrhages constitute a problem in diagnosis and management. In young patients whose vision is retained at good levels and the abnormality spontaneously regresses, a diagnosis of central retinal vein occlusion (see above) is usually made, without disclosure of underlying inflammation, hyperviscosity, or coagulopathy.

When disc swelling seems disproportionate to other hemorrhagic features, the vague term "papillophlebitis" is clinically applied, admittedly with little or no evidence of actual inflammatory disease. Although the course may be protracted (up to 18 months), the outcome is benign and apparently is unaltered by corticosteroid therapy. In a series of 40 patients with this diagnostic rubric,[107] some 7 cases of mitral valve prolapse were found, and 8 of 23 patients studied hematologically showed an increase in platelet coagulant activity concerned with the initiation of early stages of intrinsic coagulation. Nine patients had macular edema that contributed to lowered acuity, at times worse than 20/200, and "all patients had a fluorescein angiogram that was consistent with a central retinal vein occlusion of the nonischemic type." So-called papillophlebitis may be associated with retinal arterial occlusions and may possibly represent a form of idiopathic vasculitis or a coagulation defect of pregnancy.[108]

In contrast to this benign form of papillary or retinal "vasculitis," Cogan[109] documented a "severe vasculitis" category, including cases of periarteritis nodosa, Behçet's disease, multiple sclerosis, and granulomatous vasculitis. The cause in patients without systemic disease is speculative, but Cogan demonstrated in his patients with "severe vasculitis" that there was round cell infiltration of the venular walls.

The question of retinal arteritis, vasculitis, and autoimmune mechanisms was admirably reviewed by M. D. Sanders,[110] who presented clinical information on 150 cases examined at St. Thomas' Hospital, London. Retinal vasculitis should be considered when inflammatory changes (focal or extensive sheathing or occlusion of vessels; retinal infiltrates and hemorrhages; cellular debris in vitreous; vascular leakage of fluorescein) occur in relation to retinal vessels. Diagnostic categories include the following: infectious (tuberculosis, syphilis, herpes simplex, cytomegalovirus [CMV]); multiple sclerosis with phlebitis; polyarteritis nodosa, lupus erythematosus, Wegener's and Goodpasture's syndromes, sarcoidosis, Behçet's disease; autoimmune vasculitis without systemic disease, polymyositis, dermatomyositis, polyarteritis nodosa, Whipple's disease, and ulcerative colitis. Despite these purported associations, in well patients with *primary retinal vasculitis* and no medical history suggestive of underlying systemic disease, results of diagnostic batteries are meager, and follow-up data do not suggest subsequent manifestations of specific causes.[111] Although it is admittedly unrewarding, minimal evaluation would include complete blood count, ESR, urinalysis, fluorescent treponemal antibody absorption test, rapid plasma reagent, and chest roentgenogram.[111]

Retinal vasculitis exceptionally is associated with CNS vasculitis (angiitis). In 1882, Eales described a variety of retinal periphlebitis characterized by "retinal hemorrhage associated with epistaxis and constipation" seen in young men in southern England. Patients present with recurrent, usually monocular, vitreous hemorrhages that may persist for years and ultimately involve the second eye. Neurologic complications must be rare, but subacute myelopathies, chronic lymphocytic meningitis, and middle cerebral artery stroke have been reported.[112] Distinction from the retinal vasculitides discussed above is problematic, and "Eales' disease" remains a diagnosis of exclusion.

Microangiopathy of the brain, retina, and inner ear (Susac's syndrome) is a rare disorder predominantly affecting women of child-bearing age, but without a specific origin or systemic manifestations. An immune or coagulopathic background is unproved. Patients present with the following: vision loss due to branch retinal arteriolar occlusions with vessel hyperfluorescence on fluorescein angiography, and delayed leakage; hearing loss; multiple CNS infarctions.[113] Efficacy of treatment with corticosteroids and immunosuppressive agents is uncertain, but hyperbaric oxygenation has been beneficial in a single case, with rapid visual improvement.[114]

Other infrequent causes of multifocal segmental retinal vasculitis, co-mingled with neuroretinitis and choroiditis, include Lyme disease,[115] *Rochalimaea* infection (cat-scratch disease),[116] and intraocular lymphoma.[117] Without neurologic or systemic implications, a syndrome of retinal vasculitis, with aneurysmal dilatation of arterioles, capillary non-perfusion, and exudative neuroretinitis with marked decrease in acuity, has been described, with an age range of 9 to 49 years and a female preponderance; oral corticosteroids had no beneficial effects.[118] Ten patients with isolated retinal vasculitis with family history of multiple sclerosis, or positive HLA-B7 typing, underwent MRI, which showed white matter lesions resembling those of multiple sclerosis in 3 instances, suggesting a causative relationship.[119]

UVEO-MENINGEAL SYNDROMES

As noted, surprising numbers of etiologically diverse diseases simultaneously or sequentially involve the retina, uvea, and brain. Of these, the Vogt-Koyanagi-Harada syndrome is best known, characterized by bilateral diffuse granulomatous panuveitis, whitening (poliosis) especially of eyebrows and lashes, skin depigmentation (vitiligo), alopecia, meningismus with headache and CSF pleocytosis, rarely focal CNS signs, tinnitus, hearing loss, and vertigo. Autoimmune inflammation directed

TABLE 5–5. Uveo-meningeal Syndromes

Infections
  Syphilis, Lyme borreliosis, tuberculosis, fungal infections
  Cytomegalovirus, herpes simplex, herpes zoster, rubeola, subacute sclerosing panencephalitis
  Toxoplasmosis, Whipple's disease
Chronic inflammations
  Sarcoidosis
  Vogt-Koyanagi-Harada syndrome
  Behçet's syndrome
  Lupus erythematosus
Multiple sclerosis
Malignancies
  Reticulum cell sarcoma
  Lymphomas: B or T cell
  Metastatic carcinoma
Miscellaneous disorders
  Acute posterior pigment epitheliopathy
  Acute zonal occult outer retinopathy
  Sympathetic ophthalmia
  Inflammatory bowel disease

against melanocytes seems the basic mechanism, with an epidemiologic predilection for pigmented racial groups, especially in Japan and other parts of Asia; it is uncommon in whites. Prolonged corticosteroid and other immunosuppressive therapy is effective.[120]

Ureitis, including periphlebitis ("venous sheathing"), and pars planitis, is infrequently discovered in association with multiple sclerosis. Delay between onset of neurologic and ocular symptoms occurs, and the possibility of a shared genetic factor is raised.[120a]

Zonal outer retinopathies (AZOOR, see above) can show choroidal changes and are reported with CSF pleocytosis, cervical myelopathy, and periventricular white matter lesions on MRI, abnormal ERG, perivenous sheathing, and retinal pigment migration.[121] Posterior placoid pigment epitheliopathy (APMPPE, see above) also is reported to occur in association with headaches, CSF aseptic cellular reaction, TIAs, inner ear symptoms, and multiple strokes, requiring immunosuppressive agents for presumed cerebral vasculitis.[122] The classification found in Table 5–5 highlights the difficult diagnostic dilemma posed by these diverse disorders.

HUMAN IMMUNODEFICIENCY VIRUS INFECTION AND AIDS

The spectrum of ocular, orbital, and CNS involvement with human immunodeficiency virus (HIV) infection, and subsequent acquired immune deficiency syndrome (AIDS), is vast and complicated, characterized by peculiar neoplasia and a host of opportunistic infectious agents that invade the retina, optic nerve, leptomeninges, and brain, at times mimicking other neurologic syndromes. Co-existing manifestations in the eye and brain present confounding factors for neuro-ophthalmologic

localization. The usual parsimonious medical expectation that a single basic disorder encompasses all manifestations of an illness is inoperative in the patient with severely depressed cellular immunity, and, indeed, unrelated problems may be mislabeled. Ocular findings are detected in the majority of patients with AIDS at sometime in the course of the disease, the most common being relatively asymptomatic noninfectious microangiopathy consisting principally of microinfarcts ("cotton-wool spots") admixed with small hemorrhages, occurring in at least 50% of patients with AIDS, 34% of those with AIDS-related complex, and 3% of persons with asymptomatic HIV infection.[123] Interestingly, there is distinct evidence[124] of abnormal visual function (contrast sensitivity function, automated perimetry, color sense) in HIV-positive patients without ophthalmoscopic evidence of retinopathy, with normal global neuropsychologic function, and unrelated to disease state as determined by markers including CD4 T-lymphocyte count. It is speculated that such visual function may be related to HIV infection at some level of the visual pathways, or it may be an effect of antiviral or other therapeutic agents. Morphometric techniques[125] have demonstrated markedly lower mean axonal populations in AIDS-affected optic nerves, possibly reflecting a form of primary optic neuropathy (see the discussion in Chapter 5, Part II for optic neuropathies in AIDS).

Opportunistic infections, particularly CMV retinitis, are major causes of severe visual loss and blindness; CMV retinitis is estimated to occur in 37% of patients with AIDS.[126] CMV retinitis is a relatively late manifestation of the basic disease and is associated with CD4 T-cell counts of less than 0.10×10^9/L. Other tissues are affected, including the brain, lungs, and gastrointestinal tract. CMV retinitis presents as patches of opaque retina with intraretinal hemorrhages and exudative borders of advancing necrosis, which may eventuate in retinal detachment. Intravenous or intraocular ganciclovir and intravenous foscarnet are effective in controlling (virostatic) CMV retinitis, but they do not eliminate the virus.[126]

Other opportunistic fundus infections include the following: toxoplasmosis (retinochoroiditis, at times also involving optic nerve[127]), frequently accompanied by toxoplasmic encephalitis, the most common cause of focal CNS dysfunction in AIDS; varicella-zoster virus, producing acute retinal necrosis[128]; herpes simplex; and *Pneumocystis carinii* choroidopathy. Central retinal vein occlusions are documented, with pathologic examination disclosing no histologic evidence of HIV, a finding suggesting other hemorheologic factors.[129] The protean manifestations of AIDS are exemplified by a case of sudden blindness in a 50-year-old man who showed, at autopsy, simultaneous CMV infection of the retina, herpes simplex in the optic nerve, and non-Hodgkin's lymphoma of the optic tract.[130]

TOXIC RETINOPATHIES

Given the vast array of pharmaceutical agents and their extensive usage, and ingenious "recreational" drug usage, toxic effects on the retina only infrequently are encountered (see Chapter 5, Part II for Toxic Optic Neuropathies). Aside from the well-known problems with observable pigmentary maculopathies secondary to long-term intake of the antipsychotic phenothiazines, and hydroxychloroquine[131] (for rheumatoid arthritis, lupus erythematosus), and the acute systemic response to methanol poisoning, included here is retinal toxicity with peculiar symptoms or a clinical course that could be misconstrued in neuro-ophthalmologic context.

Ocular symptoms of the *cardiac glycosides* have been recognized since the time of Withering, who wrote on "foxglove" in 1785. Visual anomalies include blurring, pericentral scotoma, abnormal dark adaptation, xanthopsia ("yellow vision"), a peculiar sensation of whitish glare described at times as "frosting," and other aberrations of color perception. Symptoms may be continuous or intermittent and are reversible with diminished dosage levels, although other systemic signs of digitalis toxicity may be absent, and, indeed, serum levels may be well within the normal therapeutic range.[132] Although this condition is classically attributed to optic nerve dysfunction, evidence provided by ERG and color vision data implicate a cone dysfunction syndrome, likely related to inhibition of adenosine triphosphate in rod outer segments, or ganglion cell intoxication.[132] Pain on eye movement is also reported.[133] Fisher[134] recorded visual disturbances in five elderly patients who were receiving *quinidine* therapy, disturbances that were at first attributed to transient ischemic episodes, consisting of temporary dark shadows or bright afterimages noted only on awakening, and lasting a few minutes to less than 1 hour. Four of these patients were also receiving digoxin, and a synergistic effect cannot be dismissed. Although the long-term effect of quinine on retinal ganglion cells is well known, causing severe visual field contraction, optic atrophy, and narrowing of retinal arteries, Fisher considered these morning scotomas to be symptoms of transient failure of retinal light adaptation.

The oral antiestrogen agent *tamoxifen,* used for breast cancer, even at high daily doses has infrequent ocular side effects, including the deposition of fine crystalline deposits in the retina and occasional macular edema,[135] and intra-arterial *cisplatin* for glioblastoma may produce severe retinotoxic effects.[136] *Interferon* produces retinopathy characterized by hemorrhages and cotton-wool spots.[137] In patients undergoing renal transplantation, to prevent organ rejection, a murine monoclonal antibody, *OKT3,* is used and is associated with profound and irreversible visual loss at the retinal level.[138]

Most dramatically, temporary blindness occurs following transuretheral prostate resection (TURP), during which a non-electrolyte, non-conducting irrigating fluid (*glycine*) is absorbed through prostatic venous sinuses into the systemic circulation.[139] The TURP syndrome consists of confusion, bradycardia, nausea, hypertension, convulsions, and visual disturbance (even to no light perception) lasting minutes to several hours, and it may be related to hyponatremia, glycine retinal toxicity, or cortical edema. *Retinol* (vitamin A) is fat soluble, absorbed in the small intestine, and stored in the liver; deficiency occurs in malnutritional situations, liver dysfunction, and malabsorption states,[140] including mastocytosis,[141] and it is characterized by night blindness, visual loss, and abnormal ERG findings.

Along with other remote effects of carcinoma on the nervous system must be included an immune-mediated retinal photoreceptor degeneration, *cancer-associated retinopathy* (CAR). Described initially, and most commonly, with small cell carcinoma of the lung, visual disturbances include usually subacute loss of acuity and field depression, color anomalies, narrowed arterioles, pigment epithelial disturbances, and vitreous cells. The ERG is severely diminished, and pathologic examination discloses loss of rods and cones and thinning of the outer nuclear layer of the retina, but only mild disruption of inner retinal layers. Antiretina antibodies have been isolated in sera from patients with CAR syndrome, and rising titers of CAR antigen prove useful in identifying this disorder.[142] Acute night blindness and sensations of shimmering lights have been reported as paraneoplastic effects of *melanoma* (MAR), with ERG and other psychophysical responses consistent with interruption of bipolar rod function and selective disruption of magnocelluler neurons.[143] Thirkill[144] provided a review of the CAR syndrome and noted the evidence of elaboration of autoantibodies reactive with the 23 kDa retinal CAR antigen, located within the photoreceptors. Although paraneoplasia antibodies can be reduced by plasmapheresis and immunosuppressants, only questionable results are reported, and controversy persists over consequences of reducing the immune competence of cancer patients. Intravenous immunoglobulin is an alternative treatment option.[144a] In the setting of cancer, especially with rapid visual loss and *normal ERG,* the likelihood of *carcinomatous meningitis* should be considered, as well as the possibility of complications of chemotherapy. Autoimmune retinopathy may occur without evidence of cancer, but with typical photopsias, field depression, ERG abnormality, and sera containing antiretinal antibodies directed against *inner plexiform layer,* as opposed to CAR.[145]

CONGENITAL HAMARTOMA SYNDROMES

The "neurophakomatoses" are a diverse group of disorders nosologically related by the presence of hamartomatous lesions, and, indeed, the term "hereditary hamartomatosis" is a more accurate description. However, whereas neurofibromatosis, tuberous sclerosis, and von Hippel-Lindau disease are transmitted with irregular dominance and considerable variation in penetrance, no hereditary basis of Sturge-Weber or angio-osteohypertrophy (Klippel-Trenaunay-Weber) syndrome has been established.

A *hamartoma* is a tumor of anomalous origin composed of elements normally present in the tissue in which it originates and with a limited capacity for proliferation. The following tumors may be classified as hamartomas: (1) in neurofibromatosis: optic gliomas (see Chapter 6), neurofibromas, and ganglioneuromas; (2) in tuberous sclerosis: retinal and cerebral astrocytomas, cutaneous angiofibromas ("adenoma sebaceum"), rhabdomyomas, and leiomyomas; (3) in von Hippel-Lindau disease: hemangioblastomas of the cerebellum and retina (including optic nerve head) and renal hypernephromas or cysts; (4) in Sturge-Weber disease: facial and choroidal cavernous hemangiomas and meningeal angiomatous malformations; and (5) in Klippel-Trenaunay-Weber syndrome: cutaneous nevi, visceral and limb hemangiomas, and orbitofacial venous varices.

If all disorders with neurocutaneous manifestations are considered, the term phakomatoses (Greek, *phakos,* "spot," "birthmark") is appropriate, and the catalog of "related" disorders becomes cumbersome. The Phakomatoses, Volume 14 of Vinken and Bruyn's *Handbook of Clinical Neurology,* is extraordinarily complete and serves as a source of detailed clinical descriptions of these diseases.[146] Syndromes characterized by vascular hamartomas, that is, retinal-cerebellar angiomatosis (von Hippel-Lindau), and other angiomatous malformations, are discussed in Chapter 17.

Tuberous Sclerosis

Tuberous sclerosis, so-called because of cerebral *tubers* (potatoes), is a multiorgan complex that often shows the stigmata of retinal astrocytic hamartomas in

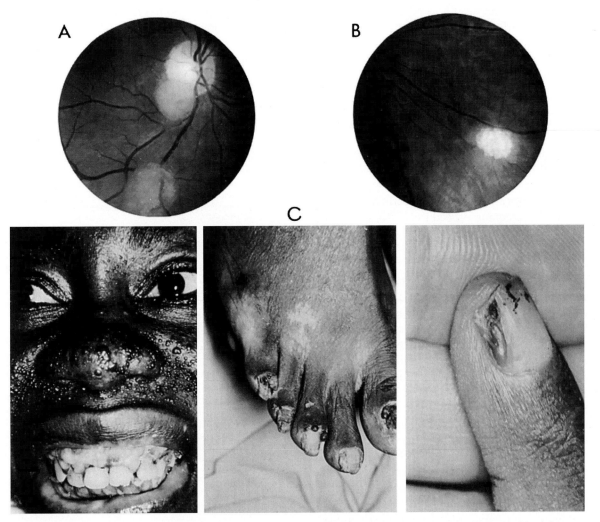

Fig. 5–10. Tuberous sclerosis. Retinal astrocytic hamartomas in epipapillary, parapapillary, and peripheral sites. **A.** Superficial translucent lesions through which retinal vessels may be seen. **B.** Peripheral calcified "mulberry" lesion. **C.** Cutaneous stigmata include facial fibroma ("adenoma sebaceum") and periungual fibroma of the toes and fingers.

epipapillary and parapapillary locations, as well as in the retinal periphery (Fig. 5–10; see Plate 5–1B). These characteristic lesions appear as elevated semitransparent domes in the nerve fiber layer of the retina and may undergo calcification as the patient ages. The calcified hamartomas, when on or near the optic disc, have been termed "giant drusen." These tumors should not be confused with the much more common drusen (hyaline bodies; see Chapter 5, Part II, Optic Nerve) within the substance of the nerve head, which are non-hamartomatous lesions and are not characterized by astrocytic hyperplasia. There is no evidence to support the suggestion that hyaline bodies of the optic disc are minor manifestations of tuberous sclerosis.

The retinal hamartomas are said to occur in approximately half of patients with tuberous sclerosis. Though rarely symptomatic themselves, they are of great help in establishing diagnosis in the setting of seizures, facial angiofibromas and variable mental retardation. Seizures and EEG abnormalities are present in 80% to 90%, adenoma sebaceum in 80%, mental retardation in 60%, intracranial calcifications in 50%, as well as cardiac rhabdomyomas or hamartomas.[147] Because of ventricular obstruction by giant cell astrocytomas, papilledema may develop and consequently visual loss.[148] On rare occasions abnormal capillaries on optic disc astrocytomas may abruptly alter vision because of intravitreal hemorrhage.[149] Familial occurrence in first-degree relatives should be sought, but some 60% of cases arise as new mutations.

Neuroimaging in tuberous sclerosis demonstrates subependymal (periventricular) nodules, calcifications, and parenchymal hamartomas (cortical tubers); although calcifications are difficult to discern, MRI is considered a better screening procedure.[150]

Neurofibromatosis

Neurofibromatosis embraces at least two disease entities. General neurofibromatosis (NF-1; von Recklinghausen's disease) is characterized by café-au-lait skin lesions, neurofibromas, schwannomas, optic-chiasmatic gliomas, and Lisch's nodules on the iris. NF-1 is the most commonly inherited CNS disorder, with an estimated prevalence of 1 in 3000 in Western countries, with gene locus at chromosome region 17q11.2. Lesions of the fundus are rare in neurofibromatosis, although some authors believe that the astrocytic hamartomas typical of tuberous sclerosis also occur in patients with neurofibromatosis. Although there is said to be an increased incidence of medullated retinal nerve fibers, no convincing evidence exists. Multiple gray-brown to yellow, placoid choroidal nevi may be seen at the posterior pole,[151] representing a proliferation of Schwann's cells and occurring in 50% of patients with neurofibromatosis.[152] Other stigmata include neurofibroma and neurilem-

moma of the orbit and lid, neuronal hamartomas of the iris (Lisch's nodules) and trabecular meshwork, congenital glaucoma, and sphenoid wing dysplasia with pulsating enophthalmos or exophthalmos.

Neurofibromatosis-2 (NF-2) is an autosomal dominant trait characterized by bilateral acoustic schwannomas associated with other neurofibromas, gliomas, and schwannomas. NF-2 is caused by a mutation in the chromosome region 22q12, with a prevalence rate of only 0.1 in 100,000.[147] Cutaneous lesions such as café-au-lait spots and neurofibromas are also found in NF-2. Various cataracts, posterior subcapsular or cortical, are described, as well as small tuberous sclerosis–type retinal nerve fiber and pigment epithelial hamartomas and macular epiretinal membranes, but not Lisch's iris nodules, as found in NF-1.[153] A limited study[154] of the behavior of optic nerve gliomas in NF-1 versus those in NF-2 suggests that there is better survival rate with less likelihood of tumor progression in NF-1. In addition, in NF-1 tumors are located more anteriorly, that is, in the orbit and chiasm, than in the optic tract or hypothalamus. Optic gliomas are discussed subsequently in Chapter 5, Part II.

REFERENCES

1. Gass JDM: Acute zonal occult outer retinopathy. J Clin Neuroophthalmol 13:79, 1993
2. Jacobson SG, Morales DS, Sun XK et al: Pattern of retinal dysfunction in acute zonal occult outer retinopathy. Ophthalmology 102:1187, 1995
3. Balazs AG, Rootman J, Drance SM et al: The effect of age on the nerve fiber population of the human optic nerve. Am J Ophthalmol 97:760, 1984
4. Weale RA: The aging retina. Geriatrics 3:425, 1985
5. Jonas JB, Schneider U, Naumann GOH: Count and density of human retinal photoreceptors. Graefes Arch Clin Exp Ophthalmol 230:505, 1992
6. Bird AC: Retinal photoreceptor dystrophies: Edward Jackson Memorial Lecture. Am J Ophthalmol 119:543, 1995
7. Trobe JD, Bergsma DR: Atypical retinitis pigmentosa masquerading as nerve fiber bundle lesion. Am J Ophthalmol 79:681, 1975
8. Abedin S, Simmons RJ, Hirose T: Simulated double Bjerrum's scotomas by retinal pigment epithelium and receptor degeneration. Ann Ophthalmol 13:1117, 1981
9. Grover S, Fishman GA, Brown J: Frequency of optic disc or parapapillary nerve fiber layer drusen in retinitis pigmentosa. Ophthalmology 104:295, 1997
10. Lambert SR, Taylor D, Kriss A: The infant with nystagmus, normal appearing fundi, but an abnormal ERG. Surv Ophthalmol 34:173, 1989
11. Enevoldson TP, Sanders MD, Harding AE: Autosomal dominant cerebellar ataxia with pigmentary macular dystrophy: a clinical and genetic study of eight families. Brain 117:445, 1994
12. Rabiah PK, Bateman JB, Demer JL, Perlman S: Ophthalmic findings in patients with ataxia. Am J Ophthalmol 123:108, 1997
13. To KW, Adamian M, Jakobiec FA, Berson EL: Olivopontocerebellar atrophy with retinal degeneration: an electroretinographic and histopathologic investigation. Ophthalmology 100:15, 1993
14. Abe T, Abe K, Aoki M et al: Ocular changes in patients with spinocerebellar degeneration and repeated trinucleotide expansion of spinocerebellar ataxia type 1 gene. Arch Ophthalmol 115:231, 1997
15. Yokota T, Shiojiri T, Gotoda T et al: Friedreich-like ataxia with

retinitis pigmentosa caused by the His-101 Gln mutation of the α-tocopherol transfer protein gene. Ann Neurol 41:826, 1997

16. Gibson TJ, Koonin EV, Musco G et al: Friedrich's ataxia protein: phylogenetic evidence for mitochondrial dysfunction. Trends Neurosci 19:465, 1996

17. Ortiz RG, Newman NJ, Shoffner JM et al: Variable retinal and neurologic manifestations in patients harboring the mitochondrial DNA 8993 mutation. Arch Ophthalmol 111:1525, 1993

18. Chang TS, Johns DR, Walker D et al: Ocular clinicopathologic study of the mitochondrial encephalopathy overlap syndromes. Arch Ophthalmol 111:1254, 1993

19. Fang W, Huang CC, Lee CC et al: Ophthalmologic manifestations of MELAS syndrome. Arch Neurol 50:977, 1993

20. Rummelt V, Folberg R, Ionasescu V et al: Ocular pathology of MELAS syndrome with mitochondrial DNA nucleotide 3243 point mutation. Ophthalmology 100:1757, 1993

21. Small KW, Gehrs K: Clinical study of a large family with autosomal dominant progressive cone degeneration. Am J Ophthalmol 121:1, 1996

22. Miyake Y, Horiguchi M, Tomita N et al: Occult macular dystrophy. Am J Ophthalmol 122:644, 1996

23. Jacobson DM: Acute zonal outer retinopathy and central nervous system inflammation. J Neuroophthalmol 16:172, 1996

24. Cunningham ET, Schatz H, McDonald HR et al: Acute multifocal retinitis. Am J Ophthalmol 123:347, 1997

25. Bullock JD, Fletcher RL: Cerebrospinal fluid abnormalities in acute multifocal placoid pigment epitheliopathy. Am J Ophthalmol 84:45, 1977

26. Zhang K, Nguyen THE, Crandall A et al: Genetic and molecular studies of macular dystrophies: recent developments. Surv Ophthalmol 40:51, 1995

27. Goldberg MF, Cotlier E, Fichenscher LG et al: Macular cherry-red spot, corneal clouding, and β galactosidase deficiency: clinical, biochemical and electron microscopy study of a new autosomal recessive storage disease. Arch Intern Med 128:387, 1971

28. van Bael M, Natowicz MR, Tomczak J et al: Heterozygosity for Tay-Sachs disease in non Jewish Americans with ancestry from Ireland or Great Britain. J Med Genet 33:829, 1996

29. Hund E, Grau A, Fogel W et al: Progressive cerebellar ataxia, proximal neurogenic weakness and ocular motor disturbances: hexosaminidase A deficiency with late clinical onset in four siblings. J Neurol Sci 145:25, 1997

30. Mugikura S, Takahashi S, Higano S et al: MR findings in Tay-Sachs disease. J Comput Assist Tomogr 20:551, 1996

31. Goebel HH. The neuronal ceroid-lipofuscinoses. Semin Pediatr Neurol 3:270, 1996

32. Tyynela J, Suopanki J, Santavuori P et al: Variant late infantile neuronal ceroid-lipofuscinosis: pathology and biochemistry. J Neuropathol Exp Neurol 56:369, 1997

33. Autti T, Raininko R, Santavuori P et al: MRI of neuronal ceroid lipofuscinosis II. Postmortem MRI and histopathologic study in 16 cases of juvenile and late infantile type. Neuroradiology 39:371, 1997

34. Lane SC, Jolly RD, Schmechel DE et al: Apoptosis as the mechanism of neurodegeneration in Batten's disease. J Neurochem 67:677, 1996

35. Goldberg MF, Duke JR: Ocular histopathology in Hunter's syndrome: systemic mucopolysaccharidosis type II. Arch Ophthalmol 77:503, 1967

36. Kenyon KR, Quigley HA, Hussels IE et al: The systemic mucopolysaccharidoses: ultrastructural and histochemical studies of conjunctiva and skin. Am J Ophthalmol 73:811, 1972

37. Beck M, Cole G: Discoedema in association with Hunter's syndrome: ocular histopathologic findings. Br J Ophthalmol 68:590, 1984

38. Shinomiya N, Nagayama T, Fujioka Y et al: MRI in mild type of mucopolysaccharidosis II (Hunter's syndrome). Neuroradiology 38:483, 1996

39. Mailer C: Gargoylism associated with optic atrophy. Can J Ophthalmol 4:266, 1969

40. Goldberg MF, Scott CI, McKusick VA: Hydrocephalus and papilledema in the Maroteaux-Lamy syndrome (mucopolysaccharidosis type II). Arch Ophthalmol 77:503, 1967

41. Sogg RL, Steinman, Rathjen B et al: Cherry-red spot–

42. Muci-Mendoza R, Arruga J, Edward WO, Hoyt WF: Retinal fluorescein angiographic evidence for atheromatous microembolism. Stroke 11:154, 1980

43. Slavin ML, Glaser JS: Segmental arteriolar sheathing: a sign of retinal emboli. Neuroophthalmology 6:215, 1986

44. Fisher CM. Observations of the fundus oculi in transient monocular blindness. Neurology 9:333, 1959

45. David NJ, Klintworth GK, Friedberg SJ et al: Fatal atheromatous cerebral embolism associated with bright plaques in the retinal circulation. Neurology 13:708, 1963

46. McBrien DJ, Bradley RD, Ashton N: The nature of retinal emboli in stenosis of the internal carotid artery. Lancet 1:697, 1963

47. Zimmerman LE: Embolism of the central retinal artery. Arch Ophthalmol 73:822, 1965

48. Cogan DG, Kuwabara T, Moser H: Fat emboli in the retina following angiography. Arch Ophthalmol 71:308, 1964

49. Mitchell P, Wang JJ, Li W et al: Prevalence of asymptomatic retinal emboli in an Australian urban community. Stroke 28:63, 1997

50. Brown C, Margargal L: Central retinal artery obstruction and visual acuity. Ophthalmology 89:14, 1983

51. Wilson LA, Warlow CP, Russell RWR: Cardiovascular disease in patients with retinal artery occlusion. Lancet 1:292, 1979

52. Smit RLM, Baarsma GS, Koudstaal PJ: The source of embolism in amaurosis fugax and retinal artery occlusion. Int Ophthalmol 18:83, 1994

53. Burger SK, Saul RF, Selhorst JB et al: Transient monocular blindness caused by vasospasm. N Engl J Med 325:870, 1991

54. Kosmorsky GS, Rosenfeld SI, Burde RM: Transient monocular obscuration—?amaurosis fugax: a case report. Br J Ophthalmol 69:688, 1985

55. Adams HP, Putman SF, Corbett JJ et al: Amaurosis fugax: results of arteriography in 59 patients. Stroke 14:742, 1983

56. Ellenberger C, Epstein AD: Ocular complications of atherosclerosis: what do they mean? Semin Neurol 6:185, 1986

57. Muller M, Wessel K, Mehdorn E et al: Carotid artery disease in vascular ocular syndromes. J Clin Neuroophthalmol 13:175, 1993

58. O'Farrell CM, FitzGerald DE: Prognostic value of carotid ultrasound lesion morphology in retinal ischaemia: results of a long term follow up. Br J Ophthalmol 77:781, 1993

59. Eliasziw M, Rankin RN, Fox AJ et al: Accuracy and prognostic consequences of ultrasonography in identifying severe carotid artery stenosis. Stroke 26:1747, 1995

60. Furlan A, Whisnant J, Kearns T: Unilateral visual loss in bright light: an unusual symptom of carotid artery occlusive disease. Arch Neurol 36:675, 1979

61. Levin LA, Mootha VV: Postprandial transient visual loss: a symptom of critical carotid stenosis. Ophthalmology 104:397, 1997

62. Mizener JB, Podhajsky P, Hayreh HH. Ocular ischemic syndrome. Ophthalmology 104:859, 1997

63. Rubin JR, McIntyre KM, Lukens MC et al: Carotid endarterectomy for chronic retinal ischemia. Surg Gynecol Obstet 171:497, 1990

64. Winterkorn JMS, Beckman RL: Recovery from ocular ischemic syndrome after treatment with verapamil. J Neuroophthalmol 15:209, 1995

65. North American Symptomatic Endarterectomy Trial Collaborators: Beneficial effect of carotid endarterectomy in symptomatic patients with high grade carotid stenosis. N Engl J Med 325:445, 1991

66. Striefler JY, Eliasziew M, Benavente OR et al: The risk of stroke in patients with first-ever retinal vs hemispheric transient ischemic attacks and high grade carotid stenosis. Arch Neurol 52:246, 1995

67. Goldstein LB, McCrory DC, Landsman PB et al: Multicenter review of perioperative risk factors for carotid endarterectomy in patients with ipsilateral symptoms. Stroke 25:1116, 1994

68. Asymptomatic Carotid Atherosclerosis Study: Clinical advisory: carotid endarterectomy for patients with asymptomatic

myoclonus syndrome. Trans Am Acad Ophthalmol 86:1861, 1979

internal carotid artery stenosis. Special report. Stroke 25:2523, 1994

69. Cohen S: Carotid endarterectomy for asymptomatic disease. J Stroke Cerebrovasc Dis 6:180, 1997

70. Hankey GJ, Slattery JM, Warlow CP: Prognosis and prognostic factors of retinal infarction: a prospective cohort study. BMJ 302:499, 1991

71. Antiplatelet Trialists' Collaboration: Collaborative overview of randomized trials of antiplatelet therapy. I. Prevention of death, myocardial infarction, and stroke by prolonged antiplatelet therapy in various categories of patients. BMJ 308:81, 1994

72. Bousser MG, Eschwege E, Haguenau M et al: "AICLA" controlled trial of aspirin and dipyridamole in the secondary prevention of atherothrombotic cerebral ischemia. Stroke 14:5, 1983

73. Ramirez-Lassepas M, Cipolle RJ: Medical treatment of transient ischemic attacks: does it influence mortality? Stroke 19:397, 1988

74. Trobe JD: Who needs carotid endarterctomy (circa 1996)? Ophthalmol Clin North Am 9:513, 1996

75. Natuzzi ES, Stoney RJ: Fibromuscular disease of the carotid artery. In Ernst C, Stanley JC (eds): Current Therapy in Vascular Surgery, 3rd ed, p 114. St. Louis, Mosby–Yearbook, 1995

76. Silbert PL, Mokri B, Schievink WI: Headache and neck pain in spontaneous internal carotid and vertebral dissection. Neurology 45:1517, 1995

76a. Biousse V, Touboul PJ, D'Anglejan-Chatillon J et al. Ophthalmologic manifestations of internal carotid artery dissection. Am J Ophthalmol 126:565, 1998

77. Schievink WI, Mokri B, Piepgras DG: Spontaneous dissection of the cervicocephalic arteries in childhood and adolescence. Neurology 44:1607, 1994

78. Lewis JR, Glaser JG, Scharz NJ et al: Pulseless (Takayasu) disease with ophthalmic manifestations. J Clin Neuroophthalmol 13:242, 1993

79. Williamson TH, Harris A: Color Doppler ultrasound imaging of the eye and orbit. Surv Ophthalmol 40:255, 1996

80. Mawn LA, Hedges TR, Rand W et al: Orbital color Doppler imaging in carotid occlusive disease. Arch Ophthalmol 115:492, 1997

81. Dexter DD, Whisnant JP, Connolly DC et al: The association of stroke and coronary heart disease: a population study. Mayo Clin Proc 62:1077, 1987

82. Bergen RL, Cangemi FE, Glassman R: Bilateral arterial occlusion secondary to Barlow's syndrome. Ann Ophthalmol 14:673, 1982

83. Lesser RL, Yeinemann M-H, Borkowski H et al: Mitral valve prolapse and amaurosis fugax. J Clin Neuroophthalmol 1:153, 1981

84. McKinsey DS, Ratts TE, Bisno AL: Underlying cardiac lesions in adults with infective endocarditis: the changing spectrum. Am J Med 82:681, 1987

85. Mangat HS: Retinal artery occlusion. Surv Ophthalmol 40:145, 1995

86. Brown GC, Magargal LE, Shields JA et al: Retinal arterial obstruction in children and young adults. Ophthalmology 88:18, 1981

87. Greven CM, Slusher MM, Weaver RG: Retinal arterial occlusions in young adults. Am J Ophthalmol 120:776, 1995

88. Wisotsky BJ, Engel HM: Transesophageal echocardiography in the diagnosis of branch retinal artery obstruction. Am J Ophthalmol 115:653, 1993

89. Johnson MW, Thomley ML, Huang SS et al: Idiopathic recurrent branch retinal artery occlusion: natural history and laboratory evaluation. Ophthalmology 101:480, 1994

90. Vine AK, Samama MM: The role of abnormalities in the anticoagulant and fibrinolytic systems in retinal vascular occlusions. Surv Ophthalmol 37:283, 1993

91. Wenzler EM, Rademakers AJJM, Boers GHJ et al: Hyperhomocysteinemia in retinal artery and vein occlusion. Am J Ophthalmol 115:162, 1993

92. Saver JL: Emerging risk factors for stroke: patent foramen ovale, proximal aortic atherosclerosis, antiphospholipid anti-bodies, and activated protein C resistance. J Stroke Cerebrovasc Dis 4:167, 1997

93. Glacet-Bernard A, Bayani N, Chretian P et al: Antiphospholipid antibodies in retinal vascular occlusions: a prospective study of 75 patients. Arch Ophthalmol 112:790, 1994

94. Selhub J, Jacques PF, Bostom AG et al: Association between plasma homocysteine concentrations and extracranial carotid artery stenosis. N Engl J Med 332:286, 1995

95. Lightman DA, Brod RD: Branch retinal artery occlusion associated with Lyme disease. Arch Ophthalmol 109:1198, 1991

96. Ruby AJ, Jampol LM: Crohn's disease and retinal vascular disease. Am J Ophthalmol 110:349, 1990

97. Haskjold E, Froland S, Egge K: Ocular polyarteritis nodosa: report of a case. Acta Ophthalmol 65:749, 1987

98. Petitti DB, Sidney S, Bernstein A et al: Stroke in users of low-dose oral contraceptives. N Engl J Med 335:8, 1996

99. Becker WJ: Migraine and oral contraceptives. Can J Neurol Sci 24:16, 1997

100. Schmidt D, Schumacher M, Wakhloo AK: Microcatheter urokinase infusion in central artery occlusion. Am J Ophthalmol 113:429, 1992

101. Eye Disease Case-Control Study Group: Risk factors for central retinal vein occlusion. Arch Ophthalmol 114:545, 1996

102. Biousse V, Newman NJ, Sternberg P: Retinal vein occlusion and transient monocular visual loss associated with hyperhomocystinemia. Am J Ophthalmol 124:257, 1997

103. Wiechens B, Schroder JO, Potzsch B et al: Primary antiphospholipid antibody syndrome and retinal occlusive vasculopathy. Am J Ophthalmol 123:848, 1997

104. Larsson J, Olafsdottir E, Bauer B: Activated protein C resistance in young adults with central retinal vein occlusion. Br J Ophthalmol 80:200, 1996

105. Fong ACO, Schatz H: Central retinal vein occlusion in young adults. Surv Ophthalmol 37:393, 1993

106. Wolter JR, Birchfield WJ: Ocular migraine in a young man resulting in unilateral blindness and retinal edema. J Pediatr Ophthalmol 8:173, 1971

107. Sanborn GE, Magargal L: Papillophlebitis: an update. In Smith JL (ed): Neuro-ophthalmology Enters the Nineties, p 47. Hialeah, FL, Dutton, 1988

108. Humayun M, Kattah J, Cupps TR et al: Papillophlebitis and arteriolar occlusion in a pregnant woman. J Clin Neuroophthalmol 12:226, 1992

109. Cogan DG: Retinal and papillary vasculitis. In Cant JS (ed): The William MacKensie Centenary Symposium on Ocular Circulation in Health and Disease, p 249. London: Kimpton, 1969

110. Sanders MD: Retinal arteritis, retinal vasculitis and autoimmune retinal vasculitis. Eye 1:441, 1987

111. George RK, Walton RC, Whitcup SM et al: Primary retinal vasculitis: systemic associations and diagnostic evaluation. Ophthalmology 103:384, 1996

112. Gordon MF, Coyle PK, Golub B: Eales' disease presenting as stroke in the young adult. Ann Neurol 24:264, 1988

113. O'Halloran HS, Pearson PA, Lee WB, Susac JO et al: Microangiopathy of the brain, retina, and cochlea (Susac syndrome). A report of five cases and a review of the literature. Ophthalmol 105:1038, 1998

114. Li HK, Dejean BJ, Tang RA: Reversal of visual loss with hyperbaric oxygen treatment in a patient with Susac syndrome. Ophthalmology 103:2091, 1996

115. Balcer LJ, Winterkorn JMS, Galetta SL: Neuro-ophthalmic manifestations of Lyme disease. J Neuroophthalmol 17:108, 1997

116. Ormerod LD, Skolnick KA, Menosky MM, Pavan PR et al: Retinal and choroidal manifestations of cat-scratch disease. Ophthalmology 105:1024, 1998

117. Brown SM, Jampol LM, Cantrill HL: Intraocular lymphoma presenting as retinal vasculitis. Surv Ophthalmol 39:133, 1994

118. Chang TS, Aylward GW, Davis JL et al: Idiopathic retinal vasculitis, aneurysms, and neuroretinitis. Ophthalmology 102:1089, 1995

119. Gass A, Graham E, Moseley IF et al: Cranial MRI in idiopathic retinal vasculitis. J Neurol 242:174, 1995

120. Moorthy RS, Inomata H, Rao NA: Vogt-Koyanagi-Harada syndrome. Surv Ophthalmol 39:265, 1995

120a. Biousse V, Trichet C, Bloch-Michel et al: Multiple sclerosis associated with uveitis in two large clinic-based series. Neurol 52:179, 1999

121. Jacobson DM: Acute zonal occult outer retinopathy and central nervous system inflammation. J Neuroophthalmol 16:172, 1996

122. Comu S, Verstraeten T, Rinkoff JS et al: Neurologic manifestations of acute posterior multifocal placoid pigment epitheliopathy. Stroke 27:996, 1996

123. Jabs DA: Ocular manifestations of HIV infection. Trans Am Ophthalmol Soc 93:623, 1995

124. Mueller AJ, Plummer DJ, Dua R et al: Analysis of visual dysfunctions in HIV-positive patients without retinitis. Am J Ophthalmol 124:158, 1997

125. Tenhula WN, Xu SZ, Madigan MC et al: Morphometric comparisons of optic nerve axon loss in acquired immunodeficiency syndrome. Am J Ophthalmol 113:14, 1992

126. Jabs DA: Acquired immunodeficiency syndrome and the eye. Arch Ophthalmol 114:863, 1996

127. Grossniklaus HE, Specht CS, Allaire G et al: Toxoplasma gondii retinochoroiditis and optic neuritis in acquired immune deficiency syndrome: report of a case. Ophthalmology 97:1342, 1990

128. Holland GN and Executive Committee of the American Uveitis Society: Standard diagnostic criteria for the diagnosis of the acute retinal necrosis syndrome. Am J Ophthalmol 117:663, 1994

129. Friedman SM, Margo CE: Bilateral central retinal occlusions in patient with acquired immunodeficiency syndrome: clinicopathologic correlation. Arch Ophthalmol 113:1184, 1995

130. Zimmer C, Nieuwenhuis I, Danisevski M et al: Sudden blindness in an AIDS patient: simultaneous infection with cytomegalovirus and herpes simplex viruses and development of malignant non Hodgkin lymphoma. Klin Monatsbl Augenheilkd 199:48, 1991

131. Weiner A, Sandberg MA, Gaudio AR et al: Hydroxychloroquine retinopathy. Am J Ophthalmol 112:528, 1991

132. Piltz J, Wertenbaker C, Lance S et al: Digoxin toxicity: recognizing the varied visual presentations. J Clin Neuroophthalmol 13:275, 1993

133. Mermoud A, Safran AB, de Stoutz N: Pain upon eye movement following digoxin absorption. J Neuroophthalmol 12:41, 1992

134. Fisher CM: Visual disturbances associated with quinidine and quinine. Neurology 31:1569, 1981

135. Nayfield SG, Gorin MB: Tamoxifen-associated eye disease: a review. J Clin Oncol 14:1018, 1996

136. Wu HM, Lee AG, Lehane DE et al: Ocular and orbital complications of intrarterial cisplatin. J Neuroophthalmol 17:195, 1997

137. Guyer DR, Tiedman J, Yannuzzi LA et al: Interferon-associated retinopathy. Arch Ophthalmol 111:350, 1993

138. Dukar O, Barr CC: Visual loss complicating OKT3 monoclonal antibody therapy. Am J Ophthalmol 115:781, 1993

139. Barletta JP, Fanous MM, Hamed LM: Temporary blindness in the TUR syndrome. J Neuroophthalmol 14:6, 1994

140. Newman NJ, Capone A, Leeper HF et al: Clinical and subclinical ophthalmic findings with retinol deficiency. Ophthalmology 101:1077, 1994

141. Lesser RL, Brodie SE, Sugin SL: Mastocytosis-induced nyctalopia. J Neuroophthalmol 16:115, 1996

142. Thirkill CE, Roth AM, Keltner JL: Cancer-associated retinopathy. Arch Ophthalmol 105:372, 1987

143. Wolf JE, Arden GB: Selective magnocellular damage in melanoma-associated retinopathy: comparison with congenital stationary nightblindness. Vision Res 36:2369, 1996

144. Thirkill CE: Cancer associated retinopathy: the CAR syndrome. Neuro-ophthalmology 14:297, 1994

144a. Guy J, Aptsiauri N: Treatment of paraneoplastic visual loss with intravenous immunoglobulin. Report of 3 cases. Arch Ophthalmol 117:471, 1999

145. Mizener JB, Kimura AE, Adamus G et al: Autoimmune retinopathy in the absence of cancer. Am J Ophthalmol 123:607, 1997

146. Vinken PJ, Bruyn GW (eds): Handbook of Clinical Neurology. The Neurophakomatoses, vol. 14. New York, American Elsevier, 1972

147. Gomez MR: Neurocutaneous Diseases. In Bradley WG, Daroff RB, Fenichel GM et al (eds): Neurology in Clinical Practice, p 1566. Boston, Butterworth-Heineman, 1996

148. Dotan SA, Trobe JD, Gebarski SS: Visual loss in tuberous sclerosis. Neurology 41:1915, 1991

149. Kroll AJ, Ricker DP, Robb RM et al: Vitreous hemorrhage complicating retinal astrocytic hamartoma. Surv Ophthalmol 26:31, 1981

150. Altman NR, Purser RK, Post MJD: Tuberous sclerosis: characteristics at CT and MR imaging. Radiology 167:527, 1988

151. Savino PJ, Glaser JS, Luxemberg MN: Pulsating enophthalmos and choroidal hamartomas: two rare stigmata of neurofibromatosis. Br J Ophthalmol 61:483, 1977

152. Lewis RA, Riccardi VM: Von Recklinghaussen neurofibromatosis: incidence of iris hamartomata. Ophthalmology 88:348, 1981

153. Ragge NK, Baser ME, Klein J et al: Ocular abnormalities in neurofibromatosis 2. Am J Ophthalmol 120:634, 1995

154. Deliganis AV, Geyer JR, Berger MS: Prognostic significance of type 1 neurofibromatosis (von Recklinghausen disease) in childhood optic glioma. Neurosurgery 38:1114, 1996

Part II. The Optic Nerve

Congenital Optic Disc Dysplasias and Anomalies
Nerve Hypoplasia
Colobomas and Pits
Dysversions and Crescents
Anomalous Disc Elevations: Pseudopapilledema and Hyaline Bodies
Heredodegenerative Optic Atrophies
Recessive Optic Atrophy
Simple
Complicated
Wolfram's Syndrome and Juvenile Diabetes
Dominant (Juvenile) Optic Atrophy
Leber's Disease
Neurodegenerative Syndromes
Acquired Optic Nerve Disease: An Overview
Clinical Characteristics
Neuroimaging Techniques
The "Swollen Disc": Differential Diagnosis
Papilledema with Raised Intracranial Pressure
Pseudotumor Cerebri Syndrome
Primary: Idiopathic Intracranial Hypertension
Secondary Pseudotumor Cerebri Syndrome
Inflammatory Optic Neuropathies: Optic Neuritis
Demyelinative Disease
Immune-mediated and Atypical Optic Neuritides
Infective Neuropathies

Slowly Progressive and "Chronic" Optic Neuritis
Contiguous Inflammations
Ischemic Optic Neuropathies
Common (Arteriosclerotic, Non-arteritic) Ischemic Optic Neuropathy
Cranial (Giant Cell) Arteritis
Diabetes Mellitus Papillopathy
Infrequently Associated Disorders
Glaucoma and Pseudoglaucoma
Neoplasms and Related Conditions
Masses of the Optic Disc
Optic Gliomas
Perioptic Meningiomas
Secondary Neoplasms: Carcinoma and Lymphomas
Paranasal Sinus Disease
Orbitopathies: Graves' Disease
Vascular Compression: Aneurysms
Nutritional and Toxic Optic Neuropathies
Vitamin Deficiencies and "Tobacco-Alcohol Amblyopia"
Drugs and Toxins
Central Scotoma Syndromes
Traumatic Optic Neuropathies
Orbito-cranial Injuries
Radiation and Thermal Burns

My lad asked me to look up a word in the French Dictionary and I could not make out the letters because of the bouncing grey dots. The next day I could see peripheral colours but the central zone of vision was covered with what seemed like a grey asbestos mat that occluded all light. The next day saw a further deterioration, loss of colour and general darkening. . . . In three days all visual response had been lost.

High on the right of my circle of vision, through the murk, I could make out my fingers fluttering after two weeks of blackness. "Hello, Cobalt Blue!" Response to the ophthalmoscope. Strong white light was blue. . . .

It was a thrill to see the cloud and identify its shape at such distance even though that mid-grey was as near as I could get to white. . . . A friend brought me a plant with red flowers. . . . "You may have difficulty with reds." . . . Another pot of flowers but what fascinated me was the pointilist-like disintegration of each detail . . . At home. The grey flicks are still there but . . . I add this ironic homage . . . "You won't notice any difference but a doctor could tell."

Artist Peter MacKarell went blind in one eye and then recovered, no doubt due to optic neuritis.
New Scientist, February, 1982

The optic nerve, roughly the diameter of thick spaghetti, is subject to a staggering variety of congenital anomalies and acquired disorders. Or perhaps it is even more remarkable that most persons are born without and re-

main free of optic nerve disease over a long lifetime. From simple myopia, optic neuritis, glaucoma, infarcts, and even its unfavorable location in the crowded skull base, the second numbered cranial nerve is victim to the widest spectrum of developmental malformations and disease processes. Consider the gross anatomic relationships (Fig. 5–11): at the nerve head, the peculiarities of vascular supply and ocular tissue tension (intraocular pressure) are unique; in the orbit, the nerve may be compromised by muscle enlargement or soft tissue tumors; the optic canal is flimsy protection from fractures or sinus inflammations; and the neighborhood relationship with the pituitary gland and arterial circle is clearly an evolutionary disadvantage. Indeed, malfunctions of the optic nerves and chiasm, taken together as the anterior visual pathways, constitute a large portion of all neuro-ophthalmologic diagnostic and management challenges.

CONGENITAL OPTIC DISC DYSPLASIAS AND ANOMALIES

Considerable variation in optic disc size exists, influenced at least in part by refractive error. At times, it is difficult to determine ophthalmoscopically when the size

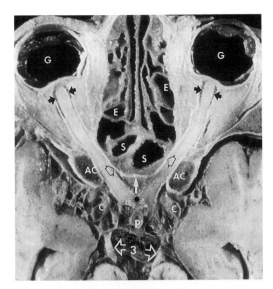

Fig. 5–11. Axial anatomic section of the course of the optic nerves. *G,* globes; *small black arrows* just behind globes show the subarachnoid space within the optic nerve sheaths; *S,* sphenoid and *E,* ethmoid air cells; *AC,* anterior clinoids with dark bone marrow; *open black arrows* on the canalicular segments of the optic nerves indicate the thin bony medial optic canal wall shared with the sphenoid sinus; *white arrow* indicates the tuberculum of the planum sphenoidale; *asterisk* indicates chiasm bordered by carotid arteries, *C*; *P,* pituitary stalk; oculomotor nerves, 3 with *open arrows.* (Courtesy of Dr. Renate Unsold)

of the disc falls outside the limits of normal. Megalopapilla, other than those disc variants occurring in myopia or with frank colobomatous malformations, must be exceedingly rare, but micropapilla (disc hypoplasia) is not and warrants inclusion in the diagnostic dilemma of the child with poor vision in one or both eyes. Other congenital disc malformations are accompanied by field defects mistaken for acquired disease, or they are regularly misinterpreted as nerve head swelling.

Among those benign conditions mistaken for new disease is *aberrant myelination* of the retinal nerve fiber layer on and around the disc, which presents a funduscopic picture of intensely white patches with feathered edges (see Color Plate 5–1A). Said to occur in less than 1% of ophthalmologic patients, slightly more common in men, and bilateral in 20%, such myelination is anecdotally linked to numerous conditions, but it may be associated with the triad of amblyopia, strabismus, and myopia.[1]

Nerve Hypoplasia

Hypoplasia of the optic disc may be unilateral or bilateral, marked or minimal (see Color Plate 5–1C), and associated with good or poor visual function. The condition may occur in isolation or may accompany other ocular or forebrain malformations. This anomaly has

alternately been termed micropapilla, partial aplasia, or, incorrectly, aplasia. Literature related to optic disc hypoplasia has been for years almost exclusively composed of isolated case reports, but recognition of associated endocrine and central nervous system (CNS) anomalies and the relative ease of magnetic resonance imaging (MRI) have provoked considerable rewakened interest. This is especially true when optic hypoplasia is not simply part of gross ocular maldevelopment, but rather is discovered as a cause of diminished vision, strabismus, nystagmus, or growth retardation, in various combinations. Some authors[2,3] contend that increased abuse of alcohol and drugs has contributed to an increased prevalence of optic nerve hypoplasia (ONH), but surely also there is heightened awareness of this funduscopic anomaly and its systemic ramifications.

When hyperplasia is bilateral and is accompanied by poor vision and nystagmus, most patients harbor other developmental abnormalities, but such defects occur in only about 20% of unilateral or segmental cases of hypoplasia.[4] When the nerve head is slightly or segmentally reduced, especially in the presence of normal acuity, fundus diagnosis may be supported by careful side-by-side comparison of disc photographs (Fig. 5–12), or calculation from photographs of the ratio of the disc center-to-fovea distance (DM), to disc diameter (DD); this ratio (DM/DD) is significantly higher in hypoplasia than in normal fundi, a ratio greater than 3.0 being considered diagnostic.[5] Otherwise, optic disc dimensions may be assessed using the Goldmann three-mirror contact lens and adjustable slit-lamp beam to measure vertical and horizontal disc diameters and applying the formula for area of an ellipse, according to the method of Jonas et al.[6] In eyes with minimal spherical refractive error, Zeki et al[7] found that a ratio of disc-to-macula to DD of 2.94 provides an 95% population upper limit, whereas disc hypoplasia has a mean ratio of 3.57.

Field defects with ONH are variable and include central depressions, nasal and temporal wedges and hemianopias, inferior "altitudinal" loss, and generalized constrictions.[8,9] Disc hypoplasia need not be accompanied by severe diminution of visual acuity, but, as a rule, the smaller the disc, the worse is the vision. The size of the optic disc may also be diminished in albinism, aniridia, and in other disc anomalies such as inferior scleral crescents and in the "crowded" elevated discs of pseudopapilledema (see below).

Maternal diabetes has been implicated in simple ONH, but especially in segmental hypoplasia of the superior portion of the nerve head.[10] Otherwise incriminated as teratogenic are a variety of toxic agents, including phenytoin, quinine, alcohol, lysergic acid,[2] and cocaine.[11]

ONH may be the result of a spectrum of malformations occurring at several sites along the developing visual system, from the retinal ganglion cells and nerve

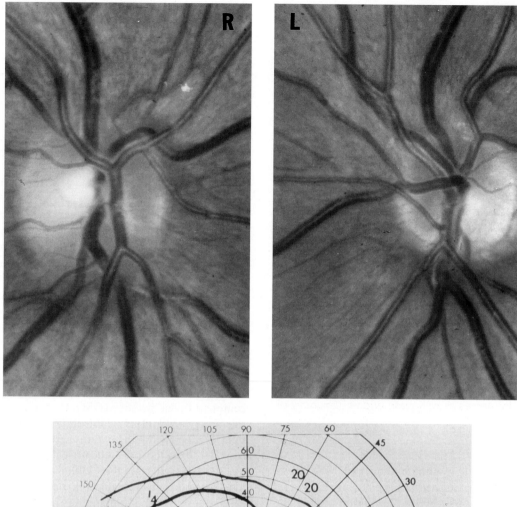

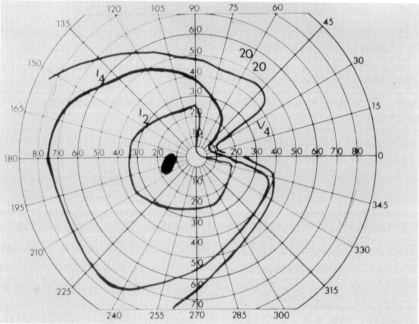

Fig. 5–12. Relative optic nerve hypoplasia. **Top.** *R,* right optic disc; *L,* left optic disc. Note smaller left disc, with otherwise normal morphology and no peripapillary pigment disturbance. **Bottom.** Left visual field shows a dense nasal wedge defect. A left afferent pupil defect was present, and the case misdiagnosed as optic neuritis due to multiple sclerosis.

head through the chiasm to occipital cortex.[12] Hoyt et al[13] described "bow-tie" hypoplasia (homonymous hemioptic hypoplasia) in eyes *opposite* congenital cerebral hemisphere lesions, with simple ONH in the homolateral fundus, resulting from transsynaptic retrograde axonal degeneration.

The congenital syndrome of *septo-optic dysplasia* (de Morsier's syndrome) may be recognized by the clinical triad of short stature, nystagmus, and optic disc hypoplasia. Neuroimaging demonstrates a single anterior ventricle (holoprosencephaly) without a midline partition; that is, the septum pellucidum is absent (Fig. 5–13). Other important but variable aspects include the following: neonatal hypotonia, seizures, and prolonged bilirubinemia; growth hormone, corticotropin, and antidiuretic hormone deficiencies; and mental retardation. Brodsky et al[14] reported sudden death in patients with corticotropin deficiency, diabetes insipidus, and thermoregulatory disturbances, aggravated by fever and dehydration. The forebrain dysplasia is important to recognize because accompanying growth hormone deficiency (and often diabetes insipidus) may be corrected, resulting in resumption of normal skeletal growth patterns.[15] Septo-optic dysplasia is not necessarily a strictly separate entity, and various radiologic findings and endocrine deficiencies carry specific prognostic clinical implications. MRI[16] is essential in identifying several clinical subgroups of ONH, as follows: isolated ONH; absence of septum pellucidum; posterior pituitary ectopia (posterior pituitary bright spot absent or ectopic hyperintense focus in tuber cinereum, absence of infundibulum, and especially growth hormone deficiency and diabetes insipidus); hemispheric migration anomalies (schizencephaly, cortical heterotopia); and intrauterine or perinatal hemispheric injuries (*e.g.,* periventricular leukomalacia).

Dysplastic disc development may accompany congenital tumors that involve the anterior visual pathways, such as optic glioma and craniopharyngioma, such nerve heads being described as hypoplastic, truncated, or irregularly oval.[17] Other investigators[18] have reported *enlarged* discs with optic glioma.

It seems rational that patients with bilateral ONH should undergo neuroradiologic imaging, preferably MRI, and endocrinologic assessment, and that patients with unilateral ONH, or with segmental disc hypoplasia, in whom growth and development are normal, should undergo regular ophthalmologic and pediatric examinations. Children with unilateral ONH and reduced vision may undergo a trial of occlusion therapy to discover the additional role of amblyopia.

True *aplasia of the optic nerves* is an exceedingly rare condition, only some 30 cases reported in the world literature, with no evidence of a hereditary tendency or consistent environmental factors.[19] In an otherwise healthy infant, bilateral aplasia of optic nerves, chiasm, and tracts is documented.[20]

Colobomas and Pits

Optic nerve colobomas (Greek, meaning mutilation or curtailment) or pits are congenital malformations that enlarge or distort the nerve head circumference and assume several forms (Fig. 5–14; see also Chapter 13, Fig. 13–4): enlarged discs with deep excavation; enlarged, relatively round disc filled with retained embryonic glial and vascular remnants, at times projecting forward as a funnel ("morning glory syndrome" of Kindler); discs posteriorly displaced within excavated peripapillary staphylomas; dysplastic, excavated, vertically oblong discs contiguous with retinochoroidal colobomas, located especially inferiorly; and slightly enlarged, irregular discs containing *pits* within the borders of the nerve head (see below). In most instances, the expanded

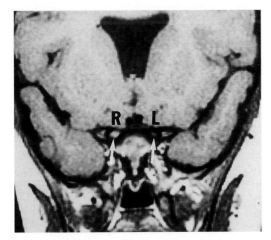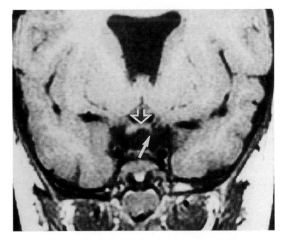

Fig. 5–13. Septo-optic dysplasia: magnetic resonance coronal images. **Left.** Absent septum pellucidum with a single midline ventricle; *arrows* indicate prechiasmal optic nerves: *L,* left nerve is hypoplastic (compare with right, *R*). **Right.** At chiasm (*open arrow*) note the hypoplastic left nerve contribution (*arrow*).

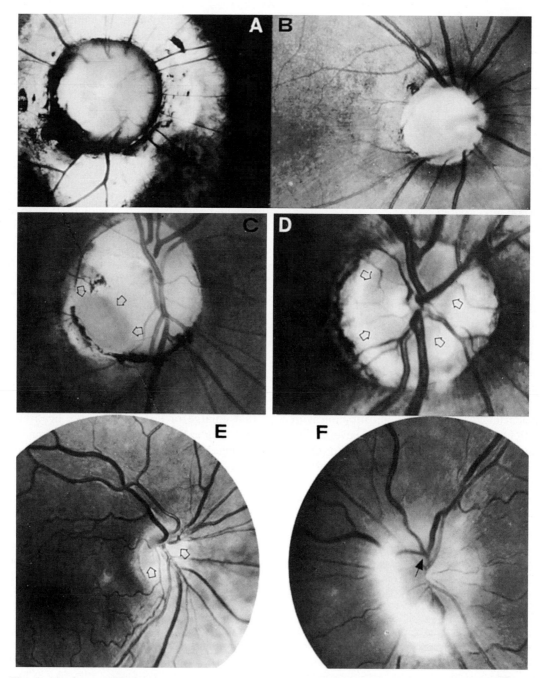

Fig. 5–14. Congenital anomalies of the optic disc. **A.** Large disc coloboma is surrounded by staphylomatous sclera. The disc is partially filled with dysplastic glial tissue. The patient had a transsphenoidal encephalocele that presented as a nasopharyngeal mass. **B.** Moderate-sized disc coloboma with a central cavity. **C.** Typical optic pit (*arrows*) in the inferotemporal aspect of an enlarged disc. **D.** Unilateral anomalous disc. Nerve substance (outlined by *arrows*) is truncated nasally and surrounded by a scleral ring. The patient complained of transient visual loss lasting minutes. Vision was 20/20 (6/6) with a mild superotemporal field defect (see also Fig. 5–15). **E.** Inferior crescent (Fuchs' coloboma; tilted disc). The actual disc substance (*arrows*) is hypoplastic, with a large inferonasal scleral crescent. Note hypopigmentation in the inferonasal retinal pigment epithelium and choroid (see field defect in Fig. 5–16) and anomalous trifurcation of the inferior retinal artery. **F.** Myelinated nerve fibers on an anomalously elevated disc with no central cup. Note anomalous venous trifurcation (*arrow*) (see Color Plate 5–1A).

peripapillary area is irregularly pigmented and is crossed by numerous anomalous vessels (Fig. 5–14A). These conditions probably represent different degrees of dysplasia in the spectrum of optic nerve malformations possibly related to faulty closure of the embryonic ventral (fetal) fissure of the optic stalk and cup.[21] Rare instances of coloboma show momentary dynamic changes in the surrounding peripapillary staphyloma, described as "contractile" or "pulsatile," and possibly related to mesodermal fat or smooth muscle replacing the optic meninges.[22,23]

Savell and Cook[24] recorded a family with 15 members affected by bilateral colobomas and a pattern of autosomal dominant inheritance, but most colobomatous dysplasias are unilateral and sporadic, especially the morning glory type.[3,22] Gopal et al[25] categorized several variants of disc position and morphology in the spectrum of coloboma, the majority of discs being included in the retinochoroidal defect itself. Simple disc colobomas may be accompanied by a variety of systemic disorders,[3] including Aicardi's syndrome, CHARGE association (congenital heart disease, choanal atresia), oculo-auricular dysplasia (Goldenhar), linear sebaceous nevus, and orbital cyst. Bilateral disc coloboma is reported in association with bilateral retro-bulbar arachnoid cysts,[26] and with Dandy-Walker cyst[27]; unilateral coloboma is recorded with basal vascular system lesions that include carotid occlusions, moya-moya collateralization with dolichoectasia, and absent ophthalmic artery.[28]

Of great clinical importance is the association of disc malformations, especially morning glory,[29] and congenital forebrain anomalies, including *basal encephaloceles.* Herniated brain tissue may present as pulsating exophthalmos (spheno-orbital encephalocele, most commonly in neurofibromatosis), hypertelorism with a pulsatile nasopharyngeal mass (transsphenoidal encephalocele), or a frontonasal mass, with or without hypertelorism (fronto-ethmoidal encephalocele) or other mid-facial malformation. The physical findings of transsphenoidal or transethmoidal basal encephalocele are listed below:

Midline facial anomalies
  Broad nasal root
  Hypertelorism
  Midline lip defect
  Wide bitemporal skull diameter
  Cleft palate
Nasopharyngeal mass
  Midline pharyngeal space
  Pulsatile
  Symptoms of nasal obstruction
  "Nasal polyp" (true polyp rare in infancy)
  Hypopituitarism/dwarfism
Ocular
Congenital disc anomalies (colobomatous dysplasias)
  Chiasmal field defects, poor vision
  Exotropia

Neuroimaging of the skull base, the chiasm, and the inferoanterior brain structures affirms the diagnosis. Biopsy or attempted resection of posterior nasopharyngeal masses should be vigorously deprecated because these "masses" invariably are encephalomeningoceles, and surgical manipulation may result in meningitis with tragic outcome. Patients with congenital disc malformations may complain of transient obscurations of vision lasting seconds to minutes, but the mechanism of visual disturbance is unknown (Figs. 5–14D and 5–15).

Pits of the optic disc are usually definable ophthalmoscopically as intrapapillary pearly gray dimples or slits containing filmy pale glial material, located typically just within the scleral rim of the disc margin, extending about 2 clock hours or one-third of the disc diameter. The disc border is frequently distorted and may be highlighted by contiguous mild pigment epithelial changes (see Fig. 5–14C), and cilioretinal vessels may traverse the depression.[30] Pits usually occur singly in a temporal location, less frequently centrally, or in an inferior, superior, or nasal quadrant, but they may be multiple and bilateral in perhaps some 15% of patients. They are rarely familial, but an autosomal dominant inheritance pattern is possible. Indeed, Ragge et al[31] suggested that there is evidence that cavitary anomalies of the disc form a spectrum ranging from pits to colobomas, and the existence of persons with pits in one eye and contralateral coloboma implies that these anomalies are variations of the same genetic or environmental insult; moreover, pedigrees are reported that contain the various phenotypic expressions of the cavitary anomalies, some related to mutations of the *PAX2* gene.

The association of temporal pits with serous detachment of the macula, and consequent diminished acuity, is well known, with an incidence perhaps in some 50%[32] of patients and presenting in young adulthood. Otherwise, stable visual field changes take the form of dense nerve fiber bundle defects that extend from the blind spot, especially toward fixation in the papillomacular zone.[33] In contrast to congenital disc pits, acquired pits are part of the spectrum of glaucomatous excavation, perhaps more frequent with normal ocular tension, typically with dense field depressions in the central portion of the visual field.[34] Pulsatile communication of fluid between the vitreous cavity and a retro-bulbar cyst via an optic pit has been demonstrated.[35]

Dysversions and Crescents

Field defects associated with congenital dysversions of the optic disc ("tilted discs," situs inversus) and accompanying depigmented peripapillary crescents may be confused with the bitemporal hemianopia of acquired chiasmal lesions. The most common variety of crescent is that located inferiorly (inferior conus, Fuchs' coloboma), first described by Fuchs in 1882 (see Color Plate 5–1D; see Fig. 5–14E). Not only is the disc hypoplastic,

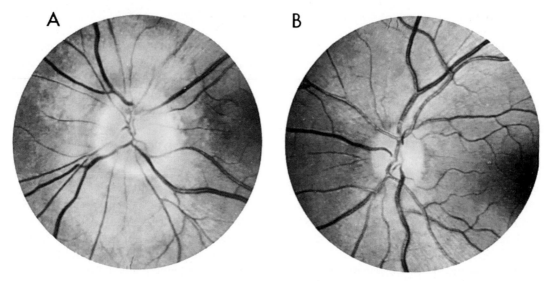

Fig. 5–15. A young woman complained of transient obscurations of right vision lasting 15 seconds. **A.** Right optic disc is large and surrounded by staphylomatous sclera. The retinal vessels are somewhat attenuated. The remainer of ocular examination is unremarkable. **B.** Normal left disc. (Courtesy of Dr. Peter Rosen)

ovoid, and vertically truncated, but also the fundus in the sector contiguous to the crescent takes on a semialbinotic or tigroid appearance because of hypopigmentation of pigment epithelium and choroid. Because the inferonasal retinal quadrant is involved most frequently, relative superior temporal field defects are found (Fig. 5–16), and they may simulate bitemporal hemianopia.[36] As a rule, inferior crescents are associated with moderate myopia with astigmatism (usually manifest in the same axis as the dysversion of the disc, that is, between 90° and 110° in right eyes and between 90° and 70° in left eyes), slightly reduced corrected visual acuity, and abnormal foveal reflex. During field testing, failure to properly correct for optical anomalies enhances the refractive scotoma that is most profound at and above the area of the blind spot. Riise[37] provided an excellent monograph on this entity. Disc abnormalities in craniofacial disorders, including hypertelorism, Crouzon's and Apert's syndromes, show a spectrum of forms: simple pallor, tilt and inferior conus, and coloboma, some with widespread fundus hypopigmentation.[38]

Anomalous Disc Elevations: Pseudopapilledema and Hyaline Bodies

Anomalous elevation of the optic nerve head, with or without ophthalmoscopically detectable hyaline bodies, is a major cause of unnecessary alarm and misdirected diagnostic procedures. Because this funduscopic appearance somewhat resembles acquired disc swelling, including papilledema of raised intracranial pressure, in previous decades patients were subjected to cerebral arteriography, pneumoencephalography, and even craniotomy for innocent headaches, vertigo, or more trivial

symptoms. Nowhere in neuro-ophthalmology is funduscopic differentiation more critical, for once a pronouncement of "papilledema" is made, a course of neurodiagnostic procedures becomes inevitable, and the patient, usually a child or young adult, as well as family members, endure the suspicion of brain tumor.

Congenitally elevated discs have been termed *pseudopapilledema* or *pseudoneuritis,* but, when possible, more specific funduscopic characteristics should be described (*e.g.,* intrapapillary hyaline bodies, simple hyperopia, persistent hyaloid tissue). It is likely that most cases of anomalous elevation are associated with hyaline bodies of the nerve head (alternately, *drusen;* because the term "drusen" is more frequently applied to the common multiple punctate pigment epithelial, subretinal lesions at the posterior pole, perhaps the term "hyaline bodies" is less confusing, histopathologic tinctorial niceties aside).

Disc hyaline bodies are acellular laminated concretions of unknown source, often partially calcified, and possibly related to accumulation of axoplasmic derivatives of degenerating retinal nerve fibers, in which orthograde axoplasmic flow is obstipated at an abnormally narrow scleral canal.[39,40] Hyaline bodies slowly become (more) visible as they enlarge toward the disc surface and margins, but the overlying retinal nerve fibers also becomes progressively thinner. Anomalously elevated discs in children usually do not show ophthalmoscopically detectable hyaline bodies (said to be "buried"), which insidiously emerge by the early teens. Hoover et al[41] reported first evidence in one or both eyes at a mean age of 12.1 years in 40 children, and other series included a low age range of 6 years.[42]

The occurrence of overt hyaline bodies in parents of children with anomalously elevated discs, but without

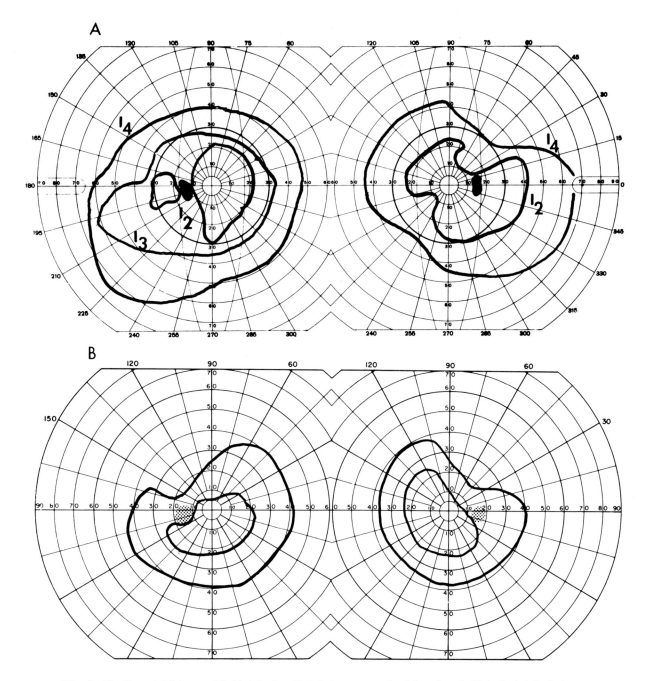

Fig. 5–16. Pseudobitemporal field defects with inferior crescents of the disc. **A.** Note that defects have vertices at or near the blind spots and the vertical meridian is not a limiting border. (RE: −7.00 +1.50 cx 155°; LE: −8.00 +3.00 cx 87°). **B.** Superior temporal defects slope across vertical meridian. Defects are slight (2, 3/1000 w) and relative.

apparent hyaline bodies, attests to both the progressive and the heredofamilial nature of this disorder. Indeed, some family members have visible hyaline bodies, whereas others have only elevated discs (see Plate 5–1E). Examination of family members is ideal when the distinction between true papilledema and pseudopapilledema is in doubt.

According to the genetic analysis of Lorentzen,[43] disc hyaline bodies are inherited as an autosomal ir-

regular dominant trait. Additionally, there appears to be a distinct tendency for occurrence in fair Caucasians.[42,44]

Although one disc may be more elevated than the other, both with or without apparent hyaline bodies, there is a tendency toward some degree of bilaterality. Lorentzen's[43] figure for bilaterality in ophthalmoscopically visible hyaline bodies is 73%, and that of Rosenberg et al[44] is 69%. Mustonen[45] studied 184 patients and found hyaline bodies to occur bilaterally in 66.9%, strictly unilateral in 25.5%, and with the contralateral eye showing disc elevation without hyaline bodies in 7.6%. There is no significant relationship between hyaline bodies and refractive error,[44,45] a factor further minimized in light of unilateral occurrence. With the infrequent exception of retinitis pigmentosa,[46] and angioid streaks (with and without pseudoxanthoma elasticum),[47] there appears to be no statistically significant association of hyaline bodies with the numerous and diverse ocular and neurologic disorders (including tuberous sclerosis) with which they have been described.[44,45]

Hyaline bodies may become symptomatic by virtue of either insidious field loss or spontaneous hemorrhage, at times associated with choroidal neovascular membrane formation, even in children.[41,48] Field defects usually take the form of blind spot enlargement, arcuate or other nerve fiber bundle patterns, or irregular peripheral contraction[49,50] (Fig. 5–17). These deficits typically progress exceedingly slowly, with a predilection to involve the inferior nasal quadrant. Because enlarged blind spots occur in both pseudopapilledema and true papilledema, this finding is of no differential diagnostic significance. Loss of central field, that is, diminished acuity, should not usually be attributed to disc drusen unless it is due to hemorrhagic complications such as bleeding from submacular fibrovascular membranes (Color Plate 5–2D), arterial occlusions, or ischemic disc infarction[51,52] or is associated with profound loss of peripheral field, which may occur rarely without obvious additional fundus findings.[53]

It is not uncommon to elicit a history of transient obscurations of vision in patients with hyaline bodies,[43] and this symptom may further serve to confuse the clinical differentiation from true papilledema. These episodes may last seconds to hours, and vision may be profoundly affected during the episode.[54] Sarkies and Sanders[55] have documented the extraordinary history of 26 years of recurrent episodic visual loss associated with ischemic disc swelling, perhaps related to anomalous vasculature.

Pseudopapilledema, with or without visible intrapapillary hyaline bodies, is not an uncommon condition. Friedman et al[56] cited the following figures for incidence of hyaline bodies: in Lorentzen's clinical study, 3.4/1000; in histologic series, 10 and 20.4/1000 (the latter figure indicating a frequency of 6 times that of the clinical diagnosis). Therefore, it should not be surprising that other ophthalmoscopic changes occur, but they need not be statistically related. I have seen a 54-year-old woman with long-standing bilateral hyaline bodies who developed mild but distinct disc swelling associated with a massive right hemispheral glioblastoma. In addition, a 15-year-old girl presented with bilateral pseudopapilledema and typical unilateral papillitis that recovered spontaneously.

Ophthalmoscopic criteria that distinguish between true and pseudopapilledema are listed below and are elaborated in Color Plates 5–1E and F and Color Plates 5–2A, B, and C.

1. The central cup is absent; the disc diameter tends toward small.

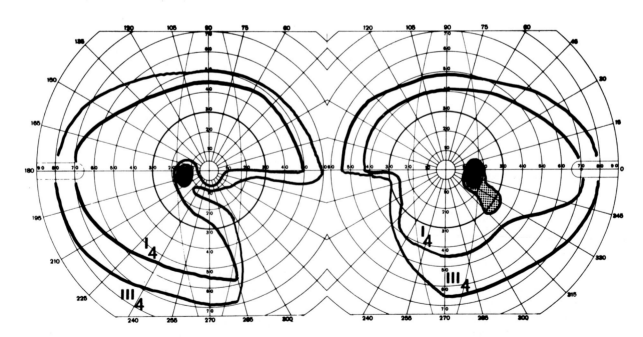

Fig. 5–17. Defects with hyaline bodies (drusen) of the nerve head. Irregular enlargement of blind spots is frequent and may be accentuated with derangement of peripapillary pigment epithelium (see Color Plates 5–2A and B). Nerve fiber bundle defects commonly course inferonasally; irregular, general peripheral contraction and wedge defects are also seen.

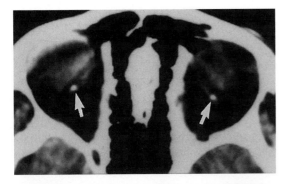
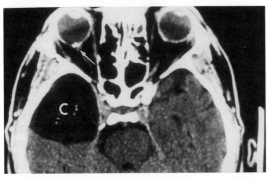
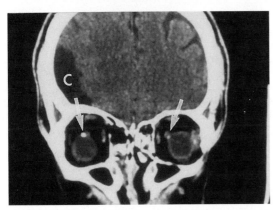

Fig. 5–18. Hyaline bodies (*arrows*) of optic discs on computed tomography. Note the incidental arachnoid cyst (*C*) of the temporal fossa, in **middle** and **bottom.**

2. Vessels arise from the central apex of the disc.
3. Anomalous branching of vessels occurs; an increased number of major disc vessels is noted; venous pulsation is present.
4. The disc may be transilluminated with a focal light source of the ophthalmoscope or slit beam, with a glow of hyaline bodies when present.
5. The disc margins are irregular with derangement of peripapillary retinal pigment epithelium.
6. Superficial capillary telangiectasia is absent.
7. No hemorrhages (rare exceptions) are seen.
8. No exudates or cotton-wool spots are present.

If difficulty in fundus diagnosis persists, the following rules may prove valuable: a spontaneous venous pulsation militates strongly against papilledema of increased cerebrospinal fluid (CSF) pressure; if the patient is otherwise thriving, it is probably not papilledema; computed tomography (CT) scan[57] and ultrasonography can reveal buried hyaline bodies (Fig. 5–18).

HEREDODEGENERATIVE OPTIC ATROPHIES

Among the causes of insidious, bilateral, and symmetric loss of central vision must be considered the heredodegenerative optic atrophies. Although it is seemingly a simple task to uncover familial incidence, in many cases such patterns cannot easily be established or are confounded by variations in phenotypic expression. Optic abiotrophies may occur as monosymptomatic isolated bilateral central visual defects, or they may accompany other nervous system degenerations involving motor, sensory, and auditory function. Optic atrophy also evolves secondarily in heritable storage disorders, in which accumulation of abnormal material in retinal ganglion cells results in consecutive disc pallor (*e.g.,* Tay-Sachs disease; see Chapter 5, Part I). Retinitis pigmentosa and other retinal dystrophies, including Leber's congenital amaurosis, show variable degrees of optic atrophy, but the primary disorder is the retinal degeneration.

Simple or complicated optic atrophies occur in various patterns of transmission and with graded symptomatology, such that a vast and heterogenous literature has accrued. Table 5–6 is an attempt at pragmatic clinical classification.

Recessive Optic Atrophy

Simple

Isolated optic atrophy of recessive inheritance must represent a relatively rare entity, the very existence of which has been called into question.[58] In older literature citations, most such instances were not clinically well documented, where consanguineous parentage was roughly coupled with congenital or early childhood optic atrophy, and most cases were reported without electroretinography (ERG) recording, much less modern techniques that assess mitochondrial genome mutations. Those cases originally described by Behr in 1909 as complicated optic atrophy (see below) seem too heterogeneous for analysis, and citation search of the *Index Medicus* and *Medline* since 1968 reveals no clearly documented cases.[58]

Complicated

The previous reservations notwithstanding, instances are described of a form of complicated optic atrophy, also called *infantile recessive atrophy,* or Behr's syndrome. In 1909, Behr described six boys in whom optic

TABLE 5–6. Heredofamilial Optic Atrophies

	Dominant	Recessive			Cytoplasmic
	Juvenile (infantile)	Early infantile (congenital); simple	Behr's type; complicated*	With diabetes mellitus; ± deafness	Leber's disease
Age at onset	Childhood (4–8 hr)	Early childhood† (3–4 yr)	Childhood (1–9 hr)	Childhood (6–14 yr)	Early adulthood (18–30 yr; up to sixth decade)
Visual impairment	Mild/moderate (20/40–20/200)	Severe (20/200–HM)	Moderate (20/200)	Severe (20/400–FC)	Moderate/severe (20/200–FC)
Nystagmus	Rare‡	Usual	In 50%	Absent	Absent
Optic disc	Mild temporaral pallor; ± temporal excavation	Marked diffuse pallor (± arteriolar attenuation)§	Mild temporal pallor	Marked diffuse pallor	Moderate diffuse pallor; nerve fiber prominent especially in acute phase
Color vision	Blue-yellow dyschromatopsia	Severe dyschromatopsia/achromatopsia	Moderate to severe dyschromatopsia	Severe dyschromatopsia	Dense central scrotoma for colors
Course	Variable slight progression	Stable	Stable	Progressive	Acute visual loss, then usually stable; may improve/worsen

FC, finger counting; HM, hand motions.
* See discussion of heredodegenerative neurologic syndromes.
† Difficult to assess in infancy, but visual impairment usually manifests by age 4 years.
‡ Presence of nystagmus with poor vision and earlier onset suggests separate form or associated vestibulopathy.
§ Distinguished from tapetoretinal degenerations by normal electroretinogram.

atrophy was associated with mild mental deficiency, spasticity, hypertonia, and ataxia. Subsequent reports have indicated no sex predilection, although all of Behr's original patients were male. The disorder purportedly has its onset in childhood (1 to 9 years) and stabilizes after a variable period of progression. Pallor of the disc tends to be temporal; nystagmus is present in one-half the patients and strabismus in two-thirds, according to Francois.[59] It is generally thought that Behr's infantile complicated optic atrophy may represent a transitional form between simple hereditary optic atrophy and the hereditary cerebellar ataxias of the Marie type. Two sisters with Behr's syndrome have been reported,[60] including the autopsy findings of atrophy of the optic nerves, tracts and lateral geniculate, and mild changes in visual radiations and cortex. Also consistent with Behr's syndrome, a constellation of recessively inherited infantile optic atrophy, ataxia, extrapyramidal dysfunction (choreiform movements), variable cognitive function, and juvenile spastic paresis is reported among Iraqi Jews with elevated urinary excretion of 3-methylglutaconic acid.[61]

Axonal motor and sensory neuropathy is also documented in association with optic atrophy, with presumed autosomal inheritance.[62] Occurring almost exclusively in the Finnish population is the PEHO syndrome (progressive encephalopathy, subcutaneous limb edema, hypsarrhythmia, and optic atrophy), presenting as intractable seizures, and infantile hypotonia, attributed to an autosomal recessive infantile cerebello-optic atrophy.[63] Optic atrophy is also reported in autosomal recessive familial dysautonomia.[64]

Wolfram's Syndrome and Juvenile Diabetes

The association of early childhood–onset optic atrophy with diminished vision usually in the 20/200 range and juvenile diabetes is known as Wolfram's syndrome, and is recalled by the mnemonic DIDMOAD (diabetes insipidus, diabetes mellitus, optic atrophy, and deafness).[65] The disc pallor is not directly related to degree of diabetic retinopathy and, indeed, is found even without background retinopathy. Lessell and Rosman[66] reported an experience of 9 cases that included other associated manifestations, including ptosis, ataxia, nystagmus, seizures, mental retardation, abnormal ERG, elevated spinal fluid protein and cells, and small stature. Other systemic anomalies include ureterohydronephosis and neurogenic bladder. In the United Kingdom, the prevalence rate is 1/770,000, with median age at presentation of diabetes at 6 years and optic atrophy at 11 years; cerebellar ataxia and myoclonus tend to evolve in the fourth decade, and median age at death is 30 years (range, 25 to 49 years).[67]

Neuropathologic examination[68] has disclosed the following: atrophy of olfactory bulbs and tracts, optic nerves, and chiasm; loss of neurons in small cell layers of the lateral geniculate; atrophy of the superior colliculus; fiber loss in the cochlear nerve and cochlear nuclei; olivopontocerebellar atrophy; and pyramidal tract demyelination. Other neurologic features include central apnea and respiratory failure, startle myoclonus, axial rigidity, and Parinaud's syndrome.[69] MRI may show striking brain stem atrophy, especially of the pons and midbrain (Fig. 5–19).

The possibility of a mitochondrial defect has been raised, with rare patients that present with Leber-type visual loss (see below) and 11778 DNA mutation,[70] and other studies demonstrate heteroplasmic 8.5-kb deletion in mitochondrial DNA[71] and clusters of nucleotide exchanges at positions 4216 (similar to Leber-type optic atrophy), but with other distinct haplotype exchange variants.[72] For these reasons, the Wolfram genotype may not be homogeneous.

To reiterate, the simple autosomal recessive optic atrophies are not common, and patients previously categorized as having recessive congenital or infantile optic atrophy may indeed have suffered from retinal dysplasias or other unrecognized hereditary patterns. Of the more complicated situations in which optic atrophy is associated with clinical manifestations in organs unrelated functionally or embryologically, the possibility of mitochondrial defects is now strongly implicated.

Dominant (Juvenile) Optic Atrophy

The monograph on dominant optic atrophy by Poul Kjer[73] published in 1959 was an important milestone in nosologic analysis of the heritable optic atrophies, defining the clinical parameters and providing further evidence for distinction from Leber's hereditary optic atrophy, with which it had previously been confused.

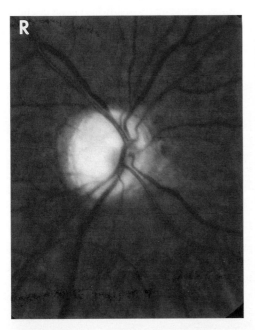
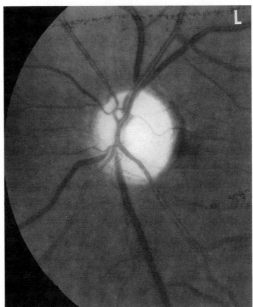
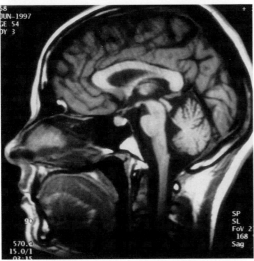

Fig. 5–19. Wolfram's syndrome. A 23-year-old woman with diabetes mellitus, visual acuity 20/400 OU, and severe ataxia. **Top.** R, right and L, left optic discs with profound atrophy. **Bottom.** Magnetic resonance imaging (T1-weighted, sagittal section) shows severe atrophy of cerebellum, brain stem, and spinal cord.

Kjer distinguished two dominant forms, separated primarily by the presence of nystagmus. Damien Smith[74] provided an additional admirable review of dominant optic atrophy and defined diagnostic criteria and clinical variants, emended here with data from a study of 21 families from the Genetic Clinic of Moorfields Hospital[75]: (1) dominant autosomal inheritance; (2) insidious onset between the ages of 4 and 8 years; (3) moderately reduced visual acuity, from 20/30 to 20/70, but rarely so poor as 20/200, with some considerable asymmetry of acuities possible, and modest deterioration with age; (4) temporal pallor of optic discs, at times with temporal sectoral excavation, and striking thinning in the papillomacular nerve fiber layer (Fig. 5–20); other discs show diffuse atrophy; (5) centrocecal enlargement of the blind spot or mid-zonal temporal depressions, at times mimicking temporal central hemianopia (Figs. 5–21 and 5–22); (6) full peripheral fields but elevated threshold for motion detection; (7) acquired blue-yellow dyschromatopsia, which is pathognomonic when present (about 8%), but also with nonspecific or mixed color-confusion

axes; and (8) reduced amplitude and delayed evoked potentials and reduced N95 component of pattern ERG.

Kjer[73] and others[75] have noted that many patients are ignorant of the familial nature of their disease and, indeed, had themselves not been aware of visual defects. Frequently, no special schooling is required for these patients, nor are vocations regularly limited. These phenomena attest to the insidious onset in childhood, mildly progressive course, and usual mild degree of visual dysfunction. From Kjer's data (and those of the Moorfields Hospital study), there is some evidence of disease progression, because patients less than 15 years of age did not show vision worse than 20/200, whereas 10% of patients 15 to 44 years old, and 25% of patients 45 years and older, had visual function less than 20/200; none of Kjer's patients had vision reduced to hand-motion or light-perception levels, although the Moorfields data do include such low levels. Other familial studies[76,77] also suggest a less sanguine visual outcome, with many patients experiencing insidious visual decline even to levels of legal blindness by middle age. In a three-generation

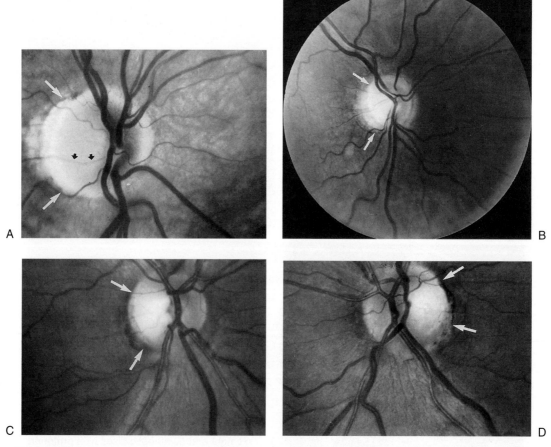

Fig. 5–20. Dominant optic atrophy. *White arrows* indicate circumscribed temporal atrophy. **A.** Right eye with focal temporal atrophy and excavation (see vessel depression, *black arrows*). **B.** Right eye of the son of the patient in (**A**). **C** and **D.** Patient with right eye acuity of 20/80 and left eye acuity of 20/100; see D-15 color test and Humphrey visual fields (see Fig. 5–21).

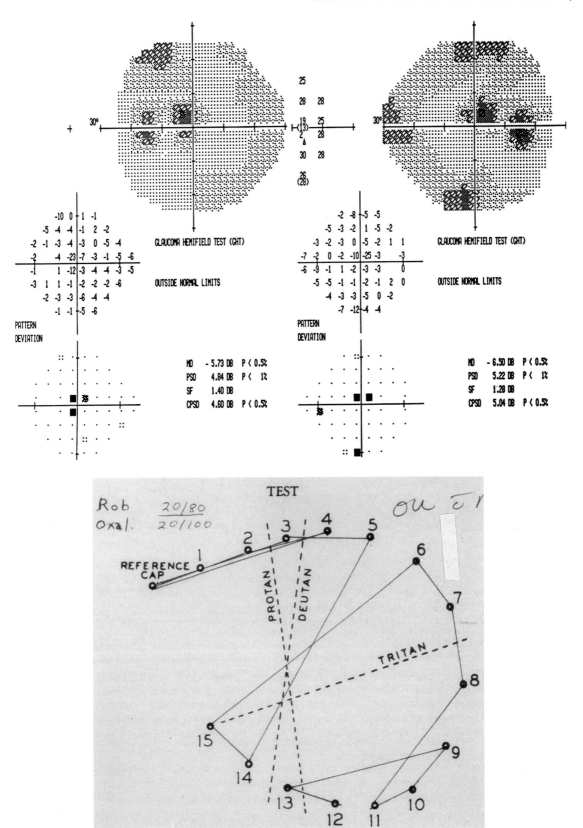

Fig. 5–21. Dominant optic atrophy. For patient fundi, see Figure 5–20C and D. **Top.** Humphrey 30-2 visual field with cecocentral depressions mimicking chiasmal disease. **Bottom.** Plot of D-15 color vision score. Note the error pattern aligned at the tritan axis.

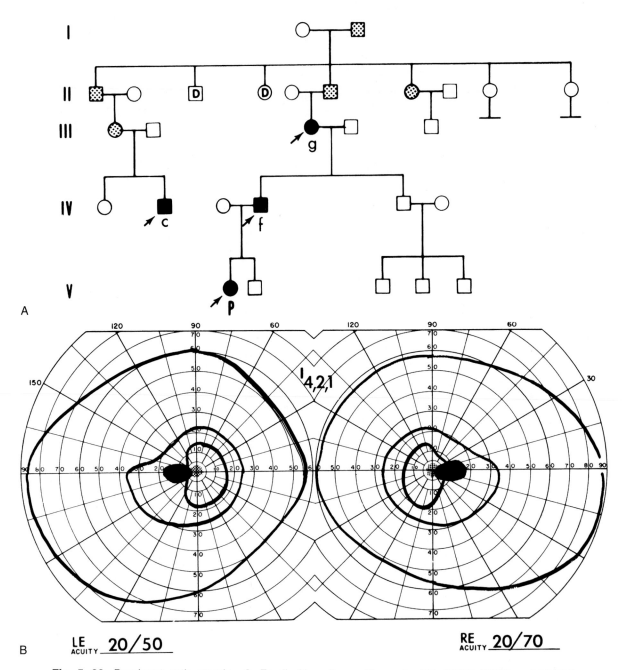

Fig. 5–22. Dominant optic atrophy. **A.** Family H pedigree. Proposita (*P*): 20/70 (6/21) and 20/100 (6/30) acuity and tritanopia. Father (*f*): 20/40 (6/12) and 20/50 (6/15) acuity and mild unclassified dyschromatopsia. Grandmother (*g*): 20/30 (6/9) and 20/40 (6/12) acuity and tritanopia. Cousin (*c*): 20/70 and 20/100 acuity and undetermined color defect. *Arrows* indicate persons examined. Other family members (*stippling*) have reportedly poor vision. **B.** Visual field in dominant optic atrophy. Note cecocentral scotomas and superotemporal depression of internal isopters I-2,1, which simulates the bitemporal pattern of chiasmal interference.

Danish analysis,[78] over a mean follow-up of 14 years (range, 1 to 38 years), one-third of patients showed no progression, whereas in two-thirds, visual deterioration occurred, at times quickly; presenting visual acuities in offspring were not worse than in parents, nor was there a gender difference. Genomic DNA linkage mapping has identified a genetic homogeneity at chromosome region 3q27-3q28.[76–78]

Regarding nystagmus, interestingly, none of Kjer's patients was unequivocally demonstrated to have the combination of optic atrophy and nystagmus. However, C.S. Hoyt[79] reported nystagmus with sensorineural hearing loss in 2 families, and Grehn et al[80] carefully documented autosomal dominant optic atrophy of severe degree, hearing loss with mutism, deuteranomalous color defects, no nystagmus, and normal ERG when this test was conducted. Twenty-three members of a large kindred[81] demonstrated progressive optic atrophy, acuity of 20/30 to 20/400, variable a- and b-wave ERG amplitude reductions (without pigmentary retinopathy), ptosis and moderate gaze palsies, hearing loss beginning in the second decade, and ataxia; CT scan and CSF results were normal. Other associated syndromes include a dominant form of relatively asymptomatic hereditary motor and sensory neuropathy (HMSN type IV) with optic atrophy.[82] Thus, there is an obvious spectrum of dominantly inherited optic atrophies not encompassed by the relatively benign Kjer type.

Johnston et al[83] described a pathologic study, including diffuse atrophy of the retinal ganglion cell layer, normal inner and outer nuclear layers, and thinning of the papillomacular nerve fiber bundle; the optic nerves showed non-inflammatory demyelination and loss of temporal disc substance. In addition, in a pathologic study of one of Kjer's original patients,[84] there was ganglion cell loss in retina and geniculate body, normal cortex, and some axonal loss in both vestibulo-auditory nerves. These authors concluded that evidence pointed to primary retinal ganglion cell degeneration.

Sufficient case material has accrued to indicate that dominant (juvenile-onset) optic atrophy is the most common heredofamilial simple (monosymptomatic) optic atrophy. Visual dysfunction in this disorder is considerably milder than in either Leber's hereditary optic neuropathy (LHON) or any form of recessive optic atrophy. As a rule, progression is minimal, and prognosis good, but, in some instances, relatively rapid deterioration may occur, even after years of stable visual function.

Leber's Disease

In 1871, Leber described a nosologically distinct hereditary form of optic neuropathy that now bears his name. Leber's hereditary optic neuropathy (LHON) is characterized by sudden and severe loss of visual acuity associated with large, dense central scotomas, sequentially bilateral, occurring mostly in the second and third decades of life, affecting young males primarily. The disorder is inherited strictly in the maternal line (Fig. 5–23), but with incomplete penetrance, and affected males do not transmit the trait. Although most patients with LHON are otherwise healthy, some show cardiac conduction defects, and also well documented[85,86] are major and minor neurologic abnormalities including dystonia, spasticity, ataxia, encephalopathic episodes and psychiatric disturbances, and a syndrome mimicking multiple sclerosis (MS). The degree of symmetry, high rate of failure to remit, mostly painless onset, and typical

disc appearance serve to distinguish most cases of Leber's optic neuropathy from the retro-bulbar neuritis of MS. Nonetheless, MRI should be considered to rule out demyelinative disease, for which therapeutic trials are now available (see below). T2-weighted fast spin echo MRI does not show signal changes in the optic nerves in the acute stage of LHON.[87]

During the acute phase of visual loss, the nerve head usually appears hyperemic and swollen, as do the dense arcuate retinal nerve fiber bundles above and below the disc, accompanied by tortuosity of large and small peripapillary vessels (see Color Plate 5–2F). Variable arteriolo-venular shunting is best demonstrated by fundus fluorescein angiography (Fig. 5–24). Nikoskelainen et al[88,89] demonstrated that this characteristic peripapillary microangiopathy occurs also in the presymptomatic phase of involved eyes and in a high number of asymptomatic offspring in the female line. Increased peripapillary capillary shunting and disc hyperemia herald the acute phase of visual loss; slowly, marked disc pallor evolves. Peripapillary and subhyaloid hemorrhage is quite rare. Thus, telangiectatic microangiopathy is a hereditary "marker" and signifies increased risk of acute optic neuropathy, with a phase of visual loss triggered by as yet unclear environmental or metabolic factors.

The strict maternal transmission is determined by inheritance of defective cytoplasmic mitochondrial DNA from the mother, that is, a nucleotide mutation that substitutes adenine for guanine, affecting the organelle's capacity to manufacture adenosine triphosphate.[90] Mitochondrial mutations at nucleotide position 11778 (Wallace mutation) account for an estimated 50% to 76% of LHON probands, the 3460 point mutation for 7% to 30%, and at point 14484 for about 10% to 31%, with some ethnic variability.[88] In the series of Newman et al,[91] 82% of patients with the 11778 mutation were males, but in a large British series,[92] male-to-female ratios were as follows: for mtDNA mutation 11778, 2.5:1; for 3460, 2:1; and for 14484, 5.7:1. Apparently, patients with the 14484 mutation may show a greater tendency for spontaneous recuperation of vision,[92,93] which correlates also with younger age onset, especially less than age 15 years[88]; other analyses suggest that final acuity may be most favorable with the 3460 mutation.[88] Although the disc remains diffusely pale, remarkable visual recovery includes recuperation from finger-counting levels to eventual 20/20 acuity. It is suggested that women with the 11778 mutation may suffer particularly severe visual loss, even to levels of only light perception, and that an MS-like illness may be observed in a large proportion in this group.[92]

Instances of apparently non-familial cases ("singleton") are not rare, and the relative ease and accessibility of mitochondrial testing may disclose occult cases of LHON among otherwise undiagnosed chronic or acute, but bilateral, optic neuropathies. False-positive results

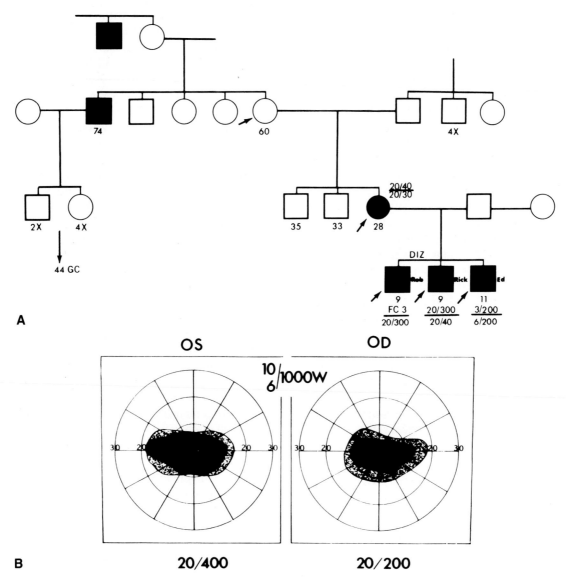

Fig. 5–23. Leber's optic atrophy. **A.** Family B pedigree. Three young sons with useful vision in one of six eyes. Mother, age 28 years, suffered acute bilateral loss of vision at age 14 years, with slowly progressive recovery over 6 years. Maternal uncle, age 74, suffered acute bilateral loss of vision at age 18. Note oblique transmission in the female line. *Arrows* indicate persons examined. **B.** Typical dense central field defects.

for the 11778 mutation may occur and can be verified by concomitant loss of restriction endonuclease SfNI and MaeIII marker sites.[94] Otherwise, point mutations at 11778, 3460, and 14480 have not been detected in normal control subjects.

Combined data indicate age at onset to be usually in the second or third decade, typically in the late teens to middle twenties, but ranging from 5 years well into the sixth and even seventh decades. In the analysis by Riordan-Eva et al,[92] visual loss developed between ages 11 and 30 years in 69%, with no significant differences between point mutation groups or gender. There are data[88] that marginally support a slightly later age-onset incidence in females, but variable age of onset in some

families contrasts with remarkably constant age of onset for other sibships. Asymmetry of onset is difficult to assess because of patient subjectivity, but some interval of weeks to a few months would appear to be the rule. According to Nikoskelainen et al,[88] 40% of patients are unsure of the interval between eyes, but second eye onset was less than 2 months in 23%, from 2 to 6 months in 32%, and more than 6 months in only 6%. Newman et al[91] reported simultaneous onset in 55% of patients with 11778 mutation and an inter-eye interval of 1.8 months, whereas in the British study,[92] visual loss was simultaneous in 22% and sequential in 78%, with a median inter-eye delay of 8 weeks. Individual variations in severity and tempo may be confusing, but entirely

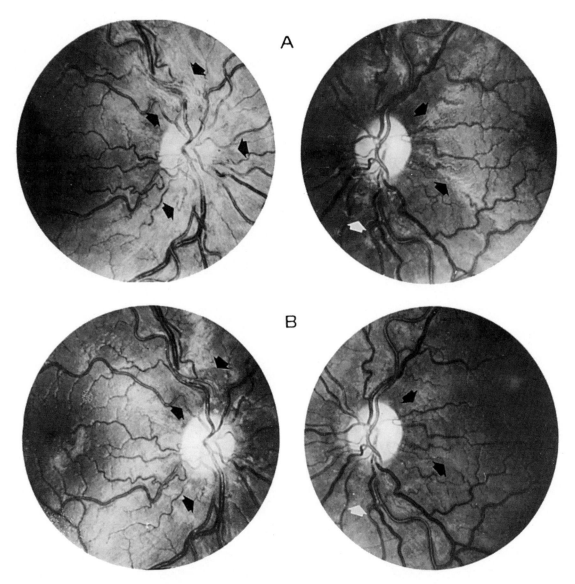

Fig. 5–24. Leber's optic atrophy. **A.** In the acute "neuritic" stage the disc appears hyperemic, the nerve fiber layer is prominent and opacified (compare *arrows* in right eye, **A** and **B**), and the retinal internal limiting membrane is wrinkled (compare *arrows* in left eye, **A** and **B**). **B.** Pseudoedema recedes over months, leaving a flat pale disc.

unilateral cases are distinctly rare[88,91,92]; one case with the 11778 mutation was considered unilateral for 16 years.[88] Of interest, monozygotic ("identical") twins homoplastic for mitochondrial mutations 4216, 13708, and 11778 are reported, one with typical visual loss at age 34 years, the second with normal visual function and unremarkable optic discs after more than 6 years of observation.[95]

There are no known effective therapeutic measures, medical or surgical, although succinate and co-enzyme Q, co-factors for normal mitochondrial function, may be easily used. The role of endogenous and external epigenetic "trigger" factors has been questioned. It is reasonable to counsel individuals at risk to at least guard against potential toxins such as tobacco and alcohol. An entire issue of *Clinical Neuroscience* (Volume 2, 1994) is given over to LHON and is a rich source of additional specific information.

Neurodegenerative Syndromes

There is considerable overlapping of syndromes variously combining progressive degeneration of cerebellar and pyramidal systems, deafness, and optic atrophy. To add to the nosologic confusion, familial progressive polyneuropathies of the Charcot-Marie-Tooth type have occasionally been associated with optic atrophy[96] or abnormal visual-evoked potentials.[97] The association of optic atrophy with spinocerebellar degenerations, familial bulbospinal neuronopathy,[98] cerebellar ataxia with

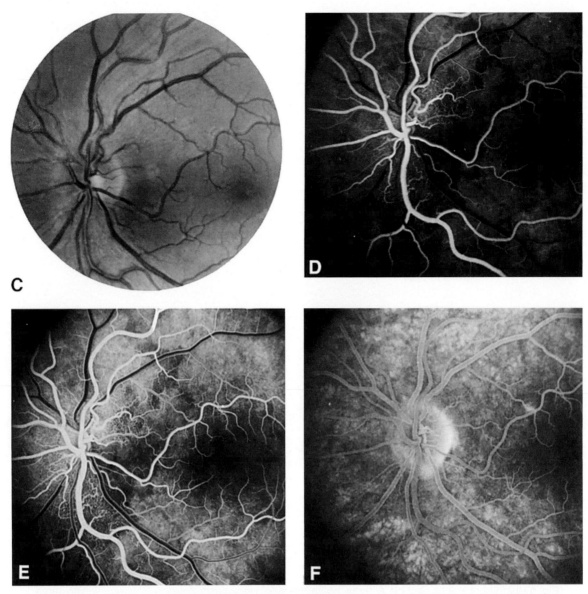

Fig. 5–24. (*continued*) **C.** Left optic disc of a 17-year-old boy with Leber's optic neuropathy. **D** through **F.** Fluorescein angiography demonstrates peripapillary microangiopathy, with mildly dilated retinal arterioles (**D**), capillary shunts in arteriovenous phase (**E**). The late phase (**F**) shows no fluorescein leakage from disc tissue.

sensorineural deafness (CAPOS syndrome),[99] and familial dysautonomia[64,100] is also well established. Optic nerve dysfunction, though not necessarily symptomatic, is documented in Friedreich-type and hereditary spastic ataxia.[101] As previously noted, optic atrophy associated with neurologic signs may take the form of an acute optic neuritis, at least superficially resembling Leber's disease, or may occur as a recessive optic atrophy in childhood, associated with ataxia (Behr's syndrome). Other ocular findings associated with cerebellar ataxia include ophthalmoplegia with slow saccades, retinal pigmentary degenerations with primary or consecutive optic atrophy.

This frequent intermingling of spinocerebellar degenerations, heredoataxias, motor and sensory neuropa-

thies, deafness, and optic atrophy strongly suggests a complex genetic continuum in which finite distinctions are not yet possible (Fig. 5–25). Transmission may be dominant, as in Charcot-Marie-Tooth polyneuropathy, some cases of Friedreich's ataxia, and in CAPOS syndrome, recessive, as in most cases of Marie's disease, or may not conform to strict mendelian rules, or as yet disclosed mitochondrial mutations.

ACQUIRED OPTIC NERVE DISEASE: AN OVERVIEW

In neuro-ophthalmologic practice, many patients are victims of lesions of the prechiasmal visual pathways.

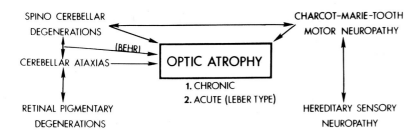

Fig. 5–25. Continuum of heredodegenerative syndromes associated with optic atrophy. Behr's syndrome may represent a transitional form between simple (monosymptomatic) hereditary optic atrophy and the heredoataxias. Acoustic nerve degeneration is another frequent concomitant.

These disorders are both varied and numerous and therefore constitute a common diagnostic challenge. The clinical distinction of optic neuropathies from maculopathies and other retinal disorders is elaborated in Chapter 2 and in Chapter 5, Part I.

Clinical Characteristics

The typical and characteristic symptomatic deficits of visual function with optic nerve disease may be summarized as follows:

1. Monocular deficits are the rule unless, of course, both optic nerves are involved. Hereditary atrophies and toxic-nutritional neuropathies are bilateral, but they may be asymmetric. Optic neuritis is occasionally bilateral and simultaneous, most frequently in childhood.
2. Defects in central field function include diminished acuity, desaturation of color perception, a sense of reduced brightness, and sluggish direct pupillary light reaction.
3. Field defects include central depression and nerve fiber bundle defects. Altitudinal defects are more usually vascular in origin. Optic disc disease (*e.g.,* glaucoma, ischemic neuropathy, hyaline bodies) typically shows inferior nasal predilection.
4. The appearance of disc pallor depends on the nature of the offending lesion, the time interval, the degree of axonal attrition, and, to some extent, the distance of the lesion from the optic nerve head. Disc swelling is discussed below.

Acquired optic nerve disease is usually heralded by acute, or subacute progressive, dimming of central vision. Abrupt onset of monocular visual dysfunction in the age group up to the fifth decade, with a normal-appearing optic disc, is highly suggestive of *retro-bulbar neuritis,* especially if accompanied by dull orbital pain or discomfort of the globe itself. Otherwise, pain is not generally a symptom of optic neuropathies. In the older age group, the single most common optic nerve disease that presents as apoplectic loss of vision is *ischemic infarct* of the disc, almost always with disc swelling during the acute phase, for which reason the term *anterior ischemic optic neuropathy* (anterior ION) has been popularly applied. Retro-bulbar disease producing abrupt

to subacute loss in the elderly includes *cranial arteritis* (CA) and *meningeal metastases.* Slowly progressive monocular visual loss over many months, in neuro-ophthalmologic context, typifies chronic tumoral compression of the optic nerve in its prechiasmal portion.

Insidious bilateral, but not necessarily symmetric, central, or cecocentral scotomas are hallmarks of intrinsic optic nerve disease, resulting from *nutritional deficiencies,* intake of *toxins,* or *heredofamilial atrophies.* Rarely, demyelinative disease runs such a slowly progressive course.

When a central field defect is found in one eye, careful search of the temporal field of the contralateral eye is mandatory to rule out the possibility of junctional (nerve and chiasm) compression (see Fig. 6–1A and C). Most prechiasmal optic neuropathies are due to *inflammatory or vascular disease,* whereas practically all chiasmal syndromes are due to *pituitary adenomas, other neoplasms, or aneurysm compression.*

Visual loss may be subjectively misinterpreted as sudden under circumstances in which the better eye is momentarily closed or obstructed, or when the involved eye is used unaccustomarily for monocular viewing (*e.g.,* microscope, telescope, gunsight).

Optic atrophy, with few exceptions, is generally a nonspecific clinical observation, and ophthalmoscopic criteria that permit a retrospective etiologic diagnosis, without other clinical clues, may include arterial attenuation in vascular causes. However, Frisen and Claesson[102] quantitatively demonstrated a reduction in central retinal artery caliber of 17% to 24% in non-ischemic descending (retro-bulbar nerve, chiasm lesions) optic atrophy. Likewise, focal narrowing of retinal vessels correlates best with age and may be seen with a wide variety of optic nerve diseases, including glaucoma.[103]

Neuroimaging Techniques

With the exception of lesions or fractures of skull bones, MRI has supplanted CT in the elucidation of occult optic nerve disease. By clinical criteria, suspicion may fall on a particular segment of the nerve, such as intraorbital, intracanalicular, or prechiasmal (intracranial), and special anatomic attention should be addressed accordingly. Standard "brain" studies may provide few sections of orbital or basal skull structures. Therefore, the clinician should provide precise and specific instructions to the radiologist or technician. Relatively thin-section techniques (*e.g.*, 3 mm) are required especially for adequate visualization of the optic canal, paraclinoidal and prechiasmatic portions of optic nerves, with and without gadolinium enhancement. Ideally, high-resolution (1 to 1.5 Tesla unit magnet systems) T1- and T2-weighted views should include axial, coronal, and sagittal sections; oblique views aligned with the long axis of the optic nerve (oblique sagittal) are of dubious value. The fat tissue of the orbit permits excellent contrast because fat appears bright (hyperintense) on T1-weighted images, whereas muscles, vessels, and nerves are darker (hypointense). Moreover, the optic nerve shares MRI characteristics with myelinated white matter of the brain. Blood vessels appear dark because of proton "flow voids."[104] Protocols that delineate optic nerves from orbital fat and minimize eye movement artifacts, such as fat-suppression fast spin-echo,[105] are more effective than conventional T1- or T2-weighted images (see Figs. 14–19 and 14–20). Subsequent illustrations of specific studies follow; a more exhaustive discussion of technical details is beyond the scope of this work, and the reader is referred to available comprehensive reviews.[106]

Ultrasonography (echography) is a practical, noninvasive adjunct to evaluate anatomic characteristics of optic nerve morphology. Standardized echography is useful in disclosing the presence of perineural fluid, highly suggestive of inflammatory optic neuritis. In addition, perineural fluid accumulation in papilledema may be confirmed and monitored.[107]

THE "SWOLLEN DISC": DIFFERENTIAL DIAGNOSIS

Active or passive edematous swelling of the optic disc provides compelling objective evidence of perturbed distal optic nerve function, but by appearance alone it is rarely specific. The causes of optic disc "swelling" are legion, as outlined in Table 5–7. It is imperative to separate *papilledema,* that is, disc swelling due to increased intracranial pressure as defined in the following section, from all other causes of acquired disc edema. Disc swelling is usually interpreted as such a compelling sign of intracranial mass lesion that diagnostic studies often take an inappropriate, if no longer uncomfortable, course.

The distinction of congenitally elevated discs, that is, pseudopapilledema, from papilledema has already been elaborated. It should be recalled that true papilledema, even in the fully developed form, does *not* reduce acuity (unless the macula is encroached), nor does it present with field defects other than enlarged blind spots. Therefore, confusion should not arise in distinguishing papilledema from inflammatory papillitis or from ION

TABLE 5–7. Etiology of the "Swollen" Disc

Congenital	Disc tumors
Anomalous elevation	Hemangioma
Hyaline bodies (drusen)	Glioma
Gliotic dysplasia	Metastatic
Ocular disease	Vascular
Uveitis	Ischemic neuropathy
Hypotony	Arteritis, cranial
Vein occlusion	Arteritis, collagen
Inflammatory	Juvenile diabetes
Papillitis	Proliferative retinopathies
Neuroretinitis	Orbital tumors
? Papillophlebitis	Perioptic meningioma
Infiltrative	Glioma
Lymphoma	Sheath "cysts"
Reticuoendothelial	Retrobulbar mass
Systemic disease	Graves' disease
Anemia	Elevated intracranial pressure
Hypoxemia	Mass lesion
Hypertension	Pseudotumor cerebri
Uremia	Hypertension

(Table 5–8), two common causes of disc edema that regularly are associated with acute loss of acuity or field and diminished direct light reaction of the ipsilateral pupil.

Disc edema accompanying local ocular diseases, including uveitis, central retinal vein occlusion, or postoperative hypotony, should represent no diagnostic problem. Even simple posterior vitreous detachment[108] may be associated with disc and peripapillary hemorrhage and edema.[109] Primary nerve head tumors (melanocytoma, glioma, astrocytic hamartoma, hemangioma) are rare and usually are definable by ophthalmoscopy. Metastatic disc tumors, other than those arising in the adjacent choroid and retina, are extremely infrequent and are characterized by massive hemorrhagic elevation of the disc and peripapillary retina and drastic reduction of vision. Occasionally, the optic nerve head may be infiltrated by leukemia or similar hematologic process, usually with rapidly progressive visual loss.

Orbital mass lesions characteristically produce proptosis, but they may present as chronic, unilateral disc edema with insidiously advancing field loss. As a general rule, *unilateral disc swelling should be considered a local vascular or inflammatory disorder of the nerve head or the result of a chronic perioptic mass lesion in the orbit* (*e.g.*, nerve sheath meningioma). On rare occasions, papilledema from increased intracranial pressure, including pseudotumor cerebri,[110] may be remarkably asymmetric or even strictly unilateral. When any diagnostic dilemma arises, enhanced CT scan or MRI of brain and orbital optic nerves is mandatory and should be performed sooner rather than later, but obviously after thorough history-taking and meticulous examination.

As noted, thin-section (ideally 1.5 mm) contrast-enhanced CT scan or especially fat-suppression MRI dis-

TABLE 5–8. Clinical Characteristics of Optic Neuritis, Papilledema, and Ischemic Optic Neuropathy

	Optic neuritis	Papilledema	Ischemic neuropathy
Symptoms			
Visual	Rapidly progressive loss of central vision; acuity rarely spared	No visual loss; ± transient obscurations	Acute field defect, commonly altitudinal; acuity variable
Other	Tender globe, pain on motion; orbit or brow ache	Headache, nausea, vomiting; other focal neurologic signs	Usually none; cranial arteritis to be ruled out
Bilateral	Rarely in adults; may alternate in MS; frequent in children, especially papillitis	Always bilateral, with extremely rare exceptions; may be asymmetric	Typically unilateral in acute stage; second eye involved subsequently with picture of "Foster-Kennedy" syndrome
Signs			
Pupil	No anisocoria; diminished light reaction on side of neuritis	No anisocoria; normal reactions unless asymmetric atrophy	No anisocoria; diminished light reaction on side of disc infarct
Acuity	Usually diminished	Normal acuity	Acuity variable; severe loss (including NLP) common in arteritis
Fundus	Retrobulbar: normal; Papillitis: variable degree of disc swelling, with few flame hemorrhages; cells in vitreous variable	Variable degrees of disc swelling, hemorrhages, cytoid infarcts	Usually pallid segmental disc edema with few flame hemorrhages
Visual prognosis	Vision usually returns to normal or functional levels	Good, with relief of cause of increased intracranial pressure	Poor prognosis for return; second eye ultimately involved in one third of idiopathic cases

MS, multiple sclerosis; *NLP*, no light perception.

plays fine details of optic nerve anatomy on both axial and coronal views, and increase or distortion of nerve diameter is regularly detected. Standardized A-scan ultrasonography[107] also defines the morphologic characteristics (normal vs. enlarged, solid vs. sheath fluid) of various optic neuropathies; this technique can effectively distinguish among causes of chronic optic neuropathy (perioptic tumor mass vs. remote neuropathy) and disc edema (tumor vs. inflammatory neuritis vs. ischemic neuropathy). Conditions that enlarge the optic nerves include optic neuritis, papilledema of raised CSF pressure, Graves' orbitopathy, direct or indirect trauma, perioptic inflammatory pseudotumor and sarcoid, optic glioma, perioptic meningioma, and infrequent infiltrations.

PAPILLEDEMA WITH RAISED INTRACRANIAL PRESSURE

Although it is admittedly an arbitrary decision, in this discussion the term "papilledema" is reserved for the following situation: passive disc swelling associated with increased intracranial pressure, almost always bilateral, and without visual deficit (at least in those stages of development that precede atrophy). It is intended that this rather circumscribed usage will prevent confusion when other forms of disc swelling are considered or when ophthalmologists offer opinions to neurologists and neurosurgeons. Furthermore, this definition should take into account the possibility of brain tumor and must also include the urgent need for neurodiagnostic procedures (contrast-enhanced CT scan, MRI, lumbar puncture) to exclude or discover mass lesions.

The pathogenesis of papilledema is a confused and controversial issue. Elevation of intracranial pressure in acute and chronic experiments have provided variable results and conclusions, but it seems reasonable that raised pressure is transmitted in the vaginal sheaths of the optic nerves[111] with resultant (or attendant?) stagnation of the venous return from the retina and nerve head. That nerve sheath pressure is critical has been demonstrated by Hayreh, who showed reversal of disc swelling by opening the nerve sheath, and subsequently Tso and Hayreh[112] established that there is stasis of both fast and slow axoplasm flow at the lamina cribrosa of the nerve head. In essence, optic nerve fibers are compressed in the subarachnoid space of the intraorbital portion of the optic nerve because of an elevation of CSF pressure. The subsequent obstipation of intra-axonal fluid mechanics results in leakage of water, protein, and other axoplasmic contents into the extracellular space of the prelaminar region of the optic disc. This protein-rich fluid adds to the osmotic pressure of the extracellular space of the disc substance. Venous obstruction and dilation, and nerve fiber hypoxia and vascular telangiectasis of the disc, are secondary events. Therefore, it is likely that papilledema is primarily a mechanical rather than a vascular phenomenon. It has been suggested[113] that the distal retro-bulbar portion of the optic nerve sheath is bulbous and distensible, and that movement of the globe in the orbit normally milks sheath fluid posteriorly, thus reversing flow and completing the circulation of CSF into the intracranial subarachnoid space. Therefore, perturbation of this pumping mechanism may also play a role in the evolution of papilledema.

No simple mechanistic explanation serves to include

other circumstances in which papilledema develops. Patients with cyanotic congenital heart disease may show papilledema with markedly tortuous retinal vessels, in the absence of elevated CSF pressure.[114] Decreased arterial oxygen saturation and polycythemia are believed to be etiologic factors, which similarly may play a role in the production of papilledema in sleep apnea.[115] Other conditions include spinal cord tumors (with and without elevated CSF protein),[116] thoracic disc herniation,[117] syringomyelia without hydocephalus,[118] inflammatory polyneuritis,[119] thyrotoxicosis,[120] and neurocysticercosis.[121]

The various underlying mechanisms that raise CSF pressure may be summarized as follows: intracranial mass lesions; increased CSF production (e.g., choroid plexus papilloma); decreased CSF absorption, the presumed cause of pseudotumor cerebri; high protein content or cellular debris that obstructs CSF absorption at arachnoidal granulations; obstructive hydrocephalus; increased cerebral blood volume (arteriovenous shunts and malformations[122,123]); and obstruction of cranial venous outflow (venous sinus thrombosis,[124] neck surgery,[125] and jugular vein compression[126]).

The clinical picture of *chronic unilateral* disc swelling most commonly results from obstruction of the subarachnoid space of the ipsilateral nerve by an intraorbital process such as sheath meningioma (with modest visual loss in the early stage and normal CSF pressure). As noted, on rare occasions, true unilateral papilledema does evolve from increased CSF pressure, including in the pseudotumor cerebri syndrome[127]; with respect to intracranial mass lesions, unilateral papilledema has no consistent lateralizing value. Previous optic atrophy may prevent disc swelling of one side, with papilledema developing on the other (the so-called Foster Kennedy syndrome, attributed to subfrontal masses). It is also speculated that a congenital nerve sheath anomaly may obstruct transmission of pressure such that the disc remains flat despite elevated intracranial pressure. However, Muci-Mendoza et al[128] demonstrated by CT scan bilateral optic nerve sheath distention in two cases of pseudotumor cerebri, with *unilateral* papilledema, thus raising the question of mechanisms at the *distal* portion of the optic nerve.

Although usually associated with slow-growing or subacute mass lesions, papilledema may develop within hours from subarachnoid or intracerebral hemorrhage,[129] but curiously, papilledema seemingly is relatively rare in acute elevation of pressure that is due to spontaneous intracranial hemorrhage or craniocerebral trauma.[130] Once the intracranial space is decompressed, venous congestion of the disc diminishes rapidly, but disc edema, hemorrhages, and exudates resolve more slowly. Well-developed papilledema resulting from mass lesions takes 6 to 10 weeks to regress after lowering of intracranial pressure.

Early, and even well-developed, papilledema may not be symptomatic. Neither visual field nor acuity is affected unless retinal hemorrhage, edema, or exudate involves the macular area. Enlargement of the blind spot is of no help in early diagnosis because ophthalmoscopically overt disc swelling precedes, and actually accounts for, this typical field change. The major clinical concept that separates papilledema of intracranial origin from other forms of acquired disc swelling is that *visual acuity, field, and pupillary reactions are typically normal,* whereas visual function (acuity, field, pupillary reaction) is almost always defective with papillitis (neuritis) or ION. When papilledema has existed for many weeks or months, nerve fiber attrition results in progressive field loss in the form of irregular peripheral contraction and nerve fiber bundle defects (as in Fig. 5–17). This is the atrophic stage of chronic papilledema, which can ultimately lead to severe visual loss and even blindness (Fig. 5–26).

Patients with well-developed papilledema experience brief transient obscurations of vision. "Gray-outs," "black-outs," or other momentary dimming of vision may involve one or both eyes at a time, last seconds, and clear completely. Sudden changes in posture may precipitate such obscurations, or they can occur spontaneously. The cause of these visual disturbances is unknown, but it is probably related to transient fluctuations in nerve head perfusion as determined by the influence of increased intracranial pressure on cerebral blood flow mechanisms. Obscurations are unrelated to the location or nature of space-occupying lesions and occur with great regularity in the pseudotumor cerebri syndrome. The frequency of obscurations appears to be most closely correlated with high intracranial pressure (at least at the moment of the obscurations) and advanced degree of disc swelling. Transient obscurations *without papilledema,* but resolved by relief of intracranial pressure, are reported.[131] It is problematic that a prognosis of ultimate visual function is related to the frequency or intensity of these episodes.

Other signs and symptoms associated with papilledema are related to the underlying pathologic processes that produce the increased intracranial pressure. Headache, nausea and vomiting, and diplopia resulting from lateral recti weakness are typical but nonspecific symptoms of raised CSF pressure, whereas hemiparesis, hemianopias or other field defects, seizures, or specific ocular motility disturbances all have localizing value.

It is helpful ophthalmoscopically to "stage" papilledema, which on occasion has considerable clinical value. As suggested by Jackson in 1871, papilledema may be classified into four temporal types: early, fully developed, chronic, and atrophic. The early phase of papilledema refers to the incipient disc changes that occur before the development of obvious disc swelling. Blurring of the nerve fiber layer and obscuration of the superior and inferior disc margins are early changes that may actually precede venous engorgement (see Color

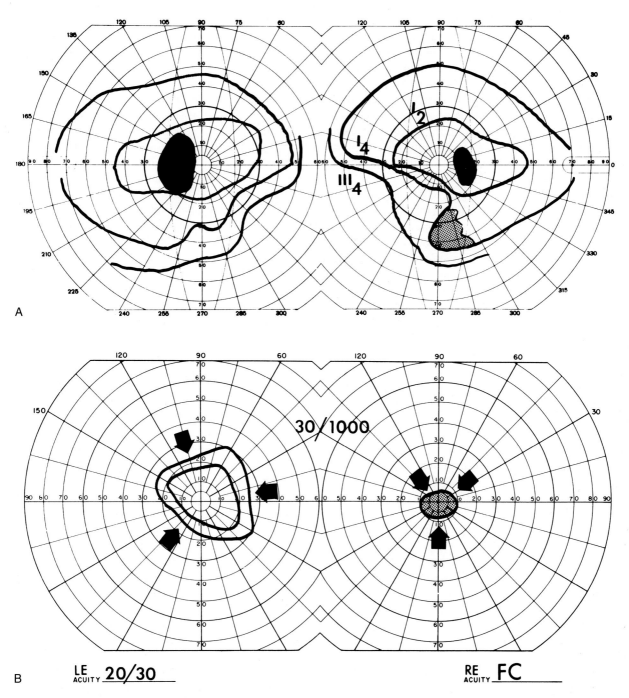

Fig. 5–26. Visual defects with papilledema. **A.** Long-standing papilledema in pseudotumor cerebri. Blind spots may be of sufficient size to mimic bitemporal hemianopia. Field is generally constricted with preferential involvement of inferior nasal areas. **B.** Extreme loss of peripheral field with long-standing frontal glioma. Note retention of the central field in the left eye (*LE*). *RE*, right eye.

Plate 5–1F and Color Plates 5–4A and B). The use of red-free light (green filter) in the ophthalmoscopic may further delineate early nerve fiber layer changes in incipient papilledema. The veins of the retina ultimately become engorged, tortuous, and dusky, but usually not until disc swelling is well under way.

Spontaneous pulsation of major disc veins is anticipated in approximately 80% of eyes, and its presence militates against the possibility of raised CSF pressure. It is estimated that spontaneous venous pulsation ceases when intracranial pressure exceeds 200 ± 25 mm H_2O, but the absence or presence of pulsation is not a consistently useful sign.[132]

The occurrence of splinter hemorrhages in the nerve fiber layer at or just beyond the disc margin is a major confirmatory finding, especially in the course of repeated fundus observations. However, as noted previously, hemorrhages may infrequently occur with intra-papillary hyaline bodies or in chronic glaucoma, posterior vitreous separation, or for no apparent reason in the elderly.

In early papilledema, as well as in the more fully developed stage, the optic cup is retained. In fact, absence of the central cup is much more likely to be seen in pseudopapilledema than in incipient disc swelling. In the more chronic stage of papilledema, the central cup is likely to be slowly obliterated.

As edema progresses, the surface of the disc becomes elevated above the plane of the retina. Nerve fiber layer opacification obscures the scleral disc margins, and minor or major vessels are buried as they course off the disc. At this stage, that is, fully developed papilledema, disc elevation is consistently accompanied by multiple flame hemorrhages, nerve fiber layer infarcts ("cotton-wool" spots), serpentine tortuosity of veins, and marked disc hyperemia and hypervascularity attributable to telangiectatic dilatation of the superficial capillary bed of the disc surface (see Color Plates 5–4C and D). Swelling of the nerve fiber layer extends laterally into the retina, so that the area of the nerve head appears enlarged. The retina is raised up from pigment epithelium, and circumferential retinal folds (Paton's lines) may be seen around the swollen disc, representing the concentric lateral displacement of retina; these may extend even to the macula. Rarely, retinal exudates radiate spoke-like from the fovea in the form of a star (or half-star between the disc and fovea), with the apex toward the fovea (see Color Plate 5–D). If intracranial pressure remains elevated, the acute hemorrhagic and exudative components resolve, and the disc progressively takes on the appearance of the dome of a champagne cork (see Color Plates 5–F and 5–4E). The central cup remains obliterated, but peripapillary retinal edema resorbs. Small, round glistening "hard exudates" (axoplasm or protein remnants?) on the surface of the disc may simulate hyaline bodies. This stage of chronic papilledema indicates that disc swelling has been present for months. Nerve fiber attrition is predictable, leading to progressive field loss (see Fig. 5–26). As the disc detumesces, pallor slowly emerges, with apparent "sheathing" of vessels but no real loss of disc substance. Although the disc usually has a milky gray appearance ("secondary optic atrophy") (see Color Plate 5–4E), at times it appears remarkably crisp and white. Even with fairly rapid detumescence of pre-atrophic papilledema, retinal exudates, changes in the foveal pigment epithelium secondary to edema or subretinal hemorrhage may permanently reduce central acuity.[133]

Choroidal folds, with and without acquired hyperopia, are described in association with papilledema, with neuroimaging that strongly suggests that these striae are likely related to distention of the most distal patulous portion of the optic nerve sheath, which flattens and foreshortens the posterior wall of the globe. It is reported[134] that such folds may precede actually disc swelling.

The appearance of the optic discs, sequence of funduscopic changes, and ultimate visual outcome are dependent on variations of intracranial pathology, surgical interventions, and obscure hemodynamic events involving both the disc and the retro-bulbar visual pathways. Acute and drastic visual loss in the form of ischemic infarction of the disc is documented,[135] as well as central retinal artery occlusion.[136] In the presence of well-developed, usually chronic, papilledema, cranial decompression, including shunt procedures or ventriculography, is followed by visual loss that is abrupt or progressive over weeks. Such tragic outcome is neither understood nor predictable, and it may not be prevented even if shunting procedures precede decompression of the primary mass. This event may be related to arterial hypotension provoked by intracranial decompression, especially with the patient in a seated position (e.g., for posterior craniectomy), or to an increase in CSF pressure precipitated by anesthesia. A question of perfusion insufficiency of the distal optic nerve has been raised,[137] but the precise mechanism(s) remain elusive.

Although much has been written regarding the use of fluorescein angiography in the diagnosis of papilledema, in instances of ophthalmoscopically definable papilledema, fluorescein fundus angiography is usually superfluous. In eyes in which disc changes are truly debatable, fluorescein angiography may be inconclusive and should not be considered the single indication for further complicated diagnostic studies. Thin-section CT views and fast spin-echo MRI,[138] as well as standardized A-scan ultrasonography,[107] are useful in confirming distended perioptic meninges, and the latter provides a convenient technique to monitor the effects of therapy on nerve sheath size.

For the ophthalmologist or neurologist, the finding of bilateral papilledema is, of course, an indication for immediate action. Following adequate history-taking, including queries regarding the use of pharmaceuticals associated with pseudotumor cerebri (see below), and otherwise competent neuro-ophthalmologic assessment including *blood pressure evaluation,* CT scan or MRI is mandatory to determine the state of the ventricular system and the potential presence of a mass lesion.

Pseudotumor Cerebri Syndrome

Pragmatically, ophthalmologists may distinguish perhaps three major clinical types of pseudotumor cerebri syndrome: purely *idiopathic intracranial hypertension* (IIH); a condition in which *venous sinus thrombosis* is demonstrable; and a condition in which other *identifi-*

able toxic or mechanical mechanisms secondarily cause raised intracranial pressure.

Primary: Idiopathic Intracranial Hypertension

IIH without discernable origin, perhaps somewhat inaccurately equated with a more general syndrome of "pseudotumor cerebri," is strictly a diagnosis of exclusion, although in obese female patients it is a frequently anticipated cause of well-developed, often florid papilledema (see Color Plate 5–4C) and headaches. Other neurologic deficits, with the exception of nonspecific signs of raised CSF pressure (see below), are inconsistent with this diagnosis or, at least, occur so infrequently that a thorough investigation beyond simple contrast-enhanced neuroimaging is essential.

Although various factors (Table 5–9) are implicated in the production IIH, most cases reveal no clearly identifiable underlying cause, although there is a distinct female preponderance from the teens through the fifth decade, that is, the hormonally active, child-bearing years. In fact, there is no apparent gender difference for IIH in children or a tendency to obesity.[139,140] Otherwise, these indisputable characterizations strongly imply an "endocrine connection," although studies of hormonal function in IIH, including patients with radiologic empty sella or with long-standing raised CSF pressure, do not show significant abnormalities of the anterior or posterior pituitary or of the peripheral target glands.[141]

IIH affects about 1 to 2/100,000 in the general population, but 19 to 21/100,000 of obese women of reproductive age.[142] The relative percentage of men with pseudotumor ranges from 17% to 35% in large series, with the Iowa study citing 16% in male patients older than 16 years of age,[143] and including obesity and hypertension as risk factors, but discounting the roles of tetracyclines, steroids, vitamin A, or head trauma. More recently, the antiarrhythmic drug amiodarone[144] and the androgen danazol[145] were reported to induce pseudotumor cerebri, joining the classic list of steroid usage or withdrawal, nalidixic acid, hypervitaminosis A, tetracyclines, the insecticide chlordecone (Kepone),[146] and lithium.[147] The association with anovulatory agents (especially Norplant) may be fortuitous, these being so commonly used in the population at risk. Ironically, IIH has been reported without elevated CSF pressure,[148] but in a typical obese, hypersomnolent young woman, with papilledema and headaches, normal MRI, and responding to standard therapy.

General symptoms and signs of increased CSF pressure include the following: daily diffuse or frontal headache; transient visual obscurations ("black-outs") asso-

TABLE 5–9. Conditions Associated with Papilledema and Increased Intracranial Pressure (Excluding Space-Occupying Lesions)

Renal diseases	Viral diseases	Miscellaneous diseases
Chronic uremia	Poliomyelitis	Gastrointestinal hemorrhage
Developmental diseases	Acute lymphocyte meningitis	Lupus erythematosus
Syringomyelia	Coxsackie B virus encephalitis	Sarcoidosis
Craniostenosis	Inclusion-body encephalitis	Syphilis
Aquaductal stenosis (adult type)	Recurrent polyneuritis	Subarachnoid hemorrhage
Toxic conditions	Guillain-Barré syndrome	Status epilepticus
Heavy-metal poisoning:	Parasitic diseases	Paget's disease
Lead, arsenic	Sandfly fever	Opticochiasmatic arachnoiditis
Hypervitaminosis A	Trypanosomiasis	Neoplastic diseases
Tetracycline therapy	Torulosis	Carcinomatous "meningitis"
Nalidixic acid therapy	Neurocysticercosis	Leukemia
Prolonged steroid therapy	Metabolic endocrine conditions	Spinal-cord tumors
Steroid withdrawal	Eclampsia	Hematologic diseases
Lithium	Hypoparathyroidism	Infectious mononucleosis
Allergic diseases	Addison's disease	Idiopathic thrombocytopenic purpura
Serum sickness	Scurvy	Pernicious anemia
Allergies	Oral progestational agents	Polycythemia
Infectious diseases	Diabetic ketoacidosis	Iron-deficiency anemia
Bacterial	Menarche	Hemophilia
Subacute bacterial endocarditis	Obesity	Circulatory diseases
Meningitis	Menstrual abnormalities	Congestive heart failure
Chronic mastoiditis (lateral-sinus thrombosis)	Pregnancy	Mediastinal neoplasm
Brucellosis	Thyrotoxicosis	Congenital cardiac cyanosis
Radical neck surgery	Degenerative diseases	Hypertensive encephalopathy
	Schilder's disease	Pulmonary emphysema
	Muscular dystrophy	Dural-sinus thrombosis
	Head trauma	Chronic pulmonary hypoventilation
		Sleep apnea

Adapted from Buchheit WA, Burton C, Haag B et al: Papilledema and idiopathic intracranial hypertension: report of a familial occurrence. N Engl J Med 280:938, 1969

ciated with usually florid bilateral papilledema (rarely unilateral[127]); neck stiffness; shoulder, arm, or leg pain, likely representing transmission of CSF pressure to dural sleeves of radicular spinal nerve roots; pulsatile tinnitus, related to transmitted increased pressure in the scala tympani of the inner ear; and diplopia due to sixth nerve palsy. Unusual ocular motor disturbances are infrequently encountered, including internuclear ophthalmoplegia, external ophthalmoplegia, vertical gaze palsies, and supranuclear palsies.[149]

Neuroimages of the brain are categorically normal, their role being to exclude other causes of raised CSF pressure: CT or MRI shows undisplaced normal or small ventricles and no signs of mass lesions. Dural venous sinuses may show evidence of thrombosis or slowed flow in an unknown proportion of otherwise idiopathic cases, but otherwise neither CT nor MRI has revealed much evidence in regard to pathogenesis; rarely, increase in brain white matter signal, representing a prolongation of the T2 relaxation time, indicates a general increased water content,[150] consistent with previous theories of intracellular and extracellular edema.

Authoritative consensus dictates that lumbar puncture is vital in affirming a diagnosis of IIH, the only supportive finding being raised CSF pressure, but without abnormalities in protein level or cell count. Curiously, low-pressure pseudotumor is reported,[148] as is IIH without papilledema.[151] CSF pleocytosis or increased protein content suggests chronic inflammatory meningitis or encephalitis, or lupus arteritis. Corbett[151a] provided the figure 200 to 250 mm H_2O for the upper limit of normal for CSF opening pressure, especially in the obese patient (Fig. 5–27).

Although headaches may easily be controlled, the possibility of visual loss is real and demands regular monitoring, in children[140] as in adults.[152] Visual field defects relate to progressive nerve fiber atrophy consecu-

tive to chronic papilledema, with fundus evidence of special predilection for thinning in the superior temporal arcuate nerve fiber bundles.[153] Field defects take the form of blind spot enlargement, generalized field depression, arcuate nerve fiber bundle defects, and nasal contraction (see Fig. 5–26A). There is histopathologic evidence of axonal loss, especially in the peripheral rather than axial portions of the optic nerves, which may be as extensive as 80% to 90% attrition.[154] Automated field strategies[152] within the central 30° and along the nasal horizontal meridian disclose visual loss in more than 75% of involved eyes. Ultimately, the potential for visual loss is the single most serious complication of IIH, and proper management demands *meticulous ophthalmologic surveillance.*

That IIH is a *self-limited* disorder, with brief and transient manifestations, must be in considerable doubt. The precise pathophysiologic mechanism is not yet clarified, but various theoretical considerations include the following[142]: increased resistance to CSF outflow; vasogenic brain edema; and increased intracranial blood volume. Noteworthy is the relative rarity of IIH beyond middle age, suggesting either an endocrine transition or the mitigating effect of age-related brain atrophy. Whereas pathogenesis is confused, the efficacy of medical management is well established. Therapy commonly begins with the carbonic anhydrase inhibitor acetazolamide (Diamox), 500 mg twice daily; side effects include perioral and hand paresthesias, anorexia, metallic taste, and rarely renal stones or aplastic anemia and transient myopia with choroidal detachments.[155] Furosemide (Lasix), 2 mg/kg three times daily, or thiazide diuretics are alternatives. It is not clear whether diuretics are effective by decreasing central plasma volume or by suppressing CSF production. Corticosteroids may be less useful considering the side effects of fluid retention, hypertension, and elevation of intraocular tension. However, in in-

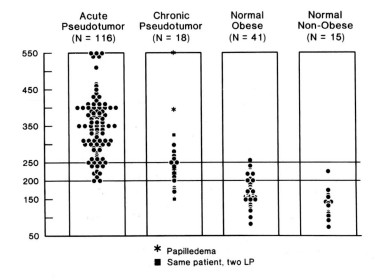

Fig. 5–27. Cerebrospinal fluid pressures in normal obese, normal nonobese, and acute or chronic pseudotumor cerebri. (From Corbett JJ: Problems in the diagnosis and treatment of pseudotumor cerebri. Can J Neurol Sci 10:221, 1983)

stances of relatively acute visual loss associated with florid papilledema, high-dose intravenous methyprednisolone may quickly reduce edema and may rapidly improve vision.[156] The importance of a weight-reduction program bears emphasis; Johnson et al[157] have suggested that as little as 6% weight loss may be critical to the success of standard acetazolamide therapy. Multiple lumber punctures may be effective but painful, and patient compliance is understandably tenuous. Therapeutic success is determined by relief of headaches, diminished frequency of transient visual obscurations, regression of papilledema, stability or improvement of field defects, and weight reduction.

When various optimum medical therapies fail, and disc swelling with field loss is progressing, operative decompressions are necessary. Lumbar-peritoneal shunts are undertaken frequently and are successful in acutely lowering intracranial pressure, but accumulated data[158] indicate a high rate of shunt failure requiring multiple revisions. Shunting usually relieves headaches, but it may paradoxically produce headaches related to low CSF pressure. More importantly, delayed shunt failure may go undetected with recrudescence of intracranial hypertension and insidious papilledema with slow or sudden visual loss.[159] Peculiarly, shunt failure may present with visual loss without papilledema.[160]

Direct fenestration of the optic nerve sheaths via medial or lateral orbitotomy has evolved as an effective and relatively simple procedure for relief of papilledema and stabilization of visual function.[161,162] Nonetheless, such surgical manipulation may worsen vision through vascular events[163] or neural damage.[164] Interestingly, bilateral disc detumescence may follow unilateral optic sheath opening, and headache may be relieved, but to what extent the intracranial subarachnoid compartment is decompressed is debatable (see Chapter 14, Part II).

The co-existence of IIH with *pregnancy* is likely fortuitous, but perinatal hypercoagulable states are known to play a role in cerebral, pelvic, and deep vein thromboses. Although teratogenicity is debatable, acetazolamide may be safely used after 20 weeks, that is, beyond the critical teratogenic period. Peculiarly, some unknown proportion of patients with chronic daily headaches, *without papilledema* and with normal neuroimaging, may show elevated CSF pressures (range, 230 mm to 450 mm H$_2$O); when treated with acetazolamide or furosemide, headache control improves.[151,165] Of extraordinary interest is *familial* idiopathic pseudotumor, of which more than a dozen cases have been reported, including in siblings, but also in successive generations, strongly suggesting a hereditary disposition.[166]

Secondary Pseudotumor Cerebri Syndromes

With the advent of MRI, cerebral dural *venous sinus thrombosis* or venous outflow obstruction is demon-

strated with increasing frequency. Such cases of dural sinus hypertension include surgical neck dissection, ligation of sigmoid sinus, thrombosed central intravenous catheters, tumoral compression or invasion of dural sinuses, and arteriovenous malformations.[167] Indeed, it may be that elevated intracranial venous pressure is a universal mechanism in pseudotumor cerebri of various causes.[124] The importance of otitis media, mastoiditis, and lateral sinus thrombosis in childhood pseudotumor is, of course, well known.[139] Purvin et al[168] have characterized the neuro-ophthalmic manifestations of cerebral venous obstruction, listing cases of noncompressive (Behçet's disease, mastoiditis, thrombogenic factors), compressive (dural sinus meningioma, glomus tumor, cervical masses), and iatrogenic surgical ligation of dural sinuses or during neck surgery. Other underlying risks for hypercoagulable states include paroxysmal nocturnal hemoglobinuria.[169]

Various *toxic or mechanical factors* are incriminated in the pseudotumor syndrome (see Table 5–9), some of which are unsubstantiated; that is, *association* does not necessarily imply *cause*. *Oral contraceptives* are reported as a likely risk factor for migraine and vascular disease in the child-bearing population, and purportedly for venous thrombosis and pseudotumor cerebri, but in the absence of other risk factors (smoking, diabetes, hypertension obesity, hyperlipidemia), no substantial evidence exits.[170,171] In children or young adults, growth hormone replacement,[172] Addison's disease (primary hypoadrenalism),[173] long-term corticosteroid use or withdrawal,[139,174] vitamin A intoxication,[175] nalidixic acid, minocycline,[175a] and thyroid replacement[139] all seem to be genuine determinants. Chronic pulmonary insufficiency with pickwickian syndrome (obesity, hypoventilation, and somnolence) produces hypercapnia, increased cerebral blood flow, and increased CSF pressure.[176]

Skull growth anomalies such as achondroplasia[177] or with craniosynostosis[178] may be associated with insidious and severe visual failure related to chronic raised intracranial pressure and papilledema. In addition, many different abnormalities in CSF composition, as in the infections cryptococcosis, cysticercosis, and neurosarcoidosis, or in residual subarachnoid blood, may serve to obstruct absorption of CSF by arachnoidal villi, producing a secondary form of pseudotumor cerebri.[179]

INFLAMMATORY OPTIC NEUROPATHIES: OPTIC NEURITIS

The medical rubric "optic neuritis" is perhaps more a clinical syndrome than a topical disease. By the suffix "-itis" is understood *inflammation* of the nerve, but this modest definition fails to convey the complex nosologic spectrum that embraces the following conditions: demyelinative, other immune-mediated, infective, and idiopathic optic neuritides; inflammatory diseases of the adjacent paranasal sinuses, brain and meninges, cranial base, and orbit, which contiguously involve the optic nerves; granulomatous infiltrations such as sarcoidosis; and infections shared with the retina.

When the optic nerve is damaged by vascular, compressive, or unknown mechanisms, the more general term "optic neuropathy" is preferable. "Papillitis" refers to the intraocular form of optic neuritis in which disc swelling of variable degree is observed. The clinical distinction among "papilledema," that is, passive disc edema associated with increased intracranial pressure, papillitis, and ischemic neuropathy with disc edema is summarized in Table 5–8.

The general clinical characteristics of non-infective optic neuritis may be summarized as follows:

1. Relatively acute impairment of vision, progressing rapidly for hours or days; visual function usually reaches its lowest level by 1 to 2 weeks after onset, but it may actually be improving by that time.

2. The typical episode involves one eye only, although in children especially it is not unusual for bilateral neuritis (with disc swelling) to follow viral illnesses, including measles, mumps, and chickenpox.

3. Tenderness of the globe and deep orbital or brow pain, especially with eye movements, may precede or coincide with visual impairment.

4. Visual function is depressed over the entire field, but most markedly involves the central 20°, with variable diminution of acuity, color sense, and contrast sensitivity; normal or near-normal acuity may be preserved.

5. Perimetric findings include admixtures of central and cecocentral scotomas, nerve fiber bundle and altitudinal defects, and general constrictions (Fig. 5–28).

6. In the majority of cases, especially in demyelinating

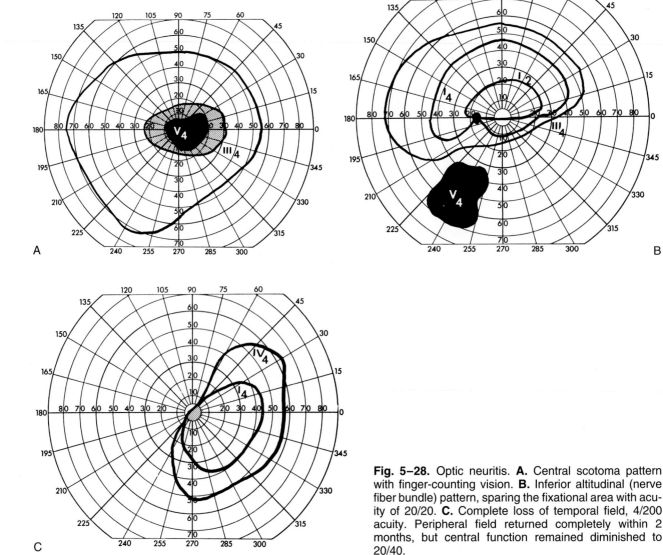

Fig. 5–28. Optic neuritis. **A.** Central scotoma pattern with finger-counting vision. **B.** Inferior altitudinal (nerve fiber bundle) pattern, sparing the fixational area with acuity of 20/20. **C.** Complete loss of temporal field, 4/200 acuity. Peripheral field returned completely within 2 months, but central function remained diminished to 20/40.

disease, visual function begins to improve in the second or third week, and many patients enjoy normal or near-normal vision by the fourth to fifth week; in others, following a fairly rapid improvement to modest levels of acuity (20/60 to 20/40), vision slowly but steadily improves over several months.

7. In a small percentage of cases, vision does not improve to functional levels, and, even more rarely, vision does not improve at all after the initial precipitous loss.

Visual symptomatology in optic neuritis is related to the nature of neural conduction defects, which may be subjectively approximated by viewing through a neutral density filter or dark lens before the eye. In addition to diminished central acuity and field loss, the following symptoms are typical: drabness (desaturation) of colored objects, although specialized color vision testing[180] suggests mixed types of dyschromatopsia without correlation with acuity, and fluctuations over time; apparent dimness of light intensities (e.g., room lighting appears reduced when viewed with affected eye); impairment of binocular depth perception (stereo-illusion), especially with moving objects (Pulfrich's phenomenon[181]), attributed to inter-eye disparity of light sense or retinal illumination; and increase in visual deficit with exercise (Uhthoff's symptom[182]) or other elevations of body temperature, typically noticed in the chronic or recovered phase. These visual defects may persist after return of reading acuity to normal levels, and thus patients continue to be visually symptomatic in spite of good acuity and field.

From the Optic Neuritis Treatment Trial (ONTT),[183] visual field defects included the following: diffuse depression occurred in about 48%, and especially vertical altitudinal half and quadrant localized defects; strictly central or cecocentral scotomas constituted less than 10%; various single or double arcuate defects were reported; and unilateral nasal or temporal hemianopias were recorded, as well as chiasmal and retro-chiasmal patterns. At ONTT entry, field defects were found in two-thirds of fellow (non-acute) eyes.

In the common retro-bulbar form of optic neuritis, the fundus is unchanged during the acute episode, and subsequent pallor may range from profound to imperceptible. Papillitis, that is, disc swelling caused by local inflammatory processes of the nerve head, may be thought of as an intraocular form of optic neuritis, although etiologic considerations are not parallel. In children, papillitis is the common presentation of optic neuritis. In the Kennedy-Carroll series,[184] 22 of 26 children less than 15 years of age showed acute disc swelling. In addition, simultaneous bilateral neuritis is by far more common in children than adults. This latter point may be attributable to two factors: children with unilateral visual loss are less likely to complain than those with bilateral visual loss; the incidence of viral diseases (mumps, chickenpox, nonspecific fevers, and upper respiratory infections) is high in childhood, and these systemic disorders may be more prone to provoke symmetric optic neuritis than other demyelinative or inflammatory causes.

The role of vaccination and infections preceding optic neuritis in childhood was noted in a Scandinavian study,[185] in which 8 of 11 children had bilateral nerve involvement; in this series, 10 patients eventually developed definite MS, implying that associated immune mechanisms may be risk factors for MS. From the Mayo Clinic study[186] of 79 children less than 16 years old with isolated optic neuritis (39% unilateral, 57% bilateral, 3% recurrent), 13% had clinical MS by 10 years of follow-up, and 26% by 40 years; gender, age of onset, fundus findings, or acuity level had no predictive value, but the presence of bilateral sequential or recurrent optic neuritis increased the risk of MS, whereas the presence of infection within the 2 preceding weeks decreased the risk. It is likely that some degree of parainfectious encephalomyelitis (acute disseminated encephalomyelitis) exists in a subset of children with optic neuritis, as evidenced by the frequency of headache, nausea and vomiting, spinal fluid lymphocytosis, and some MRI abnormalities are indeed reported.[187]

Papillitis is frequently accompanied by cells in the vitreous especially just anterior to the disc, and deep retinal exudates may form a star figure at the macula, or half-star between the disc and fovea, termed Leber's stellate maculopathy (Fig. 5–29). When edema spreads to the peripapillary nerve fiber layer, the term neuroretinitis is applied. This fundus appearance is not likely to be associated with subsequent disseminated sclerosis (see below). In certain patients, especially following febrile illnesses, a viral agent may be suspected. We have seen three instances of children with unilateral papillitis, with temporally related mumps in siblings. Otherwise, even recurrent neuroretinitis with mixed visual outcome, and no discoverable systemic cause, is not a harbinger of MS.[188]

Visual prognosis with papillitis or uncomplicated neuroretinitis is surprisingly good, even in the presence of massive disc edema and hemorrhages or with initial severe loss of visual function. However, progressive atrophy may ensue regardless of therapeutic intervention, and good visual outcome is not guaranteed. In hopes of favorably influencing visual outcome, corticosteroids are used orally, but, as with retro-bulbar neuritis, there is no substantive evidence that eventual visual function is affected by therapy. In patients with neuroretinal edema or cellular debris in the vitreous, a short-term course of steroids seems reasonable.

Discussed previously (Chapter 5, Part I), but noted in passing here, optic neuritis, expressed in variable degrees of disc swelling, may accompany inflammation primarily of the uvea, retina, or sclera. The ocular signs

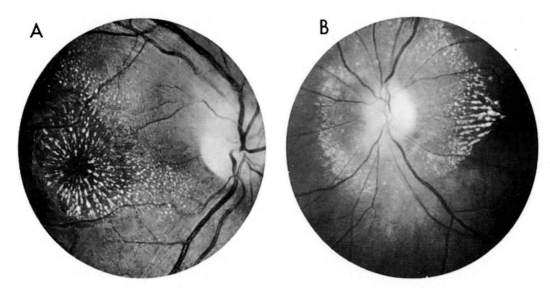

Fig. 5–29. Papillitis; neuroretinitis. **A.** Fundus of an 8-year-old boy who complained of visual loss 2 weeks after his 4-year-old sister developed mumps. Note mild disc swelling and deep retinal exudates in the form of a macular star. Vision of 20/80 (6/24) ultimately cleared to 20/15 (6/5) with no therapy. **B.** Acute loss of vision in a 27-year-old healthy woman. Prepapillary haze is due to cells in the vitreous. Arteries are narrowed, and the peripapillary retina is thick and elevated. Retinal exudates surround the disc and form a macular hemistar. Vision did not recover (20/200) (6/60) despite multiple retro-bulbar steroid injections.

and symptoms, cellular debris in the vitreous, and fundus characteristics are sufficient to establish a local, if nonspecific, cause of the neuritis. In such cases, reduced central vision may be due to cystoid macular edema rather than the papillitis, or a combination of both.

In clinical practice, the largest proportions of cases of optic neuritis present as a monosymptomatic event without clinically obvious cause. By history or physical examination alone, only rarely is a specific cause deduced (Table 5–10). History-taking should include the following points: symptoms of a preceding viral illness (*e.g.,* upper respiratory or gastrointestinal infection, febrile illness); subjective sinus disease; previous or co-existing neurologic signs and symptoms (*e.g.,* paresthesias, clumsiness of limbs, ataxia, diplopia, urinary incontinence); and concurrent viral illness in the family (especially children) or other close contacts. The presence of *painful eye movement* is an especially useful symptom,

TABLE 5–10. Causes of Optic Neuritis

Unknown origin
Multiple sclerosis
Viral infections of childhood (measles, mumps, chicken pox) with or without encephalitis
Postviral, paraviral infections
Infectious mononucleosis
Herpes zoster
Contiguous inflammation of meninges, orbit, sinuses
Granulomatous inflammations (syphilis, tuberculosis, cryptococcosis, sarcoidosis)
Intraocular inflammations

occurring in more than 90% of patients with optic neuritis.[189] The minute details of disc swelling in some instances may be helpful in the distinction of optic neuritis from *anterior ION* (see below), the presence of altitudinal or pallid edema, hemorrhages, or arterial attenuation suggesting the latter diagnosis,[190] but of course pain and younger age of onset favor neuritis.

The standard workup of patients with monosymptomatic optic neuritis, who are otherwise in good health and with an unremarkable medical history, is controversial. Unfortunately, many instances of isolated optic neuritis represent the clinical onset, or *forme fruste,* of disseminated demyelinating disease, that is, MS (see below). Even in a seemingly typical case of optic neuritis, neuroimaging studies, specifically MRI, are no longer considered superfluous, not only to rule out potential occult structural defects, but to detect brain white matter lesions. These most commonly take the form of discrete or confluent lesions contiguous with the ventricles (periventricular) (Fig. 5–30), but also in the anterior and posterior forceps, subcortical white matter, internal capsule, temporal lobes, and pons. On entry in the ONTT, fully 49% of patients had abnormal brain MRIs. With fat-suppression MRI techniques (Fig. 5–31), increased signal intensities in optic nerves may be found in 80% to 100% of patients with optic neuritis.[191] Dunker and Wiegand,[192] using short-time inversion recovery MRI technique suggested that optic nerve lesions greater than 17.5 mm in length, or lesions involving the intracanalicular segment, are more likely associated with incomplete or partial visual recovery.

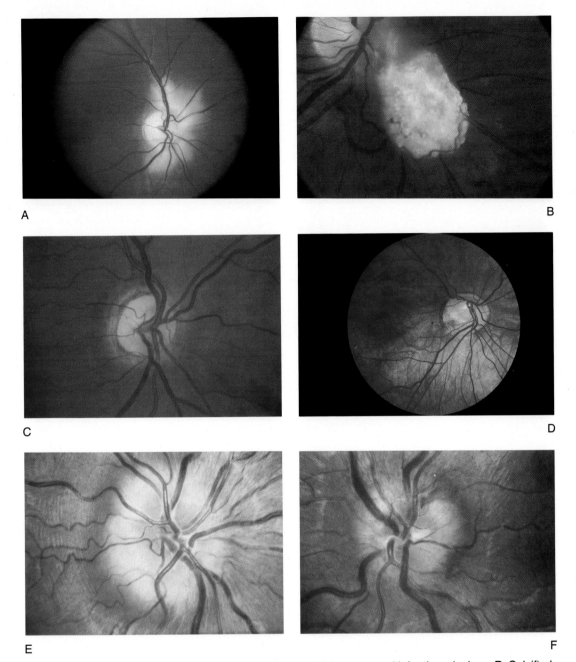

Color Plate 5–1. **A.** Myelinated nerve fibers. Retina is white, opaque, with feathered edges. **B.** Calcified astrocytic hamartoma of retinal nerve fiber layer in tuberous sclerosis. **C.** Hypoplasia of the optic nerve. Disk is small and with pigment rim and surrounding paler ring. Disk vessels appear disproportionately large. **D.** Inferior crescent. Disk is small and horizontally oval with scleral crescent at lower border. Contiguous inferior fundus sector is hypopigmented and appears albinotic; foveal reflex is indistinct. **E.** Pseudopapilledema; congenital elevated disk (compare with true papilledema, **F**). Note absence of central cup, vessels arise at disk apex. Vascular anomalies include excessive number of major disk vessels and multiple bifurcations. Nerve fiber layer does not obscure vessels at disk margins. **F.** Chronic moderate papilledema (compare with pseudopapilledema in **E.**). Note retention of central cup, flame hemorrhage at superior border, absence of anomalous vessel pattern, small arterioles are obscured in nerve fiber layer.

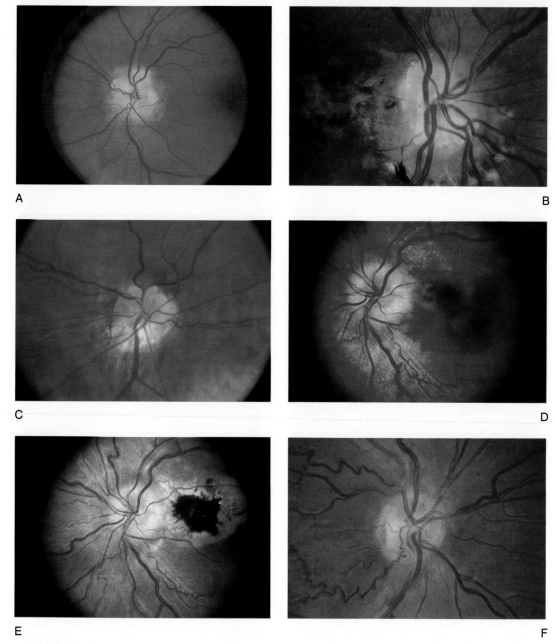

Color Plate 5–2. A. Hyaline bodies (drusen) of optic nerve. Note crystalline "rock candy" appearance. **B.** Hyaline bodies. Note anomalous arterial branching and marked reaction of pigment epithelium. **C.** Hyaline bodies in hypoplastic disk associated with inferior scleral crescent syndrome. **D.** Anomalous elevated disk (? Buried hyaline bodies) with spontaneous sub-retinal hemorrhage, in 5 year old child. Father had visible hyaline bodies. **E.** Resolution of hemorrhage **(D)**, with proliferation of pigment epithelium and permanent visual loss. **F.** Leber hereditary optic neuropathy with typical tortuous vessels and nerve fiber layer thickening.

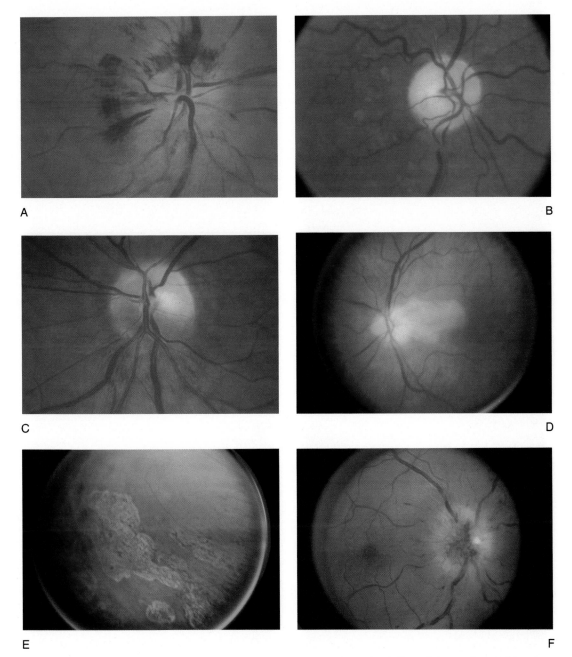

Color Plate 5–3. A. Ischemic optic neuropathy with disk edema and "flame" hemorrhages in nerve fiber layer. **B.** Disk atrophy after ischemic optic neuropathy. Note arteriolar narrowing. **C.** Superior segmental atrophy after disk infarct, with inferior field defect. Inferior half of disk appears hyperemic. **D.** Cranial arteritis. Milk pale edema of disk extending into macula. **E.** Cranial arteritis. Pigmentary changes 3 months after choroidal infarcts. **F.** Diabetic papillopathy. Note florid telangiectasia of disk capillaries and cyst at fovea.

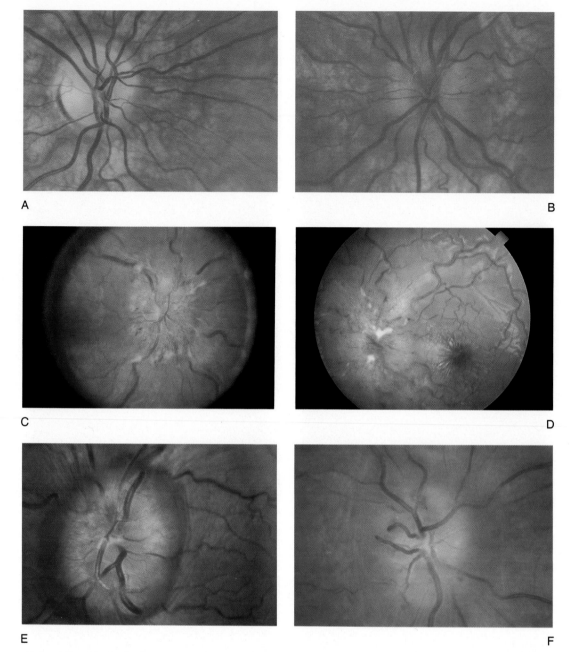

Color Plate 5–4. A. Papilledema of raised intracranial pressure. In patient with frontal astrocytoma, right disk shows early edema of superior pole. **B.** Left disk of same patient shows more advanced edema, yet absence of hemorrhages, exudates, or engorgement. **C.** Fully developed papilledema in a case of pseudotumor cerebri. Multiple superficial infarcts of nerve fiber layer ("cotton-wool spots"). Veins are dilated and tortuous. The disk diameter appears enlarged by edema that spreads laterally into, and elevates, the retinal nerve fiber layer. Center of disk relatively spared. **D.** Severe papilledema associated with dural venous sinus thrombosis in young boy. Note exudative partial "star" figure at fovea. **E.** Chronic papilledema of many months duration. "Champagne cork" appearance after resolution of hemorrhages. **F.** Chronic papilledema after detumescence of edema, revealing pallor and formation of retinochoroidal venous shunts.

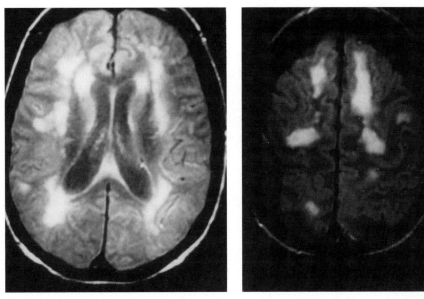

Fig. 5–30. Magnetic resonance imaging (TR 2000, TE 30) in multiple sclerosis. **Left.** Periventricular and subcortical hyperintense white matter lesions. **Right.** White matter lesions in cortical gyri.

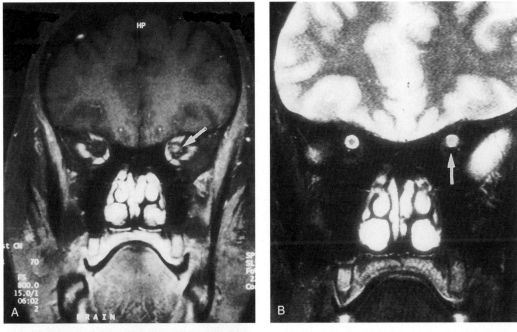

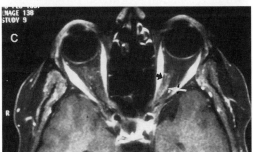

Fig. 5–31. Optic neuritis. A 45-year-old woman with left eye acuity 20/100, eye movement pain, and normal optic disc: magnetic resonance imaging. **A.** Fat-suppression T1-weighted scan, with contrast, high-intensity signal of the left optic nerve (*arrow*). **B.** T2-weighted, FLAIR sequence shows a hyperintense left nerve (*arrow*); compare with the right nerve, with central dark nerve surrounded by hyperintense cerebrospinal fluid. **C.** Fat-saturated T1-weighted image with gadolinium shows a hyperintense signal of nerve (between *arrows*).

Vision rapidly regains acuity levels of 20/20 to 20/40 often within a few weeks and in 75% of cases by 6 months; recovery is only marginally influenced by corticosteroid treatment during the first 2 weeks, but without significant therapeutic effect on all parameters of visual function at 1 year.[189] Paradoxically, in the ONNT, the regimen of oral steroids alone not only proved without benefit, but it was associated with an increased rate of new attacks (30%, compared with 14% in the group treated with intravenous methylprednisolone, and 16% recurrence rate in the group receiving placebo). The only predictor of poor visual outcome was very low vision at ONTT study entry, with 8 of 160 patients with acuity of 20/200 or worse still at that level at 6 months; remarkably, of 30 patients with initial vision of only light perception or worse, 20 (67%) nonetheless recovered to 20/40 or better.

Of great interest are the results of applying the same visual testing procedures to clinically unaffected eyes contralateral to acute optic neuritis[193]: 14% show diminished acuity, 15% abnormalities of contrast sensitivity, 22% dyschromatopsia, and 48% field defects. Intuitively, these phenomena infer the presence of bilateral optic neuropathy and the likelihood of disseminated demyelinative lesions, although in patients without subjective history of previous optic neuritis, this conclusion is debatable. (The details of tests of visual function, including color sense, contrast sensitivity, and evoked potentials are described in Chapter 2).

In spite of recovery to good levels of reading acuity, and failure to uncover specific defects by standardized techniques,[194] loss of contrast at medium spatial frequencies and disordered depth and motion perception (see above, Pulfrich's stereo-illusion phenomenon) best correlate with subjective symptoms. Extraordinary complaints include phosphenes, photopsias, and subjectively better vision under dim (scotopic) levels of illumination.[195,196]

Demyelinative Disease

As noted above, the association of optic neuritis, usually of the retro-bulbar type, with demyelinating disease is well recognized. In fact, optic neuritis, internuclear ophthalmoplegia, and various nystagmus patterns are the most common ocular complications of MS. In the individual patient with a first episode of monosymptomatic optic neuritis and a normal MRI study, it is not yet possible to predict with precision the future development of MS. According to the ONTT,[197] of 388 patients with acute optic neuritis, but without probable or definite MS, 5-year cumulative probability of definite MS was 30%, and it did not differ by treatment group. Neurologic impairment was generally mild. In 89 patients with 3 or more MRI abnormal white matter signals, 51% developed definite MS; 35% of patients with one or 2 lesions developed MS, as did 16% of 202 patients even with normal baseline MRI. Another study analysis[198] showed 42 of 74 patients (57%) with isolated monosymptomatic optic neuritis to have multiple white matter changes on MRI, but all clinically asymptomatic lesions; during 5.6 years mean follow-up, 28% developed MS (of which 76% had initially abnormal MRIs); of 53 patients who did not develop clinically symptomatic MS, 26 (49%) had initially abnormal MRIs; this study found that abnormal CSF immunoglobulin G levels correlated more strongly than did abnormal MRIs with subsequent clinically definite MS. According to the ONTT,[189] additional tests, including laboratory studies for lupus or syphilis, chest radiography, and lumbar puncture, proved of no diagnostic or prognostic value; white patients predominated, 77% of patients were women, and mean age was 32 years.

From the British experience at Moorfields Eye Hospital,[199] after a mean follow-up of nearly 12 years, it was found that 57% of 101 patients presenting with optic neuritis had developed MS, almost all with clinically "definite" disease. With life-table analysis, the probability of developing MS was 75%, 15 years after initial optic neuritis, and the presence of HLA-DR2 or DR3 increased the overall risk. In a population-based study[200] of 116 patients with monosymptomatic optic neuritis (80% women), 55% had 3 or more lesions on MRI (all with at least 1 periventricular white matter locus), 9% had 1 to 2 lesions, and 35% had normal imaging; of 143 patients, oligoclonal immunoglobulin G bands were demonstrated in the CSF of 72%; and of 146 patients, 47% carried the DR15,DQ6,Dw2 haplotype; laboratory screening for syphilis and *Borrelia* were entirely unproductive. Only 4 patients with strongly positive MRI findings were negative for oligoclonal bands. (In the absence of oligoclonal bands so typical of MS, some clinicians caution that another diagnosis must be considered.) During the study period (mean follow-up, 2.2 years), 36% developed definite MS, but there was no significantly higher risk among women, supporting the lack of gender risk in evolution of MS as in the ONTT.[197]

Retinal *venous sheathing* (periphlebitis retinae) accompanying optic neuritis may serve as an additional "marker" for MS, as well as providing some pathophysiologic insight. Lightman et al[201] found retinal vascular abnormalities in 14 of 50 patients with optic neuritis; MS developed in 8 of these 14 and in 5 of 32 patients without retinal vasculitis. The occurrence of perivenular sheathing or fluorescein leakage in tissues free of myelin and oligodendrocytes provides evidence that vascular changes may be the primary event in the formation of new demyelinative lesions. A Danish study[202] found 27 instances of retinal periphlebitis among 135 cases of MS, and those patients with such fundus findings suffered a more severe neurologic course. Of note is the association of MS with uveitis, usually mild "pars planitis,"[203] and also of positive MRI in a minority of patients with retinal vasculitis with a positive family history of MS.[204]

Other granulomatous inflammations such as syphilis, sarcoid, tuberculosis, and Behçet's disease must be considered as causes of uveitis and CNS disorders (see Chapter 5, Part I, Ureomeningeal Syndromes).

It is apparent that *the longer the follow-up of patients with optic neuritis, the greater the incidence of subsequent demyelinative signs and symptoms, and MRI is a major predictor of such development.* Identification of risk factors, especially MRI white matter lesions and presence of oligoclonal bands in CSF, provides guidelines for therapy. For example, patients receiving a course of intravenous corticosteroids show a slower rate of progression to MS; that is, there is a distinct 2-year delaying influence on subsequent signs and symptoms,[189] and, arguably, even in patients with isolated first-event optic neuritis, this treatment should be considered when MRI shows diagnostic changes. In acute optic neuritis, CSF changes, with the exception of oligoclonal banding, do not predict development of MS independently of baseline MRI characteristics.[205]

The early and accurate identification of patients with occult MS is vital. The long-term treatment of MS is evolving, with clinical trials of naturally occurring and recombinant interferons (antiviral proteins from T lymphocytes), co-polymers, oral myelin, and other immune-stimulating and immune-suppressing agents.

Neuromyelitis optica (Devic's disease) is a curious variant of demyelinative disease of indeterminate nosology. This syndrome is characterized by rapid or subacute, severe unilateral or bilateral visual loss accompanied by transverse myelitis and paraplegia. MRI lesions are more rare in the brain than in MS, and there is a propensity for necrotizing myelopathy of the cervical and upper thoracic spinal cord associated with thickened blood vessels.[206] Organ-specific antibodies may be detected, spinal cord lesions extend beyond one segment by MRI, and remissions are much less likely than in MS.[207]

Immune-mediated and Atypical Optic Neuritides

Many different inflammatory conditions afflict the optic nerves, confounding nonchalant differential considerations beyond simple MS. These causes embrace an exhausting range of possibilities (see Table 5–10) that tax determinations of specific clinical diagnosis. However, some physical features may prove useful. For example, optic disc edema may eventuate in fundus patterns of precipitates radially arranged in the macula, pointing toward the fovea (see Fig. 5–29) and termed a "macular star." As noted previously, this is a nonspecific retinal feature found even in diabetes and hypertension, less frequently in papilledema of raised intracranial pressure, and rarely in ION. It does suggest inflammation of the disc itself (papillitis, neuroretinitis), including causes such as various viruses, cat-scratch disease, spirochetal disease, and even sarcoidosis.[208] However, the presence of macular exudates militates strongly against MS.

Acute disseminated encephalomyelitis may follow viral infections, including measles, mononucleosis, mumps, varicella, and pertussis. Acute disseminated encephalomyelitis mimics experimental acute encephalitis induced by sensitization to myelin basic protein. Especially in childhood, this disorder may cause bilateral optic neuropathy, with headache, seizures, or meningeal signs, including CSF lymphocytosis and raised CSF pressure.[209] Encephalitis with optic neuritis may develop subsequent to vaccination for polio, measles-mumps-rubella, hepatitis, or diphtheria-tetanus-pertussis, for example.[185,187,210]

Of special interest are reports of optic neuritis after influenza vaccination,[211,212] attributed to allergic cross-reaction to viral antigens or to immune-mediated vasculitis. Other acute inflammatory demyelinating polyneuropathies, such as Guillain-Barré syndrome, follow immune upsets, but optic neuropathy with Guillain-Barré syndrome must be rare (as well as auditory neuritis), extraordinary case reports,[213,214] notwithstanding.

Optic neuropathies following chickenpox,[215] rubella, rubeola, mumps, herpes zoster, and mononucleosis[216] may be *formes frustes* of acute disseminated encephalomyelitis or are referred to as *parainfectious,* as opposed to direct tissue infiltration by microbiologic agents. Indeed, an undoubtedly immune-mediated form of bilateral optic neuritis is reported following bee sting.[217] In such instances, visual loss is typically bilateral and severe, occurring 10 days to 2 weeks after dermatologic signs (or envenomization), such delay suggesting an autoimmune cascade mechanism. In general, complete visual recovery is anticipated, although corticosteroid therapy may be indicated.[209,210]

The association of optic neuritis with systemic lupus erythematosus and other autoimmune states (*e.g.,* mixed connective tissue disease, Sjögren's syndrome) is well-known, if relatively rare. The principal pathologic process is one of inflammation and necrosis of blood vessel walls and, as such, is best classified as a variety of ION, discussed subsequently. Without the necessary criteria for classification as systemic lupus erythematosus, a small subset of patients are considered to suffer from a form of "autoimmune optic neuritis," which is roughly characterized by more severe visual loss and resistance to corticosteroid therapy than is typical of idiopathic or demyelinative types. At times, diagnostic criteria are circuitous and, in the absence of substantial clinical or laboratory support (hematuria, serum antinuclear antibodies, erythrocyte sedimentation rate [ESR], abnormal complement levels), a vague relationship with immune-mediated processes is insinuated, especially in young women (see below).

Infective Neuropathies

Of those optic neuritides in which infectious agents are more readily apparent, the impact of human immu-

TABLE 5–11. Optic Neuropathies in Immunodeficiency

Papilledema (raised cerebrospinal fluid pressure)
   Cryptococcal meningitis
   Toxoplasmosis
   Lymphoma
Optic neuritis
   Cryptococcosis
   Syphilis (perineuritis form)
   Cytomegalovirus
   Pneumocystis carinii
   Human immunodeficiency virus ?
   Histoplasmosis
   Varicella

nodeficiency virus (HIV) infection and acquired immune deficiency syndrome (AIDS) has most palpably altered the modern etiologic spectrum. HIV-associated optic nerve disease may be related to tumoral compression, infiltrations such as lymphoma, vasculitides, inflammations, and especially secondary infections. As noted in Chapter 5, Part I, opportunistic infectious agents regularly invade the retina, optic nerve, meninges, and brain, and co-existing multiple infections further confound diagnosis and management. Neurologic symptoms are said to occur in 40% of cases, CNS pathologic findings in 70% to 80%, ocular manifestations in 50% to 70%, and neuro-ophthalmologic signs in at least 3% to 8%.[218,219] Optic nerve complications of immunodeficiency are included in Table 5–11.

AIDS-related optic neuropathies generally reflect direct infestations of viral, spirochetal, or fungal organisms, but grossly diminished axonal counts may indicate a primary AIDS optic neuropathy.[220] Otherwise, cytomegalovirus retinitis with spread to the nerve, or as an initial papillitis, is associated with poor visual outcome even with therapy.[221] Likewise, cryptococcosis (Fig. 5–34) may be associated with chronic optic meningitis, with insidious or rapid vision loss related to fulminant nerve necrosis.[222] Optic nerve sheath decompression for raised CSF pressure in cryptococcal meningitis has been reported to improve function.[223] Other infectious agents include *Toxoplasma gondii,*[224] varicella-zoster,[225,226] and *Histoplasma capsulatum.*[227]

The role of HIV itself as an etiologic agent in optic nerve disease is imprecise, but the virus has been isolated from all ocular tissues, it is neurotropic, and is implicated in cases of meningitis (including with *Cryptococcus*), encephalitis, and peripheral neuropathies.[228] Indeed, HIV-seropositive patients are reported with recoverable bilateral optic neuropathies without other infectious or neoplastic processes, suggesting a primary role of HIV infection.[229] Berger et al[228] described a neurologic disease clinically indistinguishable from MS, including mostly bilateral optic neuritis, occurring with HIV; indeed, histopathologic features of the CNS were consistent with MS.

By 1990, the incidence of primary and secondary syphilis in the United States increased 34% to 18.7/100,000 persons, and serologic testing is indicated in many cases of optic neuropathy without other clearly discernable cause, but especially in patients with, or at risk for, AIDS. Co-infection alters the natural history and increases the propensity for a more aggressive course and rapidly evolving neurosyphilis. Moreover, even in biopsy-confirmed syphilis, treponemal and nontreponemal tests may be negative in HIV infection.[219] Corticosteroids, so frequently used in optic neuritis, are contraindicated until infectious causes are ruled out, including CSF assessment, especially when HIV is suspected. Empiric penicillin treatment for neurosyphilis may be considered.[229] Modern laboratory tests include the fluorescent treponemal antibody absorption (FTA-ABS) test and microhemagglutination assay.

Syphilitic neuroretinitis, papillitis, and "perineuritis" are clinical manifestations of secondary stage and neurorecurrence, whereas slowly progressive atrophy evolves in the tertiary stage; simple papilledema of raised pressure may herald meningoencephalitis.[230] Uncomplicated "retro-bulbar" neuritis, so common otherwise, must be extremely rare in syphilis, although Zambrano[231] reported bilateral overnight blindness in association with AIDS. Optic "perineuritis" purportedly inflames primarily the optic meninges, with relative sparing of the central core of the nerve and preservation of central field function, including acuity; disc swelling is characteristic, but papilledema of increased pressure and meningitis are ruled out by lumbar puncture. Color vision and evoked potentials may be normal.[232] Late "descending" optic atrophy is a sign of tertiary neurosyphilis, classically seen in taboparesis.

Arruga et al[233] reviewed neuroretinitis in acquired, secondary syphilis, with funduscopically evident clouding of the central retina, vasculitis, hemorrhages, pigment epithelial disarray, and disc swelling; most cases are bilateral, and vitreous cellular debris is present.

Lyme borreliosis must be an uncommon cause of optic neuropathies, or of any other ocular manifestation, according to authoritative reviews[234] of neurologic manifestations of the disease. In the early disease, a nonspecific follicular conjunctivitis occurs in about 10% of patients, and flu-like symptoms are common along with the typical *erythema migrans* rash, itself noted in only 60% to 80% of cases. Uveitis is extremely rare, as is neuroretinitis. Schmutzhard et al[235] included two young women with "optic neuritis," and Pachner and Steere[236] cited no optic nerve involvement among 38 cases of Lyme meningitis. The case report of Wu et al[237] of "optic disc edema" seemingly occurred in the setting of a 7-year-old boy with stiff neck and CSF pleocytosis. Strominger et al[238] reported worsening of Lyme neuroborreliosis, including optic neuritis, following ceftriaxone therapy. In the *early disseminated phase,* aseptic mening-

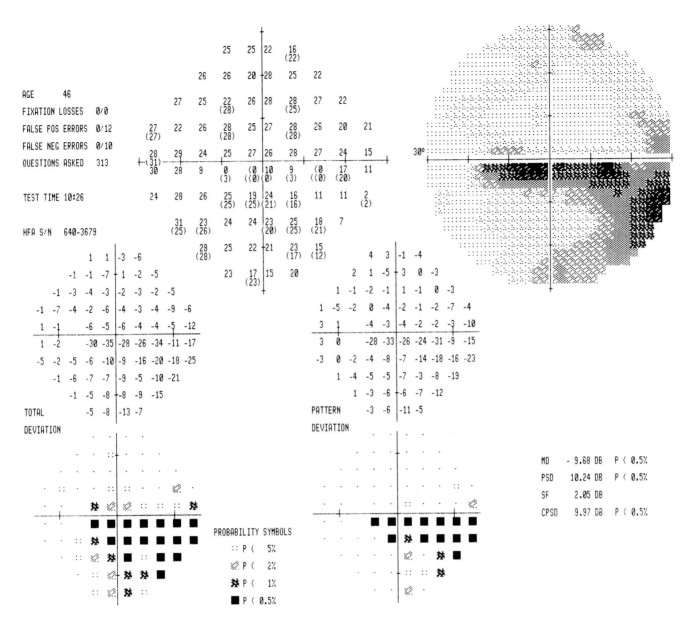

Fig. 5–32. Left visual field in optic neuritis; cecocentral scotoma pattern and nasal depression (see case description in Fig. 5–31).

itis, cranial neuropathies (facial palsy being the most common), and radiculoneuritis occur. Indirect immunofluorescence antibody (IFA) and enzyme-linked immunosorbent assays (ELISA) are used to detect antibodies, but even for patients with the pathognomonic cutaneous manifestation of erythema migrans, in a Connecticut study the overall sensitivity of serology was 30% to 45% by IFA and 24% to 32% for ELISA.[239] At present, seropositivity alone does not distinguish between past exposure and active infection, and false-positive results are common. Polymerase chain reaction techniques are currently being evaluated.[235] In the early stages, doxycycline or penicillins are used, and ceftriaxone is used for neurologic or ophthalmic disease.[235]

Cat-scratch disease is an infection caused by *Bartonella (Rochalimaea) henselae* and *R. quintana,* gram-negative bacilli implicated in subacute regional lymphadenitis, conjunctivitis (at times with pre-auricular adenopathy), intermediate uveitis, retinal vasculitis, serous retinal detachment (see also Chapter 5, Part I), papillitis with retinal exudates, and aseptic meningitis.[240,241] Disease evolves days to weeks after cat scratch or bite, and it is thought that almost 50% of domestic cats, and their fleas, are the persistent reservoir of these organisms. Visual acuity is variable, and papillitis may be bilateral. IFA of serum is positive in the majority of patients, but serologic assays are also positive in some 3% of the healthy population. Although cat-scratch disease is considered a self-limited and relatively benign infectious disorder, and no optimal therapy is yet defined, various antibiotics are usually administered to maximize visual outcome.[241] Reed et al[242] suggested the use of doxycycline and rifampin.

Toxacara canis[243] is also documented to cause inflammatory papillitis with vitreous cellular reaction. *Toxoplasma gondii* (the agent of toxoplasmosis), a relatively frequent cause of posterior uveitis in the United States, with characteristic pigmented chorioretinal scars, is an uncommon but eradicable agent that can produce neuroretinitis characterized by retinal edema with macular star exudates. Serologic tests include IFA titers and ELISA, and sulfamethoxazole, sulfadiazine, or clindamycin therapy is indicated, usually coupled with corticosteroids.[244] Familial Mediterranean fever (recurrent polyserositis), an autosomal recessive disorder, is reported to produce uveitis, retinal detachment, or optic neuritis.[245]

Slowly Progressive and "Chronic" Optic Neuritis

Although it is undoubtedly true that certain inflammatory conditions such as sarcoidosis, syphilis, tuberculosis, or other chronic meniningitides may be responsible for insidiously progressive loss of vision, the diagnosis of "chronic optic neuritis" is otherwise only rarely applicable. Most such clinical enigmas are eventually disclosed as compressive lesions such as meningiomas (intracanalicular or tuberculum sellae), pituitary tumors, or paraclinoid aneurysms. Moreover, because it is uncommon for demyelinative optic neuritis to run a relentless course, this clinical rubric demands precise neuroimaging procedures (MRI) and spinal fluid investigations. A salutary visual response to systemic corticosteroids may *not* be interpreted as positive evidence of inflammatory causes because vision may also be improved when mass lesions actually exist (see Chapter 6).

Covert visual loss, both unilateral and bilateral, that progresses at a slow uniform rate is documented in MS,[246] and indeed it may be the presenting symptom. Insidious depression of visual acuity is the rule, although central scotoma patterns may be indiscernible in severe field loss. Such chronic central or cecocentral scotomas must be considered *extremely rare* in compressive lesions (see Chapter 6). Other associated neurologic signs and symptoms, CSF protein abnormalities, and typical white matter signals with MRI provide evidence in favor of a demyelinative cause.

Eidelberg et al[247] studied the clinical, electrophysiologic, and MRI features of 20 patients 12 to 77 years of age with *chronic unilateral progressive visual failure* lasting a minimum of 6 months. Extrinsic mass lesions were disclosed in 8 patients, intrinsic nerve or sheath tumors in 5; in 7 patients, short-time inversion recovery MRI sequences revealed altered signals in symptomatic nerves, and T2-weighted sequences showed periventricular white matter lesions.

Perineuritis, an idiopathic inflammatory cuffing of the orbital and intracranial optic nerve, does occur,[248] with or without pain or other orbital signs, and it may radiologically mimic nerve sheath meningioma.[249] Bilateral instances are recorded,[250] and other features include nerve enlargement and retinal vascular occlusions.[251] Such instances of perineuritis may be caused by syphilis.[252]

Sarcoidosis frequently involves the nervous system and can present as abrupt or chronic visual loss, with or without disc changes. The cranial nerves, most commonly the facial and optic, the meninges, hypothalamus, and pituitary gland are frequent sites. In a series of 11 patients with sarcoidosis of the optic nerve,[253] ranging in age from 16 to 48 years, only 2 patients were previously known to have the disorder. Four patients showed disc granulomas, 4 had optic nerve granulomas, and 3 mimicked retro-bulbar neuritis. Chest film findings were characteristic in 8 of 11, but only one-third of these cases had elevated serum angiotensin-converting enzyme levels.

Sarcoid granulomas may elevate the optic disc or may inflame retro-bulbar nerves and chiasm (see Fig. 6–10), presenting as optic atrophy. Chorioretinopathy, uveitis, and perivascular infiltrates ("candle-wax spots") are well-recognized fundal signs of sarcoid.[254] Leptomeningeal sarcoid may present as secondary pseudotumor cerebri resulting from dural sinus thrombosis.[255] Modern MRI now regularly discloses enlarged anterior visual pathway sites, and lymph node or, more rarely, optic nerve or chiasm, biopsy provides histologic affirmation. Therapy is based on corticosteroids and immunosuppressives such as methotrexate. Current inclusive reviews are available elsewhere.[256,257]

Other causes of optic meningeal or nerve enlargement and chronic visual loss include perioptic meningioma, optic glioma, perioptic idiopathic inflammation, and Wegener's granulomatosis[258] (see below). The cautionary comment of David Cogan again bears repetition: "Probably no branch of neuro-ophthalmology has to its discredit the abundance of erroneous diagnoses as has optic neuritis."

Contiguous Inflammations

The optic nerve may be secondarily involved by various inflammatory lesions of adjacent tissues, including the orbit, paranasal sinuses, and intracranial meninges. With orbital cellulitis or nonspecific inflammatory pseudotumor, it is not clear whether true optic neuritis is present or visual deficits are caused by pressure effect. In orbital inflammatory pseudotumor, especially in the subacute or chronic forms, visual loss may be accompanied by variable degrees of disc swelling, a finding suggesting actual optic neuritis or perineuritis, as noted above. Rarely is visual impairment an initial symptom, and other clinical signs (proptosis, diplopia, conjunctival chemosis) usually have evolved before vision is disturbed. Systemic steroids are frequently beneficial.

Decades ago, many instances of optic neuritis were attributed to acute or chronic sinusitis. This popular concept was not far-fetched, especially when the close anatomic relationship of the optic nerve with the ethmoid and sphenoid sinuses is considered (see Figs. 4–5 and 5–11). The pendulum has now swung far in the other direction, and indeed rarely can the paranasal sinuses be directly incriminated in cases of optic neuritis.

Acute, severe, and irreversible visible loss may occur from spheno-ethmoiditis and contiguous cellulitis at the orbital apex.[259] Visual loss occurs before, and often out of proportion to, overt signs of orbital inflammation. To be ruled out are Wegener's granulomatosis (see below), opportunistic fungal infections, and acute compression by mucopyocele.

Mucoceles of the sphenoid sinus may be associated with chronic progressive visual loss and ocular motor nerve palsies. However, on rare occasions, a clinical picture consistent with optic neuritis may be encountered, as exemplified by the following case:

A 16-year-old boy complained of progressive loss of central vision of 6 weeks' duration. For 6 months, the patient had noted mucopurulent nasal discharge, pain, and tenderness of the brows, and for 3 weeks, deep orbital ache increased on eye movement. Examination revealed corrected acuities of 20/40, right, and 20/70, left. Fields demonstrated a central scotoma in the left eye and a similar defect with superior extension in the right field (Fig. 5–33). The nerve heads showed mild but distinct hyperemia and edema. Frontal tomography demonstrated massive enlargement of the sphenoid sinuses. Following transnasal evacuation of a chronic pyomucocele, vision and discs returned to normal.

Optic neuritis may accompany acute or chronic meningitis in children or adults. Purulent leptomeningitis spreads to involve the optic nerve sheaths, primarily in the optic canal, or the substance of the nerve itself. Disc swelling may be present. Optic atrophy can follow severe neuritis, but as a rule, vision returns to functional levels, even after several months. In cases complicated by hydrocephalus or opticochiasmatic arachnoiditis, field loss may be progressive.

The optic nerves may also be involved in focal basal granulomas[260] or diffuse granulomatous or infectious meningitis, including fungal infections such as cryptococcosis,[261] syphilis, and tuberculosis (Fig. 5–34). The therapy is that of the primary infectious process, but ultimate visual outcome is guarded.

As noted, optic neuritis is not rare in the viral disorders of childhood, which may be associated with symptomatic or asymptomatic meningoencephalitis. As a rule, bilateral disc swelling is seen, resulting from either papilledema or optic neuritis. Both viral and bacterial meningitis may cause visual complications that fall into three anatomic categories: (1) papillitis, retro-bulbar interstitial, or perineuritis (leptomeningitis); (2) cortical blindness (usually with cortical venous thromboses); and (3) progressive optic atrophy as a result of opticochiasmatic arachnoiditis or hydrocephalus.

On rare occasions, herpes zoster ophthalmicus, the trigeminal dermatologic reactivation of varicella-zoster virus (human herpes virus-3), may be associated with optic neuritis, either in the retro-bulbar form or with a severe ischemic papillitis. In immune-compromised patients, varicella-zoster optic neuropathy may precede retinal necrosis,[262] or it is more usually delayed.[263] The efficacy of acyclovir and corticosteroids is variable. With perineuritis and perivasculitis as pathologic substrate, poor visual outcome is the rule, from which the following case is an extraordinary exception:

A 7-year-old boy experienced right earache followed by vesiculation in the cutaneous distribution of the ophthalmic trigeminal nerve (Fig. 5–35). Vision was recorded as "light perception only," and corticosteroids were injected into the right orbit. Ultimate visual outcome while the patient received systemic steroids was 20/25, within 2 weeks. Within 9 days of onset, two siblings developed chickenpox.

Histopathologically, zoster involves the optic nerve as an inflammatory arteritis with associated mild leptomeningitis. With these lesions in mind, it was believed that the recovery of vision in the patient in the above case was directly attributable to intraorbital and systemic steroids.

Diffuse idiopathic perioptic meningeal thickening (cranial fibrosclerosis; hypertrophic pachymeningitis) is a relatively rare cause of progressive visual loss, with or without associated systemic multifocal fibrosclerosis.[264] Signs and symptoms include chronic headaches, optic disc atrophy or edema, meningeal thickening on MRI (Fig. 5–36), CSF pleocytosis and protein elevation, dural sinus thrombosis, and cranial nerve palsies producing ophthalmoplegia, hearing loss, and facial palsies. Other causes of pachymeningitis must be ruled out, including sarcoidosis, tuberculosis, syphilis, rheumatoid arthritis, dural carcinomatosis, meningioma-en-plaque, and plasmacytoma. These conditions may be distinguished by accompanying clinical findings and definitive meningeal biopsy. Corticosteroid and immunosuppressive agents are undoubtedly useful.

ISCHEMIC OPTIC NEUROPATHIES

Infarction of the optic disc, and rarely of the retro-bulbar portion of the optic nerve, unrelated to inflammation, demyelination, neural infiltration or metastasis, compression by mass lesion, or diffuse orbital congestion, is a poorly understood but well-recognized and

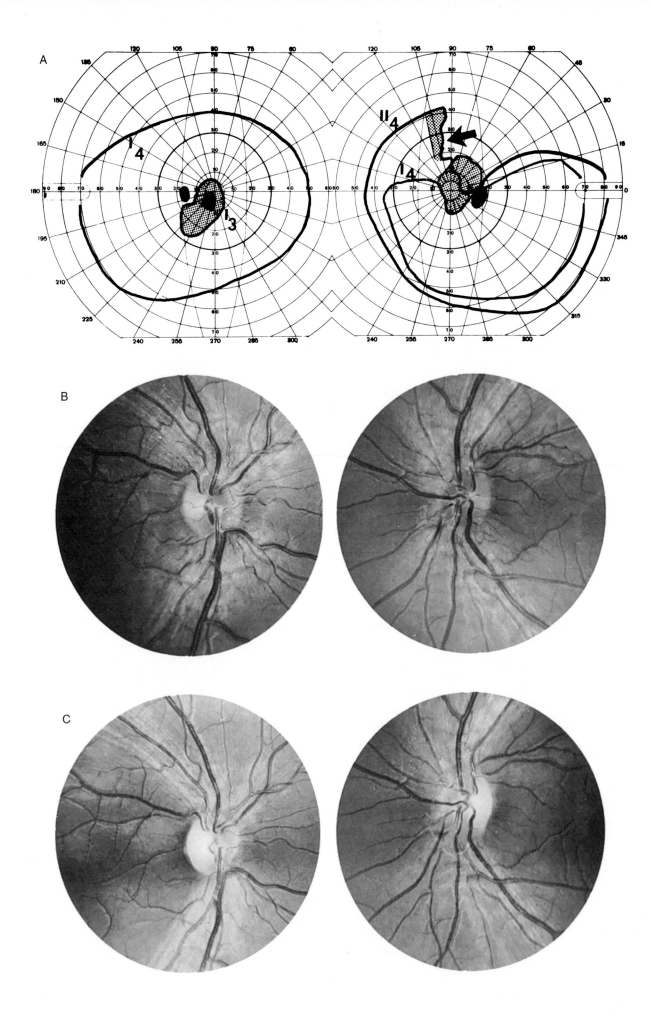

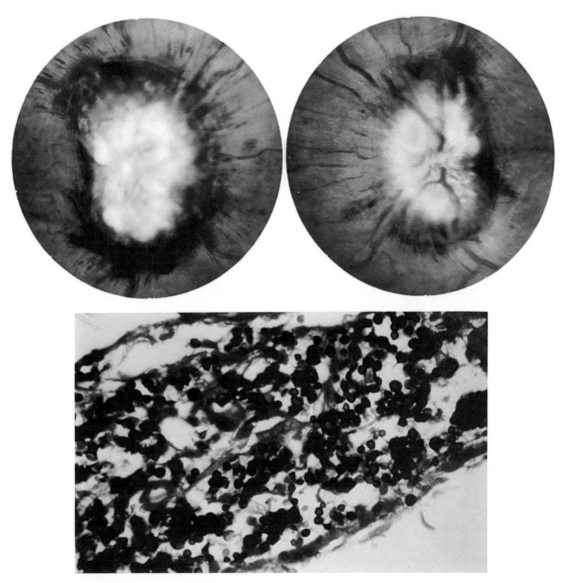

Fig. 5–34. Cryptococcosis with severe hemorrhagic disc swelling. Visual function of hand movement in each eye. At autopsy, organisms were found within the meninges and substance of the optic nerve.

unfortunately *common* cause of sudden loss of vision, especially in the presenescent and elderly population. Primary ION is the most frequent basis of disc swelling in adulthood after 50 years of age. By "ischemic," we also include other diverse subsets only infrequently associated with ION, including severe hypertensive episodes, juvenile diabetes, acute blood loss, collagen arteritis, delayed radionecrosis, and paraneural inflammation. However, when more specific mechanisms are evident, the clinical situation with regard to therapies and outcome differs substantially from the typical idiopathic, or perhaps "arteriosclerotic," form of ION.

A brief anatomic review of the vascular supply of the optic nerve may be summarized. The nerve fiber layer at the surface of the disc is supplied by small papillary capillaries of the central retinal artery branches, whereas the major prelaminar disc substance is nourished by

Fig. 5–33. Optic neuritis associated with sphenoidal pyomucocele. **A.** Field defects are essentially central scotomas. Visual acuity: 20/40 (6/12), right; 20/70 (6/21), left. The right eye has a superior defect as well, which is relative (*arrow*) and crosses the vertical meridian. **B.** Optic discs before sinus surgery. Note bilateral disc hyperemia, edema, and venous engorgement. **C.** Six weeks after evacuation of mucocele, visual function and fundi are normal. There were no signs or symptoms of meningitis.

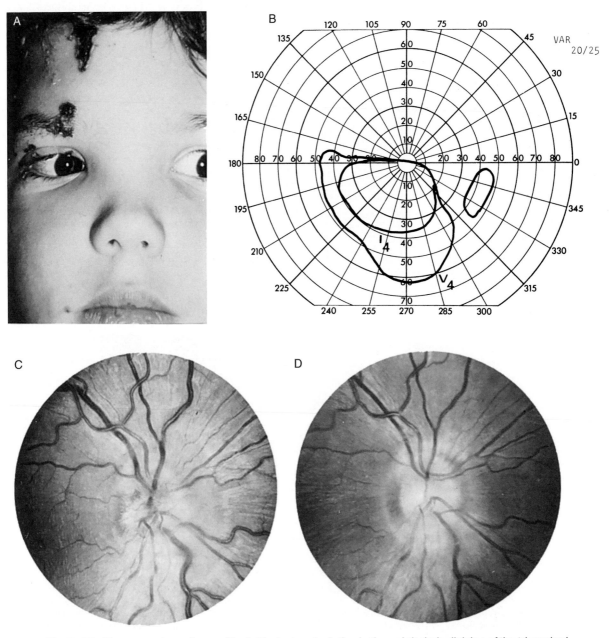

Fig. 5–35. Herpes zoster optic neuritis. **A.** Typical vesiculation in the ophthalmic division of the trigeminal nerve. **B.** Light perception only, returned to 20/25 vision and field as indicated. **C.** Acute disc swelling. **D.** Disc 5 days later, after orbital and systemic steroid therapy.

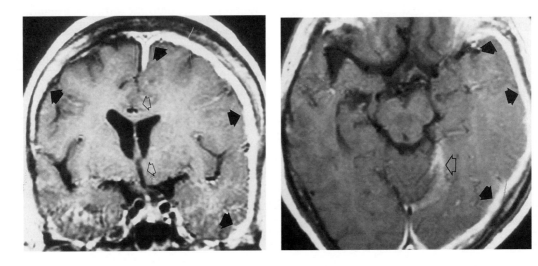

peripapillary choroidal arterioles from the elliptic anastomotic annulus formed from the short posterior ciliary arteries (see Fig. 4–4).[265,266] The perforated lamina cribrosa of the scleral wall, and this section of the optic nerve, is also supplied by centripetal arterioles of the partial arterial circle (Zinn-Haller) formed by branches of the posterior choroidal arteries. Consensus dictates that the central retinal artery does not contribute in any significant way to these anterior portions of the nerve. The immediate retro-laminar segment is supplied by recurrent pial arterioles of the peripapillary circulation, and pial capillaries of the central retinal artery running in the fibrous supportive septa of the nerve. Venous drainage is principally via the central retinal vein and variable peripapillary optociliary collaterals. These latter vessels may enlarge in conditions of chronic nerve sleeve obstruction, such as papilledema and meningeal infiltration, forming ophthalmoscopically visible shunts at the disc perimeter (see Color Plate 5–4F). The orbital and canalicular segments of the optic nerve are supplied by penetrating capillaries of the peripheral pial plexus of the ophthalmic artery and, to some extent, by the intra-axial central retinal artery circulation. The likely influence of these vascular patterns is discussed below.

Common (Arteriosclerotic, Non-arteritic) Ischemic Optic Neuropathy

In contrast to inflammatory or demyelinative retrobulbar optic neuritis, ION characteristically involves the prelaminar portion of the optic nerve with a constant ophthalmoscopic appearance of disc swelling (thus, the alternate term "anterior" ION) (Fig. 5–37 and Color Plate 5–3A). In fact, the absence of disc swelling with acute monocular loss of vision makes a diagnosis of "simple" ischemic infarction untenable. The rare exception to this rule is retro-bulbar ION associated with cranial arteritis (see below). Otherwise, abrupt visual loss in the elderly patient with a *normal* optic disc should bring to mind the possibility of other lesions, including rapidly expanding basal tumors or carcinomatous infiltration of the optic nerve sheaths.

Common ION may be generally characterized as follows:[267–269] age- and sex-adjusted incidence rate as high as 10/100,000; slight male predominance (about 62%) and extremely uncommon in black persons; peak median age 66[268] or 72 years,[267] but on rare occasions ION may occur in the late forties; hypertension in more than

40% to 50% and diabetes in 25%, these risk factors being of greater importance with onset in the slightly younger subset; many, perhaps most, patients noting visual symptoms on awakening; sudden onset of altitudinal[267,270] or other field defects (see Fig. 5–6), usually, but not invariably, involving the central fixational area and producing reduced acuity, ranging from 20/20 to no light perception, with one-half of patients seeing better than 20/60, and one-third seeing 20/200 or worse; visual deficits typically maximal at onset, but deterioration may progress for a few days to several weeks[270,271]; recurrent disc infarcts in the same eye are considered relatively rare.[272]

Results of the Ischemic Optic Neuropathy Decompression Trial[271] indicate that untreated eyes show a spontaneous improvement rate of three or more optotype lines in 43%, and visual deterioration in 12%; other studies[273] provide variable results (see below). Unlike infarction with cranial arteritis, premonitory ocular symptoms do not occur, and significant eye or brow discomfort, or headache, is exceptional, perhaps in about 10%, unlike optic neuritis, in which orbital ache or pain on eye movement is a prominent symptom (see above).

The optic disc is swollen to some degree (Fig. 5–37), usually in a sector with small flame hemorrhages, and edema typically extends only a short distance beyond the border of the disc. It has been suggested that altitudinal swelling, pallor, arterial attenuation, and hemorrhage are found more commonly in anterior ION than in optic neuritis.[190] In addition, a presymptomatic phase of disc swelling may be observed[274]; for example, a patient presents with characteristic ION with visual loss in one eye, and disc edema with good visual function surprisingly is found in the contralateral fundus; after a brief delay, disc edema progresses, and vision usually declines. Perhaps this odd situation is related to chronic or subacute nerve ischemia with obstipation of axoplasm flow, but without significant nerve fiber infarction.

Clinical and experimental studies[275] indicate that ION is precipitated by insufficiency in posterior ciliary artery circulation, more likely resulting from a reduction in critical perfusion pressure than from embolism or thrombosis, and that branches of the peripapillary choroidal arterial system become ischemic, with consequent infarction of retinal nerve fiber bundles in the disc substance anterior to the lamina cribrosa. Olver and associates[276] studied the morphology of the microvasculature

Fig. 5–36. Chronic idiopathic pachymeningitis in a 64-year-old woman with headaches, bilateral visual loss, and left disc edema: magnetic resonance T1-weighted image with gadolinium. **Left.** Coronal section shows massive hypertrophic thickening of the meninges (*black arrows*), and rightward shift of the midline structures (*open arrows*) because of edema of the left hemisphere. **Right.** Axial section shows infiltration of the meninges and tentorium (*open arrow*); note also diffuse hemispheral edema. (From ref. 264)

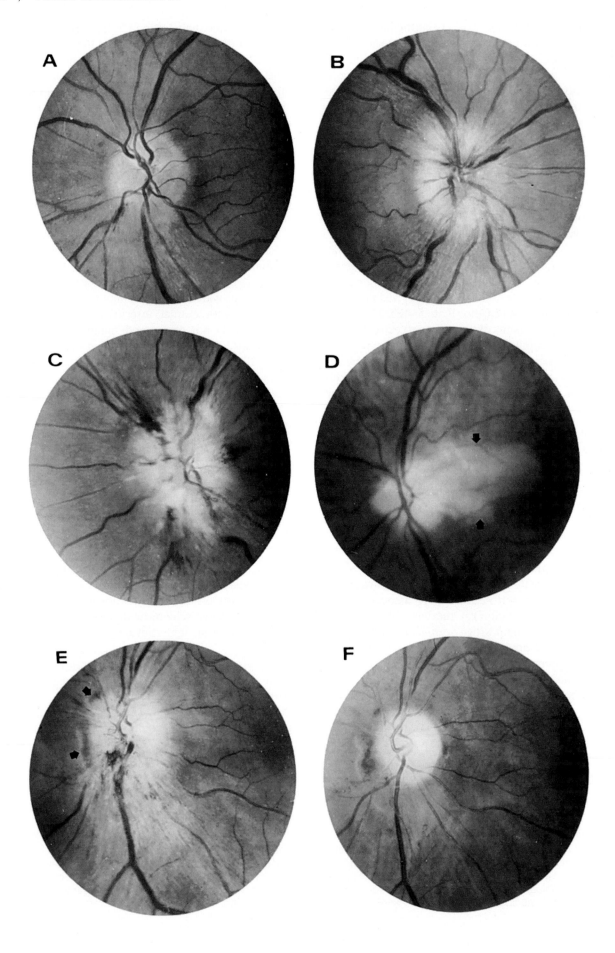

of the retro-laminar area of the human optic nerve and described an elliptic anastomosis ("circle of Zinn-Haller") of branches of the medial and lateral para-optic short posterior ciliary arteries. This ellipse is divided into superior and inferior portions by the entry points of these branches into the eye, providing potential superior and inferior "altitudinal" blood supplies to the retro-laminar optic nerve that may play a role in the pathogenesis of the upper- or lower-half patterns of visual field defects frequently found in ION. Fundus fluorescein angiography in 41 instances of non-arteritic ION, less than 3 weeks after onset, showed delay in prelaminar optic disc capillary dye filling, but neither onset nor completion of filling of peripapillary choroid was delayed when compared with control subjects; frequency of delayed filling within peripapillary choroidal watershed zones was also not increased, nor was there consistent correlation by quadrant between disc filling delay, choroidal filling delay, optic disc swelling or hyperfluorescence, and visual field defect.[277] The role of carotid embolic or occlusive disease is considered below.

Although some small case series imply that chronic raised intraocular tension may play a role in ION, in larger series,[278] no evidence was found to support this hypothesis. Pre-existing chronic glaucoma in the involved or fellow eye must be considered a *rare condition.* Hayreh et al[279] emphasized the role of nocturnal hypotension and failure of disc autoregulatory mechanisms, predisposed by hypotensive medications often taken at bedtime. Again, the early morning subjective symptoms support this hypoperfusion hypothesis; indeed, Hayreh believed that more than 70% of patients note the new visual symptoms on awakening or shortly thereafter, and that ION develops more often in summer than in winter months.

The visual field defects in ION vary but usually take the form of arcuate scotomas or "altitudinal hemianopias" of the superior or inferior half-fields (see Fig. 5–6). These altitudinal or nasal pseudo-quadrantic defects are dense and are easily discovered by hand or finger-counting confrontational field techniques. The localizing value of the position of the "vertex" of quadrantic and wedge-shaped defects has been emphasized by Kestenbaum: when the wedge originates at, or points toward, the blind spot, the defect is due to disease at the nerve head or just behind it. The differential diagnosis of such arcuate scotomas (*i.e.*, with curvilinear or radial borders originating at the blind spot) includes branch retinal artery occlusion, glaucoma, ION, optic neuritis, hyaline bodies (drusen) of the optic disc, congenital optic pit, juxtapapillary inflammation, and, *very rarely,* chiasmal interference. Central scotomas are the predominant field defects in about one-sixth to one-fourth[280] of cases of common ION.

Optic atrophy ensues as disc edema resolves (see Fig. 5–37 and Color Plate 5–3B), and some small loss of disc tissue may be evident; increase in cup size is observed, but rarely is glaucomatous excavation mimicked.[281] The ophthalmoscopic criteria that permit a retrospective diagnosis of optic atrophy of ischemic origin include arterial attenuation,[282] although Frisen and Claesson[283] have quantitatively demonstrated a reduction in central retinal artery caliber of 17% to 24% in non-ischemic, descending (retro-bulbar nerve, chiasm lesions) optic atrophy.

Following ischemic infarction of one disc, there is great likelihood of second eye involvement, generally believed to sequentially occur in approximately 30% to 40%. Beri and associates[284] provided the following figures for 10-year cumulative incidence rates: for patients 45 to 64 years of age, 55.3%; for patients 65 years old or older, 34.4%; for patients younger than age 45, 75.9%; for patients with diabetes mellitus, 72.2%; for patients with arterial hypertension, 42.2%; for patients with diabetes and hypertension, 60.6%. When ION occurs in the second eye, there is no consistent agreement on correlation of final visual function outcomes.[285,286]

In common ION *simultaneous* bilateral disc infarction is practically unknown, and an underlying systemic disease such as cranial arteritis or severe renovascular hypertension must be suspected. The occurrence of *consecutive* disc infarction with fresh disc swelling in one eye, when combined with contralateral previous optic atrophy, mimics the ophthalmoscopic combination popularized as the "Foster Kennedy syndrome,"[287] but there are obvious functional differences that separate acute disc infarction from papilledema of raised pressure (see Table 5–8). Ironically, then, the celebrated "diagnostic sign" of Foster Kennedy is most typical of alternating, consecutive ION and is exceedingly infrequent as a sign

Fig. 5–37. Ischemic optic neuropathy. **A.** Minimal swelling of inferior disc border with a few fine superficial linear hemorrhages. Arteries are narrowed. **B.** Diffuse disc swelling with pallid edema of the nerve fiber layer. Veins are slightly engorged. **C.** Massive disc swelling with hemorrhages and microinfarcts. **D.** Milky disc infarct without hemorrhages, extending into the retina in the distribution of the cilioretinal artery (*arrows*). The other eye was *simultaneously* involved, with similar fundus appearance. The patient had vision of hand movement in both eyes, erythrocyte sedimentation rate, 123 mm/hour, and a painful temporal artery. **E.** Acute infarction of the disc. Note subretinal hemorrhage at the nasal margin (*arrows*). **F.** Fundus in **E** 2 months later. The disc is atrophic, and the arteries are strikingly narrowed. The subretinal blood is incompletely resorbed.

of intracranial frontal fossa masses with raised intracranial pressure.

Although the precise roles of diabetes and hypertension are not known, certainly the prevalence of these systemic disorders is significantly greater in patients with ION than in comparable age-matched groups[268,269]; as noted, correlations with these systemic risk factors seem to be greater in patients less than 45 years old. Likewise, the association of cerebral and cardiac vascular disease seems to be circumstantial, and that simple ION, uncomplicated by chronic diabetes or hypertension, may be taken for a harbinger of future vascular events is moot. Although ipsilateral carotid disease does not seem to be a risk factor for ION,[288] analysis of MRI of the brain in a small series of patients with ION (8 of 13 with hypertension) suggests an increased number (mean, 4.0 vs. 1.4 in age-matched controls) of ischemic white matter lesions.[289] Giuffre[290] reported that serum cholesterol, triglycerides, and glucose are elevated in ION, and other investigators have found a correlation of elevated concentrations of immunoglobulin G anticardiolipin antibody in patients with arteritic ION, but not in common ION.[291] Various coagulopathic states have been implicated, including activated protein C resistance, as well as antithrombin III and antiphospholipid antibody syndromes.[292] Smoking, elevated cholesterol, and serum fibrinogen >3.6 g/l are also risk factors.[293]

A series of funduscopic analyses addressed the question of the cup-to-disc ratio as a possible morphologic factor in the pathogenesis of common ION, culminating in the article by Beck and associates.[294] By observing the disc appearance of the normal fellow eyes of patients with ION, it is apparent that the optic cup is small or absent at a significant rate in common ION (but not in *arteritic* ION). Furthermore, one study[295] suggested that both the horizontal disc diameter and disc area are smaller in fellow eyes with ION than in controls ($p<.05$), and there is evidence[296] of a modest protective role of myopia versus hyperopia. Possibly, ischemic axons in the "crowded" setting of a small scleral canal are predisposed to infarction. However, because patients with common ION may have variably sized contralateral physiologic cups, and patients with arteritic ION may show contralateral cupless discs, no strong diagnostic distinction should be placed on the state of fellow eye cup-to-disc ratio.

No medical therapies have proved to be effective in restoring vision in acute ION, although systemic corticosteroid usage could theoretically reduce the focal impact of edema and free radical production; therefore, short-term therapeutic trials are not unreasonable. The untoward effects of corticosteroids on diabetes, hypertension, intraocular tension, and general well-being must be taken into account. Hyperbaric oxygen is considered ineffective,[297] and levodopa/carbidopa[298] is under investigation. Regarding aspirin (ASA), in a retrospective study of 431 patients[299] (153 treated with ASA), the 2-year cumulative probability of ION in second eye was 7% in the ASA-treated group and 15% in the untreated; 5-year cumulative rates were 17% and 20%, respectively, thereby suggesting at least a short-term advantage, but the total 5-year cumulative risk of only 19% in this study seems lower than most reported incidences of fellow eye occurrence. Kupersmith et al[300] suggest that ASA taken two or more times per week decreases the risk of second eye involvement, regardless of other risk factors.

As noted, spontaneous significant recovery of vision after ION indeed occurs. Movsas and associates[271] documented that, of 116 eyes with acuity of 20/60 or worse, 21% improved by 3 or more lines, and of 126 eyes with acuity better than 20/60, 23% improved by 3 or more lines. In a small series,[273] 5 of 21 eyes improved acuity, even from 10/400 to 20/30.

Optic nerve sheath fenestration for drainage of perineural subarachnoid CSF has been systematically investigated by the Ischemic Optic Neuropathy Decompression Trial[301] in a large series of patients with both progressive and stable common (non-arteritic) ION: whereas visual function worsened spontaneously in 12% of 125 eyes, vision worsened in 24% of 119 eyes subjected to decompressive surgery. These results were in keeping with the poor surgical outcomes in the University of Miami study[302] of 47 eyes, and Indiana University study[303] of 18 operated eyes; indeed, in the latter series, 23 of 71 eyes without surgery had increased acuity of 2 or more optotype lines.

Although intense interest in therapies for common ION continues, the actual incidence of this disorder is imprecise. Two limited surveys suggest an age-adjusted annual incidence in the white population 50 years old and older of 2.77[304] and 10.2[267] per 100,000 individuals; by extrapolation, it is estimated that 5700 new cases would occur each year in the white population of the United States. Tobacco usage has also been implicated[305] in ION, especially in the slightly younger subset of patients. After onset of common ION, patients with both hypertension and diabetes show higher rates of subsequent cerebrovascular disease.

Cranial (Giant Cell) Arteritis

The most common vasculitis responsible for neuro-ophthalmologic symptoms and signs is cranial arteritis, and the frequent presentation is a usually severe form of ION, occurring in a slightly older age group than *common* ION, and usually with devastating visual loss (Table 5–12). Even a *tentative diagnosis* must be treated as a true *ophthalmologic emergency*. Arteritis may result in a *retro-bulbar* form of nerve infarction in about 7% of patients with ocular symptoms, according to Hayreh et al,[306] or it may produce a picture of central or branch retinal artery occlusion (about 14%); these authors also

TABLE 5–12. Ischemic Optical Neuropathy

	Common: arteriosclerotic	Cranial arteritis
Age peak	60–65 yr	70–80 yr
Visual dysfunction	Minimal-severe	Usually severe
Second eye*	≈40%	≈75%
Fundus, acute	Swollen disc, often segmental	Swollen, normal disc, or central artery occlusion
Systemic manifestations	Hypertension ≈50%	Malaise, weight loss, fever, polymyalgia, head pain
ESR (mm/h)	≤40	Usually high (50–120)
Response to steroids	None	Systemic symptoms +; return of vision ±

* Stimultaneous bilateral visual loss is highly suggestive of arteritis and practically excludes common type. Acute massive blood loss with hypotension may produce bilateral nerve infarction.

noted an appreciable incidence of fleeting premonitory visual symptoms (31%), similar to amaurosis fugax from carotid atheromatous emboli. Such episodes may be precipitated by changes from the supine to upright head position and suggest impending nerve infarction; bed rest with lowering of the head to flat or dependent levels is an important maneuver, of course, along with hospitalization for intensive corticosteroid therapy (see below).

Few cases of biopsy-proved CA occur in patients younger than age 50 years, and instances of "juvenile temporal arteritis" represent focal and benign lesions limited to branches of the external carotid artery,[307] without the systemic implications of CA in the aging population. The precise origin of CA is not clear, but reports of presence in first-degree relatives, a distinct predilection for occurrence in whites, and an association with HLA-DR1 all suggest a genetic link.[308] Apparently, in response to antigens residing in arterial walls, helper T lymphocytes infiltrate and proliferate *in situ,* and interferon gamma produced by T cells is the key cytokine in the inflammatory cascade, including macrophage activation.[309]

In the population age 50 years or older, annual *incidence* rates for CA are estimated at as high as 15 to 30/100,000[310]; age-specific *prevalence* rate between ages 60 and 69 years is 33/100,000, and more than age 80 years, 844/100,000.[311] Most large series report a female-to-male preponderance of about 3 to 4:1, and this disorder is most prevalent in the white population of European origin.

The nosologic relationship of CA (temporal or giant cell) with *polymyalgia rheumatica* (PMR) is unsettled, although differences are more quantitative than qualitative, with the important exception of the perceived risk of visual loss, varying widely in the literature between 6% and 70%.[306] Certainly, both syndromes share clinical features, laboratory abnormalities, arterial histopathologic features, and potential for serious adverse outcomes.[312] Perhaps CA and PMR represent a spectrum

of the same basic disease, but patients with simple PMR seem successfully managed without the high-dose steroid therapy usually justified in instances of CA, in which blindness is considered more likely. Interestingly, Turnbull[312] suggested that the yearly incidence of both CA and PMR has increased because of diagnostic awareness, but that the incidence of severe visual loss has decreased (for the same reason), resulting in a spurious amelioration of disease severity.

Visual loss with arteritic ION tends to be more profound than with common ION[313]; levels of finger-counting to no perception of light are not uncommon. At times, the optic disc is characterized by a milk-pale edema that may extend into the retina,[306] some considerable distance away from the optic nerve (see Fig. 5–37D and Color Plate 5–3D), and central retinal artery occlusion with "cherry-red spot" also occurs. As mentioned, bilateral simultaneous ION is suggestive of CA, and both therapy and laboratory investigations are bent toward that diagnosis. In 50 cases of arteritic ION,[314] 19 of the 20 patients who had *bilateral* vision loss had both eyes involved by the time of initial visits; in the Iowa series,[306] of 27 patients with *bilateral* loss, 17% were simultaneous, and second eye loss was delayed 1 to 7 days in 46%, 8 to 14 days in 8%, 15 to 30 days in 8%, and more than 6 months in 8%. Therefore, when second eye infarction occurs in CA, it usually does so within days to weeks, longer intervals being exceptional. The general prognostic value of this point bears emphasis: if the second eye is not yet involved, and patients are under adequate systemic corticosteroid therapy, the likelihood of bilateral visual loss becomes more remote (though not assured) with each passing week.

Other signs of orbital hypoxia include evidence of anterior segment ischemia: hyperemia of the conjunctival and episcleral vessels, mild-to-moderate corneal edema, lowered intraocular tension, anterior chamber cellular reaction, iris rubeosis, and rapidly progressive cataract. Irregular streaks and patches of chorioretinal pigmentary disturbances secondary to *choroidal isch-*

emia may appear weeks after visual loss (see Color Plate 5–3E), and considerable disc cupping may rapidly ensue, at times mimicking extensive cupping of glaucoma.[306,315] Mild visual symptoms associated with punctate retinal infarcts ("cotton-wool spots") may herald the onset of ocular ischemia,[316] and in a series of seven such cases (six biopsy-positive), the authors concluded that prompt corticosteroid therapy led to preservation of vision in all. Diplopia is infrequent, less than 6% in the Iowa series,[306] probably reflecting diffuse ischemia of extraocular muscles,[317] but preceding symptomatic ophthalmoplegia of any degree may be obscured by the more dramatic occurrence of severe visual loss.

Ocular pneumotonography, which measures the ocular pulsation induced by perfusion pressure in choroidal (posterior ciliary) and ophthalmic arteries, has been used[318] to distinguish common ION from arteritic ION. In patients with arteritic ION, ocular pulse amplitude was only 4% of pulse amplitude of patients with arteritis *but without ION* and only 6% of pulse amplitude of patients with *non-arteritic ION*. Moreover, half the patients with arteritic ION showed pulsation loss in the non-infarcted contralateral eye. Return of pulse amplitudes to a normal range can occur rapidly with systemic corticosteroid therapy, although in some cases the pulse does not revert to normal levels. Bosley and associates[319] suggested that ocular pneumoplethysmography, measuring ocular pulse amplitude that reflects the volume changes in the globe with each cardiac cycle, provides a diagnostic accuracy of 94% for CA, rivaling the accuracy of ESR determination or even of temporal artery biopsy.

Fluorescein fundus angiography has proved helpful in distinguishing between the common and arteritic forms of ION. Siatkowski et al[320] demonstrated that delayed retinal arterial appearance of dye beyond 15 seconds after arm injection, or without full choroidal dye filling (*i.e.,* choroidal *non-perfusion*) by 18 seconds (Fig. 5–38), is highly suggestive of the diffuse orbital and choroidal circulation involvement associated with arteritic, but not with common ION, in which mean retinal arterial appearance time was 11.29 seconds, and mean choroidal filling time was 12.9 seconds. Slavin et al[321] reported visual loss in three patients caused by choroidal ischemia, established by fluorescein angiography, preceding anterior ION in giant cell arteritis. Color Doppler ultrasound hemodynamics are also demonstrably altered in CA, including reduced central retinal and short posterior ciliary artery mean flow velocities and increased vascular resistance values.[322] Most recently, color duplex ultrasonography of temporal arteries demonstrated a typical hypoechoic dark halo around the perfused lumen of stenotic or thrombosed temporal arteries; this halo was said to be reversible following corticosteroid therapy.[323] These adjunctive clinical studies are especially helpful when systemic signs and symptoms are minimal or absent and the ESR is non-pathologic, when CA is occult or atypical.

Other ophthalmic manifestations of CA include the following[310]: anterior segment ischemia with corneal

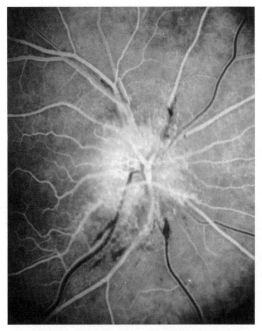
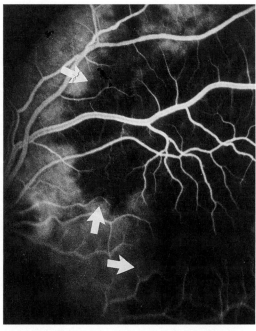

Fig. 5–38. Fluorescein angiography in ischemic optic neuropathy (ION). **Left.** Common ION; at 16 seconds, arteriovenous phase shows telangiectasia of disc capillaries and normal choroidal background fluorescence. **Right.** Arteritis ION; even by 34 seconds, note dark, non-perfused choroid (*arrows*).

edema, aqueous cells and protein flare, hypotony, and rapidly advancing cataract; retinal central and branch artery occlusion, retinal infarcts ("cotton-wool spots" or "cherry-red spot"), choroidal infarcts; orbital cellulitis and facial swelling. Rare instances of *posterior* ION in arteritis, with infarction occurring in retro-laminar portions of the optic nerve,[306,310] show no fundus abnormalities during the acute phase. This clinical possibility is always a *diagnosis of exclusion,* and a search for nonvascular causes must be conducted, including exquisite neuroimages of the anterior visual pathways and cranial meninges, for example.

It is critical to discover, when possible, instances of ION due to CA because prompt steroid therapy may be effective in restoring some degree of vision (see below), averting similar visual deficit in the other eye, and potentially improving long-term systemic morbidity and mortality, although several analyses showed no statistically significant effect of arteritis on survivorship rates.[312,324] Patients with CA/PMR may complain of weakness, weight loss, and fever. Myalgia of the large muscle masses of the shoulders, neck, thighs, and buttocks is variable, and, indeed, these symptoms constitute PMR (previously believed to represent a variant of *rheumatoid arthritis,* but more properly termed *polymyalgia arteritica,* as in some Scandinavian countries). PMR and CA are best viewed as facets of a common disease spectrum with variable risk outcome, with PMR often responding to lower doses of steroids, whereas fear of blindness dictates the use of higher doses in CA.[312] Other common complaints include chronic suboccipital headache (frequently mistakenly attributed to cervical osteoarthritis, so common in this age group), and pain or tenderness of the scalp of the forehead or temples. A palpable, often non-pulsatile, temporal artery should be sought as a likely biopsy site.

Pain in the jaw muscles precipitated by eating or talking (masseter or jaw "claudication") is apparently an extraordinarily specific symptom, noted in 55% of patients with visual loss in the Mayo series[325] and 53% in the Bascom Palmer series.[326] Remarkably, according to the Iowa study[327] of 363 patients undergoing temporal artery biopsy, the odds of a positive biopsy are increased by 9-fold in the presence of *jaw claudication,* by 3.4 times with neck pain, by 3.2 times with C-reactive protein (CRP) levels greater than 2.45 mg/dl, and only by a factor of 2 for elevated ESR of 47 mm to 107 mm per hour. To reiterate, jaw, tongue, and swallowing claudication are highly specific and sensitive symptoms of CA.

The Westergren ESR has been considered the most consistently helpful laboratory test in the confirmation of the diagnosis of arteritis. Cullen,[328] in comparing arteritic versus "arteriosclerotic" (common, idiopathic) ION, found only 3 of 19 patients in the latter group with ESR greater than 30 mm per hour (mean, 26 mm), whereas only 3 of 25 patients with biopsy-positive arteri-

tis had ESRs of 50 mm and less (mean, 84 mm; 70 mm or more in 80%). In the Iowa study[327] mean ESR was 84.9±33.4 mm per hour (range, 4 mm to 140 mm) in 106 biopsy-positive patients, and 14±10.7 (range, 1 to 59) in age-matched controls; CRP mean was 6.6±6.7 mg/dl (range, 0.5 to 34.7) in biopsy-positive, and <0.5±0.5 (range, <0.5 to 3.3) in controls.

It is clear that ESR increases with age and is "elevated" (*i.e.,* greater than 20 mm/hour) in apparently healthy elderly subjects. Miller and Green[329] provide the following rule for calculation of the maximum normal ESR at a given age: in men, (age in years)/2; in women, (age in years plus 10)/2. We agree with the aforementioned authors and personally use 35 mm to 40 mm/hour (Westergren) as the upper limit of normal for the ESR in the elderly. Hayreh et al[327] contribute data that suggest cutoff criteria of 33 mm/hour in men and 35 in women, providing a sensitivity of 92% and specificity of 92%. The ESR reflects red cell aggregation, which is fostered by plasma fibrinogen or globulins ("acute-phase reactants" of inflammatory or infectious states), and may be elevated in diabetes, nephrotic syndrome, connective tissue disorders, and neoplasm.[330]

As noted above, CRP may be more specific. From the Iowa study,[327] it is clear that CRP is elevated along with ESR in patients with CA, but not in control subjects with elevated ESR. The specificity and sensitivity of CRP in detecting CA were 100% and 83% in men and 100% and 79% in women, respectively. The authors therefore found CRP to be highly useful for both diagnosis and for monitoring therapy.

The affirmation provided by a positive artery biopsy is obviously helpful when instituting long-term corticosteroid therapy in an elderly patient. However, Klein and associates established the presence of "skip lesions" in temporal artery biopsies from patients with unequivocal CA.[331] They also pointed out that a temporal artery that is normal to palpation may show histologic signs of inflammation and that patients with "skip lesions" do not have a more benign form of the disease. Biopsy is usually performed on a frontal branch of the superficial temporal artery ipsilateral to head pain or visual loss, and the specimen should be of maximal length; *bilateral* biopsies increase the diagnostic yield.[310] Given the implications of long-term therapy, multiple biopsies may be considered, especially in the "occult" form of CA, with no systemic signs or symptoms and normal or minimally elevated ESR; Hayreh et al[306] estimated this *occult* variant to represent some 20% of cases of giant cell arteritis. With the phenomenon of skip lesions in mind, a negative biopsy does not militate strongly against a diagnosis of arteritis. Therefore, it may be argued that arterial biopsy is often superfluous because diagnosis or treatment is not altered by the results, especially in the full-blown case of CA accompanied by significant ESR elevation, with or without symptoms of PMR. Other typically involved sites may be considered for biopsy, such as the suboccipital arteries. Wegener's granulomatosis is reported rarely to show temporal vasculitis,[332] and focal non-caseating granuloma of sarcoid is documented.[333]

In the appropriately aged patient with systemic or cranial signs or symptoms, and normal or (usually) elevated ESR, systemic corticosteroid therapy (*e.g.,* oral prednisone 80 to 100 mg/day, or intravenous methyl-prednisolone 250 mg every 6 hours) should be instituted immediately on presumed diagnosis. To reiterate: *When arteritis is suspected, therapy should not be delayed for results of ESR, other laboratory investigations or biopsy.* Although reversal of visual loss is not predictable, the general symptomatic response to steroids may be dramatic within 24 hours, with relief of headache, myalgias, and malaise.

No precise information may be deduced regarding the risk of visual loss in CA/PMR, with values ranging from as little as 7% to as high as 60% (average 36%), and rates of simultaneous or consecutive bilaterality loss from one-third to three-fourths.[325,326,334] ION is the single most frequent clinical presentation, reflecting the predilection for diffuse inflammation of orbital arteries, and especially of posterior ciliary circulation.[335] Although recovery of vision is considered rare, sanguine outcomes are substantiated,[310,325,326,334] some examples being the following: from finger-counting and 20/400–100 levels, to as good as 20/25–40 following steroid therapy; these recovery rates range from 15% to 34%, with some support for intensive intravenous therapy as opposed to smaller oral dosage schedules.[326] On the other hand, unfortunately some visual deteroration may continue while patients are receiving apparently adequate therapeutic doses.[336] It is difficult to be more (or less) dogmatic about route of administration or level of steroid dosage, no strictly controlled trials being yet available. In the elderly patient, however, hospitalization is justifiable, especially to monitor the untoward effects of large steroid doses on blood glucose, serum potassium, and blood pressure and to maintain a lowered head position. Most patients experience greater or lesser side effects of steroid medication and, indeed, sudden death, cardiac arrhythmia, and anaphylaxis are reported.[337]

Prolonged therapy should be dictated by symptomatic response to steroids and anticipated depression of the ESR. It is suggested that high oral dosage be maintained for approximately 4 to 8 weeks, then tapered so long as the patient remains symptom free and the ESR is less than 40 mm per hour (see above). Complications of prolonged steroid usage are well known and include gastric ulcers, hyperglycemia, osteoporosis, hypoadrenalism, and recrudescence of tuberculosis. Corticosteroids in this age group can produce severe and rapid myopathy, including proximal muscle weakness and myalgia, which may be mistakenly construed as continuing or worsening symptoms of PMR, paradoxically sug-

gesting that dosage should be increased. Again, after initial presentation and commencement of therapy, it should be recalled that the risk of delayed visual loss,[306] or benefit to general well-being, may be overestimated.[312] In most patients, about 88%,[338] the disease is clinically inactive at a mean follow-up of more than 7 years.

Biopsy specimens of temporal arteries from patients with CA/PMR with ongoing or recurrent manifestations may show pathologic changes regardless of steroid dosage or duration; that is, biopsy positivity rate is not directly related to prior therapy, the resolution of vessel inflammation being governed by incompletely understood factors. As an alternative to corticosteroid therapy, or when side effects are intolerable, methotrexate (7.5 to 20.0 mg/week) is of limited effect, as are other immunosuppressive agents.[310] In a randomized, double-blind study,[339] patients begun on prednisone and then randomized to receive methotrexate or placebo showed no effect on remissions or relapses; that is, there was no demonstrable steroid-sparing effect of weekly methotrexate. Dapsone has been suggested, but with considerable side effects, including agranulocytosis.[340]

Diabetes Mellitus Papillopathy

It is currently unclear whether a direct relationship exists between diabetes and acquired optic neuropathies, other than as an apparent risk factor for common ION, especially in the slightly younger age group. As previously discussed (see above), a genetically determined progressive optic atrophy may be associated with juvenile diabetes (Wolfram's syndrome), but the incidence in diabetes of inflammatory retro-bulbar neuritis or papillitis is probably no higher than in the non-diabetic population. Skillern and Lockhart[341] collected 14 cases of "optic neuritis" in patients with poorly controlled diabetes. Apparently, slowly progressive loss of vision was a common symptom (as opposed to the frequently apoplectic onset of ION), and visual fields showed central scotomas or peripheral contraction. No mention was made of altitudinal defects, and only 2 patients demonstrated diabetic retinopathy. Of greater importance is the report by Lubow and Makley[342] of teenage patients with long-standing juvenile diabetes who presented with hemorrhagic swelling of one or both optic discs, mimicking papilledema of increased intracranial pressure (Fig. 5–39 and Color Plate 5–3G).

Barr et al[343] reported a series of 21 eyes in 12 patients with juvenile diabetes and outlined a clinical profile consisting of symptoms of slightly blurred vision, minimal acuity and field deficits, general salutary outcome, and no consistent correlation with clinical control of hyperglycemia; diabetic retinopathy is usually of modest degree, and prognosis for proliferative retinopathy is uncertain. Neurodiagnostic studies are not indicated,

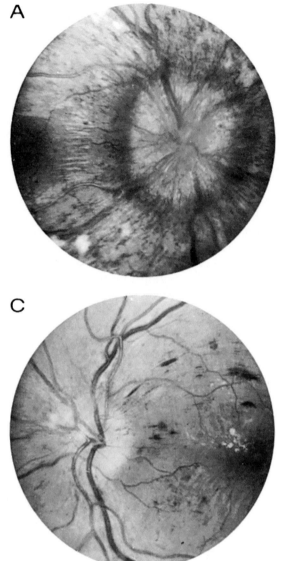

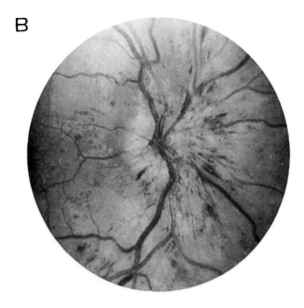

Fig. 5–39. Papillopathy in diabetes. **A.** Florid hemorrhagic disc swelling, vision 20/25 (6/7.5), found during routine examination of a 16-year-old girl with a 9-year history of diabetes. Spontaneous regression occurred. Right **(B)** and left **(C)** discs of a 16-year-old who had had diabetes since the age of 3 years. Vision was normal.

and corticosteroid administration upsets diabetic control without providing any known therapeutic effect. A study[344] of 27 eyes in 19 diabetic patients showed an age range of 17 to 79 years (mean, 50 years), two-thirds of patients with type II diabetes, disc swelling resolving slowly (average, 3.7 months), macular edema in 70% of eyes, with only 4 eyes with final acuity less than 20/50 (these all with prominent macular edema); acute visual fields showed enlarged blind spots or general depression, but not altitudinal defects. Widespread retinal capillary non-perfusion was found in 52% of eyes studied with fluorescein angiography, yet with a conspicuous lack of progressive diabetic retinopathy.

The transient nature, frequent bilaterality, benign outcome, and low incidence of subsequent disc atrophy are all features that leave unanswered the question of precise pathophysiology, despite evidence of retinal hypoperfusion. Although likely related to hypoxia of the pre-papillary capillaries or unidentified metabolic substances, "diabetic papillopathy" enjoys a much better visual prognosis than do most other types of ION. This form of bilateral disc edema, with normal acuity and minimal field change, may be confused with papilledema of raised intracranial pressure, however.

Infrequently Associated Conditions

In 1973, Carroll originally called attention to a form of ischemic optic papillopathy occurring after uncomplicated *cataract extraction,* with sudden visual loss from 4 weeks to 15 months postoperatively.[345] In Carroll's series, about half the patients with initial eye affected had visual loss following operation on the second eye; three patients were in their fifties, and the disc infarction occurred with either retro-bulbar or general anesthesia; no patient experienced a loss of vision in a second eye unless subjected to cataract extraction; neither corticosteroids nor anticoagulants are effective therapies.

Sufficient data fail to incriminate simple postoperative rise in ocular tension, although discs with marginal perfusion could be vulnerable. Hayreh's suggestion of lowering ocular tension when second eyes are at risk seems reasonable.[346] This subtype of optic neuropathy following cataract extraction represents a distinct variant characterized by a circumscribed onset time course and high incidence of consecutive bilaterality, to the point of predictability, when the second eye is operated on (even in the fifth and sixth decades).[347]

Acute disc edema with visual loss, in patients not yet old enough to be included in what may comfortably be called the "vasculopathic" age group, and without compelling risk factors of diabetes or severe hypertension, falls into categories in which *collagen vascular or autoimmune arteritis* are suspected (see below) or in which inflammatory neuritis may not be ruled out clinically. This rare, idiopathic ION of the "young" tends to be bilateral and recurrent.[348] The question of retinal arterial vasospasm or thrombophilic states is unanswered, and, indeed, both unilateral and sequential bilateral disc infarctions have been reported in *migraine*[349,350] and during cluster headache.[351] On the other hand, migraine is an extremely common disorder, and any association with optic neuropathies may be fortuitous.

Other varieties of ischemic disc swelling occur following marked or recurrent *blood loss*,[352] most frequently from the gastrointestinal tract, but with visual symptoms peculiarly delayed by days to weeks. Williams et al[353] provided a complete overview (for anesthesiologists) of the subject of visual loss following *non-ophthalmic* surgical procedures. These intraoperative or postoperative visual events occurred in 77 cases culled from the literature, of which 27 were related to occipital cortical strokes, in 22 instances following cardiopulmonary bypass (CPB) or cardiac valve surgery. Anterior ION occurred in 19 cases, 14 of which followed CPB; posterior ION occurred in 17 cases, 4 following CPB, 5 after neck dissections; other procedures followed by anterior or posterior ION included rhinoplasty, sinus surgery, abdominal and thoracic resections, and other common procedures. Likewise, ION has occurred after lengthy spinal procedures without evidence of intra-operative globe compression related to head support in the prone position (the "head-rest syndrome" of Hollenhorst,[354] originally described in neurosurgical procedures), but instead attributed to prolonged anesthesia, deliberate or incidental hypotension, and relative anemia due to blood loss.[355] In my experience, prolonged globe compression produces variable degrees of *choroidal infarction,* which eventually causes widespread reaction of pigment epithelium distinguishable by funduscopy from optic nerve ischemia alone. Delayed and, at times, progressive ION may follow CPB or other general surgical procedures in which continuous postoperative red blood cell destruction decrementally drops hemoglobin levels[356]; visual loss has been reversed apparently by blood replacement.

Frequently enough, *both* eyes are involved, and bilateral *retro-bulbar infarcts* with mild disc edema have been documented histologically.[357] Risk factors apparently include systemic hypertension, diabetes, coronary artery disease, pre-existing anemia, and occasionally renal failure with uremia. In three cases of acute *non-surgical* hypotensive episodes, including unduly rapid correction of malignant hypertension, and during renal dialysis, five eyes had anterior ION with partial recovery on immediate reversal of hypotension; pre-existing anemia was present (hematocrit range of 23% to 28%).[358] Prolonged CPB and low perioperative hematocrits[359] during open heart surgery are well-documented causes of ION. Cardiac arrest has also precipitated ION.[360] *One may conclude that intraoperative hypotension, usually coupled with low hematocrit, is the single most common cause of genuine posterior ION.*

Knox and associates[361] reported a variety of *uremic* optic neuropathy characterized by bilateral visual loss with disc swelling in patients with severe renal disease manifested by uremia, anemia, and hypertension. Improvement followed hemodialysis, except in one case of actual cryptococcal meningitis. However, Hamed and associates[362] contended that "uremic optic neuropathy" does not constitute a single pathophysiologic entity, but rather a heterogeneity of pathophysiologic processes that include complications of raised CSF pressure, severe consecutive anterior ION, and adverse reaction to hemodialysis itself. Bilateral ION was reported in a young woman with optic disc drusen and chronic hypotension while she was undergoing renal dialysis.[363] These risk factors, that is, pre-existing hypertension, anemia, and uremia, taken collectively likely interfere with vital autoregulation of arterial perfusion at the disc or retrobulbar nerve in ways not yet completely understood.

Carotid artery disease does not seem to play any regular role in ION; in fact, retinal arterial embolization and ION are mutually exclusive findings, except in the rarest of situations. Waybright and associates[364] documented 3 instances of typical ION with ipsilateral carotid occlusions, with retrograde filling of the ophthalmic artery by external carotid branches, perhaps indicating hypoperfusion of the nerve head, and Brown[365] reported a single case of abrupt visual loss at first with a normal disc, then with pale edema, in an eye with chronic hypoxia from complete carotid occlusion. From a series of 612 patients with acute ischemic hemispheric strokes resulting from internal carotid occlusions with "reversed flow in the ophthalmic artery," only 3 cases of simultaneous optic nerve infarction were uncovered.[366] Pulseless disease (Takayasu's disease) has been complicated by ION.[367,368] In addition, in a patient with atrial fibrillation,[369] emboli were found in the posterior ciliary arteries at autopsy, and Tomsak[370] recorded 3 patients with ION accompanied by retinal emboli, following coronary artery bypass surgery and cardiac catheterization.

Acute disc swelling attributed to ION has occurred in eclampsia,[371] porphyria,[372] and pseudoxanthoma elasticum with platelet hyperaggregability.[373] Sickle cell disease is reported rarely to cause anterior[374] and posterior ION,[375] in single case documentations.

Although cranial (giant cell) arteritis is clearly the most commonly encountered vasculitis of neuro-ophthalmic importance, other arteritides do involve the anterior pathways with some regularity, with disc swelling, retro-bulbar neuropathy, or chiasmal inflammation. MRI of vasculitis-induced retro-bulbar ischemia in *lupus arteritis, rheumatoid arthritis,* and *Sjögren's syndrome* has demonstrated[376] enlargement and gadolinium enhancement of orbital and prechiasmal segments of optic nerves, and especially of the chiasm (Fig. 5–40). Childhood lupus is reported as a cause of bilateral, simultaneous optic neuropathy.[377] When lupus is suspected, assay of antinuclear antibody and anti–double-stranded DNA antibody titers are diagnostic clues, and there is evidence that antiphospholipid antibodies are associated with neurologic and ophthalmic complications of lupus.[378] In addition, Sjögren's syndrome is recognized as an autoimmune-mediated cause of dysfunction of salivary gland (xerostomia) and lacrimal gland (xerophthalmia), and rarely with extraglandular manifestations, including optic neuropathy and CNS disease.[379] Primary Sjögren's syndrome is characterized by female preponderance, pulmonary fibrosis, glomerulonephritis, thyroiditis, presence of high titers of antinuclear antibody, anti-SSA(Ro), and anti-SSB(La); this disorder should be distinguished from MS, lupus, and antiphospholipid syndrome, for which labial salivary gland biopsy is essential. Otherwise, polyarteritis nodosa[380] and relapsing polychondritis[381] are rare vasculitic causes of ION, as is Takayasu's arteritis[378,382] (see also the discussion in Chapter 5, Part II on retinal arterial occlusions).

As ION with disc swelling (*i.e., anterior*) does not constitute a single nosologic disorder, neither does retro-bulbar (*i.e., posterior*) optic nerve ischemia connote a distinctive origin, but it represents a rare consequence of various diseases. This "posterior" ION variant consists of abrupt unilateral, rarely bilateral, visual loss without disc edema; other compressive, inflammatory, toxic, traumatic, or infiltrative causes must be rigorously excluded. Isayama and associates[383] reported 14 patients with posterior ION, aged 20 to 73 years (6 less than 54 years), with hypertension, diabetes, and infrequent carotid stenosis, and also documented is an instance of acute internal artery occlusion.[384]

When other specific mechanisms of ischemic damage to the retro-bulbar optic nerves are evident, for example, as a delayed complication of radiation therapy, the term posterior ION may be only loosely applied, although no doubt vasculitic ischemia plays a role. In those subsets of ION in which a degree of inflammation is implicated, the use of systemic corticosteroid therapy seems reasonable.

GLAUCOMA AND PSEUDOGLAUCOMA

Although admittedly glaucoma is not an appropriate topic for extensive coverage here, nor is this rubric even a single entity, certain salient points bear emphasis in neuro-ophthalmologic context. In general, the diagnosis of glaucoma is usually made on the classic triad of characteristic *patterns of visual field defects,* typical morphologic *loss of optic disc substance* ("cupping"), at times in association with focal changes of peripapillary pigment epithelium, and *variable elevation of intraocular tension,* although not in itself a requisite for diagnosis. Pathophysiologic mechanisms aside, at times this common ophthalmologic diagnosis may prove elusive when field defects are atypical, disc substance loss is minimal, and intraocular pressure is not recorded in an abnormal range or when there are dissociations among the key criteria. Susceptibility to nerve damage varies greatly, and one-sixth to one-half of patients with glaucoma have initial pressure readings of less than 21 mmHg,[385] nor does intraocular tension reliably predict disc damage. The development of reproducible glaucomatous field loss is characteristic of advanced, not early, glaucoma; in early stages, optic nerve head *morphology* is a more sensitive marker of disease, and in later stages, perimetry is a more sensitive technique to monitor damage.[386] As a rule, the hallmark features of glaucomatous damage are loss in the dense superior and inferior arcuate retinal nerve fiber bundles and prolonged sparing of the central papillomacular area that subserves acuity. Therefore, with field loss in the centrocecal area, that is, the papillomacular bundle, a "neurologic lesion" may be suspected. Indeed, disc cupping may further compound the diagnostic confusion,[282] for example, from chronic compression of the optic nerve by tumor or aneurysm.[387] Greenfield et al[388] compared the optic discs of 52 eyes with glaucoma and the discs of 28 patients with compressive lesions of the anterior visual pathways and concluded that corrected acuity less than 20/40 was 77% specific for *non-glaucomatous cupping,* and eyes with glaucoma had significantly less neuroretinal rim pallor, that is, pallor of the remaining disc tissue militated strongly *against* glaucoma; in glaucoma, there was greater tissue loss in the vertical axis of the cup and higher frequency of peripapillary pigment epithelial atrophy, more frequent disc edge hemorrhages (isolated small flame or punctate hemorrhage without disc edema,

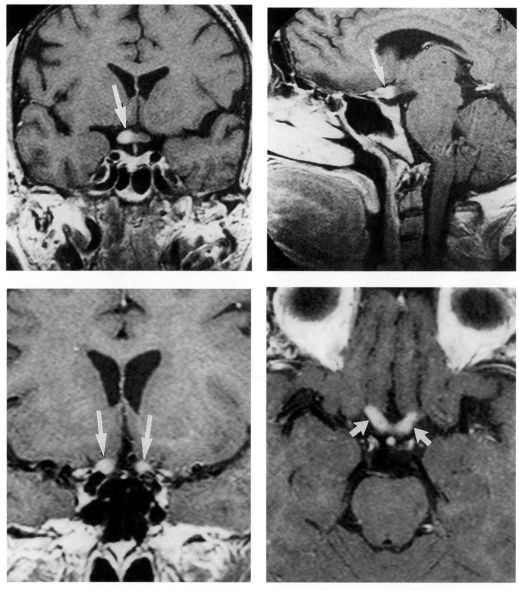

Fig. 5–40. Vasculitis-induced optic neuropathies: magnetic resonance T1-weighted imaging with gadolinium enhancement. **Top.** A 54-year-old woman with rheumatoid arthritis and no light perception in the right eye. *Left,* coronal and *right,* sagittal sections show enlargement and contrast enhancement of the right optic nerve *(arrow).* **Bottom.** A 62-year-old woman with Sjögren's disease and visual loss. *Left,* coronal and *right,* axial sections, show contrast enhancement of both optic nerves. (From ref. 376)

the so-called "Drance" hemorrhage, associated with field defect increase[389]), and age greater than 50 years. However, simple glaucoma occasionally does produce cecocentral field defects and may thus mimic neurologic optic atrophy (Fig. 5–41). Reduction of visual acuity, often unilateral, is encountered in these patients; therefore, the field defects tend to be asymmetric, but accompanying peripheral field defects, especially nasal steps, often serve to distinguish these central field defects from deficits of other chronic optic neuropathies.

Conversely, progressive visual defects may be attributed to "glaucoma" when no such condition exists.

Here, the interpretation of visual field defects is critical, and the judicious use of radiologic studies is mandatory. Greenfield et al[388] found that only 2 of 31 patients diagnosed initially with glaucoma had neuroradiologic evidence of mass lesions, and in both instances other neuro-ophthalmic signs had been overlooked, including optic disc neural rim pallor. Defects that preferentially involve the nasal field, but without a hemianopic character (aligned on the vertical meridian) are most likely due to glaucoma or ION. Bilateral nasal field defects that are truly hemianopic must be extraordinarily rare. Otherwise, binasal defects may be associated with chronic

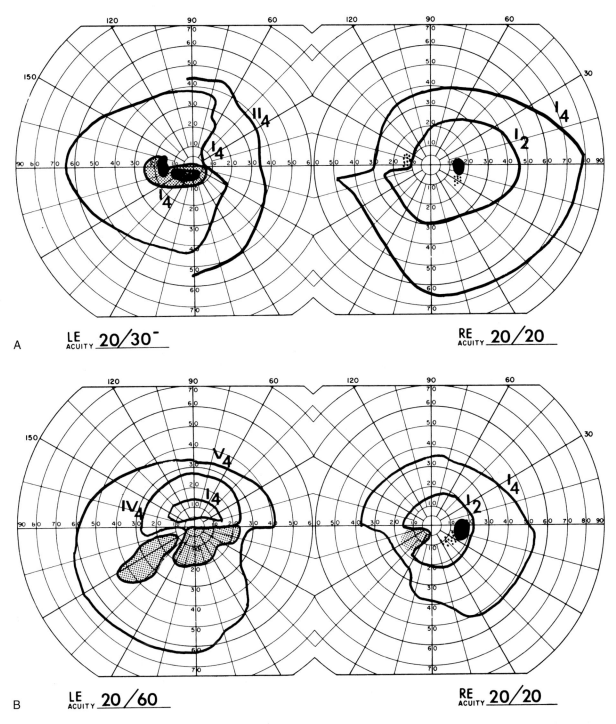

Fig. 5–41. Central defects in glaucoma. **A.** A 62-year-old woman with slowly progressive visual loss in the left eye. Optic canal laminography were negative. Tonographic outflow values were 0.04 and 0.06. Note the centrocecal scotoma of the left eye and bilateral nasal defects. **B.** A 66-year-old man with long-standing reduced vision in left eye, previously diagnosed as amblyopia. Headache and left Gunn's pupil raised the question of a neurologic lesion. Findings were suggestive of glaucomatous discs. Fields show nasal step in the right eye, a central altitudinal nerve fiber bundle, and nasal step in the left eye. Co-efficients of outflow were 0.25 and 0.11. *LE,* left eye; *RE,* right eye.

papilledema or hyaline bodies of the nerve head, either of which should be discernible by ophthalmoscopy.

NEOPLASMS AND RELATED CONDITIONS

Given the diversity of anatomic environments (the globe, orbit, adjacent paranasal sinuses, optic canal, skull base, and prechiasmal subarachnoid space) traversed by the optic nerves in their lengthy course to the chiasm (see Fig. 5–11), a comprehensive spectrum of potential mass lesions may be proposed. These include neoplasms of the nerve itself (gliomas) or its sheaths (meningiomas), or masses arising in contiguous tissues of the orbit, paranasal sinuses, pituitary gland and parasellar structures, and at the base of the middle cranial fossa. In addition, distant malignancies may metastasize to the nerve and its coverings. Saccular and fusiform aneurysms of the internal carotid artery also simulate neoplastic masses, as do basal infiltrative and inflammatory lesions.

Masses of the Optic Disc

These often fascinating lesions provoke controversy related to funduscopic and fluorescein angiographic differential characteristics, but the neuro-ophthalmic dilemma is reduced from "Where?" to "What?" Congenital elevations (pseudopapilledema and hyaline bodies), epipapillary astrocytomas, and acquired disc swelling are discussed previously, to which is added mention of glial and vascular remnants of the primitive embryonic hyaloid system that take the form of thinly curved membranes or gray pearl-like nodules attached to the disc face. Vascular hamartomas include the capillary and cavernous hemangiomas and the racemose malformations of the Wyburn-Mason syndrome (see Chapter 17). Melanocytomas are deeply pigmented disc tumors with limited growth potential, not to be confused with juxtapapillary choroidal melanomas that extend into the disc. Retinoblastomas may also secondarily invade the optic nerve, but with a characteristic fundus appearance.

Metastatic carcinoma, lymphoblastic and myeloblastic leukemic infiltrates, and sarcoid granulomas may present at the disc, usually with severe and sudden loss of vision. Indeed, in general, secondary tumors are more common than all primary optic nerve tumors. Brown and Shields[390] have provided an excellent one-stop monograph, *Tumors of the Optic Nerve Head*.

Optic Gliomas

Primary astrocytic tumors of the anterior visual pathways assume two major clinical forms: the relatively benign gliomas (hamartomas) of childhood and the rare malignant glioblastoma of adulthood. With the exception of visual loss and anatomic location, these two lesions have little in common, and the assumption that the progressive malignant form stems from the static childhood form is untenable. The major clinical characteristics of these tumors are contrasted in Chapter 6.

Optic gliomas represent almost 20% of orbital tumors of childhood and 65% of all intrinsic optic nerve tumors; about 25% of optic gliomas involve the nerve alone, in which case there may be a small female preponderance.[391] It is estimated that as many as 70% of childhood optic pathway gliomas are associated with neurofibromatosis-1 (NF-1), an autosomal dominant disorder, and that such lesions may be uncovered incidentally in this disease.[392] Optic nerve gliomas may also occur sporadically and do occur with neurofibromatosis-2 more rarely. These NF-1 low-grade neoplasms are best termed "pilocytic astrocytoma of the optic pathway" and are essentially indistinguishable from hypothalamic or thalamic diencephalic glioma; invasive and aggressive behavior is rare. The incidence of *symptomatic* optic glioma in NF-1 is 2% to 8%, although neuroimaging studies imply a higher incidence.[392] Typically, most childhood optic gliomas present in the first 6 years, median age being 4.9 years, and some 90% before age 20 years.

With childhood optic glioma, clinical presentation is predicated on location and extent of tumor. Optic gliomas account for only a small percentage of children presenting with proptosis, but they present as insidious proptosis of variable degree, and, although vision is usually diminished, remarkably good visual function is not uncommon.[392] Strabismus, disc pallor, or disc swelling may be observed. Progressive proptosis, even if abrupt, or increased visual deficit does *not* imply aggressive activity of the tumor, hemorrhage, or necrosis. In a patient with such rapid increase in proptosis and concurrent loss of vision, Anderson and Spencer[393] elucidated the following histopathologic features: (1) microcystic areas of tumor are neither necrotic nor degenerated but composed of highly differentiated glial cells; (2) the "microcysts" are extracellular accumulations of periodic acid–Schiff–positive mucosubstance, presumably synthesized by tumor cells; (3) the space around axons is distended by mucosubstance, with a tendency to collect in central areas of the glioma; and (4) the hydrophilic property of mucosubstance may contribute to rapid expansion of the glioma (simulating "growth"), with concurrent loss of visual function or increase in proptosis. Vision may fluctuate, abruptly worsen, or even spontaneously improve.[391]

The optic disc may appear normal, pale, or swollen, and congenital enlargement is described, as well as vein occlusion.[391,394] Approximately 70% of orbital gliomas involve the anterior aspect of the optic canal, best appreciated by bone-window settings on CT or by thin-section MRI (Fig. 5–42). Paradoxically, canal enlarge-

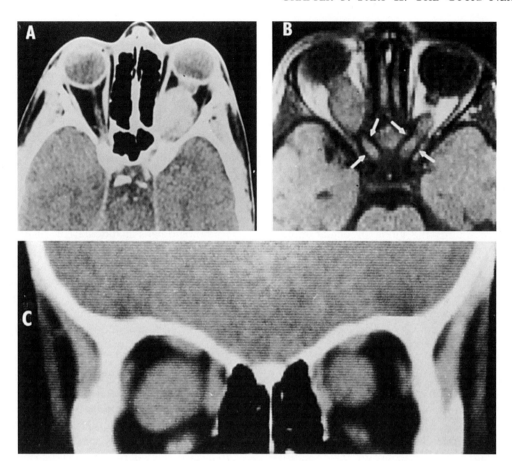

Fig. 5–42. Optic nerve glioma. **A.** Computed tomography (CT) axial section shows smoothly fusiform enlargement of one optic nerve; chronic mass effect has expanded the orbit diameter. **B.** Magnetic resonance T1-weighted axial section; note moderate enlargement of both optic canals (*arrows*). **C.** CT coronal section of bilateral optic nerve gliomas.

ment does not categorically imply gliomatous change in the nerve but may represent arachnoidal proliferation. Regarding the concept of "extension" of orbital gliomas to involve the intracranial visual pathway or aggressive orbital and transcranial surgery to prevent such "extension," the following points must be made: (1) incomplete resection of gliomas leads to no recurrence (although rarely arachnoidal hyperplasia may mimic regrowth of tumor), and such patients do spectacularly well over long periods of observation; (2) incomplete excision is not accompanied by malignant transformation, nor has it ever been documented that childhood gliomas undergo malignant degeneration; (3) documented instances[395] wherein a previously normal optic canal subsequently enlarged must be extremely rare[392] (large canals likely represent congenital bony change in concord with congenital large optic nerve); and (4) subsequent visual symptoms in the opposite eye, or of a chiasmal nature, do not necessarily imply "extension" because many gliomas initially reside in one nerve plus chiasm or chiasm plus both intracranial nerves.

Of course, modern MRI is prerequisite for baseline staging of all cases, and regular follow-up is indicated, but it is clear from accumulated data[392] that only a small minority of children with isolated orbital gliomas and NF-1 will exhibit tumor progression 5 to 10 years after diagnosis. It is suggested that physical examination and sequential MRI be performed 3 months after initial detection of orbital gliomas and yearly thereafter, and radiation therapy should be reserved primarily for patients with useful residual vision, but with evidence of visual deterioration or radiographic progression; there is no evidence to support the efficacy of chemotherapy for isolated optic nerve gliomas.[392]

MRIs of optic nerve gliomas in NF-1 show typical double-intensity tubular thickening characteristic of perineural arachnoidal gliomatosis (the perineural layer with signal characteristics similar to water or CSF), elongation of the nerves, and vertical kinking in the midorbit.[396,397] Precise MRI studies, echography (regular, homogeneous, low to medium reflectivity[398]), and the constellation of clinical signs and symptoms obviate the question of routine lateral orbital exploration for histologic confirmation, although orbital meningiomas in the first 2 decades of life may behave as aggressive lesions, and collateral hyperplasia of the nerve sheath may be mistaken for meningioma. Because gliomas do not erode through dura, whereas meningiomas do, extradural tumor extension should raise the suspicion of meningioma, and such tissue may undergo biopsy for diagnostic purposes. Ganglioglioma, an extremely rare CNS tumor, may mimic a rapidly expanding orbital glioma.[399]

If proptosis of a blind or near-blind eye is cosmetically unacceptable, frontal resection of the tumor from the globe to the orbital apex, and judicious canal unroofing, seems to be logical. Care should be taken not to injure the motor nerves at the apex or the posterior ciliary nerves at the globe. Enucleation and exenteration are categorically not indicated, nor is complete excision if such a procedure injures the globe or ocular motor mechanism. The efficacy of radiation therapy for orbital glioma is variable,[392,400] and conservativism cannot be faulted. Chiasmal and hypothalamic gliomas of childhood and malignant optic glioma of adulthood are discussed in Chapter 6.

Perioptic Meningiomas

Meningiomas arise from meningothelial cells of the arachnoid, at multiple intracranial sites, in the optic canals, and from the intradural tissue that invests the optic nerves in the orbit. Meningiomas of the anterior and middle cranial fossae, and those of the perineural orbital portion and optic canal, are of major neuro-ophthalmologic interest because of the progressive signs and symptoms, typically insidious visual deterioration, and some degree of proptosis. There is a distinct female predilection for meningiomas (60% to 75%), and the intracranial variety occurs predominantly in middle-aged and elderly adults.

Although most meningiomas that involve the orbit derive from the adjacent posterior position of the sphenoid bone, or within the optic canal, intraorbital perioptic meningiomas, arising from the nerve sheath, account for only 1% to 2% of all meningiomas, but for one-third of primary optic nerve tumors.[401] In this location, perioptic meningiomas tend to occur at a younger age, perhaps because of earlier onset of visual symptoms. Karp et al[402] noted that 10 of 25 primary intraorbital meningiomas occurred in patients less than 20 years of age, and 6 patients were in the first decade. Dutton[401] reported a mean age at presentation of 40.8 years (range, 2.5 to 78 years), and bilateral (multifocal vs. contiguous?) cases are documented. Meningiomas presenting in youth may be associated with neurofibromatosis.[401] Orbital meningiomas that do not arise from the nerve sheath, that is, "ectopic" tumors, must be extremely rare.

The optic nerves may be involved via several mechanisms, as follows. Intraorbital meningiomas arising from the nerve sheath produce slowly progressive axial proptosis or loss of vision. The retro-bulbar mass may further manifest by increasing hyperopia and the appearance on ophthalmoscopy of retinochoroidal striae. At first, the disc may appear normal, but optic atrophy or chronic disc swelling ensues (Fig. 5–43). The clinical triad of the presence of optociliary venous shunts on the disc, when accompanied by diffuse disc edema (eventually replaced slowly by pallor), and insidious visual loss, is highly suggestive of indolent nerve sheath meningiomas, even in those patients without proptosis or when the posterior aspect of the optic canal may be principally involved. Pain is distinctly rare, but transient visual obscurations may occur, and ocular motor defects imply extension to the orbital apex or dural penetration with invasion of orbital soft tissues.

Radiologic signs include narrow fusiform or irregular tubular enlargement of the optic nerve (see Fig. 5–43), at times with calcification detectable by CT or ultrasonography[107]; the central neural tissue may be outlined by parallel perioptic thickening, giving the appearance of railroad ("tram") tracking. Similar "tracking" has been reported in isolated optic nerve sarcoid.[403] Unless the posterior aspect of the tumor involves the orbital apex or optic canal, no bony abnormalities are seen. Gadolinium-enhanced T1-weighted MRI usually shows marked enhancement of intracanalicular and intracranial meningiomas, but in the orbit, the tumor signal is less distinct from adjacent fat; fat-suppression protocols resolve this physical obstacle.[401,404,405]

In adults, delay in diagnosis is the rule, and, although inexorable blindness is an unsettling prospect, any surgical procedure is ineffective and all too frequently ruins what vision remains. Therefore, with radiologically indolent tumors, there may be no advantage to any form of surgical intervention, either by an orbital approach or by transfrontal craniotomy, although disfiguring proptosis or prevention of intracranial extension may force a decision for judicious frontal craniotomy. Radiation therapy is believed by some to delay recurrence after resection, and precision primary, fractional (5400 cGy at 180 cGy/day) irradiation does show some promise.[401,406,407]

Intracanalicular meningiomas usually represent either extensions of posterior orbital tumors or invasion into the canal by periforaminal meningiomas arising in the area of the anterior clinoids or tuberculum sellae. Posterior periforaminal, clinoidal, and tuberculum sellae meningiomas comprise the majority of meningiomas that produce prechiasmal (optic nerve) visual deficits. The monotonous presentation is a complaint of slowly progressive monocular loss of vision, with all the signs and symptoms of an optic nerve conduction defect. With suprasellar extension, these tumors produce chiasmal interference, with variations on a bitemporal theme (see Chapter 6). Pallor of the disc is usually less than that anticipated in view of the visual deficit. It is with posterior periforaminal and tuberculum meningiomas that thin-section gadolinium-enhanced MRI techniques are especially productive.

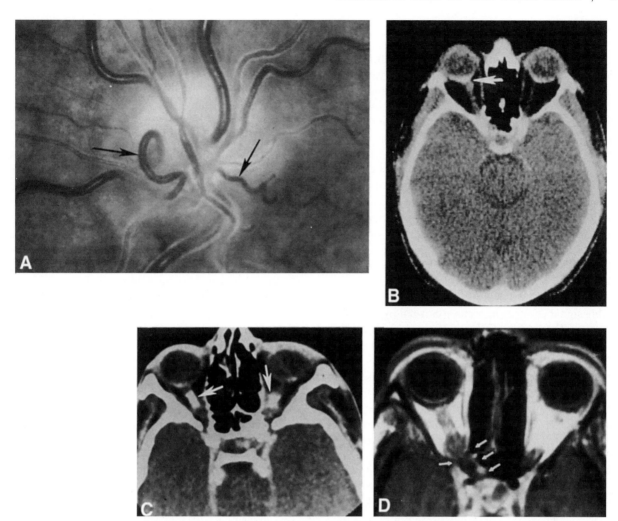

Fig. 5–43. Optic nerve sheath (perioptic) meningioma. **A.** Chronic disc edema with progressive atrophy and retinociliary venous shunts (*arrows*). **B.** Computed tomography (CT) axial section of nerve (from **A**) shows irregular thickening of the sheath (*arrow*). **C.** CT axial section disclosed bilateral bone-density calcification (*arrows*). **D.** Magnetic resonance axial section (TR, 900 msec; TE, 20 msec, gadolinium-enhanced). Note evidence of meningioma spread in the canal area (*arrows*).

Meningiomas of the *sphenoidal wing* present as proptosis and reactive hyperostosis evident on CT or MRI. These slow-growing tumors may eventually involve the optic nerve, early in their course if medially located, and as a relatively late complication if the mass predominantly involves the lateral aspect of the sphenoid ridge and middle cranial fossa (pterional meningioma).

The higher incidence of meningiomas in women, increased growth rate during pregnancy, and possible association with breast carcinoma all suggest an influence of female sex hormones. The presence of progesterone-receptor staining suggests a more favorable prognosis, but effective medical therapy is unproved.[408]

Secondary Neoplasms: Carcinomas and Lymphomas

As noted, the optic nerves are more frequently involved by exogenous tumors and malignant infiltrations than by primary neural neoplasms. These secondary causes include contiguous spread of intraocular melanoma and retinoblastoma, hematologic malignancies, leptomeningeal infiltration, and direct invasion by metastatic systemic cancer. Of course, orbital, sinus, and skull base masses may compromise the anterior visual pathways, and these do so with some frequency. Aside from extrinsic basal masses, such as pituitary adenomas, meningiomas, and paraclinoidal carotid aneurysms, other lesions are relatively uncommon yet present as "retrobulbar neuritis" with a normal fundus appearance.

When a systemic malignancy is previously diagnosed, abrupt visual loss not attributable to fundus lesions is *prima facie* evidence of meningeal carcinomatosis. In two reviews of carcinomatosis,[409,410] the incidence of ocular symptoms was striking; either as the presenting complaint or as a subsequent development, visual loss or double vision comprised the largest group of symptomatic cranial nerve deficits. Rapidly consecutive contralateral visual loss, other cranial nerve palsies, including facial, spinal root symptoms, and headache are also ominous features. Adenocarcinoma of the breast and lung are the most frequent tumors to metastasize diffusely to the leptomeninges and subarachnoid space. Lymphoma, including reticulum cell sarcoma, and melanoma are also relatively common sources of meningeal seeding.[411] McFadzean et al[412] have suggested that the combination of headaches, rapidly progressive visual loss, sluggish pupil reactions, and normal optic discs (or at least delayed pallor), with usually normal neuroimages, should bring to mind the diagnosis of leptomeningeal carcinomatosis.

Leptomeningeal deposits are not easily uncovered by radiologic techniques. In a comparative study of CT and MRI, enhanced CT detected meningeal tumor in only 39% of 23 cases with positive CSF cytology and focal CNS defects, and non-enhanced MRI detected the tumor in only 23%; furthermore, MRI failed to show discernable signal changes in areas abnormal by enhanced CT criteria.[413] Multiple CSF fluid samples may be required and cytocentrifuge technique applied to acquire cytologic confirmation.

The pathophysiologic mechanisms of visual loss with meningeal carcinomatosis include "tumor cuffing" in the perioptic meninges accompanied by localized demyelination, direct tumor infiltration into the substance of the nerve, and demyelination out of proportion to sparse tumor cell infiltrate. With regard to the concept of optic myelopathy as a remote complication of distant malignancy, paraneoplastic syndrome with optic neuropathy has been associated with anti-CV2 antibodies, with resolution following excision of primary small cell carcinoma of the lung.[413a]

The outcome of carcinomatosis of the meninges is uniformly grim, with death ensuing within months. However, a substantiated diagnosis precludes unnecessary and uncomfortable neurodiagnostic studies.

The optic nerves may be involved by *diffuse infiltrative lesions* of diverse origin, including the lymphoma-reticuloendothelioses,[414-416] the histiocytoses, plasmacytomas,[417] and others. Infiltrative disorders more or less share a common clinical profile of subacute or rapid visual loss in one or both eyes. Disc swelling is seen on occasion, indicating infiltration of the nerve head itself. It should be recalled that chronic granulomas, such as sarcoid (see above), may mimic neoplasia.

Leukemia may produce disc swelling via several mechanisms. These include meningeal infiltrate or intracranial hemorrhagic diathesis resulting in obstruction of CSF and increased intracranial pressure, pseudotumor cerebri syndrome associated with prolonged corticosteroid therapy, disc edema associated with severe anemic retinopathy, and actual leukemic permeation of disc tissue; pallid disc edema may be due to massive infiltrates,[418] and prompt irradiation may reverse visual loss.[419] Although chronic lymphocytic leukemia is said

only infrequently to cause neurologic symptoms, meningitis, confusional states, cranial nerve abnormalities, cerebellar dysfunction, and optic neuropathy are all reported.[420]

Although lymphoma may represent up to 10% of orbital malignancies, direct involvement of the optic disc or retina is rare. Of intraocular lymphoma, reticulum cell (histiocytic lymphoma, microgliomatosis) is most frequent, and this malignancy has been reported to involve the intracranial optic nerve.[421] The syndrome of posterior uveitis associated with reticulum cell sarcoma (microgliomatosis) of the brain has become well established.[422] I have personally seen two middle-aged men with myocosis fungoides whose systemic lymphoma was heralded by a picture of acute optic neuritis with disc swelling and severe acute visual loss.

Visual loss in leukemia and lymphoma may also be due to opportunistic infections of the CNS, including cryptococcosis, toxoplasmosis, or herpes zoster infection. Chemotherapeutic agents such as vincristine may be implicated, and the optic nerve complications of cisplatin, carboplatin in combination with cyclophosphamide, carmustine, and bone marrow transplant are well recognized.[423-424] In patients with noncarcinomatous (*e.g.,* leukemia, lymphoma, myeloma) neoplastic infiltration of the optic nerves, radiation therapy often results in rapid return of vision to useful levels,[419] whereas treatment directed at the systemic disorder may have little effect on visual function.

Enlargement of the orbital segment of the optic nerve may be the result of a wide spectrum of pathologic processes (Table 5–13), which at least may be anatomically localized as the focal cause of visual loss, specific radiologic characteristics (some pathognomonic) and accompanying clinical signs and symptoms, aside. It goes without saying that historical medical data, review of systemic diseases and of previous surgical procedures, physical findings, precise neuroimaging of the orbits and skull base, laboratory investigations, and at times CSF examination and tissue biopsy procedures must all be part of a judiciously considered differential diagnosis.

Paranasal Sinus Disease

Diseases of the paranasal sinuses, although perhaps disproportionately invoked in years past, are not to be overlooked as a cause of visual loss, proptosis, diplopia, or headache. Ocular motor disturbances with nasopharyngeal tumors and sphenoidal mucoceles are discussed in Chapter 12. This discussion considers the visual complications of inflammatory disorders, mucoceles, and carcinoma of the paranasal sinuses.

The anatomic relationships with the posterior ethmoid and sphenoidal paranasal sinuses (see Fig. 5–11) place the optic nerves in peculiarly disadvantageous positions, not only in regard to neighboring lesions, but

TABLE 5-13. Enlargement of the Optic Nerve

Inflammatory	Neoplasia	Miscellaneous

Optic neuritis
  Demyelinative (MS), viral, or idiopathic
Perioptic neuritis:
  Idiopathic pseudotumor
  Syphilis
Sarcoid
Toxoplasmosis
Cryptococcosis
	Optic glioma
	Perioptic meningioma
	Hemangioblastoma
	Metastasis
	Leukemia
	Lymphoma
	Ganglioglioma
		Anatomic variant,
		  patulous sheaths
		Papilledema of raised
		  cerebrospinal pressure
		Graves' orbitopathy
		Trauma, hematoma
		Arachnoid cyst
		Globoid leukodystrophy

MS, multiple sclerosis.

also in harm's way of endoscopic surgical manipulations. Anatomic variability notwithstanding, studies of fine bony details provided by thin-section coronal CT views[425] show that the course of the optic canal is directly adjacent to the posterior ethmoid wall in 3%, the majority being in the lateral or superior wall of the sphenoid sinus, 15% indenting the sinus wall, and 6% passing through the sinus cavity; bone dehiscence of the optic canal is found in fully 25%, directly exposing the nerves to thin sinus mucosa. Buss et al[426] reported instances of ophthalmic complications of sinus surgery, including blindness resulting from orbital hematoma and optic nerve transection, nor is the chiasm itself entirely safe during endoscopic procedures.[427]

Mucoceles are cystic bony expansions of the paranasal sinuses that contain mucoid and epithelial debris as a result of obstruction of normal drainage through ostia. These arise in the frontal, ethmoidal, or sphenoidal sinuses and present as effects of mass lesions. With sphenoidal mucocele (posterior ethmoidosphenoidal), the optic nerves are liable to damage as the mass enlarges laterally to involve the optic canals; actually, inflammation alone without bony distortion may result in irreversible blindness.[259] Visual loss is usually monocular and slowly progressive, and optic atrophy attests to chronicity. Field defects take the form of central scotomas, with or without peripheral depressions, but chiasmal syndromes (*e.g.,* monocular blindness plus contralateral temporal hemianopia) are infrequent.[428] Rapid unilateral or bilateral visual loss with severe headache may mimic pituitary apoplexy.

The radiologic findings with sphenoidal mucocele include expansion of the sphenoid sinus (Fig. 5–44), elevation of the tuberculum sellae and chiasmatic sulcus, obliteration of optic canal and superior orbital fissure, and lateral displacement of medial orbital walls. An anterior clinoid variant of sphenoidal mucocele has been described, with visual loss mimicking retro-bulbar neuritis.[429] In general, the presence of anterior clinoid pneumatization is associated with bone dehiscence and exposure of the optic nerve.[425] For mucocele, rhinologic surgery is the treatment of choice, usually by endonasal decompression, and some return of vision may be anticipated unless optic atrophy is advanced.

Indolent fungal infections with minimal sinusitis may present as orbital apex syndrome, including rapidly advancing or chronic, progressive optic neuropathy. Of these, mucormycosis[430] (with or without diabetes) and aspergillosis[431] are most frequent, at times mimicking cranial arteritis, with facial pain, retinal vascular occlusions, or ophthalmoplegia, for which aggressive corticosteroid therapy may prove disastrous. Early transnasal endoscopic exploration for biopsy is vital.

Wegener's granulomatosis ("lethal midline granuloma") is a necrotizing vasculitis with a predilection for the upper respiratory tracts, at times heralded by nasal and sinus congestion and discharge, and destruction of midline nasal cartilage. Pulmonary nodules or infiltrates and glomerulonephritis with hematuria fulfill the other clinical criteria, and orbital inflammation is common. Isolated retro-bulbar neuropathy has been documented,[258] and ocular signs may signal this disorder in up to 17% of cases.[432] Ophthalmic complications include the following: episcleritis and scleritis; corneal ulceration; uveitis; retinal vasculitis and optic neuropathy; and granulomatous inflammation of lacrimal glands, salivary glands, orbital soft tissue, and paranasal sinuses. Meningocerebral inflammation, a form of pachymeningitis detectable by enhanced MRI, produces headache, seizures, and cranial neuropathies.[433] Antineutrophilic cytoplasmic antibody (c-ANCA) assay provides highly specific laboratory confirmation, but absence does not rule out this disorder, and biopsy of nasal or sinus tissues commonly shows typical vasculitic, granulomatous inflammation.[422] Corticosteroids and immunosuppressants such as methotrexate are the usual therapies. Intranasal cocaine abuse can produce a type of chronic ischemic mucoperichondritis and osteolytic sinusitis, at times with nasoseptal perforation, and variably associated with signs of orbital inflammation and contiguous inflammatory optic neuropathy.[434]

Tumors of the nasopharynx and paranasal sinuses rarely present primarily as visual loss, but may eventually involve the optic nerve when the posterior ethmoidal or sphenoidal sinus is invaded. Occurring predominantly in men at least in the sixth decade of life, squamous cell carcinoma is the most common type, typically in the maxillary sinus, less frequently the ethmoid complex, and

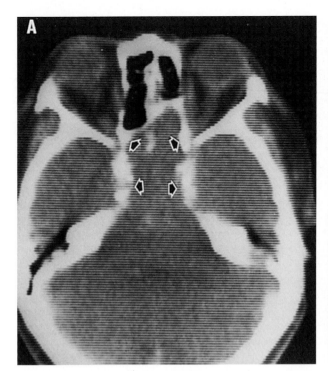
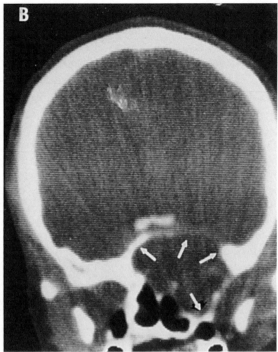

Fig. 5–44. Sphenoethmoidal mucocele with visual loss. Computed tomography (CT) axial section (**A**) and CT coronal section (**B**) demonstrate expansion and deformation of sinus walls (*arrows*).

rarely the frontal or sphenoid sinuses. From the excellent review of Harbison et al,[435] in sphenoidal malignancies, headache and diplopia (cranial nerves III, IV, VI, and V) are more usual complaints than visual loss, which involved only 5 of 42 patients in the Harbison series. Visual loss is subacute or rapidly progressive to blindness. Other signs and symptoms, that is, facial pain or anesthesia, radiologic findings, and biopsy usually confirm the diagnosis. Esthesioneuroblastoma, a malignant neuroectodermal tumor originating in olfactory nasal mucosa, is reported to produce rapidly progressive visual loss,[436] although presenting symptoms more commonly include nasal obstruction, epistaxis, facial numbness, diplopia, and proptosis. In patients subjected to radiation therapy for malignant nasopharyngeal tumors, loss of vision months after therapy may be attributable to delayed radionecrosis of the optic nerve (see below), but recurrence and spread of tumor must be considered.

Orbitopathies: Graves' Disease

A variety of orbital disease, including inflammations, trauma, and tumor, may produce optic nerve dysfunction. The ophthalmopathy of Graves' disease is not only a frequently overlooked cause of spontaneous diplopia, but visual loss due to orbital congestion may be mistakenly attributed to corneal exposure and tear film problems (see Chapter 14). By mechanisms not yet entirely elucidated, the optic nerve may participate in the orbitopathy associated with dysthyroid states or even in apparent euthyroidism. Extraocular muscles are enlarged by endomysial fibrosis, mucopolysaccharide deposition, and perivascular lymphocyte and plasmacyte infiltration. Morphologically, the optic nerves are encroached on by swollen muscles at the tight orbital apex,[437,438] and on the basis of ultrasonography and CT, or MRI, it is indeed likely that the optic nerve is compressed by the confluence of enlarged recti muscles in the posterior orbit, but prolapse of orbital fat through the superior orbital fissure is also a possible mechanism.[439] There is a loss of large-type axons in the proximal segment of the orbital portion of the optic nerves, associated with mild astrocyte increase, but the nerve and meninges are not inflamed.[440] It is estimated that optic nerve dysfunction occurs in some 6% of patients with Graves' orbitopathy.[441]

As a rule, at the onset of optic neuropathy, many patients are clinically euthyroid, having been treated previously for hyperthyroidism. Middle-aged patients with otherwise well-developed, but not necessarily severe, ophthalmopathy present with usually insidious loss of central vision in one or both eyes. Ocular motility is frequently restricted at this stage, and corneal exposure may be minimal. Care should be taken not to attribute a disproportionate visual loss to minor corneal complications and ignore the potentially blinding optic neuropathy, the tests for which have been outlined (see Chapter 2).

Acuity may be as poor as finger-counting or only minimally diminished, but color sense is uniformly faulty. Visual fields demonstrate central scotomas, often combined with inferior nerve fiber bundle defects (Fig. 5–45). The latter defects may be confused with those of glaucoma, especially if intraocular pressure is spuriously elevated by restrictive myopathy (see Chapter 14). The ocular fundus may be entirely normal, or various degrees of disc swelling may be observed (Fig. 5–46), but, apart from profound atrophy, the state of the disc has little prognostic correlation with eventual visual outcome.[442]

The natural course of dysthyroid optic neuropathy is not entirely benign. In a subject review,[442] it was noted that more than 20% of cases documented in the literature had eventual acuity of 20/100 or less, including vision of finger-counting and worse. Initial therapy consists of systemic corticosteroids in large doses, orbital decompressive procedures, and irradiation. For example, medical therapy may commence with 80 mg prednisone per day orally, and if no response (acuity, fields) is demonstrable within 2 weeks, the dosage is increased or delivered by intravenous pulse (*e.g.,* methylprednisolone 250 mg every 6 hours) over 3 to 5 days of hospitalization. As a rule, patients do not tolerate well such high levels of corticosteroids, and few care to continue this regimen beyond 6 to 8 weeks. If visual function is severely impaired or is worsening despite medical therapy, radiation therapy or surgical orbital decompression is indicated. The use of intraorbital steroid injections has not been effective, and there is little reason to recommend this route of administration otherwise.

Radiation therapy (*e.g.,* 2000 cGy delivered by posteriorly angled apposed lateral ports, 200 cGy/session)[443] for dysthyroid optic neuropathy is generally effective, even as an initial form of treatment. Indeed, in patients refractory to large doses of corticosteroids, dramatic recovery of vision has followed administration of 1500 to 2000 rads.[442] Regarding orbital decompressive surgery, it would seem that the transantral, inferior septal, medial, and lateral approaches are variably successful, as long as there is adequate decompression of the posterior aspect of the orbit floor (see Chapter 14). It is problematic whether massive doses of corticosteroids, surgical orbital decompression, or modest doses of radiation are least harmful to the individual patient, and, at times, all three approaches may be necessary. Other orbital processes that involve the optic nerve are discussed in Chapter 14.

Vascular Compression: Aneurysms

As the intracranial portion of the optic nerve ascends from the canal to the chiasm, it lies immediately above the initial supracavernous segment of the internal carotid artery (Figs. 4–1 and 12–20). The anterior cerebral artery passes dorsal to the nerve, often in direct contact, then turns rostrally in the prechiasmatic notch, where it is joined to the opposite anterior cerebral artery via the anterior communicating artery. Thus, the prechiasmal portion of the optic nerve and the anterior angle of the chiasm are intimately related to the major arteries that form the anterior aspect of the basal circle of Willis. These vessels become tortuous and dilated with increasing age and on infrequent occasions may be responsible for progressive visual loss.

Ectatic dilation ("fusiform aneurysm") of the intracranial segment of the internal carotid artery may compress the optic nerve from below, elevating it against the unyielding periforaminal dura, anterior clinoid, and anterior cerebral artery. Jacobson et al[444] demonstrated by MRI that contact between the supraclinoid portion of the carotid artery and one or both optic nerve occurs in 70% of asymptomatic patients, depending also on the diameter of the vessel and with advancing age. Therefore, it is problematic to attribute occult optic neuropathy (*e.g.,* normal tension glaucoma) simply to the intimate anatomic relationship of the carotid artery and the adjacent optic nerves. Pathologically, arterial grooving does occur and may result in atrophy of contiguous axons,[445] to which the evolution of slowly progressive central, nasal, and arcuate field defects may be attributed (Fig. 5–47).[446] Interestingly, a 34-year-old woman with progressive, painless monocular visual loss was reported[447] with compression of the ipsilateral nerve by a dolichoectatic carotid artery, with recovery within 1 month of craniotomy for optic canal decompression. Of course, a diagnosis of ischemic nerve or chiasm compression by dolichoectatic arteries may be entertained only after mass lesions or other pathologic causes are categorically excluded.

Aneurysms at the skull base, in proximity to the optic nerve, also may present as insidious or rapid visual loss *mimicking retro-bulbar neuritis,* as exemplified by the patient reported by Miller et al,[448] underscoring three vital points: (1) even if it is true that a carotid-ophthalmic aneurysm must be 10 mm in diameter before it causes visual symptoms, such an aneurysm nevertheless may not be detected by MRI, and if aneurysms less than 10 mm can in fact cause visual symptoms, there is even a greater probability that such an aneurysm would be undetected by MRI; (2) rather than presenting as dramatic subarachnoid hemorrhage, the sacculation of unruptured cranial aneurysms may grow by thrombus organization, intimal proliferation, and ischemia of the aneurysm wall with subsequent thickening and scar formation; and (3) an atypical clinical course, including progression of monocular visual loss, or evolving chiasmal syndrome, demands re-investigation.

The common anterior communicating artery aneurysm does not usually present with neuro-ophthalmic signs, but on rare occasions may produce acute monocular blindness by downward compression from above,

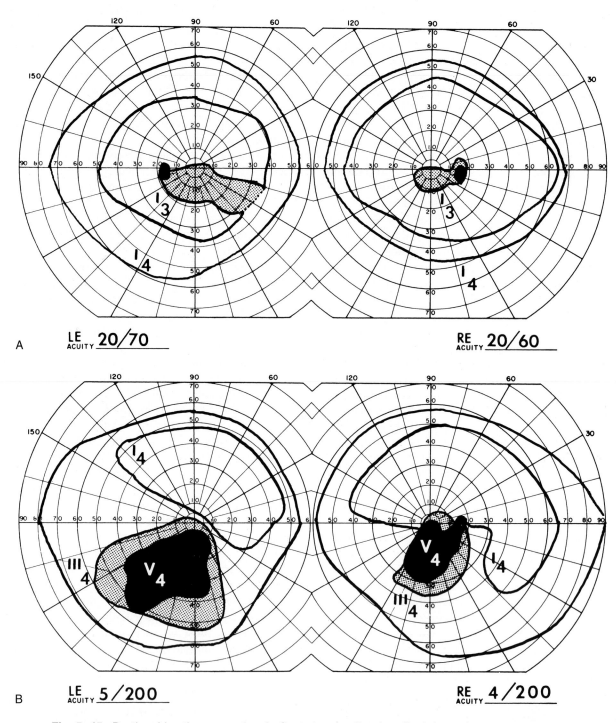

Fig. 5–45. Dysthyroid optic neuropathy. **A.** Central nerve fiber bundle defects. An arcuate pattern in the left field mimics glaucoma. The patient was a 53-year-old woman with moderate bilateral proptosis and lid retraction, who noted slowly progressive loss of color appreciation. Visual defects cleared rapidly and completely on large doses of systemic corticosteroids. Discs were at all times normal. **B.** A 57-year-old woman with moderate congestive ophthalmopathy experienced diminution of vision from 20/25 OU to 20/100 OU in 6 weeks and 4/200 to 5/200 by 10 weeks. The right disc was swollen and elevated with several hemorrhages; the left disc was normal. Massive doses of systemic steroids resulted in slow improvement to 20/200 and 20/400. *LE,* left eye; *RE,* right eye.

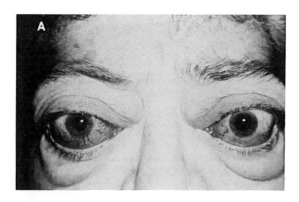

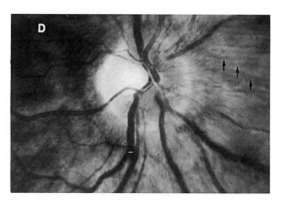

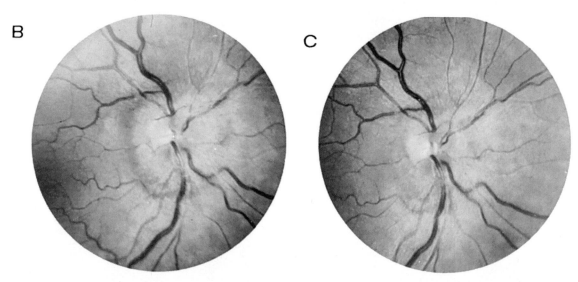

Fig. 5–46. Dysthyroid optic neuropathy. **A.** Patient with 4 years of stable ophthalmopathy noted progressive right visual loss to 20/80. **B.** Right disc is edematous and elevated. Lateral orbital decompression with floor fracture was performed. Within 48 hours, vision was 20/25, and the disc detumesced **(C)**. **D.** The fundus of a different patient demonstrates a hyperemic, edematous disc and retinochoroidal folds (*arrows*).

adherence to, and eventual hemorrhage into the optic nerve.[449] Aneurysmal compression of the chiasm is considered in Chapter 6.

NUTRITIONAL AND TOXIC OPTIC NEUROPATHIES

Insidious and slowly progressive bilateral loss of function in the central fields, with resultant diminished acuity, decreased color sense, and central scotomas, should alert the physician to the possibility of intrinsic optic nerve disease related to dietary deficiencies, exposure to toxins, or adverse reaction to pharmaceuticals. At onset, diagnosis is confounded by optic discs that are usually unremarkable, with optic atrophy eventually evolving. In the same clinical setting, atypical centrocecal field loss with glaucoma, macular cone dystrophy, and primary hereditary optic atrophy must also be considered. No distinction is made between central and

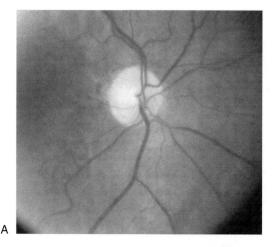

Fig. 5–47. Optic neuropathy with carotid dolichoectasia in a 74-year-old man with progressive dimming of right eye vision: acuity of right, 20/30, and left, 20/20. **A.** Right optic disc shows a saucer-like excavation diagnosed as "normal tension glaucoma."

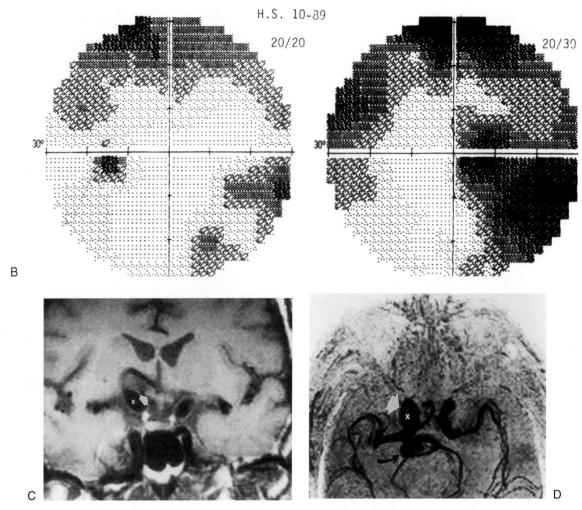

Fig. 5–47. (*continued*) **B.** Visual fields. **C.** Magnetic resonance imaging shows elevation and distortion of the right side of the chiasm (*arrows*) by fusiform dilation of the internal carotid artery (*x*). **D.** Magnetic resonance angiogram demonstrates an ectatic right (*x*) carotid artery (*arrow*); the basilar artery (curved artery) is also ectatic.

cecocentral visual field defects, for which a differential diagnosis is outlined below.

A. Deficiency states
    1. Thiamine ("tobacco-alcohol amblyopia")
    2. Vitamin B_{12} (pernicious anemia; ? "tobacco amblyopia")
B. Drugs/toxins
    1. Ethambutol
    2. Chloramphenicol
    3. Streptomycin
    4. Isoniazid
    5. Chlorpropamide
    6. Digitalis
    7. Chloroquine
    8. Vigabatrin
    9. Disulfiram
    10. Heavy metals
    11. Yohimbine
C. Hereditary optic atrophies
    1. Dominant (juvenile)
    2. Leber's
    3. Associated with heredodegenerative neurologic syndromes
    4. Recessive, associated with juvenile diabetes
D. Demyelinative
E. Graves' orbitopathy
F. Atypical glaucoma
G. Macular dystrophies and degenerations

Vitamin Deficiencies and "Tobacco-Alcohol Amblyopia"

Regarding the origin of nutritional neuropathies, the great weight of clinical evidence overwhelmingly favors a dietary deficiency of B-complex vitamins (predominantly thiamine) rather than the direct toxic effects of tobacco or chronic alcoholism. Even when "tobacco amblyopia" is touted as the common variety of abuse-related optic neuropathy, multiple factors seem to converge: patients are often elderly men with diets poor in protein and B vitamins; vitamin B_{12} absorption may be defective; alcoholic consumption is variable; rough grades of pipe tobacco are smoked.

Of greater practical importance, there are no clinical differences among "tobacco amblyopia," and "tobacco-alcohol amblyopia," optic neuropathy in chronic alcoholism, or malnutrition optic neuropathy. It appears that dietary deficiency is the common denominator, and thiamine improves the condition in spite of continuing abuse of alcohol or tobacco.[450]

It goes without saying that alcoholic patients tend not to disclose accurate daily consumption figures, and history-taking from relatives and friends may be more reliable, including details of diet. Although the patient may staunchly deny alcohol abuse, at the slit lamp, the examiner may be only too acutely aware of the odor of alcoholic breath. Normal body weight, much less obesity, is uncommon in this group. Bankers, lawyers, and even physicians are not immune, although the following case history is more common:

> A 72-year-old widower presented with visual complaints related to reading and driving of 2 to 3 months' duration. Acuity was 20/200 and 20/60, and bilateral central scotomas were elicited (Fig. 5–48); the fundi were normal. The patient drank half a pint whiskey each day and smoked 10 to 12 cigars. He lived alone in a mobile home and "didn't bother cooking for myself." Daily meals usually consisted of peanut butter and jelly sandwiches for breakfast, no lunch, and "some crackers" for supper. This menu had not changed for well over a year. Serum vitamin B_{12}, folate, and lead levels were all normal. Brewer's yeast tablets and the preparation of meals by a neighbor resulted in improvement of vision to 20/40 and 20/30 within 2 months and disappearance of demonstrable field defects.

Bilateral, relatively symmetric centrocecal scotomas, with preservation of the peripheral field, are the characteristic field defects encountered in nutritional-toxic neuropathy. Although minor variations in the scotomas have been said to distinguish between "alcohol" and "tobacco" amblyopia, no real distinctions may be made between central and cecocentral depressions; precise threshold techniques tend to disclose patches of defective field between the blind spot and the fixational area. The defects are characterized by "soft" margins that are difficult to define for white stimuli, but are larger and easier to plot for colored targets, especially red, on the tangent screen. A dense "nucleus" may at times be found between the blind spot and the fixational area, but nerve fiber bundle defects do not occur. Visual acuity is usually reduced to 20/200 levels but may be surprisingly good despite a symptomatic central defect, in which case the scotoma may be demonstrable with red targets only.

On occasion, bilateral cecocentral scotomas may mimic the bitemporal depression of chiasmal interference. The following features should distinguish the field of nutritional neuropathies from that of chiasmal interference: visual acuity is diminished; the defects extend across the vertical meridian, especially demonstrable with red targets; there is no peripheral hemianopic depression; and as the defects progress, they appear more cecocentral and less hemianopic.

As a rule, the fundus appears perfectly normal, but a small percentage of patients may show splinter retinal hemorrhages on or off the disc (Fig. 5–49) or minimal disc edema. Frisen[451] described bilateral evanescent dilation and tortuousity of small capillaries in the arcuate nerve fiber bundles. With the retinal hemorrhages, these changes imply a retinal ganglion cell disorder (in addition to neuropathy), as suggested by evoked potential studies.[452]

A case of severe visual loss with bilateral disc edema and retinal hemorrhages was reported,[453] in a patient with ulcerative colitis, reversed by subcutaneous thiamine injections. Also documented is vitamin B_{12} deficiency from malabsorption with initial hematologic manifestations reversed by folic acid, and then cecocentral scotomas that cleared with vitamin B_{12} administration.[454]

In elderly patients especially, the possibility of vitamin B_{12} or *folate* deficiency should not be overlooked. Central scotoma disease may precede the classic neurologic syndrome of subacute dysfunction of the dorsal and lateral spinal columns, and, in fact, optic nerve and neurologic deficits may be well established before macrocytic anemia is present. Hematologic consultation, including elucidation of vitamin B_{12} absorption, is warranted in the investigation of cases of bilateral progressive central scotomas, especially in the presence of normal hematocrit. The field defects of pernicious or pre-pernicious anemia are identical to those of the other toxic-nutritional optic neuropathies, and evoked potential abnormalities may be found in pernicious anemia even without visual symptoms.[455]

The inter-relationships of nutritional deficiency, vitamin B_{12} malabsorption, serum cyanide-thiocyanate level (from cigar and pipe smoking), and therapeutic response to hydroxocobalamin are controversial issues.[456] To confound the inter-relationship of malnutrition and extrinsic factors further, in 1991 to 1993, it was reported in Cuba that some 50,000 persons, mostly men, were affected by epidemic bilateral optic neuropathy, variable sensory neuropathy, and sensorineural hearing loss. Tobacco use was considered an associated risk, and recovery occurred following parenteral and oral B-complex vitamins.[457] This experience may be contrasted with that in the 1969 Nigeria civil war, and in Mozambique in 1981, when diets consisting of cassava roots and leaves

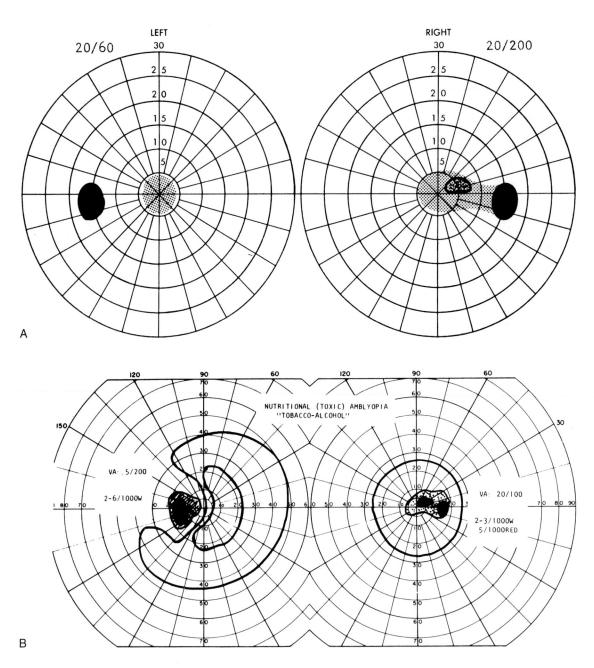

Fig. 5–48. Nutritional optic neuropathy. **A.** Bilateral central field defects most marked to color. **B.** More pronounced defects may superficially simulate chiasmal interference.

caused a syndrome of bilateral optic neuropathy, nerve deafness, and sensory ataxia, associated with a rise in serum cyanocobalamin levels.[458]

For uncomplicated cases of nutritional deficiencies, prognosis for recovery of vision is excellent for all but the most chronic cases. Treatment consists of a well-balanced diet and B-complex vitamin supplement. Among the least expensive preparations is baking yeast, either in powder form (*e.g.*, Fleischmann's Dried Yeast) or tablets (500 mg, 20 tablets per day; Squibb). Intramuscular thiamine may also be used.

Methanol intoxication is quite a different story, causing severe metabolic acidosis, progressive cerebral dysfunction, and variable visual loss associated with disc edema, at times with cystoid macular edema.[459] The four cases studied histopathologically by Sharpe et al[460] demonstrated myelin damage with axonal preservation in the retro-laminar portion of the optic nerve, probably caused by histotoxic anoxia. Acute treatment consists of intravenous bicarbonate and ethyl alcohol.

A most peculiar relatively rapid, bilateral optic atrophy termed "Jamaican optic neuropathy" afflicts young

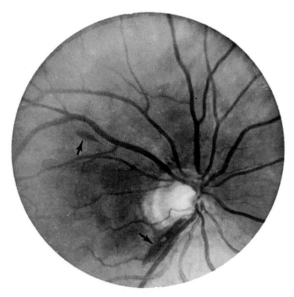

Fig. 5–49. Nutritional optic neuropathy. Slightly hyperemic disc with nerve fiber layer hemorrhages (*arrows*). The upper hemorrhage at some distance from the disc raises the question of a toxic process not limited to the nerve. There was no anemia.

West Indian blacks. This paradoxical disorder defies characterization in terms of an infective, hereditary, toxic, or nutritional origin. Vision is reduced to 20/200 levels, and dense central scotomas are demonstrable. I have seen this syndrome in young Bahamians, Haitians, Cubans, Puerto Ricans, and Jamaicans who have lived in the United States for years preceding loss of sight. They are well nourished, non-intoxicated, and non-reactive on syphilis serologic tests (FTA-ABS), with inconsequential family histories. A British series[461] included West African as well as Caribbean immigrants, and, thus, a genetic factor seems rational. No form of therapy affords relief.

Drugs and Toxins

Insidiously progressive or subacute onset of central field defects may occur as complications of medical therapy or of exposure to specific toxins. The catalog of potentially neurotoxic substances of ophthalmologic significance compiled in Grant's *Toxicology of the Eye*[462] should be consulted for more complete indices, but certain agents deserve emphasis here. The antituberculous agents isoniazid and ethambutol hydrochloride (Myambutol) have been clearly incriminated in dose-dependent insidious or subacute optic neuropathies, usually reversible over many months, but not always so.[463] Incidence in patients receiving 15 to 25 mg/kg/day is estimated at 2% to 15%.[464] After several months, acuity fails and field defects are typically cecocentral, but occasional

bitemporal hemianopic depression infers also a chiasmal interference (Fig. 5–50). The relative influences of age, renal function, and serum zinc levels are unclear. Electrophysiologic studies suggest that both retina and optic nerve are involved (ERG and visual-evoked potentials); visual-evoked potentials, color vision tests, and contrast sensitivity measurements[465] have proved helpful in detecting subclinical effects, and are more sensitive than simple acuity. Other antituberculous agents such as isoniazid and streptomycin are also rarely associated causes of optic neuropathy.[464]

Extensive clinical and epidemiologic evidence, primarily from Japan, has linked a neurologic syndrome that includes optic atrophy (subacute myelo-optic neuropathy) with the halogenated hydroxyquinolines.[466] These preparations include iodochlorhydroxyquin (Entero-Vioform), iodoquinol (Diodoquin), and clioquinol, the use of which should probably be reserved for acrodermatitis enteropathica or asymptomatic amebiasis. Certainly, the use of these agents is to be deprecated in inflammatory bowel disease or nonspecific diarrhea, especially in children.[467]

Other potentially optic neurotoxic agents include chloramphenicol, especially in children with cystic fibrosis,[468] D-penicillamine,[469] toluene from glue sniffing,[470] 5-fluorouracil,[471] intracarotid BCNU (carmustine),[472] hexachlorophene,[473] and cyclosporine.[474] The antianginal antiarrhythmic amiodarone has been associated with disc edema that mimics ION or papilledema of raised intracranial pressure.[475,476] Toxic effects of chemotherapeutic agents (*e.g.,* cisplatin, cyclophosphamide[423]) are discussed above. Interferon-alpha has been reported to cause abrupt visual loss with disc edema.[423a] Digitalis and quinine effects are discussed in Chapter 5, Part II.

Central Scotoma Syndromes

It is with the greatest of care and attention that the physician must probe for factors possibly related to the onset of what constitutes a bilateral central scotoma syndrome. As well as drug intake and family history, the patient should be carefully questioned regarding exposure to toxins (heavy metals, fumes, solvents). In the absence of any identifiable specific origin, the investigation of bilateral central scotomas, excluding maculopathies (which may require fluorescein angiography and focal foveal cone ERG[477]) should include the following:

1. Family history.
2. Medical history.
3. Drug history.
4. Diet history.
5. Work history; exposure to toxins.
6. Serum: vitamin B_{12}, folate.
7. Serum lead.
8. Hemogram, including mean corpuscular volume.

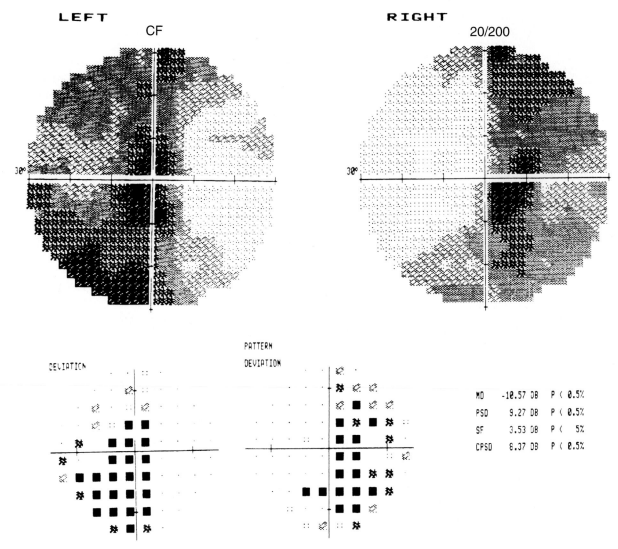

Fig. 5-50. Visual loss in ethambutol optic neuropathy. The patient was treated with excessive dosage for pulmonary atypical mycobacillus. Note the bitemporal pattern inferring chiasmal disturbance.

9. Hematology consult; B_{12} absorption tests.
10. Contrast-enhanced CT or MRI; thin sections of anterior visual pathways.

When possible, all previous medications should be discontinued; the patient should be placed on a high-protein diet with supplemental B-complex vitamins. If pernicious anemia is suspected, the aid of a competent hematologist should be sought before any parenteral medications are administered.

TRAUMATIC OPTIC NEUROPATHIES

Injury to the optic nerve may take many forms, the most common of which is a direct penetrating wound of the orbit or indirect injury as result of orbitofacial or cranial trauma. As a rule, the appropriate diagnosis is suggested by history alone, but apparently insignificant events may be overlooked. Surgeons may contribute to optic nerve morbidity during operative procedures of the lids or orbit, of the paranasal sinuses, or during general anesthesia with the patient in a face-down position and prolonged compression of the globe.

Orbito-cranial Injuries

Penetrating injuries of the orbit, accidental or the result of altercations, may result in transection or contusion of the nerve. When possible, it is imperative that visual function, including pupillary reactions (direct and consensual), and the fundus be evaluated *before* any surgical procedures are undertaken. For example, therapy directed primarily at repair of an orbital floor fracture is ill advised in the presence of severely impaired vision likely resulting from insult to the optic nerve. Medicolegal implications are obvious. Radiologic studies for orbito-cranial fractures or ocular and orbital foreign bodies are mandatory, but evidence of a retained foreign body alone is *not* an indication for surgical intervention. Neuroimaging should establish whether penetrating transorbital injuries violate the intracranium through the superior orbital fissure or orbital roof; thin-section CT scans with bone-window techniques are usually considered superior for disclosing bone fractures, and they may reveal vital optic canal fracture sites. In closed-head trauma or when penetrating injuries are suspected, baseline neurologic assessment is essential.

Blunt trauma to the eye and adnexa may result in severe visual loss, not accounted for by visible injury to the globe; when trauma is trivial, the cause of stable or progressive optic atrophy, at times with loss of disc substance, may be puzzling. Seemingly insignificant eye or lid injury can result in disproportionate optic nerve damage, and meticulous search for any evidence of lid or conjunctival penetration should be made. The mechanism of neural damage in many instances is speculative, but direct contusion necrosis or compressive ischemia of retro-bulbar axons is likely, and visual recovery is guarded; as yet, there is no convincing form of therapy (see below).[478] Hemorrhage within the nerve substance or sheaths may be disclosed by enhanced CT scanning or by standardized A-scan ultrasonography,[107,479] and evulsion of the distal end of the nerve usually assumes a typical fundus picture of peripapillary hemorrhage and disruption of the choroid. Protracted post-traumatic disc swelling with slowly increasing vision is described.[480] Optic atrophy is not immediately apparent because descending degeneration, even with complete transection, takes 3 to 6 weeks, as evidenced by progressive disc pallor.[481]

Loss of vision following orbital surgery is a well-documented tragedy, likely related to intraoperative or postoperative orbital hemorrhage, tight pressure dressings, or manipulation of the nerve itself; preoperative anemia or intraoperative hypotension may play a role (see the discussion of ION after surgical procedures). Visual loss may follow repair of orbital floor fractures using subperiosteal implants or after simple rhinoplasty.[482] Callahan[483] reviewed 68 cases of visual loss following simple blepharoplasty and concluded that intraoperative or postoperative orbital hemorrhage is the universal cause. Of course, the indications for cosmetic surgical procedures should be carefully weighed, especially in the elderly hypertensive patient. Postoperatively, the physician and nursing staff should be alerted for the complaint of acute severe pain, which may herald the onset of orbital hemorrhage. Pressure bandages should be avoided because they add to orbital tissue tension, they obscure lid and conjunctival signs of retro-bulbar bleeding, and pupillary reactions cannot be monitored.

Needle positioning during standard retro-bulbar anesthesia may injure the optic nerve, directly or by perineural or orbital hemorrhaging, usually producing immediate decreased vision discovered in the postoperative interval, with an afferent pupil reaction and usually normal fundus. Such nerve lesions may be confirmed by MRI[484]; in one instance, MRI confirmed an enlarged nerve, but sheath fenestration with release of hemorrhagic distention failed to reverse severe visual loss.[485] Liu et al[486] demonstrated, in an elegant and precise MRI analysis of the optic nerve configuration and location in extremes of gaze, that the standard Atkinson position (the eye directed upward and nasally) places the optic nerve in close proximity to the needle path, and that a downward and inward gaze position is optimal. Recall that the orbital segment of optic nerve takes a sinuous course, its length being 25 mm to 30 mm, whereas the orbit is relatively shallow, with a long axis of only 18 mm. The present practice of subtenon (peribulbar) injection techniques may prove less hazardous.

During orthopedic or neurosurgical procedures with the patient in a face-down position, such as for cervical laminectomy or posterior craniectomy, malposition of the face on the headrest may inadvertently tamponade the globe, on which the entire weight of the head is supported for hours at a time.[487] Resulting retinochoroidal infarction with severe visual deficit is noted on recovery from anesthesia; facial or lid edema may be present, and other signs of secondary ocular ischemia such as iridocyclitis and prolonged ocular hypotony have also been reported.[488]

During orbitofacial or closed-head trauma, the optic nerve is subjected to a variety of forces. In the orbit, as noted above, the nerve is redundant and is cushioned by orbital fat, for which reasons it is less liable to indirect injury. However, the nerve is strongly tethered to bone at the orbital opening of the optic canal, in the canal itself, and at the intracranial entrance of the canal. Moreover, the optic canal has a mean subdural cross-sectional space of only 1.84 mm², through which traverses an extremely delicate vasculature.[489] Thus, even small amounts of bleeding or edema may infarct the nerve, and how much more so an actual fracture with bone displacement. At both ends of the canal, the nerve is also subjected to shearing forces, because the brain and orbital contents are free to move, but the intracanalicular portion of the nerve is not.

As a rule, indirect injury to the optic nerve follows anterofrontal impact with rapid deceleration of the head, such as occurs in automobile accidents, falls from bicycles, motorcycles, skateboarding, or other frontal trauma. The visual deficits are usually instantaneous and of a marked degree. Lessell[490] noted that the severity of visual loss does not correlate well with level of consciousness or presence of craniofacial fractures.

The management of indirect optic nerve injuries is

controversial, with no clear consensus. Documented outcomes include spontaneous recovery and improvement with corticosteroids, and after a variety of sugical decompressions, but irreversible severe visual loss is the rule.[478] The use of intravenous dexamethasone in high doses (*e.g.,* more than 1 mg/kg/day), either as an alternative or as an adjunct to surgery, is based on acute spinal cord injury studies, and no carefully controlled prospective data are yet conclusive.[478,491] Extracranial techniques using either transethmoidal or transsphenoidal approaches are rational and may prove advantageous, considering the demonstrated pathologic changes in the intracanalicular segment of optic nerves. When perineural fluid collection is demonstrable in the orbital segment, sheath decompression may be considered, and subperiosteal or intraorbital hemorrhages associated with optic neuropathy are relative indications for surgical evacuation, especially if vision is worsening.

Radiation and Thermal Burns

The optic nerves are subject to direct effects of ionizing radiation, usually secondary to conventional radiation therapy of malignant lesions of the paranasal sinuses or of pituitary tumors, and of stereotactic radiosurgery of perichiasmal tumors. Despite the large number of patients undergoing therapeutic irradiation, the clinical incidence of radionecrosis of the nervous system is small. Visual loss attributed at first to tumor recurrence is now clearly radiologically distinguishable from radiation effects to the nerves and chiasm. Radionecrosis of the orbital optic nerve has been confirmed histologically,[492] consisting of proliferation of endothelial cells and thickening of vessel walls with fibrinoid necrosis, obliterated vessel lumina, and necrosis of retro-laminar nerve substance with reactive astrocytosis. Shukovsky and Fletcher[493] reported three instances of progressive visual loss with optic atrophy occurring between 4 and 5 years, following megavoltage radiation to the ethmoidal sinuses and nasal cavity. Delayed radionecrosis of the optic nerves and chiasm and potential therapies are discussed at length in Chapter 6.

A rare and peculiar delayed type of optic neuropathy has occurred following thermal burns of the body. Salz and Donin[494] reported such a case and reviewed the literature. Neither septicemia nor circulatory failure appears to play a role in the pathogenesis, and bilaterality of the disorder in all patients suggests a "burn neurotoxin," which may be elaborated 2 to 3 weeks after initial thermal injury. The burns need not be extensive. All reported patients have been infants, children, or young adults. Otherwise, visual loss may be an early complication of burns, attributed to diffuse cerebral edema and hypoxia and accompanied by other signs and symptoms of encephalopathy.

REFERENCES

1. Lee MS, Gonzalez C: Unilateral peripapillary myelinated retinal nerve fibers associated with strabismus, amblyopia and myopia. Am J Ophthalmol 125:554, 1998
2. Lambert SR, Hoyt CS, Narahara MH: Optic nerve hypoplasia. Surv Ophthalmol 32:1, 1987
3. Brodsky MC: Congenital optic disk anomalies. Surv Ophthalmol 39:89, 1994
4. Skarf B, Hoyt CS: Optic nerve hypoplasia in children: association with anomalies of the endocrine and CNS. Arch Ophthalmol 102:62, 1984
5. Alvarez E, Wakakura M, Khan Z et al: J Pediatr Ophthalmol Strab 25:151, 1988
6. Jonas JB, Papastathopoulos K: Ophthalmoscopic measurement of the optic disc. Ophthalmology 102:1102, 1995
7. Zeki SM, Dudgeon J, Dutton GN: Reappraisal of the ratio of disc to macula/disc diameter in optic nerve hypoplasia. Br J Ophthalmol 75:538, 1991
8. Peterson RA, Walton DS: Optic nerve hypoplasia with good visual acuity and visual field defect: a study of children of diabetic mothers. Arch Ophthalmol 95:254, 1977
9. Buchanan TA, Hoyt WF: Temporal visual field defects associated with nasal hypoplasia of the optic disc. Br J Ophthalmol 65:636, 1981
10. Brodsky MC, Schroeder GT, Ford R: Superior segmental optic hypoplasia in identical twins. J Clin Neuroophthalmol 13:152, 1993
11. Good WV, Ferriero DM, Golabi M et al: Abnormalities of the visual system in infants exposed to cocaine. Ophthalmology 99:341, 1992
12. Novakovic P, Taylor DSI, Hoyt WF: Localising patterns of optic nerve hypoplasia-retina to occipital lobe. Br J Ophthalmol 72:176, 1988
13. Hoyt WF, Rios-Montenegro EN, Behrens MM et al: Homonymous hemioptic hypoplasia: funduscopic features in standard and red-free illumination in three patients with congenital hemiplegia. Br J Ophthalmol 56:537, 1972
14. Brodsky MC, Conte FA, Taylor D et al: Sudden death in septo-optic dysplasia: report of of 5 cases. Arch Ophthalmol 115:66, 1997
15. Margalith D, Tze WJ, Jan JE: Congenital optic nerve hypoplasia with hypothalamic-pituitary dysplasia. Am J Dis Child 139:361, 1985
16. Brodsky MC, Glasier CM: Optic nerve hypoplasia: clinical significance of associated central nervous system abnormalities on magnetic resonance imaging. Arch Ophthalmol 111:66, 1993
17. Taylor D: Congenital tumours of the anterior visual system with dysplasia of the optic disc. Br J Ophthalmol 66:455, 1982
18. Grimson BS, Perry DD: Enlargement of the optic disc in childhood optic nerve tumors. Am J Ophthalmol 97:627, 1984
19. Howard MA, Thompson JT, Howard RO: Aplasia of the optic nerve. Trans Am Ophthalmol Soc 91:267, 1993
20. Scott IU, Warman R, Nolan A: Bilateral aplasia of the optic nerves, chiasm, and tracts in an otherwise healthy infant. Am J Ophthalmol 124:409, 1997
21. Apple DJ, Rabb MF, Walsh PM: Congenital anomalies of the optic disc. Surv Ophthalmol 27:3, 1982
22. Pollock S: The morning glory disc anomaly: contractile movement, classification, and embryogenesis. Doc Ophthalmol 65:439, 1987
23. Vuori M-L: Morning glory disc anomaly with pulsating peripapillary staphyloma: a case history. Acta Ophthalmol 65:602, 1987
24. Savell J, Cook JR: Optic nerve colobomas of autosomal dominant heredity. Arch Ophthalmol 94:395, 1976
25. Gopal L, Badrinath SS, Kumar KS et al: Optic disc in fundus coloboma. Ophthalmology 103:2120, 1996
26. Slamovits TL, Kimball GP, Friberg TI et al: Bilateral optic disc

colobomas with orbital cysts and hypoplastic optic nerves and chiasm. J Clin Neuroophthalmol 9:172, 1989

27. Orcutt JC, Bunt AH: Anomalous optic discs in a patient with Dandy-Walker cyst. J Clin Neuroophthalmol 2:43, 1982
28. Hanson MR, Price RL, Rothner AD et al: Developmental anomalies of the optic disc and carotid circulation. J Clin Neuroophthalmol 5:3, 1985
29. Eustis HS, Sanders MR, Zimmerman T: Morning glory syndrome in children. Arch Ophthalmol 112:204, 1994
30. Theodossiadis GP, Kollia AK, Theodossiadis PG: Cilioretinal arteries in conjunction with a pit of the optic disc. Ophthalologica 204:115, 1992
31. Ragge NK, Ravine D, Wilkie AOM: Dominant inheritance of optic pits. Am J Ophthalmol 125:124, 1998
32. Brown GC: Congenital pits of the optic nerve head. II. Clinical studies in humans. Ophthalmology 87:51, 1980
33. Adelung K, Aulhorn E, Thiel H-J: Funktionsstorungen bei Grubenpapille. Klin Monatsbl Augenheilk 191:1, 1987
34. Cashwell LF, Ford JG: Central visual field changes associated with acquired pits of the optic nerve. Ophthalmology 102:1270, 1995
35. Friberg TR, McLellan TG: Vitreous pulsations, relative hypotony, and retrobulbar cyst associated with a congenital optic pit. Am J Ophthalmol 114:767, 1992
36. Giuffre G: The spectrum of the visual field defects in the tilted disc syndrome: clinical study and review. Neuroophthalmology 6:239, 1986
37. Riise D: The nasal fundus ectasia. Acta Ophthalmol Suppl 126, 1975
38. Margolis S, Siegel IM: The tilted disc syndrome in craniofacial diseases. In Smith JL (ed), Neuro-ophthalmology Focus 1980, p 97. Masson, 1980
39. Spencer WH: Drusen of the optic disc and aberrant axoplasmic transport. Am J Ophthalmol 85:1, 1978
40. Tso MOM: Pathology and pathogenesis of drusen of the optic nerve head. Ophthalmology 88:1066, 1981
41. Hoover DL, Robb RM, Peterson RA: Optic disc drusen in children. J Pediatr Ophthalmol Strab 25:191, 1988
42. Mansour AM, Hamed LM: Racial variation of optic nerve diseases. Neuroophthalmology 11:319, 1991
43. Lorentzen SE: Drusen of the optic disc: a clinical and genetic study. Acta Ophthalmol 90:1, 1966
44. Rosenberg MA, Savino PJ, Glaser JS: A clinical analysis of pseudopapilledema. I. Population, laterality, acuity, refractive error, ophthalmoscopic characteristics, and coincident disease. Arch Ophthalmol 97:65, 1979
45. Mustonen E: Pseudopapilledema with and without verified optic disc drusen: a clinical analysis I. Acta Ophthalmol 61:1037, 1983
46. Novack RL, Foos RY: Drusen of the optic disc in retinitis pigmentosa. Am J Ophthalmol 103:44, 1987
47. Pierro L, Brancato R, Minicucci M et al: Echographic diagnosis of drusen of the optic nerve head in patients with angioid streaks. Ophthalmologica 208:239, 1994
48. Brown SM, Del Monte MA: Choroidal neovascular membrane associated with optic nerve head drusen in a child. Am J Ophthalmol 121:215, 1996
49. Savino PJ, Glaser JS, Rosenberg MA: A clinical analysis of pseudopapilledema. II. Visual field defects. Arch Ophthalmol 97:71, 1979
50. Mustonen E: Pseudopapilledema with and without verified optic disc drusen: a clinical analysis II. Visual fields. Acta Ophthalmol 61:1057, 1983
51. Gittinger JW, Lessell S, Bondar RL: Ischemic optic neuropathy associated with disc drusen. J Clin Neuroophthalmol 4:79, 1984
52. Beck RW, Corbett JJ, Thompson HS et al: Decreased visual acuity from optic disc drusen. Arch Ophthalmol 103:1155, 1985
53. Moody TA, Irvine AR, Cahn PH et al: Sudden visual field constriction associated with optic disc drusen. J Clin Neuroophthalmol 13:8, 1993
54. Sadun A, Currie JN, Lessell S: Transient visual obscurations with elevated optic discs. Ann Neurol 16:489, 1984

55. Sarkies NJC, Sanders MD: Optic disc drusen and episodic visual loss. Br J Ophthalmol 71:537, 1987
56. Friedman AH, Beckerman B, Gold DH et al: Drusen of the optic disc. Surv Ophthalmol 21:375, 1977
57. Mullie MA, Sanders MD: Computed tomographic diagnosis of buried drusen of the optic nerve head. Can J Ophthalmol 20:114, 1985
58. Moller HU: Recessively inherited, simple optic atrophy: does it exist? Ophthalmic Paediatr Genet 13:31, 1992
59. Francois J: Heredity in Ophthalmology. St. Louis, CV Mosby, 1961
60. Horoupian DS, Zucker DK, Moshe S et al: Behr syndrome: a clinicopathologic report. Neurology 29:323, 1979
61. Costeff H, Elpeleg O, Apter N et al: 3-Methylglutaconic aciduria in "optic atrophy plus." Ann Neurol 33:103, 1993
62. Chalmers RM, Riorden-Eva P, Wood NW: Autosomal recessive inheritance of hereditary motor and sensory neuropathy with optic atrophy. J Neurol Neurosurg Psychiatry 62:385, 1997
63. Shevell MI, Colangelo P, Treacy E et al: Progressive encephalopathy with edema, hypsarryhthmia, and optic atrophy (PEHO syndrome). Pediatr Neurol 15:337, 1996
64. Rizzo JF, Lessell S, Liebman SD: Optic atrophy in familial dysautonomia. Am J Ophthalmol 102:463, 1986
65. Cremers CWRJ, Wijdeveld PGAB, Pinkers AJLG: Juvenile diabetes, optic atrophy, hearing loss, diabetes insipidus, atonia of the urinary tract and bladder, and other abnormalities (Wolfram syndrome): a review of 88 cases from the literature with personal observations on 3 new patients. Acta Paediatr Scand Suppl 264, 1977
66. Lessell S, Rosman NP: Juvenile diabetes mellitus and optic atrophy. Arch Neurol 34:759, 1977
67. Barrett TG, Bundey SE, Macleod AF: Neurodegeneration and diabetes: UK nationwide study of Wolfram (DIDMOAD) syndrome. Lancet 346:1458, 1995
68. Genis D, Davalos A, Molins A, Ferrer I: Wolfram syndrome: a neuropathologic study. Acta Neuropathol (Berl) 93:426, 1997
69. Scolding NJ, Kellar-Wood HF, Shaw C et al: Wolfram syndrome: hereditary diabetes mellitus with brainstem and optic atrophy. Ann Neurol 39:352, 1996
70. Pilz D, Quarell OW, Jones EW: Mitochondrial mutation commonly associated with Leber's hereditary optic neuropathy observed in a patient with Wolfram syndrome (DIDMOAD). J Med Genet 31:328, 1994
71. Barrientos A, Casademont J, Saiz A et al: Autosomal recessive Wolfram syndrome associated with an 8.5-kb mtDNA single deletion. Am J Genet 58:963, 1996
72. Hofmann S, Bezold R, Jaksch M et al: Wolfram (DIDMOAD) syndrome and Leber hereditary optic neuropathy (LHON) are associated with distinct mitochondrial haplotypes. Genomics 39:8, 1997
73. Kjer P: Infantile optic atrophy with dominant mode of inheritance: a clinical and genetic study of 19 Danish families. Acta Ophthalmol Suppl 54, 1959
74. Smith DP: Diagnostic criteria in dominantly inherited juvenile optic atrophy: a report of 3 new families. Am J Optom 49:183, 1972
75. Votruba M, Fitzke FW, Holder GE et al: Clinical features in affected individuals from 21 pedigrees with dominant optic atrophy. Arch Ophthalmol 116:351, 1998
76. Brown J, Fingert JH, Taylor CM et al: Clinical and genetic analysis of a family affected with dominant optic atrophy (OPA1). Arch Ophthalmol 115:95, 1997
77. Johnston RL, Seller MJ, Behman JT et al: Dominant optic atrophy. Refining the clinical diagnostic criteria in light of genetic linkage studies. Ophthalmol 106:123, 1999
78. Kjer B, Eiberg H, Kjer P, Rosenberg T: Dominant optic atrophy mapped to chromosome 3q region. II. Clinical and epidemiologic aspects. Acta Ophthalmol Scand 74:3, 1996
79. Hoyt CS: Autosomal dominant optic atrophy: a spectrum of disability. Ophthalmology 87:245, 1980
80. Grehn F, Kommerell G, Ropers H-H et al: Dominant optic atrophy with sensorineural hearing loss. Ophthalmic Paediatr Genet 1:77, 1982

81. Treft RL, Sanborn GE, Carey J et al: Dominant optic atrophy, deafness, ptosis, ophthalmoplegia, dystaxia, and myopathy: a new syndrome. Ophthalmology 91:908, 1984

82. Chalmers RM, Bird AC, Harding AE: Autosomal dominant optic atrophy with asymptomatic peripheral neuropathy. J Neurol Neurosurg Psychiatry 60:195, 1996

83. Johnston PB, Gaster RN, Smith VC et al: A clinicopathologic study of autosomal dominant optic atrophy. Am J Ophthalmol 88:868, 1979

84. Kjer P, Jensen OA, Klinken L: Histopathology of eye, optic nerve and brain in a case of dominant optic atrophy. Acta Ophthalmol 61:300, 1983

85. Kellar-Wood H, Robertson N, Govan GG et al: Leber's hereditary optic neuropathy mitochondrial DNA mutations in multiple sclerosis. Ann Neurol 36:109, 1994

86. Newman NJ: Optic neuropathy. Neurology 46:315, 1996

87. Mashima Y, Oshitari K, Imamura Y, Momoshima S et al: Orbital high resolution magnetic resonance imaging with fast spin echo in the acute stage of Leber's hereditary optic neuropathy. J Neurol Neurosurg Psychiat 64:124, 1998

88. Nikoskelainen EK, Huoponen K, Juvonen V et al: Ophthalmologic findings in Leber hereditary optic neuropathy, with special reference to mtDNA mutations. Arch Ophathalmol 103:504, 1996

89. Nikoskelainen E, Hoyt WF, Nummelin K et al: Fundus findings in Leber's hereditary optic neuroretinopathy. III. Fluorescein angiographic studies. Arch Ophathalmol 102:981, 1984

90. Newman NJ: Leber's hereditery optic neuropathy: new genetic considerations. Arch Neurol 50:540, 1993

91. Newman NJ, Lott MT, Wallace DC: The clinical characteristics of pedigrees of Lebers' hereditary optic neuropathy with the 11778 mutation. Am J Ophthalmol 111:750, 1991

92. Riordan-Eva P, Sanders MD, Govan GG et al: The clinical features of Leber's hereditary optic neuropathy defined by the presence of a pathogenic mitochondrial DNA mutation. Brain 118:319, 1995

93. Johns DR, Heher KL, Miller NR et al: Leber's hereditary optic neuropathy: clinical manifestations of the 14484 mutation. Arch Ophthalmol 111:495, 1993

94. Mashima Y, Hiida Y, Saga M et al: Risk of false-positive molecular genetic diagnosis of Leber's hereditary optic neuropathy. Am J Ophthalmol 119:245, 1995

95. Johns DR, Smith KH, Miller NR et al: Identical twins who are discordant for Leber's hereditary optic neuropathy. Arch Ophthalmol 111:1491, 1993

96. Hoyt WF: Charcot-Marie-Tooth disease with primary optic atrophy: report of a case. Arch Ophthalmol 64:925, 1960

97. Bird TD, Griep E: Pattern reversal visual evoked potentials: studies in Charcot-Marie-Tooth hereditary neuropathy. Arch Neurol 38:739, 1981

98. Paradiso G, Micheli F, Taratuto AL et al: Familial bulbospinal neuronopathy with optic atrophy: a distinct entity. J Neurol Neurosurg Psychiatry 61:196, 1996

99. Nicolaides P, Appleton RE, Fryer A: Cerebellar ataxia, areflexia, pes cavus, optic atrophy, and sensorineural hearing loss (CAPOS): a new syndrome. J Med Genet 33:419, 1996

100. Groom M, Kay MD, Corrent GF: Optic neuropathy in familial dysautonomia. J Neuroophthalmol 17:101, 1977

101. Livingston IR, Mastaglia FL, Edis R et al: Visual involvement in Friedreich's ataxia and hereditary spastic ataxia: a clinical and visual evoked response study. Arch Neurol 38:75, 1981

102. Frisen L, Claesson M: Narrowing of the retinal arterioles in descending optic atrophy: a quantitative clinical study. Ophthalmology 94:1020, 1984

103. Papastathopoulos K, Jonas JB: Focal narrowing of retinal arterioles in optic nerve atrophy. Ophthalmology 102:1706, 1995

104. Ettl A, Kramer J, Daxer A et al: High resolution magnetic resonance imaging of neurovascular orbital anatomy. Ophthalmology 104:869, 1997

105. Mukhenji SK, Tart RP, Fitzsimmons J et al: Fat-suppressed MR of the orbit and cavernous sinus: comparison of fast spin-echo and conventional spin-echo. AJNR Am J Neuroradiol 15:1707, 1994

106. Davis PC, Newman NJ: Advances in neuro-imaging of the visual pathways. Am J Ophthalmol 121:690, 1996

107. Byrne SF, Green RL: Ultrasound of the Eye and Orbit. St. Louis, CV Mosby, 1992

108. Katz B, Hoyt WF: Intrapapillary and peripapillary hemorrhage in young patients with incomplete posterior vitreous detachment. Ophthalmology 102:349, 1995

109. Kokame GT: Intrapapillary, papillary, and vitreous hemorrhage: letters, and reply. Ophthalmology 102:1003, 1995

110. Sher NA, Wirtschafter J, Shapiro SK et al: Unilateral papilledema in "benign" intracranial hypertension (pseudotumor cerebri). JAMA 250:2346, 1983

111. Liu D, Michon J: Measurement of the subarachnoid pressure of the optic nerve in human subjects. Am J Ophthalmol 119:81, 1994

112. Hayreh SS: Pathogenesis of optic disc oedema. In Kennard C, Rose FC (eds): Physiological Aspects of Clinical Neuro-Ophthalmology, p 431. Chicago, Year Book, 1988

113. Liu D, Kahn M: Measurement and relationship of subarachnoid pressure of the optic nerve to intracranial pressure in fresh cadavers. Am J Ophthalmol 116:548, 1993

114. Peterson RA, Rosenthal A: Retinopathy and papilledema in cyanotic congenital heart disease. Pediatrics 49:243, 1972

115. Bucci FA, Krohel GB: Optic nerve swelling secondary to the obstructive sleep apnea syndrome. Am J Ophthalmol 105:428, 1988

116. Hardten DR, Wen DY, Wirtschafter JD et al: Papilledema and intraspinal lumbar paraganglioma. J Clin Neuroophthalmol 12:158, 1992

117. Michowiz SD, Rappaport HZ, Shaked I et al: Thoracic disc herniation associated with papilledema. J Neurosurg 61:1132, 1984

118. Marks SJ, Schick A, Charney JZ et al: The association of papilledema with syringomyelia: case report. Mt Sinai J Med 55:333, 1988

119. Ropper AH, Marmarou A: Mechanism of pseudotumor in Guillain-Barré syndrome. Arch Neurol 41:259, 1984

120. Stern BJ, Gruen R, Koeppel J et al: Recurrent thyrotoxicosis and papilledema in a patient with communicating hydrocephalus. Arch Neurol 41:65, 1984

121. Scharf D: Neurocysticercosis: two hundred thirty-eight cases from a California hospital. Arch Neurol 45:777, 1988

122. Chimowitz MI, Little JR, Awad IA et al: Intracranial hypertension associated with unruptured cerebral arteriovenous malformations. Ann Neurol 27:474, 1990

123. Verm A, Lee AG: Bilateral optic disk with macular exudates as the manifesting sign of a cerebral arteriovenous malformation. Am J Ophthalmol 123:422, 1997

124. Karahalios DG, Rekate HL, Khayata MH et al: Elevated intracranial venous pressure as a universal mechanism in pseudotumor cerebri of varying etiologies. Neurology 46:198, 1996

125. Marr WG, Chambers RG: Pseudotumor cerebri syndrome following unilateral neck dissection. Am J Ophthalmol 51:605, 1961

126. Graus F, Slatkin NE: Papilledema in the metastatic jugular foramen syndrome. Arch Neurol 40:816, 1983

127. Strominger MB, Weiss GB, Mehler MF: Asymptomatic unilateral papilledema in pseudotumor cerebri. J Clin Neuroophthalmol 12:238, 1992

128. Muci-Mendoza R, Arruga J, Hoyt WF: Distensión bilateral del espacio subaracnoideo perioptico en el pseudotumor cerebral con papiledema unilateral: su demonstración a traves de la tomografia computarizada de la orbita. Rev Neurol 39:11, 1981

129. Pagani LF: The rapid appearence of papilledema. J Neurosurg 30:247, 1969

130. Steffen H, Eifert B, Aschoff A et al: The diagnostic value of optic disc elevation in acute elevated intracranial pressure. Ophthalmology 103:1229, 1996

131. Hilton-Jones D, Ponsford JR, Graham N: Transient visual obscurations, without papilledema. J Neurol Neurosurg Psychiatry 45:832, 1982

132. Hedges TR, Baron EM, Hedges TR et al: The retinal venous pulse: its relation to optic disc characteristics and choroidal pulse. Ophthalmology 101:542, 1994

133. Carter SR, Seifrf SR: Macular changes in pseudotumor cerebri before and after optic nerve sheath fenestration. Ophthalmology 102:937, 1995
134. Jacobson DM: Intracranial hypertension and syndrome of acquired hyperopia and choroidal folds. J Neuroophthalmol 15:178, 1995
135. Corbett JJ, Savino PJ, Thompson HS et al: Visual loss in pseudotumor cerebri: follow-up of 57 patients from five to 41 years and a profile of 14 patients with permanent severe visual loss. Arch Neurol 39:461, 1982
136. Baker RS, Buncic JR: Sudden visual loss in pseudotumor cerebri due to central retinal artery occlusion. Arch Neurol 41:1274, 1984
137. Beck RW, Greenberg HS: Post-decompression optic neuropathy. J Neurosurg 63:196, 1985
138. Mashima Y, Oshitari K, Imamura Y et al: High-rsolution magnetic resonance imaging of the intraorbital optic nerve and subarachnoid space in patients with papilledema and optic atrophy. Arch Ophthalmol 114:1197, 1996
139. Lessell S: Pediatric pseudotumor cerebri (idiopathic intracranial hypertension). Surv Ophthalmol 37:155, 1992
140. Cinciripini GS, Donahue S, Borchert MS: Idiopathic intracranial hypertension in prepubertal pediatric patients: characteristics, treatment, and outcome. Am J Ophthalmol 127:178, 1999
141. Sorensen PS, Gjerris F, Svenstrup B: Endocrine studies in patients with pseudotumor cerebri: estrogen levels in blood and cerebrospinal fluid. Arch Neurol 43:902, 1986
142. Radhakrishnan K, Ahlskog JE, Garrity JA et al: Idiopathic intracranial hypertension. Mayo Clin Proc 69:169, 1994
143. Digre KB, Corbett JJ: Pseudotumor cerebri in men. Arch Neurol 45:866, 1988
144. Borruat FX, Regli F: Pseudotumor cerebri as a complication of amiodarone therapy. Am J Ophthalmol 116:776, 1993
145. Hamed LM, Glaser JS, Schatz NJ et al: Danazol-induced pseudotumor cerebri. Arch Ophthalmol 100:1000, 1989
146. Sanborn GE, Selhorst JB, Calabrese VP et al: Pseudotumor cerebri and insecticide intoxication. Neurology 29:1222, 1979
147. Saul RF, Hamburger HA, Selhorst JB: Pseudotumor cerebri secondary to lithium carbonate. JAMA 253:2869, 1985
148. Green JP, Newman NJ, Stowe ZN et al: "Normal pressure" pseudotumor cerebri. J Neuroophthalmol 16:241, 1996
149. Friedman DI, Forman S, Levi L, Lavin PJ et al: Unusual ocular motility disturbances with increased intracranial pressure. Neurol 50:1893, 1998
150. Moser FG, Hilal SK, Abrams G et al: MR imaging of pseudotumor cerebri. AJNR Am J Neuroradiol 9:39, 1988
151. Wang SJ, Silberstein SD, Patterson S, Young WB: Idiopathic intracranial hypertension without papilledema. A case-control study in a headache center. Neurol 51:245, 1998
151a. Corbett JJ: Problems in the diagnosis and treatment of pseudotumor cerebri. Can J Neurol Sci 10:221, 1983
152. Wall M, George D: Visual loss in pseudotumor cerebri: incidence and defects related to visual field strategy. Arch Neurol 44:170, 1987
153. Hedges TR, Legge RH, Peli E et al: Retinal nerve fiber layer loss in idiopathic intracranial hypertension. Ophthalmology 102:1242, 1995
154. Gu XZ, Tsai JC, Wurdeman A et al: Pattern of axonal loss in longstanding papilledema due to idiopathic intracranial hypertension. Curr Eye Res 14:173, 1995
155. Fan JT, Johnson DH, Burk RR: Transient myopia, angle closure and choroidal detachments after oral acetazolamide. Am J Ophthalmol 115:813, 1993
156. Liu GT, Glaser JS, Schatz NJ: High-dose methylprednisolone and acetazolamide for visual loss in pseudotumor cerebri. Am J Ophthalmol 118:88, 1994
157. Johnson LN, Krohel GB, Madsen RW et al: The role of weight loss and acetazolamide in the treatment of idiopathic intracranial hypertension (pseudotumor cerebri). Ophthalmology 105:2313, 1998
158. Burgett RA, Purvin VA, Kawasaki A: Lumboperitoneal shunting for pseudotumor cerebri. Neurology 49:734, 1997
159. Liu GT, Volpe NJ, Schatz NJ et al: Severe sudden visual loss caused by pseudotumor cerebri and lumboperitoneal shunt failure. Am J Ophthalmol 122:129, 1996
160. Lee AG: Visual loss as the manifesting symptom of ventriculoperitoneal shunt malfunction. Am J Ophthalmol 122:127, 1996
161. Corbett JJ, Nerad JA, Tse DT et al: Results of optic nerve sheath fenestration for pseudotumor cerebri: the lateral orbitotomy approach. Arch Ophthalmol 106:1391, 1988
162. Spoor TC, McHenry JG: Long-term effectiveness of optic nerve sheath decompression for pseudotumor cerebri. Arch Ophthalmol 111:632, 1993
163. Rizzo JF, Lessell S: Choroidal infarction after optic nerve sheath fenestration. Ophthalmology 101:1622, 1994
164. Mauriello JA, Shaderowsky P, Gizzi M et al: Management of visual loss after optic nerve sheath decompression in patients with pseudotumor cerebri. Ophthalmology 102:441, 1995
165. Mathew NT, Ravishankar K, Sanin LC: Coexistence of migraine and idiopathic intracranial hypertension without papilledema. Neurology 46:1226, 1996
166. Magnante DO, Bullock JD: Familial pseudotumor cerebri: occurrence in a mother while pregnant with a subsequently affected daughter. (personal communication)
167. Lam BL, Schatz NJ, Glaser JS et al: Pseudotumor cerebri from cranial venous obstruction. Ophthalmology 99:706, 1992
168. Purvin VA, Trobe JD, Kosmorsky G: Neuro-ophthalmic features of cerebral venous obstruction. Arch Neurol 52:880, 1995
169. Hauser D, Barzilai N, Zalish M et al: Bilateral papilledema with retinal hemorrhages in association with cerebral venous sinus thrombosis and paroxysmal nocturnal hemoglobinuria. Am J Opthalmol 122:592, 1996
170. Ireland B, Corbett JJ, Wallace R: The search for causes of idiopathic intracranial hypertension. Arch Neurol 47:315, 1990
171. FDA Medwatch and Spontaneous Reporting System. Norplant 1991–1993. Obstet Gynecol 85:538, 1995
172. Malozowski S, Tanner LA, Wysowski DK et al: Benign intracranial hypertension in children with growth hormone deficiency treated with growth hormone. J Pediatr 126:996, 1995
173. Alexandrakis G, Filatov, Walsh T: Pseudotumor cerebri in a 12-year-old boy with Addison's disease. Am J Ophthalmol 116:650, 1993
174. Liu GT, Kay MD, Bienfang DC et al: Pseudotumor cerebri associated with corticosteroid withdrawal in inflammatory bowel disease. Am J Ophthalmol 117:352, 1994
175. Sirdofsky M, Kattah J, Macedo P: Intracranial hypertension in a dieting patient. J Neuro-ophthalmol 14:9, 1994
175a. Chiu AM, Chuenkongkaew WL, Cornblath W, et al: Minocycline treatment and pseudotumor cerebri syndrome. Am J Ophthalmol 126:116, 1998
176. Jennum P, Borgesen SE: Intracranial pressure and obstructive sleep apnea. Chest 95:279, 1989
177. Landau K, Gloor BP: Therapy resistant papilledema in achondroplasia. J Neuroophthalmol 14:24, 1994
178. Stavrou P, Sgouros S, Willshaw HE et al: Visual failure caused by raised intracranial pressure in craniosynostosis. Childs Nerv Syst 13:64, 1997
179. Johnston I, Hawke S, Halmagyi M et al: The pseudotumor syndrome: disorders of cerebrospinal fluid circulation causing intracranial hypertension without ventriculomegaly. Arch Neurol 48:740, 1991
180. Katz B: The dyschromatopsia of optic neuritis. Trans Am Ophthalmol Soc 93:685, 1995
181. Mojon DS, Rösler KM, Oetliker H: A bedside test to determine motion stereopsis using the Pulfrich phenomenon. Ophthalmol 105:1337, 1998
182. Selhorst JB, Saul RF: Uhthoff and his symptom. J Neuroophthalmol 15:63, 1995
183. Keltner JL, Johnson CA, Spurr JO et al: Visual field profile of optic neuritis: one-year follow-up in the optic neuritis treatment trial. Arch Ophthalmol 112:946, 1994
184. Kennedy C, Caroll FD: Optic neuritis in children. Trans Am Acad Ophthalmol Otolaryngol 64:700, 1960
185. Riikonen R: The role of infection and vacination in the genesis of optic neuritis and multiple sclerosis in children. Acta Neurol Scand 80:425, 1989
186. Lucchinetti CF, Kiers L, O'Duffy A et al: Risk factors for

developing multiple sclerosis after childhood optic neuritis. Neurology 49:1413, 1997

187. Hamed LM, Silbiger J, Guy J et al: Parainfectious optic neuritis and encephalomyelitis: a report of two cases with thalamic involvement. J Clin Neuroophthalmol 13:18, 1993

188. Purvin VA, Chioran G: Recurrent neuroretinitis. Arch Ophthalmol 112:365, 1994

189. Beck RW, Cleary PA, Trobe JD et al: The effect of corticosteroids for acute optic neuritis on the subsequent development of multiple sclerosis. N Engl J Med 329:1764, 1993

190. Warner JEA, Lessell S, Rizzo JF et al: Does optic disc appearance distinguish ischemic optic neuropathy from optic neuritis. Arch Ophthalmol 115:1408, 1997

191. Guy J, Mao J, Bidgood WD et al: Enhancement and demyelination of the intraorbital optic nerve: fat suppression magnetic resonance imagining. Ophthalmology 99:713, 1992

192. Dunker S, Wiegand W: Prognostic value of magnetic resonance imaging in monosymptomatic optic neuritis. Ophthalmology 103:1768, 1996

193. Beck RW, Kupersmith MJ, Cleary PA et al: Fellow eye abnormalities in acute unilateral optic neuritis. Ophthalmology 100:691, 1993

194. Cleary PA, Beck RW, Bourque LB et al: Visual symptoms after optic neuritis: results from the Optic Neuritis Treatment Trial. J Neuroophthalmol 17:18, 1997

195. Jacobs L, Karpik A, Bozian D et al: Auditory-visual synesthesia. Arch Neurol 38:211, 1981

196. Safran AB, Kine LB, Glaser JS: Positive visual phenomena in optic nerve and chiasm disease: photopsias and photophobia. In Glaser JS (ed): Neuro-ophthalmology, Vol X, p 225. St. Louis, CV Mosby, 1980

197. Kaufman DI, Beck R, ONTT Study Group: The 5-year risk of MS after optic neuritis: experience of the Optic Neuritis Treatment Trial. Neurology 49:1404, 1997

198. Jacobs LD, Kaba SE, Miller CM et al: Correlation of clinical: magnetic resonance imaging, and cerebrospinal fluid findings in optic neuritis. Ann Neurol 41:392, 1997

199. Francis DA, Compston DA, Batchelor JR et al: A reassessment of the risk of multiple sclerosis developing in patients with optic neuritis after extended follow-up. J Neurol Neurosurg Psychiatry 50:6, 1987

200. Soderstom M, Ya-Ping J, Hillert J et al: Optic neuritis. Prognosis for multiple sclerosis from MRI, CSF, and HLA findings. Neurology 50:708, 1998

201. Lightman S, McDonald WI, Bird AC et al: Retinal venous sheathing in optic neuritis: its significance for pathogenesis of multiple sclerosis. Brain 100:405, 1987

202. Engell T: Neurological disease activity in multiple sclerosis patients with periphlebitis retinae. Acta Neurol Scand 73:168, 1986

203. Malinowski SM, Pulido JS, Folk JC: Long-term visual outcome and complications associated with pars planitis. Ophthalmology 100:818, 1993

204. Gass A, Graham E, Moseley IF et al: Cranial MRI in idiopathic retinal vasculitis. J Neurol 242:174, 1995

205. Cole SR, Beck RW, Moke PS et al: The predictive value of CSF oligoclonal banding for MS 5 years after optic neuritis. Optic Neuritis Study Group. Neurol 51:885, 1998

206. Mandler RN, Davis LE, Jeffrey DR et al: Devic's neuromyelitis optica: a clinocopathologic study of 8 patients. Ann Neurol 34:162, 1993

207. O'Riordan JI, Gallagher HL, Thompson AJ et al: Clinical, CSF and MRI findings in Devic's neuromyelitis optica. J Neurol Neurosurg Psychiatry 60:382, 1996

208. Brazis PW, Lee AG: Optic disk edema with a macular star. Mayo Clin Proc 71:1162, 1996

209. Ellis BD, Kosmorsky GS, Cohen BH. Medical and surgical management of acute disseminated encephalomyelitis. J Neuroophthalmol 14:210, 1994

210. Hamed LM, Silbiger J, Guy J et al: Parainfectious optic neuritis and encephalomyelitis. J Neuroophthalmol 13:18, 1993

211. Kawasaki A, Purvin VA, Tang R: Bilateral anterior ischemic optic neuropathy following influenza vaccination. J Neuroophthalmol 18:56, 1998

212. Hull TP, Bates JH: Optic neuritis after influenza vaccination. Am J Ophthalmol 124:703, 1997

213. Pall HS, Williams AC: Subacute polyradiculopathy with optic and auditory nerve involvement. Arch Neurol 44:885, 1987

214. Borruat FX, Schatz NJ, Glaser JS, Forteza A: Central nervous system involvement in Guillain-Barré–like syndrome: clinical and magnetic resonance imaging evidence. Eur Neurol 38:129, 1997

215. Miller DH, Kay R, Schon F et al: Optic neuritis following chickenpox in adults. J Neurol 233:182, 1986

216. Selbst RG, Selhorst JB, Harbison JW et al: Parainfectious optic neuritis. Arch Neurol 40:347, 1983

217. Berrios RR, Serrano LA: Bilateral optic neuritis after a bee sting. Am J Ophthalmol 117:677, 1994

218. Keane J. Neuro-ophthalmologic signs of AIDS: 50 patients. Neurology 41:841, 1991

219. Nichols JW, Goodwin JA: Neuro-ophthalmologic complications of AIDS. Semin Ophthalmol 7:24, 1992

220. Tenhula WN, Xu SZ, Madigan MC et al: Morphometric comparisons of optic nerve axon loss in acquired immunodeficiency syndrome. Am J Ophthalmol 113:14, 1992

221. Patel SS, Rutzen AR, Marx JL et al: Cytomegalovirus papillitis in patients with acquired immune deficiency syndrome. Ophthalmology 103:1476, 1996

222. Cohen DB, Glasgow BJ: Bilateral optic nerve cryptococcosis in sudden blindness in patients with acquired immune deficiency syndrome. Ophthalmology 100:1689, 1993

223. Garrity JA, Herman DC, Imes R et al: Optic nerve sheath decompression for visual loss in patients with acquired immunodeficiency syndrome and cryptococcal meningitis with papilledema. Am J Ophthalmol 116:472, 1993

224. Grossniklaus HE, Specht CS, Allaire G et al: *Toxoplasma gondii* retinochoroiditis and optic neuritis in acquired immune deficiency syndrome: report of a case. Ophthalmology 97:1342, 1990

225. Shayegani A, Odel JG, Kazim M et al: Varicella-zoster virus optic neuritis in a patient with human immunodeficiency virus. Am J Ophthalmol 122:586, 1996

226. Lee MS, Cooney EL, Stoessel KM et al: Varicella zoster virus retrobulbar optic neuritis in patients with acquired immunodeficiency syndrome. Ophthalmology 105:467, 1998

227. Yau TH, Rivera-Velazquez, Mark AS et al: Unilateral optic neuritis in a patient with the acquired immunodeficiency syndrome. Am J Ophthalmol 121:324, 1996

228. Gabuzda DH, Hirsch MS: Neurologic manifestations of infection with human immunodeficiency virus. Ann Intern Med 107:383, 1987

229. Burton BJL, Leff AP: Plant steroid–responsive HIV optic neuropathy. J Neuroophthalmol 18:25, 1998

230. Margo CE, Hamed LM: Ocular syphilis. Surv Ophthalmol 37:203, 1992

231. Zambrano W, Perez GM, Smith JL: Acute syphilitic blindness in AIDS. J Clin Neuroophthalmol 7:1, 1987

232. Toshniwal P: Optic perineuritis with secondary syphilis. J Clin Neuroophthalmol 7:6, 1987

233. Arruga J, Valentines J, Mauri F et al: Neuroretinitis in acquired syphilis. Ophthalmology 92:262, 1985

234. Balcer LJ, Winterkorn JMS, Galetta SL: Neuro-ophthalmic manifestations of Lyme disease. J Neuroophthalmol 17:108, 1997

235. Schmutzhard E, Pohl P, Stanek G: Involvement of *Borrelia burgdorferi* in cranial nerve affection. Zentrabl Bakt Hyg A 263:328, 1986

236. Pachner AR, Steere AC: The triad of neurologic manifestations of Lyme disease: meningitis, cranial neuritis, and radiculoneuritis. Neurology 35:47, 1985

237. Wu G, Lincoff H, Ellsworth RM et al: Optic disc edema and Lyme disease. Ann Ophthalmol 18:252, 1986

238. Strominger MB, Slamovits TL, Herskovitz S et al: Transient worsening of optic neuropathy as a sequela of the Jarisch-Herxheimer reaction in the treatment of Lyme disease. J Neuroophthalmol 14:77, 1994

239. Lyme disease: Connecticut. JAMA 259:1147, 1988

240. Wong MT, Dolan MJ, Lattuada CP et al: Neuroretinitis, aseptic meningitis, and lymphadenitis associated with *Bartonella*

henselae infection in immunocompetent patients and patients infected with human immunodeficiency virus type 1. Clin Infect Dis 21:352, 1995

241. Golnik KC, Marotto ME, Fanous MM et al: Ophthalmic manifestations of *Rochalimaea* species. Am J Ophthalmol 118:145, 1994

242. Reed JB, Scales DK, Wong MT et al: *Bartonella henselae* neuroretinitis in cat scratch disease: diagnosis, management, and sequelae. Ophthalmology 105:459, 1998

243. Cox TA, Haskins GE, Gangitano JL et al: Bilateral *Toxacara* optic neuropathy. J Clin Neuroophthalmol 3:267, 1983

244. Fish RH, Hoskins JC, Kline LB: Toxoplasmosis neuroretinitis. Ophthalmology 100:1177, 1993

245. Lossos A, Eliashiv S, Ben-Chetrit E: Optic neuritis associated with familial Mediterranean fever. J Clin Neuroophthalmol 13:141, 1993

246. Ormerod IEC, McDonald WI: Multiple sclerosis presenting with progressive visual failure. J Neurol Neurosurg Psychiatry 47:943, 1984

247. Eidelberg D, Newton MR, Johnson G et al: Chronic unilateral optic neuropathy: a magnetic resonance study. Ann Neurol 24:3, 1988

248. Fay AM, Kane SA, Kazim M et al: Magnetic resonance imaging of optic perineuritis. J Neuroophthalmol 17:247, 1997

249. Dutton JJ, Anderson RL: Idiopathic inflammatory perioptic neuritis simulating optic nerve sheath meningioma. Am J Ophthalmol 100:424, 1985

250. Hykin PG, Spalton DJ: Bilateral perineuritis of the optic nerves. J Neurol Neurosurg Psychiatry 54:375, 1991

251. Winterkorn JM, Odel JG, Behrens MM et al: J Neuroophthalmol 14:157, 1994

252. Frohman L, Wolansky L: Magnetic resonance imaginging of syphilitic optic perineuritis. J Neuroophthalmol 17:57, 1997

253. Beardsley TL, Brown SVL, Sydnor CF et al: Eleven cases of sarcoidosis of the optic nerve. Am J Ophthalmol 97:62, 1984

254. Vrabec TR, Augsburger JJ, Fisccher DH et al: Taches de bougie. Ophthalmology 102:1712, 1995

255. Akova YA, Kansu T, Duman S: Pseudotumor cerebri secondary to dural sinus thrombosis in neurosarcoidosis. J Clin Neuroophthalmol 13:188, 1993

256. Beck AD, Newman NJ, Grossniklaus HE et al: Optic nerve enlargement and chronic visual loss. Surv Ophthalmol 38:555, 1994

257. Newman LS, Rose CS, Maier LA: Sarcoidosis. N Engl J Med 336:1224, 1997

258. Belden CJ, Hamed L, Mancuso AA: Bilateral isolated retrobulbar optic neuropathy in limited Wegener's granulomatosis. J Clin Neuroophthalmol 13:119, 1993

259. Slavin M, Glaser JS: Acute severe irreversible visual loss with sphenoethmoiditis: "posterior" orbital cellulitis. Arch Ophthalmol 105:345, 1987

260. Kodsi SR, Younge BR, Leavitt JA et al: Intracranial plasma cell granuloma presenting as an optic neuropathy. Surv Ophthalmol 38:70, 1993

261. Ofner S, Baker RS: Visual loss in cryptococcal meningitis. J Clin Neuropophthalmol 7:45, 1987

262. Lee MS, Cooney EL, Stoessel KM et al: Varicella zoster virus retrobulbar optic neuritis preceding retinitis in patients with acquired immunodeficiency syndrome. Ophthalmology 105:467, 1998

263. Borruat FX, Herbort CP: Herpes zoster ophthalmicus: anterior ischemic optic neuropathy and acyclovir. J Clin Neuroophthalmol 12:37, 1992

264. Lam BL, Barrett DA, Glaser JS et al: Visual loss from idiopathic intracranial pachymeningitis. Neurology 44:694, 1994

265. Hayreh SS: The optic nerve head circulation in health and disease. Exp Eye Res 61:259, 1995

266. Onda E, Ciofi GA, Bacon DR, van Buskirk EM: Microvasculature of the human optic nerve. Am J Ophthalmol 120:92, 1995

267. Hattenhauer MG, Leavitt JA, Hodge DO et al: Incidence of nonarteritic anterior ischemic optic neuropathy. Am J Ophthalmol 123:103, 1997

268. IONDT Study Group: Characteristics of patients with nonarteritic anterior ischemic neuropathy eligible for the ischemic optic neuropathy decompression trial. Arch Ophthalmol 114:1366, 1996

269. Hayreh SS, Joos KM, Podhajsky PA et al: Systemic diseases associated with nonarteritic anterior ischemic optic neuropathy. Am J Ophthalmol 118:766, 1994

270. Kline LB: Progression of visual field defects in ischemic optic neuropathy. Am J Ophthalmol 106:199, 1988

271. Movsas T, Kelman SE, Elman MJ et al: The natural course of non-arteritic ischemic optic neuropathy. Invest Ophthalmol Vis Sci 42:951, 1991

272. Borchert M, Lessell S: Progressive and recurrent nonarteritic anterior ischemic optic neuropathy. Am J Ophthalmol 106:443, 1988

273. Arnold AC, Hepler RS: Natural history of nonarteritic anterior ischemic optic neuropathy. J Neuroophthalmol 14:66, 1994

274. Gordon RN, Burde RM, Slamovits T: Asymptomatic optic disc edema. J Neuroophthalmol 17:29, 1997

275. Hayreh SS: Acute ischemic disorders of the optic nerve: pathogenesis, clinical manifestations, and management. Ophthalmol Clin North Am 9:407, 1996

276. Olver JM, Spalton DJ, McCartney ACE: Microvascular study of the retrolaminar optic nerve in man: the possible significance in anterior ischemic optic neuropathy. Eye 4:7, 1990

277. Arnold AC, Hepler RS: Fluorescein angiography in acute nonarteritic anterior ischemic optic neuropathy. Am J Ophthalmol 117:222, 1994

278. Kalenak JW, Kosmorsky GS, Rockwood EJ: Nonarteritic anterior ischemic optic neuropathy and intraocular pressure. Arch Ophthalmol 109:660, 1991

279. Hayreh SS, Podhajsky PA, Zimmerman B: Nonarteritic anterior ischemic optic neuropathy: time of onset of visual loss. Am J Ophthalmol 124:641, 1997

280. Rizzo JF, Lessell S: Optic neuritis and ischemic optic neuropathy: overlapping clinical profiles. Arch Ophthalmol 109:1668, 1991

281. Trobe JD, Glaser JS, Cassady JC et al: Nonglaucomatous excavation of the optic disc. Arch Ophthalmol 98:1046, 1980

282. Trobe JD, Glaser JS, Cassady JC: Optic atrophy: differential diagnosis by fundus observation alone. Arch Ophthalmol 98:1040, 1980

283. Frisen L, Claesson M: Narrowing of the retinal arterioles in descending optic atrophy: a quantitative clinical study. Ophthalmology 91:1342, 1984

284. Beri M, Klugman MR, Kohler JA et al: Anterior ischemic optic neuropathy. VII. Incidence of bilaterality and various influencing factors. Ophthalmology 94:1020, 1987

285. Boone MI, Massry GG, Frankel RA et al: Visual outcome in bilateral nonarteritic anterior ischemic optic neuropathy. Ophthalmology 103:1223, 1996

286. WuDunn D, Zimmerman K, Sadun AA, Feldon SE: Comparison of visual function in fellow eyes after bilateral nonarteritic anterior ischemic optic neutropathy. Ophthalmology 104:104, 1997

287. Lepore FE, Yarian DL: A mimic of the "exact diagnostic sign" of Foster Kennedy. Ann Ophthalmol 17:411, 1985

288. Fry CL, Carter JE, Kanter MC et al: Anterior ischemic optic neuropathy is not associated with carotid artery atherosclerosis. Stroke 24:539, 1993

289. Arnold AC, Hepler RS, Hamilton DR, Lufkin RB: Magnetic resonance imaging of the brain in nonarteritic ischemic optic neuropathy. J Neuroophthalmol 15:158, 1995

290. Giuffre G: Hematologic risk factors for anterior ischemic optic neuropathy. Neuroophthalmology 10:197, 1990

291. Watts MT, Greaves M, Rennie IG et al: Antiphospholipid antibodies in the aetiology of of ischaemic optic neuropathy. Eye 5:75, 1991

292. Worrall BB, Moazami G, Odel JG et al: Anterior ischemic optic neuropathy and activated protein C resistance: a case report and review of the literature. J Neuroophthalmol 17:162, 1997

293. Talks SJ, Chong NH, Gibson JM, Dodson PM: Fibrinogen, cholesterol and smoking as risk factors for non-arteritic anterior ischemic optic neuropathy. Eye 9:85, 1995

294. Beck RW, Servais GE, Hayreh SS: Anterior ischemic optic

neuropathy. IX. Cup-to-disc ratio and its role in pathogenesis. Ophthalmology 94:1503, 1987

295. Mansour AM, Shoch D, Logani S: Optic disk size in ischemic optic neuropathy. Am J Ophthalmol 106:587, 1988

296. Katz B, Spencer WH: Hyperopia as a risk factor for nonarteritic anterior ischemic optic neuropathy. Am J Ophthalmol 116:754, 1993

297. Arnold AC, Hepler RS, Lieber M, Alexander JM: Hyperbaric oxygen therapy for nonarteritic anterior ischemic optic neuropathy. Am J Ophthalmol 122:535, 1996

298. Johnson LN, Gould TJ, Krohel GB: Effect of levodopa and carbidopa on recovery of visual function in patients with nonarteritic anterior ischemic optic neuropathy of longer than six months' duration. Am J Ophthalmol 121:77, 1996

299. Beck RW, Hayreh SS, Podhajsky PA et al: Aspirin in nonarteritic anterior ischemic optic neuropathy. Am J Ophthalmol 123:212, 1997

300. Kupersmith MJ, Frohman L, Sanderson M et al: Aspirin reduces the incidence of second eye NAION: a retrospective study. J Neuroophthalmol 17:250, 1997

301. Ischemic Optic Neuropathy Decompression Trial Research Group: Optic nerve decompression surgery for nonarteritic anterior ischemic optic neuropathy (NAION) is not effective and may be harmful. JAMA 273:625, 1995

302. Glaser JS, Teimory M, Schatz NJ: Optic nerve sheath fenestration for progressive ischemic optic neuropathy. Arch Ophthalmol 112:1047, 1994

303. Yee RD, Selky AK, Purvin VA: Outcomes of surgical and nonsurgical management of nonarteritic ischemic optic neuropathy. Trans Am Ophthmalol Soc 91:227, 1993

304. Johnson LN, Arnold AC: Incidence of nonarteritic and arteritic anterior ischemic optic neuropathy. J Neuroophthalmol 14:38, 1994

305. Chung SM, Gay CA, McCrary JA: Nonarteritic ischemic optic neuropathy: the impact of tobacco use. Ophthalmology 101:779, 1994

306. Hayreh SS, Podhajsky PA, Zimmerman B: Ocular manifestations of cranial arteritis. Am J Ophthalmol 125:509, 1998

307. Tomlinson FH, Lie JT, Nienhuis BJ et al: Juvenile temporal arteritis revisited. Mayo Clin Proc 69:445, 1994

308. Weyand CM, Bartley GB: Giant cell arteritis: new concepts in pathogenesis and implications for management. Am J Ophthalmol 123:392, 1997

309. Wagner AD, Bjornsson J, Bartley GB et al: Interferon gamma–producing T cells in giant cell vasculitis represent a minority of tissue-infiltrating cells and located distant from the site of pathology. Am J Pathol 148:1925, 1996

310. Ghanci FD, Dutton GN: Current concepts in giant cell (temporal) arteritis. Surv Ophthalmol 42:99, 1997

311. Hauser WA, Ferguson RH, Holley KE et al: Temporal arteritis in Rochester, Minnesota, 1951 to 1967. Mayo Clin Proc 46:597, 1971

312. Turnbull J: Temporal arteritis and polymyalgia rheumatica: nosographic and nosologic considerations. Neurology 46:901, 1996

313. Hayreh SS, Podhajsky P: Visual field defects in anterior ischemic optic neuropathy. Doc Ophthalmol Proc Ser 19:53, 1979

314. Beri M, Klugman MR, Kohler JA et al: Anterior ischemic optic neuropathy. VII. Incidence of bilaterality and various influencing factors. Ophthalmology 94:1020, 1987

315. Sebag J, Thomas JV, Epstein EL et al: Optic disc cupping in arteritic anterior ischemic optic neuropathy resembles glaucomatous cupping. Ophthalmology 93:357, 1986

316. Melberg NS, Grand MG, Diekert JP et al: Cotton-wool spots and early diagnosis of giant cell arteritis. Ophthalmology 102:1611, 1995

317. Barricks ME, Traviesa DB, Glaser JS, Levy IS: Ophthalmoplegia in cranial arteritis. Brain 100:209, 1977

318. Bienfang DC: Loss of the ocular pulse in the acute phase of temporal arteritis. Acta Ophthalmol Suppl 191:35, 1989

319. Bosley TM, Savino PJ, Sergott RC et al: Ocular pneumoplethysmography can help in the diagnosis of giant-cell arteritis. Arch Ophthalmol 107:379, 1989

320. Siatkowski RM, Gass JDM, Glaser JS et al: Fluorescein angiography in the diagnosis of giant cell arteritis. Am J Ophthalmol 115:57, 1993

321. Slavin ML, Barondes MJ: Visual loss caused by choroidal ischemia preceding anterior ischemic optic neuropathy in giant cell arteritis. Am J Ophthalmol 117:81, 1994

322. Ho AC, Sergott RC, Regillo CD et al: Color Doppler hemodynamics of giant cell arteritis. Arch Ophthalmol 112:938, 1994

323. Schmidt WA, Kraft HE, Vorpahl K et al: Color duplex ultrasonography in the diagnosis of temporal arteritis. N Engl J Med 337:1336, 1997

324. Andersson R, Malvall BE, Bengtsson BA: Long-term survival in giant cell arteritis including remporal arteritis and polymyalgia rheumatica. Acta Med Scand 220:361, 1986

325. Aiello PD, Trautman JC, McPhee TJ et al: Visual prognosis in giant cell arteritis. Ophthalmology 100:550, 1993

326. Liu GT, Glaser JS, Schatz NJ, Smith JL: Visual morbidity in giant cell arteritis: clinical characteristics and prognosis for vision. Ophthalmology 101:1779, 1994

327. Hayreh SS, Podhajsky PA, Raman R, Zimmerman B: Giant cell arteritis: validity and reliability of various diagnostic criteria. Am J Ophthalmol 123:285, 1997

328. Cullen JF: Ischemic optic neuropathy. Trans Ophthalmol Soc UK 87:759, 1967

329. Miller A, Green M: Simple rule for calculating normal erythrocyte sedimentation rate. BMJ 286:266, 1983

330. Gruener G, Merchut MP: Renal causes of elevated sedimentation rate in suspected temporal arteritis. J Clin Neuroophthalmol 12:272, 1992

331. Klein RG, Campbell RJ, Hunder GG, Carney JA: Skip lesions in temporal arteritis. Mayo Clin Proc 51:504, 1976

332. Nishino H, DeRemee RA, Rubino FA et al: Wegener's granulomatosis associated with vasculitis of the temporal artery: report of five cases. Mayo Clin Proc 68:115, 1993

333. Levy MH, Margo CE: Temporal artery biopsy and sarcoidosis. Am J Ophthalmol 117:409, 1994

334. Goodman BW: Temporal arteritis. Am J Med 67:839, 1979

335. Wilkinson IMS, Russell RWR: Arteries of the head and neck in giant cell arteritis: a pathological study to show the pattern of arterial involvement. Arch Neurol 27:378, 1972

336. Cornblath WT, Eggenberger ER: Progressive visual loss from giant cell arteritis despite high-dose intravenous methylprednisolone. Ophthalmology 104:854, 1997

337. Gardiner PVG, Griffiths ID: Sudden death after treatment with pulsed methylprednisolone. BMJ 300:125, 1990

338. Matteson EL, Gold KN, Bloch DA et al: Long-term survival of patients with giant cell arteritis in the American College of Rheumatology giant cell arteritis criteria cohort. Am J Med 100:193, 1996

339. van der Veen MJ, Dinant HJ, Vam Booma-Frankfort C et al: Can methotrexate be used as a steroid sparing agent in the treatment of polymyalgia rheumatica and giant cell arteritis? Ann Rheum Dis 55:218. 1996

340. Demaziere A: Dapsone in the long-term treatment of temporal arteritis. Am J Med 87:3, 1989

341. Skillern PG, Lockhart G: Optic neuritis and uncontrolled diabetes mellitus in 14 patients. Ann Intern Med 51:468, 1959

342. Lubow M, Makley TA: Pseudopapilledema of juvenile diabetes mellitus. Arch Ophthalmol 85:417, 1971

343. Barr CC, Glaser JS, Blankenship G: Acute disc swelling in juvenile diabetes: clinical profile and natural history of 12 cases. Arch Ophthalmol 98:2185, 1980

344. Regillo CD, Brown GC, Savino PJ et al: Diabetic papillopathy: patient characteristics and fundus findings. Arch Ophthalmol 113:889, 1995

345. Carroll FD: Optic nerve complications of cataract extraction. Trans Am Acad Ophthalmol Otolaryngol 77:623, 1973

346. Hayreh SS: Anterior ischemic optic neuropathy. IV. Occurrence after cataract extraction. Arch Ophthalmol 98:1410, 1980

347. Serrano LA, Behrens MM, Carroll FD: Postcataract extraction ischemic optic neuropathy. Arch Ophthalmol 100:1177, 1982

348. Hamed LM, Purvin V, Rosenberg M: Recurrent anterior ischemic optic neuropathy in young adults. J Clin Neuroophthalmol 8:239, 1988

349. O'Hara M, O'Connor PS: Migrainous optic neuropathy. J Clin Neuro Ophthalmol 4:85, 1984

350. Katz B: Bilateral sequential migrainous ischemic optic neuropathy. Am J Ophthalmol 99:489, 1985

351. Toshniwal P: Anterior ischemic optic neuropathy secondary to cluster headache. Acta Neurol Scand 73:213, 1986

352. Hayreh SS: Anterior ischemic optic neuropathy. VIII. Clinical features and pathogenesis of post-hemorrhagic amaurosis. Ophthalmology 94:1488, 1987

353. Williams EL, Hart WM, Tempelhoff R: Postoperative ischemic optic neuropathy. Anesth Analg 80:1018, 1995

354. Hollenhorst RW, Svein HJ, Benoit CF: Unilateral blindness occurring during anesthesia for neurosurgical operations. Arch Ophthalmol 52:819, 1954

355. Katz DM, Trobe JD, Cornblath WT, Kline LB: Ischemic optic neuropathy after lumbar spine surgery. Arch Ophthalmol 112:925, 1994

356. Jaben SL, Glaser JS, Daily M: Ischemic optic neuropathy following general surgical procedures. J Clin Neuroophthalmol 3:239, 1983

357. Johnson MW, Kincaid MC, Trobe JD: Bilateral retrobulbar optic nerve infarctions after blood loss and hypotension: a clinicopathologic case study. Ophthalmology 94:1577, 1987

358. Connolly SE, Gordon KB, Horton JC: Salvage of vision after hypotension-induced ischemic optic neuropathy. Am J Ophthalmol 117:235, 1994

359. Shapira OM, Kimmel WA, Lindsey PS et al: Anterior ischemic optic neuropathy after open heart operations. Ann Thorac Surg 61:660, 1996

360. Slavin ML: Ischemic optic neuropathy after cardiac arrest. Am J Ophthalmol 104:435, 1987

361. Knox DL, Hanneken AM, Hollows FC et al: Uremic optic neuropathy. Arch Ophthalmol 106:50, 1988

362. Hamed LM, Winward KE, Glaser JS et al: Optic neuropathy in uremia. Am J Ophthalmol 108:30, 1989

363. Michaelson C, Behrens M, Odel J: Bilateral anterior ischemic optic neuropathy associated with optic disc drusen and systemic hypotension. Br J Ophthalmol 73:767, 1989

364. Waybright EA, Selhorst JB, Combs J: Anterior ischemic optic neuropathy with internal carotid artery occlusion. Am J Ophthalmol 93:42, 1982

365. Brown GC: Anterior ischemic optic neuropathy occurring in association with carotid artery obstruction. J Clin Neuroophthalmol 6:39, 1986

366. Bogousslavsky J, Regli F, Zografos L et al: Optico-cerebral syndrome: simultaneous hemodynamic infarction of optic nerve and brain. Neurology 37:263, 1987

367. Leonard TJK, Sanders MD: Ischaemic optic neuropathy in pulseless disease. Br J Ophthalmol 67:389, 1983

368. Hall S, Barr W, Lie JT et al: Takayasu arteritis: a study of 32 North American patients. Medicine 64:89, 1985

369. Liebermann MF, Shahi A, Grenn WR: Embolic ischemic optic neuropathy. Am J Ophthalmol 86:206, 1978

370. Tomsak RL: Ischemic optic neuropathy associated with retinal embolism. Am J Ophthalmol 99:590, 1985

371. Beck RW, Gamel JW, Willcourt RJ et al: Acute ischemic optic neuropathy in severe preeclampsia. Am J Ophthalmol 90:342, 1980

372. DeFrancisco M, Savino PJ, Schatz NJ: Optic atrophy in acute intermittent porphyria. Am J Ophthalmol 87:221, 1979

373. Manor RS, Axer-Siegal R, Cohenn S et al: Bilateral anterior ischemic optic neuropathy, pseudoxanthoma elasticum, and platelet hyperaggregability. Neuroophthalmology 6:173, 1986

374. Slavin ML, Barondes MJ: Ischemic optic neuropathy in sickle cell disease. Am J Ophthalmol 105:212, 1988

375. Perlman JI, Forman S, Gonzalez ER. Retrobulbar ischemic optic neuropathy associated with sickle cell disease. J Neuroophthalmol 14:45, 1994

376. Sklar EML, Schatz NJ, Glaser JS et al: MR of vasculitis-induced optic neuropathy. AJNR Am J Neuroradiol 17:121, 1996

377. Ahmadieh H, Roodpeyma S, Azarmina M et al: Bilateral simultaneous optic neuritis in chidhood systemic lupus erythematosus. J Neuroophthalmol 14:84, 1994

378. Frohman LP, Lama P: Annual review of systemic diseases: 1995–1996. I. J Neuroophthalmol 18:67, 1998

379. Tesar JT, McMillan V, Molina R et al: Optic neuropathy and central nervous system disease assoiciated with Sjögren's syndrome. Am J Med 92:686, 1992

380. Hutchinson CH: Polyarteritis nodosa presenting as posterior ischemic optic neuropathy. J R Soc Med 77:1043, 1984

381. Massry GG, Chung SM, Selhorst JB: Optic neuropathy, headache, and diplopia with MRI suggestive of cerebral arteritis in relapsing polychondritis. J Neuroophthalmol 15:171, 1995

382. Schmidt MH, Fox AJ, Nicolle DA: Bilateral anterior ischemic optic neuropathy as a presentation of Takayasu's disease. J Neuroophthalmol 17:156, 1997

383. Isayama Y, Takahashi T, Inoue M et al: Posterior ischemic optic neuropathy. III. Clinical diagnosis. Ophthalmologica 187:141, 1983

384. Sawle GV, Sarkies NJC: Posterior ischaemic optic neuropathy due to internal artery occlusion. Neuroophthalmology 7:349, 1987

385. Sommer A, Tielsch JM, Katz J et al: Relationship between intraocular pressure and primary open-angle glaucoma among white and black Americans. Arch Ophthalmol 109:10980, 1991

386. Caprioli J: Recognizing structural damage to the optic nerve head and nerve fiber layer in glaucoma. Am J Ophthalmol 124:516, 1997

387. Kalenak JW, Kosmorsky GS, Hassenbusch SJ: Compression of the intracranial optic nerve mimicking unilateral normal-pressure glaucoma. J Clin Neuroophthalmol 12:230, 1992

388. Greenfield DS, Siatkowski RM, Glaser JG et al: The cupped disc: who needs neuroimaging? Ophthalmology 105:1866, 1998

389. Siegner SW, Netland PA: Optic disc hemorrhages and progression of glaucoma. Ophthalmology 103:1014, 1996

390. Brown GC, Shields JA: Tumors of the optic nerve head. Surv Ophthalmol 29:239, 1985

391. Dutton JJ: Gliomas of the anterior visual pathway. Surv Ophthalmol 38:427, 1994

392. Listernick R, Louis DN, Packer RJ et al: Optic pathway gliomas in children with neurofibromatosis 1: consensus statement from NF1 Optic Pathway Glioma Task Force. Ann Neurol 41:143, 1997

393. Anderson DR, Spencer WH: Ultrastructural and histochemical observations of optic nerve gliomas. Arch Ophthalmol 83:324, 1970

394. Grimson BS, Perry DD: Enlargement of the optic disk in childhood optic nerve tumors. Am J Ophthalmol 97:627, 1984

395. McDonnell P, Miller NR: Chiasmatic and hypothalamic extension of optic nerve glioma. Arch Ophthalmol 101:1412, 1983

396. Imes RK, Hoyt WF: Magnetic resonance imaging signs of optic nerve gliomas in neurofibromatosis 1. Am J Ophthalmol 111:729, 1991

397. Brodsky MC: The "pseudo-CSF" signal of orbital optic glioma on magnetic resonance imaging: a signature of neurofibromatosis. Surv Ophthalmol 38:213, 1993

398. Gans MS, Frazier Byrne S, Glaser JS: Standardized a-scan echography in optic nerve disease. Arch Ophthalmol 105:1232, 1987

399. Sadun F, Hinton DR, Sadun AA: Rapid growth of an optic nerve ganglioglioma in a patient with neurofibromatosis 1. Ophthalmology 103:794, 1996

400. Jenkin D, Angyalfi S, Becker L et al: Optic glioma in children: surveillance, resection or irradiation. Int J Radiat Oncol Biolm Phys 25:215, 1993

401. Dutton JJ: Optic nerve sheath meningiomas. Surv Ophthalmol 37:167, 1992

402. Karp LA, Zimmerman LE, Borit A et al: Primary intraorbital meningiomas. Arch Ophthalmol 91:24, 1974

403. Ing EB, Garrity JA, Cross SA et al: Sarcoid masquerading as optic nerve sheath meningioma. Mayo Clin Proc 72:38, 1997

404. Zimmerman CF, Schatz NJ, Glaser JS: Magnetic resonance imaging of optic nerve meningiomas. Ophthalmology 97:585, 1990

405. Lindblom B, Truwit CL, Hoyt WF: Optic nerve sheath meningioma: definition of intraorbital, intracanalicular, and intracranial

components with magnetic resonance imaging. Ophthalmology 99:560, 1992

406. Eng TY, Albright NW, Kuwahara G et al: Precision radiation therapy for optic nerve sheath meningiomas. Int J Rad Oncol Biol Phys 22:1093, 1992

407. Lee AG, Woo SY, Miller NR et al: Improvement in visual function in an eye with presumed optic nerve sheath meningioma after treatment with three-dimensional conformal radiation therapy. J Neuroophthalmol 16:247, 1996

408. Hsu DW, Efird JT, Hedley-White ET: Progesterone and estrogen receptors in meningiomas: prognostic considerations. J Neurosurg 86:113, 1997

409. Olsen ME, Chernik NL, Posner JB: Infiltration of the leptomeninges by systemic cancer: a clinical and pathologic study. Arch Neurol 30:122, 1974

410. Little JR, Dale AJD, Okazaki H: Meningeal carcinomatosis. Arch Neurol 30:138, 1984

411. Christmas NJ, Mead MD, Richardson EP, Albert DM: Secondary optic nerve tumors. Surv Ophthalmol 36:196, 1991

412. McFadzean R, Brosnahan D, Doyle D et al: A diagnostic quartet in leptomeningeal infiltration of the optic nerve sheath. J Neuroophthalmol 14:175, 1994

413. Krol G, Sze G, Malkin M et al: MR of cranial and spinal meningeal carcinomatosis: comparison with CT and myelography. AJNR Am J Neuroradiol 9:709, 1988

413a. de la Sayette V, Bertran F, Honnorat J et al: Paraneoplastic cerebellar syndrome and optic neuritis with anti-CV2 antibodies: clinical response to excision of the primary tumor. Arch Neurol 55:405, 1998

414. Siatkowski RM, Lam BL, Schatz NJ et al: Optic neuropathy in Hodgkin's disease. Am J Ophthalmol 114:625, 1992

415. Strominger MB, Schatz NJ, Glaser JS: Lymphomatous optic neuropathy. Am J Ophthalmol 116:774, 1993

416. Kashani AA, Kerman BM: Central nervous system malignant B-cell lymphoma identified with standardized echography of the optic nerve. J Neuroophthalmol 17:243, 1997

417. Kodsi SR, Younge BR, Leavitt JA et al: Intracranial plasma cell granuloma presenting as an optic neuropathy. Surv Ophthalmol 38:70, 1993

418. Nikaido H, Mishima H, Ono H et al: Leukemic involvement of the optic nerve. Am J Ophthalmol 105:294, 1988

419. Kaikov Y: Optic nerve head infiltration in acute leukemia in children: an indication for emergency optic nerve radiation therapy. Med Pediatr Oncol 826:101, 1996

420. Cramer SC, Glaspy JA, Efird JT et al: Chronic lymphocytic leukemia and the central nervous system: a clinical and pathologic study. Neurology 46:19, 1996

421. Purvin V, vanDyk HJL: Primary reticulum cell sarcoma of the brain presenting as steroid-responsive optic neuropathy. J Clin Neuroophthalmol 4:15, 1984

422. Wagoner MD, Gonder JR, Albert DM: Intraocular reticulum cell sarcoma. Ophthalmology 87:724, 1980

423. Khawly JA, Rubin P, Petros W et al: Retinopathy and optic neuropathy in bone marrow transplantation for breast cancer. Ophthalmology 103:87, 1996

423a. Purvin, V: Anterior ischemic optic neuropathy secondary to interferon-alpha. Arch Ophthalmol 113:1041, 1995

424. Caraceni A, Martini C, Spatti G et al: Recovering optic neuritis during systemic cisplatin and carboplatin chemotherapy. Acta Neurol Scand 96:260, 1997

425. DeLano MC, Fun FY, Zinreich SJ: Relationship of the optic nerves to the posterior paranasal sinuses: a CT anatomic study. AJNR Am J Neuroradiol 17:669, 1996

426. Buss DR, Tse Dt, Farris BK: Ophthalmic complications of sinus surgery. Ophthalmology 97:612, 1990

427. Hayman, Carter K, Schiffman JS et al: A sellar misadventure: imaging considerations. Surv Ophthalmol 41:252, 1996

428. Goodwin JA, Glaser JS. Chiasmal syndrome in sphenoid sinus mucocele. Ann Neurol 4:440, 1978

429. Johnson LN, Hepler RS, Yee RD et al: Sphenoid sinus mucocele (anterior clinoid variant) mimicking diabetic ophthalmoplegia and retrobulbar neuritis. Am J Ophthalmol 102:111, 1986

430. Dooley DP, Hollsten DA, Grimes SR et al: Indolent orbital

431. Hutnik, Nicolle DA, Munoz DG: Orbital aspergillosis: a fatal masquerader. J Neuroophthalmol 17:257, 1997

432. Frohman LP, Lama P: Annual review of systemic diseases: 1995–1996. J Neuroophthalmol 18:67, 1998

433. Newman NJ, Slamovits TL, Friedland S et al: Neuro-ophthalmic manifestations of meningocerebral inflammation from the limited form of Wegener's granulomatosis. Am J Ophthalmol 120:613, 1995

434. Goldberg RA, Weisman JS, McFarland JE et al: Orbital inflammation and optic neuropathies associated with chronic sinusitis of intranasal cocaine abuse: possible role of contiguous inflammation. Arch Ophthalmol 107:831, 1989

435. Harbison JW, Lessell S, Selhorst JB: Neuro-ophthalmology of sphenoid sinus carcinoma. Brain 107:855, 1984

436. Berman EL, Chu A, Wirtschafter JD et al: Esthesioneuroblastoma presenting as sudden unilateral visual loss. J Clin Neuroophthalmol 12:31, 1992

437. Neigel JM, Rootman J, Belkin RI et al: Dysthyroid optic neuropathy: the crowded orbital apex syndrome. Ophthalmology 95:1515, 1988

438. Glatt HJ: Optic nerve dysfunction in thyroid eye disease: a clinician's perspective. Radiology 200:26, 1996

439. Birchall D, Goodall KL, Noble JL et al: Graves' ophthalmopathy: intracranial prolapse on CT as an indicator of optic nerve compression. Radiology 200:123, 1996

440. Hufnagel TJ, Hickey WF, Cobbs WH et al: Immunohistochemical and ultrastructural studies on the exenterated orbital tissues of a patient with Graves' disease. Ophthalmology 91:1411, 1984

441. Bartley GB, Fatourechi V, Kadrmas EF et al: Clinical features of Graves' ophthalmopathy in an incidence cohort. Am J Ophthalmol 121:284, 1996

442. Trobe JD, Glaser JS, LaFlamme P: Dysthyroid optic neuropathy: clinical profile and rationale for management. Arch Ophthalmol 179:285, 1978

443. Kao SCS, Kendler DL, Nugent RA et al: Radiotherapy in the management of thyroid orbitopathy: computed tomography and clinical outcomes. Arch Ophthalmol 111:819, 1993

444. Jacobson DM, Warner JJ, Broste SK: Optic nerve contact and compression by the carotid artery in asymptomatic patients. Am J Ophthalmol 123:677, 1997

445. Lindenberg R, Walsh FB, Sacks JG: Neuropathology of Vision: An Atlas. Philadelphia, Lea & Febiger, 1973

446. Golnik KC, Hund PW, Stroman GA et al: Magnetic resonance imaging in patients with unexplained optic neuropathy. Ophthalmology 103:515, 1996

447. Colapinto EV, Cabeen MA, Johnson LN: Optic nerve compression by a dolichoectatic internal carotid artery: case report. Neurosurgery 39:604, 1996

448. Miller NR, Savino PJ, Schneider T: Rapid growth of an intracranial aneurysm causing apparent retrobulbar optic neuritis. J Neuroophthalmol 15:212, 1995

449. Chan JW, Hoyt WF, Ellis WG et al: Pathogenesis of acute monocular blindness from leaking anterior communicating artery aneurysms: report of six cases. Neurology 48:680, 1997

450. Samples JR, Younge BR: Tobacco-alcohol amblyopia. J Clin Neuroophthalmol 1:213, 1981

451. Frisen L: Fundus changes in acute malnutritional optic neuropathy. Arch Ophthalmol 101:577, 1983

452. Kupersmith MJ, Weiss PA, Carr RE: The visual-evoked potential in tobacco-alcohol and nutritional amblyopia. Am J Ophthalmol 95:307, 1983

453. van Noort BAA, Bos PJM, Klopping C et al: Optic neuropathy from thiamine deficiency in a patient with ulcerative colitis. Doc Ophthalmol 67:45, 1987

454. Stambolian D, Behrens MM: Optic neuropathy associated with B12 deficiency. Am J Ophthalmol 83:465, 1977

455. Troncoso J, Mancall EL, Schatz NJ: Visual evoked responses in pernicious anemia. Arch Neurol 36:168, 1979

456. Rizzo JF, Lessell S: Tobacco amblyopia. Am J Ophthalmol 116:84, 1993

457. Cuba Neuropathy Field Investigation Team: Epidemic optic

neuropathy in Cuba: clinical characterization and risk factors. N Engl J Med 333:1176, 1955

458. Freeman AG: Optic neuropathy and chronic cyanide toxicity. Lancet 1:441, 1986

459. McKellar MJ, Hidajat RR, Elder MJ: Acute ocular methanol toxicity: clinical and electrophysiologic features. Aust N Z J Ophthalmol 3:225, 1997

460. Sharpe JA, Hostovsky M, Bilbao JM et al: Methanol optic neuropathy: a histopathological study. Neurology 32:1093, 1982

461. Fasler JJ, Rose FC: West Indian amblyopia. Postgrad Med J 56:494, 1980

462. Grant WM: Toxicology of the Eye. Springfield, IL, Charles C Thomas, 1986

463. Kumar A, Sandramouli S, Verma L et al: Ocular ethambutol toxicity: is it reversible? J Clin Neuroophthalmol 13:15, 1993

464. Helm G, Holland G: Ocular tuberculosis. Surv Ophthalmol 38:230, 1993

465. Salmon JF, Carmichael TR, Welsh NH: Use of contrast sensitivity measurement in the detection of subclinical ethambutol toxic optic neuropathy. Br J Ophthalmol 71:192, 1987

466. Ricoy JR, Ortega A, Cabello A: Subacute myelo-optic neuropathy (SMON). J Neurol Sci 53:241, 1982

467. Pittman FE, Westphal MC: Optic atrophy following treatment with diiodohydroxyquin. Pediatrics 53:81, 1974

468. Godel V, Nemet P, Lazar M: Chloramphenicol optic neuropathy. Arch Ophthalmol 98:1417, 1980

469. Klingele TG, Burde RM: Optic neuropathy associated with penicillamine therapy in a patient with rheumatoid arthritis. J Clin Neuroophthalmol 4:75, 1984

470. Ehyai A, Freemon FR: Progressive optic neuropathy and sensorineural hearing loss due to chronic glue sniffing. J Neurol Neurosurg Psychiatry 46:349, 1983

471. Adams JW, Bofenkamp TM, Kobrin J et al: Recurrent acute toxic optic neuropathy secondary to 5-FU. Cancer Treat Rep 68:565, 1984

472. Pickrell L, Purvin V: Ischemic optic neuropathy secondary to intracarotid infusion of BCNU. J Clin Neuroophthalmol 7:87, 1987

473. Slamovits TL, Burde RM, Klingele TG: Bilateral optic atrophy caused by chronic oral ingestion and topical application of hexachlorophene. Am J Ophthalmol 89:676, 1980

474. Coskuncan NM, Jabs DA, Dunn JP et al: The eye in bone marrow transplantation. VI. Retinal complications. Arch Ophthalmol 112:372, 1994

475. Gittinger JW, Asdourian GK: Papillopathy caused by amiodarone. Arch Ophthalmol 105:349, 1987

476. Garrett SN, Kennedy JJ, Schiffman JS: Amiodarone optic neuropathy. J Clin Neuroophthalmol 8:105, 1988

477. Matthews GP, Sandberg MA, Berson EL: Foveal cone electroretinograms in patients with central visual loss of unexplained etiology. Arch Ophthalmol 110:1568, 1992

478. Steinsapir KD, Goldberg RA: Traumatic optic neuropathy. Surv Ophthalmol 38:487, 1994

479. Kline LB, McCluskey MM, Skalka HW: Imaging techniques in optic nerve evulsion. J Clin Neuroophthalmol 8:281, 1988

480. Brodsky MC, Wald KJ, Chen S et al: Protracted posttraumatic optic disc swelling. Ophthalmology 102:1628, 1995

481. Quigley HA, Davis EB, Anderson DR: Descending optic nerve degeneration in primates. Invest Ophthalmol Vis Sci 16:861, 1977

482. Cheney ML, Blair PA: Blindness as a complication of rhinoplasty. Arch Otolaryngol Head Neck Surg 113:768, 1987

483. Callahan MA: Prevention of blindness after blepharoplasty. Ophthalmology 90:1047, 1983

484. Horton JC, Hoyt WF, Foreman DS et al: Confirmation by magnetic resonance imaging of optic nerve injury after retrobulbar anesthesia. Arch Ophthalmol 114:351, 1996

485. Devoto MH, Kersten RC, Zalta AH et al: Optic nerve injury after retrobulbar anesthesia. Arch Ophthalmol 115:687, 1997

486. Liu C, Youl B, Moseley I: Magnetic resonance imaging of the optic nerve in extremes of gaze: implications for the positioning of the globe for retrobulbar anaesthesia. Br J Ophthalmol 76:728, 1992

487. Hollenhorst RW, Svien HJ, Benold CF: Unilateral blindness occurring during anesthesia for neurosurgical operations. Arch Ophthalmol 52:819, 1954

488. Jampol LM, Goldbaum M, Rosenberg M, Bahr R: Ischemia of ciliary arterial circulation from ocular compression. Arch Ophthalmol 93:1311, 1975

489. Chou P-I, Sadun AA, Lee H: Vasculature and morphometry of the optic canal and intracanalicular optic nerve. J Neuroophthalmol 15:186, 1995

490. Lessell S: Indirect optic nerve trauma. Arch Ophthalmol 107:382, 1989

491. Cook MW, Levin LA, Joseph MP et al: Traumatic optic neuropathy: a meta-analysis. Arch Otolaryngol Head Neck Surg 122:389, 1996

492. Ross HS, Rosenberg S, Friedman AH: Delayed radiation necrosis of the optic nerve. Am J Ophthalmol 76:683, 1973

493. Shukovsky LJ, Fletcher GH: Retinal and optic nerve complications in a high dose irradiation technique of ethmoid sinus and nasal cavity. Radiology 104:629, 1972

494. Salz JJ, Donin JF: Blindness after burns. Can J Ophthalmol 7:243, 1972

CHAPTER 6

Topical Diagnosis: The Optic Chiasm

Joel S. Glaser

Clinical Manifestations
Neuroimaging Procedures: General Considerations
Congenital Chiasmal Dysplasias
Neoplasms and Related Conditions
  Pituitary Tumors
    Adenomas
    Acromegaly
    Pituitary "Apoplexy"
    Imaging of Pituitary Tumors
  Meningiomas
  Craniopharyngiomas
  Optic and Hypothalamic Gliomas

Dysgerminomas
Suprasellar Aneurysms
Demyelinative Disease and Inflammations
Miscellaneous Chiasmal Lesions
  Arachnoidal and Epithelial Cysts
  Metastatic Diseases and Other Mass Lesions
  Sphenoidal Mucoceles
  Trauma
  Complications of Radiation Therapy
  Hydrocephalus
  Pregnancy
Empty Sella Syndrome

> The modern neurosurgeon has come to deal largely with lesions that mechanically affect the central apparatus of vision, while the ophthalmic surgeon limits his operative procedure to the intra-orbital portion of the apparatus. One in a sense is extracranial, the other an intracranial ophthalmic surgeon, neither of them venturing to trespass much beyond the narrows of the optic foramina.
>
> Harvey Cushing (1930)

The optic chiasm is the crossroads of the visual sensory system, containing some 2.4 million afferent axons, and it is also the conjunction of at least 4 major medical disciplines: neurosurgery, neurology, endocrinology, and, of course ophthalmology. Many of the disease processes that involve the intracranial portions of the optic nerves likewise involve the chiasm. Because of the relationship of the nerves and chiasm with the basal structures of the anterior and middle cranial fossae (see Chapter 12, Figs. 12–20 and 12–21), pituitary adenomas, meningiomas, and aneurysms frequently encroach on the anterior visual pathways. Failure of early diagnosis in chiasmal disorders endangers the life of the patient and lessens the likelihood of reversal of visual and hormonal deficits.

The anatomy of the chiasm is addressed in some detail in Chapter 4, but the following points deserve emphasis in the context of topical diagnosis. The chiasm is situated

J. S. Glaser: Departments of Neurology and Ophthalmology, Bascom Palmer Eye Institute, University of Miami School of Medicine Miami; and Neuro-ophthalmology, Cleveland Clinic Florida, Ft. Lauderdale, Florida

in the suprasellar arachnoidal cistern and forms the floor of the anteroinferior midline recess of the third ventricle. The inferior aspect of the chiasm is usually 8 mm to 13 mm above the nasotuberculum line (*i.e.*, the plane of the diaphragma sellae or clinoid processes). The intracranial portion of the optic nerves is inclined as much as 45° from the horizontal and measures 17 ± 2.5 mm in length (see Fig. 4–6). The lateral aspects of the chiasm are embraced by the supraclinoid portions of the internal carotid arteries, and the anterior cerebral arteries pass over the dorsal surface of the optic nerves as they converge. The optic nerves are fixed at the intracranial exit from the optic canals, the dorsal aspect of which is formed by an unyielding falciform fold of dura.

From the preceding description of the position of the chiasm, it should be clear that basal mass lesions, even of moderate size, need not encroach on the chiasm. For example, pituitary adenomas must extend well above the confines of the sella turcica in order to contact the chiasm. The corollary is that, in the presence of chiasmal visual field defect, advanced suprasellar extension of an adenoma may be predicted. Small tumors are detected clinically only when signs of unilateral optic nerve compression evolve or endocrinologic symptoms prevail.

It is not clear whether field defects are due to direct compression of visual fibers or to interference with vasculature; the midline section of the chiasm may be most vulnerable because of watershed vasculature. At any rate, at craniotomy, major stretching, distortion, and thinning of the nerves and chiasm are commonly encountered, shedding little light on the mechanism of impairment of function or the nature of visual recovery.

CLINICAL MANIFESTATIONS

Most chiasmal syndromes are caused by extrinsic tumors, classically pituitary adenomas, suprasellar meningiomas, and craniopharyngiomas, or by carotid aneurysms. With few exceptions, these slow-growing tumors produce insidiously progressive visual deficits in the form of variations on a bitemporal theme (Fig. 6–1). Asymmetry of field loss is the rule, such that one eye may show advanced deficits, including reduced acuity, whereas only relative temporal field depression is found in the contralateral field. Until acuity is diminished in one or both eyes, patients' visual symptoms are vague, such as "trouble seeing to the side," a history of fender-bending, or finding that, when passed by another automobile, the overtaking vehicle suddenly appears directly ahead. The first clue to the presence of a hemianopic defect may be revealed during monocular reading of acuity charts; with the right eye only the left letters are seen, and with the left eye only the right letters are seen (see Fig. 2–2). That is, optotypes that fall into defective hemifields may be ignored or blurred. Although compression by mass lesions is typified by a pattern of relentless, slow depression of monocular or binocular function, pituitary adenomas, craniopharyngiomas, or aneurysms may provoke sudden worsening or fluctuations in vision that mimic optic neuritis, at times with confounding improvement during corticosteroid therapy.

Peculiar sensory phenomena are experienced by some patients with usually well-developed field defects, consisting of a *non-paretic* form of diplopia and clumsiness in visual tasks requiring depth perception (*e.g.,* seating the tip of a screwdriver, threading a needle). Loss of portions of normally superimposed binocular field results in absence of corresponding points in visual space (or on the retinas) and subsequently in diminished fusional capacity. In essence, the patient is subjected to two "free-floating" nasal hemifields without interhemispheral linkage to keep them aligned. Vertical and horizontal slippage produces doubling of images, gaps in otherwise continuous visual panorama, and steps in horizontal lines.

Elkington[1] noted that the preoperative symptoms in a series of 260 patients with pituitary adenoma included some degree of double vision in 98 patients, but a demonstrable ocular palsy was present in only 14. In addition, without temporal fields, objects beyond the point of binocular fixation fall on non-seeing nasal retina, so that a blind area exists, with extinction of objects beyond the fixation point. These bitemporal hemianopic sensory phenomena are discussed at length by Nachtigaller and Hoyt.[2]

The association of extraocular muscle palsies with chiasmal field defects implies involvement of the structures in the cavernous sinus, usually a sign of rapid expansion of a pituitary adenoma (see Chapter 12). Except in children, only rarely is tumor diagnosis delayed sufficiently for obstruction of the ventricular system to occur, with elevation of intracranial pressure and lateral rectus weakness.

Pallor of the optic discs, although an anticipated physical sign of chiasmal interference, is not a requisite in diagnosis. In a series of 156 cases of pituitary tumors, Chamlin et al[3] found optic atrophy in only 155 of 312 eyes (50%). Wilson and Falconer[4] also found unequivocal disc pallor in only 28 of 50 patients; they pointed out that optic atrophy may not be present even when visual symptoms have lasted as long as 2 years. Even extensive field loss in chiasmal syndromes may be associated with normal or minimally pale discs. Therefore, it is unwise to rely on the presence of optic atrophy as an indication of chiasmal interference; disc pallor is corroborative evidence at best, greater weight being placed on carefully evaluated visual fields.

It is risky to predict on the basis of disc appearance the ultimate level of vision anticipated following chiasmal decompression. As a rule, the more atrophic the disc, and the greater the duration of visual symptoms, the less likely is the return of function in defective areas of field, but recuperation of vision to surprisingly good levels, in spite of relatively advanced disc pallor, does indeed occur.

Suprasellar tumors of presumed prenatal origin, such as optic gliomas or craniopharyngiomas, may be associated with congenitally dysplastic optic discs. These disc anomalies include variable hypoplasia, tilted or "irregularly oval" nerve heads,[5] or enlarged discs.[6]

Techniques for the screening or elaboration of field defects are discussed in Chapter 2. The importance of establishing that the vertical meridian forms the central border of the temporal defect is paramount in distinguishing true chiasmal interference from temporal field depression that simulates temporal hemianopias. Those conditions that can mimic chiasmal field defects include the following (see Chapter 5, Part II):

1. Tilted discs (inferior crescents, nasal fundus ectasia).
2. Nasal sector retinitis pigmentosa.
3. Bilateral cecocentral scotomas.
4. Papilledema with greatly enlarged blind spots.
5. Overhanging redundant upper lid tissue.
6. Dominant optic atrophy.
7. Ethambutol toxic optic neuropathy.

Trobe et al[7] have devised a visual field technique that selectively explores the vertical meridian as a "strategy" in screening for chiasmal defects, reducing testing time, and increasing efficiency. This system employs both ki-

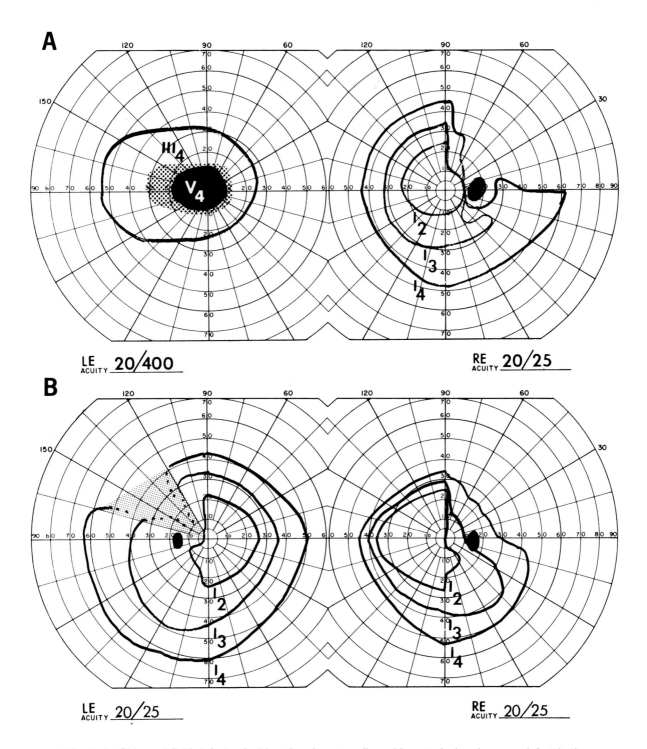

Fig. 6–1. Chiasmal field defects. **A.** "Junctional scotoma" combines typical optic nerve defect in the left field (*LE*) with temporal hemianopia in the right (*RE*) (see also *C*). **B.** Classic bitemporal hemianopia. Riddoch's phenomenon (motion perception) is demonstrable in the shaded area of the left field.

netic and static suprathreshold stimuli on the Goldmann perimeter, emphasizing especially the 15° perifixational area. Using the Haag-Streit 940 ST automated perimeter with a screening strategy that charts two isopters at about 10° and 15° of nasal eccentricity, and determining

subjective symmetry across the vertical meridian, Frisen[8] found the earliest visual field defects in mid-chiasmal compression to be bitemporal depressions of central isopters, usually more pronounced superiorly and *often lacking a clear vertical step.* Apparently, for points of

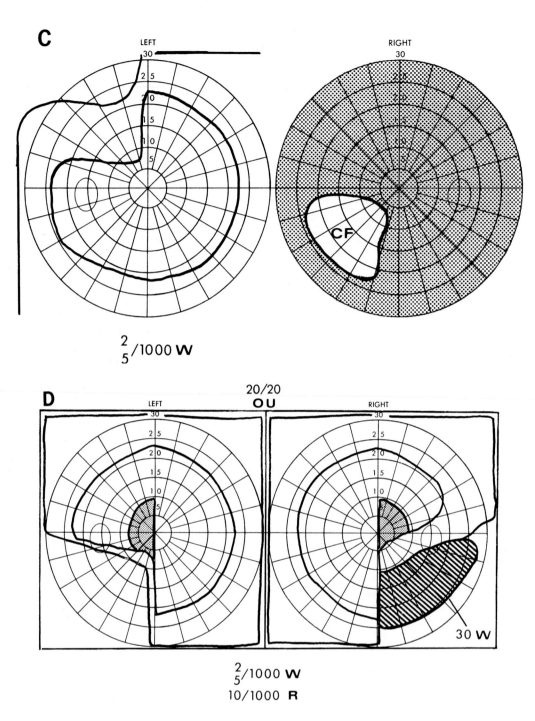

Fig. 6–1. (*continued*) **C.** Asymmetric progression, with severe visual deficit in the right eye and early superior temporal depression on the left. **D.** Defect characteristic of posterior chiasmal notch lesion. Note the central hemianopic scotomas and inferior quadrant defects.

equal eccentricity in the central visual field, temporal thresholds are normally higher than nasal thresholds. Of great practical import are Frisén's conclusions: screening can be limited to careful charting of one single kinetic isopter of small radius (*e.g.,* 8° to 12°), complemented with rapid assessment of symmetry of subjective color saturation across the vertical meridian; if this critical central isopter plot is normal, no further diagnostic

evidence accrues by determining additional peripheral isopters (see also Chapter 2).

Central and cecocentral scotomas are compelling evidence of *intrinsic* optic nerve disease (see Chapter 5, Part II). Rare cases are reported[9] of "atypical" bilateral scotomas attributed to suprasellar mass lesions: intrinsic histiocytosis of the chiasm, a chiasmal glioma, and a cystic craniopharyngioma; thus, two lesions were indeed

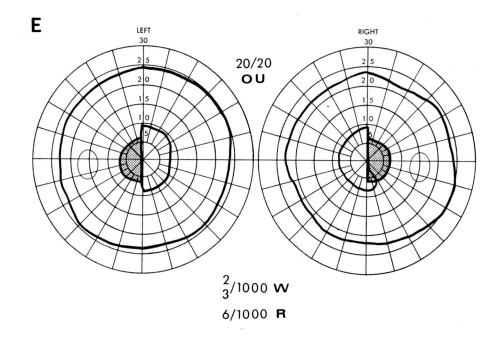

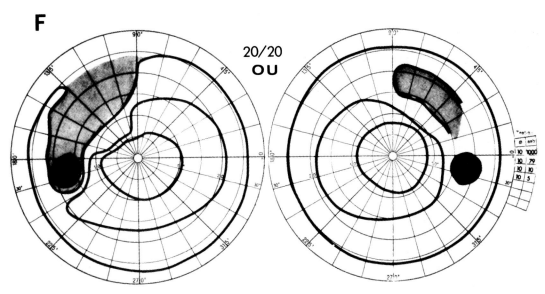

Fig. 6–1. (*continued*) **E.** Central hemianopic scotomas typical of posterior chiasmal interference. **F.** Temporal hemianopic arcuate scotomas. The patient sustained head trauma, with resultant field defects and diabetes insipidus.

intrinsic. The anterior knee of Wilbrand, that is, a forward looping of decussating fibers 1 mm to 2 mm into the contralateral optic nerve, is probably an artifact[10] and does not account for the pattern of central depression in one eye and contralateral superior temporal hemianopic depression (see Fig. 6–1A).

Well documented are examples of "posterior chiasmal angle" lesions that produce homonymous hemianopias with depression selectively of the *inferior temporal field near fixation* (see Fig. 6–1D); for example, two presumed dysgerminomas and a presumed craniopharyngioma caused these posterior chiasmal defects,

at the junction with one optic tract.[11] Such patients, unlike posterior pathway hemianopias, have visual acuity diminished in one or both eyes, and usually asymmetric optic atrophy is observed (see Chapter 7).

NEUROIMAGING PROCEDURES: GENERAL CONSIDERATIONS

Errors of *omission,* that is, failure to perform timely radiologic procedures, constitute a major shortcoming in the practice of ophthalmology. Of equal importance are errors of *commission,* whereby inappropriate, inadequate, or incomplete imaging studies are obtained; these errors are compounded when such investigations are interpreted as "normal," providing a false sense of security and further delaying definitive diagnostic investigations. It is imperative that the physician on clinical grounds make an informed topical diagnosis and then ask two questions: (1) What studies are appropriate to visualize the appropriate anatomy? (2) Are the neuro-images (computed tomography [CT], magnetic resonance imaging [MRI], angiography, ultrasonography) obtained of sufficient quality to provide definitive information? Moreover, timely acquisition of well-performed neurodiagnostic studies is vital in ultimate outcome. For example, of 149 patients with pituitary adenoma treated at the National Hospital, London,[12] nearly one-fourth had visual complaints for 2 to 10 years without definitive diagnosis, a finding that underscores the continuing failure of the medical community to assess cases of "unexplained" visual loss appropriately.

The details of neuroradiologic techniques and their interpretations are beyond the intent of this work, but certain specific concepts may be commented on here. More detailed clarifications are included under discussions of specific lesions, to follow. Plain views of the skull and optic canals must now be considered strictly preliminary studies in the investigation of the patient with non-ocular visual loss. This is not to disparage the use of uncomplicated procedures, but only limited information is available from plain film studies, and subtle changes in the canals and bony structures of the sella are regularly overlooked and are, at any rate, better visualized by CT using "bone-window" settings. Measurements of the sella, whether linear or volumetric, are not in and of themselves important. In marginal cases, such measurements are unreliable; in obvious cases, they are superfluous, and in neither instance is the question of suprasellar extension resolved.

Whether plain film abnormalities are detected or not, especially in patients with chiasmal syndrome, more refined neuroimaging techniques, such as CT with iodinated contrast or gadolinium-enhanced MRI, and cerebral arteriography in selected cases, must be applied. Some generalizations may be enunciated here, with special reference to the optic chiasm and related structures.

As a rule, CT provides greater definition than MRI for bone destruction or erosion (*e.g.,* craniopharyngioma, meningioma) and hyperostosis, (*e.g.,* meningioma), as well as for vascular or tumoral calcifications (*e.g.,* craniopharyngioma) or acute hemorrhages, but MRI more clearly demonstrates vascular encasement (*e.g.,* meningioma), extent of involvement of structures adjacent to masses, invasion of cavernous sinus, presence of aneurysms, configuration of gliomas, degree of expansion into the suprasellar cistern, central nervous system (CNS) infarcts, and demyelinative lesions. Thin-section MRI is equal to, or better than, enhanced CT in de-

picting large pituitary adenomas, although CT may be more sensitive in detecting microadenomas that do not enlarge the sella. The intracanalicular portion of optic nerves is seen to best advantage with MRI, but bony changes are exquisitely delineated by CT "bone-window" settings. The use of gadolinium-enhanced MRI, with fat-suppression protocols, is especially appropriate for orbital studies, and *cerebral arteriography* must be included, especially when radiologic and, in some instances, surgical intervention is contemplated. MRI is relatively contraindicated in the presence of, for example, cerebral aneurysm clips, cardiac pacemaker, or ferro-magnetic foreign bodies. At this time, gas pneumoencephalography, radionuclide brain scan, and metrizamide cisternography must be considered obsolete.

High-resolution MRI (1.5 Tesla magnet strength, 3-mm thick sections) provides accurate coronal measurements of intracranial optic nerves (height, 3.5 $\pm$ 0.06 mm; width, 6.01 $\pm$ 0.1 mm),[13] and chiasm (height, 2.69 $\pm$ 0.08 mm; width, 14.96 $\pm$ 0.33 mm; area, 43.7 $\pm$ 5.21 mm^2).[13,14] Both advanced age and optic atrophy diminish the height and width of the chiasm.[13–15]

CONGENITAL CHIASMAL DYSPLASIAS

The chiasm is infrequently the site of developmental anomalies that, at times, are related to malformations of other diencephalic midline structures, including the third ventricle. Embryonic dysgenesis results in abnormal growth of the primitive optic vesicles that produces unilateral or bilateral anophthalmos or useless microphthalmic cysts. Such gross ocular anomalies may occur in isolation or may be associated with a spectrum of neural defects, including major malformations that preclude survival.

Of greater clinical impact are the more subtle ocular dysplasias that accompany those anterior forebrain malformations that are compatible with long life. Specific congenital anomalies of the optic discs may indicate the presence of otherwise occult forebrain malformations. Optic disc hypoplasia and colobomatous dysplasias are therefore not simply fundus curiosities, but often they are ophthalmoscopic clues to associated brain and endocrine defects. These symptom complexes are discussed in Chapter 5, Part II, with congenital anomalies of the optic discs.

NEOPLASMS AND RELATED CONDITIONS

Most cases of chiasmal interference are due to mass lesions, either tumors or aneurysms. Although certain patterns of visual failure may suggest the location and type of lesion, such niceties often prove fallible in the face of neuroradiologic procedures or at craniotomy. At any rate, the diagnostic evaluation of all non-traumatic chiasmal syndromes is stereotyped: to rule in or out the presence of a potentially treatable mass lesion. Aneurysms are discussed briefly below, but in somewhat greater detail in Chapter 17, along with vascular tumors, and arteriovenous malformations that involve the chiasm.

Pituitary Tumors

Tumor of the pituitary gland is the single most common intracranial neoplasm that produces neuro-ophthalmologic symptomatology, and chiasmal interference is overwhelmingly the most frequent presentation. Pituitary adenomas constitute some 12% to 15% of clinically symptomatic intracranial tumors.

Adenomas

Kernohan and Sayre[16] reported that asymptomatic adenomas occur in more than 20% of pituitary glands examined at autopsy, and some degree of adenomatous hyperplasia can be found in almost every pituitary gland. A post-mortem study[17] composed of pituitary glands removed from 120 persons without clinical evidence of pituitary tumors revealed a 27% incidence of microadenomas, of which 41% stained for prolactin (PRL), without a gender difference. To generalize, more than 1 in 10 persons in the general population dies harboring a prolactinoma. Moreover, some 15% of microadenomas, that is, smaller than 10 mm in diameter and confined within the sella, and frequently uncovered as incidental findings, become significantly enlarged.[18] The incessant parade of this clinical syndrome is therefore not surprising.

Symptomatic adenomas occur infrequently in persons younger than 20 years, but they are common from the fourth through the seventh decades. The classic histologic designation as chromophobic, eosinophilic, or basophilic on the basis of light microscopy is obsolete, and adenomas are now classified according to the hormones they secrete. A functional nomenclature based on immunocytologic and ultrastructural characteristics has evolved[19]:

A. Adenomas with clinically manifest endocrine activity
   1. Somatotropes (growth hormone [GH]; acromegaly)
   2. Lactotropes (PRL; amenorrhea, galactorrhea; Forbes-Albright syndrome)
   3. Corticotropes (adrenocorticotropin [ACTH]; Cushing's or Nelson's syndromes)
   4. Thyrotropes (hyperthyroidism or hypothyroidism)
   5. Gonadotropes (follicle-stimulating hormone, luteinizing hormone)
   6. Multiple hormones (GR, PRL, ACTH)

B. Adenomas without clinically manifest endocrine activity
   1. Inactive oncocytoma
   2. Null cell
   3. PRL without galactorrhea
   4. Low amounts of normal hormones (GH, PRL)

Endocrine-inactive tumors fail to produce clinical manifestations of any secretory product when a normal hormone is produced in amounts too small to be detected, when an abnormal hormone is produced but not recognized by biologic receptor sites or detected by radioimmunoassay, or when formerly endocrine-active cells have lost the ability to produce hormone as a result of degeneration. Of 1000 pituitary tumors surgically treated by Wilson,[20] 226 were endocrine-inactive, and 774 were secretory, as follows: PRL, 410; GH, 195; ACTH, 167; thyroid-stimulating hormone, 2. Non-secretory adenomas, which consist mostly of null-cell adenomas, tend to be larger at presentation than do secretory tumors, with a median age of 57 years, and male predominance.[21]

Non-ocular symptoms, as previously discussed, include chronic headaches (severe or mild) in more than two-thirds of patients,[1] fatigue, impotence or amenorrhea, sexual hair change, or other signs of gonadal, thyroidal, or adrenal insufficiency. The typical sequence of hormonal deficiencies associated with large adenomas is early loss of GH and gonadotropin, later loss of thyrotropin and corticotropin. With the increasing application of neuroimaging and sensitive assays for abnormal hormones, the incidence of ophthalmologic presentation is decreasing, whereas the incidence of neuro-endocrine findings is increasing. Signs and symptoms, visual or otherwise, nonetheless may exist for months to years before so much as a visual field or plain skull film is obtained.[4]

Visual failure with pituitary tumors assumes a limited number of field patterns. As suprasellar extension evolves, a single optic nerve may be compromised, with resultant progressive monocular visual loss in the form of a central scotoma. More frequently, as the tumor splays apart the anterior chiasmal notch, superotemporal peripheral hemianopic defects occur. However, this well-touted superior bitemporal hemianopia is almost always accompanied by minor or major hemianopic scotomas approaching the fixational area along the vertical meridian (see Fig. 6–1). Asymmetry of field defects is the rule, the eye with the greater deficit likely showing diminished visual acuity. Marked asymmetry is not uncommon, such that one eye may be nearly blind while the other shows a temporal hemianopic defect (see Fig. 6–1C); this combination is as exquisitely localizing to the chiasm as is classic bitemporal hemianopia. Adenomas extending posteriorly produce incongruous hemianopias (see Fig. 6–5) by optic tract involvement; central vision is usually diminished, at least in the ipsilateral eye, and optic atrophy evolves.

On extremely rare occasions, arcuate Bjerrum's scotomas extend from the blind spot into the nasal field[22] or terminate at the vertical meridian.[23] Such defects are usually monocular and are difficult to distinguish from glaucoma by perimetry alone. With progression, especially if the temporal field of the other eye becomes involved, a more typical field pattern evolves. In late stages of visual loss, the only suggestion of the chiasmal character of field defects may be minimal preservation of the nasal field of one eye (see Fig. 6–1C). The importance of serial examinations is obvious, but, when doubt exists, neuroimaging is mandatory.

The absence of field defects, for example, in patients undergoing evaluation for amenorrhea, galactorrhea, or sellar enlargement incidentally discovered, does not imply the absence of an adenoma. Obviously, patients with microadenomas, that is, confined within the sella, do not have field defects. From a study[24] of 50 cases of pituitary adenomas with chiasmal syndrome, it was concluded that visual disturbance occurs when the chiasm is displaced approximately 10 mm upward (see also Fig. 4–6).

The modern management of pituitary adenomas should involve several disciplines: current neuroradiologic studies detect microadenomas and provide precise delineation of gross morphology and status of neighboring structures, and mixed MRI signals suggest new or old hemorrhage, cysts, and so forth (Fig. 6–2); radioimmunoassay techniques assay PRL and other endocrine levels; oral neuropharmacologic agents, such as bromergocryptine, provide a "medical adenomectomy" for hyperprolactinemia and acromegaly; transsphenoidal surgery, including high-illumination microscopical procedures, televised radiofluoroscopic monitoring, and infection control, has all but replaced transcranial approaches; immunohistochemistry techniques have replaced the anachronistic tinctorial designations (*e.g.*, chromophobe, basophilic) with a functional classification.

PRL-secreting adenomas are the single most common type of pituitary tumor and occur more frequently in women than in men.[20] Most of these tumors are microadenomas, although tumors confined to the sella are relatively rare in men. In women, amenorrhea and galactorrhea are the symptoms that provoke investigation, whereas in men, symptoms include loss of libido, impotence, gynecomastia, galactorrhea, and hypopituitarism.[25]

These various clinical manifestations occur with or without visual loss, depending on the volume of the adenoma; that is, the degree of suprasellar extension and compression of the chiasm. As a rule, true prolactinomas are associated with serum PRL levels higher than 150 to 200 ng/ml, and they usually range from 700 to 7000 ng/ml; the larger the tumor, the greater the serum PRL

and, therefore, radiologically large adenomas with PRL levels lower than 200 ng/ml are probably non-secreting and are not likely to respond to medical therapy (see below).

Hyperprolactinemia up to 100 ng/ml may be due to simple physiologic causes, including stress, sexual intercourse, nipple stimulation, and exercise, or it may be secondary to pharmacologic agents such as phenothiazines, tricyclic antidepressants, calcium channel blockers, and cimetidine.[25] However, other lesions in and around the pituitary gland and hypothalamus that compromise the pituitary stalk may present as "pseudoprolactinomas." Immunohistochemical studies performed on 97 tissue specimens in patients operated on for presumed prolactinomas at the Mayo Clinic in Rochester, Minnesota[26] revealed 65% to be microadenomas, but null-cell tumors accounted for 4 of 5 pseudoprolactinomas; these tended to be large at diagnosis, but with minor PRL elevation. Suprasellar cystic lesions can also cause hyperprolactinemia with field defects,[27] as can carotid suprasellar aneurysms.[28] Unlike true prolactinomas, non–PRL-secreting suprasellar tumors, with secondary hyperprolactinemia due to pituitary stalk compression, do not show a correlation between size and PRL level.[29]

With the advent of the ergot-derived dopamine agonist bromocriptine, there is a pharmacologic alternative (or adjunct) to surgery for prolactinomas. Bromocriptine (2-bromo-alpha-ergocryptine) is representative of a class of ergot derivatives that, since the early 1970s, have been known to inhibit pituitary gonadotropic function, reduce PRL secretion, and diminish the size of pituitary tumors (see Fig. 6–2). Such ergot derivatives are structurally related to dopamine, a PRL-inhibitory factor elaborated by hypothalamic dopaminergic neurons. It is likely that bromocriptine acts in two ways: dopamine turnover in tubero-infundibular neurons is depressed, thereby increasing hypothalamic dopamine; dopamine receptors of the pituitary are inhibited, reducing both spontaneous PRL secretion and the release of PRL provoked by thyrotropin-releasing hormone. At any rate, bromocriptine decreases PRL production and secretion, with resultant reduction in lactotrope size and subsequent diminution of tumor volume, often rapidly, within 1 to 2 hours of initiation of treatment.[25]

Spark et al,[30] among others, reported the efficacy of bromocriptine in reducing tumor size; it was demonstrated that bromocriptine lowered PRL, reduced GH in acromegaly, and reversed visual field defects. However, patients with extrasellar extension or with high PRL levels did less well. The great weight of evidence now clearly shows that most microadenomas (intrasellar) are demonstrably reduced in size,[31] in about 3 months at an average dose of 5 mg per day, but cystic necrosis may develop, and adenomas may increase in volume if bromocriptine is discontinued.

The tumor-reducing effect of bromocriptine on pro-

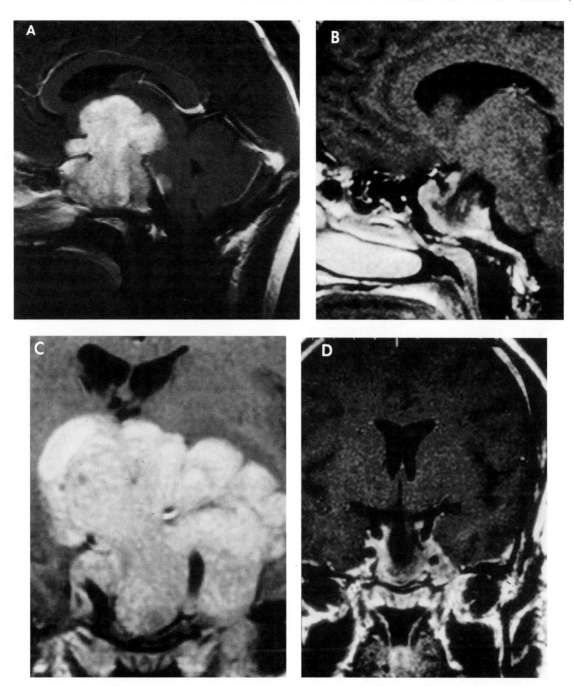

Fig. 6–2. Large prolactinoma. Original vision in the right eye (*RE*) was 8/200, left eye (*LE*) 1/200, with serum prolactin of 26,000 ng/ml and galactorrhea. Four months of bromocriptine reduced prolactin to 661 ng/ml, vision improved to RE 20/40, LE 20/50. At 3 years, vision was as follows: RE 20/30, LE 20/20; prolactin was 25.9 ng/ml. Enhanced magnetic resonance imaging. Sagittal **(A)** and coronal **(C)** images at diagnosis. Sagittal **(B)** and coronal **(D)** images at 2-year follow-up, showing dramatic shrinkage of the mass.

lactinomas has been tested on 5 types of large, extrasellar pituitary tumors.[32] Twenty patients were treated prospectively for up to 4.5 years with bromocriptine 30 mg or 60 mg per day (2 patients received 15 mg and 160 mg, respectively), and the effect on the size of the pituitary tumors was quantitated by planimetry of CT scans be-

fore and during treatment. The immediate success rate was 16 of 20 tumors, and 11 non-secreting tumors were reduced by a median of 32%, with an immediate success rate of 9 of 11. Nine secreting tumors (4 that secreted PRL; 3, GH; 1, ACTH; and 1, thyroid-stimulating hormone) were reduced by a median of 51%. The reduction in tumor size was significantly associated with pre-treatment volume, but not with the hormonal serum concentrations or with previous radiation treatment. Moreover, bromocriptine treatment did not cause any pituitary insufficiency other than the desired suppression of PRL.

The clinical course of 10 patients with macroprolactinomas at the Wills Eye Hospital in Philadelphia was carefully documented[33] after treatment with bromocriptine in daily doses ranging from 7.5 to 30 mg. Nine patients enjoyed improvement in acuity and fields quite rapidly, often within a few days, including the following: hand movements to 20/20 within 1 month, counting fingers to 20/20 or 20/30 within 7 to 12 days, and dramatic recovery of field defects. There was also a demonstrable decrease in tumor size by CT criteria, and lowering of serum PRL. Four patients subsequently required transsphenoidal decompression, for conditions including failure of visual improvement, cerebrospinal fluid (CSF) rhinorrhea, and medication intolerance. The authors cautioned that the long-term effects of bromocriptine therapy are not known, and prompt tumor regrowth is to be anticipated when the drug is discontinued. It was recommended that patients who are to undergo surgical decompression should be treated preoperatively to decrease tumor size and "to facilitate surgical removal," and that residual tumor with elevated PRL should be treated with bromocriptine. A similar patient[34] with a large pituitary tumor, hyperprolactinemia, bitemporal fields defects, and invasion of one cavernous sinus (involving the fifth and sixth cranial nerves) was treated with bromocriptine 7.5 mg per day,[35] with marked reduction in the tumor size and resolution of field defects and cranial nerve dysfunction over a 6-month period, at which point the sella appeared empty.

Other dopamine agonists are available or under investigation, including long-acting bromocriptine (Parlodel), cabergoline, and CV-205-502; some prolactinomas resistant to standard dopamine agonists may respond to more potent agents such as cabergoline.[35] Ophthalmic results in patients with macroprolactinomas treated with dopamine agonists show generally good results, with few instances of pituitary necrosis.[25,36] Indeed, it may be that these newer pharmaceuticals should be the *treatment of choice* in patients with large pituitary tumors with extrasellar extensions.

These unquestionable successes notwithstanding, there remain unanswered questions concerning dopamine agonist therapy: Is long-term medical therapy preferable to simple transsphenoidal surgery? Can such patients ever be weaned from medical therapy? What about the ultimate outcome of tumors not characterized by PRL secretion? Should large, asymmetric (invasive?) adenomas be pre-treated to make surgical removal easier? Based on an extensive experience, Wilson[20] recommended microsurgical transsphenoidal removal of macroprolactinomas, with presurgical bromocriptine

treatment of tumors larger than 2 cm. The details of neurosurgical procedures are beyond the scope of this present work, but Wilson's review and other sources[37] should be consulted. Varying within the spectrum of surgical experiences, complications of transsphenoidal procedures include anterior pituitary insufficiency (about 20%), diabetes insipidus (about 18%), CSF rhinorrhea (about 4%), and, rarely, loss of vision or diplopia.[38] Infrequent untoward results include hydrocephalus secondary to subarachnoid blood, cerebral ischemia related to vasospasm, meningitis with or without CSF leak, and death associated with intraoperative or postoperative hemorrhage.[20,38]

Radiation therapy is currently used as an integral part of postoperative treatment in patients with incompletely resected non-functional adenomas. External-beam conventional protocols delivering median total dosage of 45 Gy are considered highly effective in preventing recurrence of hormonally inactive tumors, but they may compound relative hypopituitarism.[39] Young patients with total tumor removal, or without MRI evidence of recurrence, may be safely observed with radiation therapy held in reserve. The role of stereotactic radiosurgery (single-fraction high-dosage) of pituitary adenomas is not yet clear, preliminary results notwithstanding.[40]

Following uncomplicated surgical decompression, visual acuity and fields may return with dramatic speed or improve weekly. Such restoration is dependent on duration of visual morbidity and, to some extent, the degree of pallor of the optic discs. Preoperatively, if careful ophthalmoscopy reveals attrition of the retinal nerve fiber layer, corresponding field defects are permanent. For the most part, what vision returns does so by 3 to 4 months, if not sooner, but many months may pass before maximum recovery is attained. Not all surgical procedures are successful, and visual function may worsen, especially after frontal craniotomy for large adenomas with massive suprasellar extension. Visual deterioration at or immediately following surgery is related to intrasellar hematoma formation, edema of tumor remnants, or direct surgical manipulation of optic nerves or chiasm and adjacent vasculature. Arterial injuries, for example, 21 instances in more than 1800 cases, produce intraoperative hemorrhage, delayed epistaxis, carotid arterial occlusion, and pseudoaneurysm.[41] Postoperative packing of the sella with muscle or subcutaneous fat may compress the optic nerves and chiasm, for which reason MRI is warranted when vision is worsened or does not recover quickly within a few days.[42]

After surgical, medical, or radiation therapy, the visual fields should be assessed as soon as possible to determine baseline function. In uncomplicated cases, monthly intervals during the first 3 months should suffice, then at 6 months, and subsequently yearly follow-up are usually adequate. Recurrence of visual failure may be caused by regrowth of tumor, arachnoidal adhesions associated with a progressive "empty sella syndrome" (see below), or delayed radionecrosis (see below). Tumor recurrence is by far the most common mechanism of visual deterioration, but field examination alone may not make this distinction. With prolactinomas, serum PRL levels may be monitored, and, indeed, prolactinomas have a higher recurrence rate than non-secreting tumors.[43]

Although it is not known for certain which factors influence risk of recurrence, certainly the original size of the tumor does, as well as PRL activity. In one series,[44] the rate of recurrence in 56 patients with large adenomas, all but 1 having received postoperative irradiation, was 20% (11/56), occurring between 6 months and 6 years. Again, it was not clear that original tumor size was related to more aggressive growth or high recurrence rate, but no histologic differences were found between tumors that were large and relapsing and those that were smaller and did not recur. In another series[45] of 100 non-functioning pituitary tumors, of which 82% were null-cell adenomas, symptomatic recurrence developed in 6 patients, and 10 demonstrated radiographic recurrence during 48 to 100 months (mean, 73.4 months) of observation after transsphenoidal surgery; the effect of radiation therapy was moot.

The follow-up of treated adenomas has been problematic, from the standpoint of detecting recurrence. As adenomas must be large initially to cause visual defects, so must recurrences be substantial before defects again evolve. Although progressive visual failure may be the incontestable impetus for re-operation or irradiation, consecutive perimetry may not be counted on to reveal "early" tumor recurrence. An anatomic assessment, as provided by CT scanning or MRI with coronal views, provides the most sensitive technique for monitoring tumor regrowth. In addition, measurement of serum PRL levels in the immediate postoperative period and at regular intervals is a rational way to determine recurrence of prolactinomas.

Pituitary adenomas may act more aggressively on occasion, invading the laterally adjacent cavernous sinuses and producing acute or chronic cranial nerve palsies (see Chapter 12). Potential markers for aggressive biologic behavior include p53, MIB-1, PCNA, RB, and H-ras; a high MIB-1 antibody index indicates active proliferation, as does positive p53.[46] Indeed, prolactinomas may metastasize. A case of "sinusoidal adenoma" invading the skull base, pterygoid, and orbit of a 12-year-old boy was reported[47]; the cytologic picture suggested "a higher degree of malignancy than usual," but it did not appear to be an undifferentiated carcinoma. Another rare instance of an invasive pituitary adenoma was described also in a 12-year-old boy who presented with severe headache, vomiting, rapid loss of monocular acuity, and sixth nerve palsy[48]; histologically, there was absence of cellular pleomorphism or of mitosis despite the invasive course. Histologic criteria apparently are not sufficient to indicate invasive tendencies, and local extension is not evidence of malignancy. Seeding of the subarachnoid space and spread outside the cranium are extremely rare complications that indicate biologic malignancy.

Malignant lesions of the pituitary may be initially mistaken for simple adenomas, including sellar plasmacytoma, lung, and breast metastases[49]; atypical features suggesting malignancy include rapidly progressive visual loss, ocular motor palsies, and facial numbness (see also below, Metastatic Diseases and Other Mass Lesions). In addition, benign and rare vascular malformations of the sella fossa are reported.[50]

Acromegaly

Other adenomas secrete ACTH or thyroid-stimulating hormone or are "mixed" (most commonly PRL- and GH-secreting), but they are principally of endocrinologic interest and relate to neuro-ophthalmology only when extrasellar extension produces field defects. However, acromegaly requires further elaboration.

Acromegaly is the clinical condition associated with excess GH either from autonomous pituitary adenoma secretion or from hypothalamic production of GH-releasing factor with subsequent GH hypersecretion. Many GH-secreting tumors contain a mutant form of the chain of G_S protein in the somatotrope. This represents a relatively rare endocrinopathy, although in Wilson's surgical series[20] of 1000 transssphenoidal procedures, there were 195 cases of GH-secreting adenomas, and 228 cases of acromegaly were found among 1000 adenomas seen at the Mayo Clinic from 1935 to 1972.[51] Clinical features include bone and soft tissue enlargement, especially of hands, feet, and face, visceromegaly, arthritis and carpal tunnel syndrome, hypertension, diabetes, hyperhidrosis, weakness, arthralgias, tooth malocclusion, headaches, impotence, menstrual irregularities, and abnormal glucose tolerance test results. Adenomas associated with acromegaly seem not to expand beyond the sella with the regularity typical of prolactinomas or non-secretory tumors. This phenomenon may be attributable to earlier detection as a consequence of prominent clinical manifestations. Nonetheless, 144 of 228 patients with acromegaly in the Mayo Clinic series[51] had visual field defects, a finding that may reflect delay in diagnosis in a series commenced 6 decades ago.

The use of octreotide and other long-acting analogs of somatostatin are indicated as follows: for the treatment of patients with active disease when surgery or radiation therapy has failed or is contraindicated; while awaiting the clinical effects of radiation therapy; as primary treatment in the elderly and medically incapacitated.[52] Long-term octreotide therapy reduces serum levels of GH and insulin-like growth factor-1, and it reduces tumor size.[53] Ablation of GH-adenomas is also achieved with various forms of radiation therapy, but more or less immediate remission is best accomplished by transsphenoidal resection.

Pituitary "Apoplexy"

Pituitary "apoplexy" refers to an acute change in volume of a pituitary adenoma as a result of spontaneous hemorrhage, edematous swelling, or necrosis. Postpartum infarction or hemorrhage in non-tumorous glands does occur, as firmly established in the obstetric literature as "Sheehan's syndrome,"[54] but chiasmal compression is a rare event. Even in clinically silent cases, adenoma necrosis with cystic liquefaction and evidence of previous bleeding is encountered commonly enough and may be identified by radiologic criteria (see below). Gross or microscopic hemorrhagic necrosis is apparently independent of endocrine activity or neoplastic pattern. In a review[55] of 320 verified adenomas, with a high incidence in giant or recurrent large adenomas (41%), evidence of hemorrhage was found in 58 cases (18%). Mean age was 50 years, and clinical courses included the following: acute apoplexy, 7 cases; subacute apoplexy, 11 cases; recent silent hemorrhages, 13 cases; old silent hemorrhage, 27 cases. That is, in 58 cases of hemorrhage in adenomas, 40 were symptomatically silent. From a series[56] of 453 operated adenomas, 45 (10%) demonstrated hemorrhage, but only 13 of these patients had acute symptoms of pituitary apoplexy; the authors correlated hemorrhage with marked suprasellar extension. Wilson[20] concluded that most massive pituitary tumors are prolactinomas, and there is "evidence of necrosis in most prolactinomas"; spontaneous necrosis or hemorrhage is related to indolent tumor growth; that is, tumor cell population expands or contracts at a rate determined by the balance of cell production and cell death.

Hemorrhage into adenomas is documented following head trauma,[57] after cardiopulmonary bypass,[58] and subsequent to tests of pituitary function using thyroid-releasing hormone, gonadotropin-releasing hormone, and insulin.[59] Additionally, uncomplicated pregnancy, bleeding disorders, radiation therapy, adrenalectomy, and physical exertion are all reported predisposing factors in pituitary "apoplexy."[60] Indeed, pituitary hemorrhage may occur in adolescence,[61] principally in prolactinomas.

Clinical signs and symptoms include the following: acute onset of severe headache, often sickening frontal or retro-bulbar cephalgia, or other less disabling change in headache pattern; acute or rapidly progressing unilateral or bilateral (usually asymmetric) ophthalmoplegia due to rapid expansion into cavernous sinuses (see also Chapter 12); epistaxis or CSF rhinorrhea when the mass ruptures or erodes into the sphenoid sinus; complications of blood or necrosis debris in the CSF, with "pseudomeningitis"; rapid neurologic deterioration and obtundation, although patients need not be stuporous; and, greater or lesser degrees of hypopituitarism.[62,63] Selective expansion laterally into the cavernous sinus may produce ophthalmoplegia without visual loss; selective expansion superiorly may produce visual loss without ophthalmoplegia. Almost without exception, enlargement of the sella is found even on plain skull film views; both CT and MRI detect fresh hemorrhage (Fig. 6–3), but MRI may fail to demonstrate acute hemorrhage unless specific sequences are employed (hemorrhage may be isointense on T_1-weighted images and hypointense on T_2-weighted images; in the subacute phase, extracellular methemoglobin should appear bright on both T_1 and T_2 sequences). Corticosteroid replacement and other supportive measures may be critical, and, in most instances, decompression through the sphenoid sinus is advisable, sooner rather than later. Bromocriptine has been suggested as a temporizing measure when signs and symptoms are modest and not progressing,[64] and there are advocates[65] for conservative management consisting of intravenous dexamethasone, so long as visual deficits are minimal or rapidly improve; otherwise decompressive surgery is required. Given the regularity with which pituitary apoplexy is often a delayed diagnosis, being confused with ruptured aneurysm or meningitis, for example, and that transsphenoidal surgery is a relatively simple undertaking, further procrastination in decompression of the compromised visual pathways is to be avoided.

Imaging of Pituitary Tumors

In addition to the radiologic implications mentioned previously, specific points should be emphasized. Contrast-enhanced CT and, especially, MRI have replaced all previous radiologic techniques in the detection and anatomic assessment of sellar and juxtasellar lesions. MRI has also the inherent advantage of using no radiation, nor does it require iodinated contrast injections. Although thin-section contrasted CT does indeed disclose most lesions, bone changes, and recent hemorrhage, MRI is superior in delineating distortions of optic nerves and chiasm, in displaying arteries, and in revealing fat, hemorrhage, or cyst (see Figs. 6–3E through M). Indeed, in a prospective study of normal volunteers, gadolinium-enhanced MRI disclosed pituitary adenomas (3 mm to 6 mm in diameter, *i.e.*, microadenomas) in 10% of adults aged 18 to 60 years.[66] T_2-weighted fast spin-echo MRIs are currently the most precise sequence for demonstrating the optic nerves and chiasm, even when these structures are severely distorted by suprasellar tumor extension.[67]

The question of invasion or displacement of the cavernous sinus has been studied by MRI technique,[68] with

Fig. 6–3. Neuroimaging of pituitary adenomas. **A.** Axial computed tomography (CT) section shows a round tumor mass filling the suprasellar cistern; ring enhancement (*arrows*) indicates subcapsular hemorrhage. **B.** Contrast-enhanced coronal CT section through a large invasive adenoma. Note encasement of the carotid artery (*arrows*) and the position of the middle cerebral artery above (*arrowheads*). **C.** Axial CT section shows lateral expansion into the cavernous sinuses (*white arrows*) and a necrotic cyst (*black arrow*). **D.** Subfrontal superior extent of the mass. Note the middle cerebral arteries.

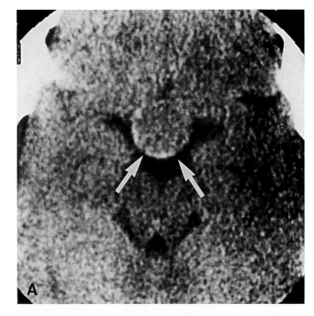

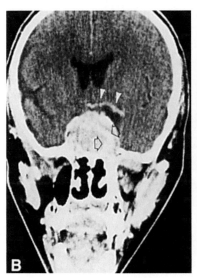
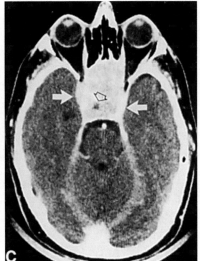
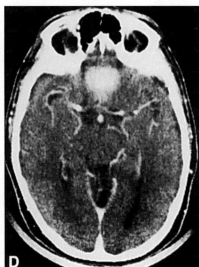

the following conclusions: the normal cavernous sinuses are usually symmetric but vary in size; the lateral dural margins are easily recognized as linear, discrete, low-intensity structures; the medial dural margin (pituitary capsule) is rarely discernible; sensitivity of predicting cavernous sinus invasion is only 55%; no features permit certain distinction between invasive and noninvasive adenomas, because the medial wall of the cavernous sinus is not reliably identified; the most specific sign of invasion is carotid artery encasement. Normal pituitary glands extend laterally into the cavernous sinus in 29% of microanatomic dissection specimens.[69]

A study[70] of the CT appearance of pituitary masses after transsphenoidal surgery showed that the superior limits do *not* return to normal immediately despite complete tumor removal, but only gradually regress in 3 to 4 months. This phenomenon is variably due to blood clot in the sella, to muscle or fat used as packing material, and to adhesions between the diaphragma sellae or tumor and brain tissue above. Therefore, neuroimaging in the immediate postoperative period may be misleading, and baseline radiologic evaluation may be delayed for 3 to 4 months, unless otherwise indicated.

Meningiomas

Posterior perioptic foraminal, medial sphenoid ridge, and tuberculum sellae meningiomas produce prechiasmal (optic nerve) or chiasmal compression, as do olfactory groove and planum masses that extend posteriorly. Visual deficits usually take the form of slowly progressive *monocular* loss of vision, and, when both fields are involved, there is a distinct tendency toward marked assymetry, frequently with extensive visual deficit on

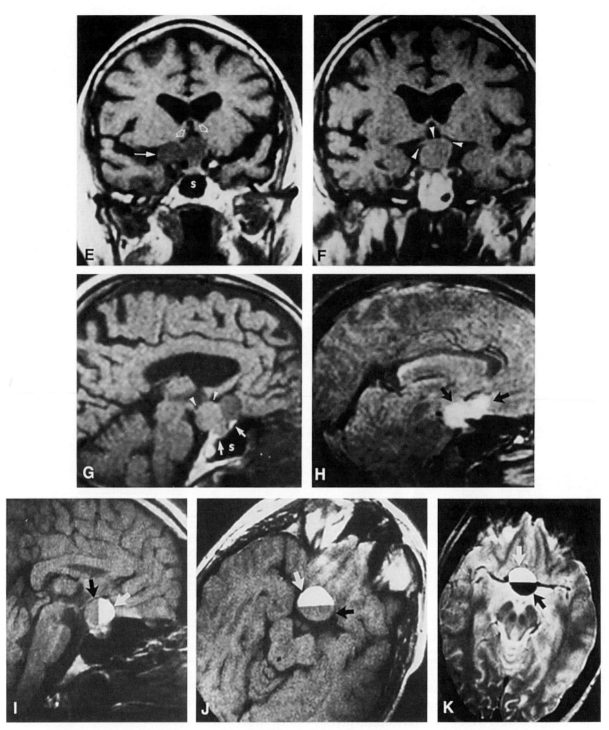

Fig. 6–3. (*continued*) **E.** Magnetic resonance imaging of a large lobulated prolactinoma, with suprasellar extension. Note the distortion of the third ventricle (*open arrows*) and extension toward the temporal lobe (*long arrow*); the tumor has not involved the sphenoidal sinus (*s*). **F.** Chiasm (*arrowheads*) is draped on the superior surface of the tumor (TR, 550 milliseconds; TE, 26 milliseconds). **G.** Sagittal section shows suprasellar growth with the chiasm above (*arrowheads*); the sella (*arrows*) and sphenoidal sinus (*s*) are normal (TR, 850 milliseconds; TE, 26 milliseconds). **H.** Hyperintense signal (TR, 2000 milliseconds; TE, 60 milliseconds) indicates the partial cystic character. Sagittal **(I)** and axial **(J)** sections with head tilt to the right, in case of a large cystic adenoma with an interface level between newer blood (*white arrow*) and older blood (*black arrow*) (TR, 800 milliseconds; TE, 30 milliseconds). **K.** Signal difference is intensified (TR, 2100 milliseconds; TE, 80 milliseconds).

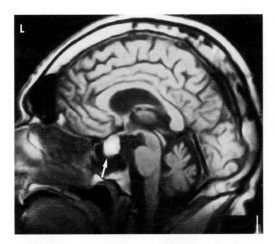
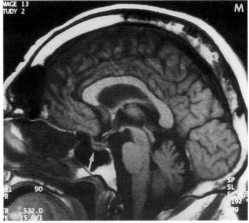

Fig. 6–3. (*continued*) **L.** Hemorrhage (bright signal, *arrow*) in a pituitary adenoma with headache and bitemporal field depressions. **M.** Without interventions, 2-month follow-up showed spontaneous involution, with normal pituitary gland (*arrow*), stalk, and chiasm.

one side before the contralateral field becomes involved. Slow growth across the tuberculum eventuates in contralateral optic nerve or chiasmal interference. There is a distinct predilection for meningiomas to occur in middle-aged women, and enlargement during pregnancy, as well as possible association with breast cancer, supports evidence for the role of estrogen and progesterone receptors.[71]

Although nonspecific headaches are a common feature of suprasellar meningiomas, most patients present with monosymptomatic failure of vision and are thus likely to present initially to the ophthalmologist. Although relentless deterioration of vision is the rule, fluctuations over weeks or months may mimic optic neuritis.[72] Slavin[73] documented an exceptional case of acute, bilateral central scotomas developing over 2 weeks, in the presence of a gigantic meningioma that extended into the ethmoid sinuses and under the frontal lobes. In a series of suprasellar meningiomas,[74] the time interval from the onset of unilateral visual loss to subjective bilateral defects, was 1 to 8 years; simultaneous bilateral onset was not documented. Although periocular pain made worse by eye movement is typical of inflammatory optic neuritis, Ehlers and Malmros[75] reported this symptom with suprasellar meningiomas.

Asymmetric optic disc pallor is a relatively "late sign," normal discs being fully compatible with visual loss over many months. The much-touted Foster Kennedy syndrome, that is, optic atrophy with contralateral papilledema due to large subfrontal meningiomas, remains a distinct rarity.[75] Anosmia, also classically considered an important finding with olfactory meningiomas, is much overrated and is difficult to assess. Delayed diagnosis of large tumors results in frontal lobe compression and edema causing mental changes or hydrocephalus due to obstruction of the ventricular system.

In previous decades, chiasmal interference with optic atrophy, but "normal" plain skull films, was referred to as "Cushing's syndrome of the chiasm," caused by meningiomas, aneurysms, or other non-calcified suprasellar lesions. The modern neuroimaging techniques of enhanced CT, "bone-window" protocols, and gadolinium-contrasted MRI are now exceedingly sensitive in disclosing meningiomas or other parachiasmal masses (Fig. 6–4). At present, contrast-enhanced CT or MRI precisely demonstrate extra-axial tumor configuration; CT is superior in disclosing calcification or bone changes, but it is inferior for assessing suprasellar or intrasellar extension, postsurgical changes, and vascular displacement or encasement.[76] Whether MRI or even MR angiography obviates standard selective arteriography, especially when surgical intervention is contemplated, is moot.

In a large surgical series,[77] 257 patients underwent 338 craniotomies for meningiomas at diverse intracranial locations. Of these, there were 35 sphenoid wing, 20 olfactory groove, 12 tuberculum sellae, and 2 orbitocranial meningiomas; that is, about 27% of tumors were of potential neuro-ophthalmologic interest. For the entire series, average observed survival was 9 years, and recurrence rate was 22% overall. At the Massachusetts General Hospital in Boston,[78] of 225 patients operated on for meningioma, parasellar tumors constituted 12%; only half of these were considered grossly "completely excised," but with a 5-year probability of recurrence or progression of 19%. No radiation therapy was applied in this series.

Rosenberg and Miller[79] analyzed the visual results in 16 patients following modern microsurgical removal of meningiomas involving the intracranial optic nerves or chiasm. Median age at diagnosis was 56.5 years, and median duration of visual symptoms was 19.5 months. Visual acuity improved in 12 of 32 eyes, worsened in 8 (3 optic nerves were transected; 5 eyes showed an average

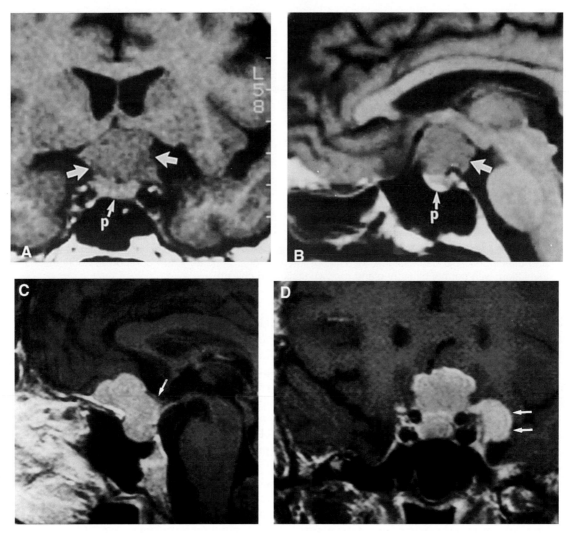

Fig. 6–4. Magnetic resonance imaging of a suprasellar meningioma (TR, 600 milliseconds; TE, 20 milliseconds). **A.** Coronal section of a large meningioma (*large arrows*), isodense to brain. **B.** Sagittal section. Note the normal sella and pituitary gland (*p*). Sagittal **(C)** and coronal **(D)** sections of a planum meningioma, extending into the sella. Note the upward deflection of the chiasm (*arrow* in **C**) and extension to the cavernous sinus (*arrows* in **D**).

drop of 2.6 lines in acuity), and 10 eyes retained normal function. Visual outcome appeared to be related most closely to duration of symptoms.

The response of meningiomas to irradiation has not been clearly established. In general, growth and re-growth rates are extremely slow, compounding the problem of assessing the question of radiotherapeutic efficacy. In a series of 12 incompletely resected meningiomas (8 sphenoidal, 2 petrosal, 1 each orbital and parasagittal), patients were subjected to 4800 to 6080 cGy (median dose, 5490 cGy) in 6 weeks[80]; median post-radiation follow-up was 54.5 months (range, 20 to 120 months), and 9 patients were said to remain free of clinical or radiologic signs of tumor progression. Recurrent lesions were discovered at 4, 6, and 9 years, and the authors concluded that postoperative radiation therapy is indicated for incompletely excised meningiomas.

Carella et al[81] reviewed the experience with 68 patients, 49 women and 19 men, divided into 3 groups: (A) 43 patients who had surgery (42 with known residual tumor) followed by irradiation; (B) 14 patients who had radiation for recurrence, of whom 11 underwent subtotal resection before radiation therapy; (C) 11 patients who had radiation as primary treatment. In Group A, 41 of 43 patients were alive, most doing well neurologically after 1 to 10 years; in Group B, 5 were dead of meningioma (all within 3 years), and 7 patients were considered "stable"; in Group C, all were alive at 3 to 6 years, 9 with neurologic improvement, and 4 with CT evidence of tumor shrinkage with central necrosis.

Conventional fractionated radiation therapy continues to provide mixed results,[82,83] and stereotactic radiation therapy with single-fraction dosage has enthusiastic advocates, but relatively short-term follow-up data.[84]

Undoubtedly, external-beam radiation therapy has a role as an effective adjunctive treatment in the control of meningioma recurrence, but the possibility of collateral damage, including radionecrosis (see below) of vital neural structures, must be considered.

With reference specifically to results of radiation therapy of meningiomas involving the anterior visual pathway, Kupersmith et al[85] analyzed 4 patients treated by irradiation alone and 16 treated in combination with tumor excision. Improvement in visual function occurred in 13 patients, 2 showed temporary improvement, and 5 maintained stable function for up to 9.5 years; follow-up CT did not disclose reduction in tumor size. The study by Kennerdell et al,[86] dealing primarily with optic nerve sheath meningiomas, inferred a distinct salutary effect of irradiation alone or as a supplement to partial microsurgical resection.

The management of menigiomas involving the intracranial optic nerves and chiasm may be summarized as follows: surgery remains the principal initial endeavor, in some instances with efforts intended only at judicious gross "de-bulking"; postoperative radiation therapy at least appears to increase the recurrence-free interval in cases of incompletely resected tumors; radiation therapy alone (dosage range, 5000 to 5500 cGy) is an acceptable alternative in patients considered poor surgical risks, especially where tumor has encased major arteries or invaded the skull base or when neuroimaging demonstrates surgically inaccessable optic nerves or chiasm. Complications arise when adhesions of tumor to portions of nerves or chiasm, or to vessels, are agressively manipulated in attempts at "complete removal."

Progesterone receptor sites are expressed in 81% of women and 40% of men with meningiomas,[71,84] with 96% of benign and 40% of malignant meningiomas containing progesterone receptor–positive nuclei, but without correlation between progesterone receptor index and age or histologic subtype.[71] Moreover, the efficacy of antiprogesterone agents such as mifepristone has proved disappointing.[87] At present, immunotherapy in the form of interferon-alpha is under investigation.[88] Treatment options, or the absence thereof, must be considered in light of the glacial growth rate of most meningiomas. For example, Olivero et al[89] found that 78% of 60 asymptomatic meningiomas followed for over 2.5 years demonstrated no growth, and the remaining 22% showed a mean growth rate of only 0.24 cm in maximum diameter per year. Therefore, judicious observation may prove the best option, especially in the elderly or in patients with considerable risk for surgical intervention.

Recurrence or regrowth of tumor is best monitored by contrast-enhanced CT and gadolinium-enhanced MRI. After initial postoperative baseline visual field plotting, consecutive perimetry discloses visual failure only as a relatively late sign of tumor enlargement.

Perioptic meningioma of the intraorbital portion of the optic nerve is considered in Chapter 5, Part II.

Craniopharyngiomas

Craniopharyngiomas are tumors that arise from vestigial epidermoid remnants of Rathke's pouch, scattered as cell rests in the infundibulo-hypophyseal region. These tumors are usually admixtures of solid cellular components and variable-sized cysts containing oily composites of degenerated blood and desquamated epithelium or necrotic tissue (and blood) with cholesterol crystals. Dystrophic calcification of this debris is detectable with plain films and CT imaging and is an important radiologic sign estimated to be seen in more than 80% of childhood craniopharyngiomas. These tumors are congenital (dysontogenic) and, in rare instances, may present in the neonate. There is a more or less bimodal age incidence, peaking in the first 2 decades and again in the years 50 to 70 (Fig. 6–5). These predominantly suprasellar tumors account for 2% to 4% of all intracranial tumors regardless of age group, but the incidence is 8% to 13% in children. Of all suprasellar masses, craniopharyngiomas comprise 54% in children, and 20% in adults, and show two clinicopathologic and pathogenetic separate types: adamantinous (predominantly cystic, in childhood) and squamous-papillary (predominantly solid, adulthood).[90]

Presentation in childhood is commonly related to hydrocephalus and endocrinopathies, consisting of variable degrees of hypopituitarism with or without diabetes insipidus; obesity and somnolence also attest to hypo-

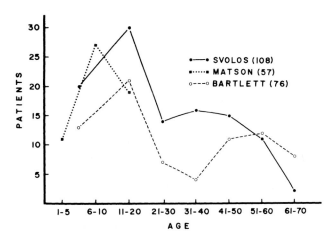

Fig. 6–5. Age distribution of craniopharyngioma. (Data from Svolos D: Craniopharyngiomas: a study based on 108 verified cases. Acta Chir Scand Suppl 403:1, 1969; Matson DD, Crigler JF: Management of craniopharyngioma in childhood. J Neurosurg 30:377, 1969; and Bartlett JR: Craniopharyngiomas: an analysis of some aspects of symptomatology, radiology and histology. Brain 94:725, 1971. The Matson series was limited to children younger than 16 years.)

thalamic disturbance. Gonadotropic hormone deficit results in retarded or absent sexual development, and precocious puberty is rare. In children, progressive visual loss goes unnoticed until a level of severe bilateral impairment is reached, or unless headache, vomiting, and behavioral changes occur. Increased intracranial pressure produces papilledema in about 65%, and optic atrophy is observed in roughly 60%.[91]

In adults, visual deterioration is the universal symptom that demands investigation, although occult endocrine dysfunction may be uncovered; hypopituitarism, diabetes insipidus, amenorrhea, and galactorrhea inconstantly eventuate. Visual field defects are frequently asymmetric bitemporal hemianopias or a homonymous pattern with reduced acuity (Fig. 6–6) when the optic tract is compressed.[92]

CT scanning retains special relevance to craniopharyngioma diagnosis, currently superior to MRI in detection of calcification and cyst formation (Fig. 6–7A to C); however, the extent of involvement of adjacent structures, that is, the optic chiasm, third ventricle, and intracavernous carotid artery, is more clearly delineated by MRI (Fig. 6–7D and E).[93] Craniopharyngioma fluid collections are found to be uniformly bright on T_2-weighted sequences, but on T_1-weighted images, the signal intensity may range from hypointense to hyperintense, reflecting the heterogeneous contents of cysts. Because calcification and cyst formation are hallmarks of craniopharyngiomas, CT is more specific than MRI.

At times, intrinsic infiltration of tumor may thicken the chiasm and contiguous optic nerve, a radiologic configuration that mimics glioma.[94] Likewise, glioma may be simulated when the optic canal is invaded and enlarged, but accompanying bony erosion of the sella weighs heavily toward craniopharyngioma.

More than half a century ago, Harvey Cushing declared that craniopharyngiomas "offer one of the most baffling of surgical problems," and were "disheartening from an operative standpoint."[95] Fortunately, in the modern era, the surgical microscope, steroid replacement, radiation therapy, and valve-regulated shunts have all proved valuable adjuncts to the operative management of these masses. Since the time of Matson, a major neurosurgical school of thought was preoccupied with "complete" removal of craniopharyngiomas in preference to subtotal extirpation. Although primary total removal is no doubt ideal, this is actually only rarely accomplished. The question of "matsonian total removal" was addressed in the 1975 follow-up by Katz,[96] who analyzed the results of surgical management in 51 of Matson's patients operated upon between 1950 to 1968; there was a 25% operative mortality, a 71% 11-year mortality, and 76% of those cases examined by autopsy had residual tumor at the time of death.

A less ambitious approach consists of cyst aspiration, intracapsular dissection, cyst drainage via subcutaneous reservoir, and radiation therapy. In a series of 43 children at the Columbia-Presbyterian Medical Center in

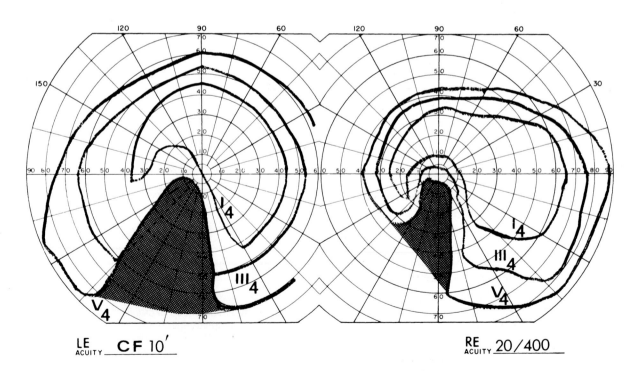

Fig. 6–6. Chiasmal-optic tract (posterior "junctional") field defect in an elderly woman with craniopharyngioma elevating the floor of the third ventricle and compressing the right optic tract. Note inferior incongruous hemianopia combined with diminished central acuity. *LE,* left eye; *RE,* right eye.

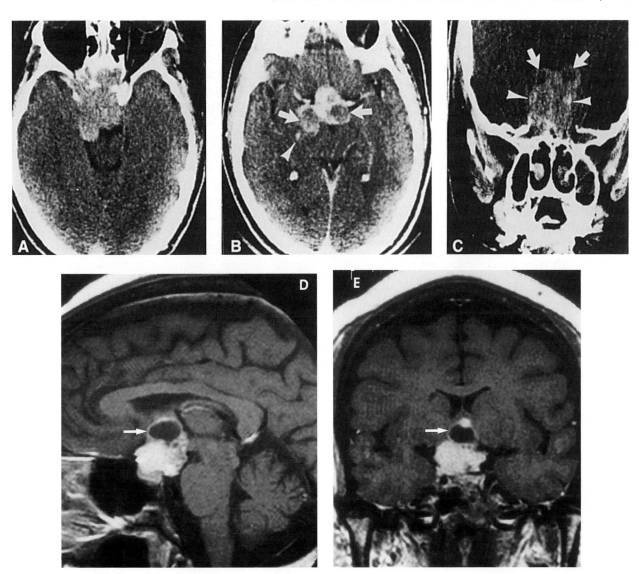

Fig. 6–7. Computed tomography scan of a large, multicystic craniopharyngioma. **A.** Axial section through the sella shows destruction of the bony skull base. Axial **(B)** and coronal **(C)** sections show cysts (*white arrows*) and calcification (*arrowheads*). Contrast-enhanced magnetic resonance imaging of the craniopharyngioma. Sagittal **(D)** and coronal **(E)** sections with gadolinium show solid and cystic (*arrows*) portions.

New York from 1952 to 1977,[97] 10-year actuarial survival rates were 52% for subtotal resection alone and 87% for subtotal plus radiation (mean, 5000 cGy). Tumors had recurred by 10 years in half of 14 children in whom removal was thought to be total, in more than 90% of those whose tumors were subtotally removed, and in less than 25% of those at risk after subtotal resection and irradiation. Recurrences were usually evident within 2 years, but more delayed after "total" resections. From a later series of 37 children cared for at Children's Hospital, Boston, from 1972 to 1981,[98] it was concluded that radiation therapy was equally, if not more, effective than attempted excision in controlling subsequent tumor growth. It is inferred that conservative surgery combined with irradiation (mean dose, 5464 cGy) offers less risk for psychosocial impairment than does tumor excision, although the delayed effects of radiation to the juvenile brain must be taken into account (see the discussion of therapy for optic glioma, below).

Craniopharyngiomas that arise low on the hypophyseal stalk are subdiaphragmatic and may be approached via the transsphenoidal route[99]; cystic recurrences may also be managed by transsphenoidal drainage, although surgical cure is unlikely. Interestingly enough, the first craniopharyngioma operated on successfully was reported in 1910, by Halstead, via the transsphenoidal approach.[100]

Regardless of surgical approach or use of radiation

therapy, endocrine replacement is anticipated in all cases, often for life.

Optic and Hypothalamic Gliomas

As noted in Chapter 5, Part I, astrocytic tumors of the anterior visual pathways present as two unrelated pathologic entities: the relatively benign and stable piloid glioma of childhood and the rare malignant glioblastoma of adulthood. Clinically and histologically, these two neoplasms have little in common, and the assumption that the malignant form stems from the indolent childhood glioma is untenable. The major clinical characteristics of these astrocytomas are contrasted in Table 6–1.

Childhood gliomas are clinically and pathologically controversial lesions, questions arising regarding natural course, growth potential, and efficacy of therapy. In 1922, Verhoeff remarked that, because most optic gliomas become manifest in early childhood, it is highly suggestive that these tumors "are really congenital in origin and due to some more or less localized abnormality in the embryonic development of the neuroglia of the nerve." Furthermore, Verhoeff believed that a glioma "does not increase in size by invading or destroying . . . but does so by causing pre-existing neuroglia in the vicinity of the growth to proliferate." Therefore, taking into account their occurrence in infancy and childhood, their indolent natural course, limited growth characteristics, histopathologic composition, and association with neurofibromatosis (see Chapter 5, Part II, and below), it is not unreasonable to make a case that optic gliomas are hereditary congenital hamartomas.

Alvord and Lofton,[101] in a literature review, uncovered 623 cases of optic gliomas with sufficient information to permit actuarial (life-table) analysis of prognosis as influenced by patients' age, tumor site, treatment, presence of concomitant neurofibromatosis, or extension into the hypothalamus or ventricle. The development of mathematical models led to the conclusion that these tumors, generally regarded histologically as low-grade astrocytomas, actually have a wide but continuous range of growth rates. Some grow rapidly enough to be explained by simple exponential doubling at a constant rate, but most behave as though their growth decelerates. This phenomenon makes comparisons of various groups of patients difficult, but no support was found for the classic hypothesis (see above) that some of these tumors may be hamartomas.

The association of von Recklinghausen's neurofibromatosis (NF), a form of congenital multiple hamartomatosis, and optic glioma is well known. The frequency of this association cannot be established with accuracy, but it is more common than generally recognized. The review by Hoyt and Baghdassarian[102] included 36 cases of anterior optic gliomas, of which 21 occurred with NF; in 1 family, 2 siblings had optic gliomas, and in a second family, gliomas occurred in a mother and child. In a large series[103] of 121 children younger than 18 years with NF (evaluated between 1953 and 1984), 17 (14%) had brain tumors, of which 9 were optic gliomas. Using MRI in 217 patients with NF aged 4 weeks to 69 years, tumors of the anterior visual pathways were uncovered in 15%, the mean age of patients with chiasmal tumors being about 15 years less than with optic nerve lesions only.[104] Other similar studies[105] of patients with NF using brain MRI showed an appreciable incidence of optic gliomas.

In the child with diminished vision, with or without proptosis, the stigmata of NF should be searched for, including café-au-lait spots, axillary freckling, iris fibromas, and peripheral nerve tumors. Family history should be carefully detailed with regard to skin manifestations, scoliosis, brain tumors, and seizures.

With regard to the indolent glioma of childhood, clinical presentation is predicated on location and extent of mass. Strictly intraorbital gliomas (see Chapter 5, Part II) present as insidious proptosis of variable degree, and although vision is usually diminished, remarkably good visual function is not uncommon. Orbital gliomas may be contiguous with astrocytic proliferation that extends posteriorly into the optic canal, the intracranial optic nerve, and the chiasm itself, that is, in the configuration of an "opto-chiasmatic" glioma. Anterior visual pathway gliomas may also be part of a more extensive mass

TABLE 6–1. Primary Gliomas of Nerve and Chiasm

	Childhood	Adulthood
Age at onset of symptoms	4–8 yr	Middle age
Presentation	Visual defects, proptosis	Rapid, severe unilateral visual loss (mimics neuritis)
Course	Relatively stable, nonprogressive	Rapid bilateral visual deterioration; other intracranial signs
Prognosis	Compatible with long life	Death within months to 2 yr
Neurofibromatosis	Related in large percentage of cases	No relationship
Histology	Noninvasive, pilocytic astrocytoma	Invasive, malignant astrocytoma (glioblastoma); may metastasize

that involves the hypothalamus, that is, an "opto-hypo-thalamic" glioma, with or without a congenital or juvenile diencephalic syndrome. Posterior continuation involves optic tracts and hemispheres.

Miller et al[106] classified chiasmal gliomas into anterior and posterior, suggesting that the latter, with involvement of the hypothalamus or optic tracts, manifest a more aggressive course and show a variable response to radiation therapy; in this series of 29 patients with pathologically documented chiasmal glioma, 9 tumors were anterior and 20 were posterior. The American Cancer Society proposed a system[107] for clinical staging of optic pathway gliomas, according to standard oncologic terminology and based on visual function and anatomic location, as follows: T1, one optic nerve, intraorbital or intracranial; T2, both optic nerves; T3, optic chiasm; T4, hypothalamus or thalamus. The system for visual staging is simplistic and seems less useful.

Russell's *diencephalic syndrome* of early childhood hypothalamic glioma consists of the following: emaciation despite adequate nutritional intake, which develops after a period of normal growth; hyperactivity and euphoria; skin pallor (without anemia); hypotension; and hypoglycemia. Other notable signs include nystagmus, variable optic atrophy, sexual precocity, and laughing seizures. Layden and Edwards[108] pointed out that, in 21 of 39 patients in whom eye movements were reported, pendular or rotary nystagmus occurred. Although *spasmus nutans* (disconjugate nystagmus, head titubation, and torticollis; see below and also Chapter 13) has been associated with chiasmal gliomas, in a review[109] of 67 consecutive children with this diagnosis who underwent 29 imaging studies, none had evidence of a mass lesion, and the authors questioned the need for neuroimaging, at least on initial evaluation.

Most cases of diencephalic syndrome are due to low-grade astrocytomas of the hypothalamus or adjacent chiasm, and almost all patients present when they are less than 2 years old. From Indiana University,[110] 12 cases of opticochiasmatic glioma with diencephalic syndrome were recorded, all with "failure to thrive," but with normal linear growth, and none with NF. Clinical evidence of bilateral optic nerve involvement was seen in 10 of these 12 patients, but at operation it was not possible to determine an initial site of origin. Ten children received radiation therapy with subsequent weight gain, deposition of subcutaneous fat, and normal development. Modern neuroimaging techniques may obviate craniotomy for biopsy,[111] and dissemination in the cerebral hemisphere and to the spine has been reported.[112] Radiation therapy is widely supported.

The question of *precocious sexual development* with hypothalamic gliomas bears comment. True precocious puberty occurs as a result of the premature release of luteinizing hormone–releasing hormone from the hypothalamus, which, in turn, stimulates the secretion of the pituitary gonadotropins that stimulate the gonadal sex steroids. The differential diagnosis of true precocious puberty includes cerebral and idiopathic categories, a distinction that cannot be made endocrinologically because of similarities in pituitary gonadotropin and sex steroid levels, but it may be facilitated by neuroimaging. Of 90 children (73 girls and 17 boys) with true precocious puberty who underwent high-resolution CT scanning,[113] 34 cerebral abnormalities were demonstrated in 32 children, 16 boys and 16 girls. These lesions included 17 hypothalamic hamartomas (defined as ectopic gray matter), 1 hypothalamic astrocytoma, 4 chiasmal gliomas and 2 other chiasm lesions, 8 ventricular abnormalities (2 associated with optic gliomas, and 1 each hypothalamic astrocytoma and hamartoma), 1 arachnoid cyst, and 1 teratoma. MRI of central precocious puberty in 50 consecutive patients[114] disclosed several abnormalities of the hypothalamic-pituitary axis, including glioma and ganglioglioma, anomalous distortions of the third ventricle and hypothalamus, and small tuber cinereum masses. Habiby et al[115] found precocious puberty in 40% of children with NF-1 and optic chiasm gliomas.

Chiasmal gliomas are more common than the isolated orbital type, and they present to the ophthalmologist as unilateral or bilateral visual loss, strabismus, "amblyopia," optic atrophy or disc hypoplasia, or nystagmus. Indeed, the nystagmus may mimic spasmus nutans complete with head nodding, or it may show a gross bilateral mixed horizontal-rotary pattern, especially when vision is severely defective. In a multicenter, retrospective report[116] of 10 infants in whom acquired nystagmus was the initial sign of chiasmal or parachiasmal glioma, 9 children presented before the age of 10 months. The nystagmus, primarily described as pendular and asymmetric, was difficult to differentiate from spasmus nutans. On average, the intracranial glioma was not recognized for 8.6 months after the onset of nystagmus, and in 5 diagnosed as "spasmus nutans," the mean delay in tumor diagnosis was 14.5 months. Three associated clinical findings were present or developed in these patients that distinguish this entity from spasmus nutans: optic atrophy in all 10 patients, poor feeding due to diencephalic syndrome in 5 of 10, and increased intracranial pressure with hydrocephalus in 3 of 10. In addition, I have examined 2 infants blind from glioma who showed a see-saw nystagmus with intermittent bursts of rapid saccadic movements reminiscent of opsoclonus.

Children with extensive basal tumors frequently develop hydrocephalus or signs and symptoms of increased intracranial pressure. Hypothalamic signs include precocious puberty (see above), obesity, dwarfism, hypersomnolence, and diabetes insipidus. As a rule, the non-visual complications of large optic gliomas arise in infancy and early childhood, and onset of ventricular obstruction or of hypothalamic involvement is uncommon much beyond the age of 5 years.

Visual fields defects with chiasmatic gliomas have been analyzed,[117] without finding a consistent relationship between the pattern of deficit and the location, size, or extent of tumor; in 12 of 20 patients, the putative bitemporal pattern of chiasmal interference was absent. Central scotomas or measurable depression of the central field, including reduced acuity, occurred in 70% of eyes; therefore, the absence of bitemporal hemianopia or one of its variants cannot be interpreted as a sign that glioma *does not* involve the chiasm. This same report stressed the indolent nature of these tumors and the monotonously stable clinical course of chiasmatic gliomas.

The radiologic investigation of potential chiasmal lesions in childhood is sophisticated to the extent that "biopsy by neuroimaging" may obviate surgical exploration and actual tissue diagnosis. Biopsy may actually increase visual defects.[117] Radiologic changes typical of optic glioma include smoothly enlarged optic canal, J- or omega-shaped remodeling of the sella due to erosion or dysplasia of the chiasmatic sulcus of the tuberculum, and suprasellar mass with elevation and flattening of the floor of the third ventricle. With some reserva-tions, CT characteristics are nearly diagnostic,[118] including the following three configurations: (1) tubular thickening of the optic nerve and chiasm; (2) suprasellar tumor with contiguous optic nerve expansion; and (3) suprasellar tumor with optic tract spread (Fig. 6–8). The diagnosis of globular or otherwise irregularly configured gliomas, without optic nerve or tract involvement, cannot be made on the basis of CT criteria alone. Contrast enhancement is typical. Findings in seven children[119] included spread along optic tracts and, in five instances, involvement of lateral geniculate bodies and adjacent radiations. In fact, this propensity to track along posterior visual pathways implies the diagnosis of glioma. MRI is superior to CT in demonstrating posterior extent of optic pathway gliomas and additionally detects focal areas of hyperintensity in basal ganglia, internal capsule, cerebellum, and white matter that are not detected by CT.[120,121]

The management of chiasmal gliomas is problematic and is often confounded by the absence or presence of neurofibromatosis, the quality of neuroimages, the variability of outcome data for morbidity and mortality, and reports reflecting enthusiastic advocacy for surgery

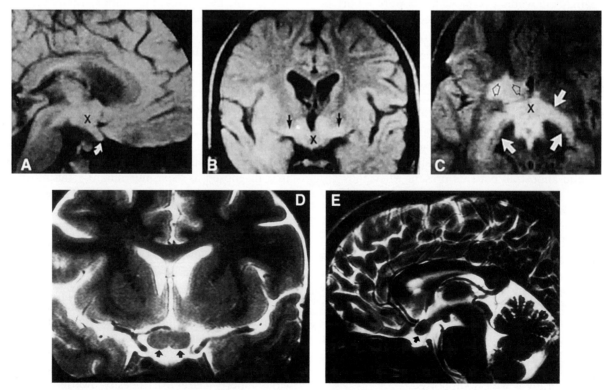

Fig. 6–8. Magnetic resonance imaging of a childhood optochiasmatic glioma. **A.** Sagittal section shows a ballooned optic nerve (*curved arrow*) and a thickened chiasm (*X*). **B.** Coronal section reveals a glioma in the chiasm (*X*), optic tracts (*arrows*), and walls of the third ventricle. **C.** T$_2$-weighted axial image (TR, 200 milliseconds; TE 60 milliseconds) with postbiopsy edema (*open arrows*) and a glioma in the chiasm (*X*) with posterior extension to both optic tracts (*white arrows*). Coronal (**D**) and sagittal (**E**) views of a glioma of the chiasm (*arrows*).

or radiation therapy. Surgical resection of chiasmal gliomas seldom improves vision or prolongs life, and, indeed, exploration and biopsy may worsen visual and general morbidity, including inducing diabetes insipidus and other hypothalamic dysfunction. An occasional intraneural cyst presents the opportunity for decompressive incision,[122] and exophytic growth is rare.[123] In infants with NF-1, a glioma may rarely develop when previous early neuroimaging disclosed normal visual pathway structures,[124] and spontaneous involution regression is exceptional but, indeed, documented.[125,126] Nonetheless, it seems reasonable that exploration should be undertaken *when doubt persists* even after modern neuroimaging and thorough assessment of associated signs and symptoms, including search for stigmata of neurofibromatosis, and lumbar puncture to assess for inflammatory cells and angiotensin-converting enzyme levels. Sarcoidosis may present with chiasmal enlargement that mimics glioma (see below). Surgical CSF shunting procedures are of obvious value when hydrocephalus exists.

That chiasmal gliomas tend to behave as relatively benign pilocytic astrocytomas with limited growth potential is a recurring thesis in large, carefully scrutinized series of cases, with appropriate follow-up intervals, exceptions to this rule notwithstanding. For example, the fate of patients with chiasmal gliomas in the original 1969 study from the University of California, was re-examined. Imes and Hoyt[127] documented the outcome of 28 patients with chiasmal gliomas, with a median follow-up of 20 years. Sixteen patients died (57%), but only 5 of causes directly related to the chiasmal mass, and 4 of these died before 1969, within 3 years of initial diagnosis; that is, the risk of death was greatest in the early period. Nine of 16 deaths occurred in patients with NF, 2 of chiasmal glioma, 7 with other malignant brain tumors or sarcomatous degeneration of peripheral tumors, but without any higher mortality rate among patients with NF. The "quality of life" of survivors was considered good, with no patient showing further decrease in visual function since the 1969 assessment. The authors concluded that the level of visual impairment present at initial diagnosis does not change appreciably thereafter, and this long-term study still affords no conclusive answers regarding the efficacy of radiation therapy.

Other series suggest more aggressive behavior of chiasmal gliomas, in adults as well as in children (see the discussion of optic glioma in Chapter 5, Part II). Therefore, there is no consensus regarding "the most appropriate management" of childhood visual gliomas, and the role of interventional radiation therapy remains peculiarly imprecise and uncertain, with ardent advocates for and against it. Data of each report must be cautiously scrutinized, especially when vision is said to benefit generally. The location and extent of tumor, age of patient,

and length of follow-up are all critical parameters in assessing treated versus untreated cases. Indeed, some instances of visual improvement and documented tumor shrinkage do occur following irradiation,[118,128–131] a finding implying that local radiation therapy results in at least transient stabilization in some patients. Visual improvement or stabilization is indeed achieved, but a high incidence of endocrine abnormalities is reported, especially GH deficiencies, as well as neuropsychiatric decline. Danoff et al[132] reported mental retardation in 4 cases, and endocrine dysfunction in 3 cases of 18 irradiated children, and Packer et al,[133] in a review of a 20-year experience at the Children's Hospital of Philadelphia, also confirmed moderate to severe intellectual compromise. The question of radiation therapy is further confounded by the risks of delayed complications that take the form of progressive dystrophic calcifying microangiopathy and demyelinization in adjacent and distant brain sites,[134] as well as large-vessel occlusions with catastrophic infarction reported in children with gliomas receiving irradiation within standard dosage range.[135] Considering the usually early age at presentation of optic gliomas, and the propensity for delayed complications, radiation therapy should not be commenced in a reflex manner.

Given these problems of irradiating immature brains, young children with newly discovered, progressive low-grade gliomas may be considered candidates for combined carboplatin and vincristine chemotherapy.[136] In addition, etoposide (VP-16) is currently under investigation.[137] It is suggested that chemotherapy has few deleterious effects and represents a useful alternative to irradiation, especially in young children. It may be emphasized that, even with the possibility of eventual tumor growth, delay in instituting radiation may lessen the adverse effects on the more matured brain.

A reasonable and rational strategy for optic chiasm gliomas must take into account the patient's age at onset of symptoms, the level of visual function, the presence of complicating hypothalamic features, ventricular obstruction, neuroradiologic baseline staging, and regular re-assessment of the various parameters of progression. Surgical exploration is required for tissue diagnosis only when doubt remains after adequate neuroimaging or when hydrocephalus is present. Radiation therapy should be commenced with caution at as advanced an age as possible, and in fractional doses of less than 200 cGy. As noted, further information is forthcoming with regard to chemotherapy as a valuable alternative.

Primary *malignant gliomas (glioblastomas)* of the visual pathways are rare tumors of adulthood, not to be confused with the relatively frequent low-grade astrocytomas of childhood, as discussed above (see Table 6–1). However, a rare case was reported in childhood[138] following radiation for a cerebellar medulloblastoma, and another presenting as pseudotumor cerebri in the extraordinary case of a 16-year-old girl with minimal papilledema and slight thalamic enlargement on MRI.[139] Hoyt et al[140] reviewed the subject and recorded 5 cases. They synthesized a syndrome of malignant optic glioma of adulthood composed of the following: usually involving middle-aged (majority, forties to fifties, range, 22 to 59 years) men (10 of 15 cases); beginning with signs and symptoms that mimic optic neuritis (rapid monocular loss of vision, retro-orbital pain, disc edema, and transient improvement with steroid therapy); progressing within 5 to 6 weeks to total blindness (may pass through chiasmal syndrome with contralateral hemianopia, then bilateral blindness); and terminating fatally within several months (3 months to 2 years). In a literature review,[141] only 30 cases had been identified since 1900, ranging in age from 22 to 79 years (mean, age 52 years), without association with neurofibromatosis. Progressive enlargement of the optic nerves and chiasm complex is documented by MRI,[142] with the tumor predominantly centered in the optic chiasm or tract, but with infiltration of surrounding structures. Thus, this syndrome represents the occurrence of a common brain tumor (glioblastoma) in an uncommon location. Albers et al[143] have suggested that combined irradiation therapy and chemotherapy offer some temporary relief.

Dysgerminomas

Primary suprasellar dysgerminomas (atypical teratoma, "ectopic pinealoma") are rare causes of chiasmal interference, but they constitute a more or less distinguishable clinical syndrome. Such tumors likely arise from cell rests in the anterior portion of the floor of the third ventricle, or they originate in the neurohypophysis; these *germ cell tumors (germinoma, embryonal carcinoma, choriocarcinoma, yolk sac tumor, and mixed tumors)* seem *not* directly related to the pineal itself, although some histologically resemble atypical pineal teratomas. Usually lacking characteristics of developed pineal parenchyma, these neoplasms may be indistinguishable from testicular seminomas, and portions of three germinal layers may be observed.

In a series of 153 patients with histologically verified lesions,[144] 78% were male, with a mean age of 16 years (range, 2 to 45 years); 78% of patients were between 6 and 24 years of age; 51% of tumors were located in the pineal region, 30% in the neurohypophysis, and the remainder in basal ganglia, cerebellopontine angle, lateral ventricle, or multiple sites. Patients with pineal masses present with symptoms and signs of aqueductal obstruction and intracranial hypertension, including vertical gaze palsies (Parinaud's syndrome) and papilledema; neurohypophyseal lesions present with diabetes insipidus and visual loss, with variable growth retardation and amenorrhea. Serum titers of human chorionic gonadotropin and alpha-fetoprotein may be elevated. Partial resection, radiation therapy, and chemotherapy result in variable survival rates.[144]

Camins and Mount[145] reviewed 58 cases and also suggested the presence of a classic triad consisting of visual field loss, at times not necessarily of a clearly chiasmatic pattern (due to intrinsic infiltration of the anterior visual pathways), diabetes insipidus, and mixed hypopituitarism; in this series, symptoms commenced at the end of the first decade or during the second decade, with growth retardation; there was an equal male-female incidence. Again, definitive diagnosis and therapy depend on confirmatory biopsy, although the clinical situation at times suggests the diagnosis (Fig. 6–9). Neuroimaging may appear similar to chiasmatic glioma.[146]

Radiation therapy (4000 to 6000 cGy) offers excellent long-term palliation, if not cure. Because subarachnoid seeding of the neuraxis is a distinct possibility, more extensive radiation may be indicated, and long-range endocrine replacement is critical.

Suprasellar Aneurysms

Aneurysms of the paraclinoidal and supraclinoidal segments of the internal carotid artery are relatively frequent causes of progressive visual loss, usually producing markedly asymmetric field defects and occurring most commonly in middle-aged women. Aneurysms and other vascular lesions that involve the chiasm are discussed in detail in Chapter 17.

DEMYELINATIVE DISEASE AND INFLAMMATIONS

Disseminated sclerosis is considered an uncommon cause of the chiasmal syndrome. Although visual field defects vary considerably, most patterns in multiple sclerosis (MS) imply that the prechiasmal portion of the optic nerves harbor the majority of lesions, but microscopic survey of the visual pathways indicates that the distribution of plaques assumes a less predictable pattern. Lumsden[147] described pronounced demyelination or axonal degeneration within the optic chiasms of 36 consecutive necropsied patients with MS; loss of neural tissue was at times so severe as to render the optic nerves "thinner than usual," even on macroscopic examination.

It is a paradox that so few clinical reports have described chiasmal visual field defects in patients with MS, despite the compelling neuropathologic evidence of the high incidence of demyelination at that site. In 1925, Traquair published "Acute Retrobulbar Neuritis Affecting the Optic Chiasm and Tract,"[148] in which the visual fields of four patients were recorded; two cases were clearly of a bitemporal pattern (one case appears to be a monocular cecocentral scotoma, and the other shows a homonymous hemianopia), and all were ascribed to MS. Indeed, Traquair believed that chiasmal

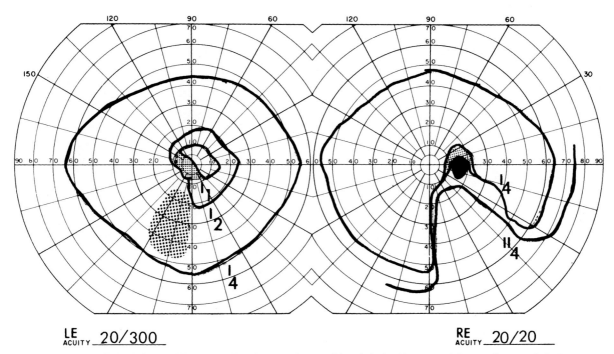

Fig. 6–9. Field defects with suprasellar dysgerminoma. Note inferior bitemporal depressions and diminished vision on the left; deficits are characteristic of posterior chiasmal interference (see Fig. 6–1, **D**). *LE,* left eye; *RE,* right eye.

neuritis would be more frequently found with more exhaustive field analysis.

Spector et al[149] reported 6 cases of chiasmal neuritis in MS, all women between 20 and 40 years of age; field defects were commonly of a "junctional" pattern, with reduction of acuity in one or both eyes. Of 12 eyes, 9 ultimately attained excellent vision, with an apparently salutary effect of systemic corticosteroids. Abnormal pneumoencephalograms were seen in 2 patients; 1 of these underwent exploratory craniotomy with visualization of a swollen chiasm and right nerve. From the Optic Neuritis Treatment Trial (see Chapter 5, Part II), field defects of chiasmal origin were also documented. According to Lindenberg et al,[150] swelling of the optic nerves and chiasm due to lymphocytic infiltration and astrocytic proliferation may mimic optic glioma. MRI is, of course, most useful in detecting white matter lesions, including the anterior visual pathways (Fig. 6–10).

The place of *neuromyelitis optica* (Devic's syndrome) in the spectrum of demyelinative syndromes included under the rubric of "multiple sclerosis" is unclear, but neither clinical nor pathologic features seem to isolate "Devic's syndrome" adequately. Usually acute in onset, there is a propensity for occurrence in children and young adults, with severe bilateral visual loss (chiasmal neuritis ?) accompanied by paraplegia due to transverse myelitis usually at a high cervical level. In the case of a 61-year-old woman without evidence of collagen or

giant cell arteritis, bilateral visual loss was followed by slowly progressive paraplegia[151]; post-mortem examination disclosed numerous areas of severe demyelination with foci of cystic degeneration extending through several cervical cord segments, with thickening and hyalinization of blood vessels and accumulation of perivascular lymphocytes; the optic chiasm and tracts were demyelinated, and small vessels showed hyalinization, but there were no other demyelinative lesions elsewhere in the hemispheres, brain stem, or cerebellum.

Other cases of chiasmal optic neuritis, other than MS, are infrequently documented.[152] Purvin et al[153] have reported chiasmal neuritis as a complication of Epstein-Barr virus infection, without polyradiculopathy. Ethchlorvynol (Placidyl) has been incriminated as a toxic cause of "chiasmal optic neuritis,"[154] and field defects with ethambutol may suggest a bitemporal pattern (see Chapter 5, Part II).

The question of *opticochiasmatic arachnoiditis* is controversial and confusing. Most cases seem complicated by previous trauma, meningitis, encephalitis, hemorrhage, arachnoidal cysts, and even familial optic neuropathies (Leber's type ?). This diagnostic consideration is always tentative, resting on exclusion of other definable mechanisms of visual loss and often requiring craniotomy for verification. Infrequent instances in which other contributing factors are excluded seem genuine. Cant and Harrison[155] reported a valid case of progressive vi-

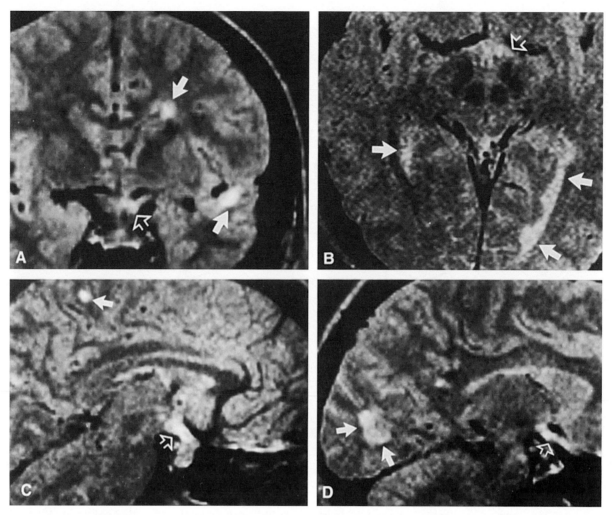

Fig. 6–10. Magnetic resonance imaging (TR, 2000 milliseconds; TE, 80 milliseconds) in multiple sclerosis. Coronal **(A)**, axial **(B)**, and parasagittal **(C)** sections show white matter demyelinative lesions of the chiasm (*open arrows*) and optic radiations (**B,** *large arrows*). **D.** Lesion in the occipital cortex (*large arrows*).

sual deterioration associated with growth failure; "the arachnoid of the optic cistern was found to be very much thickened and the brain closely adherent to the left optic nerve." Surgical lysis of adhesions resulted in rapidly improved vision. Oliver et al[156] documented two cases of pathologically verified chiasmal arachnoiditis associated with vascular disease in the form of polyarteritis and meningovascular syphilis. Iraci et al[157] documented a case of cystic, adhesive fibrous arachnoidal thickening with lymphocyte and plasma cell infiltration of no known cause. Suffice to add, this vague diagnostic category is shrinking as a result of advances in neuroimaging and spinal fluid analyses.

Infectious meningitis may produce visual loss by chiasmal arachnoidal inflammation. In 13 cases of purulent meningitis (including infections with *Diplococcus pneumoniae, Staphylococcus,* and *Pseudomonas aeruginosa*), 3 cases of cryptococcal meningitis, and 2 of tuberculous meningitis examined by autopsy at Kobe University, Japan,[158] histopathologic changes included the following: polymorphonuclear and lymphocyte infiltration along perivascular spaces in the periphery of optic nerves and chiasm, pial abscesses, and necrosis (and granulomas in cryptococcal cases); perivascular infiltration, endarteritis, necrotizing angiitis, and thrombus formation. Therefore, pathologic processes may be classified as inflammatory and vascular, both of which contribute to demyelinization and axonal degeneration. In this series, no clinical data were included. A 10-year-old girl is reported, with painful visual loss associated with an enlarged right optic nerve and chiasm, and a positive Lyme immunofluorescent immunoglobulin G titer of 1:512.[159]

With a special propensity to involve the hypothalamus and pituitary region, *sarcoidosis* infiltrates the chiasm with some regularity and is one of the chief non-neoplastic causes of chiasmal visual loss (Fig. 6–11). Decker et al[160] reported a case of severe progressive visual loss over only a 2-week interval and CT evidence of an intrasellar and suprasellar granuloma; vision improved

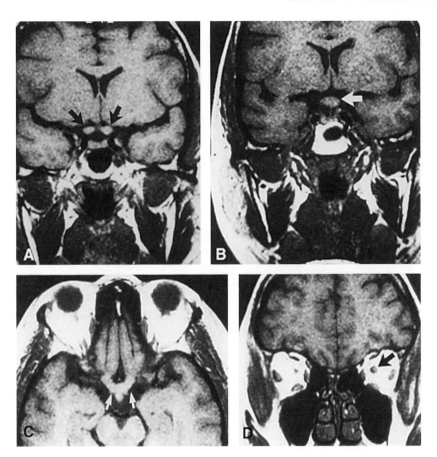

Fig. 6–11. Sarcoidosis of the optic nerves and chiasm. Bilateral insidious visual loss in a 39-year-old woman. Magnetic resonance imaging sequences (TR, 600 milliseconds; TE, 20 milliseconds). **A.** Coronal section shows bilateral enlargement of prechiasmal optic nerves (*arrows*). **B.** Enlarged chiasm (*arrrows*) in coronal section. **C.** Axial section. **D.** Midorbit section shows enlarged left optic nerve (*arrow*). (Courtesy of Dr. James Rush)

after transsphenoidal resection. Tang et al[161] recorded four patients with sarcoidosis and characteristic chiasmal defects, including profound visual loss in one eye with temporal defects in the contralateral field; in two patients, no discrete mass was visible by neuroimaging, or at craniotomy in one, implying diffuse infiltration. Sarcoidosis of the CNS need not show systemic manifestations. CNS sarcoidosis, including of the visual pathways, is usually treated with corticosteroids, or alternatively with azathioprine, cyclosporine, cyclophosphamide, chlorambucil, methotrexate, and even radiation therapy in refractory cases.[162,163]

Tuberculosis causing meningitis, basal arachnoiditis, and opto-chiasmatic neuritis is a rare event in developed countries, but it may be a complication associated with acquired immunodeficiency syndrome. It is elsewhere most common in infants in whom other tuberculous foci may be identified in the lungs, peritoneum, abdominal viscera, and lymph nodes, although the miliary form is the most frequent origin of meningeal infection.[164] Leptomeningitis and chiasmal arachnoiditis cause visual loss and optic atrophy, with general concentric contraction of the field being typical, and hydocephalus a common associated condition. Microsurgical lysis of adhesions in the chiasmatic cistern is considered essential, with good return of vision, and antituberculous treatment is indispensable.

A form of *paraneoplastic* autoimmune demyelination with acute necrotizing myelopathy of the chiasm was described,[165] associated with papillary carcinoma of the thyroid. Immunoglobulin G, myelin basic protein, and activated helper T cells were increased in the CSF.

MISCELLANEOUS CHIASMAL LESIONS

Arachnoidal and Epithelial Cysts

Arachnoidal cysts are typically serous cavities lined by neuroepithelium, but they may be of diverse origin, including trauma and inflammation. Many are asymptomatic, occupying silent compartments such as anterior to the temporal lobes (see Fig. 5–18), or they cause variable symptoms by mass effects on adjacent brain structures. Some suprasellar cysts apparently arise as congenital anomalies in the floor of the third ventricle. In children, developmental sellar cysts, a form of primary empty sella (see below), may be associated with GH or other pituitary deficiencies including precocious or delayed puberty.[166] Intrasellar cysts are apparently common findings in anatomic studies, McGrath[167] giving the figure of 33% in 83 necropsy specimens. Other cysts arise in the sella itself and are variably termed *cysts of Rathke's pouch, epithelial cysts, and colloid cysts,* depending on diverse anatomic disposition and histologic characteristics. These cysts extend into the chiasmatic cistern, variably producing visual and endocrinologic dysfunction. In the "empty sella syndrome" (see below) such intrasellar cysts communicate with the subarachnoid space.

Benes et al[168] provided an excellent review of arachnoidal cysts and their neuro-ophthalmologic implications. These investigators noted that 70% of such cysts occur in the basal portions of the cranial vault, including temporal fossa (29%), posterior fossa (21%), and parasellar region (18%). Adult patients chiefly complain of headaches (50%), blurred vision (40%), and seizures (40%); some 15% of adults, and children older than 5 years, complain of diplopia.

Rathke's cleft cysts originate in vestigial epithelial remnants of primitive stomodial ectoderm, which normally forms the anterior and intermediate lobes, and pars tuberalis of the pituitary gland. Cysts of the residual stomodial lumen (Rathke's cleft) are found in as much as 22% of autopsies and are discovered in increasing number with the advent of CT and MRI neuroimaging.[169] These cysts cause headache, amenorrhea, hypopituitarism, diabetes insipidus, and galactorrhea. They commonly present with chiasmal syndrome visual loss, requiring surgical decompression, but radiation therapy is not necessary.[170] MRI is characterized by low signal intensity on T_1-weighted images and high intensity on T_2-weighted images. By radiologic criteria alone, distinction from craniopharyngioma may prove problematic. MRI usually shows arachnoidal cysts to be characterized by a signal that is identical to CSF on all sequences (Fig. 6–12), but a hyperintense signal on T_1 is seen when protein content is greater than in CSF.

Baskin and Wilson[171] reported the results of transsphenoidal treatment of 38 non-neoplastic cysts within the pituitary fossa, excluding craniopharyngiomas and cystic adenomas. Headaches, menstrual irregularities, galactorrhea, and hyperprolactinemia were common clinical manifestations. Indications for transsphenoidal exploration include relief of chiasmal compression, in-

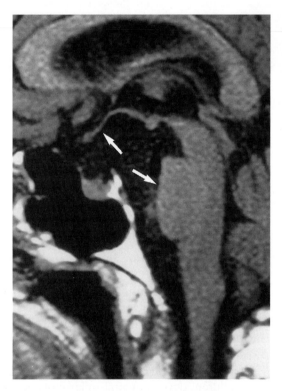
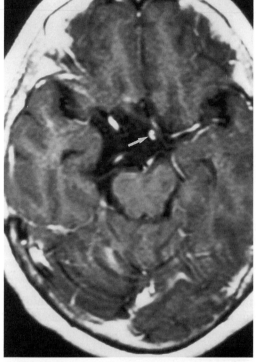
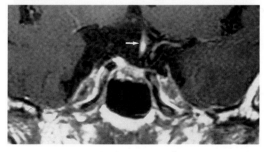

Fig. 6–12. Suprasellar cyst presenting with chronic visual loss. Magnetic resonance imaging (MRI) shows that the signal is isointense to cerebrospinal fluid. **Top.** *Left,* sagittal section demonstrates elevation of the optic chiasm and posterior deformation of the midbrain. *Right,* axial computed tomography displays leftward displacement of the pituitary stalk (*arrow*). **Bottom.** MRI shows lateral compression of the stalk (*arrow*).

terference with pituitary gland or stalk, and exclusion of other sellar neoplasms.

Metastatic Diseases and Other Mass Lesions

Awash in the basal cisterns, the optic nerves and chiasm are occasional targets for invasion by metastatic cells that have gained the subarachnoid space or have gained access via a rich network of arteries. Leptomeningeal metastases may herald diffuse meningeal carcinomatosis; the picture of rapid unilateral or bilateral visual loss mimicking retro-bulbar optic neuritis, that is, usually without optic disc swelling, and beyond the usual age range, should bring this mechanism to mind. Breast and lung represent the most common primary sites. Appen et al[172] documented pathologic changes that include plaque-like infiltration of the subarachnoid space of the optic nerves by tumor cells, with minimal alteration of myelin and normal axons. Other reports[173] showed the following: infiltrative tumor cells with degeneration and necrosis of axons and myelin; secondary inflammation, with vasculitis and endothelial proliferation; tumor cells within vessels; petechial bleeding; and occlusion of subarachnoid vessels. These findings suggest hematogenous spread or secondary dissemination through CSF.

In the patient without known malignancy, confirmation of "malignant meningitis" is difficult. A course of rapidly sequential multiple cranial nerve palsies is highly suggestive (see Chapter 12). Small meningeal deposits tend to elude radiologic detection, but contrasted CT or gadolinium-enhanced MRI can show abnormal enhancements in or adjacent to involved meninges. Multiple cytologic examinations of CSF by millipore filter technique are advisable (see also Chapter 5).

Malignant lymphoma may infiltrate the leptomeninges, septal tissue, and perivascular spaces of the optic nerves and chiasm, causing segmental demyelination.[174] Other lymphoproliferative disorders such as chronic lymphocytic leukemia also rarely involve the chiasm,[175] as does histiocytosis,[176] which may mimic chiasmal glioma (Fig. 6–13). These processes are perplexing challenges unless the primary disorder is already declared.

Pituitary metastases are uncommon manifestations of systemic cancer and may be difficult to distinguish from simple adenoma. In order to ascertain the incidence of pituitary tumors in patients with cancer, and to characterize the clinical presentations of metastases to the pituitary gland, the experience at Memorial Sloan-Kettering Cancer Center in New York during 1976 to 1979 has been reviewed[177]; additionally, the pituitary glands from 500 consecutive autopsies of cancer patients were examined. Only 4 patients had symptomatic tumors; 2 of 3 examined histologically were adenomas, and 1 was a metastasis. Radiologic evaluation, including polytomography and CT, did not reliably distinguish metasta-

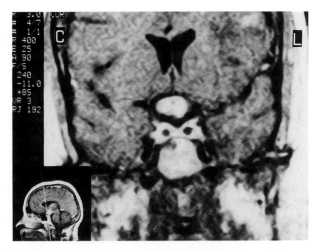

Fig. 6–13. Histiocytosis of the chiasm and hypothalamus presenting as polydipsia, polyuria, hypersomnolence, and visual loss. Laboratory data were consistent with panhypopituitarism. Biopsy of the left frontal mass showed Langerhan-type histiocytosis. Contrast-enhanced magnetic resonance imaging shows a massively enlarged chiasm. (From Job OM, Sehatz NJ, Glaser JS: Visual loss with Langerhans cell histiocytosis: multifocal central nervous system involvement. J Neuroophthalmol 19:49, 1999)

ses from adenoma, but the clinical syndromes were distinctive, with diabetes insipidus in the metastatic case. A review of the published literature of 28 symptomatic pituitary metastases revealed an incidence of diabetes insipidus of 82%, but visual loss in only 11%, because just one-fourth of affected glands are enlarged. In the autopsy series, metastases were found in 3.6% and adenomas in 1.8% of studied specimens.

Thus, the clinical manifestations of pituitary adenoma and metastasis differ, diabetes insipidus being the striking distinguishing finding in metastatic disease, whereas anterior pituitary deficiency is rare, there being a predilection for seeding of the posterior lobe of the pituitary. As a rule, pituitary metastasis occurs in patients with widely metastatic disease. It is suggested that pituitary metastases be treated with focal radiation therapy and corticosteroids even when visual loss evolves.

As noted, *malignant glioblastoma multiforme* may rarely enlarge the chiasm in adults, as established by MRI,[178] which tends to demonstrate absence of optic nerve abnormality in the canals or orbits but invasion of contiguous brain structures. Other lesions that rarely involve the chiasm include gangliogliomas,[179] hemangiopericytoma,[180] hemangioblastoma,[181] and metastatic medulloblastoma.[182]

Sphenoidal Mucoceles

Mucocele of the posterior ethmoid and sphenoid paranasal sinus complex is characterized by chronic headache and dysfunction of one or more of the cranial

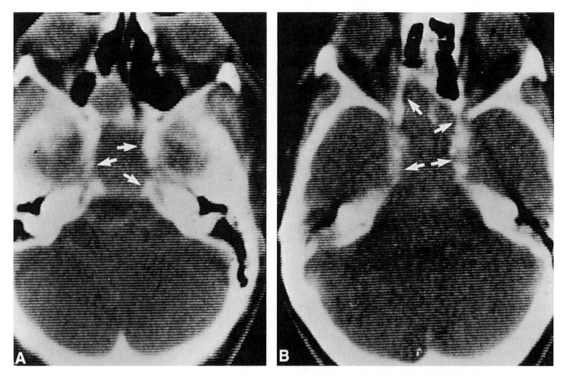

Fig. 6–14. Sphenoidal pyomucocele with visual loss. **A** and **B.** Computed tomography sections through the skull base show an expanded sphenoethmoidal sinus complex (*arrows*) and bone destruction.

nerves that pass through the orbital apex. Visual loss and field defects indicating involvement of one or both optic nerves have been adequately described, but reviews of the literature suggest that involvement of the optic chiasm is rare. Two patients with spheno-ethmoidal mucoceles are reported,[183] who developed field defects consistent with chiasmal interference; in one instance, sudden bilateral visual loss mimicked pituitary apoplexy, whereas the other patient experienced slowly progressive, bilateral central field defects.

The radiologic findings with sphenoidal mucocele include expansion of the sphenoid sinus (Fig. 6–14), elevation of the tuberculum sellae and chiasmatic sulcus, obliteration of optic canals and superior orbital fissure, and lateral displacement of medial orbital walls.[184] When the sella is expanded, an intrasellar and suprasellar mass may mimic an adenoma.[185] Otolaryngologic or neurosurgical endonasal decompression is the treatment of choice, and some return of vision is anticipated unless optic atrophy is advanced (see also Chapter 5, Part II).

Trauma

Visual loss following closed-head trauma is usually attributable to contusion or laceration of the optic nerves, which occurs acutely at the time of impact. Traumatic chiasmal syndromes are considerably less frequent, approximately 100 cases having been reported.[186] For example, of 24 patients who sustained blunt head injuries that resulted in insults to the visual system, 5 involved the optic chiasm, solely or in combination with optic nerve lesions, but only 1 case was complicated by diabetes insipidus.[187] Savino et al[188] recorded 11 patients with traumatic chiasmal injuries in which visual field defects varied from complete monocular blindness with contralateral temporal hemianopia to subtle bitemporal arcuate scotomas (see Fig. 6–1F). The degree of visual deficit was not necessarily related to the severity of the craniocerebral trauma. Transient diabetes insipidus was present in 7 of 11 patients, but, unlike the field defects, this complication improved. Other accompanying findings variably include anosmia, cranial nerve defects (III, IV, VI, V, VII, VIII), CSF rhinorrhea and otorrhea, panhypopituitarism, carotid-cavernous fistula, carotid pseudoaneurysm, and meningitis. CT may disclose sagittal midline fractures of the clivus and sella turcica, suggesting a midline separation of the skull.[185]

The precise mechanism of chiasmal trauma is problematic, with few cases meeting the essential criteria of post-traumatic visual evaluation, and subsequent surgical exploration or autopsy examination. Sagittal tearing of the chiasm associated with sphenoidal fracture, post-traumatic thrombosis of carotid artery branches that supply the chiasm, and contusion hemorrhage and necrosis are alternative, relevant theories (Fig. 6–15). In 52 cases of lethal craniocerebral trauma,[189] 36 instances of pituitary hemorrhages and 10 instances of primary and secondary chiasmal lesions were found, consisting

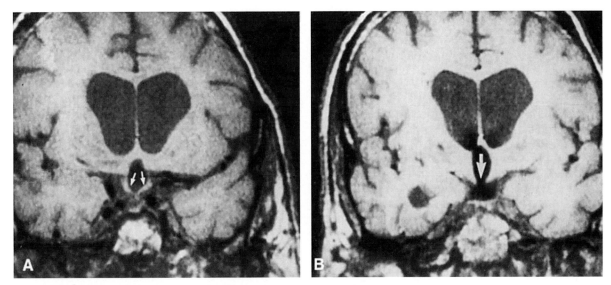

Fig. 6-15. Chiasmal trauma in closed-head injury in a 40-year-old motorcyclist with blindness and diabetes insipidus. Magnetic resonance images (TR, 1000 milliseconds; TE, 30 milliseconds). **A.** Coronal section shows a midsagittal tear and downward displacement of chiasm (*small arrows*). **B.** More posterior section shows an apparent rupture of the floor of the third ventricle (*arrow*).

of bleeding and necrosis of the central chiasmal bar. Crompton[190] found hypothalamic ischemic lesions and hemorrhages in 45 of 106 persons who died after head trauma and attributed these pathologic changes to shearing of small perforating vessels. Similar lesions may cause the usually transient diabetes insipidus.

Instances are reported[191] of traumatic avulsion of a globe and nerve, with transection at the anterior chiasm associated with contralateral temporal hemianopia. Endoscopic surgical procedures in the sphenoid sinus may also damage the chiasm.[192]

Complications of Radiation Therapy

Late cerebral radionecrosis is a relatively rare complication of radiation therapy. A precise estimate of incidence is difficult to ascertain, given the problem of differentiating tumor recurrence and postoperative scarring from radionecrosis. Therapeutic radiation is used for pituitary adenomas, parasellar and clinoidal meningiomas, suprasellar tumors, and especially malignancies of the paranasal sinuses. The cumulative data of Warman and Glaser,[193] relating time interval from completion of radiation therapy, to visual loss from radionecrosis, suggest that the 8- to 13-month period encompasses two-thirds of all cases, contrary to previous figures suggesting a peak incidence at 1 to 1.5 years[194] (see also below and Fig. 6-16).

There seems to be no correlation between patient age and interval to onset of visual symptoms. Radionecrosis of the anterior visual pathways usually manifests as a rapidly progressive loss of vision in one eye, the second eye following shortly thereafter in the majority of cases.

A rapidly relentless progression to profound visual loss evolves, frequently to total blindness. Initial visual field deficits are typically central scotoma or nerve fiber bundle defects,[193] with or without arcuate scotomas. Alternatively, a chiasmal or optic tract pattern may evolve.[195]

As noted, chiasmal radionecrosis especially may follow radiation therapy to pituitary tumors.[193,196,197] Autopsy in two such cases[196] revealed perioptic meningeal thickening with patchy demyelination of nerves and chiasm, slight axis cylinder damage, hyaline thickening and perivascular inflammatory cell infiltration of small vessels in the hypothalamus, and necrosis of frontal lobes;

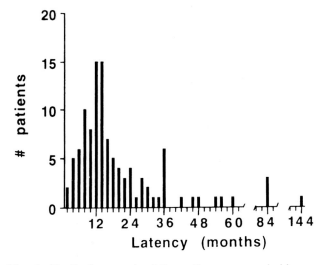

Fig. 6-16. Radionecrosis of the optic nerves and chiasm. Histogram displays latency (months) from the time of radiation therapy to the onset of visual loss. (From ref. 207)

necrosis and inflammation of portions of the sphenoid bone with endarteritis of intraosseous vessels. The newer techniques of focal stereotactic ("gamma-knife") radiosurgery are also reported[198] to produce radiation-induced optic neuropathy within 7 to 30 months (Fig. 6–17).

The optic discs initially appear normal, unless there was pre-existing atrophy due to the primary tumor process, but disc edema is occasionally observed. Eventually, marked pallor is evident within 2 months of initial visual loss. This clinical constellation, which occurs within a few months to several years, is highly evocative of radionecrosis, but adequate visualization of the optic nerves and chiasm by gadolinium-enhanced MRI is required to rule out recurrence or extension of the primary tumor. MRI shows often marked enlargement of the nerves and chiasm, and hyperintense signal on contrast-enhanced T_1-weighted sequences.[199,200] It is imperative that MRIs include thin-section axial and coronal views along the length of the orbital optic nerve segments, preferably with fat-suppression protocols, and precise visualization of the chiasm.

Hufnagel et al[201] have recorded the extraordinary occurrence of a malignant glioma of the chiasm 8 years after resection of a recurrent prolactinoma followed with supplemental radiation therapy (5500 cGy). Radiation-induced tumors or other second malignancies are extremely rare, with long latency periods.[194]

Aristizabal et al[202] concluded that, not only do total dosages in excess of 5000 cGy increase morbidity, but also that complications occur even with daily fractions in the range of 200 to 220 cGy per treatment, owing to individual variation in radiation tolerance. Analysis of radiation-induced optic neuropathy after megavoltage external-beam irradiation,[203] involving 215 optic nerves in 131 patients with extracranial head and neck tumors, revealed the following: anterior ischemic neuropathy developed in 5 nerves (mean and median times of 32 and 30 months; range, 2 to 4 years); retro-bulbar optic neuropathy in 12 nerves (mean and median times of 47 and 28 months; range, 1 to 14 years); no injuries in 106 nerves that received a total dose of less than 59 Gy; the 15-year actuarial risk of optic neuropathy after doses more than or equal to 60 Gy was 11% when treatment fraction was less than 1.9 Gy, compared with 47% with fraction sizes greater than or equal to 1.9 Gy. Data suggest increasing risk with increasing age, but the role of hormonal secretions, such as PRL, in influencing risk of radiation-induced visual damage is unknown. Patients concomitantly using chemotherapeutic agents, including lomustine (CCNU), when subjected to even low-dose whole-brain irradiation are at risk.[204]

The management of radionecrosis remains empirical; there are no prospective studies comparing different treatment modalities, nor have specific therapeutic guidelines been established. The mechanism of delayed radionecrosis is primarily active vasculitis, as noted above, with secondary ischemic anoxia leading to axonal necrosis. Fibrinoid necrosis of vessel walls, with endothelial proliferation and lumen obliteration, leads to thrombotic occlusion. Based on such pathophysiologic observations, in theory anticoagulation is a rea-

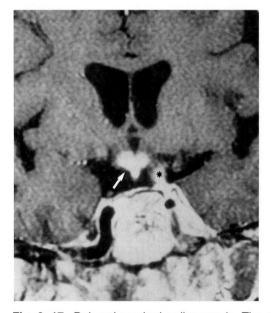
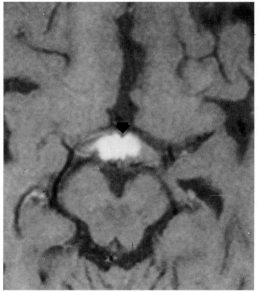

Fig. 6–17. Delayed cerebral radionecrosis. The patient was a 44-year-old woman with chronic left visual loss to 20/70 who underwent stereotactic radiosurgery (single-session gamma). At 12 months, she suddenly lost all vision in both eyes. Enhanced magnetic resonance imaging: *Left* (coronal) and *right* (axial) sections show a hyperintense signal from the optic chiasm, tracts, and pituitary stalk (*arrows*). *Asterisk,* paraclinoid mengioma.

sonable approach to minimize the damage once radionecrosis is triggered. Early anticoagulation has been proposed as an effective treatment for cerebral and spinal cord radionecrosis,[205] but with no compelling evidence of efficacy for lesions in the visual pathways. In tissues damaged by radiation, wound healing has been accelerated when subjected to hyperbaric oxygen, and this therapy is under evaluation for radiation retinopathy and radiation optic neuropathy. Borruat et al[206] reported reversal of visual loss with hyperbaric oxygen in a single patient. Subsequently, Borruat et al[207] thoroughly reviewed the world literature on 115 cases, analyzing the efficacy of various therapies compared against the natural course of radiation optic neuropathy: irradiated lesions comprised pituitary adenomas (54%), paranasal sinus tumors (13%), craniopharyngioma (7%), sellar metastases (7%), meningiomas (6%), and miscellaneous conditions; latency period ranged from 1 to 144 months, with a median delay of 13 months following cessation of radiation therapy (see Fig. 6–16); visual loss was bilateral in 74% of patients. In patients treated with hyperbaric oxygen, 2 had significant recovery of visual function, vision in 1 patient remained unchanged, and 1 continued to show visual deterioration. However, among 120 similar cases, no spontaneous improvement in vision was documented, *nor was there recovery with any other form of therapy,* including corticosteroids or anticoagulants. These data suggest that hyperbaric oxygen at a minimum pressure of 2.4 atmospheres of 100% oxygen, over 30 sessions, may be effective in reversing or stabilizing visual loss due to delayed radionecrosis, especially when commenced within a few short days of visual decline. The endocrinologic and neuropsychiatric risks of delayed effects of radiation therapy are included above, in the discussion of optic gliomas.

Hydrocephalus

With internal hydrocephalus, distention of the third ventricle is said to result in chiasmal stretching, and, thus, bitemporal field defects can constitute a "false localizing sign." The carefully detailed case description of Sinclair and Dott,[208] and the observations of Hughes,[209] leave little doubt that such a mechanism exists, albeit rarely (Fig. 6–18). Corbett[210] also documented this exceptional situation. The basic field defect pattern may be complicated by progressive optic atrophy or compression of the nerves and chiasm against the unyielding bony sellar structures or arterial circle. Unilateral amaurosis has been reported in a child with decompensated hydrocephalus, presumably because of compression of one optic nerve against the internal carotid artery.[211] Increased intracranial pressure need not

otherwise be symptomatic, nor is extreme elevation necessary for the production of field defects. Depending on the degree of atrophy, vision may recover subsequent to relief of hydrocephalus.

Pregnancy

Visual disturbances in the form of field defects during pregnancy require comment. Although the pituitary gland does undergo a small degree of enlargement during pregnancy, principally because of hypertrophy and hyperplasia of PRL cells, it must be recalled that the chiasm generally lies a full centimeter above the level of the diaphragma sellae. Therefore, in the absence of a pre-existing adenoma, no visual change may causally be related to pregnancy alone. Pregnant women with pituitary microadenomas are not at risk for chiasmal compression, although those with macroadenomas greater than 1.1 cm may develop field loss.[212] Suprasellar meningiomas may be sensitive to levels of estrogen and progesterone and may undergo a growth spurt, especially during the second half of pregnancy.[213] In general, however, one may conclude that intracranial neoplasms do not appear to present more often during pregnancy.

A disorder as common as optic neuritis eventually occurs during pregnancy, but a direct relationship remains tenuous. Likewise, there is no convincing evidence for a syndrome of "lactation optic neuritis." If such occurs, a pre-existing mass or MS must be suspected. Demyelinative disease is not regularly adversely influenced during pregnancy, but signs and symptoms may be exacerbated by labor and delivery. Indeed, most

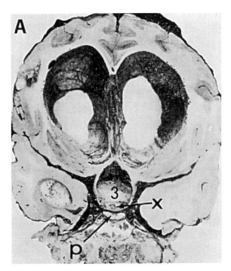

Fig. 6–18. Effect of internal hydrocephalus. **A.** Coronal section of the brain and basal structures from a patient with a cerebellar tumor and optic atrophy. The third ventricle (*3*) is dilated, the chiasm (*X*) is stretched, and the sella with the pituitary (*P*) is compressed.

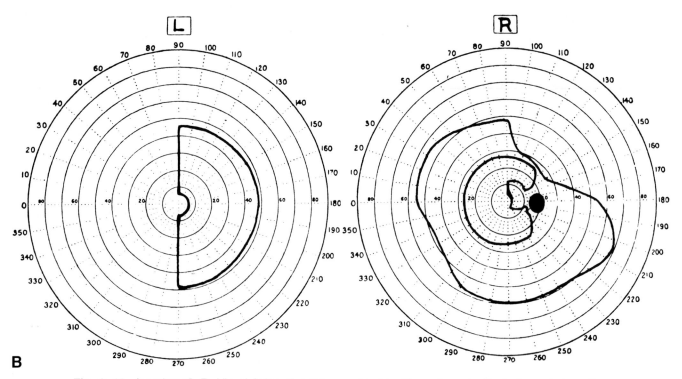

Fig. 6–18. (*continued*) **B.** Visual fields of a 17-year-old girl with post-meningitic hydrocephalus. At surgery, the ballooned third ventricle was seen to stretch the chiasm; ventriculostomy through the anterior wall of the third ventricle relieved hydrocephalus with improvement in field defects. (From ref. 208)

studies report a decrease in disease activity during gestation and an *increase* in relapses during the post-partum period, likely reflecting a relative immunosuppressive state during gestation.[214]

Lymphocytic adenohypophysitis is a distinct disease process characterized by diffuse lymphocytic infiltration of the pituitary gland, predominantly affecting women, presenting during late pregnancy or in the first post-partum year. The association with Hashimoto's thyroiditis and the variable presence of antipituitary antibodies strongly suggest an autoimmune-mediated disorder.[215] The size of the inflamed pituitary is variable, as are endocrine deficiencies, defects in corticotroph and thyrotroph being most frequent, with PRL elevation in about 40%, but posterior lobe function being relatively spared. Weight loss, weakness, and anemia are common, and chiasmal compression may evolve. Response to steroid therapy is not consistent, but spontaneous resolution and, at times, involution occur, suggesting a possible mechanism of some instances of empty sella syndrome.

Distinction must be made between spuriously contracted fields or vague temporal depressions of a functional nature and true temporal hemianopic defects. Pregnancy and the post-partum interval are times of physiologic and psychologic stress; the possibility of non-organic visual complaints, or corneal and fundus alterations, should be kept in mind. "The Pregnant Woman's Eye," by Sunness,[216] is a useful review.

EMPTY SELLA SYNDROME

Extension of the subarachnoid space into the sella turcica through a deficient sellar diaphragm may manifest as an incidental radiographic finding, consisting of a normal-sized or slightly enlarged bony sella, not empty

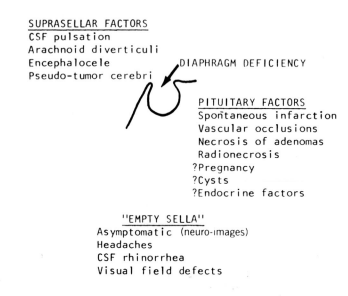

Fig. 6–19. "Empty sella." Summary of potential factors. (After Obrador S: The empty sella and some related syndromes. Neurosurgery 36:162, 1972)

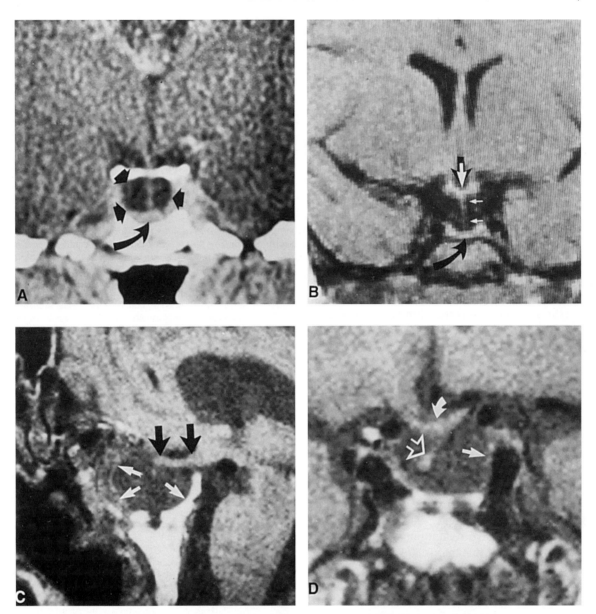

Fig. 6–20. Neuroimaging of empty sella. **A.** Computed tomography scan of a 46-year-old woman with a vague headache complex. Coronal section shows a dark empty sella (*arrows*) with a preserved midline hypophyseal stalk and flattened remnant of the pituitary gland (*curved arrow*). **B.** T$_1$-weighted magnetic resonance imaging (MRI) shows the flattened pituitary (*curved arrow*), the midline stalk (*small white arrows*), and the chiasm above (*large white arrow*). **C.** MRI (TR, 800 milliseconds; TE, 26 milliseconds); sagittal section shows a large, remodeled sella (*white arrows*) with moderate prolapse of the optic nerves and chiasm (*black arrows*). **D.** Coronal section through the sella; *solid arrow* on remaining dural wall, *open arrow* on distorted pituitary stalk, with the chiasm above (*small curved arrow*).

but filled with CSF; a flattened residual pituitary gland may remain. Kaufman[217] defines the empty sella as nontumorous remodeling that results from a combination of incomplete diaphragma sellae and CSF. Bergland et al[218] reaffirmed previous observations that diaphragmal openings are indeed common; they found defects greater than 5 mm in diameter in 39% of 225 normal autopsy specimens. Bergland's material also revealed that an empty sella need not be enlarged, and normal volume is fairly common. *Primary* empty sella occurs

spontaneously and may be associated with pseudotumor cerebri, arachnoidal cyst, lymphocytic hypophysitis, or possibly infarction of the diaphragma and pituitary gland. Sellar cysts in childhood (see above) are likely developmental and associated with hypothalamic-pituitary disorders.[188] Reversible empty sella, that is, reappearance of the pituitary gland, has been suggested as an indicator of successful therapy for idiopathic intracranial hypertension.[219] *Secondary* empty sella follows pituitary surgery or radiation therapy (Fig. 6–19).

The clinical and radiographic characteristics of primary empty sella were thoroughly reviewed by Neelon et al,[220] the following features being notable: obese women predominate (27 women, 4 men), ranging in age from 27 to 72 years, with a mean age of 49 years; headache is a common symptom; in the Duke University study there was no instance of visual impairment due to chiasmal interference; an enlarged sella was found serendipitously on plain skull films obtained for evaluation of headaches, syncope, or other symptoms; pseudotumor cerebri was present in 4 women; 20 patients had normal pituitary function, and 8 demonstrated endocrine disturbances that included panhypopituitarism, or GH, gonadotropin, and thyrotropin deficiency.

Hyperprolactinemia may occur in patients with intrasellar cisternal herniation without evidence of pituitary tumor, but the elevation of serum PRL is usually moderate. For example, in a study[221] of 47 patients with empty sella, hyperprolactinemia was found in 6, with a range of 39 to 123 ng/L. Of course, adequate neuroimaging with enhanced CT or MRI (Fig. 6–20) will resolve the question of empty sella vs. mass lesion. Children are rarely included in this diagnostic category, but they are reported[222] with primary empty sella and associated congenital anomalies, including delayed puberty, anosmia, diabetes insipidus, delayed growth, and optic atrophy.[223]

In a series of 19 patients with primary empty sella at the University of Michigan,[224] the following features were noteworthy: all were women; 12 patients complained initially of headache; in 7 patients, visual disturbances were prominent subjective symptoms (blurred vision, diplopia, micropsia); 3 had bilateral papilledema and were believed to have pseudotumor cerebri; and 2 patients demonstrated minimal relative hemianopias without obvious cause. Although it is speculated that the high female preponderance noted in all series implies a mechanism related to physiologic hypertrophy and subsequent involution of the pituitary gland during pregnancy, there was no significant relationship between the number of pregnancies and sellar volume in the Duke University series.

In the *secondary* form of empty sella that occurs following pituitary surgery or irradiation, adhesions may form between tumor "capsule" (or sellar diaphragm) and the optic nerves and chiasm. Retraction of these adhesions may draw the visual system downward into the empty sella, with resulting visual defects.[225,226] Packing the sellar cavity prophylactically to elevate the diaphragma has been proposed,[224] or "chiasmapexy" when chiasmal herniation is observed at surgical re-exploration.[227]

REFERENCES

1. Elkington SG: Pituitary adenoma: preoperative symptomatology in a series of 260 patients. Br J Ophthalmol 52:322, 1968
2. Nachtigaller H, Hoyt WF: Storungen des Scheindruckes bei bitemporaler Hemianopsie und Verschiebung der Sehachsen. Klin Monatsbl Augenheilkd 156:821, 1970
3. Chamlin M, Davidoff LM, Feiring EH: Ophthalmologic changes produced by pituitary tumors. Am J Ophthalmol 40:353, 1955
4. Wilson P, Falconer MA: Patterns of visual failure with pituitary tumours: clinical and radiological correlations. Br J Ophthalmol 52:94, 1968
5. Taylor D: Congenital tumours of the anterior visual system with dysplasia of the optic discs. Br J Ophthalmol 66:455, 1982
6. Grimson BS, Perry DD: Enlargement of the optic disc in childhood optic nerve tumors. Am J Ophthalmol 97:627, 1993
7. Trobe JD, Acosta PC, Krischer JP: A screening method for chiasmal visual field defects. Arch Ophthalmol 99:264, 1981
8. Frisen L: The earliest visual field defects in midchiasmal compression. Doc Ophthalmol 42:14, 1985
9. Gutman I, Behrens M, Odel J: Bilateral central and centrocaecal scotomata due to mass lesions. Br J Ophthalmol 68:336, 1984
10. Horton JC: Wilbrand's knee of the primate optic chiasm is an artefact of monocular enucleation. Trans Am Ophthalmol Soc 95:579, 1997
11. Suckling RD: Visual fields in posterior chiasmal angle lesions. Trans Ophthalmol Soc N Z 36:23, 1984
12. Symon L, Jakubowski J: Transcranial management of pituitary tumours with suprasellar extension. J Neurol Neurosurg Psychiatry 42:123, 1979
13. Parravano JG, Toledo A, Kucharczyk W: Dimensions of the optic nerves, chiasm, and tracts: MR quantitative comparison between patients with optic atrophy and normals. J Comput Assist Tomogr 17:688, 1993
14. Wagner AL, Murtagh FR, Hazlett KS et al: Measurement of the normal optic chiasm on coronal images. AJNR Am J Neuroradiol 18:723, 1997
15. Iwata F, Patronas NJ, Caruso RC et al: Association of visual field, cup-disc ratio, and magnetic resonance imaging of optic chiasm. Arch Ophthalmol 115:729, 1997
16. Kernohan JW, Sayre GP: Tumors of the pituitary gland and infundibulum. In Atlas of Tumor Pathology, series 1, fascicle 36. Washington, DC, Armed Forces Institute of Pathology, 1956
17. Burrow GN, Wortzman G, Rewcastle NB et al: Microadenomas of the pituitary and abnormal sellar tomograms in an unelected autopsy service. N Engl J Med 304:156, 1981
18. Donovan LE, Corenblum B: The natural history of the pituitary incidentaloma. Arch Intern Med 155:181, 1995
19. Thapar K, Kovacs K, Horvath E: Morphology of the pituitary in health and disease. In Becker KL, Bilezikian JP, Bremner WJ et al (eds): Principles and Practice of Endocrinology and Metabolism, p 103. Philadelphia, JB Lippincott, 1995
20. Wilson CB: A decade of pituitary microsurgery: the Herbert Olivecrona lecture. J Neurosurg 61:814, 1984
21. Ebersold MJ, Quast LM, Laws ER et al: Long-term results in transsphenoidal removal of nonfunctioning pituitary adenomas. J Neurosurg 64:713, 1986
22. Kearns TP, Rucker CW: Arcuate defects in the visual fields due to chromophobe adenoma of the pituitary gland. Am J Ophthalmol 45:505, 1958
23. Trobe JD: Chromophobe adenoma presenting with a hemianopic temporal arcuate scotoma. Am J Ophthalmol 77:388, 1974
24. Ikeda H, Yoshimoto T: Visual disturbances in patients with pituitary adenoma. Acta Neurol Scand 92:157, 1995
25. Katznelson L, Klibanski: Prolactin and its disorders. In Becker KL, Bilezikian JP, Bremner WJ et al (eds): Principles and Practice of Endocrinology and Metabolism, p 140. Philadelphia, JB Lippincott, 1995
26. Randall RV, Laws ER, Abboud CF et al: Transsphenoidal microsurgical treatment of prolactin-producing pituitary adenomas: results in 100 patients. Mayo Clin Proc 58:108, 1983
27. Woodruff WW, Heinz ER, Djang WT et al: Hyperprolactenemia: an unusual manifestation of suprasellar cystic lesions. AJNR Am J Neuroradiol 8:113, 1987
28. Kahn SR, Leblanc R, Sadikot AF et al: Marked hyperprolactinemia caused by carotid aneurysm. Can J Neurol Sci 24:64, 1997
29. Kruse A, Astrup J, Gyldensted C et al: Hyperprolactinemia in

patients with pituitary adenomas: the pituitary stalk compression syndrome. Br J Neurosurg 9:453, 1995

30. Spark RF, Baker R, Bienfang DC, Bergland R: Bromocriptine reduces pituitary tumor size and hypersecretion. JAMA 247: 311, 1982

31. Bonneville JF, Poulignot D, Catin F et al: Computed tomographic demonstration of the effects of bromocriptine on pituitary microadenoma size. Radiology 143:451, 1982

32. Wollesen F, Anderson T, Karle A: Size reduction of extrasellar pituitary tumors during bromocriptine treatment: quantitation of effect on different types of tumors. Ann Intern Med 96:281, 1982

33. Moster ML, Savino PJ, Schatz NJ et al: Visual function in prolactinoma patients treated with bromocriptine. Ophthalmology 92:1332, 1985

34. King LW, Molitch ME, Gittinger JW et al: Cavernous sinus syndrome due to prolactinoma: resolution with bromocriptine. Surg Neurol 19:280, 1083

35. Colao A: Prolactinomas resistant to standard dopamine agonists respond to chronic cabergoline treatment. J Clin Endocrinol Metab 82:876, 1997

36. Grochowski M, Khalfallah Y, Vighetto A et al: Ophthalmic results in patients with macroprolactinomas treated with a new prolactin inhibitor CV 205–502. Br J Ophthalmol 77:785, 1993

37. Saito K, Kuwayama A, Yamamoto N et al: The transsphenoidal removal of nonfunctioning pituitary adenomas with suprasellar extensions: the open sella method and intentionally staged operation. Neurosurgery 36:668, 1995

38. Ciric I, Ragin A, Baumgartner C et al: Complications of transsphenoidal surgery: results of a national survey, review of the literature, and personal experience. Neurosurgery 40:225, 1997

39. Tsang RW, Brierly JD, Panzarella T et al: Radiation therapy for pituitary adenoma: treatment outcome and prognostic factors. Int J Radiat Oncol Biol Phys 30:557, 1994

40. Seo Y, Fukuoka S, Takanashi M et al: Gamma knife surgery for Cushing's disease. Surg Neurol 43:170, 1995

41. Raymond J, Hardy J, Czepko R et al: Arterial injuries in transspenoidal surgery for pituitary adenoma: the role of angiography and endovascular treatment. AJNR Am J Neuroradiol 18:655, 1997

42. Slavin ML, Lam BL, Decker RE et al: Chiasmal compression from fat packing after transsphenoidal resection of intrasellar tumor in two patients. Am J Ophthalmol 115:368, 1993

43. Baskin DS: Neurosurgical management of pituitary-hypothalamic neoplasms. In Becker KL, Bilezikian JP, Bremner WJ et al (eds): Principles and Practice of Endocrinology and Metabolism, p 238. Philadelphia, JB Lippincott, 1995

44. Valtonen S, Salmi J: Operative management of chromophobe pituitary tumour recurrences. Acta Neurochir (Wien) 62:233, 1982

45. Ebersold MJ, Quast LM, Laws ER et al: Long-term results in transsphenoidal removal of nonfunctioning pituitary adenomas. J Neurosurg 64:713, 1986

46. Thapar K: Proliferative activity and invasiveness among pituitary adenomas and carcinomas: an analysis using the MIB-1 antibody. Neurosurgery 38:99, 1996

47. Sammartino A, Bonavolonta G, Pettinato G, Loffredo A: Exophthalmos caused by an invasive pituitary adenoma in a child. Ophthalmologica 179:83, 1979

48. De Divitiis E, De Chiara A, Benvenuti D et al: Adenome invasif hypophysaire chez un enfant. Neurochirurgie 26:405, 1980

49. Juneau P, Schoene WC, Black P: Malignant tumors in the pituitary gland. Arch Neurol 49:555, 1992

50. Gould TJ, Johnson LN, Colapinto EV et al: Intrasellar vascular malformation mimicking a pituitary macroadenoma. J Neuroophthalmol 16:199, 1996

51. Hollenhorst RW, Younge BR: Ocular manifestations produced by adenomas of the pituitary gland: analysis of 1,000 cases. In Kohler PO, Ross GT (eds): Diagnosis and Treatment of Pituitary Tumors, p 53. New York, Elsevier, 1973

52. Merimee TJ, Grant MB: Growth hormone and its disorders. In Becker KL, Bilezikian JP, Bremner WJ et al (eds): Principles and Practice of Endocrinology and Metabolism, p 129. Philadelphia, JB Lippincott, 1995

53. Lundin P, Engstom E, Karlsson FA et al: Long-term octotide

54. Rolih CA, Ober P: Pituitary apoplexy. Endocrinol Metab Clin North Am 22:291, 1993

55. Symon L, Mohanty S: Haemorrhage in pituitary tumours. Acta Neurochir (Wien) 65:41, 1982

56. Fraioli B, Esposito V, Palma L et al: Hemorrhagic pituitary adenomas: clinicopathological features and surgical treatment. Neurosurgery 27:741, 1990

57. Holness RO, Ogundino FA, Langille RA: Pituitary apoplexy following closed head trauma. J Neurosurg 59:677, 1983

58. Savage EB, Gugino L, Starr PA et al: Pituitary apoplexy following cardiopulmonary bypass: considerations for a staged cardiac and neurosurgical procedure. Eur J Cardiothorac Surg 8:333, 1994

59. Masago A, Ueda Y, Kanai H et al: Pituitary apoplexy after pituitary function test: a report of two cases and review of the literature. Surg Neurol 43:158, 1995

60. Reid RL, Quigley ME, Yen SSC: Pituitary apoplexy: a review Arch Neurol 42:712, 1985

61. Poussaint TY, Barnes PD, Anthony DC et al: Hemorrhagic pituitary adenomas in adolescence. AJNR Am J Neuroradiol 17: 1907, 1996

62. McFadzean RM, Doyle D, Rampling R et al: Pituitary apoplexy and its effect on vision. Neurosurgery 29:669, 1991

63. Bonicki W, Kasperlik-Zaluska A, Koszewski W et al: Pituitary apoplexy: endocrine, surgical and oncological emergency. Incidence, clinical course and treatment with reference to 799 cases of pituitary adenomas. Acta Neurochir (Wien) 120:118, 1993

64. Brisman MH, Katz G, Post KD: Symptoms of pituitary apoplexy rapidly reversed with bromocriptine: case report. J Neurosurg 85:1153, 1996

65. Maccagnan P, Macedo CL, Kayath MJ et al: Conservative management of pituitary apoplexy: a prospective study. J Clin Endocrinol Metab 80:2190, 1995

66. Hall WA, Luciano MG, Doppman JL et al: Pituitary magnetic resonance imaging in normal human volunteers: occult adenomas in the general population. Ann Intern Med 120:817, 1994

67. Wolansky LJ, Rao SB, Schulder M et al: Extrasellar extension of pituitary lesions: comparison of T2 weighted fast spin echo MRI with T1 weighted sequences. Int J Neuroradiol 2:147, 1996

68. Scotti G, Yu CY, Dillon WP et al: MR imaging of cavernous sinus involvement by pituitary adenomas. AJNR Am J Neuroradiol 9:657, 1988

69. Destrieux C, Kakou MK, Velut S et al: Microanatomy of the hypophyseal fossa boundaries. Neurosurgery 88:743, 1998

70. Teng MMH, Huang CI, Chang T: The pituitary mass after transsphenoidal hypophysectomy. AJNR Am J Neuroradiol 9:23, 1988

71. Hsu DW, Efird JT, Hedley-White ET: Progesterone and estrogen receptors in meningiomas: prognostic considerations. J Neurosurg 86:113, 1997

72. Rucker CW, Kearns TP: Mistaken diagnosis in some cases of meningioma. Am J Ophthalmol 51:15, 1961

73. Slavin ML: Acute, severe, symmetric visual loss with cecocentral scotomas due to olfactory groove meningioma. J Clin Neuroophthalmol 6:224, 1986

74. Gregorius FK, Hepler RS, Stern WE: Loss and recovery of vision with suprasellar meningiomas. J Neurosurg 42:69, 1975

75. Ehlers N, Malmros R: The suprasellar meningioma: a review of the literature and presentation of a series of 31 cases. Acta Ophthalmol Suppl 121:1, 1973

76. Yeakley JW, Kulkarni MV, McArdle CB et al: High-resolution MR imaging of juxtasellar meningiomas with CT and angiographic correlation. AJNR Am J Neuroradiol 9:279, 1988

77. Chan RC, Thompson GB: Morbidity, mortality and quality of life following surgery for intracranial meningiomas: a retrospective study in 257 cases. J Neurosurg 60:52, 1984

78. Mirimanoff RO, Dosoretz DE, Linggood RM et al: Analysis of recurrence and progression following neurosurgical resection. J Neurosurg 62:18, 1985

79. Rosenberg LF, Miller NR: Visual results after microsurgical removal of meningiomas involving the anterior visual system. Arch Ophthalmol 102:1019, 1984

80. Petty AM, Kun LE, Meyer GA: Radiation therapy for incompletely resected meningiomas. J Neurosurg 62:502, 1985
81. Carella RJ, Ransohoff J, Newall J: Role of radiation therapy in the management of meningioma. Neurosurgery 10:332, 1982
82. Maire JP, Caudry M, Guerin J et al: Fractionated radiation therapy in the treatment of intracranial meningiomas: local control, functional efficacy, and tolerance in 91 patients. Int J Radiat Oncol Biol Phys 33:315, 1995
83. Haie-Meder C, Brunel P, Cioloca C et al: Role of radiotherapy in the treatment of meningioma. Bull Cancer Radiother 82:35, 1995
84. Black PM: Hormones, radiosurgery and virtual reality: new aspects of meningioma management. Can J Neurol Sci 24:302, 1997
85. Kupersmith MJ, Warren FA, Newall J et al: Irradiation of meningiomas of the intracranial anterior visual pathway. Ann Neurol 21:131, 1987
86. Kennerdell JS, Maroon JC, Malton M et al: The management of optic nerve sheath meningiomas. Am J Ophthalmol 106:450, 1988
87. Grunberg SM, Weiss MH, Spitz IM et al: Treatment of unresectable meningiomas with the antiprogesterone agent mifepristone. J Neurosurg 74:861, 1991
88. Kyritsis AP: Chemotherapy for meningiomas. J Neurooncol 29:269, 1996
89. Olivero WC, Lister R, Elwood PW: The natural history and growth rate of asymptomatic meningiomas: a review of 60 patients. J Neurosurg 83:222, 1995
90. Burger PC, Scheithauer BW, Vogel FS: Surgical Pathology of the Nervous System and its Coverings, 3rd ed, p 536. New York, Churchill Livingstone, 1991
91. McLone DG, Raimondi AJ, Naidich TP: Craniopharyngiomas. Childs Brain 9:188, 1982
92. Savino PJ, Paris M, Schatz NJ et al: Optic tract syndrome: a review of 21 patients. Arch Ophthalmol 96:656, 1978
93. Eldevik OP, Blaivas M, Gabrielson TO et al: Craniopharyngioma: radiologic and histologic findings and recurrence. AJNR Am J Neuroradiol 17:1427, 1996
94. Brodsky MC, Hoyt WF, Barnwell SL et al: Intrachiasmatic craniopharyngioma: a rare cause of chiasmal thickening. Case report. J Neurosurg 68:300, 1988
95. Cushing HW: Papers Relating to the Pituitary Body, Hypothalamus, and Parasympathetic Nervous System. Springfield, IL, Charles C Thomas, 1932
96. Katz E: Late results of radical excision of craniopharyngioma in children. Neurosurgery 42:86, 1975
97. Carmel PW, Antunes JL, Chang CH: Craniopharyngiomas in children. Neurosurgery 11:382, 1982
98. Fischer EG, Welsh K, Belli JA et al: Treatment of craniopharyngioma in children 1972–1981. J Neurosurg 62:496, 1985
99. Laws ER: Transsphenoidal microsurgery in the management of craniopharyngioma. J Neurosurg 52:661, 1980
100. Halstead AE: The operative treatment of tumors of the hypophysis. Surg Gynecol Obstet 10:494, 1910
101. Alvord EC Jr, Lofton S: Gliomas of the optic nerve or chiasm: outcome by patient's age, tumor site, and treatment. J Neurosurg 68:85, 1988
102. Hoyt WF, Baghdassarian SA: Optic glioma of childhood: natural history and rationale for conservative management. Br J Ophthalmol 53:793, 1969
103. Blatt J, Jaffe R, Deutsch M et al: Neurofibromatosis and childhood tumors. Cancer 57:1225, 1986
104. Lewis RA, Gerson LP, Axelson KA et al: Von Recklinghausen neurofibromatosis. II. Incidence of optic gliomata. Ophthalmology 91:929, 1984
105. Bognanno JR, Edwards MK, Lee TA et al: Cranial MR imaging in neurofibromatosis. AJNR Am J Neuroradiol 9:461, 1988
106. Miller NR, Iliff WJ, Green WR: Evaluation and management of gliomas of the anterior visual pathways. Brain 97:743, 1974
107. McCullough DC, Epstein F: Optic pathway tumors: a review with proposals for clinical staging. Cancer 56:1789, 1985
108. Layden WE, Edwards WC: Ocular manifestations of the diencephalic syndrome. Am J Ophthalmol 73:78, 1972
109. Arnoldi KA, Tychsen L: Prevalence of intracranial lesions in children originally diagnosed with disconjugate nystagmus (spasmus nutans). J Pediatr Ophthalmol Strabismus 32:296, 1995
110. DeSousa AC, Kalsbeck JE, Mealey J, Fitzgerald J: Diencephalic syndrome and its relation to optico-chiasmatic glioma: review of twelve cases. Neurosurgery 4:207, 1979
111. Poussaint TY, Barnes PD, Nichols K et al: Diencephalic syndrome: clinical features and imaging findings. AJNR Am J Neuroradiol 18:1499, 1997
112. Perlongo G, Carollo C, Salviati L et al: Diencephalic syndrome and disseminated juvenile pilocytic astrocytomas of the hypothalamic-optic chiasm region. Cancer 80:142, 1997
113. Rieth KG, Comite F, Dwyer AJ et al: CT of cerebral abnormalities in precocious puberty. AJR Am J Roentgenol 148:1231, 1987
114. Bronen RA, Fulbright RK, Reynders CS et al: Magnetic resonance imaging of central precocious puberty: the importance of hypothalamic abnormalities. Int J Neuroradiol 1:145, 1995
115. Habiby R, Silverman B, Listernick R et al: Precocious puberty in children with neurofibromatosis type 1. J Pediatr 126:364, 1995
116. Lavery MA, O'Neill JF, Chu FC et al: Acquired nystagmus in early childhood: a presenting sign of intracranial tumor. Ophthalmology 91:425, 1984
117. Glaser JS, Hoyt WF, Corbett J: Visual morbidity with chiasmal glioma: long-term studies of visual fields in untreated and irradiated cases. Arch Ophthalmol 85:3, 1971
118. Fletcher WA, Imes RK, Hoyt WF: Chiasmal gliomas: appearance and long-term changes demonstrated by computerized tomography. J Neurosurg 65:154, 1986
119. Lourie GL, Osborne DR, Kirks DR: Involvement of posterior visual pathways by optic nerve gliomas. Pediatr Radiol 16:271, 1986
120. Patronas NJ, Dwyer AJ, Papathanasiou M et al: Contributions of magnetic resonance imaging in the evaluation of optic gliomas. Surg Neurol 28:367, 1987
121. Menor F, Marti-Bonmati L: CT detection of basal ganglion lesions in neurofibromatosis type 1: correlation with MRI. Neuroradiology 34:305, 1992
122. Albright AL, Sclabassi RJ: Use of the Cavitron ultrasonic aspirator (CUSA) and visual evoked potentials for chiasmal gliomas of children. J Neurosurg 63:138, 1985
123. Coppeto JR, Monteiro ML, Uphoff DF: Exophytic suprasellar gliomas: a rare cause of chiasmatic compression. Case report. Arch Ophthalmol 105:28, 1987
124. Massry GG, Morgan CF, Chung SM: Evidence of optic pathway gliomas after previously negative neuroimaging. Ophthalmology 104:930, 1997
125. Parazzini C, Triulzl F, Bianchini E et al: Spontaneous involution of optic pathway lesions in neurofibromatosis type 1: serial contrast MR evaluation. AJNR Am J Neuroradiol 16:1711, 1995
126. Leisti EL, Pyhtinen J, Poyhonen M: Spontaneous decrease of a pilocytic astrocytoma in neurofibromatosis type 1. AJNR Am J Neuroradiol 17:1691, 1996
127. Imes RK, Hoyt WF: Childhood chiasmal gliomas: update on the fate of patients in the 1969 San Francisco study. Br J Ophthalmol 70:179, 1986
128. Pierce SM, Barnes PD, Loeffler JS et al: Definitive radiation therapy in the management of symptomatic patients with optic glioma: survival and long-term effects. Cancer 65:45, 1990
129. Kovalic JJ, Grigsby PW, Shepard MJ et al: Radiation therapy for gliomas of the optic nerve and chiasm. Int J Radiat Oncol Biol Phys 18:927, 1990
130. Tao ML, Barnes PD, Billet AL et al: Childhood optic chiasm gliomas: radiographic response following radiotherapy and long-term clinical outcome. Int J Radiat Oncol Biol Phys 39:579, 1997
131. Erkal HS, Serin M, Cakmak A: Management of optic pathway and chiasmatic-hypothalmic gliomas in children with radiation therapy. Radiother Oncol 45:11, 1997
132. Danoff BF, Cowchock FS, Marquette C et al: Assessment of the long-term effects of primary radiation therapy for brain tumors in children. Cancer 49:1580, 1982
133. Packer RJ, Savino PJ, Bilaniuk LT et al: Chiasmatic gliomas of childhood: a reappraisal of the natural history and effectiveness of cranial irradiation. Childs Brain 10:393, 1983
134. Davis PC, Hoffman JC, Pearl GS et al: CT evaluation of effects of cranial radiation therapy in children. AJNR Am J Neuroradiol 7:639, 1986
135. Beyer RA, Paden P, Sobel DF et al: Moyamoya pattern of

vascular occlusion after radiotherapy for gliomas of the optic chiasm. Neurology 36:1173, 1986

136. Packer RJ, Ater J, Allen J et al: Carboplatin and vincristine chemotherapy for children with newly diagnosed progressive low-grade gliomas. J Neurosurg 86:747, 1997

137. Chamberlain MC: Recurrent chiasmatic-hypothalamic glioma treated with oral etoposide. Arch Neurol 52:509, 1995

138. Safneck JR, Napier LB, Halliday WC: Malignant astrocytoma of the optic nerve in a child. Can J Neurol Sci 19:498, 1992

139. Aroichane M, Miller NR, Eggenberger ER: Glioblastoma multiforme masquerading as pseudotumor cerebri: case report. J Clin Neuroophthalmol 13:105, 1993

140. Hoyt WF, Meshel LG, Lessell S et al: Malignant optic glioma of adulthood. Brain 96:121, 1973

141. Taphoorn MJB, de Vries-Knoppert WAEJ, Ponssen H et al: Malignant optic glioma in adults. J Neurosurg 70:277, 1989

142. Millar WS, Tartaglino LM, Sergott RC et al: MR of malignant optic glioma of adulthood. AJNR Am J Neuroradiol 16:1673, 1995

143. Albers GW, Hoyt WF, Forno LS et al: Treatment response in malignant optic glioma of adulthood. Neurology 38:1071, 1988

144. Matsutani M, Sano K, Takakura K et al: Primary intracranial germ cell tumors: a clinical analysis of 153 histologically verified cases. J Neurosurg 86:446, 1997

145. Camins MB, Mount LA: Primary suprasellar atypical teratoma. Brain 97:447, 1974

146. Wilson JT, Wald SL, Aitken PA et al: Primary diffuse chiasmatic germinomas: differentiation from optic chiasm gliomas. Pediatr Neurosurg 23:1, 1995

147. Lumsden CE: The neuropathology of multiple sclerosis. In Vinken PJ, Bruyn GW (eds): Handbook of Neurology, Vol 9, p 217. Amsterdam, North Holland, 1970

148. Traquair HM: Acute retrobulbar neuritis affecting the optic chiasm and tract. Br J Ophthalmol 9:433, 1925

149. Spector RH, Glaser JS, Schatz NJ: Demyelinative chiasmal lesions. Arch Neurol 37:757, 1980

150. Lindenberg R, Walsh FB, Sacks JG: Neuropathology of Vision: An atlas, p 250. Philadelphia, Lea & Febiger, 1973

151. Lefkowitz D, Angelo JN: Neuromyelitis optica with unusual vascular changes. Arch Neurol 41:1103, 1984

152. Waespe W, Haenny P: Bitemporal hemianopia due to chiasmal optic neuritis. Neuroophthalmology 7:69, 1987

153. Purvin V, Herr GJ, De Myer W: Chiasmal neuritis as a complication of Epstein-Barr virus infection. Arch Neurol 45:458, 1988

154. Reynolds WD, Smith JL, McCrary JA: Chiasmal optic neuritis. J Clin Neuroophthalmol 2:93, 1982

155. Cant JS, Harrison MT: Chiasmatic arachnoiditis with growth failure. Am J Ophthalmol 65:432, 1968

156. Oliver M, Beller AJ, Behar A: Chiasmal arachnoiditis as a manifestation of generalized arachnoiditis in systemic vascular disease: clinico-pathological report of 2 cases. Br J Ophthalmol 52:227, 1968

157. Iraci G, Giordano R, Gerosa M et al: Cystic suprasellar and retrosellar arachnoiditis. Ann Ophthalmol 8:1175, 1979

158. Takahashi T, Isayama Y: Chiasmal meningitis. Neuroophthalmology 1:19, 1980

159. Scott IU, Silva-Lepe A, Siatkowski RM: Chiasmal optic neuritis in Lyme disease. Am J Ophthalmol 123:136, 1997

160. Decker RE, Mardayat M, Marc J et al: Neurosarcoidosis with computerized tomographic visualization and transsphenoidal excision of a supra- and intrasellar granuloma. J Neurosurg 50:814, 1979

161. Tang RA, Grotta JC, Lee KF et al: Chiasmal syndrome in sarcoidosis. Arch Ophthalmol 101:1069, 1983

162. Agbogu BN, Stern BJ, Sewell C et al: Therapeutic considerations in patients with refractory neurosarcoidosis. Arch Neurol 52:875, 1995

163. Stelzer KJ, Thomas CR, Berger MS et al: Radiation therapy for sarcoid of the thalamus/posterior third ventricle: case report. Neurosurgery 36:1188, 1995

164. Navarro IM, Peralta VR, Leon JM et al: Tuberculous optochiasmatic arachnoiditis. Neurosurgery 9:654, 1981

165. Kuroda Y, Miyahara M, Sakemi T et al: Autopsy report of acute necrotizing opticomyelopathy associated with thyroid cancer. J Neurol Sci 120:29, 1993

166. Zucchini S, Ambrosetto P, Carla G et al: Primary empty sella: differences and similarities between children and adults. Acta Paediatr 84:1382, 1995

167. McGrath P: Cysts of sellar and pharyngeal hypophyses. Pathology 3:123, 1971

168. Benes SL, Kansu T, Savino PJ et al: Ocular manifestations of arachnoid cysts. In Glaser JS (ed): Neuro-Ophthalmology: Symposium of the University of Miami, Vol 10, p 107. St. Louis, CV Mosby, 1980

169. Sumida M, Uozumi T, Mukada K et al: Rathke cleft cysts: correlation of enhanced MR and surgical findings. AJNR Am J Neuroradiol 15:525, 1994

170. Rao GP, Blyth CPJ, Jeffreys RV: Ophthalmic manifestations of Rathke's cleft cysts. Am J Ophthalmol 119:99, 1995

171. Baskin DS, Wilson CB: Transsphenoidal treatment of non-neoplastic intrasellar cysts: a report of 38 cases. J Neurosurg 60:8, 1984

172. Appen RE, deVenecia G, Selliken JM, Giles LT: Meningeal carcinomatosis with blindness. Am J Ophthalmol 86:661, 1978

173. Takahashi T, Murase T, Isayama Y: Clinicopathological findings in the chiasmal region with reference to carcinomatous optic neuropathy cases. In Shimizu K, Oosterhuis JA (eds): Ophthalmology, Vol 2, p 1124. Amsterdam, Excerpta Medica, 1979

174. Takahashi T, Yoshimasa I: Pathological findings in the chiasmal region with reference to malignant lymphoma. Folia Ophthalmol Jpn 31:1118, 1980

175. Howard RS, Duncombe AS, Owens C et al: Compression of the optic chiasm due to a lymphoreticular malignancy. Postgrad Med J 63:1091, 1987

176. Tabarin A, Corcuff JB, Dautheribes M et al: Histiocytosis X of the hypothalamus. J Endocrinol Invest 14:139, 1991

177. Max MB, Deck F, Rottenberg DA: Pituitary metastases: incidence in cancer patients and clinical differentiation from pituitary adenoma. Neurology 31:998, 1981

178. Woiciechowsky C, Vogel S, Meyer R et al: Magnetic resonance imaging of a glioblastoma of the optic chiasm: case report. J Neurosurg 83:923, 1995

179. Liu GT, Galetta SL, Rorke LB et al: Gangliogliomas involving the optic chiasm. Neurology 46:1669, 1996

180. Morrison DA, Bibby K: Sellar and suprasellar hemangiopericytoma mimicking pituitary adenoma. Arch Ophthalmol 115:1201, 1997

181. Balcer LJ, Galetta SL, Curtis M: von Hippel-Lindau disease manifesting as a chiasmal syndrome. Surv Ophthalmol 39:302, 1995

182. Teixeira F, Penagos P, Lozano D et al: Medulloblastoma presenting as blindness of rapid evolution: a case report. J Clin Neuroophthalmol 11:250, 1991

183. Goodwin JA, Glaser JS: Chiasmal syndrome in sphenoid sinus mucocele. Ann Neurol 4:440, 1978

184. Valvassori GE, Putterman AM: Ophthalmologic and roentgenographic findings in sphenoidal mucoceles. Trans Am Acad Ophthalmol Otolaryngol 77:703, 1973

185. Abla AA, Maroon JC, Wilberger JE et al: Intrasellar mucocele simulating pituitary adenoma: case report. Neurosurgery 18:197, 1986

186. Heinz GW, Nunery WR, Grossman CB: Traumatic chiasmal syndrome associated with midline basilar skull fractures. Am J Ophthalmol 117:90, 1994

187. Elisevich KV, Ford RM, Anderson DP et al: Visual abnormalities with multiple trauma. Surg Neurol 22:565, 1984

188. Savino PJ, Glaser JS, Schatz NJ: Traumatic chiasmal syndrome. Neurology 30:963, 1980

189. Ess T, Weiler G: Histomorphologische Befunde and Chiasma opticum bei Schadel-Hirntrauma. Z Rechtsmed 82:257, 1979

190. Crompton MR: Hypothalamic lesions following closed head injury. Brain 94:165, 1971

191. Arkin MS, Rubin AD, Bilyk JR et al: Anterior chiasmal optic nerve avulsion. AJNR Am J Neuroradiol 17:1777, 1996

192. Hayman A, Carter K, Schiffman JS et al: A sellar misadventure: imaging considerations. Surv Ophthalmol 41:252, 1996

193. Warman R, Glaser JS: Radionecrosis of optico-hypothalamic glioma. Neuroophthalmology 9:219, 1989
194. Kline LB, Kim JV, Ceballos R: Radiation optic neuropathy. Ophthalmology 92:1118, 1985
195. Ebner R, Slamovits TL, Friedland S et al: Visual loss following treatment of sphenoid sinus carcinoma. Surv Ophthalmol 40:62, 1995
196. Atkinson AB, Allen IV, Gordon DS et al: Progressive visual failure in acromegaly following external pituitary irradiation. Clin Endocrinol 10:469, 1979
197. Hammer HM: Optic chiasmal radionecrosis. Trans Ophthalmol Soc UK 103:208, 1983
198. Girkin CA, Comey CH, Lunsford LD et al: Radiation optic neuropathy after stereotactic radiosurgery. Ophthalmology 104:1634, 1997
199. Zimmerman CF, Schatz NJ, Glaser JS: Magnetic resonance imaging of radiation optic neuropathy. Am J Ophthalmol 110:389, 1990
200. Hudgins PA, Newman NJ, Dillong WP et al: Radiation-induced optic neuropathy: characteristics on gadolinium-enhanced MR. AJNR Am J Neuroradiol 13:235, 1992
201. Hufnagel TJ, Kim JH, Lesser R et al: Malignant glioma of the optic chiasm eight years after radiotherapy for prolactinoma. Arch Ophthalmol 106:1701, 1988
202. Aristizabal S, Caldwell WL, Avila J: The relationship of time dose fractionation factors to complication in the treatment of pituitary tumors by irradiation. Int J Radiat Oncol Biol Phys 2:667, 1977
203. Parsons JT, Bova FJ, Fitzgerald CR et al: Radiation optic neuropathy after megavoltage external-beam irradiation: analysis of time-dose factors. Int J Radiation Oncol Biol Phys 30:755, 1994
204. Wilson WB, Perez GM, Kleinschmidt-Demasters BK: Sudden onset of blindness in patients treated with oral CCNU and low-dose cranial irradiation. Cancer 59:901, 1987
205. Glantz MJ, Burger PC, Friedman AH et al: Treatment of radiation-induced nervous system injury with heparin and warfarin. Neurology 44:2020, 1994
206. Borruat FX, Schatz NJ, Glaser JS et al: Visual recovery from radiation-induced optic neuropathy: the role of hyperbaric oxygen therapy. J Clin Neuroophthalmol 13:98, 1993
207. Borruat FX, Schatz NJ, Glaser JS: Radiation optic neuropathy: report of cases, role of hyperbaric oxygen therapy, and literature review. Neuroophthalmology 16:255, 1996
208. Sinclair AHH, Dott NM: Hydrocephalus simulating tumour in the production of chiasmal and other parahypophysial lesions. Trans Ophthalmol Soc U K 51:232, 1931
209. Hughes EBC: Some observations on the visual fields in hydrocephalus. J Neurol Neurosurg Psychiatry 9:30, 1946
210. Corbett JJ: Neuro-ophthalmologic complications of hydrocephalus and shunting procedures. Semin Neurol 6:111, 1986
211. Calogero JA, Alexander E: Unilateral amaurosis in a hydrocephalic child with an obstructed shunt: case report. J Neurosurg 34:236, 1971
212. Kupersmith MJ, Rosenberg C, Kleinberg D: Visual loss in pregnant women with pituitary adenomas. Ann Intern Med 121:473, 1994
213. Roelvink NCA, Kamphorst W, van Alphen HAM et al: Pregnancy-related primary brain and spinal tumors. Arch Neurol 44:209, 1987
214. Abramsky O: Pregnancy and multiple sclerosis. Ann Neurol 36:38, 1994
215. Cosman F, Post KD, Holub DA et al: Lymphocytic hypophysitis: report of three new cases and review of the literature. Medicine 68:240, 1989
216. Sunness JS: The pregnant woman's eye. Surv Ophthalmol 32:219, 1988
217. Kaufman B: The "empty" sella turcica, a manifestation of the intrasellar subarachnoid space. Radiology 90:931, 1968
218. Bergland RM, Ray BS, Torack RM: Anatomical variations in the pituitary gland and adjacent structures in 225 human autopsy cases. J Neurosurg 28:93, 1968
219. Zagardo MT, Cail WS, Kelman SE et al: Reversible empty sella in idiopathic intracranial hypertension: an indicator of successful therapy. AJNR Am J Neuroradiol 17:1953, 1996
220. Neelon FA, Goree JA, Lebovitz HE: The primary empty sella: clinical and radiographic characteristics and endocrine function. Medicine 52:73, 1973
221. Brismar K: Prolactin secretion in the empty sella syndrome in prolactinomas and in acromegaly. Acta Med Scand 209:397, 1981
222. Tremoulet M, Petrus M, Bonafe A, Rochiccioli P: La selle turcique vide de l'enfant. Rev Otoneuroophthalmol 54:405, 1982
223. Wilkinson IA, Duck SC, Gager WE, Daniels DL: Empty-sella syndrome: occurrence in childhood. Am J Dis Child 136:245, 1982
224. Berke JP, Buxton LF, Kokmen E: The "empty sella." Neurology 25:1137, 1975
225. Olson DR, Guiot G, Derome P: The symptomatic empty sella: prevention and correction via the transsphenoidal approach. J Neurosurg 37:553, 1972
226. Bursztyn EM, Lavyne MH, Aisen M: Empty sella syndrome with intrasellar herniation of the optic chiasm. AJNR Am J Neuroradiol 4:167, 1983
227. Kaufman B, Tomsak RL, Kaufman BA et al: Herniation of the suprasellar visual system and third ventricle into empty sellae: morphologic and clinical consideration. AJNR Am J Neuroradiol 10:65, 1989

CHAPTER 7

Retrochiasmal Visual Pathways and Higher Cortical Function

Matthew Rizzo and Jason J. S. Barton

Cerebral Visual Loss: An Overview of Causes
Lesions of the Retino-Geniculo-Striate Pathway
  Optic Tracts
  Lateral Geniculate Nucleus
  Optic Radiation
  Lesions of Striate Cortex
    Visual Field Defects from Striate Lesions
    Cerebral Blindness
    Anton's Syndrome
    Blindsight and Residual Vision
    Abnormalities in the Remaining Visual Field
Disorders of the Occipito-Temporal Pathway
  Cerebral Dyschromatopsia
  Visual Agnosia
    Prosopagnosia
    Other Disorders of Face Perception
  Acquired Alexia
    Pure Alexia (Alexia without Agraphia)
    Hemialexias
    Alexia with Agraphia
    Secondary Alexia
      Visual Loss and Reading
      Attention and Reading

      Eye Movements and Reading
      Central Dyslexias
      Assessment of Reading
Disorders of the Occipito-Parietal Pathway
  Bálint's Syndrome and Related Processing Deficits
  Cerebral Akinetopsia
Positive Visual Phenomena
  Visual Perseveration
    Palinopsia
    Cerebral Polyopia
  Visual Hallucinations
    Release Hallucinations, Charles Bonnet Syndrome
    Visual Seizures
    Migrainous Hallucinations
    Other Hallucinatory States
      Peduncular Hallucinations
      Hallucinations during Eye Closure
  Dysmetropsia
    Micropsia
    Macropsia
    Metamorphopsia
Recovery and Rehabilitation

"Me? I don't read books!"
"What do you read, then?"
"Nothing. I've become so accustomed to not reading that I don't even read what appears before my eyes. It's not easy: they teach us to read as children, and for the rest of our lives we remain the slaves of all the written stuff they fling in front of us. I may have had to make some effort myself, at first, to learn not to read, but now it comes quite naturally to me. The secret is not refusing to look at the written words. On the contrary, you must look at them intensely, until they disappear."

If On a Winter's Night a Traveler
Italo Calvino

M. Rizzo: Departments of Neurology and Engineering; and Visual Function Laboratory, Division of Behavioral Neurology and Cognitive Neuroscience, University of Iowa College of Medicine, Iowa City, Iowa

J. J. S. Barton: Departments of Neurology and Ophthalmology, Beth Israel Deaconess Medical Center; and Harvard Medical School, Boston, Massachusetts

The retino-geniculo-striate pathway forms the first component of the processing of visual information, from retina to optic nerve, and then beyond the optic chiasm. While visual modulation occurs at each step of this pathway, it functions chiefly as a serial relay of visual information to striate cortex. The retino-geniculate segment of this pathway contains axons of the retinal ganglion cells, traveling in the optic nerve, chiasm, and tract. It contains two major subdivisions, the parvocellular (P) and magnocellular (M) pathways (see Chapters 2 and 4). The geniculo-striate segment (optic radiations) contains axons projecting from the lateral geniculate nucleus to the occipital cortex. The striate cortex (area V1) is the main terminus of these parallel subcortical pathways, and occupies both banks of the calcarine fissure (see Fig. 4–11).

Only a small minority of retinal ganglion cells do not project to the lateral geniculate nucleus and on to striate cortex. Some leave the optic chiasm to innervate the suprachiasmatic nucleus of the hypothalamus, providing visual input for hormonal circadian rhythms.[1,2] Others project to visuomotor brainstem areas such as the superior colliculus and accessory optic system, or to the pretectal nuclei for the pupillary light reflex (see Chapter 15). Of the geniculate neurons, almost all project to striate cortex, with a small number innervating extrastriate cortex directly.

Lesions of the retino-geniculo-striate pathway and striate cortex cause characteristic visual field defects. Because of the serial nature of this pathway, these visual defects affect all types of visual perception in a nonspecific manner. These deficits are restricted to certain portions of the visual field, particularly with partial lesions, because of the topographic arrangement of this pathway. The decussation of the retino-geniculate axons in the optic chiasm leads to segregation of visual information by hemifield rather than by eye of origin. Lesions beyond the chiasm—of the optic tracts, the lateral geniculate nucleus (LGN), the optic radiations, or striate cortex—cause visual hemifield defects that are binocular, contralateral, and homonymous. More recent studies have raised questions of residual visual functions or "blindsight" in the scotoma due to striate lesions (see below), but these phenomena seem rare, difficult to demonstrate, and of questionable utility.

The second post-chiasmal component is the extrastriate cortical visual system. There are numerous extrastriate visual areas with specialized roles in visual perception: in the monkey, over 40 different regions have been identified. In humans these areas are located in the association cortex of the occipital lobe and adjacent temporal and parietal regions. Unlike the retino-geniculo-striate pathway, extrastriate cortex is not a serial sequence of stages. Rather, visual inputs are dispersed, condensed, and recombined in multiple secondary visual maps that process different aspects of vision, with parallel inputs and outputs, back-projections from higher to lower areas, and interconnections between areas at a similar hierarchical level.[3] Thus visual information fans out through multiple parallel and distributed extrastriate pathways. Furthermore, the retinotopic partitioning of the retino-geniculo-striate pathway become progressively degraded at successive levels in the extrastriate hierarchy; the receptive fields of individual neurons become larger and larger, with some eventually spanning the entire ipsilateral and contralateral visual field.

Lesions of extrastriate cortex cause deficits that differ greatly from those due to lesions of the retino-geniculo-striate pathway. Because of parallel processing, some types of visual perception (i.e., color, form, motion) are affected but others are intact. The pattern of loss varies with the location and extent of each individual lesion. These deficits are less localized regionally in the visual field, and in many cases are only severe when there are bilateral lesions (see also Chapters 2 and 4, and Fig. 4–12).

One useful model of extrastriate processing conceives of two visual subsystems, known as *What* and *Where* pathways.[4] A What pathway for object recognition, also known as the ventral or temporal pathway, includes areas V4 and inferotemporal cortex in monkeys. These receive a mixture of subcortical M and P inputs. The equivalent region in humans likely extends from below the calcarine fissure (ventral areas 18 and 19) into the adjacent medial temporal lobe (e.g., areas 21, 37). Damage to these regions causes agnosia, alexia, and achromatopsia.

The Where pathway for locating objects in space, also known as the dorsal or parietal pathway, includes the middle temporal and medial superior temporal areas, and various regions of posterior parietal cortex in monkeys. The middle temporal area receives mainly M inputs. In humans, this pathway likely extends from the dorsal bank of the calcarine fissure onto the superior and lateral surfaces of the hemisphere, including the occipito-parietal and temporo-parieto-occipital junctions (dorsolateral 18, 19; and areas 39 and 37). These structures are involved in motion perception, spatial vision, and visuospatial attention. Damage causes akinetopsia, or cerebral motion blindness, elements of Bálint's syndrome (simultanagnosia, optic ataxia, ocular apraxia) and hemispatial neglect.[5–8]

In contrast to the precise lesions made in monkey studies, human brain lesions often cross boundaries between areas and pathways, producing unique and varied combinations of visual field defects and selective perceptual impairments that respect neither distinctions between subcortical, striate, and extrastriate segments nor What vs. Where cortical pathways. Also, there are functional interactions between pathways that obscure such distinctions. For example, the inferotemporal cortex in the ventral stream is sensitive to object form, but can also respond to shapes that are only visible because of regional differences in visual motion, even though motion perception is considered a function of the dorsal What pathway. Nevertheless, the model of two visual systems is a reasonable concept for understanding the visual disabilities in patients.

CEREBRAL VISUAL LOSS: AN OVERVIEW OF CAUSES

The brain regions that process vision cover a broad portion of the posterior cerebral hemispheres, and cerebral lesions frequently produce visual disturbances. The most frequent cause is *cerebrovascular disease*, particularly embolic or thrombotic infarction in the posterior cerebral artery territory[9,10] (see Fig. 4–15). Several other vascular mechanisms are possible but less common (Table 7–1). Transient ischemia may also play a role in the aura of classic migraine, though permanent migrainous visual deficits are rare.

Trauma is another frequent cause of visual cortical lesions. Direct injury to visual areas occurs from open head injury with penetration of the skull from falls, falling objects, knives, bullets, or blows. Closed head injury may involve rapid acceleration and deceleration of the head, as in a fall or when the head strikes the dashboard in a car accident. The brain continues forward due to inertia, then moves back in the opposite direction. A *coup* injury produces bruising on the side of the impact and a *contre-coup* injury on the opposite side. Thus trauma to visual areas may follow a blow to either the occiput or the forehead.

Both cerebrovascular and traumatic brain injury can indirectly injure visual areas through cerebral edema. As the skull is a closed compartment, edema can result in *herniation syndromes*. Tentorial herniation of the uncus may compress the posterior cerebral arteries, infarcting one or both occipital lobes, with severe and permanent visual deficits in survivors.

There are many other causes of retrogeniculate visual loss (Table 7–1). Vision impairment is frequent in Alz-heimer's, the most common cause of dementia in older adults, and can even be the presenting complaint in patients with the visual variant of this disorder. This group may perplex the eye specialist, unaware of such manifestation of Alzheimer's and without appropriate tools for measuring the relevant visuoperceptual and cognitive impairments. Creutzfeldt-Jakob disease, a rare, rapidly progressive and incurable disorder, may likewise present with visual complaints prior to dementia, myoclonus, and the development of triphasic waves on electroencephalogram (EEG). In such cases, concerns have been raised about transmitting the infectious agent to other patients through inadequate sterilization of instruments.

Finally, in addition to increased incidence of pathologic impairments of the eye and brain in the elderly, visual performance is also reduced through normal aging. Reduction in the speed of neural processing in the central nervous system results in cognitive slowing, reduced attention capacity, and shrinkage in the useful field of view despite apparently normal visual fields by conventional perimetry. Such visual impairment can affect daily activities such as reading, route finding, face recognition, and driving, and may increase the risk of injury from car accidents and hip fractures.

LESIONS OF THE RETINO-GENICULO-STRIATE PATHWAY

Knowledge of the gross anatomic relations, vascular supply, and retinotopic and functional microanatomy of the retino-geniculo-striate pathway is essential to understand the visual defects and associated signs from lesions of these structures. These are discussed in Chapter 4.

Optic Tracts

The optic tract is the continuation of the anterior visual system from the optic chiasm to the LGN. Only the contralateral hemifield is represented in the tract. At first the decussated nasal retinal fibers are not closely aligned topographically with the other eye's temporal retinal fibers, but these gradually achieve an approximate retinal correspondence at their termination in the LGN. The retinotopic map is also tilted in the optic tracts, so that the macula is represented dorsally, inferior retina (superior visual field) laterally, and superior retina (inferior visual field) medially (see Fig. 4–9). Recent data suggest a segregation of magnocellular and parvocellular axons in the tract also, with the magnocellular axons located more ventrally.[11] Both of these topographies are mirrored in the LGN. The main arterial supply of the optic tract is the anterior choroidal artery.

The contralateral visual field defects of optic tract lesions have several important features reflecting functional anatomy. First, partial lesions of the optic tract will cause contralateral homonymous defects, but the

TABLE 7–1. Causes of Cerebral Visual Loss

Cerebrovascular disease
  Ischemia
    Embolism
    Vertebrobasilar atherosclerosis
    Hypotensive watershed infarction (middle cerebral artery–posterior cerebral artery)
    Migraine
  Hemorrhage
    Amyloid angiopathy
    Coagulopathy
    Hypertension
    Arteriovenous malformation
    Cortical vein thrombosis
  Cerebral edema
    Hypertensive encephalopathy
    Toxemia
Trauma
Herniation syndrome
Tumor
Degeneration
  Alzheimer's disease
  Creutzfeldt-Jakob disease
Infection
  Bacterial abscess
  Fungal infection (aspergillosis)
  Viral encephalitis
  AIDS
  Progressive multifocal leukoencephalopathy
Toxins
  Carbon monoxide
  Organic mercurial compounds
  Chemotherapy

incomplete topographic alignment in the retinal maps of the two eyes results in *incongruity*, with different patterns of visual loss in the two eyes[12,13] (Figs. 7–1 and 7–2, and Color Plates 7–1 and 7–2). Marked incongruity in partial hemianopia indicates a tract lesion, since lesions of the optic radiations cause only mild incongruity at most, and striate lesions are highly congruous. Of course, complete transection of the optic tract will lead to congruous, complete hemianopia, though this is less frequent than partial lesions. Although some reports claim reduced acuity, this usually indicates either bilateral tract damage or extension of the lesion to the optic chiasm or optic nerves.[13–15] As yet there are no data on whether the putative segregation of M and P streams in the tract is reflected in visual dissociations after lesions.

Second, because the axons in the optic tract originate from retinal ganglion cells, damage to the tract over time will cause *optic atrophy* and segmental defects in the retinal nerve fiber layer. This will be present in both eyes, but because only half of the axons of each eye will be affected at most, the atrophy is less marked than with other optic neuropathies. Also, the pattern of optic disc atrophy will differ between the eyes. In the eye with temporal field loss, the axons from the nasal retina are affected. The fibers from the nasal periphery enter the disc nasally, while those from the nasal fovea and parafoveal region enter the disc temporally in the papillomacular bundle. These nasal and temporal wedges of the disc show atrophy, but the superior and inferior sectors are spared, because they contain fibers from the temporal retina. The result is a bow-tie pattern of optic atrophy (Color Plate 7–1). The eye with nasal field loss will have atrophy in the superior and inferior wedges as well as the papillomacular bundle, but sparing the nasal wedge, looking much like the temporal pallor of optic neuropathy (Color Plates 7–1 and 7–2). Another distinctive disc picture occurs in the eye with temporal field loss when a mass lesion causes both optic tract compression and papilledema. Disc swelling occurs in the superior and temporal disc but not in the atrophic bow-tie regions: this is so-called twin-peaks papilledema[16,17] (see Color Plate 7–2).

Third, because fibers for the pupillary reflex also travel in all but the most distal segment of the optic tract, there is often a *relative afferent pupil defect* (RAPD). With a significantly incongruous hemianopia, the RAPD may be in the eye with greater visual loss. However, even with complete and congruous hemianopia, a tract lesions will be associated with RAPD in the eye with temporal field loss.[13,18] This is attributed to the greater size of the temporal visual field, and a slightly larger number of axons from the nasal than temporal retina (ratio 53 : 47). The RAPD is a useful sign of retinal ganglion cell dysfunction in optic tract hemianopia, as it may be present at a time when optic atrophy is not apparent[19] (see Chapter 15).

Other reported pupillary abnormalities include Behr's pupil, which is an anisocoria with the larger pupil in the contralateral eye, and Wernicke's hemianopic pupil, which is an intra-ocular afferent pupil defect, with less pupillary constriction when a small focused beam of light is shone upon the hemianopic hemiretina, compared to when the light is shone upon the intact hemiretina. Behr's pupil sign is largely discredited now. Wernicke's hemianopic pupil is difficult to elicit at the bedside because of the effects of intra-ocular light scatter,[12] though it may be seen with computerized pupillometry (Fig. 7–3).

This combination of optic atrophy, RAPD, and field incongruity are important to recognize in a patient with homonymous hemifield defects, because the differential diagnosis of optic tract lesions differs greatly from that of lesions of the optic radiations or striate cortex. While most of the latter result from vascular disease and other intra-cerebral pathology, most optic tract lesions are compressive extrinsic masses, with a differential diagnosis similar to that for optic chiasmal lesions (see Chapter 6). Patients with combined damage to the optic tracts, chiasm, and nerve are not rare.[13,20–23] Hence, pituitary adenomas, giant aneurysms of the internal carotid artery, meningiomas, and craniopharyngiomas are the chief causes of damage to the optic tract. The investigation of choice is magnetic resonance imaging of the parasellar region, with coronal and axial sections and contrast administration.

Less common lesions include inflammatory conditions such as multiple sclerosis and sarcoidosis[12,21,24–26] (Fig. 7–1 and Color Plate 7–1). Intrinsic optic pathway gliomas may occur in the optic tracts, and their radiologic appearance may be mimicked by craniopharyngiomas.[22] Vascular lesions are rare, but there are occasional reports of cavernous angiomata or arteriovenous malformations.[20,27,27a] Trauma can affect the optic tract.[12] Optic tract infarction can complicate anterior temporal lobectomy, possibly from vasospasm of the anterior choroidal artery.[28] Radiotherapy of pituitary tumors may be followed years later by optic tract necrosis.[23] Optic tract dysfunction is a side effect of α-interferon.[29] On occasion there is congenital absence of the optic tract; such patients are often unaware of their hemianopia until it is found on an eye examination.[30]

Associated abnormalities are unusual.[12] These include endocrine disturbances from hypothalamic dysfunction and memory impairment from temporal lobe involvement, reflecting the proximity of the optic tracts to these structures[14] (see Chapter 4).

Lateral Geniculate Nucleus

The LGN is a subnucleus in the ventro-postero-lateral corner of the thalamus. Neighboring thalamic subnuclei include the medial geniculate nucleus ventromedially, the ventral posterior nucleus dorsomedially, and the pulvinar superiorly and dorsally. The medial geniculate nucleus, a relay nucleus in the auditory pathway, gives rise to the acoustic radiations, which pass by the dorsomedial aspect of the LGN on their way to the auditory cortex in the temporal lobe. The optic radiations arise from the dorsolateral surface of the LGN. Ventrally, the hippocampus and parahippocampal gyrus face the LGN across the ambient cistern and the inferior horn of the lateral ventricle. The LGN has a dual blood supply: the anterior choroidal artery, a branch of the internal carotid artery; and the lateral choroidal artery, a branch of the posterior cerebral artery. The anatomy of the vascular territories within the LGN has been debated. Initial studies suggested that the anterior choroidal artery supplied the medial LGN as well as the optic tract and the lateral choroidal artery supplied the lateral LGN. However, experience with surgical arterial lesions concluded that the anterior choroidal artery supplies both the lateral and medial aspects and the lateral choroidal artery supplies the hilus and mid-zone of the LGN (see Fig. 4–7).

Although the LGN is traditionally thought of as a simple relay nucleus, it is also the site of considerable modulation of visual information, by back-projections from visual cortex and afferent projections from the brainstem reticular formation and superior colliculus.[31–33] Some of the corticofugal input influences the stimulus selectivity of LGN neurons.[32] Others postulate that these non-retinal inputs play a role in gating visual transmission through the LGN, and thus participate in selective attention.[31]

The LGN is a triangular-shaped structure with six roughly horizontal layers containing segregated inputs from the two eyes (see Fig. 4–8). The ventral two layers are the magnocellular layers, whereas the other four layers are the parvocellular component; these differ in many structural and functional aspects (see Chapter 4). The LGN has a retinotopic pattern, which is a continuation of that found in the optic tract. The macula is represented in a dorsal wedge, including the hilum, and projecting posteriorly, whereas the most peripheral fibers are located ventrally. Superior retinal fibers (contralateral inferior visual quadrant) are in the medial horn and inferior retinal fibers (contralateral superior visual quadrant) are in the lateral horn.

Because the LGN is small and relatively secluded, lesions here are rare. Its intimate relation to the optic tract and optic radiation make it difficult to be certain that a visual defect is due solely to LGN damage rather than damage to the adjacent tract or radiation. Indeed, visual field defects from purported LGN lesions resemble visual field defects from optic tract or optic radiation lesions.

Three main types of hemianopic defects have been described with LGN lesions. The first is an *incongruous hemianopia*, much like that seen with optic tract lesions, reflecting the continued segregation of ocular inputs in the LGN. The other two patterns are *sectorial hemi-anopias*, reflecting the unusual territorial division between the anterior and lateral choroidal arterial supplies. With lateral choroidal ischemia, the hilum and middle zone of the LGN are affected, causing a wedge-shaped visual defect straddling the horizontal meridian[34] (Fig. 7–4). With anterior choroidal ischemia, the lateral and medial tips of the LGN are infarcted, resulting in the reverse defect, *i.e.,* loss of the superior and inferior aspects of the contralateral hemifield with sparing around the horizontal meridian.[35] Unusual cases of presumed bilateral LGN damage have presented with an hourglass shape to either the visual field defect or the region of spared vision.[36,37]

Optic atrophy often accompanies LGN lesions. If there is damage to almost all the LGN, the optic atrophy will have a similar appearance to that seen with optic tract lesions. If there is partial damage causing sectorial hemianopias, then the optic atrophy may be more subtle and restricted to the relevant sectors of the disc.[34,35] However, because the afferent fibers subserving the pupillary light reflex have already departed for the pretectum, there is no RAPD with lesions of the LGN. With incongruous hemianopia and optic atrophy, this is the only feature that permits distinction between optic tract and LGN lesions.

A variety of pathologies have been reported with LGN lesions. Infarction is the most likely cause of sectoranopia, given the dependence of such defects upon the vascular anatomy, but astrocytomas and arteriovenous malformations are also reported.[34,35] The LGN also appears to be a target of central pontine myelinolysis, a syndrome associated with excessively rapid correction of hyponatremia.[36,37] LGN damage is even a para-infectious complication of traveler's diarrhea.[38]

Optic Radiation

The optic radiation may be affected anywhere in its course (see Chapter 4); the pattern of visual field defect reflects the site of damage. Ischemic or hemorrhagic lesions of the internal capsule affect the optic radiation while it is still a relatively compact bundle, usually causing a complete homonymous hemianopia. A similar defect can arise from damage close to the termination in striate cortex (Fig. 7–5). Lesions of the ventral fibers in the anterior temporal lobe cause a contralateral *superior visual quadrant* defect (Fig. 7–6). Most often this defect aligns on the vertical meridian, with variable extension toward the horizontal meridian and central vision.[39] Lesions of the dorsal fibers in the parietal lobe cause an *inferior visual quadrant* defect (Fig. 7–7). Because there is no sharp demarcation of the dorsal fibers from the ventral fibers in this portion of the posterior pathway, the defect seldom aligns along the horizontal meridian.[39] Overall, quadrantanopia is more frequent with lesions of striate cortex.[39] Lesions of the temporal lobe more than 8 cm posterior to its anterior tip can affect both upper and lower radiations. Small lesions may also affect certain portions of the radiations and spare others; for example, damage to the mid-portion of the optic radiation can mimic the *sectoranopias* of LGN lesions (Fig. 7–8).[40] While there can be some incongruity to the visual field defects of optic radiation lesions, this is less marked than the incongruity with optic tract lesions.

Unlike lesions of the retino-geniculate pathway or the LGN, lesions of the geniculostriate axons do not lead to optic atrophy (with the exception of some congenital lesions, through transsynaptic degeneration) or pupillary defects. However, there are frequently other signs of cerebral damage, especially if the lesion is large.[39] Thus, temporal lobe lesions cause superior quadrantic defects and sometimes also complex partial seizures, auditory or complex visual hallucinations (some of which may be seizures also), memory problems, or a Wernicke's aphasia if the dominant hemisphere is involved. Parietal lesions with mainly inferior quadrantic defects may cause cortical sensory disturbances, such as impaired two-point discrimination and graphesthesia, and impaired smooth pursuit toward the side of the lesion. With dominant hemisphere lesions, Gerstmann's syndrome (acalculia, finger anomia, right-left disorientation, and agraphia) may occur, as may a variety of aphasic syndromes, including alexia with or without agraphia, Wernicke's aphasia, or global aphasia.

The differential diagnosis of optic radiation lesions reflects the variety of cerebral hemispheric pathologies. Unlike lesions of the optic tract, most are infarcts in either the posterior cerebral or middle cerebral artery territories. Tumors, vascular malformations, infections, and leukodystrophies are also possibilities. The temporal profile of the illness will often be the major clue to the etiology.

Lesions of Striate Cortex

The primary visual area in the medial occipital lobe goes by several names: Brodmann's area 17, visual area 1 (V1), calcarine cortex, and striate cortex (see Chapter 4) The exact position of striate cortex varies between individuals. While the parieto-occipital fissure forms a reasonably reliable anterior dorsal boundary, the posterior limit containing the macular representation is more variable, extending from the medial occipital surface over the first one or two centimeters of the posterior surface of the occipital lobe (see Figs. 4–10 and 4–11).

The main vascular supply of striate cortex derives from the posterior cerebral artery (see Fig. 4–15). A parieto-occipital branch supplies the superior calcarine bank, a posterior temporal branch supplies its inferior bank, and a calcarine branch supplies the central region posteriorly. Individual variation exists, however.[41] Perhaps most importantly, the occipital pole is at the junction (watershed zone) of the vascular territories of the

posterior and middle cerebral arteries, and there is again marked variation as to which artery supplies the foveal representation in striate cortex.[41]

The retinotopic arrangement in striate cortex is well known (see Chapter 4), and confirmed with recent imaging studies of lesions.[42] The foveal representation is posterior, at the occipital pole, and the far peripheral field is anterior, on the medial occipital surface.[43,44] The superior bank of the calcarine fissure receives input from the inferior visual field, while the inferior bank contains the representation of the superior visual field. The most anterior part of striate cortex represents the monocular temporal crescent, the region of temporal field in the contralateral eye that lies beyond the limits of the nasal field (60°) of the ipsilateral eye. As in most of the visual system, there are fewer neurons devoted to peripheral vision than to central vision: over half of striate cortex is devoted to the central 10° (cortical magnification).[42,45] Occipital cortex contains a mixture of monocular and binocular cells arranged in ocular dominance columns, but large separations between the inputs of the two eyes are not present.

Visual Field Defects from Striate Lesions

Focal destruction of striate cortex produces a homonymous contralateral visual hemifield defect. Unlike the scotomata from lesions of the optic radiations and especially the optic tracts, the hemianopic defects from striate lesions are highly congruent, with virtually identical defects in the two eyes.

Complete destruction of striate cortex causes complete visual loss in the contralateral visual hemifield. Because this involves not only peripheral vision but also the contralateral half of the foveal region, it is called a *macula-splitting* homonymous hemianopia. This may occur with posterior cerebral artery ischemia in a patient whose entire striate cortex is supplied by that artery. Macula-splitting hemianopias can occur with complete lesions anywhere along the retro-chiasmal visual pathways, and thus lack localizing value (Fig. 7–5). Other signs may help in localization, such as optic atrophy and the relative afferent pupillary defect with optic tract lesions, and significant hemiparesis, hemisensory loss, aphasia, or hemi-neglect, which frequently accompany optic radiation damage that is large enough to cause complete hemianopia.

Partial lesions of the striate cortex are frequent. With posterior cerebral infarcts, a *macula-sparing hemianopia* occurs in patients with adequate collateral circulation of the macula region (occipital pole) from the middle cerebral artery[41,46] (Fig. 7–9). Previously, macula sparing was thought due to bilateral representation of a small stripe flanking the vertical meridian, which expanded to as much as 3° at the fovea. However, studies of monkey V1 do not find bilateral representation of the hemimaculae,[47] and computed tomography (CT) and magnetic resonance imaging (MRI) studies in humans with hemianopia document the correlation of macula sparing with sparing of the occipital pole.[48,49] Macula sparing has some localizing value, since it is rarely encountered with lesions outside of striate cortex.

The upper and lower banks can also be involved separately. Ischemia can do this because the banks have separate blood supplies. Upper bank infarcts cause homonymous contralateral *inferior quadrantanopia* (Fig. 7–10) and lower bank infarcts cause *superior quadrantanopia*. Although altitudinal defects have been reported occasionally, most quadrantic defects do not align at the horizontal meridian, because the upper field merges without interruption into the lower field in the depths of the calcarine fissure.[50,51] Thus, it has been argued that quadrantic defects that respect the horizontal meridian are due to involvement of area V2, the surrounding striate cortex; this remains controversial.[42] Quadrantanopias are three times more common with striate lesions than with optic radiation lesions.[39] Striate quadrantanopias are more frequently isolated signs but can be associated with other signs of higher cortical visual dysfunction, such as pure alexia or hemiachromatopsia, whereas optic radiation quadrantanopias are usually accompanied by hemiparesis, dysphasia, or amnestic problems.[39]

Selective lesions can also occur along the anterior-posterior extent of striate cortex. A lesion of the occipital pole alone causes homonymous *central hemi-scotomata*[49,52] (Fig. 7–11). This can occur with watershed infarcts during systemic hypoperfusion. Slightly more anterior lesions in the middle zone of striate cortex cause homonymous *peripheral scotomata* (Fig. 7–12). The highly congruent, homonymous nature of these defects and their restriction to one hemifield differentiate these from ocular causes of central or paracentral visual loss. Lesions with such small field defects can be missed on CT.[48] MRI with coronal sections through the occipital lobes should be performed, although even this may miss small lesions, particularly at the occipital pole.

A near-complete lesion that spares only the most anterior portion of V1 causes a pathognomonic field defect, hemianopia with sparing of the monocular temporal crescent (Fig. 7–13). The hemianopia involves the whole nasal hemifield of the ipsilateral eye, but the temporal hemianopia of the contralateral eye spares a crescent-shaped island of vision in the far periphery.[53] This is the monocular temporal crescent, the region of the visual field that is represented in the temporal field of one eye but not the nasal field of the other. The initial sense of incongruity may raise suspicions of an optic tract lesion; however, the absence of optic atrophy and RAPD, the high congruity of the homonymous defect inside 60°, and the location of the crescent outside 60° eccentricity indicate that the lesion must be in striate cortex. The converse defect, a monocular temporal crescentic scotoma, can occur with a retrosplenial lesion, along the parieto-occipital sulcus.[54]

Most striate lesions are infarctions, mainly from posterior cerebral artery occlusion (Fig. 7–14), with sudden onset visual loss and often headache.[10] In about half, the visual field defect is the only deficit, but in others damage to medial occipito-temporal regions causes amnesia, prosopagnosia, and color perception defects.[10] A syndrome of agitated delirium and hemianopia occurs with lesions of the medial occipital lobe, parahippocampus, and hippocampus.[55–57] Brainstem signs include impaired level of consciousness, III nerve palsy, dysarthria, and hemiplegia.[10] Causes of ischemia are most frequently cardiac emboli and vertebrobasilar occlusive disease; migraine is a rare cause of permanent defects.[10] Hemorrhage, vascular malformations, and primary and secondary malignancies are much less common.[39]

Bilateral lesions of striate cortex are not rare. Focal midline lesions such as tumors or traumatic injury may affect both striate cortices concurrently, since the right and left striate cortices face each other on the medial occipital surface. The most common cause, however, is posterior circulation ischemia.[58] This can affect both striate cortices either simultaneously or sequentially, as the right and left posterior cerebral arteries have a common origin from the basilar artery[58]; 22% of patients with a unilateral occipital infarction will develop bilateral infarction over 3 years.[59] *Bilateral incomplete hemianopia* is distinguished from bilateral optic nerve or ocular disease by the high congruity of the visual fields and step defects along the vertical meridian, which indicate the hemifield nature of the visual loss[58] (Fig. 7–15). Such steps are important to seek with a skilled perimetrist, but they can be difficult to demonstrate with bilateral hemiscotomata from occipital pole lesions.[60] Bilateral quadrantanopias can occur, often in patients with prosopagnosia and achromatopsia, for example, and may mimic the altitudinal defects of optic neuropathy.[50,51]

Cerebral Blindness

Cortical blindness is a term with a history of loose usage, at times referring to visual loss from occipital lobe damage, even if the loss is incomplete; hence, hemianopia or bilateral quadrantanopia has been called cortical blindness.[51] It is best reserved for what it implies: bilateral complete or severe hemianopia, with acuity at light perception only[61] or worse, and no detectable peripheral vision. Also, since the responsible lesion may involve both gray and white matter, or in some cases only white matter, a better term may be *cerebral blindness*.[61,62]

Cerebral blindness is distinguished from ocular disease by both normal pupillary light responses and normal funduscopic examination. The normal eye examina-

(text continues on p. 258)

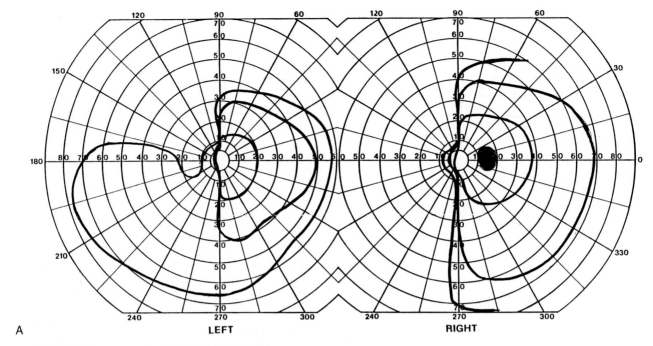

A

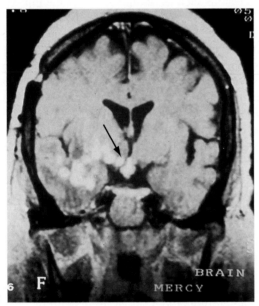

B

Fig. 7–1. Optic tract lesion. A 53-year-old woman with CNS sarcoidosis diagnosed 7 years previous with focal motor seizures. She had no visual symptoms. Acuity was 20/40 in both eyes. There was left relative afferent pupil defect. **A.** Visual fields showed incongruous left hemianopia. **B.** MRI showed enhancing lesions of right temporal lobe, infundibular region, and right optic tract (*arrow*). (From ref. 13a)

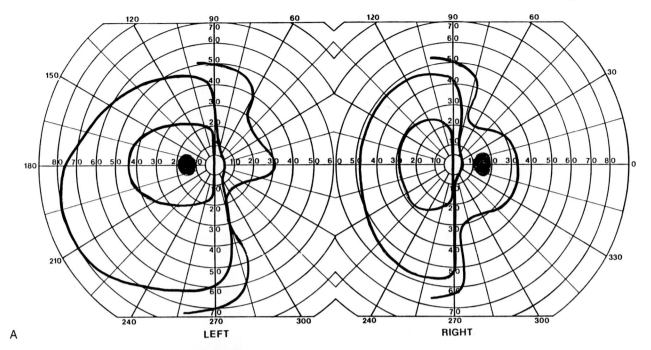

A

LEFT   RIGHT

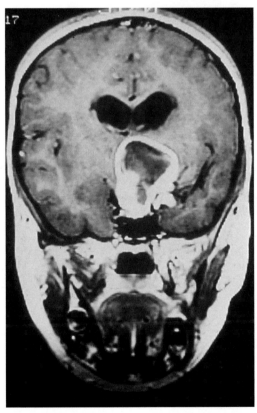

B

Fig. 7–2. Optic tract lesion. An 8-year-old girl with 1 month of headache and horizontal diplopia from right VI nerve palsy. Acuity was 20/25 in both eyes, and there was right relative afferent pupil defect. **A.** Visual fields showed mildly incongruent right hemianopia. **B.** MRI showed suprasellar mass, involving left more than right, which was a hypothalamic glioma. (From ref. 13a)

247

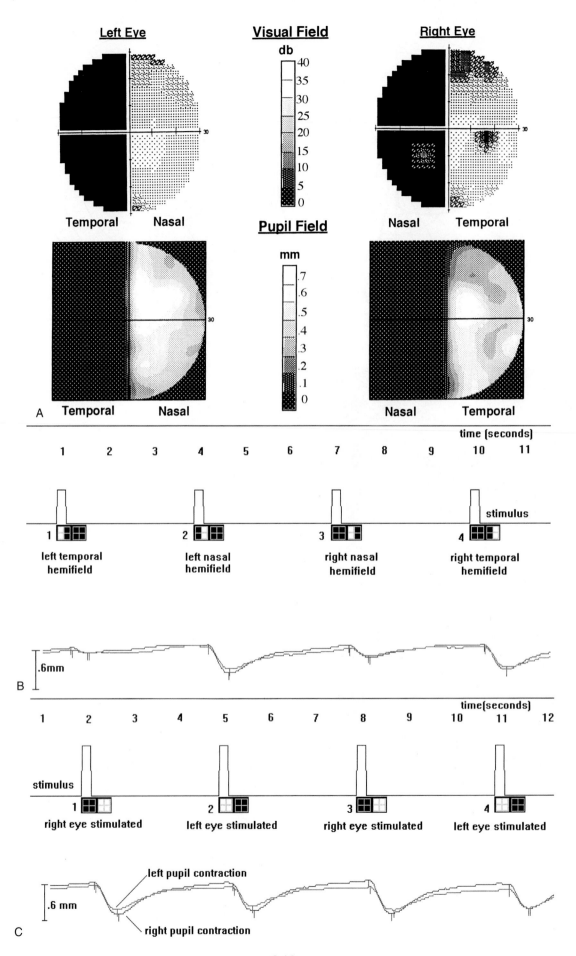

248

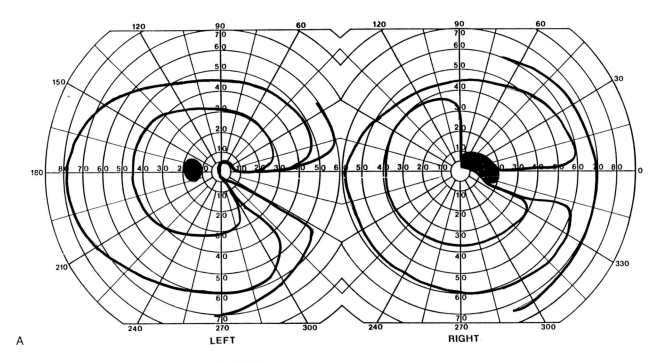

A
LEFT
RIGHT

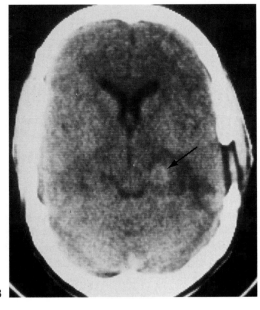

B

Fig. 7–4. Lesion of lateral geniculate nucleus (LGN) (*arrow*). **A.** Slightly incongruent right sectoranopia along the horizontal meridian. **B.** CT shows hemorrhage in the vicinity of the LGN. This field defect would result from damage to the mid-zone of the LGN. (From ref. 13a)

Fig. 7–3. A. Right optic tract lesion with left homonymous hemianopia. Pupil perimetry results (*below*) mirror the visual field defect on Humphrey perimetry (*top*). **B.** Hemifield illumination in either eye shows less response in the left field (Wernicke's hemianopic pupil). **C.** Full field illumination shows smaller response to left eye illumination (relative afferent pupil defect). (Courtesy of Dr. Randy Kardon)

249

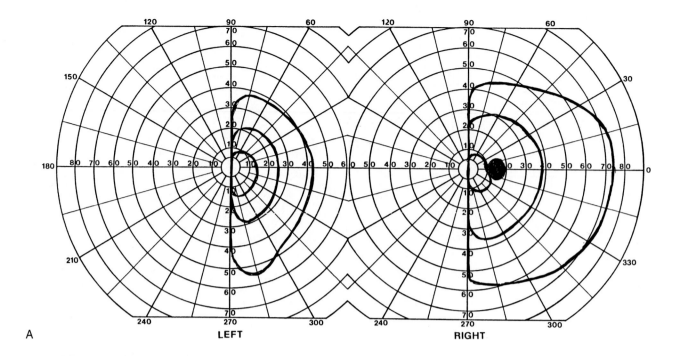

LEFT   RIGHT

A

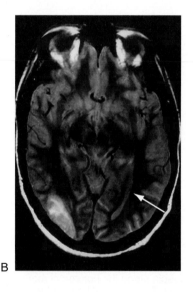

B

Fig. 7–5. Macula-splitting hemianopia. A 47-year-old man with AIDS and sudden onset of poor vision. **A**. Fields show complete left hemianopia. **B**. MRI shows lesion of right lateral occipital cortex, affecting distal optic radiations (*arrow*). Biopsy showed non-specific encephalitis.

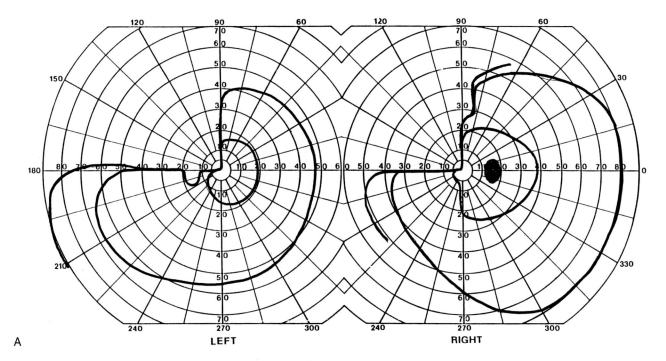

A   LEFT   RIGHT

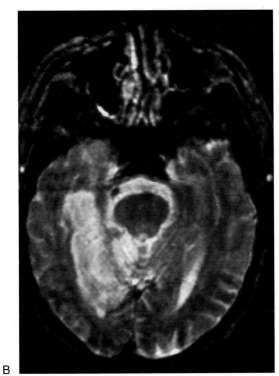

B

Fig. 7–6. Lesion of temporal optic radiation. **A.** Left superior quadrantanopia, respecting horizontal meridian, from infarct of right medial temporal lobe **(B),** in posterior cerebral artery territory. (From ref. 13a)

251

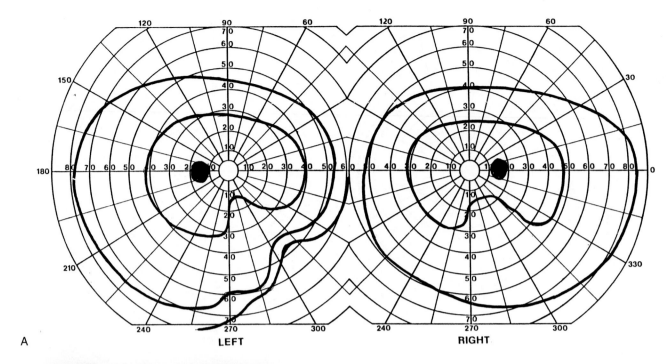

A

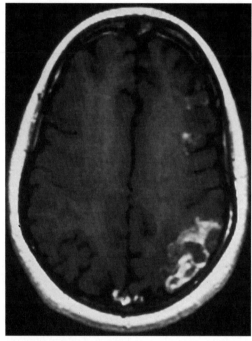

B

Fig. 7–7. Lesion of parietal optic radiation. A 35-year-old woman with 3 weeks of left-sided headache. **A.** Visual fields showed partial right inferior quadrantic defect. **B.** MRI showed infarct of parietal lobe, involving optic radiations. (From ref. 13a)

252

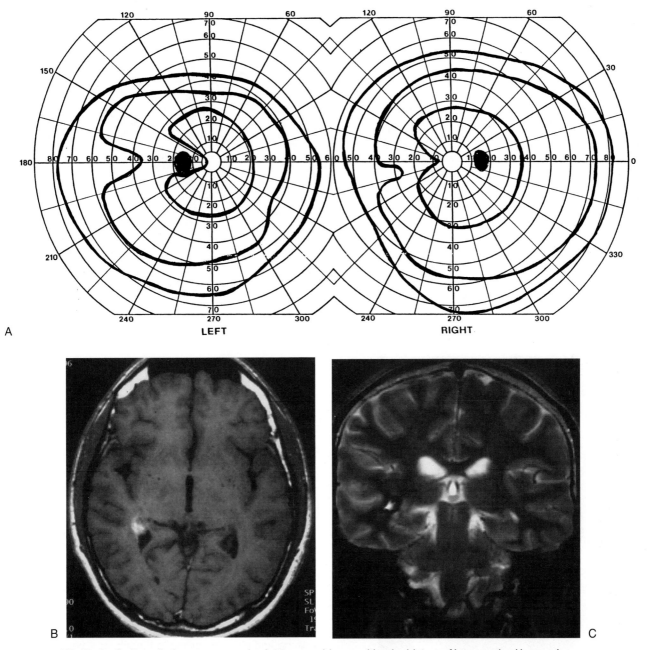

Fig. 7–8. Optic radiation sectoranopia. A 25-year-old man with prior history of intracerebral hemorrhage. **A.** With no visual symptoms, fields show subtle left sectoranopia straddling the horizontal meridian and **B, C.** MRI shows periventricular hemorrhage from a cavernous angioma, affecting the mid-portion of the optic radiations.

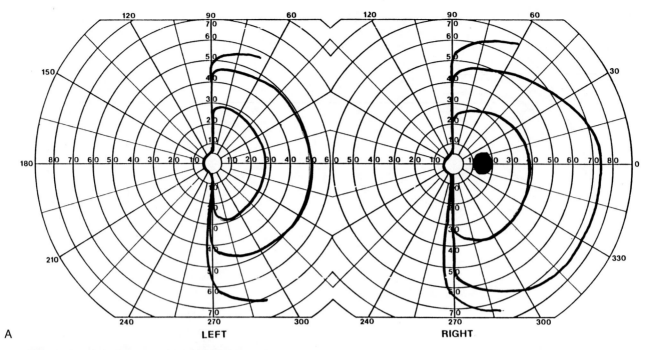

A

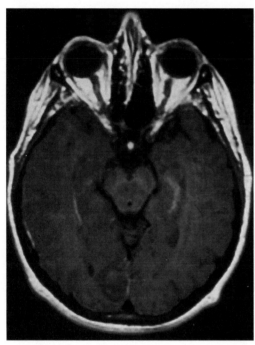

B

Fig. 7–9. Macular-sparing striate hemianopia. A 49-year-old woman with headache and difficulty seeing to the left for 1 week. **A.** Fields show left hemianopia that spares a small zone around the central fixation spot. **B.** MRI shows infarct of right striate cortex, with sparing of occipital pole. (From ref. 13a)

254

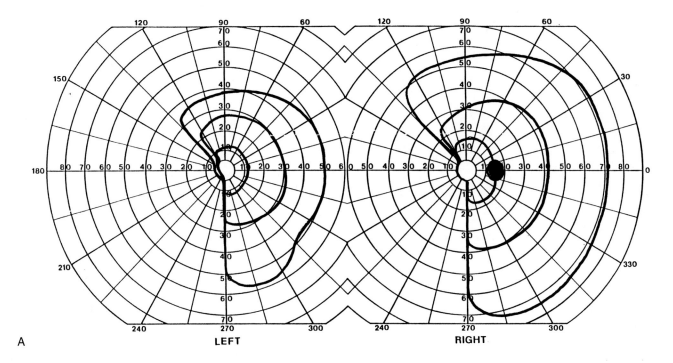

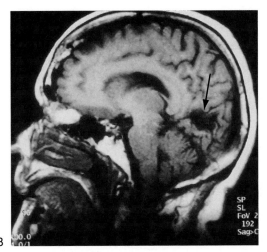

Fig. 7–10. Striate quadrantanopia. A 68-year-old woman with a stroke 3 years previous, causing left inferior quadrantanopia **(A)**. **B**. MRI shows infarct of the superior bank of the right calcarine cortex (*arrow*).

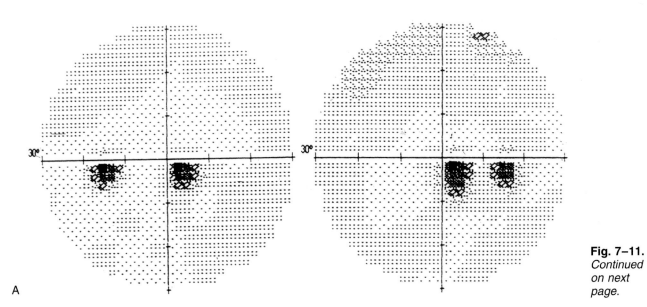

Fig. 7–11. *Continued on next page.*

255

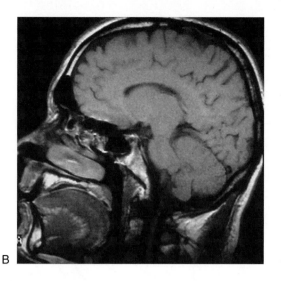

Fig. 7–11. (*continued*) Central hemi-scotomata. A 37-year-old man with sudden onset of difficulty reading. **A.** Fields show small inferior central homonymous scotomata restricted to right hemifield, respecting the vertical meridian. **B.** MRI shows subtle hypointensity at occipital pole, presumably a small infarction. (From ref. 13a)

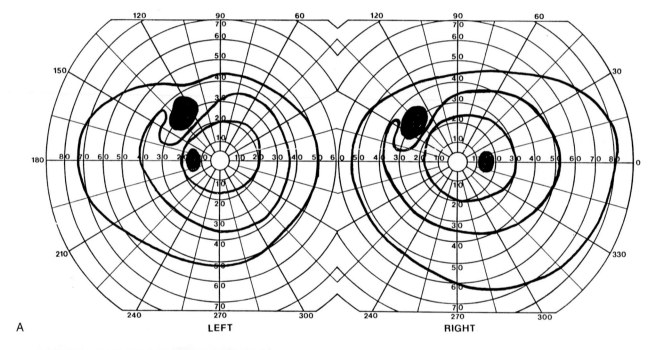

A   LEFT   RIGHT

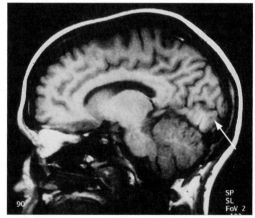

Fig. 7–12. Homonymous peripheral scotomata. A 32-year-old woman with classic migraine history. Two weeks prior she had a severe headache with transient left-sided weakness and typical blurring in left hemifield, which on this occasion did not resolve. **A.** Fields show small homonymous scotomata in left upper quadrant. **B.** MRI shows small striate infarct of the mid-zone of the inferior bank of the calcarine fissure (*arrow*).

256

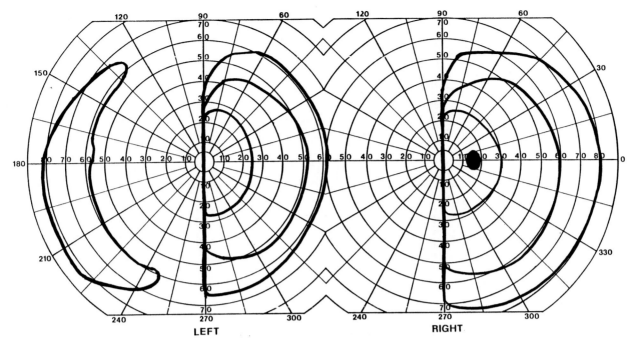

Fig. 7–13. Sparing of the monocular temporal crescent. A 65-year-old man with left hemianopia from right medial occipital infarct. Fields show complete hemianopia within an eccentricity of 60°, but sparing of the temporal field beyond 60°, which is normally only perceived in the temporal field. This indicates a striate lesion with sparing of the retrosplenial portion of calcarine cortex. (From ref. 139)

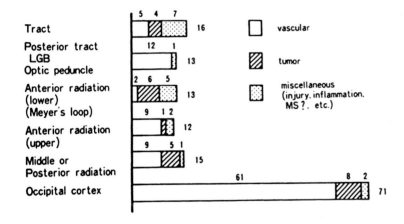

Fig. 7–14. Location and etiology of homonymous hemianopia in 140 patients. (Fujino T, Kigazawa K, Yamada R: Homonymous hemianopia. A retrospective study of 140 cases. J Neuroophthalmol 6:17, 1986. Published with permission from J Neuroophthalmol. Copyright by Aeolus Press)

257

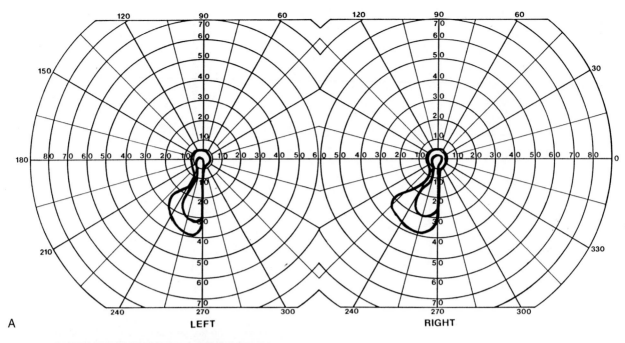

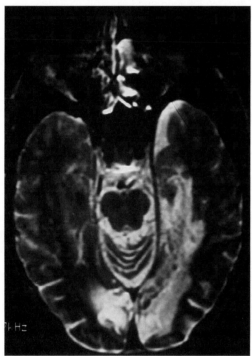

Fig. 7–15. Bilateral incomplete hemianopia. A 69-year-old man with decreased vision after prostate surgery. **A.** Fields show remaining central parafoveal vision with some sparing of inferior left quadrant. Note how the defect respects the vertical meridian. **B.** MRI shows bilateral medial occipital infarction, with sparing of the occipital poles, accounting for the macular-sparing bilaterally. (Courtesy of Dr. Lucia Vaina)

tion may lead to an erroneous diagnosis of factitious visual loss. Associated signs of damage to parietal or medial temporal structures are useful in confirming cerebral blindness but may not always be present.

Cerebral blindness can be divided into persistent and transient forms. The most frequent cause of persistent cerebral blindness is cerebrovascular infarction.[63] In addition to the common embolic or thrombotic causes, vertebrobasilar arteritis can occur in the elderly, and

subclavian steal is found in a few patients.[64–66] Infarction may be precipitated by generalized hypotension, as induced by medications like nifedipine.[67,68] Cerebral blindness is a vascular complication of cardiac surgery, due to either hemodynamic compromise or emboli.[63] A rare vascular cause of cerebral blindness is rupture of occipital mycotic aneurysms with endocarditis.[69]

Visual evoked potentials are of limited diagnostic value in cerebral blindness. They can be altered voluntarily by subjects without visual loss and yet can be normal in patients with striate lesions.[70-72] Evoked potentials cannot differentiate between blind and seeing children with neurologic disease, and normal results do not necessarily predict a good visual outcome in children.[73,74] Absent evoked responses are rare, and may only occur early in the course.[73] Absent alpha rhythm on electroencephalography is reportedly a more sensitive diagnostic sign than visual evoked potential abnormalities.[63,75,76] CT scans can be normal, but MRI with coronal images through the occipital lobe should reveal most striate or optic radiation lesions with complete and persistent visual loss. Single photon emission computed tomography (SPECT) scans may reveal bilateral functional defects in cases with only unilateral structural lesions on MRI.[77]

Among adults with infarction, blindness is permanent in 25% and residual visual field defects are common in the rest. Bi-occipital CT lucencies carry a poor prognosis for visual recovery, but abnormal visual evoked potentials do not correlate with severity or outcome.[57,63] While the abnormalities on visual evoked potentials are usually not diagnostic, they tend to improve as vision returns.[78-80]

There are many causes of a *transient cerebral blindness*, which lasts hours to days, often with full recovery (Table 7-2). Both ictal and post-ictal cerebral blindness are reported in children and adults.[81-83] Transient cerebral blindness can occur with metabolic insults, hypertensive encephalopathy, hydrocephalus, trauma, and cortical venous thrombosis.[75,84-90] Toxins are an important cause, especially chemotherapeutic agents.[61,91-94] Cerebral blindness is associated with the hyperosmolar iodinated contrast agents used in cerebral or coronary angiography; CT scans with contrast show disruption of the blood-brain barrier in the occipital lobes as early as 1 hour after angiography.[63,95-97]

The pathogenesis of transient cerebral blindness varies with the cause. Vasospasm is blamed in head trauma, eclampsia, methamphetamine abuse, and meningitis, which may also induce vasculitis.[80,98-102] Circumstantial evidence for vasospasm includes a correlation of traumatic cerebral blindness with prior migraine.[89] In other cases an association with seizures suggests that visual loss is a post-ictal deficit.[103,104] Angiographic contrast agents may cause breakdown of the blood-brain barrier under osmolar stress and subsequent neurotoxic effects, providing a rationale for dexamethasone and mannitol as specific therapy in this context.[97] Neurotoxic effects are also likely mechanisms with chemotherapeutic agents.

Pediatric cerebral blindness is not uncommon. Children may not complain of visual loss but present with agitation, disorientation, and unsteadiness.[76,98,105] During tests of vision they may not respond or may confabulate answers.[105,106] Further observation shows that they do not fix, follow, or make saccades to objects, blink to threat, or show optokinetic responses.[73,76,106] There can be an associated strabismus.[106a] Major causes include head trauma, bacterial meningitis, and hypoxia from cardiac or respiratory arrest.[79,80,102,106] Other causes include encephalitis and metabolic and toxic conditions.[86,101,103,106] (Table 7-3). Seizures are commonly associated, and mental retardation is frequent among those with meningitis.[79]

Post-traumatic transient cerebral blindness is a particular syndrome affecting children and young adults.[76,107,108] It occurs in about 1% of closed head injuries.[75,89,109] The impact is often, but not always, in the parieto-occipital region.[75,76,108,110] Headache, confusion, anxiety, nausea, and vomiting are commonly associated, and loss of consciousness at the time of injury is frequent in young children and adults, but not in adolescents.[89,108] Blindness may occur with the injury or after a short interval of minutes, or sometimes after a few hours in adolescents.[76,89,108,110] Vision recovers within 24 hours though the course in adults is more variable, with occasional residual deficits.[89,108,110] CT of the head often does not

TABLE 7-2. Causes of Transient Cerebral Blindness

Seizures (ictal or post-ictal)
Head trauma
Vascular
   Hypertensive encephalopathy
   Eclampsia
   Cerebral venous thrombosis
Toxic
   Iodinated contrast agents
   Metrizamide
   Amphetamine
   Chemotherapy
      Cisplatin
      Cyclosporine
      Vincristine
      FK506
Metabolic
   Hepatic encephalopathy
   Hypoglycemia
   Acute intermittent porphyria
Hydrocephalus

TABLE 7-3. Causes of Pediatric Cerebral Blindness

Infection
   Bacterial meningitis
   Mumps encephalitis
Head trauma
Hypoxia after cardiac/respiratory arrest
Metabolic conditions
   Hypoglycemia
   Uremia/hemodialysis dysequilibrium syndrome
Toxicity
   Methamphetamine

show occipital lesions, but EEG shows bilateral occipital slowing.[76,105,108,110] Protracted recovery, especially in children, may indicate cerebral contusions[110] or occipital lobe infarction from tentorial herniation.[110,111] There can be an association with a personal or family history of seizures and migraine.[89]

The course of cerebral blindness is variable. It can lasts hours, days, or weeks, recover fully, evolve into a hemianopia or other field defects, or be permanent.[70,74,79] If there is recovery, it usually occurs within 5 months.[74] Recovery of useful vision is more likely in children than adults.[106] The prognosis is better with hypotension during cardiac surgery than with other causes.[74] The prognosis with hypoxia is worst for preterm infants, who tend to have periventricular leukomalacia rather than parasagittal watershed infarctions; evidence of optic radiation damage on the CT or MRI is a poor sign.[112] A normal MRI in most other settings is a good prognostic sign, and significant recovery can occur if hypoxic damage is limited to the visual cortex.[74,112] Spike-and-wave discharges on EEG are associated with multiple handicaps and poor visual recovery.[74]

Transient cerebral blindness occurs in about 1% to 15% of patients with pre-eclampsia or eclampsia.[99,100,113] Antiphospholipid antibodies may be associated with infarction or venous thrombosis, and fluctuations in blood pressure with peri-partum blood loss may also contribute.[114,115] The pathogenesis is analogous to that of hypertensive encephalopathy, with development of petechial hemorrhages and focal edema from impaired cerebral vascular autoregulation, and ischemia from vasospasm.[100,116] CT scans may be normal or show bi-occipital lucencies.[100,117] MRI is more sensitive, showing T2 hyperintensities and T1 hypointensities similar to those in hypertensive encephalopathy.[116,118] Management is that of eclampsia, with magnesium sulfate, fluid restriction, and blood pressure control. The prognosis is good, with virtually all women regaining vision within a few hours to a week, rarely as long as 3 weeks.[106]

The differential diagnosis of eclamptic visual loss includes cerebral venous thrombosis and systemic hypoperfusion due to pulmonary emboli.[119,120] Eclampsia can also affect the eye, causing retinopathy with retinal detachment, edema, and vascular thrombosis, or, more rarely, anterior ischemic optic neuropathy.[121,122] Pituitary apoplexy can present with severe headache and visual loss and is a medical emergency, requiring steroid replacement, endocrinologic assessment, and sometimes surgery.

Anton's Syndrome

A small minority (perhaps 10%) of patients with cerebral blindness are not aware of their deficit, but insist that they can see (Anton's syndrome).[58,63] The origin of this denial syndrome remains obscure. Some suggest a common origin with other anosognosic syndromes, which are attributed to right hemispheric dysfunction or disconnections between the thalamus and the right parietal lobe.[123,124] Denial of blindness can also occur in patients with ocular or optic nerve disease, but lack of awareness in these patients is related to concurrent dementia or confusional states.[125] Denial of blindness with lesions of the visual cortex is not necessarily accompanied by an altered mental state. Thus, Anton's syndrome should be more specifically defined as denial of blindness in the absence of dementia or delirium. However, even this more restrictive definition is not always indicative of lesions of visual cortex, since it can be mimicked by unusual combinations of bilateral optic neuropathy with bilateral frontal lobe disease.[126]

It has even been suggested that an inverse Anton's syndrome exists.[127] These patients have incomplete visual loss but deny any ability to see. In contrast to blindsight, small islands of preserved vision can be demonstrated, and neuro-imaging in one case demonstrated residual striate cortex corresponding to the remnant visual field.[127] It was hypothesized that this "meaning stripped of its percept" (cf. the famous definition of agnosia as "a percept stripped of its meaning") resulted from disconnection of visual perception in striate cortex from attentional mechanisms in the parietal lobes.[127,128] Further reports of inverse Anton's syndrome are awaited to verify its existence and determine its mechanisms.

Blindsight and Residual Vision

Some studies claim that lesions of the geniculostriate pathway do not eliminate all visual function within the resulting scotoma. In blindsight, subjects who state that they are not aware of a visual stimulus nevertheless guess at a level better than chance when asked about some property of the stimulus. This usually requires forced-choice techniques, where subjects are asked not whether the stimulus is present or not, but whether it has property A or B (i.e., is it moving left or right?), and must respond. In residual vision, patients retain some awareness of the target within a dense visual field defect defined by perimetry, suggesting a severe but relative hemianopia.[129–132] The relation between blindsight and residual vision is not clear; one patient with residual vision had blindsight for certain types of visual stimuli, but the implications of this are not certain, since such behavior can also be mimicked by normal subjects too.[133–135]

Not all patients with cortical field defects have blindsight or residual vision, and the number of patients reported with such abilities is small. Why some patients and not others retain blindsight is unknown. Blindsight or residual vision may correlate with the degree of sparing of extrastriate cortex and subcortical projections to it.[136] Modern imaging and the emerging localization of human homologues of monkey extrastriate areas allows testing of this hypothesis; so far the results are mixed.[137–139] Sparing of extrastriate cortex may not be enough or even required for blindsight.[138–140] Age of onset may be an important factor, as children may have greater neural plasticity.[129,141,142] However, not all studies find an age effect[143] and others report that adults can be trained to show blindsight.[140,144–147] Lesion duration may be a factor, and some claim that blindsight emerges only with extensive practice over years.[148] With a few exceptions, blindsight visual abilities are degraded versions of normal perception, being less accurate, more variable, and sometimes inconsistently present.[145,146,149] Though the range of blindsight or residual visual ability reported in the literature is wide, no one has yet shown that such abilities benefit patients in daily life.

Spatial localization was studied early because of hypotheses that the spatial responses of the superior colliculus would be most likely to survive geniculostriate lesions.[150] Saccadic localization is weak and restricted to targets with eccentricities less than 30°.[149,151–153] Others have not found saccadic localization within hemianopic defects or only in patients with residual vision.[129,154–157] Localization by pointing is weak, variable, and not present in all patients, and in some studies may be an artifact of light scatter.[153,158,159] The best manual localization by a blindsight patient occurred in a region that recovered subsequently on perimetry.[136,149]

There are reports of remaining *motion perception*, including direction discrimination, optic flow direction, motion detection, and speed discrimination.[129,130,137,140,158,160,161] Rotating motion within a blind hemifield has been reported to influence the judgment of true vertical.[162] The results of some of these studies may have been artifacts.[161,162] Optokinetic nystagmus has been reported in one patient[163] with cortical blindness but not in others.[124,137] Pursuit and saccadic responses to moving stimuli were not preserved in patients with medial occipital lesions sparing the lateral human "motion area."[139]

Most studies do not find *form recognition* in blindsight, but one patient had normal discrimination of large forms and orientation.[136,149,153,161] One study found that hemianopic patients could distinguish semicircles from circles that lie halfway in the blind hemifield, but these results are invalidated by the macula sparing of the patients' hemianopia.[164] Some studies show no discrimination for *color* but others find residual color opponency in blind fields.[129,130,149,165–167] Tests of spatial and temporal *contrast sensitivity* in hemianopia were negative in one study but not others.[168–170] Interactions between blind and normal hemifields have been studied for summation

and distractor effects on response latencies, with variable results.[159,171,172]

How does blindsight arise? Most theories postulate residual visual pathways parallel to the retino-geniculo-striate system.[173] A retino-tectal pathway may subserve spatial localization, for example.[151] However, blindsight for pattern and motion are not easily explained by tectal responses alone, hence the hypothesis of input to extrastriate cortex via a retino-tecto-pulvino-extrastriate relay.[149] This requires a pathologic adaptation of pulvinar function, since visual responses in the pulvinar normally derive from visual cortex.[174,175] Blindsight for color suggests a remnant geniculo-extrastriate path, because tectal neurons lack color opponency.[165,167,173]

Persisting function of extrastriate cortex can explain the variability in blindsight among different patients. Striate lesions in humans vary in the extent of associated extrastriate damage, and the pattern of residual ability may mirror the pattern of extrastriate sparing in any given patient.[136,176] However, studies have not yet found a correlation between blindsight and lesion extent or location.[138,139,156,171] Nevertheless, residual extrastriate function has indirect support from studies of the human motion area with transcranial magnetic stimulation and functional positron emission tomography (PET) imaging.[132,177,178] Whether residual activity exists in other extrastriate regions is not known.

Against the extrastriate hypotheses are reports of blindsight in patients with hemidecortication, including saccades to targets in the blind field, variable manual localization, speed but not direction discrimination, and form perception.[141,143,150,179,180]

Other explanations of blindsight have been proposed. First, there may be surviving remnants of striate cortex[151,181,182]; at least one case with apparent blindsight had a small island of remaining vision on detailed perimetry and some striate sparing on MRI.[182] Second, blindsight is also one of a family of phenomena with dissociations between conscious reporting and unconscious behavior, including prosopagnosia, pure alexia, and amnestic syndromes. Rather than invoking separate anatomic detours for each of these effects, such dissociations may reflect partial damage to cortical networks, as some models predict.[183,184] Third, blindsight may be merely a test effect called *criterion shift,* in which subjects are conservative when asked to respond yes or no in a detection task, but base their responses on looser criteria when forced to choose A or B in a discrimination task.[181] Thus normal subjects can show blindsight-like dissociations with special stimuli.[134,135] Some have used signal detection analysis to address this problem in blindsight.[165,185] Last, test artifacts such as inadequate fixation, light scatter, non-visual cues, and non-random presentation of targets confound some blindsight studies.[181] Excluding artifact is not necessarily a trivial process. Eccentric fixation may elude eye recordings unless the head is rigorously stabilized.[186] Blindsight-like performances can be mimicked by light scatter, which cannot be adequately measured by photometers.[139,181]

Abnormalities in the Remaining Visual Field

Some patients with hemifield visual defects complain of difficulties with their remaining vision, such as visual fatigue or blurring, especially in tasks with high attentional demands like reading, finding a face in a crowd, or driving a motor vehicle. There is evidence that unilateral lesions produce not only contralateral scotomata but also deficits in both the remaining ipsilateral and contralateral visual fields. There are spatial and temporal contrast sensitivity deficits in the supposedly normal ipsilateral hemifields of patients with homonymous hemianopia.[168] There is reduced sensitivity and increased response times to signals in both hemifields and reduction in the "useful field of view" (UFOV) (see below).[187] Saccadic response times to visual targets in the ipsilateral hemifield are also reduced.[139,188]

The origins of these subtle bilateral effects of unilateral lesions are unclear. One hypothesis is that the inevitably associated white matter damage disrupts visual connections, including projections from V1 to other visual areas, callosal connections between the same or different visual areas in the two hemispheres, and feedback projections from a higher visual area to a lower one. A lesion in one area can thus affect the functioning of another, more distant area (diaschisis).[189] Disrupted connections can impair the synthesis of information from other vision areas and both hemispheres, producing long-range disturbances in both hemifields, outside the limited contralateral scotoma. Damage to extrastriate regions may have similar bilateral long-range effects, as shown in monkeys with lesions of area V4, for example.[190] Thus, associated extrastriate damage may contribute to impaired processing efficiency in the ipsilateral field of patients with hemianopia.[187]

Standard kinetic and automated static perimetry are not designed to detect such deficits. These tests ignore response speed and minimize the role of attention to get maximal estimates of sensory function, an effective approach for gauging the classic field defects due to dysfunction of the retino-geniculo-striate pathway.[191] However, the working visual capacity in elderly or brain-damaged individuals is better approximated by tests of vision under conditions of increased attentional load.[187,192,193] Measures of this UFOV have been designed, using central or peripheral distractors during perimetric tests of localization ability to gauge the effects of attention.[191] UFOV evaluation may reveal defects associated not only with hemianopia but also with aging and Alzheimer's dementia, where they may have practical import, in that UFOV reduction predicts crashes in driving simulations.[194]

DISORDERS OF THE OCCIPITO-TEMPORAL PATHWAY

Cerebral Dyschromatopsia

Color is a useful cue in object identification. Lesions in the cerebral cortex and white matter can produce a range of color deficits. Patients report that colors look different and less bright, or that objects look colorless and only appear in shades of gray.[8,195-198] *Cerebral (central) achromatopsia* refers to complete loss of color perception, whereas *cerebral dyschromatopsia* indicates some residual color perception, as is most often the case. Both are rare. *Hemiachromatopsia* and *hemidyschromatopsia* refer to color loss restricted to the contralateral hemifield, and may be more common but underrecognized.[198-201]

The pathologic correlation of cerebral color loss with inferotemporal lesions was first described in the 1880s.[202-204] Modern cases with CT and MRI confirm this and show that the lesions associated with achromatopsia occupy the lingual and fusiform gyri, in the ventromedial occipital lobe.[198,205-207] Localizations with three-dimensional MRI show a strong association of cerebral achromatopsia with damage in the middle third of the lingual gyrus and/or the white matter immediately behind the posterior tip of the lateral ventricle.[8,208] Functional neuroimaging using PET has found activation in comparable regions in normal subjects viewing color stimuli.[209] Functional MRI demonstrates activation of human areas V1 and V2 (presumed to contain ensembles of color-opponent neurons) by red-green and yellow-blue stimuli.[210] These areas provide inputs to the inferotemporal regions damaged in achromatopsia.

Both cerebral hemispheres process color, and bilateral lesions are required for cerebral achromatopsia involving the entire visual field. Unilateral lesions of either hemisphere produce color loss in the contralateral visual hemifield (hemiachromatopsia or hemidyschromatopsia). Patients with complete achromatopsia invariably complain of their loss of color vision, but those with hemiachromatopsia are often not aware of this deficit.[199-201]

Cerebral achromatopsia is commonly but not always accompanied by superior quadrantanopia, visual agnosia, and acquired alexia with left-sided lesions.[197,206,211,212] Superior quadrantanopia can occur in one or both hemifields, with the achromatopsia evident only in the lower quadrants. This indicates extension of the lesion to the inferior optic radiations or inferior calcarine cortex. Extension of the lesion anteriorly into temporal lobe may produce additional defects of memory.[197,211]

The deficits in color perception in the full syndrome

of cerebral achromatopsia can be tested with the same standardized tests used to assess patients with retinal and optic nerve disorders.[213-215] Pseudo-isochromatic plates such as the American Optical Hardy-Rand Rittler and Standard Pseudoisochromatic Plates[216,217] are useful, even in patients with alexia or aphasia, who can do this test by tracing perceived patterns with their fingers. However, some patients with achromatopsia may still pass this test, particularly if the plates are presented so distantly that the individual color dots cannot be resolved.

Color arrangement tests consist of color chips mounted in caps that can be arranged in a unique sequence. They vary in the number of chips, the difficulty of the discriminations required, and the dimension of color space they probe, such as hue, saturation, and brightness. The Farnsworth-Munsell 100 Hue evaluates hue discrimination of tokens that do not vary in luminance. The D-15 test is a shorter version that screens for severe hue discrimination loss along protan, deutan, or tritan axes. The Lanthony New Color Test similarly tests hue discrimination, but at different saturation levels, and it also asks which colors are confused with grays. The Sahlgren Saturation Test evaluates saturation discrimination by testing the ability to separate five greenish-blue and five bluish-purple caps of varying saturation.[218] The Lightness Discrimination Test consists of caps of different grays, to be ranked from dark to light.[219,220] Achromatopsic patients often have abnormal discrimination of hues and saturation, but normal perception of brightness.[8,207,221]

Anomaloscopic techniques have also been applied to study cerebral achromatopsia.[8,205] With the Nagel anomaloscope, the observer tries to match a yellow monochromatic light in one test field with a mixture of yellow-green and yellow-red lights in another, by varying the proportion in the mix. Normal observers rapidly find the unique proportion needed, whereas individuals with congenital color defects or acquired cerebral achromatopsia lack a unique solution, but have abnormal matches over a wide range.

Hemiachromatopsia is more difficult to test. Hemifield color loss can be detected by having patients report on the appearance of large color tokens moved from the ipsilesional to the contralesional hemifield. For example, a red pen may appear to turn grayish to the patient as it is moved into the aberrant field. Yet it is difficult to quantify the color loss because the standard color tests (see above) are designed for viewing within the central few degrees of vision where color vision is best. Patients with hemiachromatopsia can achieve normal color scores on these tests because of spared color vision near fixation.[8] This, coupled with the asymptomatic nature of hemiachromatopsia, suggests that color loss is often unrecognized in patients with unilateral inferior occipitotemporal lesions.

The diagnosis of cerebral achromatopsia should not depend on the ability to name colors, because color naming paradoxically may be normal in a color deficient field. The million or so colors discriminated by the visual system fall within only about a dozen categorical names in any language, and a true color deficit may be insufficient to shift color percepts across the boundaries of differently named categories.[222] Hence, color naming is not sufficiently sensitive to subtle defects in color perception, nor is it specific. Patients may fail to name color tokens because of *color anomia* or *agnosia* rather than achromatopsia.[125,223-226] The latter patients can discriminate between colors on cap-sorting tests and pseudo-isochromatic plates, but cannot name colors shown to them or point to colors when they are named by others.

The pattern of deficits on the anomaloscopic and color sorting tasks suggests that cerebral lesions produce a spectrum of color impairments affecting the processing of signals from all cone types, although there may be a greater vulnerability to color loss along the tritan (blue-yellow) axis.[8,197,206,221] Another factor requiring further investigation is the role of size; normal individuals see color less well in objects below a certain size, and this effect may be exaggerated by cerebral dyschromatopsia.

Effects on color constancy are an important issue. The wavelengths reaching the eye from an object depends on both its reflectant properties and the light illuminating the scene. Yet, the color of objects remains stable under a wide range of environmental and lighting conditions.[203,227,228] For instance, an apple continues to look red in sunlight, incandescent light, and fluorescent light, in an orchard or grocery display. This ability to discount the illuminant depends on neural computations in retina and cortex (the Retinex theory[229]). These computations likely average the spectral luminance over large regions of the surrounding background to deduce the nature of the illuminant, and this information is then taken into account to derive the true color of any object in the scene.[227,229] Zeki[203] speculated that impaired color constancy is the key defect in cerebral achromatopsia, yet if this were true, patients should report large shifts in the color appearance of objects in different environments, which they do not. Also, it is difficult to understand how a defect of color constancy could account for reports of a gray or colorless world in the most impaired individuals. A defect of color constancy may contribute, but it does not sufficiently account for all the phenomena observed in patients with cerebral achromatopsia.

Lastly, some color information appears to remain in achromatopsia. Some patients can recognize when a difference in color exists, even if they do not know the difference or the colors. Boundaries between regions of different color, but similar luminance, are detected, and this probably accounts for the ability to read pseudo-isochromatic plates.[206,207] It may reflect residual color opponent processing in striate cortex.[206] Indeed, pho-

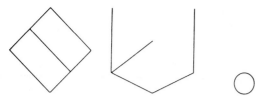

Fig. 7–16. A plate from the Benton Visual Retention Test. (Courtesy of Prof. Arthur Benton)

topic spectral sensitivity curves have shown preserved trichromacy and color opponency, indicating intact cone and parvocellular retinal ganglion cell function.[207]

Visual Agnosia

Patients with visual agnosia no longer recognize previously familiar objects nor learn to identify new objects by sight alone.[230] A historical debate centers on the necessary and sufficient impairments that generate agnosia, and the extent to which these impairments involve memory rather than perception. Teuber[128] defined agnosia as an associative disorder in which percepts are stripped of their meanings. This *associative agnosia* can be considered a selective disturbance of visual memory. In contrast, perceptual dysfunction is the main cause of disordered visual recognition in *apperceptive agnosia*.[231] However, this apperceptive/associative distinction is rarely encountered in a pure form; most patients with agnosia have a combination of impairments of visual perception and memory.

Complete assessment of patients with higher visual disorders such as agnosia begins with an examination of basic visual sensory functions like visual acuity, visual fields, and spatial contrast sensitivity. Dysfunction of basic visual processes must be excluded before a patient's complaints can be attributed to a more complex problem. Higher visual functions require more specialized neuropsychological visual tests, including tests of visual recognition, memory, reading, mental imagery,

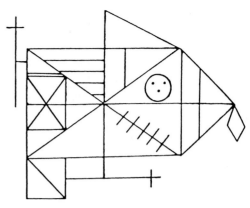

Fig. 7–18. The Rey-Osterreith Complex Figure.

visual perception, visuoconstruction, and visual attention.[232,233] Although detailed assessment of cognitive and intellectual function requires referral to a neuropsychologist, some tests can be administered easily and quickly in a neuro-ophthalmology clinic.[234,235]

The Benton Visual Retention Test (Fig. 7–16) requires a patient to reproduce 10 line drawings of geometrical designs after a brief viewing.[236] It detects impairments of visual memory, perception, and visuoconstruction. The Judgment of Line Orientation Test (Fig. 7–17) probes orientation discrimination for line segments. Visuoconstruction is assessed by drawing and writing to dictation, copying, and spontaneous writing, and by the Block Design subtest of the Wechsler Adult Intelligence Test, Revised (WAIS-R).[237] The Rey-Osterreith Complex Figure Test (CFT) (Fig. 7–18) requires subjects to copy a complex geometric figure and provides another reliable index of visuoconstructional ability.

On the Boston Naming Test (Fig. 7–19) a subject is asked to name line drawings of objects. The Visual Naming subtest of Multilingual Aphasia Exam requires

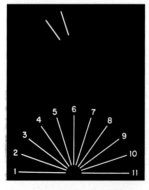

Fig. 7–17. A plate from the Judgment of Line Orientation Test. Line segments 4 and 5 match the orientations of the line segments at the top. (Courtesy of Prof. Arthur Benton)

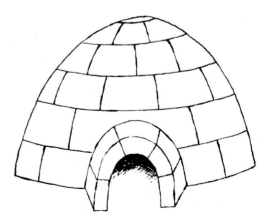

Fig. 7–19. Boston Naming Test. The patient is shown a line drawing of different items. Failure to produce the name can be caused by impairments in the domains of vision or language. (Courtesy of Prof. Harold Goodglass)

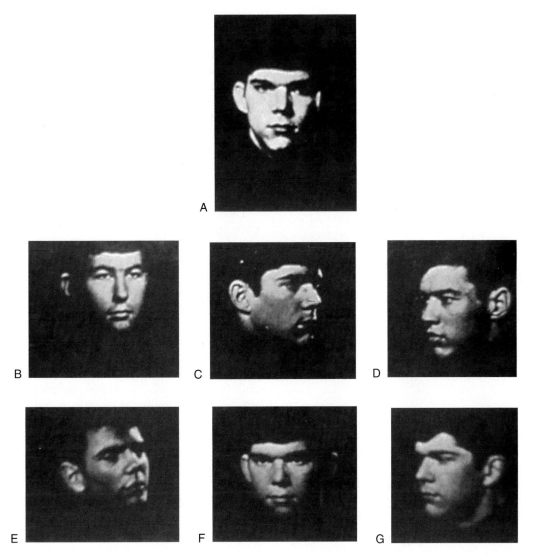

Fig. 7–20. A plate from the Benton Facial Recognition Test. (Courtesy of Prof. Arthur Benton)

the naming of photographs of objects. The Facial Recognition Test (Fig. 7–20) asks patients to select which of several pictures of faces, photographed at different angles and in different lighting conditions, match a target face.[238] As these faces are unfamiliar, this test assesses face perception rather than face recognition. Face recognition can be tested by presenting pictures of presidents, movie stars, and famous athletes.

Reading can be tested using the reading subtest of the Wide Range Achievement Test or the Chapman-Cook Speed of Reading Test (Fig. 7–21). Visual attention can be tested using a line bisection test, line cancellation test, or by having patients comment on the goings on in picture scene, such as the Cookie Theft Picture from the Boston Diagnostic Aphasia Examination.[239] Patients with hemi-neglect or simultanagnosia fail these tests (see below). General intellect is often measured

by a neuropsychologist, using the WAIS-R, and taking age and level of education into account.

The Hooper Visual Organization Test[240] (Fig. 7–22) probes mental imagery by requiring a patient to identify 30 different items (*e.g.,* shoe, fish) from cut-up, rearranged line drawings of the items. Mooney's Closure Faces Test provides information similar to the Hooper test by asking patients to judge age and sex in 44 incom-

> The woman burned herself badly while she was making soup, because she spilled a pan of cold water on herself.

Fig. 7–21. Chapman Speed of Reading Test. The patient is asked to read the sentence and pick out the word that doesn't fit.

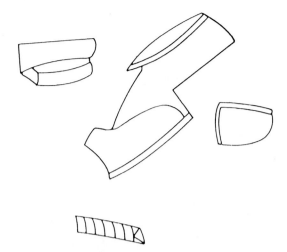

Fig. 7–22. A plate from the Hooper Visual Organization Test. (Courtesy of Western Psychological Services)

plete cartoons of faces.[241–243] Performance on this test is also dependent on memory.

Prosopagnosia

Visual agnosia may affect the identification of all classes of objects, yet there are also restricted forms of agnosia, the most important being prosopagnosia, in which patients no longer recognize the faces of previously familiar persons nor learn newly encountered faces. Because the identification of faces is crucial in daily life, prosopagnosia is a pronounced social handicap, and the patients are usually aware of their difficulty, the exception being cases with childhood onset.[244–246] To identify people, patients with prosopagnosia rely on combinations of alternative cues, including non-facial visual cues such as gait and typical mannerisms, and non-visual cues such as voice and the context in which certain people are encountered (*i.e.*, they recognize hospital staff at the hospital, but not if met on the street).[244,246,247] They are also able to recognize visually some faces that have distinctive local features, such as spectacles, hairstyle, beards, scars, or a chipped tooth. Patients with childhood onset of prosopagnosia can also be shown to rely on similar non-facial cues for identifying people. Prosopagnosic subjects may have normal recognition of other objects[248–251] or a milder visual object agnosia as well.[244,245,252]

Some patients with prosopagnosia appear to possess "covert" knowledge of familiar faces that they can no longer identify or recognize as familiar.[254] This knowledge without awareness has been demonstrated with both physiologic measurements, such as galvanic skin response[255–257] and visual evoked potentials,[251] and psychologic techniques, including the pattern of eye scanning for familiar vs. unfamiliar faces,[249] forced-choice responses for names or occupations belonging to faces,[258] and the speed of learning to pair correct vs. incorrect names with famous faces.[253,258–260] These techniques have been used to show that patients with prosopagnosia have two covert phenomena—a retained sense of which faces are familiar,[249,251,255,258] and retained knowledge of information pertaining to familiar faces, such as names and occupations.[253,256–260] However, not all prosopagnosic patients have covert recognition,[244,245,250,261] and quantitative studies suggest that covert recognition may be impaired when present.[262] No practical benefits of covert recognition are demonstrable.

Despite problems with face recognition, some patients can judge the age, gender, and emotional expression of faces and even lip-read, although alternative perceptual processes or strategies may be required.[252,250,258,259,264,265] For example, one patient relied on wrinkles to tell age, whereas normal subjects can still make age judgments without this clue.[244] Judgments about facial age, sex, emotional expression, and the direction of gaze, which is an important social signal, may also be impaired.[244–246,265]

Prosopagnosia is associated with lesions in the lingual and fusiform gyri, in medial occipito-temporal cortex.[197,266] Occasionally the lesion is in more anterior temporal cortex.[264] In one unusual case with anoxia there was no extrastriate damage; it was presumed that diffuse but specific damage in striate cortex impaired the perception of curvature, which manifest mainly as prosopagnosia.[267]

Both hemispheres process information relevant to facial perception. The idea that prosopagnosia depends on unilateral right hemispheric lesions was (1) weakened by findings of left hemisphere lesions at autopsy in some cases and absence of prosopagnosia with right hemisphere lesions until a subsequent left-sided lesion occurred; and (2) later strengthened by autopsy, CT, and MRI evidence.[247,250,262,268–279] However, bilateral lesions are most often reported in prosopagnosia as confirmed with modern neuro-imaging techniques, and produce more severe deficits.[123,197,248,249,257–259,266,280–282] One testable hypothesis is that apperceptive prosopagnosia occurs with right ventral and dorsal occipito-temporal damage, whereas an associative form occurs with bilateral ventral temporo-occipital lesions.[283] Left-sided lesions in bilateral cases may disconnect visual inputs from the right hemifields to the regions in the right hemisphere that may play the dominant role in facial recognition, with critical import in cases with left hemianopia.[284,285]

The most common causes are posterior cerebral artery infarctions, head trauma, and, to a lesser extent, viral encephalitis.[247,248,252,255–259,260,262,266,273,276,280,285–287] Tumors, hematomas, abscesses, and surgical resections are less frequently reported.[248,250,251,276,287] Impaired facial recognition also occurs with Alzheimer's dementia, or focal temporal lobar atrophy.[264,282,288] It has been reported in some patients with Parkinson's disease.[289] Developmental prosopagnosia has been described.[244–246,290] These rare patients are not aware of their problem but may come to attention because of consequent social difficulties.[246,290] They have abnormal face perception in general, with difficulty judging facial age, sex, and expressions, and slow performance of facial matching tasks.[244–246] In some cases developmental prosopagnosia may be an autosomal dominant trait, or co-exist with the Asperger syndrome of autism.[246]

Because prosopagnosia is most often reported with inferior occipital lesions, it is frequently associated with upper quadrantanopia, either left-sided or bilateral.[249,251,276,286] Right-sided lesions may also be associated with left homonymous hemianopia.[247,248,250,276] Combinations of hemianopia and upper quadrantanopia can occur, too.[248,257] Impaired memory for visual or verbal items is not uncommon, from involvement of medial temporal structures.[248,249,251,252,256,257,259,264,276]

There is also an association with achromatopsia in one or both hemifields.[244,248,249,256,257,259,276,286] Whether achromatopsia itself plays a role in object agnosia has been debated.[8,197] Object forms can be defined by chromatic borders, and inability to perceive shape from color could theoretically impair object identification. However, it has been shown that shape from color can be processed independently of color sensation, and that prosopagnosia can occur without achromatopsia, with bilateral hippocampal lesions sparing ventromedial occipital cortex.[192,241,250–252,264,291,292]

Is prosopagnosia specific for face recognition? Some argue that prosopagnosia is a general inability to identify specific members within large classes of similar items, faces being the most striking example.[123] Consequently, patients may fail to identify objects other than faces. For example, a car may be recognized as a car, yet a patient may fail to identify his or her own car, or cannot distinguish makes of cars, flowers, food, coins, or unique items such as buildings, handwriting, and personal clothing.[244,245,250,252,258,266,270,272] These phenomena may explain why some prosopagnosic patients get lost in familiar surroundings or have trouble learning their way around new surroundings, a problem called topographagnosia.[244,245,248,250,256,264,276] Topographagnosia may also be related to other disturbances that can co-exist with prosopagnosia, such as low vision, dementia, generalized amnesia, and disorders of spatial processing, as in the hemi-neglect syndrome.

Other patients with severe prosopagnosia can distinguish non-facial objects relatively well, including personal belongings, individual animals, specific places, cars, and different eyeglasses.[260,263,264,293,294] Interestingly, in prosopagnosia the discrimination of upside-down faces is relatively better than that of upright faces, suggesting that the disorder may affect a process devoted to perception of normally viewed faces.[294]

Other Disorders of Face Perception

A rare group of patients recognize people long familiar to them, but cannot learn to recognize new faces seen since the onset of their lesion.[255,295] This *anterograde prosopagnosia* occurs with bilateral damage to the amygdala, usually from surgery for epilepsy.[295] There is associated dysnomia, and patients cannot judge facial expressions or the direction of gaze, consistent with hypothesized roles for the amygdala in learning and social behavior.

Some deficits in face perception without prosopagnosia exist. Patients with right hemispheric lesions have trouble matching unfamiliar faces or determining age from faces, suggesting a disorder of face perception.[296,297] A selective defect affecting perception of facial expressions alone was localized to the left hemisphere in one study.[298] In general, these deficits seem asymptomatic and are revealed only with detailed psychological tests.

Acquired Alexia

Acquired alexia is loss of reading ability in previously literate persons. The perception and comprehension of words and letters require complex visual functions, such as pattern and form perception, as well as linguistic analysis of morphology and semantics.[299,300] To read sentences and paragraphs requires not only linguistic semantic and syntactical processing but also the deployment of basic visuospatial processes to scan lines of text, including shifts of attention and visual search with saccades. Not surprisingly, a wide variety of anatomic lesions and functional disturbances can impair reading.

Pure Alexia (Alexia without Agraphia)

Patients with pure alexia can write, but dramatically some cannot read what they have just written despite good visual acuity and oral and auditory language skills. There is a spectrum of severity. At the extreme end (global alexia), patients cannot read even numbers, letters, and other symbols, let alone words.[301] With a less pronounced deficit, patients have mildly slow reading with occasional errors, diagnosable only by comparison of reading speed with normal controls matched for educational level.[302] These patients read by deciphering words one letter at a time (letter-by-letter reading, or spelling dyslexia). The characteristic hallmark of letter-by-letter reading is that the time needed to read a word increases with the number of letters in the word.[303,304] In Japanese, which has one phonetically based writing system (kana) and another non-phonetic, ideographic one (kanji), alexia causes impaired reading of kanji but not of kana, presumably representing an equivalent of preserved letter-by-letter reading.[305]

As with prosopagnosia, studies suggest covert processing in pure alexia. Some patients can indicate whether a string of letters form a word or not, an ability that is more rapid than the laborious letter-by-letter approach they require to recognize words.[300,304,306,307] Other patients can point to words that they cannot read aloud, or identify letters more quickly when they are embedded in real words than in random letter strings.[303,308] Some patients also show covert understanding of word meaning, by categorizing words semantically (animals, plants), or matching words to objects.[304,306,309,310] Whether these demonstrations of comprehension constitute unconscious abilities or true dissociations has been challenged.[300,310] Also, as with prosopagnosia, not all patients with pure alexia show covert processing.[299,311]

Pure alexia is frequently associated with a right homonymous hemianopia or sometimes a superior quadrantanopia, which may be accompanied by hemi-achromatopsia.[312] Other associated defects include color anomia, even for items in the left hemifield; anomia for visual objects and photographs; defects of verbal memory; and other types of visual agnosia, including prosopagnosia.[125,312,313] Anomia may extend beyond visual objects, indicating an additional language disturbance.[313] A disconnection optic ataxia may occur, in which the right hand has difficulty reaching for objects in the left visual field.[312]

Almost all lesions causing pure alexia are in the left hemisphere. Most are located in the medial and inferior occipito-temporal region.[301,312] The most frequent cause is left posterior cerebral artery ischemia, but other causes include primary and metastatic tumors, arteriovenous malformations, hemorrhage, herpes simplex encephalitis, and a rare focal posterior cortical dementia.[89,300,314–319]

Classically, pure alexia is considered a "disconnection" syndrome, in which visual input from both hemifields is disconnected from language areas in the left hemisphere.[320,321] Most commonly, a left occipital lesion produces a complete right hemianopia. Anterior extension of this lesion into the splenium, forceps major, or periventricular white matter surrounding the occipital horn of the lateral ventricle interrupts callosal fibers from the right occipital lobe (i.e., left visual field information).[312] The left angular gyrus is isolated from visual input, leading to alexia and also the associated anomia for colors and sometimes objects. Support for the disconnection hypothesis derives from anatomically atypical cases, in which pure alexia results from a combination of a splenial lesion and a right hemianopia from non-occipital lesions, such as left geniculate infarction.[322,323]

Focal lesions of the left occipital white matter underlying the angular gyrus can also cause alexia, even without right hemianopia.[314,317,318,324] These subangular lesions presumably also disconnect visual input from both hemispheres to the left angular gyrus. It seems likely that the callosal fibers from the right hemisphere travel ventral to the occipital horn, though others speculate that survival of some fibers traveling dorsal to the horn may mediate the remnant letter-by-letter reading ability in patients with spelling dyslexia.[301,314,317]

Aside from the disconnectionist concept, it is argued that pure alexia may represent a type of agnosia. A perceptual defect similar to simultanagnosia has been debated.[311,325] Others have proposed that it is an associative agnosia.[311,326] The word-length effect, the letter-by-letter strategy required to read, and greater difficulties with handwritten script and briefly shown words have pointed to an inability to grasp words as a whole, and others have shown that pure alexia can be associated with problems with processing local features in texture perception.[311,327] Thus, as with prosopagnosia, pure alexia may represent the most prominent impairment of a more generalized perceptual defect, and the two may reveal lateralized differences in processing styles of the two occipito-temporal lobes.[327]

Pure (acquired) alexia must be distinguished from developmental dyslexia (often referred to simply as dyslexia), which probably has different mechanisms. Dyslexics never learn to read at a level commensurate with social and intellectual expectations because of reduced speed and efficiency of reading, transposition of letters, and other subtle difficulties. Their deficit is much less severe than the usual impairments of acquired pure alexia. The origins of developmental dyslexia remain unclear. For example, it has been attributed to impaired scanning eye movements, or to temporal processing difficulties in the nervous system, possibly related to a paucity of cells in the magnocellular layers of the dorsal LGN.[328]

Hemialexias

The disconnection hypothesis for pure alexia actually requires two disconnections of the left angular gyrus, one for each hemifield.[320,321] Each has also been described in isolation. In *left hemi-alexia*, reading is impaired in the left hemifield only, because of isolated damage to the splenium or the callosal fibers elsewhere.[89,329] *Right hemi-alexia* has been reported with a lesion of the left medial and ventral occipital lobe.[330] *Left hemiparalexia* is a rare syndrome reported with splenial damage after surgery for arteriovenous malformations.[331] Patients make substitution and omission errors for the first letter of words, much like neglect dyslexia (see below), but they do not have hemi-neglect, and have left-sided lesions with right hemianopia rather than the converse.

Alexia with Agraphia

In some patients both reading and writing are impaired but oral and auditory language is preserved.

Alexia with agraphia is associated with lesions of the left angular gyrus or sometimes the adjacent temporo-parietal junction.[320,331a,332,333] Little is known about this rare disorder. It may be accompanied by acalculia, right-left disorientation, and finger agnosia, the other elements of Gerstmann's syndrome.

Patients with Broca's aphasia from left frontal lesions have trouble with all expressive language output, and therefore also with reading aloud and writing. However, some also have marked difficulty understanding written material, in contrast to relatively preserved comprehension of spoken language.[334,335] These patients are better at occasionally grasping a whole word, while unable to name its constituent letters, hence the name *literal alexia* or letter blindness. These patients also have impaired comprehension of syntax in written or spoken language, similar to the agrammatism of their verbal output.

Secondary Alexia

Visual Loss and Reading

Bilateral loss of visual acuity will create obvious loss of reading ability and is not likely to be overlooked on ophthalmologic examination. However, visual field defects that do not affect central acuity can impair reading, too. Complete bitemporal hemianopia can cause *hemifield slide*, in which the absence of overlapping regions of binocular visual field leads to loss of binocular alignment.[336] Fusion is momentarily defective, causing episodic horizontal and vertical tropias, with transient duplication or disappearance of objects or with a vertical step in horizontal lines. Thus, letters or lines may double or disappear, but without apparent eye movement abnormalities, a non-paretic form of diplopia (see Chapter 6).

Homonymous visual field defects such as hemianopia or paracentral scotomata commonly lead to *hemianopic dyslexia* when the defect involves parafoveal vision. Patients with left hemianopia have difficulty finding the beginning of the next line (in languages written left to right), since the left margin disappears into the field defect as they scan rightward.[337] Marking their place with an L-shaped ruler helps unless there is left hemi-neglect also. Right hemianopia prolongs reading times, with prolonged fixations and reduced amplitude of reading saccades to the right.[337] Otherwise, neurologically intact individuals may turn text material 90°, with the left margin upward, and comfortably read vertically.

Attention and Reading

Left hemi-neglect, without an actual hemianopic defect, is a common neurologic syndrome, classically, but not always due to right parietal lobe lesions. Hemi-neglect for the left side of space is reflected in left-sided reading errors, known as *neglect dyslexia*.[338]

Patients omit reading the left side of lines or pages; with words, they make omissions ("bright" read as "right"), additions ("right" read as "bright") or substitutions ("right" read as "light"). Vertically printed text is not affected.[338] The impairment represents a combination of both a space-centered deficit, in which text on the left side of space is ignored, and an object-centered deficit, in which the left side of words is ignored, even if the words are on the right side of space. Neglect dyslexia is usually associated with other signs of left hemi-neglect, but it can rarely occur as an isolated manifestation.[339]

An *attentional dyslexia* has been described in which the perception of single items is adequate, but perception of several objects simultaneously is impaired.[340,341] These patients identify single words normally but not several words together, and identify single letters but cannot name the letters in a written word. When reading they make literal migration errors, in which a letter from one word is substituted into another word ("poor baby" read as "boor baby"). Letters are mistaken for others that look similar (o and c).[341] This dyslexia has been reported with lesions in the left parietal lobe or temporo-occipital junction.[340,341]

Eye Movements and Reading

Abnormal fixation and saccades may impair reading. Most unilateral cortical lesions cause subtle saccadic abnormalities and do not impair reading, but the acquired ocular motor apraxia from bilateral frontal or parietal lesions can impair reading severely.[342–345] In biparietal cases this may reflect simultanagnosia as much as the saccadic dysfunction. Brainstem or subcortical lesions may cause more severe saccadic and fixation abnormalities; reading difficulty with progressive supranuclear palsy has been attributed to square wave jerks disrupting fixation, and hypometric and slow saccades impairing scanning, but paresis of downward gaze also makes reading material inaccessible.[346]

Central Dyslexias

More subtle acquired dyslexic deficits have been described recently, and referred to as central dyslexias, as they reflect impaired central reading processes rather than attention or vision. Central dyslexias are formulated in terms of parallel processing channels in reading models from cognitive neuropsychology.[302] After letters are identified visually, there are at least two distinct means of processing, a direct phonologic route, in which generic pronunciation rules are used to convert a string of letters into sound, and an indirect lexical route, in which the whole word is perceived and identified in an internal dictionary of written words, which then generates the pronunciation of the word. Patients with *surface dyslexia* have lost the indirect route, and so are not able to pronounce correctly irregular words like "yacht" and "colonel."[346–349] Patients with *phonologic dyslexia* have lost the direct route, and so are not able to reasonably guess at the pronunciation of pseudo-words or words they have not seen before.[350–353] *Deep dyslexia* resembles phonologic dyslexia, but patients characteristically substitute words with a similar meaning for the correct one ("boat" read as "ship").[354]

Assessment of Reading

Tests of basic visual function are important, as always. However, the use of number or letter plates in testing spatial resolution or color vision must be minimized with alexic patients. Confusion can be avoided by use of simplified test forms such as the directional "E"'s of the Snellen Chart, or the tracing of paths or letters on pseudo-isochromatic plates.

Reading aloud and reading for comprehension can be assessed informally in the clinic with any available material, such as a magazine. Premorbid intellect must always be considered in determinations of alexia, and reading skills vary widely. Poor reading ability must also be referenced to other linguistic skills; more extensive dysphasia is associated with alexia, too. If the patient has also lost comprehension of spoken language, and cannot perform verbal commands from the examiner, this indicates aphasia rather than pure alexia. Writing must be tested, by having patients write a sentence to dictation and spontaneously. Overlearned segments like a signature are not an adequate test of writing. If there is difficulty in writing that is not explained by associated weakness or incoordination, the diagnosis is a more pervasive language disturbance, such as alexia with agraphia (see below).

Standard testing can help exclude aphasia [*e.g.*, Boston Diagnostic Aphasia Examination (BDAE) or Multilingual Aphasia Examination]. There are also standardized assessments of reading. The Chapman-Cook Speed of Reading Test (Fig. 7–21) requires the reading of brief paragraphs. The subject must cross out the word that spoils the meaning of the paragraph. The Wide Range Achievement (Wilmington, DE) requires reading aloud of words of increasing difficulty until the subject makes a string of errors.

Evaluation of alexia should include a reading comprehension test that does not require a verbal response (*e.g.*, BDAE Reading Sentences and Paragraphs with a pointing response), so that impaired verbal output is not confused with defective reading comprehension. Mutism doesn't mean alexia, and conversely, reading aloud does not mean comprehension, as with some patients with Alzheimer's disease. Analysis of the pattern of reading errors can be useful. The word-length effect will point to a letter-by-letter reading strategy in spelling dyslexia. Errors restricted to the left side of text or

words suggest neglect dyslexia. More specific semantic substitutions or phonologic mistakes are characteristic of the central dyslexias.[302]

DISORDERS OF THE OCCIPITO-PARIETAL PATHWAY

Bálint's Syndrome and Related Processing Deficits

Bálint[342] described a man with defects of visuospatial perception and eye-hand coordination, which he conceptualized as a triad of problems, and which Hécaen and de Ajuriaguerra[355] eventually labeled as Bálint's syndrome:

1. *Spatial disorder of attention:* the inability to perceive more than one or a few objects at a time.[255,342] Despite adequate acuity and visual fields, Bálint found constriction of the attentive field (his description would now be recognized as that of left hemi-neglect). This has been equated with *simultanagnosia*, the inability to interpret a whole scene despite preserved ability to apprehend individual parts.[356] Patients with simultanagnosia may not recognize objects and faces because of this perceptual impairment. Hence, it could be considered a type of apperceptive agnosia, though it is quite dissimilar to the usual use of agnosia in its associative sense of percepts stripped of meaning.[257,325,357] Another related term is *visual disorientation*.[358] Holmes[358] reported soldiers with occipital wounds who had trouble localizing the spatial position and distance of visual objects in their remaining visual field despite reasonable acuity and stereoacuity. Such patients have trouble counting objects, walking around obstacles, touching objects in central or peripheral vision with the hands, fixating stationary and moving objects, and scanning the environment with the eyes.[358,359]

2. *Optic ataxia:* defective hand movements under visual guidance (especially with the right hand) despite normal limb strength.[360] Bálint also discounted the effects of defective position sense (as in tabetic ataxia), because when he positioned a patient's left hand, the patient could imitate it with the right. The defect was not purely visual because, if it were, it should have equally affected both hands.

3. *Psychic paralysis of gaze:* difficulty initiating saccades to visual targets despite normal range of reflexive eye movements, including vestibulo-ocular responses and saccades to noises or suddenly appearing stimuli objects.[355,361] The gaze disorder has been considered by some to be secondary to the problem with spatial vision.[342,360] A related term is *acquired ocular motor apraxia*[361]: patients have a full range of randomly performed saccades but cannot execute saccades to command or to shift gaze between objects. Other eye movement abnormalities may be found also. *Spasm*

of fixation may contribute to the gaze difficulty; this has been defined as impaired saccadic initiation in the presence of a fixation target, but normal initiation without one.[355,361–363] Measures of latency with eye movement recordings are required to document this. Also described in some patients are gross *inaccuracies in saccadic targeting,* leading to wandering eye movements in search of targets, and difficulty maintaining fixation once targets are fixated. Impaired visual targeting of saccades has been described with bilateral damage to the inferior parietal lobules.[344,358,360]

Bálint's patient had bilateral lesions of the angular gyri, (though there was damage to other visual structures, including the corpus callosum, white matter, and pulvinar).[342] Holmes[343] deduced similar bilateral lesions of the dorsolateral cortex, likely angular gyri, from autopsy and missile trajectories in living patients. The patients of Hécaen and Ajuriaguerra[355] contribute little to localization, as they had large lesions, some affecting both frontal and parietal cortex bilaterally.

The explanations of Bálint's syndrome have been and remain varied. Holmes[343] invoked a combination of defects in spatial localization, attention to objects in the periphery, visual fixation, and visual search. He concluded that the angular gyri performed an integrative function for visual impressions from the retina and tactile and muscular sensations from the body. Hécaen and Ajuriaguerra[355] attributed sluggish visual search to "sticky fixation" and the emergence of a primitive grasp reflex of the eyes with damage in posterior parieto-occipital areas. Bifrontal involvement might cause defective search of visual information, which they termed a "bilateral pseudohemianopsia." Luria[359] felt his patient could perceive a unified structure but not an array of unrelated elements. He invoked Pavlov's theory of cortical activity in which weak cortical tonus caused each focus of excitation within visual cortex to inhibit the remainder of the visual cortex by negative induction. Limitation of visual attention, inability to combine details into a coherent whole, and piecemeal perception, were psychological consequences of this basic neurophysiologic deficit.

The validity and utility of Bálint's syndrome can be questioned.[8] Many reports of Bálint's syndrome are confounded by failure to exclude disorders of anterior visual pathways, to assess basic visual functions other than acuity, and to adequately test the visual fields. The following arguments have also been made against the concept of Bálint's syndrome:

First, Bálint's syndrome may not be a sufficiently autonomous entity. Many affected patients have additional behavioral deficits.[355] For example, elements of hemineglect lie at the core of Bálint's case and on their own could account for defective ocular search, "extinction" of objects when multiple stimuli are presented, and defective hand reaching under visual guidance.[364] On the other hand, the triad of defects are not closely bound.[355] Simultanagnosia and optic ataxia are doubly dissociable, for example. Ocular motor apraxia has been blamed on simultanagnosia but others note that some patients with ocular motor apraxia cannot make saccades to their own body parts, indicating more than just visuospatial disturbance.[343,360] Also, patients with simultanagnosia can have normal saccadic behavior.[349] Rather, each element may actually represent broad categories comprising more specific defects.[343] Simultanagnosia probably represents a combination of visual field defects and impaired attention, both of which could combine with altered spatial representations to generate optic ataxia also.

Second, the correlation between angular gyrus lesions and Bálint's syndrome is imperfect. Angular gyrus pathology can cause other deficits not included in Bálint's triad, such as hemi-neglect with right-sided lesions, aphasia and Gerstmann's syndrome with left-sided lesions, and profound defects of visual motion perception with bilateral lesions.[5,365–367] Furthermore, features of Bálint's syndrome have been reported with bifrontal and pulvinar lesions.[368,369] Simultanagnosia has been reported with lesions of the dorsal occipital lobes in Brodmann's areas 18 and 19.[249,370] Lesions of the frontal eye fields (Brodmann's areas 6 and 8) may impair voluntary saccades and ocular search, as in acquired ocular apraxia. Impaired reaching under visual guidance is associated with lesions of a wide range of areas, including Brodmann's areas 5, 7, 19, 37, 39 and cortex inferomedial to the angular gyri.[371]

Third, the theoretical foundations of Bálint's syndrome are weak. Explanations of primitive grasp reflexes or weak cortical tonus are untestable. Bálint's explanation is also weak.[355,359] His patient could neither draw a dot in the center of a circle nor perceive the error on visual inspection, suggesting that he could see either the circle or dot but not both at once. Yet, the man could identify a large object such as a person by sight alone, from which Bálint proposed an ability to see only one single object wholly at a time, no matter what size. However, we require only a few features to identify persons and objects, as can be demonstrated with degraded representations such as caricatures, silhouettes, or partial glimpses; thus, recognition never proves perception of the whole object at once.

Cases such as Bálint's are unlikely to represent the behavioral expression of a single mechanism. A compilation of two dozen cases of simultanagnosia or Bálint's syndrome indicates a diversity of assessments, deficits, lesions, and opinions, with no consensus.[372] Such cases are best understood by the precise definition of each component deficit, with anatomic correlation by modern neuroimaging.

Patients suspected to have elements of Bálint's syndrome should first be assessed with valid and reliable tests of basic visual and cognitive function. It is especially important to consider the impact of attention. Bálint's patient failed to detect objects in the periphery (more so on the left) due to constriction of the attention, the ability to focus on one of several simultaneous stimuli and withdraw from distracters.[373] The patient's visual fields were easily fatiguable, resembling effects of fatigue in normal observers in vigilance or sustained attention tasks requiring prolonged monitoring of visual displays except the effects in Bálint's patient were pathologic and did not require prolonged effort.[374–376]

Simultanagnosia can be defined operationally as an inability to report all the items and relationships in a complex visual display, despite unrestricted head and eye movements. A suitable screening tool is a picture with a balance of information in all quadrants, such as the Cookie Theft Picture from the Boston Diagnostic Aphasia Examination.[239] The patient's report can be correlated with a checklist of the items in the picture. Interpretation of a poor performance should take into account any co-existent aphasia or visual field defect. With central or paracentral scotoma, objects may seem to vanish, mimicking simultanagnosia. More extensive peripheral scotomata, or "keyhole vision," may hinder visual search and make simultaneous perception impossible.[359]

To assess optic ataxia, the examiner must again first know the visual field of the patients and ensure that they see visual targets before trying to reach them.[194] Inaccurate reaches into a hemianopic field are expected, and are not evidence of optic ataxia. The examiner presents highly visible targets such as color tokens at different distances and locations within arm's reach of the patients. The patients' head and eye movements are not restricted. They are asked to touch or grasp the target. Each hand is tested separately; the problem tends to be worse for reaches initiated with the hand and hemispace opposite the side of the lesion. In optic ataxia, patients should be accurate in reaching for parts of their own bodies, because such targets are defined by kinesthetic coordinates rather than visual coordinates. However, some patients with parietal damage may have trouble with reaching for either visual or kinesthetic targets, because of more diffuse disturbances in spatial representation.[343] Optic ataxia is differentiated from cerebellar dysmetria by its selectivity for visual targets and the lack of intention tremor or dysdiadocokinesia. Quantitative assessment of reaching, pointing, and grasping can be performed with special instrumentation (Fig. 7–23), showing increased latency of initiation, abnormal hand trajectories, increased end-point variability, tendency to reach to one side, and dissociations of distance and direction control.

Acquired ocular motor apraxia can be tested clinically

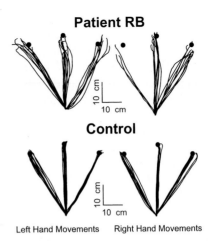

Fig. 7–23. Abnormal hand paths in a subject with damage to the visual cortex. The subject is viewed from above as he moves the head from a start position directly in front of him in the midline to targets located within arm's length to the left, right, and straight ahead. Note the inaccuracy of movements with both hands (errors in excess of 5 cm) and movement curvature. Individuals without brain lesions make such movements in almost a straight line and nearly every movement terminates on target.

by having the subject make saccades to targets on command, and contrasting the difficulty experienced on this task with the relative ease of making reflexive saccades to suddenly appearing targets in the natural environment, such as a person walking by in the hall. Inaccurate saccadic search can be observed with simple targets in the clinic, with the same caveats as for simultanagnosia regarding foreknowledge of the visual fields. The diagnosis of spasm of fixation requires more formal measurements of latency with eye movement recordings.

Cerebral Akinetopsia

Akinetopsia is an acquired defect of motion perception caused by acquired cerebral lesions. As visual motion serves many purposes, a variety of deficits can result, including defective smooth pursuit or optokinetic eye movements, impaired reaching for moving objects, and trouble perceiving objects that are distinguished from the background scene by virtue of their movement (structure-from-motion or kinetic depth).[377]

A small region in the lateral visual association cortex in monkey is important for visual motion perception. The middle temporal (MT) and medial superior temporal (MST) areas (Fig. 7–24) occupy the floor and walls of the superior temporal sulcus.[378,379] Many of their neurons are sensitive to the direction and velocity of visual images.[380,381] Lesions of MT in monkeys produce a relatively selective deficit for motion perception in the contralateral visual hemifield, which recovers within a few weeks, to a degree dependent on the size of the lesion.[382–384] The human brain likely follows a similar

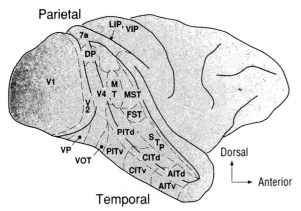

Fig. 7–24. Phylogeny of the middle temporal (MT) area is shown from lower primates (shrew) to higher primates (macaque monkey). Humans are also thought to possess an area MT. MT receives strong projections from the subcortical M pathway. Damage to this area impairs motion perception in primates and in humans is thought to result in cerebral akinetopsia, as in patient LM (see text). (From ref. 377a)

organization, and motion deficits in a few well-documented human cases are comparable to those in the monkey, except that the perceptual deficits in humans appear to last much longer, probably because human lesions are much larger, involving multiple functional regions in cortex as well as white matter tracts.[367,385,386]

Motion-blind patient L.M. is a landmark case, and has been studied extensively over two decades.[5,168,387,388] A.F. is another well-studied patient.[367] L.M. had no impression of motion in depth or of rapid motion, with fast targets appearing to jump rather than move.[5,385] On testing, L.M. perceived global coherent (first-order) motion, but her predictions of target trajectories were impaired at faster speeds, as was smooth pursuit, though her eyes could pursue a moving tactile target.[5] Her contrast sensitivity for detection of moving gratings was only mildly affected, but her perception of differences in temporal frequency or speed of gratings was impaired.[168] She could discriminate direction of movement in random dot cinematograms (RDC), but this failed with small amounts of background visual noise.[7,387] Similarly, L.M. could perceive two-dimensional (2-D) shape-from-motion and three-dimensional (3-D) structure-from-motion, but not with moderate levels of moving and stationary noise.[7]

Both A.F. and L.M. had other perceptual deficits. A.F. had a left partial hemianopia with some sparing superiorly. He had difficulties in object recognition; in tests of spatial vision such as hyperacuity, line orientation, line bisection, and spatial location; and in tests of stereopsis.[326] L.M. also has trouble perceiving 2-D shapes defined by non-motion signals including "on" and "off" transients, dynamic and static binocular disparity, and static texture cues.[7]

Both A.F. and L.M. had bilateral lesions of the lateral temporo-parieto-occipital junctions, which included significant adjacent regions and underlying white matter.[326,367,385] Nevertheless, the dorsolateral locations coincide approximately with the data from functional neuroimaging studies for a human motion processing region.[389–391] (Fig. 7–25).

Unilateral lesions of lateral occipito-temporal cortex or inferior parietal lobule cause more subtle and generally asymptomatic abnormalities of motion perception. These may result in hemi-akinetopsia, which is contralateral hemifield defects for speed discrimination, in detecting boundaries between regions with different motion, and in discriminating motion direction of complex stimuli or with background noise.[386,392–394] However, more elementary motion perceptual measures tend to be normal, such as motion detection and contrast thresholds for motion direction.[386,392] Hemi-akinetopsia may be obscured by co-existent hemianopia.

Unilateral lesions can also impair motion perception in the central visual field. Defects in identifying letters or shapes defined from the background by motion cues alone have been described.[395,396] Impaired direction discrimination is found with similar lateral occipito-temporal lesions.[394,397] Whether there is a difference between the right and left hemispheres is debated.[155,395,396] Impaired motion perception has also been found with lesions in the parietal insula and midline cerebellum, consistent with functional imaging that shows visual motion activates many areas of the brain.[398–400]

Taken together, these studies suggest that lesions of human lateral occipito-temporal cortex impair a variety of complex motion tasks, including discriminating speed, integrating motion over a video display to discern average direction and three-dimensional structure, and separating regions with different motion to discern two-dimensional structure. Elementary spatial and temporal aspects of motion perception are preserved. Furthermore, lesions elsewhere may also impair aspects of motion perception,[399] and yet other aspects of spatial analysis and object recognition may be impaired by lateral occipito-temporal lesions, as in L.M. and A.F.[7,326]

Finally, defective motion perception is also reported in Alzheimer's disease including structure-from-motion.[401–404] However, there is debate on the selectivity of motion processing deficits in Alzheimer's disease, their relationship to the stage of dementia, and where the deficit originates, ranging from the retina to visual association cortex.[403,405–408]

At present there are few clinical tests of motion perception. One way to assess motion processing deficits indirectly is by observing smooth pursuit or optokinetic eye movements, although these can be abnormal in the absence of a perceptual deficit.[155] Better testing of motion perception requires computerized stimuli that minimize clues to motion from the changes in position of a stimulus. RDCs (Fig. 7–26) present a motion signal amid

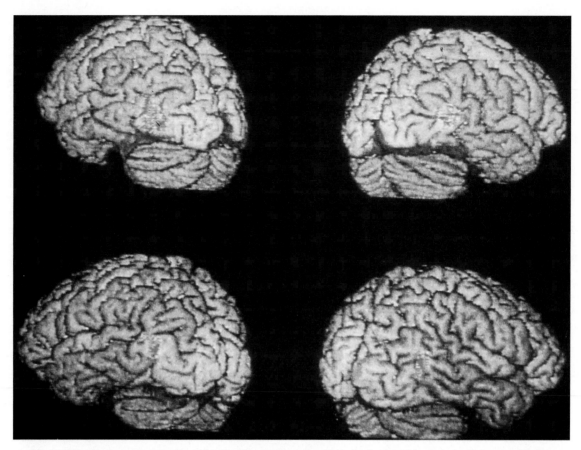

Fig. 7–25. Regional localization of activation on the lateral hemispheres of human participants viewing moving stimuli is shown. These areas are thought to contain a human area MT homologue. These areas were damaged in akinetopsia patient L.M. and are also damaged in patients with Bàlint syndrome. (From ref. 389)

spatially random background noise and allow control of spatial displacement, temporal intervals, and exposure durations. They can be designed to test a variety of motion perceptual experiences, but as yet have not attained clinical usefulness.

POSITIVE VISUAL PHENOMENA

Most often cerebral lesions affect vision by creating deficits, or negative phenomena. On occasion, they may also create positive phenomena, when false visual images are seen by the patient. These false visual images can be classified as visual perseverations, hallucinations, and distortions (dysmetropsia).

Visual Perseveration

The persistence, recurrence, or duplication of a visual image is a rare complaint in patients with cerebral lesions. Varieties include palinopsia, polyopia, and illusory visual spread. Palinopsia is the perseveration of a visual image in time.[409] Whereas visual hallucinations often consist of novel images or sometimes those from the distant past (experiential hallucinations), the palinopic vision contains elements of a more recently viewed scene, or even one that is still being viewed. Nevertheless, the difference is not always distinct and patients can have both perseverations and hallucinations.[409,410] Cerebral diplopia or polyopia is the perseveration of a visual image in space, when two or more copies of a seen object are perceived simultaneously.[411–414] In illusory visual spread, the contents or surface appearance of an object exceed the spatial boundaries of the object.[409] Thus wallpaper patterns creep beyond the surface of the wall, and cloth patterns spread from a shirt to the wearer's face.[409]

Both spatial and temporal perseveration can occur in the same patient, as in palinopic polyopia.[412,415] Some patients see multiple copies of the object in the trail of a moving object: Is this cerebral polyopia, palinopsia, or both? As yet another possible combination, Bender et al[410] argued that since palinopic images were often larger than the original images in his experience, this represented associated illusory visual spread; however, Critchley[409] thought that this combination was the exception rather than the rule.

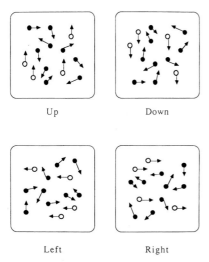

Up Down

Left Right

Fig. 7–26. Random dot cinematograms (RDCs). Testing motion perception demands stimuli that minimize inferences of movement from noticeable changes in the visual scene, the way we "see" movement of moon or stars. Suitable stimuli are computer-generated animation sequences known as RDCs. RDCs present a motion signal (*open circles*) moving in a consistent direction (*e.g.,* up, down, right, left) amid spatially random background noise (*closed circles*). By varying the ratio of signal to noise it is possible to quantify motion perception ability in patients with cerebral or retinal disorders.

Palinopsia

It is suggested that there are at least two forms of abnormal persistence of a visual image in time—an immediate and a delayed type. With the immediate type of palinopsia, an image persists after the disappearance of the actual scene, usually fading after a period of several minutes. This resembles the normal afterimage experienced after prolonged viewing of a bright object. Detailed studies of some patients have concluded that the differences between normal afterimages and such palinopic images are primarily quantitative,[415] though others disagree.[410] With the delayed type of palinopsia, an image of a previously seen object reappears after an interval of minutes to hours, sometimes repeatedly for days or even weeks.[415] Some patients have both immediate and delayed types of palinopsia.[415]

The perseverated image can occupy any location in the visual field. It may be at the same retinal location as the original image (usually the fovea) and thus move as the eyes move, much like a normal afterimage.[416] It may be translocated into a co-existent visual field defect,[409] and indeed can be a transient feature in the evolution of cerebral homonymous field defects.[409,410] At times the image is multiplied across otherwise intact visual fields.[412] On rare occasions, the location of palinopic images is contextually specific, as when the face of a television personality reappears on the faces of other people in the room, or that one shop's sign reappears over other shops.[409,412,417] While some of these cases

may be a complex form of palinopic polyopia, others may represent a constant foveal or parafoveal perseverative image that manifests itself repeatedly when the context is appropriate.

The pathophysiology of palinopsia is still unclear. Four main hypotheses have been advanced.[411] First, the immediate type of palinopsia may be an exaggeration of the normal afterimage.[415] The vividness of the palinopic image correlates with the intensity and duration of the initial stimulus, and appears as a negative (complementary color) afterimage when visualized against a light background. The palinopic image appears binocularly after monocular viewing of an object, and moves in the same direction as active eye movements but in the opposite direction when the eyes are moved passively. However, not all cases of immediate palinopsia exhibit these features; others argue that the color of palinopic images does not depend strongly on that of the original stimulus.[157,411]

Second, there is circumstantial evidence that palinopsia is an ictal manifestation. Early reports mentioned other features such as episodic loss of consciousness, tongue biting, and confusion.[409,410] More recently, epileptiform abnormalities on EEG and a good response to anti-convulsants have been reported with the immediate type of palinopsia,[418–420] and in one case with the delayed form.[418–420]

Third, palinopsia may be a non-ictal hallucinatory state.[57] Some patients have both palinopsia and co-existent non-palinopic visual hallucinations. The location of some perseverated images within visual field defects is reminiscent of release hallucinations. Drugs that induce hallucinations can cause palinopsia.[415] Cummings et al[416] suggested that delayed palinopsia with hemianopia was a release hallucination, whereas immediate palinopsia was more likely a seizure, especially in the absence of a visual field defect. This distinction requires validation.

Last, palinopsia may be psychogenic, possibly a confabulatory response to other visual dysfunction.[409] Palinopsia may occur without visual dysfunction in a psychiatric context, sometimes with other perseverative and misidentification delusions like Capgras syndrome (the belief that familiar people have been replaced by duplicates).[421]

A wide range of other symptoms can accompany palinopsia. An associated homonymous visual field defect is virtually always present, with reports of both upper and lower quadrantanopias.[276,415,417] There may be other spatial illusions of metamorphopsia, macropsia, or micropsia.[409,410,415,419] Less frequently, ventral stream deficits have been reported, such as topographagnosia, prosopagnosia, and achromatopsia.[276,410] Cummings et al[416] reported an unusual patient with perseveration in both visual and somatosensory modalities.

The differential diagnosis of palinopsia (Table 7–4) includes toxins, including both illicit hallucinogens,

TABLE 7–4. Causes of Palinopsia

Toxicity
  Illicit hallucinogens
    Mescaline, lysergic acid diethylamide, Ecstasy
  Prescription drugs
    Clomiphene
    Interleukin-2
    Trazodone
Metabolic conditions
  Non-ketotic hyperglycemia
Psychiatric conditions
  Schizophrenia
  Psychotic depression
Structural cerebral lesions

which can cause permanent palinopsia and prescribed medications, the metabolic disorder of non-ketotic hyperglycemia, and psychiatric conditions, where it is always accompanied by other signs of mental illness.[319,421–428] Once these are excluded, visual perseveration virtually always indicates a cerebral lesion. The one purported exception is a patient with bilateral optic neuritis and immediate palinopsia; however, this patient had prior brainstem symptoms, pointing to a diagnosis of multiple sclerosis, and so co-existent cerebral hemispheric lesions could not be excluded.[429]

The cerebral localizing value of palinopsia is uncertain. Right, left, and bilateral lesions are all reported, as are parieto-occipital, medial occipital, and occipito-temporal lesions.[409,410,412,417,430,431] In two cases, no lesion was found with imaging though one patient proved to have Creutzfeld-Jakob disease.[157,432]

The prognosis for palinopsia varies. Bender et al[410] considered palinopsia to be a rare transient phase in either the resolution or progression of a visual field defect, lasting days to months. Other cases of palinopsia have persisted for months to years.[157,415,416,418] Anti-convulsant medication may help some patients but not others.[416,418]

Cerebral Polyopia

Cerebral polyopia is less frequent than palinopsia. Rarely, it may occur only in certain gaze positions,[411] mimicking diplopia from ocular misalignment; however, it is not eliminated by closing one eye.[411] As a cause of *monocular diplopia or polyopia* (*i.e.*, polyopia persisting with one eye occluded), it must be distinguished from refractive abnormalities such as cataract.[433–435] However, unlike refractive polyopia, it does not resolve with viewing through a pinhole and is present with either eye viewing alone (*i.e.*, a *bilateral* monocular polyopia). The number of images reported can range to over a hundred.[414] Associated signs include visual field defects, difficulties with visually guided reaching, achromatopsia, and object agnosia,[411] but cerebral polyopia can be an isolated feature or accompanied by only a minimal field defect.[411,413,414]

Among Bender's[411] wartime cases, cerebral polyopia was usually a transient phase in the recovery of cortical blindness due to occipital missile wounds. In two cases recovery followed a progression from cortical blindness to cerebral polyopia, then cerebral diplopia. Other causes include encephalitis, multiple sclerosis, and tumors.[411]

The origins of this rare symptom are obscure. Bender[411] suggested an analogy with the monocular diplopia of strabismic patients with both a true and a false macula, in that unstable fixation causes the retinal image to shift over falsely localizing regions.[411] In support, Gottlieb noted a correlation of polyopia with eye movements into the hemianopic field, but both Meadows and Lopez have contested the need for abnormal fixation or eye movements.[413,414,436]

Visual Hallucinations

Hallucinations are perceptions without external stimulation of the relevant sensory organ. They are common in patients with dementia or confusional states.[437] They occur transiently with post-operative delirium, including after cataract surgery.[438] Drug reactions are particularly important (Table 7–5). Besides hallucinogenic street drugs such as cocaine, LSD, and marijuana, one must also consider many clinical agents, including bupropion, baclofen withdrawal, digoxin, gancyclovir, and vincristine, for example.[439–443] They are the predominant type of hallucination in alcohol withdrawal.[444] Hallucinations are not uncommon in Parkinson's disease, and may be exacerbated by the dopaminergic agonists used in its treatment.[445–447] They also occur in psychiatric disorders, though visual hallucinations are usually accompanied by hallucinations in other sensory modalities (especially auditory) and by other signs of mental illness.

Many of these disorders have other symptoms or signs that point to the correct diagnosis. When visual hallucinations happen in individuals with intact cognitive and mental function, there is often underlying neurologic or ophthalmologic disease. Isolated visual hallucinations can be categorized into three main pathophysiologic groups: release hallucinations, visual seizures, and migraine.

Release Hallucinations, Charles Bonnet Syndrome

Release visual hallucinations are associated with central or peripheral visual field defects, which are usually binocular. It is thought that these are generated in visual cortex when normal incoming sensory impulses are absent. Probably a quarter to half of patients with severe visual loss have hallucinations, but the true incidence is unknown, since many patients are reluctant to mention

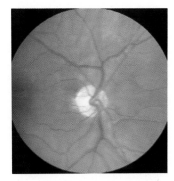 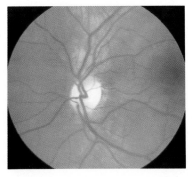

Color Plate 7–1. Optic atrophy with optic tract lesion. 53-year-old woman with CNS sarcoidosis diagnosed 7 years previous with focal motor seizures. She had no visual symptoms. Acuity was 20/40 in both eyes, and there was left relative afferent pupil defect. Note temporal and nasal pallor ("bow-tie" atrophy) in left eye and temporal pallor of right optic disk.

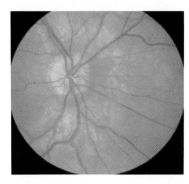 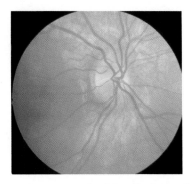

Color Plate 7–2. Optic tract lesion. 8-year-old girl with one month of headache and right VI nerve palsy. Acuity was 20/25 in both eyes, and there was right relative afferent pupil defect. Note in right eye edema at upper and lower poles of optic disk ("twin-peaks" papilledema) and nasal disc swelling in the left eye.

TABLE 7–5. Drugs Associated with Visual Hallucinations

Hallucinogens
    Dimethyltryptamine
    Harmine
    Ketamine hydrochloride
    Lysergic acid diethylamide (LSD)
    Mescaline
    Nitrous oxide
    Phencyclidine hydrochloride (PCP)
    Psilocybin
    Tetrahydrocannabinol
Stimulants
    Amphetamine
    Cocaine
    Methylphenidate
    Atropine
    Scopolamine
    Cyclopentolate
Antiparkinsonian agents
    Amantadine hydrochloride
    Anticholinergic drugs
    Bromocriptine
    Levodopa
    Lisuride
    Mesulergine
    Pergolide mesylate
Antidepressants
    Amitriptyline hydrochloride
    Amoxapine
    Bupropion hydrochloride
    Doxepin hydrochloride
    Imipramine hydrochloride
    Lithium carbonate
    Phenelzine sulfate

From Cummings JL, Miller BL: Visual hallucinations: clinical occurrence and use in differential diagnosis. West J Med 146:46, 1987

hallucinations for fear of being labeled "crazy."[75,438,448–450] In fact, these patients are mentally lucid and usually aware that the visions are not real.[450] Other sensory hallucinations are notably absent.[57] Some authors reserve the term *Charles Bonnet syndrome* for the association of visual loss with formed hallucinations, but the value of a distinction between simple and formed imagery is debatable.[451,452]

Any type of binocular visual loss can by followed by release hallucinations.[453] Cerebral disease (mainly infarctions) may be more frequent than ocular causes such as cataracts, macular degeneration, diabetic retinopathy, other retinal disease, and disease of the optic nerves and chiasm.[438,448,450,454,455] No additional lesion besides that causing the visual loss is required; the hallucinations are considered a physiologic reaction to loss of vision. With partial visual loss, the hallucinations are often confined to the blind scotoma.[456] While most series report severe visual loss in almost all patients, there are instances with minor visual impairment.[448,453,455,457] Social isolation may contribute to the hallucinations of these patients, as they can resolve with a more stimulating environment, and since hallucinations can be induced in normal subjects through sensory deprivation.[457,458]

Hallucinations can be simple or complex. Simple hallucinations include flashing spots, colored lines, or geometric shapes.[459–461] Complex hallucinations contain objects and figures, such as humans and animals.[448,453,455,462] They may be detailed, bizarre and dream-like, including dragons and policemen, and sometimes contain images from the past, like a dead relative.[450,451,455,462,463] Simple hallucinations are twice as common as complex ones, though the latter are reported in 10% to 30% of patients with visual loss.[448,451,452,459] In contrast to visual seizures (see below), the distinction between complex and simple release hallucinations is unimportant. The type of release hallucination does not indicate the site of visual loss.[455] Some patients have simple release hallucinations first, then complex ones, a progression also seen with sensory deprivation of normal subjects.[454,455,458,462]

Hallucinations often follow visual loss by days or weeks, sometimes longer, but can occur at the onset, leading to the discovery of the visual field defect.[453,462] Rarely, hallucinations may even precede hemianopia by a few days.[459] With ocular visual loss, hallucinations do not begin until the second eye loses vision.[453,454] The hallucinations can last seconds to minutes or be continuous, and they may occur several times a day or a few times per year.[450,451] They often happen in the evening and night when lighting is poor and patients are inactive or alone.[450] Hallucinations may recur for only a few days or months, but often persist for years or decades.[450,453,459,462]

Not all patients with visual loss develop release hallucinations, implying that other factors must play a role.[448,450–452,459] Most patients with hallucinations are older than 60, but this may merely reflect a greater likelihood of bilateral visual loss in the elderly; certainly, children can have release hallucinations.[450,451] Social isolation may contribute.[452,457] Associated cognitive dysfunction has been asserted by some and denied by others.[451,457] One report suggests that posterior periventricular white matter lesions on MRI correlated with hallucinations from ocular disease.[464] In contrast, preservation of visual association areas may be required for release hallucinations, as they seem not to occur after extensive damage to these areas.[57]

An ictal mechanism has been hypothesized; however, release hallucinations differ from known visual seizures by their longer duration, non-stereotyped content, and association with visual loss rather than with secondary motor or sensory epileptic events.[451,453,455,462] Entoptic phenomena (see Chapter 1) have been proposed in cases due to media opacities, but this would not explain hallucinations in patients with enucleations. Rather, the consensus is that all release hallucinations have similar origins as a physiologic reaction to visual loss, analogous to other phenomena such as the phantom limb sensation after amputation and musical hallucinations in deafness.[465] Visual experience is represented by patterns of coordinated impulses within the cortical neural network, and it may be that the brain has an inherent capacity to generate these neural patterns spontaneously, and does so during sensory deprivation from either isolation or pathologic denervation.[451,458]

Release hallucinations are usually tolerated and only require reassurance about their benign nature.[450,451] Mixed results have occurred with anticonvulsant drugs, haloperidol, and tiapride.[367,452,453,457,466,467] Increasing social contact may help.[457]

Visual Seizures

Confusion about the localizing value of hallucinations stems from failure to distinguish between release hallucinations and visual seizures. With release hallucinations, information about localization lies in the pattern of the visual field defect, not the type of hallucinatory image.[455] However, the content of visual seizures may be a useful sign.[453] Experimental stimulation in striate cortex evokes simple unformed flashes of light and colors, whereas stimulation of visual association cortex in areas 19 and temporal regions evokes complex formed images.[468,469] A similar distinction probably holds for epileptic visual hallucinations. For example, a left parieto-temporal lesion can cause hallucinations of objects and written words followed by post-ictal aphasia, whereas occipital lobe seizures cause hallucinations of colored circles and spheres, flashing or steady colored or white lights[470–472] (Fig. 7–27). Complex hallucinations from occipital lesions, likely represent spread of ictal activity into extrastriate cortex; hence the visual content at seizure onset has the most accurate localizing value.[472–474]

The distinction between visual seizures and release hallucinations can be difficult with an underlying cerebral lesion. Cogan[453] believed that release hallucinations were continuous with varying content, whereas visual seizures were brief episodes with stereotyped content. Others question this, noting that release hallucinations can be episodic and their content repetitive.[451] Associated signs are more reliable. Accompanying head or eye deviation (usually but not always contralateral), and rapid blinking are common with occipital seizures, and other signs of ictal spread should be sought, including confusion, dysphasia, tonic-clonic limb movements, and the automatisms of complex partial seizures.[472] Homonymous field defects indicate the possibility of release hallucinations, but epileptogenic lesions may also cause visual field defects. In some cases, complex hallucinations in hemianopia may be a combination of ictal and release phenomena.[475] Seizure monitoring may help but routine EEG leads often do not locate the occipital

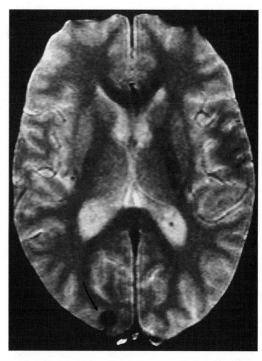

Fig. 7–27. Occipital seizures. A 50-year-old man with recently treated endocarditis. He began noting intermittent waves of colors in his vision, lasting minutes, often provoked by a sudden increase in ambient illumination. MRI shows a small right occipital hemorrhage, presumed from a septic embolus. Fields were normal.

focus, and invasive intracranial electrodes may be required.[472]

Visual seizures are uncommon in epilepsy, but can occur with a variety of cerebral lesions (Fig. 7–27). One visual seizure syndrome requiring emphasis is benign childhood epilepsy with occipital spike-waves.[476] This idiopathic epilepsy syndrome begins between ages 5 and 9 and ceases spontaneously in the teenage years. Seizures involve blindness and/or hallucinations of both simple and formed types, and may progress to motor or partial complex seizures. Some children develop nausea and headache following the visual seizure, causing confusion with migraine. The diagnosis is established by occipital spike-waves with eye closure on EEG.

Migrainous Hallucinations

Migraine causes a variety of visual symptoms, which may precede the headache (classic migraine) or occur without a headache (acephalgic migraine, or migraine equivalent).[477] Photopic images are most common, described as spots, wavy lines, or a heat-wave–like shimmering.[478] The *scintillating scotoma* is a blind region surrounded by a margin of sparkling lights (Fig. 7–28), which often slowly enlarges over time. The sparkling margin sometimes appears as a zigzag pattern of lines oriented at 60° to each other, usually in one hemifield,

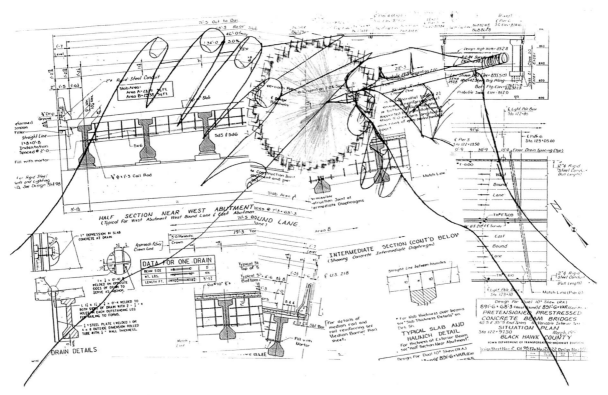

Fig. 7–28. Migrainous hallucination. Drawing by a 42-year-old professional draughtsman of his migraine aura, which has a central scotoma surrounded by a ring border of sparkling colored lights.

and on the leading edge of a C-shaped scotoma.[460] This is the fortification spectrum, or teichopsia, based on the resemblance to old European walled fortifications.[479] There may be several sets of zigzag lines in parallel, often shimmering or oscillating in brightness.[480] They may be black and white or vividly colored.[471,479,480]

These binocular congruous auras begin near the center of the visual field and expand peripherally with increasing speed over a period of about 20 minutes, with both the speed and the size of the lines increasing with retinal eccentricity. The relation of speed and size to eccentricity is predicted by the cortical magnification factor, which is a measure of the area of visual field represented in a given amount of striate cortex as a function of retinal eccentricity.[460,481] This suggests that these migrainous hallucinations are generated by a neuronal excitatory wave spreading from posterior to anterior striate cortex at a constant speed, leaving in its wake a transient neuronal depression that causes the temporary scotoma.[480] The zigzag nature of the lines may reflect the sensitivity to line orientation of striate cortex and the pattern of inhibitory interconnections within and between striate columns (see Chapter 16).[480,481]

The differential diagnosis includes occipital seizures. Although hallucinations followed by headache and vomiting can occur with both migraine and visual seizures,[482] Panayiotopoulos[472,481] has suggested that black

and white zigzag lines predominate in migraine and colored circular patterns in ictal hallucinations, an observation that requires verification. Occipital arteriovenous malformations can cause migraine-like episodes, with ipsilateral headache and contralateral visual phenomena, either field defects or fortification images.[483,484] Timing of headache with relation to the hallucination does not distinguish arteriovenous malformations from more benign migraine, and the age at onset for malformations is highly variable but often in young adulthood, similar to migraine.[484] It has been suggested that neuroimaging should be performed on all patients with migrainous auras that are always on the same side.[484]

Most migrainous hallucinations are transient, lasting 20 minutes or less, but on occasion may last up to a week. Even more rarely, some migraine patients report long-lasting simple hallucinations, often described as diffuse small particles (dots, ants, heat waves, flickerings, snow, TV static) throughout the visual field. These have lasted months to years. Investigations are usually negative, though SPECT scans occasionally show biparietal hypoperfusion.[485]

Other Hallucinatory States

Peduncular Hallucinations

Hallucinations with midbrain lesions are rare.[486,487] They have many similarities to complex release hallucinations: they can be continuous or episodic, with detailed scenes involving animals and humans, and are not stereotyped but vary between episodes.[488-493] As with release hallucinations, the hallucinations may feature scenes from the patient's past, usually with thalamic rather than midbrain infarcts.[493] Patients often have insight that the hallucinations are not real, but others do not and may interact with the hallucinations.[488,490,493-495] Similar hallucinations have been described for sounds, and there can be multimodality hallucinations involving vision, touch, sound, and even the sense of body posture.[489,490,496]

Unlike release hallucinations with visual loss, peduncular hallucinations are almost invariably associated with inversion of the sleep-wake cycle causing diurnal somnolence and nocturnal insomnia.[486,488,491-493] Other associated midbrain signs include unilateral or bilateral third nerve palsy, hemiparkinsonism, hemiparesis, and gait ataxia.[486,488,490-492,494,495] Many patients have pre-existing visual loss, but others have relatively intact vision.[488,490,494,495]

Since the original pathologic description, neuro-imaging has shown unilateral or bilateral infarction of the peduncles.[487,488,491] A detailed pathologic study showed bilateral infarction of the substantia nigra pars reticulata.[490] The correlation of neuronal activity in this structure with REM sleep stages and its connections to the pedunculopontine nucleus suggested an anatomic correlate to the disturbed sleep-wake cycle, which may underlie both the hallucinations and the sleep-wake cycle inversion. Others have postulated damage to the ascending reticular activating system with similar consequences.[495] Similar hallucinations can occur with lesions of the paramedian thalamus, which may affect the thalamic reticular nucleus.[493,495,497]

The most frequent cause is infarction, as a top-of-the-basilar syndrome.[488,490,491,495,498] It has been described as a vascular complication of angiography and transiently after microvascular decompressive surgery for trigeminal neuralgia.[498,494] Extrinsic midbrain compression by a craniopharyngioma and a medulloblastoma have been reported.[492,499] The prognosis varies with cause. With infarction, the hallucinations can persist indefinitely, though episodes may become shorter or disappear.[490,495] Hallucinations have resolved after surgical relief of compression by an extrinsic tumor.[492,499]

Hallucinations during Eye Closure

There are rare reports of hallucinations only with eye closure.[500,501] These occurred with atropine, local anesthesia, or respiratory infections with high fever. Parallels were drawn with hypnagogic hallucinations and disturbed sleep-wake cycle mechanisms.

Dysmetropsia

Illusions about the spatial aspect of visual stimuli include three main categories: micropsia, the illusion that objects are smaller than in reality; macropsia, the illusion that objects are larger than in reality; and metamorphopsia, the illusion that objects are distorted. Micropsia is most common and has several etiologies.

Micropsia

Convergence-accommodative micropsia is a normal phenomenon, in which an object appears smaller when the observer focuses at near rather than far, although there has been no change in the size of the retinal image or its spatial surround. Vergence rather than accommodation causes this effect.[502-504] Accommodative micropsia does not cause symptoms.

Psychogenic micropsia has also been reported among psychiatric patients, where it is subject to psychoanalytic interpretations, with subjects literally trying to distance themselves from environments fraught with conflict.[505-507]

Retinal micropsia occurs when the distance between foveal photoreceptors is increased, usually due to macular edema. There may be metamorphopsia also if the photoreceptor separation is irregular. Visual acuity is also reduced to a degree that correlates with psychophysical measures of micropsia.[508] Retinal micropsia is monocular or binocular, depending on the cause. Means of estimating the degree of micropsia have been developed and can monitor disease progression.[508,509] Causes of macular edema with micropsia include wrinkling of the internal limiting retinal surface membrane, central serous retinopathy, severe papilledema, macular detachment, and cystoid macular edema, though in some the edema may be subclinical.[508,509] The condition may resolve or persist for years, or retraction with scarring may transform micropsia into persistent macropsia.[509,510]

Cerebral micropsia is rare, and, in contrast to retinal micropsia, it is always binocular. Unusual variants include hemimicropsia in the contralateral hemifield.[511,512] One unusual case had hemimicropsia only for faces.[513] Given the small number of cases, the localization value of cerebral micropsia is uncertain. Occipito-temporal lesions have been reported, with either medial or lateral involvement.[512-514] Migraine-related micropsia is another variant that may be more common than appreciated; episodic micropsia or macropsia occurred in 9% of a sample of adolescents, often in the hypnagogic state or with fever, and correlated with a history of migraine.[515,516]

Macropsia

Macropsia is less frequent. *Retinal macropsia* can occur with scarring following macular edema.[510] It is a rare side effect of zolpidem.[517] *Cerebral macropsia* occurs with seizures, and hemimacropsia has been reported with a left occipital tumor and a right occipital infarct.[515,518,519] Both macropsia and micropsia are possibly migraine-related phenomena in adolescents.[516]

Metamorphopsia

Retinal metamorphopsia is more common than cerebral metamorphopsia. Most often this occurs with macular edema and micropsia, but traction upon the retina by an epi-retinal membrane may also distort the retinal map.[509,520] There is some association with the segmental buckling procedure.[521] As with retinal micropsia, retinal metamorphopsia is either monocular or binocular but different in the two eyes. Psychophysical tests of hyperacuity can quantify metamorphopsia, and the Amsler grid (see Chapter 2) can be useful at the bedside.[520]

Cerebral metamorphopsia has been described with seizures from a right parietal glioma or a right parietal arteriovenous malformation.[419,522,523] It has also occurred with posterior cerebral infarction affecting medial temporo-occipital structures, with one lesion involving only the left cingulate gyrus and retrosplenial area.[524,525] There is one report of metamorphopsia due to brainstem lesions.[525] Metamorphopsia may be limited to faces, or occur as a transient stage in the evolution of cortical blindness.[520,526]

RECOVERY AND REHABILITATION

A large database of patients with focal lesions in the occipital and adjacent temporal and parietal areas shows that one-third of stroke patients with visual impairments continue to have chronic functional deficits affecting daily life.[233,527,528,529] Cerebral visual dysfunction is often seen in rehabilitation settings also with either head injury or stroke.[233,530–533] It is associated with poorer overall outcome after rehabilitation.[193,534] Rehabilitation is most successful in patients with preserved intellect, language, memory, and executive functions, as tested neuropsychologically, and with favorable emotional, motivational, and behavioral characteristics, which often reflect the premorbid personality.[535]

In general, a scotoma that persists beyond several months is permanent. The larger and closer to fixation the scotoma, the worse the effects on daily activities such as reading and driving.[536,537] Reports that monkeys can make visual discriminations in de-striated fields have been challenged by negative studies with careful monitoring of fixation.[538,539] Even if blindsight or residual vision exists within a scotoma following a striate lesion, there is no evidence that such function is of practical use in rehabilitation. Efforts aimed at restoring the visual fields have met with considerable difficulty and

produced limited success.[540,541] However, it is possible to train individuals to scan the hemianopic field with eye movements, a strategic adaptation that also occurs without training as long as subjects do not have additional hemi-neglect.[542–546] Studies are required to determine the benefit gained by such adaptive behavior.

Regarding higher cortical deficits, attempts at retraining visual recognition in patients with visual agnosia have been ineffective, mainly because these patients also have anterograde learning deficits. Theoretically, agnosic patients could be trained to use tactile and auditory cues, and prosopagnosic patients could learn to focus on unique non-facial visual features such as gait, and local facial cues such as hair style and glasses. Many develop these abilities on their own with time. Cerebral achromatopsia is annoying but rarely disabling, because patients can still perceive object shapes and boundaries, navigate the environment, and have good spatial resolution. Certain color tasks in the environment pose special difficulties. Traffic lights are an example; however, patients can learn to use other visual cues, such as the conventional order of red being the top light and green the bottom. Patients with acquired pure alexia have a more profound disability, given the importance of literacy in our society; rehabilitation of this problem remains in its infancy.

Finally, RAND under the sponsorship of the National Eye Institute has developed the Visual Functioning Questionnaire-25 (VFQ-25). This standardized tool asks 25 questions on visual health on a 5-point scale (NEI, 1996).[547] The overall score provides an index of visual health in eye disease that is sensitive to treatment outcome. The VFQ-25 might also be applied to gauge recovery and efficacy of rehabilitation in visual dysfunction caused by cerebral lesions.

REFERENCES

1. Morin JP: The circadian visual system. Brain Res Rev 19:102, 1994
2. Czeisler CA, Shanahan TL, Klerman EB et al: Suppression of melatonin secretion in some blind patients by exposure to bright light. N Engl J Med J 332:6, 1995
3. Felleman DV, Van Essen DC: Distributed hierarchical processing in the primate cerebral cortex. Cereb Cortex 1:1, 1991
4. Ungerleider LG, Galkin TW, Mishkin M: Visuotopic organization of projections from striate cortex to inferior and lateral pulvinar in rhesus monkey. J Comp Neurol 217(2):137, 1983
5. Zihl J, von Cramon D, Mai N: Selective disturbance of movement vision after bilateral brain damage. Brain 106:3313, 1983
6. Zeki S: Cerebral akinetopsia (visual motion blindness): a review. Brain 114:811, 1991
7. Rizzo M, Nawrot M, Zihl J: Motion and shape perception in cerebral akinetopsia. Brain 118:1105, 1995
8. Rizzo M, Smith V, Pokorny J, Damasio AR: Color perception profiles in central achromatopsia. Neurology 43:995, 1993
9. Marinkovic SV, Milisavljevic MM, Lolic-Draganic V, Kovacevic MS: Distribution of the occipital branches of the posterior cerebral artery: correlation with occipital lobe infarcts. Stroke 18:728, 1987

10. Pessin MS, Lathi ES, Cohen MB et al: Clinical feature and mechanism of occipital lobe infarction. Ann Neurol 21:290, 1987

11. Tassinari G, Campara D, Balercia G, Chilosi M, Martignoni G: Magno- and parvocellular pathways are segregated in the human optic tract. Neuroreport 5:1425, 1994

12. Savino PJ, Paris M, Schatz NJ et al: Optic tract syndrome. A review of 21 patients. Arch Ophthalmol 96:656, 1978

13. Newman SA, Miller NR: Optic tract syndrome. Neuro-ophthalmologic considerations. Arch Ophthalmol 101:1241, 1983

13a. Rosen ES, Eustace P, Thompson HS, Cumming WJK (eds): Neuro-ophthalmology. London: Mosby, 1998

14. Bender MB, Bodis-Wollner I: Visual dysfunctions in optic tract lesions. Ann Neurol 3:187, 1978

15. Frisèn L: The neurology of visual acuity. Brain 13:639, 1980

16. Paul TO, Hoyt WF: Funduscopic appearance of papilledema with optic tract atrophy. Arch Ophthalmol 94:467, 1976

17. Czarnecki JS, Weingeist TA, Burton JC, Thompson HS: "Twin peaks" papilledema: the appearance of papilledema with optic tract atrophy. Can J Ophthalmol 11:279, 1976

18. Bell RA, Thompson HS: Relative afferent pupillary defect in optic tract hemianopias. Am J Ophthalmol 85:538, 1978

19. O'Connor P, Mein C, Hughes J et al: The Marcus Gunn pupil in incomplete optic tract hemianopias. J Clin Neuro Ophthalmol 2:227, 1982

20. Klein LH, Fermaglich J, Kataah J, Luessenhop AJ: Cavernous hemangioma of optic chiasm, optic nerves and right optic tract: case report and review of the literature. Virchows Arch [A] 383:225, 1979

21. Rosenblatt MA, Behrens MM, Zweufach PH et al: Magnetic resonance imaging of optic tract involvement in multiple sclerosis. Am J Ophthalmol 104:74, 1987

22. Youl BD, Plant GT, Stevens JM et al: Three cases of craniopharyngioma showing optic tract hypersignal on MRI. Neurology 40:1416, 1990

23. Tachibana O, Yamaguchi N, Yamashima T, Yamashita J: Radiation necrosis of the optic chiasm, optic tract, hypothalamus, and upper pons after radiotherapy for pituitary adenoma, detected by gadolinium-enhanced, T1-weighted magnetic resonance imaging: case report. Neurosurgery 27:640, 1990

24. Beck RW, Schatz NJ, Savino PJ: Involvement of the optic chiasm, optic tract, and geniculo-calcarine visual system in multiple sclerosis. Bull Soc Belge Ophthalmol 208:159, 1983

25. Plant GT, Kermode AG, Turano G et al: Symptomatic retrochiasmal lesions in multiple sclerosis. Clinical features, visual evoked potentials, and magnetic resonance imaging. Neurology 42:68, 1992

26. McLaurin EB, Harrington DO: Intracranial sarcoidosis with optic tract and temporal lobe involvement. Am J Ophthalmol 86:656, 1978

27. Zentner J, Grodd W, Hassler W: Cavernous angioma of the optic tract. J Neurol 236:117, 1989

27a. Kupersmith MJ, Vargas M, Hoyt WF, Berenstein A: Optic tract atrophy with cerebral arteriovenous malformations: direct and transsynaptic degeneration. Neurol 44:80, 1994

28. Anderson DR, Trobe JD, Hood TW, Gebarski SS: Optic tract injury after anterior temporal lobectomy. Ophthalmology 96:1065, 1989

29. Manesis EK, Petrou C, Brouzas D, Hadziyannis S: Optic tract neuropathy complicating low-dose interferon treatment. J Hepatol 21:474, 1994

30. Margo CE, Hamed LM, McCarty J: Congenital optic tract syndrome. Arch Ophthalmol 109:1120, 1991

31. Sherman SM, Koch C: The control of retinogeniculate transmission in the mammalian lateral geniculate nucleus. Exp Brain Res 63:1, 1986

32. Sillito AM, Murphy PC: The modulation of the retinal relay to the cortex in the dorsal lateral geniculate nucleus. Eye 2(suppl):S221, 1988

33. Harting JK, Huerta MF, Hashikawa T, van Lieshout DP: Projection of the mammalian superior colliculus upon the dorsal lateral geniculate nucleus: organization of the tectogeniculate pathways in nineteen species. J Comp Neurol 304:275, 1991

34. Frisèn L, Holmegaard L, Rosenkrantz M: Sectoral optic atrophy and homonymous horizontal sectoranopia: a lateral choroidal artery syndrome? J Neurol Neurosurg Psychiatry 41:374, 1978

35. Frisèn L: Quadruple sectoranopia and sectorial optic atrophy. A syndrome of the distal anterior choroidal artery. J Neurol Neurosurg Psychiatry 42:590, 1979

36. Donahue SP, Kardon R, Thompson HS: Hourglass-shaped visual fields as a sign of bilateral lateral geniculate myelinolysis. Am J Ophthalmol 119:378, 1995

37. Goldman JE, Horoupian DS: Demyelination of the lateral geniculate nucleus in central pontine myelinolysis. Ann Neurol 9:185, 1981

38. Greenfield DS, Siatkowski RM, Schatz NJ, Glaser JS: Bilateral geniculitis associated with severe diarrhea. Am J Ophthalmol 122:280, 1996

39. Jacobson DM: The localizing value of a quadrantanopia. Arch Neurol 54:401, 1997

40. Carter JE, O'Connor P, Shacklett D, Rosenberg M: Lesions of the optic radiations mimicking lateral geniculate nucleus visual field defects. J Neurol Neurosurg Psychiatry 48:982, 1985

41. Smith CG, Richardson WFG: The course and distribution of the arteries supplying the visual (striate) cortex. Am J Ophthalmol 61:1391, 1966

42. Horton JC, Hoyt WF: The representation of the visual field in human striate cortex: a revision of the classic Holmes map. Arch Ophthalmol 109:816, 1991

43. Inouye T: Die Sehstorungen bei Schussverletzungen der kortikalen Sesphare. Leipzig, Engelmann, 1909

44. Holmes G, Lister WT: Disturbances of vision from cerebral lesions with special reference to the cortical representation of the macula. Brain 39:34, 1916

45. McFadzean R, Brosnahan D, Hadley D, Mutlukan E: Representation of the visual field in the occipital striate cortex. Br J Ophthalmol 78:185, 1994

46. Abbie AA: The blood supply of the visual pathways. Med J Aust 2:199, 1938

47. Huber A: Homonymous hemianopia after occipital lobectomy. Am J Ophthalmol 54:623, 1962

47a. Tootell RBH, Switkes E, Silverman MS, Hamilton SL: Functional anatomy of macaque striate cortex. II. Retinoptic organization. J Neurosci 8:1531, 1988

48. McAuley DL, Russell RWR: Correlation of CAT scan and visual field defects in vascular lesions of the posterior visual pathways. J Neurol Neurosurg Psychiatry 42:298, 1979

49. Gray LG, Galetta SL, Siegal T, Schatz NJ: The central visual field in homonymous hemianopia. Evidence for unilateral foveal representation. Arch Neurol 54:312, 1997

50. Heller-Bettinger I, Kepes JJ, Preskorn SH, Wurster JB: Bilateral altitudinal anopia caused by infarction of the calcarine cortex. Neurology 26:1176, 1976

51. Rush JA: Nonbacterial thrombotic endocarditis and cortical blindness. Am J Ophthalmol 114:643, 1992

52. Spalding JMK: Wounds of the visual pathway: part II. The striate cortex. J Neurol Neurosurg Psychiatry 15:169, 1952

53. Benton S, Levy I, Swash M: Vision in the temporal crescent in occipital infarction. Brain 103:83, 1980

54. Chavis PS, Al-Hazmi A, Clunie D, Hoyt WF: Temporal crescent syndrome with magnetic resonance correlation. J Neuro-ophthalmol 17:151, 1997

55. Hornstein S, Chamberlin W, Conomy J: Infarctions of the fusiform and calcarine regions: agitated delirium and hemianopia. Trans Am Neurol Assoc 92:85, 1967

56. Medina JL, Chokroverty S, Rubino FA: Syndrome of agitated delirium and visual impairment: a manifestation of medial temporo-occipital infarction. J Neurol Neurosurg Psychiatry 40:861, 1977

57. Vaphiades MS, Celesia GG, Brigell MG: Positive spontaneous visual phenomena limited to the hemianopic field in lesions of central visual pathways. Neurology 47:408, 1996

58. Symonds C, McKenzie I: Bilateral loss of vision from cerebral infarction. Brain 80:415, 1957

59. Bougousslavsky J, van Melle G: Unilateral occipital infarction: evaluation of the risk of developing bilateral loss of vision. J Neurol Neurosurg Psychiatry 46:78, 1983

60. Halpern JI, Sedler RR: Traumatic bilateral homonymous hemianopic scotomas. Ann Ophthalmol 12:1022, 1980
61. Shutter LA, Green JP, Newman NJ et al: Cortical blindness and white matter lesions in a patient receiving FK506 after liver transplantation. Neurology 43:2417, 1993
62. Tyler HR: Neurologic disorders in renal failure. Am J Med 44:734, 1968
63. Aldrich MS, Alessi AG, Beck RW, Gilman S: Cortical blindness: etiology, diagnosis and prognosis. Ann Neurol 21:149, 1987
64. Chisholm IH: Cortical blindness in cranial arteritis. Br J Ophthalmol 59:332, 1975
65. Naito H, Kurokawa K, Kanno T et al: Status epilepticus and cortical blindness due to subclavian steal syndrome in a girl with Blalock's operation. Surg Neurol 1:46, 1973
66. Carney AL, Anderson EM: Cortical blindness and tourniquet subclavian steal. JAMA 245:572, 1981
67. Wells TG, Graham CJ, Moss MM, Kearns GL: Nifedipine poisoning in a child. Pediatrics 86:91, 1990
68. Morton C, Hickey-Dwyer M: Cortical blindness after nifedipine treatment. Br Med J 305:693, 1992
69. Lawrence-Friedl D, Bauer KM: Bilateral cortical blindness: an unusual presentation of bacterial endocarditis. Ann Emerg Med 21:1502, 1992
70. Morgan RK, Nugent B, Harrison JM, O'Connor PS: Voluntary alteration of pattern visual evoked responses. Ophthalmology 92:1356, 1985
71. Spehlmann R, Gross RA, Ho SU et al: Visual evoked potentials and postmortem findings in a case of cortical blindness. Ann Neurol 2:531, 1977
72. Celesia GG, Archer CR, Kuroiwa Y, Goldfader PR: Visual function of the extra-geniculo-calcarine system in man: relationship to cortical blindness. Arch Neurol 37:704, 1980
73. Frank Y, Torres F: Visual evoked potentials in the evaluation of "cortical blindness" in children. Ann Neurol 6:126, 1979
74. Wong VCN: Cortical blindness in children. A study of etiology and prognosis. Pediatr Neurol 7:178, 1991
75. Gjerris F, Mellemgaard L: Transitory cortical blindness in head injury. Acta Neurol Scand 45:623, 1969
76. Griffith JF, Dodge PR: Transient blindness following head injury in children. N Engl J Med 278:648, 1968
77. Drubach DA, Carmona S, Meyerrose GE et al: Brain SPECT in a case of cortical blindness. Stroke 25:1061, 1994
78. Kooi KA, Sharbrough FW: Electrophysiological findings in cortical blindness. Electroencephalogr Clin Neurophysiol 20:260, 1966
79. Duchowny MS, Weiss IP, Majlessi H, Barnet A: Visual evoked responses in childhood cortical blindness after head trauma and meningitis. A longitudinal study of six cases. Neurology 24:933, 1974
80. Tepperberg J, Nussbaum D, Feldman F: Cortical blindness following meningitis due to Hemophilus influenzae type B. J Pediatr 91:434, 1977
81. Ramani V: Cortical blindness following ictal nystagmus. Arch Neurol 42:191, 1985
82. Skolnik SA, Mizen TR, Burde RM: Transient post-ictal cortical blindness. J Clin Neuro-Ophthalmol 7:151, 1987
83. Joseph JM, Louis S: Transient ictal cortical blindness during middle age. A case report and review of the literature. J Neuro-ophthalmol 15:39, 1995
84. Miyata Y, Motomura S, Tsuji Y, Koga S: Hepatic encephalopathy and reversible cortical blindness. Am J Gastroenterol 83:780, 1988
85. Kupferschmidt H, Bont A, Schnorf H et al: Transient cortical blindness and biooccipital brain lesions in two patients with acute intermittent porphyria. Ann Intern Med 123:598, 1995
86. Mukamel M, Weitz R, Nissenkorn I et al: Acute cortical blindness associated with hypoglycemia. J Pediatr 98:583, 1981
87. Marra TR, Shah M, Mikus MA: Transient cortical blindness due to hypertensive encephalopathy. Magnetic resonance imaging correlation. J Clin Neuro-Ophthalmol 13:35, 1993
88. Tychsen L, Hoyt WF: Hydrocephalus and transient cortical blindness. Am J Ophthalmol 98:819, 1984
89. Greenblatt SH: Post-traumatic cerebral blindness: association with migraine and seizure diathesis. JAMA 225:1073, 1973

90. Patronas NJ, Argyropoulu M: Intravascular thrombosis as a possible cause of transient cortical brain lesions. CT and MRI. J Comput Assist Tomogr 16:849, 1992
91. Berman IJ, Mann MP: Seizures and transient cortical blindness associated with cisplatinum (II) diaminedichloride (PPD) therapy in a thirty-year-old man. Cancer 45:764, 1980
92. Philip PA, Carmichael J, Harris AL: Convulsions and transient cortical blindness after cisplatin. Br Med J 302:416, 1991
93. Rubin AM: Transient cortical blindness and occipital seizures with cyclosporine toxicity. Transplantation 47:572, 1989
94. Byrd RL, Rohrbaugh TM, Raney RB, Norris DG: Transient cortical blindness secondary to vincristine therapy in childhood malignancies. Cancer 47:37, 1981
95. Studdard WE, Davis DO, Young SW: Cortical blindness after cerebral angiography. Case report. J Neurosurg 54:240, 1981
96. Parry R, Rees JR, Wilde P: Transient cortical blindness after coronary angiography. Br Heart J 70:563, 1993
97. Lantos G: Cortical blindness due to osmotic disruption of the blood-brain barrier by angiographic contrast material: CT and MRI studies. Neurology 39:567, 1989
98. Eldridge PR, Punt JAG: Transient traumatic cortical blindness in children. Lancet 1:815, 1988
99. Liebowitz HA, Hall PE: Cortical blindness as a complication of eclampsia. Ann Emerg Med 13:365, 1984
100. Cunningham FG, Fernandez CO, Hernandez C: Blindness associated with preeclampsia and eclampsia. Am J Obstet Gynecol 172:1291, 1995
101. Gospe SM: Transient cortical blindness in an infant exposed to methamphetamine. Ann Emerg Med 26:380, 1995
102. DeSousa AL, Kleiman MB, Mealey J: Quadriplegia and cortical blindness in Hemophilus influenzae meningitis. J Pediatr 93:253, 1978
103. Moel DI, Kwun YA: Cortical blindness as a complication of hemodialysis. J Pediatr 93:890, 1978
104. Smirniotopoulos JG, Murphy FM, Schellinger D et al: Cortical blindness after metrizamide myelography. Report of a case and proposed pathophysiologic mechanism. Arch Neurol 41:224, 1984
105. Woodward GA: Posttraumatic cortical blindness: are we missing the diagnosis in children? Pediatr Emerg Care 6:289, 1990
106. Barnet AB, Manson JI, Wilner E: Acute cerebral blindness in childhood. Neurology 20:1147, 1970
106a. Good WV, Jan JE, DeSa L, Barkovich AJ, Groenveld M, Hoyt CS. Cortical visual impairment in children. Surv Ophthalmol 38:351, 1994
107. Hochstetler K, Beals RD: Transient cortical blindness in a child. Ann Emerg Med 16:218, 1987
108. Rodriguez A, Lozano JA, del Pozo D, Paez JH: Post-traumatic transient cortical blindness. Int Ophthalmol 17:277, 1993
109. Carmola JR, Harris BS: Transient cortical blindness: still an overlooked syndrome? N Engl J Med 282:1325, 1970
110. Kaye EM, Herskowitz J: Transient post-traumatic cortical blindness: brief versus prolonged syndromes in childhood. J Child Neurol 1:206, 1986
111. Makino A, Soga T, Obayashi M et al: Cortical blindness causes by acute general cerebral swelling. Surg Neurol 29:393, 1989
112. Lambert SR, Hoyt CS, Jan JE et al: Visual recovery from hypoxic cortical blindness during childhood. Computed tomographic and magnetic resonance predictors. Arch Ophthalmol 105:1371, 1988
113. Goodlin RC, Strieb E, Sun SF et al: Cortical blindness as the initial symptom in severe preeclampsia. Am J Ophthalmol 147:841, 1983
114. Branch DW, Andres R, Digre KB et al: The association of antiphospholipid antibodies with severe eclampsia. Obstet Gynecol 73:541, 1989
115. Seaward GR, England MJ, Nagar AK, van Gelderen CJ: Transient post-partum amaurosis. A report of four cases. J Reprod Med 34:253, 1989
116. Duncan R, Hadley D, Bone I et al: Blindness in eclampsia: CT and MR imaging. J Neurol Neurosurg Psychiatry 52:899, 1989
117. Lau SPC, Chan FL, Yu YL et al: Cortical blindness in toxemia of pregnancy: findings on computed tomography. Br J Radiol 60:347, 1987
118. Herzog TJ, Angel OH, Karram MM, Evertson LR: Use of mag-

netic resonance imaging in the diagnosis of cortical blindness in pregnancy. Obstet Gynecol 76:980, 1990

119. Beal MF, Chapman PH: Cortical blindness and homonymous hemianopia in the postpartum period. JAMA 244:2085, 1980

120. Stiller RJ, Leone-Tomaschoff S, Cuteri J, Beck L: Post-partum pulmonary embolus as an unusual cause of cortical blindness. Am J Obstet Gynecol 162:696, 1990

121. Carpenter E, Kava HL, Plotkin D: The development of total blindness as a complication of pregnancy. Am J Obstet Gynecol 66:641, 1953

122. Beck RW, Gamel JW, Willcourt RJ, Berman G: Acute ischemic optic neuropathy in severe eclampsia. Am J Ophthalmol 90:342, 1980

123. Damasio AR: Prosopagnosia. Trends Neurosci 8:132, 1985

124. Sandifer PH: Anosognosia and disorders of body scheme. Brain 69:122, 1946

125. Geschwind N, Fusillo M: Color-naming defects in association with alexia. Arch Neurol 15:137, 1966

126. McDaniel KD, McDaniel LD: Anton's syndrome in a patient with posttraumatic optic neuropathy and bifrontal contusions. Arch Neurol 48:101, 1991

127. Hartmann JA, Wolz WA, Roeltgen DP, Loverso FL: Denial of visual perception. Brain Cogn 16(1):29, 1991

128. Teuber HL: Alteration of perception and memory in man. In Weiskrantz L (ed): Analysis of Behavioral Change. New York, Harper & Row, 1968

129. Blythe IM, Kennard C, Ruddock KH: Residual vision in patients with retrogeniculate lesions of the visual pathways. Brain 110:887, 1987

130. Barbur JL, Ruddock KH, Waterfield VA: Human visual responses in the absence of the geniculo-calcarine projection. Brain 103:905, 1980

131. Barbur JL, Forsyth PM, Findlay JM: Human saccadic eye movements in the absence of the geniculocalcarine projection. Brain 111:63, 1988

132. Barbur JL, Watson JDG, Frackowiak RSJ, Zeki S: Conscious visual perception without V1. Brain 116:1293, 1993

133. Weiskrantz L, Barbur JL, Sahraie A: Parameters affecting conscious versus unconscious discrimination with damage to the visual cortex (V1). Proc Natl Acad Sci USA 92:6122, 1995

134. Meeres SL, Graves RE: Localization of unseen stimuli by humans with normal vision. Neuropsychologia 28:1231, 1990

135. Kolb FC, Braun J: Blindsight in normal observers. Nature 377:336, 1995

136. Weiskrantz L: Residual vision in a scotoma: A follow-up study of "form" discrimination. Brain 110:77, 1987

137. Perenin M-T: Discrimination of motion direction in perimetrically blind fields. NeuroReport 2:397, 1991

138. Barton JJS, Sharpe JA: Motion direction discrimination in blind hemifields. Ann Neurol 41:255, 1997

139. Barton JJS, Sharpe JA: Smooth pursuit and saccades to moving targets in blind hemifields. A comparison of medial occipital, lateral occipital, and optic radiation lesions. Brain 120:681, 1997

140. Magnussen S, Mathiesen T: Detection of moving and stationary gratings in the absence of striate cortex. Neuropsychologia 27:725, 1989

141. Perenin M-T: Visual functions within the hemianopic field following early cerebral hemidecortication in man—II. Pattern discrimination. Neuropsychologia 16:697, 1978

142. Payne BR, Lomber SG, MacNeil MA, Cornwell P: Evidence for greater sight in blindsight following damage of primary visual cortex early in life. Neuropsychologia 34:741, 1996

143. Ptito A, Lassonde M, Lepore F, Ptito M: Visual discrimination in hemispherectomized patients. Neuropsychologia 25:869, 1987

144. Zihl J: "Blindsight": improvement of visually guided eye movements by systematic practice in patients with cerebral blindness. Neuropsychologia 18:71, 1980

145. Zihl J, Werth R: Contributions to the study of "blindsight"—I. Can stray light account for saccadic localization in patients with postgeniculate visual field defects? Neuropsychologia 22:1, 1984

146. Zihl J, Werth R: Contributions to the study of "blindsight"—II. The role of specific practice for saccadic localization in patients with postgeniculate visual field defects. Neuropsychologia 22:13, 1984

147. Bridgeman B, Staggs D: Plasticity in human blindsight. Vision Res 22:1199, 1982

148. Stoerig P, Cowey A: Blindsight in man and monkey. Brain 120:535, 1997

149. Weiskrantz L, Warrington EK, Sanders MD, Marshall J: Visual capacity in the hemianopic field following a restricted occipital ablation. Brain 97:709, 1974

150. Perenin M-T, Jeannerod M: Visual functions within the hemianopic field following early cerebral hemidecortication in man—I. Spatial localization. Neuropsychologia 16:1, 1978

151. Pöppel E, Held R, Frost D: Residual visual function after brain wounds involving the central visual pathways in man. Nature 243:295, 1973

152. Sanders MD, Warrington E, Marshall J, Weiskrantz L: "Blindsight": vision in a field defect. Lancet 1:707, 1974

153. Perenin M-T, Jeannerod M: Residual function in cortically blind hemifields. Neuropsychologia 13:1, 1975

154. Meienberg O, Zangemeister WH, Rosenberg M et al: Saccadic eye movement strategies in patients with homonymous hemianopia. Ann Neurol 9:537, 1981

155. Barton JJS, Sharpe JA, Raymond JE: Directional defects in pursuit and motion perception in humans with unilateral cerebral lesions. Brain 119:1535, 1996

156. Blythe IM, Bromley JM, Kennard C, Ruddock KH: Visual discrimination of target displacement remains after damage to the striate cortex in humans. Nature 320:619, 1986

157. Blythe IM, Bromley JM, Ruddock KH et al: A study of systematic visual perseveration involving central mechanisms. Brain 106:661, 1986

158. Perenin M-T, Ruel J, Hècaen H: Residual visual capacities in a case of cortical blindness. Cortex 6:605, 1980

159. Corbetta M, Marzi CA, Tassinari G, Aglioti S: Effectiveness of different task paradigms in revealing blindsight. Brain 113:603, 1990

160. Heide W, Koenig E, Dichgans J: Optokinetic nystagmus, self-motion sensation and their after effects in patients with occipito-parietal lesions. Clin Vision Sci 5:145, 1990

161. Mestre DR, Brouchon M, Ceccaldi M, Poncet M: Perception of optical flow in cortical blindness: a case report. Neuropsychologia 30(9):783, 1992

162. Pizzamiglio L, Antonucci G, Francia A: Response of the cortically blind hemifields to a moving stimulus. Cortex 20:89, 1984

163. ter Braak JWG, Schenk VWD, van Vliet AGM: Visual reactions in a case of long-lasting cortical blindness. J Neurol Neurosurg Psychiatry 34:140, 1971

164. Torjussen T: Visual processing in cortically blind hemifields. Neuropsychologia 16:15, 1978

165. Stoerig P: Chromaticity and achromaticity. Evidence for a functional differentiation in visual field defects. Brain 110:869, 1987

166. Stoerig P, Cowey A: Wavelength sensitivity in blindsight. Nature 342:916, 1989

167. Stoerig P, Cowey A: Increment-threshold spectral sensitivity in blindsight. Evidence for colour opponency. Brain 114:1487, 1991

168. Hess RF, Pointer JS: Spatial and temporal contrast sensitivity in hemianopia. Brain 112:871, 1989

169. Weiskrantz L, Harlow A, Barbur JL: Factors affecting visual sensitivity in a hemianopic subject. Brain 114:2269, 1991

170. Barbur JL, Harlow AJ, Weiskrantz L: Spatial and temporal response properties of residual vision in a case of hemianopia. Phil Trans R Soc Lond B Biol Sci 343:157, 1994

171. Marzi CA, Tassinari G, Agliotti S, Lutzemberger L: Spatial summation across the vertical meridian in hemianopics: a test of blindsight. Neuropsychologia 24:749, 1986

172. Rafal R, Smith J, Krantz J et al: Extrageniculate vision in hemianopic humans: saccade inhibition by signals in the blind field. Science 250:118, 1990

173. Cowey A, Stoerig P: The neurobiology of blindsight. Trends Neurosci 14:140, 1991

174. Bender DB: Visual activation of neurons in the primate pulvinar depends on cortex but not colliculus. Brain Res 279:258, 1983

175. Bender DB: Electrophysiological and behavioural experiments on the primate pulvinar. Prog Brain Res 75:55, 1988

176. Weiskrantz L: The Ferrier Lecture, 1989. Outlooks for blindsight:

explicit methodologies for implicit processes. Proc R Soc Lond Ser B 239:247, 1990

177. Ffytche DH, Guy CN, Zeki S: The parallel visual motion inputs into areas V1 and V5 of human cerebral cortex. Brain 118:1375, 1995

178. Beckers G, Zeki S: The consequences of inactivating areas V1 and V5 in visual motion perception. Brain 118:49, 1995

179. Braddick O, Atkinson J, Hood B et al: Possible blindsight in infants lacking one cerebral hemisphere. Nature 360:461, 1992

180. Ptito A, Lepore F, Ptito M, Lassonde M: Target detection and movement discrimination in the blind field of hemispherectomized patients. Brain 114:497, 1991

181. Campion J, Latto R, Smith YM: Is blindsight an effect of scattered light, spared cortex, and near-threshold vision? Behav Brain Sci 6:423, 1983

182. Fendrich R, Wessinger CM, Gazzaniga MS: Residual vision in a scotoma: implications for blindsight. Science 258:1489, 1992

183. Schacter DL: Implicit knowledge: new perspectives on unconscious processes. Proc Natl Acad Sci USA 89:11113, 1992

184. Farah MJ, O'Reilly RC, Vecera SP: Dissociated overt and covert recognition as an emergent property of a lesioned neural network. Psychol Rev 100:571, 1993

185. Stoerig P, Hübner M, Pöppel E: Signal detection analysis of residual vision in a field defect due to a post-geniculate lesion. Neuropsychologia 23:589, 1985

186. Balliet R, Blood KMT, Bach-Y-Rita P: Visual field rehabilitation in the cortically blind? J Neurol Neurosurg Psychiatry 48(11):1113, 1985

187. Rizzo M, Robin D: Bilateral effects of unilateral occipital lobe lesions in humans. Brain 119:951, 1996

188. Sharpe JA, Lo AW, Rabinovitch HE: Control of the saccadic and smooth pursuit systems after cerebral henidecotication. Brain 102(2):387, 1979

189. Sherrington CS. The integrative action of the nervous system. New Haven, CT: Yale University Press, 1906, p 246

190. Desimone R, Moran J, Schein SJ, Mishkin M: A role for the corpus callosum in visual area V4 of the macaque. Vis Neurosci 10:159, 1993

191. Ball K, Roenker DL, Bruni JR: Developmental changes in attention and visual search throughout adulthood. In Enns JI (ed): Adv Psychol 69:489, 1990

192. Ball K, Owsley C, Beard B: Clinical visual perimetry underestimates peripheral field problems in older adults. Clin Vis Sci 5:113, 1990

193. Ball K, Owsley C, Sloane ME et al: Visual attention problems as a predictor of vehicle crashes in older drivers. Invest Ophthalmol Vis Sci 34:3110, 1993

194. Rizzo M, Reinach S, McGehee D, Dawson J: Simulated car crashes and crash predictors in drivers with Alzheimer's disease. Arch Neurol 54:545, 1997

195. MacKay G, Dunlop JC: The cerebral lesions in a case of complete acquired colour-blindness. Scott Med Surg J 5:503, 1899

196. Pallis CA: Impaired identification of faces and places with agnosia for colors. J Neurol Neurosurg Psychiatry 18:218, 1955

197. Meadows JC: Disturbed perception of colors associated with localized cerebral lesions. Brain 97:615, 1974

198. Damasio A, Yamada T, Damasio H et al: Central achromatopsia: behavioral, anatomic, and physiologic aspects. Neurology 30:1064, 1980

199. Albert ML, Reches A, Silverberg R: Hemianopic colour blindness. J Neurol Neurosurg Psychiatry 38:546, 1975

200. Kölmel HW: Pure homonymous hemiachromatopsia. Findings with neuroophthalmologic examination and imaging procedures. Eur Arch Psychiatr Neurol Sci 237:237, 1988

201. Paulson HL, Galetta SL, Grossman M, Alavi A: Hemiachromatopsia of unilateral occipitotemporal infarcts. Am J Ophthalmol 118:518, 1994

202. Verrey D: Hemiachromatopsie droite absolue. Arch Ophthalmol (Paris) 8:289, 1888

203. Zeki S: A century of cerebral achromatopsia. Brain 113:1727, 1990

204. Plant GT: Disorders of colour vision in diseases of the nervous system, In Cronly-Dillon JR (ed): Inherited and Acquired Colour Vision Deficiencies: Fundamental Aspects and Clinical Studies, p 173. Boca Raton, FL, CRC Press, 1991

205. Pearlman AL, Birch J, Meadows JC: Cerebral color blindness: An acquired defect in hue discrimination. Ann Neurol 5:253, 1979

206. Victor JD, Maiese K, Shapley R et al: Acquired central dyschromatopsia: analysis of a case with preservation of color discrimination. Clin Vis Sci 4:183, 1989

207. Heywood CA, Cowey A, Newcombe F: Chromatic discrimination in a cortically blind observer. Eur J Neurosci 3:802, 1991

208. Damasio H, Frank R: Three-dimensional in vivo mapping of brain lesions in humans. Arch Neurol 49:137, 1992

209. Lueck CJ, Zeki S, Friston KJ et al: The color center in the cerebral cortex. Nature 340:386, 1989

210. Engel S, Zhang X, Wandell B: Color tuning in human visual cortex measured with functional magnetic resonance imaging. Nature 388:68, 1997

211. Ogden JA: Visual object agnosia, prosopagnosia, achromatopsia, loss of visual imagery, and autobiographical amnesia following recovery from cortical blindness: case M.H. Neuropsychologia 31:571, 1993

212. Green GJ, Lessell S: Acquired cerebral dyschromatopsia. Arch Ophthalmol 95:121, 1977

213. Linksz A: An Essay on Color Vision and Clinical Color Vision Tests. New York, Grune and Stratton, 1964

214. Working Group 41, 19 NAS-NRC Committee on Vision: Procedures for Testing Color Vision. Washington, DC, National Academy Press, 1981

215. Wyszecki G, Stiles WS: Color Science: Concepts and Methods, Quantitative Data and Formulae, 2nd ed. New York, Wiley, 1982.

216. Hardy LH, Rand G, Rittler MD: AO-HRR Pseudoisochromatic Plates, 2nd ed. Chicago: American Optical Co., 1957

217. Ichikawa K, Hukame H, Tanabe S: Detection of acquired color vision defects by standard pseudoisochromatic plates, part 2. Doc Ophthalmol Proc 46:133, 1987

218. Frisèn L, Kalm P: Sahlgren's saturation test for detecting and grading acquired dyschromatopsia. Am J Ophthalmol 92:252, 1981

219. Verriest G, Uvijls A, Aspinall P et al: The lightness discrimination test. Bull Soc Belge Ophtalmol 183:162, 1979

220. Pinckers A, Verriest G: Results of shorthand lightness discrimination test. In Verriest G (ed): Color Vision Deficiencies, Vol VII, p 163. Dordrecht, The Netherlands, Martinus Nijhoff/Dr. W Junk, 1987

221. Heywood CA, Wilson B, Cowey A: A case study of cortical colour 'blindness' with relatively intact achromatic discrimination. J Neurol Neurosurg Psychiatry 50:22, 1987

222. Berlin B, Kay P: Basic Color Terms. Berkeley, University of California Press, 1969

223. Holmes G: Pure word blindness. Folia Psychiatr Neurol Neurochir Neerl 53:279, 1950

224. Oxbury JM, Oxbury SM, Humphrey NK: Varieties of color anomia. Brain 92:847, 1969

225. Davidoff JB, Ostergaard AL: Colour anomia resulting from weakened short-term colour memory. A case study. Brain 107:415, 1984

226. de Vreese LP: Two systems for color-naming defects: verbal disconnection versus colour imagery disorder. Neuropsychologia 29:1, 1991

227. Land EH, Hubel DH, Livingstone MS et al: Color-generating interaction across the corpus callosum. Nature 303:616, 1983

228. Kennard C, Lawden M, Morland AB et al: Color identification and color constancy are impaired in a patient with incomplete achromatopsia associated with prestriae lesions. Proc R Soc Lond B 260:169, 1995

229. Land EH: Recent advances in retinex theory. Vis Res 26:7, 1986

230. Damasio AR: Disorders of complex visual processing: agnosias, achromatopsia, Bálint's syndrome, and related difficulties of orientation and construction, In Mesulam M (ed): Principles of Behavioral Neurology, p 259. Philadelphia, Davis, 1985

231. Lissauer H: Ein fall von seelenblindheit nebst einern Beitrag zur Theorie deselben. Arch Psychiatr Nervenkr 21:22, 1890

232. Tranel D: Assessment of higher-order visual function. Curr Opin Ophthalmol 5:29, 1994

233. Anderson SW, Rizzo M: Recovery and rehabilitation of visual cortical dysfunction. Neurorehabilitation 5:129, 1995
234. Lezak MD: Neuropsychological Assessment, 3rd ed. New York, Oxford University Press, 1995
235. Spreen O, Strauss E: A Compendium of Neuropsychological Tests: Administration Norms and Commentary, p 157. New York, Oxford University Press, 1991
236. Benton AL, Van Allen MW: Visuoperceptual, visuospatial, and visuoconstructive disorders. In Heilman KM, Valenstein E (eds): Clinical Neuropsychology, 2nd ed, p 161. London, Oxford University Press, 1985.
237. Wechsler D: WAIS-R Manual. New York, Psychological Corporation, 1981.
238. Benton AL, Hamsher J, Varney NR et al: Contributions to Neuropsychological Assessment. New York, Oxford University Press, 1983.
239. Goodglass H, Kaplan E: The Assessment of Aphasia and Related Disorders, 2nd ed. Philadelphia, Lea and Febiger, 1983.
240. Hooper HE: The Hooper Visual Organization Test Manual. Los Angeles, Western Psychological Services, 1958.
241. Mooney CM, Ferguson GA: A new closure test. Can J Psychol 5:129, 1951
242. Lansdell H: Relation of extent of temporal removals to closure and visuomotor factors. Percept Mot Skills 31:491, 1970
243. Newcombe F: Selective deficits after focal cerebral injury. In Dimond SJ, Beanmont JG (eds): Hemisphere Function in the Human Brain, p 311. New York, Halsted Press, 1974.
244. Young AW, Ellis HD: Childhood prosopagnosia. Brain Cogn 9:16, 1989
245. de Haan EHF, Campbell R: A fifteen year follow-up of a case of developmental prosopagnosia. Cortex 27:489, 1991
246. Kracke I: Developmental prosopagnosia in Asperger syndrome: presentation and discussion of an individual case. Dev Med Child Neurol 36:873, 1994
247. Takahashi N, Kawamura M, Hirayama K et al: Prosopagnosia: a clinical and anatomic study of four patients. Cortex 31:317, 1995
248. Malone DR, Morris HH, Kay MC, Levin HS: Prosopagnosia: a double dissociation between the recognition of familiar and unfamiliar faces. J Neurol Neurosurg Psychiatry 45:820, 1982
249. Rizzo M, Hurtig R, Damasio AR: The role of scanpaths in facial recognition and learning. Ann Neurol 22:41, 1987
250. Sergent J, Villemure J-G: Prosopagnosia in a right hemispherectomized patient. Brain 112:975, 1989
251. Renault B, Signoret J-L, DeBruille B et al: Brain potentials reveal covert facial recognition in prosopagnosia. Neuropsychologia 27:905, 1989
252. de Haan EHF, Young AW, Newcombe F: Face recognition without awareness. Cogn Neuropsychol 4:385, 1987
253. de Haan EHF, Young AW, Newcombe F: Faces interfere with name classification in a prosopagnosic patient. Cortex 23:309, 1987
254. Bruyer R: Covert facial recognition in prosopagnosia: a review. Brain Cogn 15:223, 1991
255. Tranel D, Damasio AR: Knowledge without awareness: an autonomic index of facial recognition by prosopagnosics. Science 228: 1453, 1985
256. Bauer RM: Autonomic recognition of names and faces in prosopagnosia: a neuropsychological application of the guilty knowledge test. Neuropsychologia 22:457, 1984
257. Bauer RM, Verfaellie M: Electrodermal discrimination of familiar but not unfamiliar faces in prosopagnosia. Brain Cogn 8: 240, 1988
258. Sergent J, Poncet M: From covert to overt recognition of faces in a prosopagnosic patient. Brain 113:989, 1990
259. Bruyer R, Laterre C, Seron X et al: A case of prosopagnosia with some preserved covert remembrance of familiar faces. Brain Cogn 2:257, 1983
260. McNeil JE, Warrington EK: Prosopagnosia: a reclassification. Q J Exp Psychol 43A:267, 1991
261. Newcombe F, Young AW, de Haan EHF: Prosopagnosia and object agnosia without covert recognition. Neuropsychologia 27: 179, 1989
262. Schweinberger SR, Klos T, Sommer W: Covert face recognition in prosopagnosia: a dissociable function? Cortex 31:517, 1995
263. Deleted in proof
264. Evans JJ, Heggs AJ, Antoun N, Hodges JR: Progressive prosopagnosi associated with selective right temporal lobe atrophy. Brain 118:1, 1995
265. Campbell R, Heywood CA, Cowey A et al: Sensitivity to eye gaze in prosopagnosic patients and monkeys with superior temporal sulcus ablation. Neuropsychologia 28:1123, 1990
266. Damasio AR, Damasio H, van Hoesen GW: Prosopagnosia: anatomic basis and behavioral mechanisms. Neurology 32:331, 1982
267. Kosslyn SM, Hamilton SE, Bernstein JH: The perception of curvature can be selectively disrupted in prosopagnosia. Brain Cogn 27:36, 1995
268. Hécaen H, Angelargues R: Agnosia for faces (prosopagnosia). Arch Neurol 7:92, 1962
269. Assal G: Regression des troubles de la reconnaissance des physiognomies et de la mémoire topographique chez un malade opéré d'un hématome intracérébral pariéto-temporal droit. Rev Neurol 121:184, 1969
270. Whitely AM, Warrington EK: Prosopagnosia: a clinical, psychological and anatomical study of three patients. J Neurol Neurosurg Psychiatry 40:395, 1977
271. Benson DF, Segarra J, Albert ML: Visual agnosia-prosopagnosia. Arch Neurol 30:307, 1974
272. Lhermitte F, Chain F, Escourolle R et al: Étude anatomo-clinique d'un cas de prosopagnosie. Rev Neurol 126:329, 1972
273. Ettlin TM, Beckson M, Benson DF et al: Prosopagnosia: a bihemispheric disorder. Cortex 28:129, 1992
274. Benton A: Facial recognition 1990. Cortex 26:491, 1990
275. Landis T, Regard M, Bliestle A, Kleihues P: Prosopagnosia and agnosia for non-canonical views. Brain 111:1287, 1988
276. Landis T, Cummings JL, Christen L et al: Are unilateral right posterior lesions sufficient to cause prosopagnosia? Clinical and radiological findings in six additional patients. Cortex 22:243, 1986
277. de Renzi E: Prosopagnosia in two patients with CT scan evidence of damage confined to the right hemisphere. Neuropsychologia 24:385, 1986
278. Michel F, Perenin M-T, Sieroff E: Prosopagnosie sans hémianopsie après lésion unilatérale occipito-temporale droite. Rev Neurol 142:545, 1986
279. Michel F, Poncet M, Signoret JL: Les lésions responsables de la prosopagnosie sont-elles toujours bilatérales? Rev Neurol 146: 764, 1989
280. Farah MJ, Levinson KL, Klein KL: Face perception and within-category discrimination in prosopagnosia. Neuropsychologia 33: 661, 1995
281. Damasio AR: Prosopagnosia. Trends Neurosci 8:132, 1985
282. Tyrell PJ, Warrington EK, Frackowiak RSJ, Rossor MN: Progressive degeneration of the right temporal lobe studied with positron emission tomography. J Neurol Neurosurg Psychiatry 53:1048, 1990
283. Damasio AR, Tranel D, Damasio H: Face agnosia and the neural substrates of memory. Annu Rev Neurosci 13:89, 1990
284. Kay MC, Levin HS: Prosopagnosia. Am J Ophthalmol 94:75, 1982
285. de Renzi E: Prosopagnosia in two patients with CT scan evidence of damage confined to the right hemisphere. Neuropsychologia 24:385, 1986
286. Levine DN, Warach J, Farah M: Two visual systems in mental imagery: dissociation of "what" and "where" in imagery disorders due to bilateral posterior cerebral lesions. Neurology 35: 1010, 1985
287. de Renzi E, Faglioni P, Grossi D, Nichelli P: Apperceptive and associative forms of prosopagnosia. Cortex 27:213, 1991
288. Mendez MF, Martin RJ, Smyth KA, Whitehouse PJ: Disturbances of person identification in Alzheimer's disease. A retrospective study. J Nerv Ment Dis 180:94, 1992
289. Dewick HC, Hanley JR, Davies AD et al: Perception and memory for faces in Parkinson's disease. Neuropsychologia 29:785, 1991
290. McConachie HR: Developmental prosopagnosia, a single case report. Cortex 12:76, 1976
291. Heywood CA, Cowey A, Newcombe F: On the role of parvocel-

lular (P) and magnocellular (M) pathways in cerebral achromatopsia. Brain 117:245, 1994

292. Landis T, Cummings JL, Christen L et al: Are unilateral right posterior lesions sufficient to cause prosopagnosia? Clinical and radiological findings in six additional patients. Cortex 22:243, 1986

293. de Renzi E: Current issues in prosopagnosia. In Ellis HD, Jeeves MA, Newcome F, Young A (eds): Aspects of Face Processing. Dordecht, Martinus Nijhoff, 1986

294. Farah MJ, Wilson KD, Drain HM, Tanaka JR: The inverted face inversion effect in prosopagnosia: evidence for mandatory, face-specific perceptual mechanisms. Vision Res 35:2089, 1995

295. Young AW, Aggleton JP, Hellawell DJ et al: Face processing impairments after amygdalotomy. Brain 118:15, 1995

296. de Renzi E, Faglioni P, Spinnler H: The performance of patients with unilateral brain damage on face recognition tasks. Cortex 1968;4:17, 1968

297. de Renzi E, Bonacini MG, Faglioni P: Right posterior brain-damaged patients are poor at assessing the age of a face. Neuropsychologia 27:839, 1989

298. Young AW, Newcombe F, de Haan EHF et al: Face perception after brain injury. Brain 116:941, 1993

299. Behrmann M, Black SE, Bub DN: The evolution of pure alexia: a longitudinal study of recovery. Brain Lang 39:405, 1990

300. Bub DN, Arguin M: Visual word activation in pure alexia. Brain Lang 49:77, 1995

301. Binder JR, Mohr JP: The topography of callosal readin pathways. A case control analysis. Brain 115:1807, 1992

302. Black SE, Behrmann M: Localization in alexia. In Kertes A (ed): Localization and Neuroimaging in Neuropsychology, p 331. San Diego: Academic Press, 1994

303. Bub DN, Black SE, Howell J: Word recognition and orthographic context effects in letter-by-letter reader. Brain Lang 36:357, 1989

304. Coslett HB, Saffran EM, Greenbaum S, Schwartz H: Reading in pure alexia. Brain 116:21, 1993

305. Jibiki I, Yamaguchi N: The gogi (word-meaning) syndrome with impaired kanji processing: alexia with agraphia. Brain Lang 45:61, 1993

306. Albert ML, Yamadori A, Gardner H, Howes D: Comprehension in alexia. Brain 96:317, 1973

307. Coslett HB, Saffran EM: Evidence for preserved reading in pure alexia. Brain 112:327, 1989

308. Caplan LR, Hedley-White T: Cuing and memory dysfunction in alexia without agraphia: a case report. Brain 97:251, 1974

309. Landis T, Regard M, Serrat A: Iconic reading in a case of alexia without agraphia caused by a brain tumor: a tachistoscopic study. Brain Lang 11:45, 1980

310. Feinberg TE, Dyckes-Berke D, Miner CR, Roane DM: Knowledge, implicit knowledge and metaknowledge in visual agnosia and pure alexia. Brain 118:789, 1995

311. Warrington EK, Shallice T: Word-form dyslexia. Brain 103:99, 1980

312. Damasio AR, Damasio H: The anatomic basis of pure alexia. Neurology 33:1573, 1983

313. de Renzi E, Zambolin A, Crisi G: The pattern of neuropsychological impairment associated with left posterior cerebral artery infarcts. Brain 110:1099, 1987

314. Vincent FM, Sadowsky CH, Saunders RL, Reeves AG: Alexia without agraphia, hemianopia, or color-naming defect: a disconnection syndrome. Neurology 27:689, 1977

315. Uitti RJ, Donat JR, Romanchuk K: Pure alexia without hemianopia. Arch Neurol 41:1130, 1984

316. Ajax ET: Dyslexia without agraphia. Arch Neurol 17:645, 1967

317. Henderson VW, Friedman RB, Teng EL, Weiner JM: Left hemisphere pathways in reading: inferences from pure alexia without hemianopia. Neurology 35:962, 1985

318. Erdem S, Kansu T: Alexia without either agraphia or hemianopia in temporal lobe lesion due to herpes simplex encephalitis. J Neuro-ophthalmol 15:102, 1995

319. Friedman DI, Hu EH, Sadun AA: Neuro-ophthalmic complications of interleukin 2 therapy. Arch Ophthalmol 109:1679, 1991

320. Dejerine J: Contribution a l'atude anatomo-pathologique et clinique des differentes varietes de cecite verbale. Mem Soc Biol 4:51, 1892

321. Geschwind N: Disconnexion syndromes in animals and man. Brain 88:17, 1965

322. Silver FL, Chawluk JB, Bosley TM et al: Resolving metabolic abnormalities in a case of pure alexia. Neurology 38:731, 1988

323. Stommel EW, Friedman RJ, Reeves AG: Alexia without agraphia associated with spleniogeniculate infarction. Neurology 41:587, 1991

324. Iragui V, Kritchevsky M: Alexia without agraphia or hemianopia in parietal infarction. J Neurol Neurosurg Psychiatry 54:841, 1991

325. Farah MJ: Visual Agnosia. Cambridge, MA, MIT Press, 1990.

326. Vaina LM: Functional segregation of color and motion processing in the human visual cortex: clinical evidence. Cereb Cortex 5:555, 1994

327. Rentschler I, Treutwein B, Landis T: Dissociation of local and global processing in visual agnosia. Vis Res 34:963, 1994

328. Livingstone MS, Rosen GD, Drislane FW, Galaburda AM: Physiological and anatomical evidence for magnocellular defect in development dyslexia. Proc Natl Acad Sci USA 88:7943, 1991

329. Gazzaniga MS, Freedman H: Observations on visual processes after posterior callosal section. Neurology 23:1126, 1973

330. Castro-Caldas A, Salgado V: Right hemifield alexia without hemianopia. Arch Neurol 41:84, 1984

331. Binder JR, Lazar RM, Tatemichi TK et al: Left hemiparalexia. Neurology 42:562, 1992

331a. Dejerine J: Sur un cas de cecite verbale avec agraphie, suive d'autopsie. C.R. Societé du Biologie 43:197, 1891

332. Benson DF: Alexia. In Bruyn GW, Klawans HL, Vinken PJ (eds): Handbook of Clinical Neurology, p 433. New York, Elsevier, 1985

333. Kawahata N, Nagata K: Alexia with agraphia due to the left posterior inferiotemporal lobe lesion: neuropsychological analysis and its pathogenetic mechanisms. Brain Lang 33:296, 1988

334. Benson DF, Brown J, Tomlinson EB: Varieties of alexia. Word and letter blindness. Neurology 21:951, 1971

335. Benson DF: The third alexia. Arch Neurol 34:327, 1977

336. Kirkham TH: The ocular symptomology of pituitary tumors. Proc R Soc Med 65:517, 1972

337. Zihl J: Eye movement patterns in hemianopic dyslexia. Brain 118:891, 1995

338. Behrmann M, Moscovitch M, Black SE, Mozer M: Perceptual and conceptual factors in neglect dyslexia: two contrasting case studies. Brain 113:1163, 1990

339. Patterson K, Wilson B: A rose is a nose: a deficit in initial letter identification. Cogn Neuropsychol 13:447, 1990

340. Shallice T, Warrington EK: The possible role of selective attention in acquired dyslexia. Neuropsychologia 15:31, 1977

341. Levine DN, Calvanio R: A study of the visual defect in verbal alexia-simultanagnosia. Brain 101:65, 1978

342. Bálint R: Seelenlahmung des 'Schauens' optische Ataxie, raumliche Storung der Aufmerksamkeit. Monstsschr Psychiatr Neurol 25:51, 1909

343. Holmes G: Disturbances of vision caused by cerebral lesions. Br J Ophthalmol 2:353, 1918

344. Pierrot-Deseilligny C, Gray F, Brunet P: Infarcts of both inferior parietal lobules with impairment of visually guided eye movements, peripheral visual inattention, and optic ataxia. Brain 109:81, 1986

345. Husain M, Stein J: Rezso Balint and his most celebrated case. Arch Neurol 45:89, 1988

346. Friedman DI, Jankovic J, McCrary JA: Neuro-ophthalmic findings in progressive supranuclear palsy. J Clin Neuro-Ophthalmol 12:104, 1992

347. Shallice T, Warrington EK, McCarthy R: Reading without semantics. Q J Exp Psychol 35A:111, 1983

348. Patterson KE, Morton J: From orthograph to phonology: an attempt at an old interpretation. In Patterson KE, Marshall JC, Coltheart M (eds): Surface Dyslexia, p 335. London, Erlbaum, 1985

349. Cummings JL, Houlihan JP, Hill MA: The pattern of reading deterioration in dementia of the Alzheimer type. Brain Lang 29:315, 1986

350. Beauvois M-F, Derouesne J: Phonological alexia: three dissociations. J Neurol Neurosurg Psychiatry 42:1115, 1979

351. Funnell E: Phonological processes in reading: new evidence from acquired dyslexia. Br J Psychol 74:159, 1983

352. Friedman RB, Kohn SE: Impaired activation of the phonological lexicon: effects upon oral reading. Brain Lang 38:278, 1990

353. Friedman RB: Two types of phonological alexia. Cortex 31:397, 1995

354. Coltheart M: Deep dyslexia, a review of the syndrome. In Coltheart M, Patterson KE, Marshall JC (eds): Deep Dyslexia, p 22. London, Routledge & Kegan Paul, 1980

355. Hécaen H, de Ajuriaguerra J: Balint's syndrome (psychic paralysis of visual fixation) and its minor forms. Brain 77:373, 1954

356. Wolpert T: Die Simultanagnosie. Z Gesamte Neurol Psychiatr 93:397, 1924

357. Teuber HL: Alteration of perception and memory in man. In Weiskrantz L (ed): Analysis of Behavioral Change. New York, Harper and Row, 1968

358. Holmes G: Disturbances of visual orientation. Br J Ophthalmol 2:449, 1918

359. Luria AR: Disorders of simultaneous perception in a case of bilateral occipito-parietal brain injury. Brain 82:437, 1959

360. Luria AR, Pravdina-Vinarskaya EN, Yarbus AL: Disturbances of ocular movement in a case of simultanagnosia. Brain 86:219, 1962

361. Cogan DG: Congenital ocular motor apraxia. Can J Ophthalmol 1:253, 1965

362. Holmes G: Spasm of fixation. Trans Ophthalmol Soc UK 50:253, 1930

363. Johnston JL, Sharpe JA, Morrow MJ: Spasm of fixation: a quantitative study. J Neurol Sci 107:166, 1992

364. Rizzo M, Hurtig R: Visual search in hemineglect: what stirs idle eyes? Clin Vis Sci 7:39, 1992

365. Benton AL: Gerstmann's syndrome. Arch Neurol 49:445, 1992

366. Vaina LM: Selective impairment of visual motion interpretation following lesions of the right occipito-parietal area in humans. Biol Cybern 61:347, 1989

367. Vaina LM, Lemay M, Bienfang DC et al: Intact "biological motion" and "structure from motion" perception in a patient with impaired motion mechanisms. A case study. Vis Neurosci 5:353, 1990

368. Haussser CO, Robert F, Giard N: Balint's syndrome. Can J Neurol Sci 7:157, 1980

369. Ogren MP, Mateer CA, Wyler AR: Alterations in visually related eye movements following left pulvinar damage in man. Neuropsychologia 22:187, 1984

370. Rizzo M, Robin DA: Simultanagnosia: a defect of sustained attention yields insights on visual information processing. Neurology 40:447, 1990

371. Rizzo M, Rotella D, Darling W: Troubled reaching after right occipito-temporal damage. Neuropsychologia 30:711, 1992

372. Oxford University Press, p 345, 1995

373. James W: The Principles of Psychology, Vol 1, p 403. New York, Dover, 1890.

374. Mackworth NH: The breakdown of vigilance during prolonged visual search. Q J Exp Psychol 1:6, 1948

375. Broadbent DE: Perception and Communication. New York, Pergamon Press, 1958.

376. Mackworth NH, Kaplan IT, Matlay W: Eye movements during vigilance. Percept Mot Skills 18:397, 1964

377. Nakayama K: Biological image motion processing: a review. Vis Res 25:625, 1985

337a. Northcutt R, Kass J: Evolution and development of neocortex. TINS 9:378, 1995

378. Allman JM, Kaas JH: Representation of the visual field in striate and adjoining cortex of the owl monkey (Aotus trivirgatus). Brain Res 35:89, 1971

379. Dubner R, Zeki SM: Response properties and receptive fields of cells in an anatomically defined region of the superior temporal sulcus in the monkey. Brain Res 35:528, 1971

380. Maunsell JH, van Essen DC: The connections of the middle temporal visual area (MT) and their relationship to a cortical hierarchy in the macaque monkey. J Neurosci 3:2563, 1983

381. Albright TD: Direction and orientation selectivity in visual area MT of the macaque. J Neurophysiol 52:1106, 1984

382. Newsome WT, Paré EB: A selective impairment of motion perception following lesions of the middle temporal visual area (MT). J Neurosci 8:2201, 1988

383. Yamasaki DS, Wurtz RH: Recovery of function after lesions in the superior temporal sulcus in the monkey. J Neurophysiol 66:651, 1991

384. Pasternak T, Merigan HW: Motion perception following lesions of the superior temporal sulcus in the monkey. Cereb Cortex 4:247, 1994

385. Zihl J, von Cramon D, Mai N, Schmid C: Disturbance of movement vision after bilateral posterior brain damage. Further evidence and follow-up observations. Brain 114:2235, 1991

386. Plant GT, Laxer KD, Barbaro NM et al: Impaired visual motion perception in the contralateral hemifield following unilateral posterior cerebral lesions in humans. Brain 116:1303, 1993

387. Baker CL Jr, Hess RF, Zihl J: Residual motion perception in a "motion-blind" patient, assessed with limited-lifetime random-dot stimuli. J Neurosci 11:454, 1991

388. Shipp S, de Jong BM, Zihl J et al: The brain activity related to residual motion vision in a patient with bilateral lesions of V5. Brain 117:1023, 1994

389. Watson JDG, Myers R, Frackowiak RSJ et al: Area V5 of the human brain: evidence from a combined study using positron emission tomography and magnetic resonance imaging. Cereb Cortex 3:79, 1993

390. Tootell RB, Taylor JB: Anatomical evidence for MT and additional cortical visual areas in humans. Cereb Cortex 5:39, 1995

391. Barton JJS, Simpson T, Kiriakopoulos E et al: Functional magnetic resonance imaging of lateral occipitotemporal cortex during pursuit and motion perception. Ann Neurol 40:387, 1996

392. Greenlee MW, Lang HJ, Mergner T, Seeger W: Visual short-term memory of stimulus velocity in patients with unilateral posterior brain damage. J Neurosci 15:2287, 1995

393. Greenlee MW, Smith AT: Detection and discrimination of first-order and second-order motion in patients with unilateral brain damage. J Neurosci 17:804, 1997

394. Barton JJS, Sharpe JA, Raymond JE: Retinotopic and directional defects in motion discrimination in humans with cerebral lesions, Ann Neurol 37:665, 1995

395. Vaina L: Selective impairment of visual motion interpretation following lesions of the right occipito-parietal area in humans. Biol Cybern 61:347, 1989

396. Regan D, Giaschi D, Sharpe JA, Hong XH: Visual processing of motion-defined form: selective failure in patients with parieto-temporal lesions. J Neurosci 12:2198, 1992

397. Nawrot M, Shannon E, Rizzo M: Measuring visual function. Curr Opin Ophthalmol 4:30, 1993

398. Nawrot M, Rizzo M, Damasio H: Motion perception in humans with focal cerebral lesions [abstract]. Invest Ophthalmol Vis Sci 34(suppl):1231, 1993

399. Nawrot M, Rizzo M: Motion perception deficits from midline cerebellar lesions in human. Vis Res 35:723, 1994

400. Dupont P, Orban GA, de Bruyn B et al: Many areas in the human brain respond to visual motion. J Neurophysiol 72:1420, 1994

401. Gilmore GC, Wenk HE, Naylor LA, Koss E: Motion perception and Alzheimer's disease. J Gerontol 49:52, 1994

402. Silverman SE, Tran DB, Zimmerman KM, Feldon SE: Dissociation between the detection and perception of motion in Alzheimer's disease. Neurology 44:1814, 1994

403. Kurylo DD, Corkin S, Rizzo JF: Greater relative impairment of object recognition than of visuospatial abilities in Alzheimer's disease. Neuropsychology 10:74, 1996

404. Rizzo M, Nawrot M: Perception of movement and shape in Alzheimer's disease. Brain 121:2259, 1998

405. Hinton DR, Sadun AA, Blanks JC, Miller CA: Optic nerve degeneration in Alzheimer' disease. N Engl J Med 315:485, 1986

406. Sathian K: Motion perception in Alzheimer's disease. Neurology 45:1633, 1995

407. Barton JJ: Motion perception in Alzheimer's disease [letter; comment]. Neurology 45:1634, 1995

408. Silverman SE, Feldon SE: Motion perception in Alzheimer's disease. Neurology 45:1634, 1995

409. Critchley M. Types of visual perseveration: "paliopsia" and "illusory visual spread." Brain 74:267, 1951

410. Bender MB, Feldman M, Sobin AJ. Palinopsia. Brain 91:321, 1968

411. Bender MB. Polyopia and monocular diplopia of cerebral origin. Arch Neurol Psychiatry 54:323, 1945

412. Michel EM, Troost, BT. Palinopsia: cerebral localization with computed tomography. Neurol 30:887, 1980

413. Meadows JC. Observations on a case of monocular diplopia of cerebral origin. J Neurol Sci 18:249, 1973

414. Lopez JR, Adornato BT, Hoyt WF. "Entomopia:" a remarkable case of cerebral polyopia. Neurol 43:2145, 1993

415. Kinsbourne M, Warrington EK. A study of visual perseveration. J Neurol Neurosurg Psychiatr 26:468, 1963

416. Cummings JL, Syndulko K, Goldberg Z, Treiman DM. Palinopsia reconsidered. Neurol 32:444, 1982

417. Meadows JC, Munro SSF. Palinopsia. J Neurol Neurosurg Psychiatr 40:5, 1977

418. Swash M. Visual perseveration in temporal lobe epilepsy. J Neurol Neurosurg Psychiatr 42:569, 1979

419. Young WB, Heros DO, Ehrenberg BL, Hedges TR. Metamorphopsia and palinopsia. Association with periodic lateralized epileptiform discharges. Arch Neurol 46:820, 1989

420. Muller T, Buttner T, Kuhn W, Heinz A, Przuntek H. Palinopsia as sensory epileptic phenomenon. Acta Neurol Scand 91:433, 1995

420a. Lefebre C, Kölmel HW. Palinopsia as an epileptic phenomenon. Eur Neurol 29:323, 1989

421. Joseph AB. Cotard's syndrome in a patient with coexistent Capgras' syndrome, syndrome of subjective doubles, and palinopsia. J Clin Psychiatry 47:605, 1986

422. Kawasaki A, Purvin V. Persistent palinopsia following ingestion of lysergic acid diethylamide (LSD). Arch Ophthalmol 114:47, 1996.

423. McGuire PK, Cope H, Fahy TA. Diversity of psychopathology associated with use of 3,4-methylenedioxymethamphetamine ("Ecstasy"). Brit J Psychiatry 165:391, 1994

424. Purvin VA: Visual disturbances secondary to clomiphene citrate. Arch Ophthalmol 113:482, 1995

425. Hughes MS, Lessell S: Trazodone-induced palinopsia. Arch Ophthalmol 18:399, 1990

426. Johnson SF, Loge RV: Palinopsia due to non-ketotic hyperglycemia. West J Med 148:331, 1988

427. Marneros A, Korner J: Chronic palinopsia in schizophrenia. Psychopathology 26:236, 1993

428. Gates TJ, Stagno SJ, Gulledge AD: Palinopsia posing as psychotic depression. Br J Psychiatry 153:391, 1988

429. Jacome DE: Palinopsia and bitemporal visual extinction on fixation. Ann Ophthalmol 17:251, 1985

430. Cleland PG, Saunders M, Rosser R: An unusual case of visual perseveration. J Neurol Neurosurg Psychiatry 44:262, 1981

431. Lazaro RP: Palinopsia: rare but ominous symptom of cerebral dysfunction. Neurosurgery 13:310, 1983

432. Purvin V, Bonnin J, Goodman J: Palinopsia as a presenting manifestation of Creutzfeld-Jakob disease. J Clin Neuro-Ophthalmol 9:242, 1989

433. Hirst LW, Miller NR, Johnson RT: Monocular polyopia: Arch Neurol 40:756, 1983

434. Crews SJ, Gordon A, Nowakowski R: Management of monocular polyopia using an artificial iris contact lens. J Am Optom Assoc 59:140, 1948

435. Basuk WL, Zisman M, Waring GO et al: Complications of hexagonal keratotomy. Am J Ophthalmol 117:37, 1994

436. Gottlieb D: The unidirectionality of cerebral polyopia. J Clin Neuroophthalmol 12:257, 1992

437. Lerner AJ, Koss E, Patterson MB et al: Concomitants of visual hallucinations in Alzheimer's disease. Neurology 44:523, 1994

438. Olbrich HM, Engelmeier MP, Pauleikhoff D, Waubke T: Visual hallucinations in ophthalmology. Graefes Arch Clin Exp Ophthalmol 225:217, 1987

439. Ames D, Wirshing WC, Szuba MP: Organic mental disorders associated with bupropion in three patients. J Clin Psychiatry 53:53, 1992

440. Rivas DA, Chancellor MB, Hill K, Freedman MK: Neurological manifestations of baclofen withdrawal. J Urol 150:1903, 1993

441. Piltz JR, Wertenbaker C, Lance SE et al: Digoxin toxicity. Recognizing the varied visual presentations. J Clin Neuro-Ophthalmol 13:275, 1993

442. Chen JL, Brocavitch JM, Lin AY: Psychiatric disturbances associated with ganciclovir therapy. Ann Pharmacother 26:193, 1992

443. Gosh K, Sivakumaran M, Murphy P et al: Visual hallucinations following treatment with vincristine. Clin Lab Hematol 16:355, 1994

444. Platz WE, Oberlaender FA, Seidel ML: The phenomenology of perceptual hallucinations in alcohol-induced delirium tremens. Psychopathology 28:247, 1995

445. Sanchez-Ramos JR, Ortoll R, Paulson GW: Visual hallucinations associated with Parkinson's disease. Arch Neurol 53:1265, 1996

446. Lera G, Vaamonde J, Rodriguez M, Obeso JA: Cabergoline in Parkinson's disease: long-term follow-up. Neurology 43:2587, 1993

447. Zoldan J, Friedberg G, Livneh M, Melamed E: Psychosis in advanced Parkinson's disease: treatment with ondansetron, a 5-HT3 receptor antagonist. Neurology 45:1305, 1995

448. Lepore FE: Spontaneous visual phenomena with visual loss: 104 patients with lesions of retinal and neural afferent pathways. Neurology 40:444, 1990

449. Fernandez A, Lichtstein G, Vieweg VR: The Charles Bonnet syndrome: a review. J Nerv Ment Dis 185:195, 1997

450. Teunisse RJ, Cruysberg JRM, Hoefnagels WH et al: Visual hallucinations in psychological normal people: Charles Bonnet's syndrome. Lancet 347:794, 1996

451. Schultz G, Melzack R: The Charles Bonnet syndrome: "phantom visual images." Perception 20:809, 1991

452. Teunisse RJ, Cruysberg JRM, Verbeek A, Zitman FG: The Charles Bonnet syndrome: a large prospective study in The Netherlands. Br J Psychiatry 166:254, 1995

453. Cogan DG: Visual hallucinations as release phenomenon. Albrecht Graefes Arch Klin Exp Ophthalmol 188:139, 1973

454. Siatkowski RM, Zimmer B, Rosenberg PR: The Charles Bonnet syndrome. Visual perceptive dysfunction in sensory deprivation. J Clin Neuro-Ophthalmol 10:215, 1990

455. Weinberger LM, Grant FC: Visual hallucinations and their neuro-optical correlates. Arch Ophthalmol 23:166, 1940

456. Benegas NM, Liu GT, Volpe NJ, Galetta SL: "Picture within a picture" visual hallucinations. Neurology 47:1347, 1996

457. Cole MG: Charles Bonnet hallucinations: a case series. Can J Psychiatry 37:267, 1992

458. Heron W: The pathology of boredom. Sci Am 196:52, 1957

459. Kölmel HW: Coloured patterns in hemianopic fields. Brain 107:155, 1984

460. Plant GT: A centrally generated coloured phosphene. Clin Vis Sci 1:161, 1986

461. Anderson SW, Rizzo M: Hallucinations following occipital lobe damage: the pathological activation of visual representations. J Clin Exp Neurol 16:651, 1994

462. Lance JW: Simple formed hallucinations confined to the area of a specific visual field defect. Brain 99:719, 1976

463. Adair DK, Keshaven MS: The Charles Bonnet syndrome and grief reaction. Am J Psychiatry 145:895, 1988

464. Shedlack KJ, McDonald WM, Laskowitz DT, Krishnan KRR: Geniculocalcarine hyperintensities on brain magnetic resonance imaging associated with visual hallucinations in the elderly. Psychiatry Res 54:283, 1994

465. Fisman M: Musical hallucinations: report of two unusual cases. Can J Psychiatry 36:609, 1991

466. Bhatia MS, Khastgir U, Malik SC: Charles Bonnet syndrome. Br J Psychiatry 161:409, 1992

467. Badino R, Trucco M, Caja A et al: Release hallucinations and tiapride. Ital J Neurol Sci 15:183, 1994

468. Penfield W, Perot P: The brain's record of auditory and visual experience. Brain 86:595, 1963

469. Foerster O: The cerebral cortex in man. Lancet 2:309, 1931

470. Rousseau M, Debrock D, Cabaret M, Steinling M: Visual hallucinations with written words in a case of left parietotemporal lesion. J Neurol Neurosurg Psychiatry 57:1268, 1994

471. Panayiotopoulos CP: Elementary visual hallucinations in migraine and epilepsy. J Neurol Neurosurg Psychiatry 57:1371, 1994

472. Williamson PD, Thadani VM, Darcey TM et al: Occipital lobe

epilepsy: clinical characteristics, seizure spread patterns, and results of surgery. Ann Neurol 31:3, 1992

473. Lance JW, Smee RI: Partial seizures with visual disturbance treated by radiotherapy of cavernous hemangioma. Ann Neurol 26:782, 1989

474. Deleted in proof

475. Kölmel HW: Complex visual hallucinations in the hemianopic field. J Neurol Neurosurg Psychiatry 48:29, 1985

476. Gastaut H: A new type of epilepsy: benign partial epilepsy of childhood with occipital spike-waves. Clin Electroencephalogr 13:13, 1982

477. Hupp SL, Kline LB, Corbett JJ: Visual disturbances of migraine. Surv Ophthalmol 33:221, 1989

478. Lance JW, Anthony M: Some clinical aspects of migraine. A prospective survey of 500 patients. Arch Neurol 15:356, 1966

479. Plant GT: The fortification spectra of migraine. Br Med J 293:1613, 1986

480. Richards W: The fortification illusions of migraine. Sci Am 224:89, 1971

481. Grüsser O-J: Migraine phosphenes and the retino-cortical magnification factor. Vis Res 35:1125, 1995

482. Walker MC, Smith SJ, Sisodiya SM, Shorvon SD: Case of simple partial status epilepticus in occipital lobe epilepsy misdiagnosed as migraine: clinical, electrophysiological, and magnetic resonance imaging characteristics. Epilepsia 36:1233, 1995

483. Lees F: The migrainous symptoms of cerebral angiomata. J Neurol Neurosurg Psychiatry 25:45, 1962

484. Kupersmith MJ, Vargas ME, Madrid M et al: Occipital arteriovenous malformations: visual disturbances and presentation. Neurology 46:953, 1996

485. Liu GT, Schatz NJ, Galetta SL et al: Persistent positive phenomena in migraine. Neurology 45:664, 1995

486. Lhermitte J: Syndrome de la calotte du pedoncle cerebral: Les troubles psycho-sensoriels dans les lesions du mescephale. Rev Neurol (Paris) 38:1359, 1922

487. van Bogaert L: L'hallucinose pedonculaire. Rev Neurol (Paris) 43:608, 1927

488. Geller TJ, Bellur SN: Peduncular hallucinosis: magnetic resonance imaging confirmation of mesencephalic infarction during life. Ann Neurol 21:602, 1987

489. Tsukamoto H, Matsushima T, Fujiwara S, Fukui M: Peduncular hallucinosis following microvascular decompression for trigeminal neuralgia. Surg Neurol 40:31, 1993

490. McKee AC, Levine DN, Kowall NW, Richardson EP: Peduncular hallucinosis associated with isolated infarction of the substantia nigra pars reticulata. Ann Neurol 27:500, 1990

491. de la Fuente Fernandez R, Lopez JM, Rey del Corral P, de la Iglesia Martinez F: Peduncular hallucinosis and right hemiparkinsonism caused by left mesencephalic infarction. J Neurol Neurosurg Psychiatry 57:870, 1994

492. Nadvi SS, van Dellen JR: Transient peduncular hallucinosis secondary to brain stem compression by a medulloblastoma. Surg Neurol 41:250, 1994

493. Noda S, Mizoguchi M, Yamamoto A: Thalamic experiential hallucinosis. J Neurol Neurosurg Psychiatry 56:1224, 1993

494. Rozanski J: Peduncular hallucinosis following vertebral angiography. Neurology 1952;2:341, 1952

495. Feinberg WM, Rapcsak SZ: "Peduncular hallucinosis" following paramedian thalamic infarction. Neurology 39:1535, 1989

496. Cascino GD, Adams RD: Brainstem auditory hallucinosis. Neurology 36:1042, 1986

497. Serra Catafau J, Rubio F, Peres Serra J: Peduncular hallucinosis associated with posterio thalamic infarction. J Neurol 239:89, 1992

498. Caplan LR: "Top of the basilar" syndromes. Neurology 30:72, 1980

499. Dunn DW, Weisberg LA, Nadell J: Peduncular hallucinations caused by brainstem compression. Neurology 33:1360, 1983

500. Fisher CM: Visual hallucinations on eye closure associated with atropine toxicity: a neurologic analysis and comparison with other visual hallucinations. Can J Neurol Sci 19:18, 1991

501. Fisher CM: Visual hallucinations and racing thoughts on eye closure after minor surgery. Arch Neurol 48:1091, 1991

502. Heinemann EG, Tulving E, Nachmias J: The effects of oculomotor adjustments on apparent size. Am J Psychol 72:32, 1959

503. Alexander KR: On the nature of accommodative micropsia. Am J Optom Physiol Opt 52:79, 1975

504. Hollins M: Does accommodative micropsia exist? Am J Psychol 89:443, 1976

505. Myers WA: Micropsia and testicular retraction. Psychoanal Q 46:580, 1977

506. Schneck JM: Micropsia. Psychosomatics 10:249, 1969

507. Schneck JM: Psychogenic micropsia and a spontaneous auditory equivalent. Am J Clin Hypn 29:53, 1986

508. Frisèn L, Frisèn M: Micropsia and visual acuity in macular edema. A study of the neuro-retinal basis of visual acuity. Albrecht Graefes Arch Klin Exp Ophthalmol 210:69, 1979

509. Sjostrand J, Anderson C: Micropsia and metamorphopsia in the re-attached macula following retinal detachment. Acta Ophthalmol 64:425, 1986

510. Miller NR: Cerebral dysmetropsia. In Walsh and Hoyt's Clinical Neuroophthalmology, 4th ed, p 164. Baltimore, Williams and Wilkins, 1982.

511. Thièbaut F, Matavulj N: Hèmi-micropsie relative homonyme droite en quadrant infèrieur. Rev Oto-Neuro-Ophthalmol 21:245, 1949

512. Cohen L, Gray F, Meyrignac C et al: Selective deficit of visual size perception: two cases of hemi-micropsia. J Neurol Neurosurg Psychiatry 57:73, 1994

513. Ebata S, Ogawa M, Tanaka Y et al: Apparent reduction in the size of one side of the face associated with a small retrosplenial hemorrhage. J Neurol Neurosurg Psychiatry 54:68, 1991

514. Touge T, Takeuchi H, Yamada A et al: A case of posterior cerebral artery territory infarction with micropsia as the chief complaint. Rinsho Shinkeigaku 30:894, 1990

515. Wilson SAK: Dysmetropsia and its pathogenesis. Trans Ophthalmol Soc UK 36:412, 1916

516. Abe K, Oda N, Araki R, Igata M: Macropsia, micropsia, and episodic illusions in Japanese adolescents. J Am Acad Child Adolesc Psychiatry 28:493, 1989

517. Iruela L, Ibanez-Rojo V, Baca E: Zolpidem-induced macropsia in anorexic woman. Lancet 342:443, 1993

518. Brègeat P, Klein M, Thièbaut F, Bouniol: Hèmi-macropsia homonyme droite et tumeur occipitale gauche. Rev Oto-Neuro-Ophthalmol 21:245, 1949; 19:238, 1979

519. Ardile A, Botero M, Gomez J: Palinopsia and visual allesthesia. Int J Neurosci 32:775, 1987

520. Enoch JM, Schwartz A, Chang D, Hirose H: Aniseikonia, metamorphopsia and perceived entoptic pattern: some effects of a macular epiretinal membrane, and the subsequent spontaneous separation of the membrane. Ophthalmic Physiol Opt 15:339, 1995

521. Amemiya T, Iida Y, Yoshida H: Subjective and objective ocular disturbances in reattached retina after surgery for retinal detachment, with special reference to visual acuity and metamorphopsia. Ophthalmologica 186:25, 1983

522. Ida Y, Kotorii T, Nakazawa Y: A case of epilepsy with ictal metamorphopsia. Folia Psychiatr Neurol Jpn 34:395, 1980

523. Nass R, Sinha S, Solomon G: Epileptic facial metamorphopsia. Brain Dev 7:50, 1985

524. Imai N, Nohira O, Miyata K et al: A case of metamorphopsia caused by a very localized spotty infarct. Rinsho Shinkeigaku 35:302, 1995

525. Krizek GO: Metamorphopsias caused by pontine and peduncular lesions. Am J Psychiatry 142:999, 1985

526. Brau RH, Lameiro J, Llaguno AV, Rifkinson N: Metamorphopsia and permanent cortical blindness after a posterior fossa tumor. Neurosurgery 19:263, 1986

527. Palca J: Insights from broken brains. Science 248:812, 1990

528. Damasio AR: Descartes' Error: Emotion, Reason, and the Human Brain. New York, Grosset/Putnam, 1994.

529. Weinberg J, Piasetsky E, Diller L, Gordon W: Treating perceptual organization deficits in nonneglecting RBD stroke patients. J Clin Neuropsychol 4:59, 1982

530. Carlsson GS, Svardsudd K, Welin L: Long-term effects of head injuries sustained during life in three male populations. J Neurosurg 67:197, 1987

531. Mishra AV, Digre KB: Head injury: Neuro-ophthalmological disturbances. In Rizzo M, Tranel D (eds): Head Injury and Post-Concussive Syndrome. New York, Churchill Livingstone, 221–226, 1996

532. Feigenson JS, McCarthy ML, Greenberg SD et al: Factors influencing outcome and length of stay in a stroke rehabilitation unit. Stroke 8:657, 1977

533. Rossi PW, Kheyfets S, Reding MJ: Fresnel prisms improve visual perception in stroke patients with homonymous hemianopia or unilateral visual neglect. Neurology 40:1597, 1990

534. Jongbloed L: Prediction of function after stroke: a critical review. Stroke 17:765, 1986

535. Huxley AL: The Art of Seeing. Berkeley, Creative Arts Book Company, 1942; reprinted 1982.

536. Parisi JL, Bell RA, Yassein H: Homonymous hemianopic field defects and driving in Canada. Can J Ophthalmol 26(5):252, 1991

537. Szlyk JP, Brigell M, Seiple W: Effects of age and hemianopic visual field loss on driving. Optom Vis Sci 70(12):1031, 1993

538. Pasik P, Pasik T: Visual functions in monkeys after total removal of visual cerebral cortex. In Neff WD (ed): Contributions to Sensory Physiology, Vol 7. New York, Academic Press, 1982

539. Merican WH, Nealey TA, Maunsell JHR: Visual effects of lesions of cortical area V2 in macaques. J Neurosci 13:3180, 1993

540. Pommerenke K, Markowitsch JH: Rehabilitation training of homonymous visual field defects in patients with postgeniculate damage of the visual system. Restor Neurol Neurosci 1:47, 1989

541. Kerkoff G, Munßinger U, Meier EK: Neurovisual rehabilitation in cerebral blindness. Arch Neurol 51:474, 1994

542. Bruce CJ, Goldberg ME: Physiology of the frontal eye fields. Trends Neurosci 436, 1984

543. Hallett PE, Adams WD: The predictability of saccadic latency in a novel oculomotor task. Vis Res 20:329, 1980

544. Guitton D, Buchtel HA, Douglas RM: In Lennerstrand G, Zee DS, Keller EL (eds): Functional Basis of Ocular Motility Disorders, p 497. Oxford, Pergamon Press, 1982

545. Schlageter K, Gray B, Hall K et al: Incidence and treatment of visual dysfunction in traumatic brain injury. Brain Injury 7: 439, 1993

546. Behrmann M, Watt S, Black SE, Barton JJS: Impaired visual search in patients with unilateral neglect: an oculographic analysis. Neuropsychologia 35:1445, 1997

547. NEI. National Eye Institute. VFQ-25. July, 1996

CHAPTER 8

The Facial Nerve and Related Disorders of the Face

Steven L. Galetta and Mark May

Embryology
    Intramedullary Segment
    Extramedullary Segment
    Intratemporal Segment
    Anomalies
Anatomy
    Cortex and Supranuclear Pathway
    Extrapyramidal System
    Pons
    Cerebellopontine Angle
    Temporal Bone
    Extracranial Segment
    Blood Supply
Facial Nerve Function and Assessment
    Motor Evaluation
    Taste
    Tear Function
    Blink Reflex
    Physiologic Facial Synkinesis
Idiopathic (Bell's) Facial Palsy
Infectious and Immune-Mediated Neuropathies
    Herpes Zoster Cephalicus (Ramsay Hunt Syndrome)
Polyradiculopathy (Guillain-Barré Syndrome)
    Infectious Mononucleosis
    Lyme Disease

    Ear Infections
    Other Infections and Postimmunization
Trauma
Tumors
    Acoustic Neuroma
    Facial Neuroma
    Metastatic Lesions
Miscellaneous Conditions
    Sarcoidosis
    Acute Porphyrias
    Myasthenia Gravis
    Botulism
    Myotonic Dystrophy
    Progressive Hemifacial Atrophy (Parry-Romberg Syndrome)
Bilateral or Recurrent Facial Nerve Paresis
Facial Embryopathies and Childhood Palsies
Hyperkinetic Facial Disorders
    Blepharospasm
    Hemifacial Spasm
    Facial Synkinesis
    Gustatory Tearing (Crocodile Tears)
    Gustatory Sweating
    Facial Myokymia
Disorders of Eyelid Opening
Management of Facial Palsy

. . . Why Nature has given us Eye-lids? . . . I answer'd, that it was absolutely necessary for us, and all Land-animals to have Eye-lids; for if it were not so, and the Apple of our eyes were not moistened many times in the space of an hour, and all the foulness that might fall thereon, washt away, our Sight or the Tunica Cornea could be so clogg'd with filth, that we should not be able to use our Eyes; besides, the said Tunic would otherwise be parcht up or shrunk with heat, and consequently we should become Blind; whereas on the contrary, fishes living always in Water want no Eyelids, because the same Water keeps their eyes ever moist and clean . . .

Anton van Leeuwenhoek, 1704

The facial nerve, by virtue of its unique neuroanatomy and physiology, and its complex course across the skull base and face, is often involved in neuro-ophthalmologic problems. Abnormalities of lid position and defective tearing are regularly symptomatic, demanding ophthalmologic attention. This chapter provides both an anatomic and an etiologic approach to the spectrum of facial nerve disorders. The current management of facial nerve paresis and facial hyperkinetic syndromes is emphasized.

S. L. Galetta: Department of Neurology; and Division of Neuro-ophthalmology, University of Pennsylvania Medical Center, Philadelphia, Pennsylvania

M. May: Department of Otolaryngology, Head, and Neck Surgery, University of Pittsburgh, Pittsburgh, Pennsylvania

TABLE 8–1. Time During Gestation When Anatomic Structures Appear

Week of gestation	Structures noted
3rd	Collection of neural crest cells, anlage of VII cranial nerve nucleus (CNN)
5th	Chorda tympani, greater petrosal, VII motor nucleus
6th	External genu, postauricular branch, branch to posterior belly of digastric
7th	Geniculate ganglion, nervus intermedius
8th	Stapedius nerve, temporofacial and cervicofacial part of extracranial facial nerve
End of 8th	Terminal branches of VII
7th to 8th	Myoblasts that will form the facial muscles
12th	All facial muscles

EMBRYOLOGY

Normal and abnormal functions of the facial nerve can be best understood through an awareness of its embryonic development. The complexity of the nerve's course, its branching patterns, and its anatomic relationships are established during the first 3 months of prenatal life.[1] During this period, the muscles of facial expression also differentiate, become functional, and actively contract.[2] Critical phases in facial nerve development occur throughout gestation, and the nerve is not fully developed until about 4 months after birth (Table 8-1).

Intramedullary Segment

The motor nuclei of the sixth and seventh cranial nerves are initially in close proximity in the pontine subdivision of the metencephalon. As the metencephalon elongates and expands, the facial nucleus migrates ventrolaterally in relation to the abducens nucleus, displacing facial motor axons that loop dorsally in the floor of the fourth ventricle, to form the facial colliculus (Fig. 8–1). This intimate relationship between the abducens and facial motor nuclei is the anatomic substrate for the clinical findings in congenital Möbius' syndrome and in acquired inflammatory, vascular, and neoplastic lesions that involve the intramedullary segment of the facial nerve.

Extramedullary Segment

The facial nerve rootlets become distinguishable near the end of the seventh week of gestation, when the geniculate ganglion becomes well defined.[1] The nervus intermedius, which contains afferent and general visceral efferent fibers, exits the brain stem between the facial motor root and the vestibular nerve. The afferent fibers arise from the geniculate ganglion, whereas the preganglionic parasympathetic fibers originate in the superior salivatory nucleus in the brain stem (Fig. 8–2). The fact that the geniculate ganglion and the parasympathetic fibers form independently of the motor pathways allows patients with congenital facial paralysis to enjoy intact

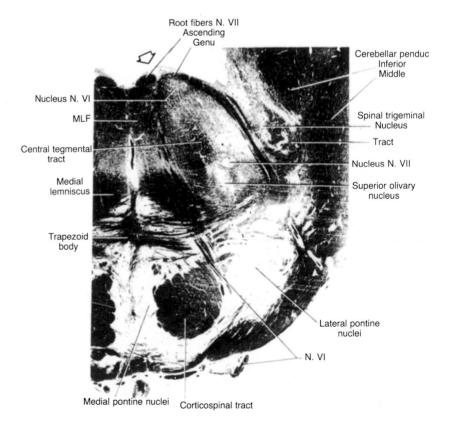

Fig. 8–1. Cross section of pons, with relationships of facial motor nucleus (*VII*), abducens nucleus (*VI*), corticospinal tract, trigeminal nucleus, and tract. Facial colliculus (*arrow*). (Carpenter M: Core Text of Neuro-Anatomy, 3rd ed, p 152. Baltimore, Williams & Wilkins, 1985)

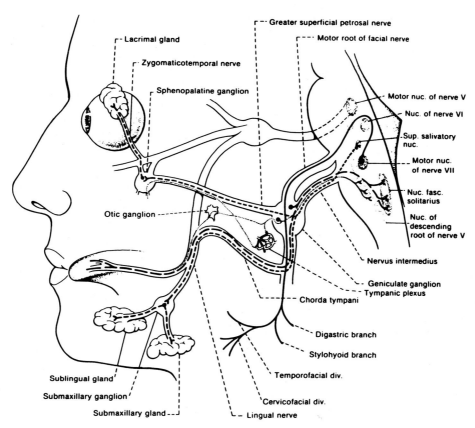

Fig. 8–2. Brain stem components and peripheral branches of facial nerve. (Dejong RN: The Neurologic Exam, 4th ed. Hagerstown, Harper & Row, 1979)

tearing and taste, but with selective impairment of the motor neurons innervating the facial muscles.

Intratemporal Segment

Small but important ganglia are scattered along the course of the facial nerve through the temporal bone.[3] These ganglia are likely composed of aberrant sensory neurons from the tympanic plexus that enter the facial nerve near the stapedial branch. Because most viruses have an affinity for afferent nerve fibers, such sensory fibers may play an important role in the development of viral-immune facial nerve palsies.

Of all the cranial nerves, the facial nerve has the largest number of communications with other nerves.[4] This situation may account for the variety of neurologic signs sometimes seen with herpes zoster cephalicus. The cutaneous branches of the second and third cervical ganglia (part of the cervical plexus of spinal nerves) are the initial nerves that establish connections with the facial nerve at its emergence from the stylomastoid foramen. In the facial palsy of herpes zoster cephalicus, these communications predict the distribution of the cutaneous eruption that involves the angle of the jaw, the back of the head, and the neck, thus following the pattern of the C2-C3 dermatome (see below).

Anomalies

The facial nerve develops within the second branchial arch during the same period that closely adjacent derivatives of the first arch, the first internal pouch and external groove, are forming the external and middle ear regions. Therefore, anomalies of the facial nerve within the temporal bone should be anticipated whenever there are associated malformations of the external or middle ear. In these cases, displacement of the facial nerve and complete absence of the bony facial canal are the most common anomalies observed. Typically, the facial nerve can be seen sagging inferiorly against the stapes bone.[5]

ANATOMY

Familiarity with the general anatomy of the neural pathways for facial function is essential for accurate diagnosis and appropriate management of the spectrum of facial neuropathies. Specific diagnostic possibilities can be implied by precise regional localization of typical lesions (Table 8–2).

Cortex and Supranuclear Pathway

The voluntary responses of facial muscles, such as smiling or grimacing on command, are dependent on

TABLE 8-2. Topical Diagnoses of Lesions of the Facial Nerve at Various Levels

Level	Signs	Probable Diagnosis
Supranuclear		
Cortex and internal capsule	Tone and upper face intact, loss of volitional movement with intact spontaneous expression, slurred speech (tongue weakness), hemiparesis on side of facial involvement. Paresis of upper extremity begins with involvement of thumb, finger, and hand movement.	Lesion of motor cortex or internal capsule on opposite side of facial involvement
Extrapyramidal	Increased salivary flow, spontaneous facial movement impaired, volitional facial movement intact, masked face of parkinsonism or dystonia, progressive hemifacial spasm	Tumor or vascular lesion of basal ganglia: parkinsonism, Meige's syndrome (cervical facial dystonia)
Midbrain	Oculomotor paresis on opposite side of lower facial paresis and hemiparesis	Syndrome of Weber
Pontine nucleus	Involvement of cranial nerves VII and VI on side of facial paresis; associated ataxia, cerebellovestibular signs, and contralateral hemiparesis	Involvement of pons at level of VII and VI nuclei by pontine glioma, multiple sclerosis, infection, infarction
	Cranial nerves VII and VI palsy noted from time of birth with or without other congenital anomalies. Facial motor involvement usually incomplete with sparing of corner of mouth or lower lip common. Another type of presentation is involvement of the lower lip with complete or partial sparing of upper face. Anomalies of the pinna, canal, or mandible associated with facial palsy indicate developmental defect of facial nerve.	Developmental facial palsy (noted at birth), oculofacial syndrome, Möbius' syndrome, thalidomide toxicity. Nondevelopmental facial or abducens nerve anomalies are most often due to infranuclear lesions.
Infranuclear		
Intracranial cerebellopontine angle	Impairment of hearing, (especially discrimination out of proportion to pure tone scores), possible ataxia, abnormalities of tearing or taste, stapes reflex decay, decreased corneal sensation, facial motor deficit (late sign)	Acoustic schwannoma
	Abnormalities in trigeminal, acoustic–vestibular, and facial nerve function, starting with facial pain or numbness. Lesion noted on CT (enhancement with contrast) may show evidence of calcification.	Meningioma
	Abnormalities of facial and acoustic–vestibular nerve function, may start with facial twitching. Erosion or lytic area evident on CT of temporal bone.	Cholesteatoma or facial schwannoma arising in temporal bone
	Abnormalities of cranial nerves VII, VIII, IX, X, XI, and XII; pulsatile tinnitus and purple–red pulsating mass bulging through the tympanic membrane	Glomus jugulare tumor
	Abnormalities of abducens nerve in addition to above	Glomus jugulare tumor extending to petrous apex to involve middle fossa
Skull base	Conductive or sensorineural hearing loss, acute or recurrent facial palsy, positive family history, abnormalities of bone density on CT	Osteopetrosis
	Multiple cranial nerve involvement in rapid succession	Carcinomatous meningitis, leukemia, Landry-Guillain-Barré, mononucleosis, diphtheria, tuberculosis, sarcoidosis, malignant external otitis
Transtemporal bone		
Internal auditory canal and labyrinthine segment of facial nerve	Ecchymosis around pinna and mastoid prominence (Battle's sign), hematotympanum with sensorineural hearing loss (tuning fork lateralizes to normal side), vertigo, nystagmus (fast component away from involved side), sudden complete facial paralysis after head trauma (usually associated with basilar skull fracture), loss of consciousness, and cerebrospinal fluid leak. Transection of facial nerve is more likely with this injury compared with longitudinal fracture.	Temporal bone fracture (transverse, longitudinal, or combination)

(continued)

TABLE 8–2. Topical Diagnoses of Lesions of the Facial Nerve at Various Levels (*continued*)

Level	Signs	Probable diagnosis
Transtemporal bone		
Geniculate ganglion	Dry eye, decreased taste and salivation. Erosion of geniculate ganglion area or middle fossa is demonstrated by pluridirectional tomography and CT of temporal bone.	Schwannoma, meningioma, cholesteatoma, hemangioma, arteriovenous malformation
	Ear pain, vesicles on pinna, dry eye, decreased taste and salivary flow, sensorineural hearing loss, nystagmus, vertigo, red chorda tympani nerve. Facial palsy may be complete or incomplete, or may progress to complete over 14 days.	Herpes zoster cephalicus (Ramsey-Hunt syndrome)
	Same as above with vesicles; no other cause evident. Facial palsy may be complete or incomplete, or may progress to complete over 10 days.	Idiopathic (Bell's) palsy (viral–inflammatory immune disorder)
	Same as above but no recovery in 6 months	Tumor
	Ecchymosis around pinna and mastoid (Battle's sign), hematotympanum, conductive hearing loss (tuning fork lateralizes to involved ear), no vestibular involvement unless stapes subluxed into vestibule (causes fluctuating sensorineural hearing loss and vertigo with nystagmus)	Longitudinal fracture of temporal bone; may be proximal or at geniculate ganglion (tearing symmetrical; tear test valid only in acute injury)
Tympanomastoid	Decreased taste and salivation, loss of stapes reflex and symmetrical tearing, sudden-onset facial palsy, which may be complete or incomplete or may progress to complete	
	Pain, vesicles, red chorda tympani	Herpes zoster cephalicus
	Pain without vesicles, red chorda tympani	Bell's palsy
	Red, bulging tympanic membrane, conductive hearing loss, usually history of upper respiratory infection. Lower face may be involved more than upper.	Acute suppurative otitis media
	Pulsatile tinnitus, purple–red pulsatile mass noted through tympanic membrane	Glomus tympanicum or jugulare
	Recurrent facial paralysis, positive family history, facial edema, fissured tongue; may present with simultaneous bilateral facial paralysis	Melkersson-Rosenthal syndrome
Extracranial	Incomplete facial nerve paresis; hearing balance, tearing, stapes reflex, taste, salivary flow spared	Penetrating wound of face; sequelae of parotid surgery; malignancy of parotid, tonsil, or oronasopharynx, rarely with benign lesion of parotid gland compressing facial nerve
	Uveitis, salivary gland enlargement, fever	Sarcoidosis (Heerfordt's syndrome), lymphoma
Sites variable	Bilateral facial paralysis from birth	Möbius' syndrome
	Bilateral facial paralysis acquired	Landry-Guillain-Barré syndrome, sarcoidosis, mononucleosis, leukemia, idiopathic (Bell's) palsy
	Facial paralysis, especially simultaneous bilateral facial paralysis with ascending areflexic quadriparesis; sensory changes usually mild, with spinal fluid typically showing albuminocytologic dissociation (elevated protein without cells)	Landry-Guillain-Barré syndrome
	Deficits of cranial nerves VI and VII or VII, VI, and III, possibly in association with marked increase in jaw jerk or gag reflex	Carcinoma of nasopharynx, metastatic carcinoma from breast, ovary, prostate; meningitis, leukemia, diabetes mellitus
Pseudobulbar palsy	Inappropriate or exaggerated laughing or crying; may be associated with marked increase in jaw jerk or gag reflex	Demyelinating, degenerative, or vascular process involving bilateral corticobulbar pathways

CT, computed tomography

discharges from the facial motor area situated in the precentral gyrus of the frontal cerebral cortex. The facial motor areas are represented with the forehead uppermost and the eyelids, midface, nose, and lips located sequentially below (Fig. 8–3). Supranuclear motor neurons from the cortical face area are carried as fascicles of the corticobulbar tract to the genu of the internal capsule, then via the cerebral peduncles to the lower pons. The portion of the facial nucleus that supplies the muscles of the upper face (frontalis, orbicularis oculi, and corrugator muscles) receives corticobulbar fibers from both right and left precentral motor cortices, but the supranuclear tracts innervating the lower face are crossed only. For this reason, the muscles that raise and wrinkle the forehead and close both eyes are bilaterally innervated. Thus, a unilateral lesion in the cortex or supranuclear pathways spares eyelid closure and forehead movement but results in paralysis of the contralatseveral lower face. This dissociation is characteristic of suranuclear lesions. However, it is also possible to show upper facial sparing with lesions of the pontine facial nucleus, with selective defects within the temporal bone, or even with an injury to nerve rootlets within the parotid gland or facial musculature. This phenomena is related to the general tendency for facial nerve function to be spatially dispersed, not only in its cortical distribution but also within the pontine nucleus and in the peripheral nerve.

Because preservation of forehead function is insufficient evidence of a cortical lesion, other neurologic signs should be sought. A cortical lesion that produces a contralateral lower facial palsy is usually associated with a motor deficit of the tongue and with weakness of the thumb, fingers, and hand on the same side as the hemifacial weakness, with lesser involvement of the leg. The cortical motor areas of the face, tongue, thumb, fingers, hand, and upper extremities lie near each other in the precentral territory nourished by the rolandic branch of the middle cerebral artery. Patients with such cortical lesions are unable to voluntarily smile, but facial expression is appropriate in response to an amusing story. Similar clinical findings may occur with lesions that involve the descending corticobulbar and corticospinal tracts.[6]

Although facial muscle tone is not significantly impaired with a supranuclear lesion, slight flattening of the nasolabial fold and drooping in the corner of the mouth may be detected contralateral to the cortical lesion.

Extrapyramidal System

The extrapyramidal system (Fig. 8–4) consists of the basal ganglia and the descending motor projections other than the fibers of the corticospinal (pyramidal) tract. Anatomically, this system appears to be a diffuse,

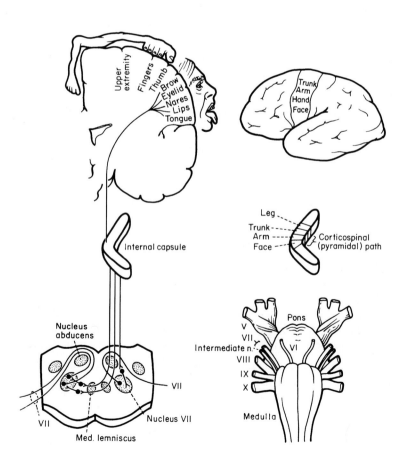

Fig. 8–3. Organization of facial motor function. Note cortical distribution, pontine nuclear connections, and relationships to other cranial nerves on ventral view of brain stem.

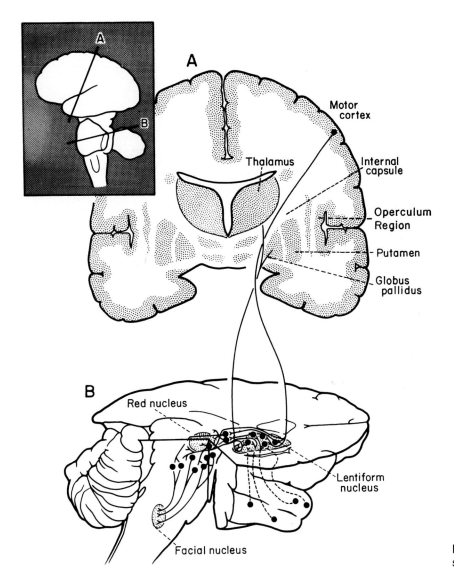

Fig. 8–4 Extrapyramidal connections for supranuclear facial pathways.

multisynaptic network that interconnects extensively with centrencephalic and brain stem structures. These pathways are not as well clarified as those of the primary (pyramidal) motor tracts. The extrapyramidal system is concerned with automatic and emotional facial language. The dull, expressionless face of parkinsonism is a well-known result of extrapyramidal pathway disease, whereas the spontaneous facial dystonia of Meige's syndrome is characterized by unilateral or, more often, bilateral blepharospasm associated with dystonic movements of the mouth and other lower facial muscles. Progression of this latter disorder may lead to chaotic contractions of the tongue and cervical muscles.

Pons

The facial motor nucleus contains about 7000 motor nuclei[7] and is located in the ventrolateral angle of the lower pontine tegmentum (see Fig. 8–1). The facial nu-

cleus can be divided into four separate cell groups that supply specific muscle groups: (1) dorsomedial (auricular and occipital muscles), (2) intermediate (frontalis, corrugator, and orbicularis oculi muscles), (3) ventromedial (platysma), and (4) lateral (buccinator and buccolabial).[8] The motor axons exit the nucleus dorsally, looping around the abducens (VI) nucleus, and form the facial genu before emerging from the lateral aspect of the pons. The superior salivatory nucleus, which is located just rostral to the facial motor nucleus, is the origin of the parasympathetic fibers that supply the sublingual, submandibular, and lacrimal glands. These salivary and lacrimal fibers join the facial nerve as the nervus intermedius in the cerebellopontine angle.

Because the facial nucleus is located ventromedial to the cochlear nuclei, and the spinal tract and nucleus of the trigeminal nerve, a lesion of the lateral pons may result in ipsilateral facial paresis, ipsilateral facial analgesia, ipsilateral Horner's syndrome, and ipsilateral

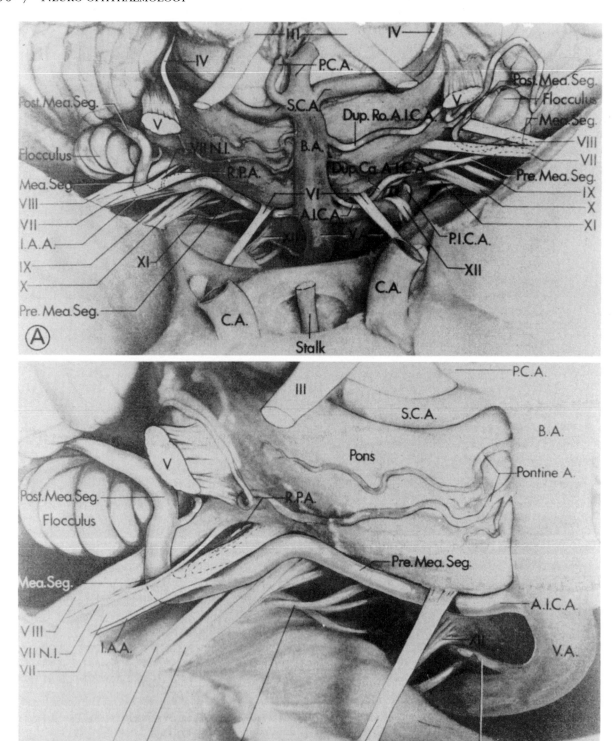

Fig. 8–5. Anatomic relationships of facial nerve trunk and brain stem structure. Anterior view of ventral aspect of brain stem and clivus, especially cerebellopontine angle. The cerebral hemispheres were removed and the oculomotor and trigeminal nerves were divided to provide this view of the anterior surface of the brain stem. **A.** The superior cerebellar arteries (*SCA*) and posterior cerebral arteries (*PCA*) arise from the superior end of the basilar artery (*BA*). The oculomotor (*III*) and trochlear (*IV*) nerves are above and the trigeminal (*V*) nerves are below the superior cerebellar arteries. The right anterior inferior cerebellar artery (*AICA*) arises from the basilar artery, courses below the abducens nerve (*VI*), and passes between the nervus intermedius (*VII NI*) and the facial motor root (*VII*) anteriorly and the vestibulocochlear nerve (*VIII*) posteriorly. The left AICA is a duplicate artery. The rostral duplicate AICA (*Dup. Ro. AICA*) is not nerve related, but the caudal AICA (*Dup. Ca. AICA*) is nerve related and

deafness (Foville's syndrome). If the lesion extends further dorsally, an ipsilateral gaze paresis would result from involvement of the sixth nerve nucleus. The combination of a unilateral sixth nerve palsy, an ipsilateral seventh nerve palsy, and a contralateral hemiparesis is known as the Millard-Gubler syndrome. Intrinsic lesions of the brain stem are usually the result of infarction, hemorrhage, tumor, or demyelination.

Cerebellopontine Angle

The facial nerve, the nervus intermedius, and the eighth (vestibuloacoustic) cranial nerve exit together from the ventrolateral aspect of the pons, surrounded by a leptomeningeal covering. In the lateral pontine cistern, the anteroinferior cerebellar artery may loop between the seventh and eighth cranial nerves as the artery courses posteriorly to supply the dorsolateral pons and cerebellum.[9] As the nervus intermedius approaches the internal auditory meatus, it joins the facial nerve. Because of the association of the facial nerve with the nervus intermedius and the vestibuloacoustic nerves at the level of the cerebellopontine angle and in the internal auditory canal, tearing, taste, submandibular saliva flow, hearing, and balance are disturbed with mass lesions at this level (Fig. 8–5).

From the brain stem to the internal auditory canal, the facial nerve is covered only by a thin layer of glia, which makes it quite vulnerable to any type of surgical manipulation but quite resistant to a slow process of stretching or compression, as might occur with an acoustic schwannoma. Large tumors that fill the cerebellopontine angle compress neighboring cranial nerves and cause defects of the 5th and, later, the 9th, 10th, and 11th cranial nerves. Lesions that occur in this area include temporal bone fractures, acoustic neuromas (schwannomas), meningiomas, and primary cholesteatomas. Hyperkinetic disorders are attributed to vascular compression of the root of the facial nerve.

Temporal Bone

The motor portion of the facial nerve and the nervus intermedius are loosely joined together as they enter

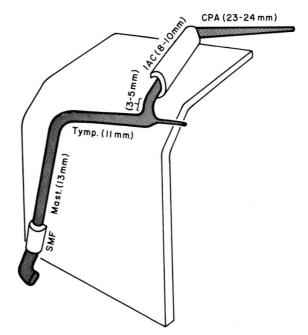

Fig. 8–6. Z-shaped course of right facial nerve, anterolateral view. *CPA*, cerebellopontine angle segment; *IAC*, internal auditory canal segment; *Tymp.*, tympanic segment in middle ear; *Mast.*, mastoid segment; *SMF*, stylomastoid foramen. Segment lengths as indicated. (Adapted from Guerrier Y: Surgical anatomy, particularly vascular supply of the facial nerve. In Fisch U (ed): Facial Nerve Surgery, pp 12–23. Birmingham, Aesculapius, 1977)

the internal auditory meatus with the acoustic nerve. In this region, the facial nerve and nervus intermedius course superiorly to the vestibuloacoustic nerve. As the facial nerve emerges from the internal auditory meatus, it departs from the vestibuloacoustic nerve to enter the fallopian (facial) canal.

The course of the facial nerve through the fallopian (facial) canal is unique; no other nerve traverses so long a distance through a canal (28 to 30 mm). The nerve follows a remarkable Z-shaped course in its intratemporal portion (Fig. 8–6).[10] Furthermore, it incorporates a sensory ganglion, the geniculate. In the fallopian canal, the nerve trunk can be divided into labyrinthine, tympanic, and mastoid segments. The labyrinthine segment

---

Fig. 8–5. (continued) passes between the facial and vestibulocochlear nerves. The left posteroinferior cerebellar artery (*PICA*) arises from the left vertebral artery (*VA*). The hypoglossal (*XII*), glossopharyngeal (*IX*), vagus (*X*), and spinal accessory (*XI*) nerves are lateral to the vertebral arteries. The carotid arteries (*CA*) and the pituitary stalk (*Stalk*) have been divided. The premeatal segments (*Pre. Mea. Seg.*) approach the nerves, the meatal segments (*Mea. Seg.*) pass between the nerves, and the postmeatal segments (*Post. Mea. Seg.*) pass above the flocculus. A recurrent perforating artery (*RPA*) and an internal auditory artery (*IAA*) arise from the right AICA. **B.** Enlarged anterosuperior view of the right cerebellopontine angle. The premeatal segment passes below the abducens nerve, the meatal segment passes between the eighth cranial nerve and the nervus intermedius, and the postmeatal segment passes above the flocculus. A recurrent perforating artery and an internal auditory artery arise from the meatal segment. Pontine arteries arise from the right side of the basilar artery. (Martin RG, Grant JL, Peace D: Microsurgical relationship of the anterior inferior cerebellar artery and the facial-vestibulocochlear nerve complex. Neurosurgery 6:483, 1980)

includes the geniculate ganglion, and it is at this level that the first branch of the facial nerve arises, the greater superficial petrosal nerve. This nerve traverses the dura of the floor of the middle cranial fossa, synapsing in the sphenopalatine ganglion; postganglionic secretory nerve fibers travel with the zygomaticotemporal nerve of the fifth nerve (V-2) and eventually join the lacrimal nerve of V-1 to innervate the lacrimal gland. Involvement of the greater superficial nerve in the middle fossa (*e.g.*, from neoplastic invasion, inflammatory processes, and trauma) impairs reflex tear secretion. When defective tearing accompanies abducens or trigeminal nerve palsy, a lesion in the middle cranial fossa is indicated. Although lacrimal fibers are classically carried by the nervus intermedius, parasympathetic neurons variably reach their destination by way of branches of the fifth or ninth cranial nerves, because there are ample opportunities for intermingling among these nerves (Fig. 8–7).

At the geniculate ganglion, the facial nerve makes a sharply angled turn posteriorly, forming a knee (genu) to enter the tympanic, or horizontal, portion of the fallopian canal. The distal tympanic segment emerges from the middle ear between the posterior wall of the auditory canal and the horizontal semicircular canal, just beneath the short process of the incus. At this point, the fallopian aqueduct makes another turn downward, forming the second genu. This marks the beginning of the mastoid segment. The nerve continues vertically downward on the anterior wall of the mastoid process to the stylomastoid foramen. The chorda tympani is the terminal branch of the nervus intermedius and usually arises from the distal third of the mastoid segment of the facial nerve. The chorda tympani nerve contains secretory motor fibers to the submaxillary and sublingual salivary glands. It also carries special sensory afferents from the anterior two thirds of the tongue (taste) and somatic sensory fibers from the posterior wall of the external auditory meatus (pain and temperature). The afferent fibers for taste synapse in the rostral nucleus solitarius of the medulla, whereas those somatic sensory fibers from the periauricular region terminate in the nucleus of the spinal tract of the fifth nerve.

Extracranial Segment

As the nerve exits the stylomastoid foramen behind the mandibular angle, and before it bifurcates, motor branches are given off to the posterior belly of the digastric, stylohyoid, and posterior auricular muscles. The main trunk of the facial nerve enters the substance of the parotid gland and then bifurcates into an upper and lower division (Fig. 8–8). These divisions can be further subdivided into the temporal, zygomatic, buccal, mandibular, and cervical branches. After emerging from the parotid gland, the facial nerve passes over the fascia of the masseter muscle. Although the course in this region is variable, there are some relationships

that are relatively constant. There are communications between the upper and lower divisions that form a variety of patterns.[11] This rich plexus of nerve filaments in the peripheral zone, just before entering the undersurface of the facial muscles, permits extensive intermingling between peripheral branches of the upper and lower divisions. These anastomoses provide the substrate for misdirected peripheral regeneration that may follow a facial nerve palsy. Such inappropriate axonal sprouting accounts for spontaneous lower facial movement upon blinking, or an eye closure provoked by smiling (facial synkinesis). Considering the number of possible routes available to each interrupted neuron, it is truly remarkable that any patients are able to voluntarily control appropriate individual muscle movement. Similarly, "crocodile tears" (see below) are the result of faulty regeneration of parasympathetic fibers that mistakenly innervate the lacrimal gland instead of the salivary glands. Thus, increased ipsilateral lacrimation associated with eating may occur after a denervating lesion of the facial nerve appears at or above the site of the geniculate ganglion, or along the course of the greater superficial petrosal nerve.

Blood Supply

The cortical motor area of the face is nourished by the rolandic branch of the middle cerebral artery. Within the pons, the facial nucleus and its motor axons receive their blood supply primarily from a combination of the anteroinferior cerebellar artery and the short and long circumferential arteries.

The extramedullary blood supply to the facial nerve as described by Nager and Nager[12] is derived from three sources: the anteroinferior cerebellar artery, which enters the internal auditory meatus in close association with the seventh and eighth cranial nerves; the petrosal branch of the middle meningeal artery, which accompanies the greater petrosal nerve; and the stylomastoid branch of the posterior auricular artery, which enters the facial canal at the stylomastoid foramen. The territories supplied by the three arteries tend to overlap at any given level. Despite the richness of the blood supply to most segments of the facial nerve, vascular compromise is likely a factor in the pathogenesis of facial palsies. The area proximal to the geniculate ganglion is especially vulnerable to ischemic compression, not only because this is the narrowest part of the fallopian canal but also because there are no anastomoses between the arterial systems immediately proximal to the geniculate ganglion.[13,14]

FACIAL NERVE FUNCTION AND ASSESSMENT

Motor Evaluation

Assessment of facial nerve motor function begins by observing the patient at rest and noting any asymmetries

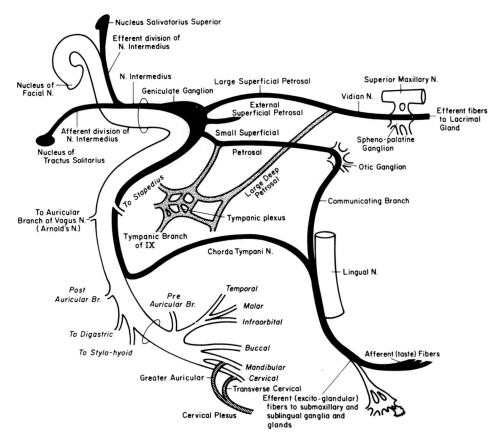

Fig. 8–7. Peripheral communications of the facial nerve. Note interconnections with cranial nerves V, IX, and X, and with the cervical plexus. (Modified from Gray's Anatomy, 36th British Edition, p 1068. Philadelphia, WB Saunders, 1980)

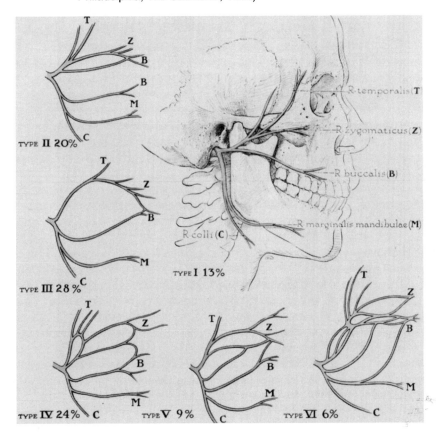

Fig. 8–8. Patterns of peripheral distribution of facial nerve. (Modified from Davis RA, Anson BJ, Puddinger JM, Kurth RE: Surgical anatomy of the facial nerve and parotid gland based upon a study of 350 cervical facial halves. Surg Gynecol Obstet 102:385, 1956)

of the face or of blink pattern. Most supranuclear and infranuclear facial nerve palsies are associated with a flattened nasolabial fold and a slightly widened palpebral fissure on the paretic side. Facial movement in response to emotional stimuli and voluntary command should also be assessed. A dissociation in response of spontaneous and voluntary movements is suggestive of supranuclear defects. Disease of the corticobulbar tracts tends to spare emotional facial responses, whereas disease of the basal ganglia preserves voluntary movements. Preservation of forehead wrinkling, seen best in attempted upward gaze, is also characteristic of supranuclear lesions (Fig. 8–9). Forced eyelid closure should be performed, and asymmetries in eyelash burying or lagophthalmos (*i.e.,* partial or total inability to close the lids) should be noted.

Taste

Taste receptors are distributed over the tongue and pharynx. Axons with cell bodies in the geniculate ganglion receive stimuli from receptors and project postganglionic afferents back to the nucleus tractus solitarius in the medulla. The seventh nerve carries taste fibers from the anterior two thirds of the tongue; taste from the posterior third of the tongue is supplied by the ninth nerve. Taste is best tested with a cotton swab dipped in a sour, sweet, or bitter solution (see Fig. 8–9). Unilateral ageusia (loss of taste) may be useful in identifying a facial lesion as peripheral, but it should be noted that bedside tests of taste are crude and often unreliable.

Tear Function

Evaluation of tear function by observation alone, without actual testing, may lead to erroneous impressions (*e.g.,* that a patient with a facial palsy is tearing excessively).

Testing for tearing is of limited diagnostic and prognostic value, unless tear production is drastically reduced or absent on the involved side. In addition, the results of actual tear testing may be similarly misleading.

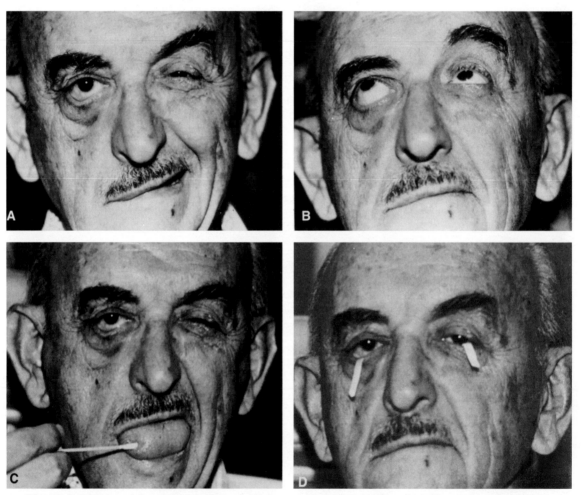

Fig. 8–9. Right peripheral facial palsy. **A.** Note paralysis of right face, including lowered eyebrow, ectropion of right lower lid with widened palpebral fissure, and flattening of nasolabial fold. **B.** During upward gaze, there is failure of the frontalis muscle to elevate eyebrow. **C.** Cotton swab is applied to anterior portion of tongue for taste testing with saline (or sugar) solution. **D.** Schirmer's test paper strips are applied to test reflex tearing (no topical anesthesia) after conjunctival tear lakes are dried.

Increased tear flow (epiphora) noted by history can be due to exposure irritation, paralytic ectropion, or failure of the lacrimal pump apparatus of the lower lid; it is not likely to be related to an irritative lesion of the greater superficial petrosal nerve. Similarly, decreased tearing, rather than suggesting a destructive process involving, for example, the greater superficial petrosal nerve, may be due to corneal hypesthesia.

Tear testing usually involves Schirmer paper strips placed in the inferior conjunctival cul-de-sacs. To avoid erroneous results from pooled tears, the conjunctival tear lake is dried before insertion of the paper strips (see Fig. 8–9). A Schirmer strip is inserted into the conjunctival sac of the uninvolved eye, and moments later a strip is placed in the involved eye. By following this sequence, the reflex blepharospasm and tearing provoked by stimulating the normal eye do not influence results in the contralateral eye.

About 10% of patients with Bell's palsy have decreased or absent corneal sensation, usually from exposure hypesthesia or as a form of adaptation.[15] In such cases, a topical anesthetic is instilled into both eyes before the Schirmer strips are placed, to eliminate the problem of selectively stimulating the eye with normal corneal sensation. The length of moistened paper is compared on the two sides after a period of 5 minutes. In the event that one of the filter strips becomes completely moistened before 5 minutes, both strips are removed and compared for results. Less than 5 mm of wetting is highly suggestive of a tear deficiency, but this finding should be viewed in the context of the patient's clinical history and the results of the slit lamp examination.

Blink Reflex

Stimulation of either cornea with a cotton wisp or tissue corner will cause a bilateral blink. The ophthalmic division of the fifth nerve (V-1) is the afferent limb of the blink reflex, with first-order neurons synapsing primarily in the chief sensory nucleus within the pontine tegmentum. Second-order neurons project from the chief sensory nucleus to both facial nerve nuclei. Thus, if the left ophthalmic division is defective, neither eye will blink to left corneal stimulation. If the right cornea is stimulated in this setting, both eyes will blink. This scenario must be contrasted with the case of a left facial nerve palsy in which only the right eye will blink fully, regardless of which cornea is stimulated.

The neural control of eyelid function, and especially of the blink reflex, is the subject of an extensive monograph by Schmidtke and Büttner-Ennever,[16] and electromyographic studies of eyelid movements are reviewed by Evinger and colleagues.[17]

Physiologic Facial Synkinesis

Classically, Bell's phenomenon results in the upward and outward deviation of each eye during lid closure against resistance. This palpebral-oculogyric reflex is particularly obvious in patients with lower motor neuron facial paresis and lagophthalmos (i.e., incomplete eye closure). Although the precise neural pathway is unknown, connections between the seventh and third nerve nuclei are implicated by this phenomenon. Francis and Loughhead[18] have found a wide variability in the character of Bell's phenomenon in normal subjects. In their series, many patients showed responses that did not conform to the typical "up and out" eye movement pattern. In addition, on repeated testing, subjects showed variable responses. Clinically, Bell's phenomenon is most useful in distinguishing infranuclear and supranuclear ocular palsies. Typically, upward deviation of the eyes with forced eyelid closure is preserved in supranuclear lesions.

In some normal persons, the external ear retracts and flattens against the mastoid with conjugate lateral gaze. This is known as the oculogyric auricular reflex and is usually greater in the ear opposite the direction of lateral gaze. The presumed neural mechanism involves proprioceptive input from the extraocular muscles to the facial nuclear complex.

In the nasolacrimal reflex, the secretion of tears may be induced by chemically stimulating the nasal mucosa by sniffing dilute solutions of ammonia or formaldehyde. The neural pathway for this reflex results from connections of the trigeminal nerve (V-1) to the greater superficial petrosal nerve. There are numerous other facial reflexes, including blinking during the sudden introduction of a bright light or loud noise, but a full description of these phenomena is beyond the scope of this text.

IDIOPATHIC (BELL'S) FACIAL PALSY

Peripheral facial paralysis is a diagnostic challenge. Every effort must be made to uncover the cause, because often a treatable lesion can be found. The causes of facial paralysis diagnosed and managed over a 24-year period are listed in Table 8–3. Of 2406 patients seen

TABLE 8–3. Causes of Facial Nerve Disorders in 2406 Patients Seen Over 24 Years by One Clinician

Cause	Patients	
	No.	%
Bell's palsy	1272	53
Trauma	502	21
Herpes zoster cephalicus	173	8
Tumor	155	7
Infection	88	4
Birth (congenital and acquired)	78	3
Hemifacial spasm	54	2
Central nervous system (axial) disease	27	1
Other	57	2
Total	2406	100

during this time, no specific cause for the paralysis could be found in 53%. Although it is tempting to label all acute facial palsies as "idiopathic" (*i.e.,* Bell's palsy), 10% of the patients referred with a diagnosis of Bell's palsy were found to have a treatable, progressive, or life-threatening lesion. It must be emphasized that Bell's palsy is a diagnosis of exclusion, reserved for cases in which all other causes of acute acquired, isolated peripheral facial paralysis have been considered and investigated if necessary.

Although Bell's palsy is a term reserved to designate an acute peripheral facial palsy of unknown cause, accumulating evidence supports a viral inflammatory-immune mechanism. In about 60% of cases, Bell's palsy is associated with a viral prodrome. The disorder is self-limiting, is nonprogressive, is not life-threatening, and spontaneously recovers; at this time it can be neither prevented nor cured. Incidence varies between 15% and 40% per 100,000 population annually.[19-22]

Subjective complaints include pain around the ear (50%), facial numbness (40%), changes in taste (50%), and numbness of the tongue (20%).[16] A family history of facial palsies is noted in 14% of patients, and the syndrome is recurrent in 12%. Of those with a history of recurrence, the same side is involved in 36%. Disturbances of the stapes reflex (dysacusis; failure to dampen the vibrating ear ossicles, as determined by middle ear function studies), loss of taste of the anterior two thirds of the tongue, and decreased sublingual and submandibular salivary secretion are most suggestive of a lesion in the tympanomastoid portion of the facial nerve.[16]

The onset of facial palsy is not in itself diagnostic. Tumors, like Bell's palsy, may present with incomplete, complete, sudden, slowly progressive, or recurrent ipsilateral peripheral facial palsy. However, when a facial nerve palsy progresses for more than 3 weeks, a tumor must be excluded. In some cases of otherwise uncomplicated Bell's palsy, examination of the spinal fluid reveals a pleocytosis and an increase in protein, without a microorganism being disclosed.[23]

In a case-control study,[24] 24.8% of patients with Bell's palsy had diabetes, compared with an age-matched control group who had a 13.1% incidence of diabetes. This difference is highly significant and implies a direct relationship between diabetes and Bell's palsy. Preservation of taste was significantly more common in patients with diabetes than in nondiabetics with Bell's palsy. This finding in diabetic patients is in accordance with previously reported studies[25] and suggests a lesion distal to the chorda tympani branch of the facial nerve.

Bell's palsy appears to have a higher incidence during pregnancy. In one study,[26] the calculated frequency in pregnant women was 45.1/100,000 births, compared with 17.4/100,000 per year in nonpregnant women of the same age group. Over 75% of the palsies occurred in the third trimester of pregnancy, and there was no apparent relationship between toxemia, primiparity, and hypertension.

Finally, there appears to be a genetic predisposition to Bell's palsy. The incidence of a positive family history for Bell's palsy in our patients was 14%. The reported frequency of a positive family history for idiopathic palsy has ranged from 2.4% to 28.6%.[27,28]

When one considers the degree of palsy and uses electromyographic data, the prognosis for recovery of facial function can be predicted with a high degree of accuracy. Ninety percent of patients will have a satisfactory recovery if the palsy is incomplete and the response to evoked electromyography (performed with supramaximal stimulation of the facial nerve at the stylomastoid foramen) remains greater than 10% of normal beyond the first 14 days after onset. Patients who do not fulfill these criteria nonetheless have at least a 50% chance of satisfactory recovery[29] (*i.e.,* complete or near complete return of facial function) (Table 8–4).[30]

Peitersen[21] studied the natural history of over 1000 patients with Bell's palsy, seen over a 15-year period, and found that in 84% recovery was satisfactory; 71% recovered without sequelae, and 13% had defects that were barely noticeable. In the remaining 16% of patients with unsatisfactory recovery of facial function, the sequelae were "crippling" in only 4% (House grade IV or worse; see Table 8–4). There was not a single patient without some recovery, and 85% began to recover facial function within 3 weeks of onset of the palsy. Peitersen concluded that the sooner recovery is noted, the better the prognosis for satisfactory function.

A variety of viral agents have been associated with idiopathic facial palsy, but the herpes group of viruses has been the one most often implicated.[31] On this basis, some authors have recommended the routine use of acyclovir in Bell's palsy patients.[32] A review of the literature on this issue found seroconversion rates of just 9.3% for varicella zoster virus and 3.7% for herpes simplex virus in patients with Bell's palsy.[31] A Swedish study of 147 patients with acute facial palsy found elevated viral titers in 9% of patients and elevated titers to *Borrelia burgdorferi* in another 11%. Despite extensive serologic testing, 67% of isolated facial palsy cases remained unexplained.[33] However, a recent study of Bell's palsy and herpes simplex virus supports a stronger viral relationship.[33a] By utilizing polymerase chain reaction techniques on endoneurial fluid and posterior auricular muscle tissue, Murakami and colleagues found herpes simplex type genomic material in 79% of patients tested.

The diagnostic evaluation of patients with acute facial palsy requires consideration of entities such as Lyme disease, HIV infection, sarcoid, herpes infection, syphilis, and a variety of meningeal processes. Magnetic resonance imaging (MRI) is not routinely performed in the evaluation of patients with Bell's palsy. However, nonspecific gadolinium enhancement of the facial nerve is

TABLE 8–4. Classification System for Reporting Results of Recovery*

Degree of Injury	Grade	Definition
Normal (1°)	I	Normal symmetric function in all areas
Mild dysfunction (barely noticeable) (1° or 2°)	II	Slight weakness noticeable only on close inspection; complete eye closure with minimal effort; slight asymmetry of smile with maximal effort; synkinesis barely noticeable, contracture, or spasm absent
Moderate dysfunction (obvious difference) (2° or 3°)	III	Obvious weakness, but not disfiguring; may not be able to lift eyebrow; complete eye closure and strong but asymmetric mouth movement with maximal effort; obvious, but not disfiguring, synkinesis, mass movement, or spasm
Moderately severe dysfunction (3°)	IV	Obvious disfiguring weakness; inability to lift brow; incomplete eye closure and asymmetry of mouth with maximal effort; severe synkinesis, mass movement, spasm
Severe dysfunction (3° to 4°)	V	Motion barely perceptible; incomplete eye closure, slight movement of corner of mouth; synkinesis, contracture, and spasm usually absent
Total paralysis	VI	No movement, loss of tone, no synkinesis, contracture, or spasm

* Recovery results noted 1 year or longer after onset.
(House JW: Facial nerve grading system. Laryngoscope 93:1056, 1983)

often observed. The severity of the facial palsy has no relationship to the findings on MRI, and the unaffected facial nerve may also show pathologic enhancement.[34]

Treatment for Bell's palsy is supportive, involving heat, massage, and facial exercises. Decompressive surgery has not been shown to alter the natural history of Bell's palsy, and the use of steroids is controversial. For instance, there is no large, well-controlled study that supports the efficacy of steroids.[35,36] At present, the decision regarding the use of steroids should be individualized. Considerations should include the patient's age, the patient's general medical condition, the duration and the completeness of the palsy, and the presence of pain. We do not use corticosteroids if it is possible that the facial palsy is caused by Lyme disease, because their administration may render this condition refractory to future antibiotic treatment. Although data is limited, the routine use of acyclovir in the treatment of Bell's palsy is becoming more widely accepted. A recent small double blind study of Bell's palsy supports the combination of acyclovir and prednisone over prednisone alone.[36a] Further study is necessary to determine whether acyclovir should be used alone in Bell's palsy.

INFECTIOUS AND IMMUNE-MEDIATED NEUROPATHIES

Herpes Zoster Cephalicus (Ramsay Hunt Syndrome)

Hunt first described the syndrome of herpes zoster cephalicus, which is characterized by a viral prodrome followed by severe pain in and around the ear, with vesicles involving the external canal and pinna.[37,38] Vesiculation may involve the ear, face, neck, tongue, larynx, or buccal mucosa. The distribution of the vesicles depends on which sensory fibers are infected. Any of the nerve branches that communicate with the facial nerve may be involved, including cranial nerves V, VIII, IX,

and X, and cervical nerves II through IV (Fig. 8–10). In the mildest form, neurologic signs are absent, whereas in severe cases there may be accompanying sensorineural hearing loss, disturbed vestibular function, and even viral encephalitis. Herpes zoster cephalicus is characterized by vesicles, a high incidence of eighth cranial nerve involvement, postherpetic pain, and a poorer prognosis for recovery of the facial palsy. The presence of hearing loss in a patient with suspected idiopathic facial palsy should strongly suggest varicella zoster virus infection.

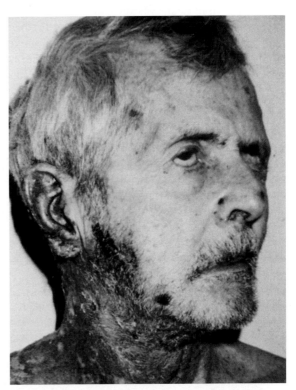

Fig. 8–10. Herpes zoster cephalicus, with Ramsay Hunt syndrome and cutaneous eruption in distribution of second, third, and fourth cervical nerves.

The natural history of herpes zoster differs from that of Bell's palsy in several ways, perhaps reflecting the difference in behavior between herpes simplex type I and the varicella-zoster viruses. Bell's palsy recurs in some 12% of cases, but herpes zoster cephalicus rarely recurs. In addition, the acute phase of the infection, as measured by electrical response and progression of facial weakness, peaks at 5 to 10 days with Bell's palsy, but at 10 to 14 days with herpes zoster cephalicus. Lastly, 84% of persons suffering from Bell's palsy have a satisfactory recovery of facial function, in contrast to 60% of those with herpes zoster cephalicus.

Treatment of herpes zoster is similar to that of Bell's palsy, but with the addition of therapeutics to control pain and vesicular eruption. Often, narcotics are required. Advances in antiviral therapy provide further avenues of treatment.[39] Small studies have supported the efficacy of acyclovir in the treatment of herpes zoster cephalicus, but its role has not been firmly established.[40,41]

POLYRADICULOPATHY (GUILLAIN-BARRÉ SYNDROME)

Guillain-Barré syndrome (GBS) is an acute inflammatory polyradiculopathy evolving as a paralytic disease. It is of unknown cause but is distinctly immune-mediated.[42] Approximately one-third of patients have evidence of campylobacter infection. The characteristic pathologic features of GBS are lymphocytic cellular infiltration of peripheral nerves and destruction of myelin. Therefore, the major complaint is weakness, the severity of which covers a wide spectrum ranging from mild ataxia to total paralysis of any or all motor and cranial nerves. In most instances, symptoms occur first in the legs, but they can begin in the arms, and tendon reflexes

are abolished in the affected areas. Facial nerve paralysis occurs in about half of the cases and is usually bilateral (Fig. 8–11).[43] Weakness can evolve to total motor paralysis, and, when the diaphragm and chest muscles become involved, respiratory embarrassment may lead to death. Abnormal cerebrospinal fluid (CSF) findings are characteristic of this disorder, although in the first few days these may be normal. After several days, the protein value begins to rise and may become very high, peaking at about 4 to 6 weeks after the onset of clinical symptoms. Cells in the CSF are typically absent, but in a small percentage of patients a mild pleocytosis may exist.[43] In the latter cases, it is important to exclude HIV infection, lymphoma, and vasculitis as possible etiologies. It is critical to recognize this disorder in its early stages so that patients can be hospitalized and closely observed for progression of neurologic defects, particularly involvement of respiratory muscles.

It has been suggested that Bell's palsy and Guillain-Barré syndrome represent a continuum of a clinical entity ranging from idiopathic unilateral facial paralysis to severe generalized polyneuropathy.[44] Evidence for this theory comes from the work of Abramsky and associates.[42] In patients with Bell's palsy and Guillain-Barré syndrome, a strong similarity in their lymphocyte response to the peripheral nerve basic protein P_1L was observed. Neither disorder showed a lymphocyte response to the other neural antigens (P_2, BE, AChR), which are commonly used to study experimental autoimmune neurologic diseases. In addition, a control group of 26 patients with a wide spectrum of neurologic disorders showed no response to the neural antigens. In our experience, the prognosis for spontaneous facial nerve recovery in Guillain-Barré syndrome is the same as for idiopathic palsy.

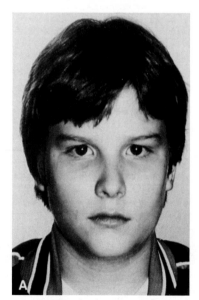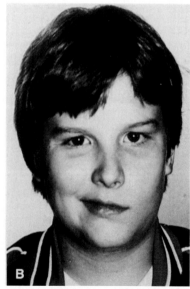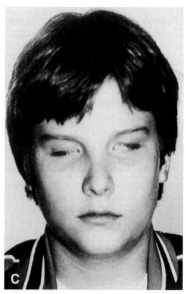

Fig. 8–11. Bulbar polyneuropathy (Guillain-Barré syndrome) with facial diplegia. **A.** At rest. **B.** Attempted smile shows some retained function on right. **C.** Attempted eye closure is incomplete (lagophthalmos).

Infectious Mononucleosis

Infectious mononucleosis (IM) is characterized by fluctuating fever, sore throat, and lymphadenopathy. Uncommonly, unilateral, recurrent, and simultaneous bilateral facial paralysis has been caused by this disorder. The syndrome of infectious mononucleosis caused by Epstein-Barr virus has a classical presentation and can often be diagnosed on clinical grounds. The prodrome lasts from 3 to 5 days and consists of headache, malaise, myalgia, and fatigue. Sore throat occurs in the first week and is the most common feature of IM. A grayish white exudative tonsillitis is practically pathognomonic, persists for 7 to 10 days, and is present in about 50% of cases. Palatine petechiae located near the border of the hard and soft palates are observed in about one third of patients, toward the end of the first week of illness. Lymph node enlargement is a hallmark of IM. The onset is gradual, and anterior and posterior cervical lymph node chains are the most commonly involved. IM resembles a number of febrile disorders characterized by fever, sore throat, adenopathy, and lymphocytosis. It may be difficult to distinguish from the early stages of other forms of febrile exudative pharyngotonsillitis, such as streptococcal infections and exudative tonsillitis of viral etiology. The differentiation depends on the results of throat cultures as well as on hematologic and serologic features characteristic of IM. An absolute increase in lymphocytes and monocytes exceeding 50% or more, and 10% atypical lymphocytes in the peripheral blood, suggests IM. Positive results of a "monospot" serologic test, a rising titer for heterophil antibodies, and development of persistent antibody against Epstein-Barr virus confirm the diagnosis.

Lyme Disease

Lyme disease may cause unilateral or bilateral facial paralysis (Fig. 8–12).[45] This disease is characterized by erythema chronicum migrans, tick-borne meningopolyneuritis, myocardial conduction abnormalities, and Lyme arthritis. The disorder was first recognized in 1975 by close geographic clustering of children with arthritis in the small community of Lyme, Connecticut. The spirochete *B. burgdorferi* is transmitted by an arthropod vector (the deer tick, *Ixodes dammini*). The skin lesion begins as a red macule or papule and expands to form a large red ring with partial central clearing. The lesion typically lasts about 3 weeks or longer (Fig. 8–13). Associated symptoms include malaise, fatigue, chills, fever, headache, myalgias, nausea, vomiting, and sore throat. Some patients develop a spectrum of neurologic symptoms and a clinical picture suggesting collagenosis, syphilis, or multiple sclerosis.

Cranial neuropathies occur frequently in Lyme disease; facial nerve palsy is the most common of these. Unilateral or bilateral facial nerve palsies occurred in

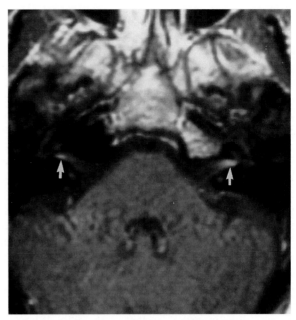

Fig. 8–12. Axial T$_1$-weighted, gadolinium-enhanced MRI showing bilateral proximal facial nerve enhancement (*arrows*) in patient with Lyme disease and facial diplegia.

11% of patients with Lyme disease in one series.[45] In the United States, facial palsy is observed in half of the patients with Lyme meningitis. The prognosis for facial nerve recovery with or without therapy is excellent, with 99.2% of patients achieving satisfactory facial function. Despite the frequent spontaneous resolution of the facial paresis, therapy should be administered to prevent the late neurologic and arthritic complications that can occur. Interestingly, facial nerve paralysis occurs with or without CSF pleocytosis. Distinguishing Lyme-associated facial palsy from idiopathic (Bell's) palsy is essen-

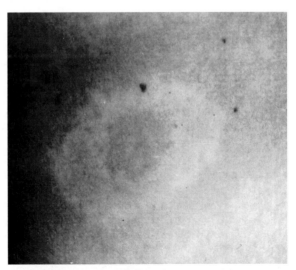

Fig. 8–13. Cutaneous lesion, erythema chronicum migrans, of tick-borne Lyme disease. (MacDonald AB: Lyme disease: a neuro-ophthalmologic view. J Clin Neuro-Ophthalmol 7: 187, 1987)

tial. Lyme disease is suggested when there is coexisting multiorgan involvement such as cardiac disease or arthritis. Nontender swelling and erythema of the face before the onset of the facial palsy may be a distinguishing feature of Lyme disease.[46]

Serologic titers using the enzyme-linked immunosorbent assay (ELISA) and Western blot techniques may help confirm the diagnosis of Lyme disease. However, both false-positive and false-negative Lyme titers are often observed.[47] Because the ELISA and Western blot techniques are not standardized, the reliability of these tests varies widely. In one study, 9 of 40 patients with Lyme disease showed reactivity to the fluorescent treponemal antibody absorption (FTA-ABS) test for syphilis at a 1:5 dilution,[48] but in these patients the Venereal Disease Research Laboratories (VDRL), rapid plasma reagin (RPR), and microhemagglutination assay— Treponema pallidum (MHATP) tests were negative. Successful treatment of early Lyme disease has been achieved with either doxycycline or penicillin. When the facial palsy is associated with meningeal inflammation, a 4-week course of intravenous ceftriaxone is recommended.

Ear Infections

In spite of the frequency of acute otitis media, particularly in children, associated facial paralysis is quite uncommon. In these cases, the facial nerve is most vulnerable as it traverses the tympanic portion of the fallopian canal. The infectious process may track along the chorda tympani nerve, the stapedius nerve, or the posterior tympanic artery to reach the facial nerve within the fallopian canal. The presence of a congenitally narrow fallopian canal is an important risk factor for the development of a facial palsy in acute otitis media.[49] Delayed facial palsy occurring several weeks after a bout of acute otitis media suggests a secondary mastoiditis. A spontaneous and satisfactory recovery is the usual course after treatment with appropriate antibiotics and myringotomy. Surgical therapy is indicated if the infection does not respond to these measures.

Chronic suppurative infection of the middle ear has a different natural history and does call for immediate surgical intervention when associated with a peripheral facial paralysis. Often the pathologic process involves compression of an exposed nerve by cholesteatoma or chronically infected granulation tissue. Abscess and osteitis are not unusual findings at the time of surgery.

In cases of complicated otitis media, localized inflammation of the petrous apex may occur, resulting in the so-called Gradenigo's syndrome.[50] This entity is characterized by facial pain associated with trigeminal, abducens, and facial nerve palsies. Neuroradiologic imaging should be performed to exclude the presence of an extradural abscess or mass lesions that might mimic Gradenigo's syndrome, such as invasive nasopharyngeal carcinoma. Treatment consists of appropriate antibiotic coverage and possible surgical debridement of the petrous bone.

A closely related disorder is the "malignant" external otitis syndrome. This infectious disorder is usually seen in elderly patients with diabetes and begins in the external auditory canal. The offending organism is Pseudomonas aeruginosa. The facial nerve may be involved at the level of the stylomastoid foramen by an associated necrotizing osteomyelitis, which may spread to involve the occipital bone, clivus, and contralateral petrous pyramid. Other complications include venous dural thromboses, meningitis, and brain abscess. Treatment should consist of broad-spectrum antibiotics effective against all strains of P. aeruginosa. Facial nerve paralysis is reversible until the nerve itself becomes necrotic.[51,52]

Other Infections and Postimmunization

Facial nerve paresis has been observed in a variety of other infectious processes, including chickenpox,[53] mumps,[53] influenza,[53] brain stem encephalitis,[54] polio,[55] enterovirus,[56] leprosy,[57] tuberculosis,[58] mucormycosis,[59,60] syphilis,[61] tetanus,[62] and diphtheria.[63] Recently, a patient with a facial palsy was found to be infected with human monocytic ehrlichiosis, an intracellular parasite that infects monoocular phagocytes.[63a] Facial paresis has also occurred after vaccination[64–66] and after the administration of tetanus antiserum.[67] Unilateral or bilateral facial palsy has been observed in HIV infection. The facial palsy associated with early HIV may spontaneously resolve and has been documented to occur at the time of HIV seroconversion.[68] In contrast, the appearance of a facial palsy in the advanced stages of HIV infection should prompt a search for other etiologies, such as meningeal lymphoma, herpes zoster, and cryptococcal meningitis.

TRAUMA

Facial nerve trauma may be accidental or iatrogenic, such as facial paralysis occurring after ophthalmologic surgical procedures where local injections are used to block the upper division of the facial nerve to achieve akinesia of the orbicularis oculi muscles.[69] The mechanism may be either direct infiltration of the nerve with the anesthetic or precipitation of an inflammatory immune disorder similar to Bell's palsy. The onset after manipulation is obvious; an unresolved facial paralysis after injection most likely is related to mechanical trauma, whereas a palsy that develops days later is likely to be of the inflammatory-immune type. Treatment is the same as for Bell's palsy (see earlier). Prognosis depends on the completeness of the palsy, electrostimulation results, and the onset of recovery.

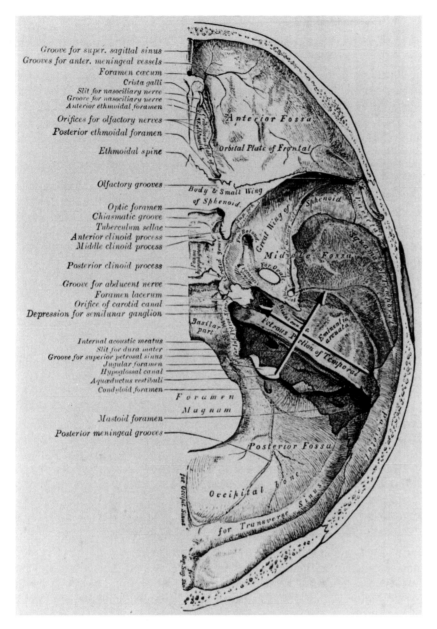

Fig. 8–14. Skull base showing transverse and longitudinal axes (*arrows*) of petrous fractures. (Gray H: Anatomy of the Human Body, 26th ed. Philadelphia, Lea & Febiger, 1955)

Facial palsies often are produced by closed-head trauma, especially when lateral skull compression has occurred. The resulting temporal bone fractures may be longitudinal or transverse to the axis of the petrous bone (Fig. 8–14). Longitudinal fractures are more common and usually spare the facial nerve, but if the facial nerve is impaired, the longitudinal fracture usually involves the segment just distal to the geniculate ganglion.[70] Paralysis typically results from compression and ischemia rather than direct injury.[71] Transverse fractures are associated with facial palsy in about 50% of cases; the facial nerve is usually impaired in the labyrinthine segment proximal to the geniculate ganglion. In transverse fractures, the paralysis is typically more severe and immediate.[71]

In a series of 90 cases of temporal bone fractures reported by Cannon and Jahrsdoerfer,[71] ecchymosis over the mastoid (Battle's sign) was present in eight patients. This sign is usually seen when the skull base is fractured and results from blood extravasated along the course of the posterior auricular artery. In longitudinal fractures, rupture of the tympanic membrane is common with associated CSF otorrhea and hemotympanum. Transverse fractures can also cause hemotympanum but are rarely associated with rupture of the tympanic membrane and bleeding from the external canal. The facial nerve is also subject to trauma as it exits the stylomastoid foramen, where it may be impaired by blunt force, knife wounds, or local infiltration of an anesthetic.

Surgical exploration and possible repair in acute traumatic paralysis are indicated in selected cases when the nerve has been crushed, stretched, or transected. Such an injury is likely in cases of temporal bone fracture that have a sudden and complete onset of paralysis, that have displacement of the temporal bone fragments noted by computed tomography (CT) scan, and that have lost the electrical response to stimulation by the fifth day. Surgical exploration in such cases should be undertaken as the patient's condition permits. If an injury occurs accidentally during surgery, repair should be performed at that time.

TUMORS

Tumors of the head and neck may envelop or invade the facial nerve in its course from the pons through the temporal bone, middle ear, and parotid gland. Intra-axial lesions involving facial function include pontine gliomas and metastatic lesions. The nerve traverses the subarachnoid space, where it may be invaded by tumor or by lymphoma that has infiltrated the meninges. In the cerebellopontine angle, the facial nerve is most commonly compromised by acoustic neuromas, facial neuromas, metastatic lesions, and meningiomas.[72] Other lesions that may affect the nerve in the temporal bone are glomus tumors[73] and epidermoids.[74] In its extracranial course through the parotid gland, the facial nerve may be involved by malignant tumors of the parotid gland; the two most common tumors are mucoepidermoid and adenoid cystic carcinoma. A facial nerve palsy is rarely associated with a benign parotid tumor.[75]

Acoustic Neuroma

Most acoustic neuromas arise from the vestibular division of the eighth nerve within the internal auditory canal. When the tumor is confined to this canal, hearing loss is the main sign; few patients have obvious involvement of the facial nerve. As the tumor expands and extends to the cerebellopontine angle, facial weakness may occur from stretching of the facial nerve. Other findings include nystagmus, decreased corneal reflex, and facial hypesthesia. In a series of 53 acoustic neuromas, only five patients had facial weakness at presenta-

tion.[76] When a patient presents with bilateral acoustic neuromas, the diagnosis of neurofibromatosis should be considered.

On CT scan, acoustic neuromas may be seen as enhancing masses in the internal auditory canal or cerebellopontine angle. For smaller tumors, gadolinium-enhanced MRI may be very helpful. On T_1-weighted gadolinium images, neuromas may appear as uniformly enhancing masses, effacing the brain stem and cerebellum with extension into the internal auditory meatus or canal. On T_2-weighted images these lesions appear hyperintense (Fig. 8–15).[77] Treatment usually consists of microsurgical excision with the use of techniques that may provide complete removal of tumor and preservation of the facial nerve. Intraoperative facial nerve monitoring during acoustic neuroma surgery may improve the preservation of facial nerve function.[78,79]

Facial Neuroma

The facial paralysis associated with facial nerve neuromas usually has a gradual onset, but it may be more rapid, simulating idiopathic facial paralysis. Indeed, the pareses may fluctuate or may be associated with hemifacial spasm. In some cases, hearing loss precedes the onset of facial weakness, thereby simulating an acoustic neuroma.[80] CT scan typically shows a uniformly enhancing mass in the fallopian canal. T_2-weighted MRI images may show a hyperintense mass in the facial canal[77] that enhances with gadolinium on T_1-weighted images (Fig. 8–16). The ultimate diagnosis of facial neuroma requires surgical exploration and biopsy. Biopsy usually results in facial paralysis. This possibility should be discussed with the patient before surgery. Facial function recovery after resection of tumor and grafting, although never normal, may include restored tone, symmetry, and weak voluntary movement. The more facial function present before surgery, the better the results with grafting. This observation must be shared with the patient, because he or she might elect to wait until facial function is lost before consenting to surgical removal.

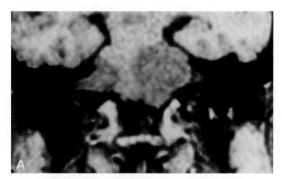
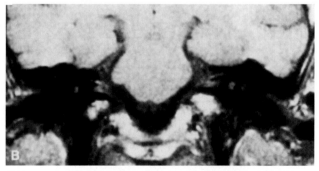

Fig. 8–15. Magnetic resonance imaging of acoustic neuroma. **A.** Coronal section through pons showing bilateral acoustic neuromas in a patient with neurofibromatosis. **B.** Normal study of same area.

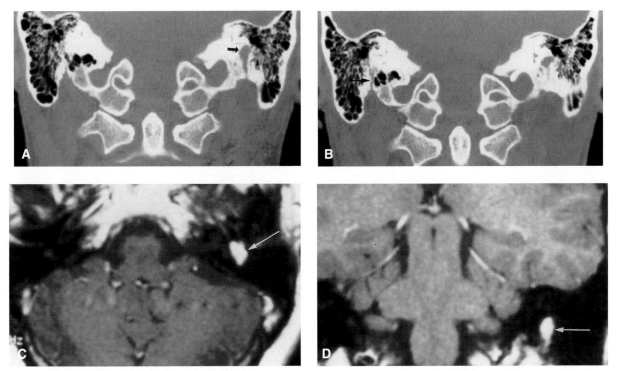

Fig. 8–16. Patient with facial neuroma. **A.** Coronal CT scan demonstrating enlarged stylomastoid foramen and facial nerve mass (*arrow*). **B.** Note size of canal in (**A,** *black arrow*) compared with normal sized canal (*open arrow*). **C.** Axial MRI scan showing an enhancing mass of tympanic segment (*arrow*). **D.** Coronal gadolinium-enhanced MRI section demonstrating same mass in mastoid segment (*arrow*).

Metastatic Lesions

A history of cancer (particularly involving the breast, lung, thyroid, kidney, ovary, or prostate) associated with a rapidly progressive facial paralysis strongly suggests a metastatic lesion. The facial nerve may be involved by a bony metastasis or by meningeal infiltration. Neuroimaging studies are indicated to search for the primary site and to localize the site of facial nerve involvement (Fig. 8–17). If these are unrevealing, serial lumbar punc-

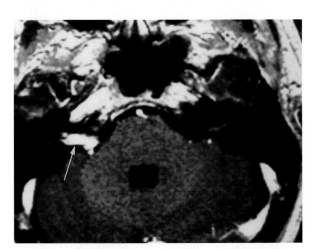

Fig. 8–17. Axial MRI scan discloses gadolinium enhancement and enlargement of right facial nerve (*arrow*) in patient with meningeal carcinomatosis.

tures may be necessary to exclude meningeal carcinomatosis. In some cases, surgical exploration of the temporal bone or of the extracranial course of the facial nerve is recommended to locate the lesion. In one study of meningeal carcinomatosis, the seventh nerve was affected in 15 of 90 patients.[81] Facial nerve involvement is often unilateral, but it occurs bilaterally in about 10% of such patients.[82]

MISCELLANEOUS CONDITIONS

Sarcoidosis

Infiltrations of the parotid glands may affect branches of the seventh nerve in their intraglandular course. As such, sarcoidosis is a distinct, if rare, cause of facial palsies.[83] However, facial palsy is the most common neurologic manifestation of sarcoidosis.[84] In a patient presenting with facial paralysis and uveitis, sarcoidosis should be strongly suspected.[85] Sarcoidosis is a granulomatous disease of undetermined origin that involves multiple organ systems. Although there is no single laboratory test that is diagnostic, sarcoidosis is characterized by an elevation in serum and urinary calcium levels, an increase in serum globulin, and an elevated serum angiotensin-converting enzyme level. Chest films commonly reveal hilar adenopathy or diffuse pulmonary infiltrates, and examination of the eyes may indicate chronic anterior or posterior uveitis. The diagnosis is made on the basis of clinical findings together with biopsy of involved tissue, which typically shows noncaseating granuloma with giant cells.

Acute Porphyrias

Bilateral facial paralysis is rarely caused by the acute porphyrias.[86] These are disorders characterized by various abnormalities in the synthesis of heme that result in an accumulation of heme precursors. Clinical manifestations usually include abdominal pain as the initial and most prominent symptom. In addition, photosensitivity and often an acute neurologic crisis may ensue, characterized by seizures, mental disturbances, cranial nerve palsies, autonomic dysfunction, and peripheral neuropathy.[86a] These crises may be precipitated by medications, including sulfonamides and barbiturates. In one series of acute intermittent porphyria,[87] the seventh nerve was affected in about 50% of patients with neuropathic crises. The diagnosis is confirmed by noting elevated urinary and stool porphyrins and a markedly elevated urinary porphobilinogen level.

Myasthenia Gravis

Myasthenia gravis is an autoimmune disorder with antibodies directed against the postsynaptic membrane of the neuromuscular junction. It is characterized clinically by fluctuating weakness of the skeletal muscles, but particularly affected are the ocular, facial, and bulbar muscles. Facial weakness may be unilateral, but it is often bilateral, manifested by paresis of both orbicularis oculi muscles and a weak, "transverse" smile in which the corners of the mouth are turned downward.

Osher and Griggs[88] have described a "peek" sign as a manifestation of orbicularis oculi weakness: with attempts at sustained gentle eyelid closure, the palpebral fissure opens slightly as the orbicularis muscle fatigues and exposes sclera, appearing as if the patient is "peeking." The diagnosis of myasthenia can be confirmed by an edrophonium (Tensilon) test. Other useful ancillary tests include electromyography, which characteristically shows a decremental response to both low and high rates of stimulation. Single-fiber electromyography of the orbicularis oculi is now the most sensitive test to confirm the facial weakness associated with myasthenia gravis.[89] Serum titers for anti–acetylcholine receptor antibodies can also be obtained.

Botulism

Bilateral facial paralysis may be caused by botulism, but this is uncommon.[90] This disease can be recognized clinically by a red parched tongue, oropharynx, hypopharynx, and larynx, associated with bilateral cranial nerve deficits. The disorder results from a neuromuscular transmission blockade by toxin that interferes with acetylcholine release at nerve terminals. Early diagnosis is critical because respiratory collapse may be imminent. The diagnosis is confirmed by isolating botulinum toxin from contaminated food or from a stool specimen from the patient. Toxin can also be demonstrated in the patient's serum by the mouse neutralization test and immunofluorescent techniques. The absence of sensory findings and the presence of normal CSF are characteristic. Electromyography typically shows an increase of the motor unit action potential amplitude to high rates of repetitive stimulation. Treatment is supportive and involves administration of the botulism equine trivalent antitoxin, and gastric lavage in early cases. Recovery is usually complete, but some patients may have residual weakness secondary to denervation atrophy.[63]

Myotonic Dystrophy

Myotonic dystrophy is a progressive distal myopathy associated with weakness of the muscles of the face, jaw, neck, and levators of the eyelids. Children with congenital myotonic dystrophy usually present at birth with facial diplegia, although without abducens paralysis; only later is the progressive nature of the myopathy evident.[91] Myotonia is conspicuously absent in the neonatal period but becomes manifest later in life. Unlike Möbius' syndrome, there is progressive muscle wasting, particularly of the sternocleidomastoid, temporal, and facial muscles. This creates an expressionless face, the so-called myopathic facies (Fig. 8–18). Other nonmus-

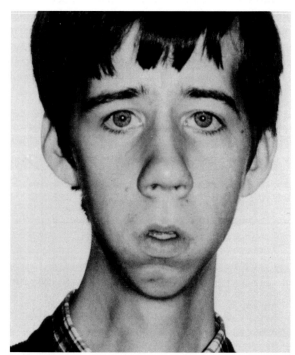

Fig. 8–18. Myotonia dystrophica. The expressionless face and swanlike neck are due to atrophy of masticatory, facial, and sternocleidomastoid muscles.

cular dystrophic anomalies, such as cataract, premature frontal baldness, and testicular atrophy, are also present. The neck is usually described as swanlike; this is due to wasting of the masticatory and sternocleidomastoid muscles.

Progressive Hemifacial Atrophy (Parry-Romberg Syndrome)

Hemifacial atrophy is an unusual condition of unknown etiology. It is characterized by spontaneous and slowly progressive atrophy of the skin and subcutaneous tissue on one side of the face and scalp (Fig. 8–19). There is a slight female predominance, and the disorder typically begins within the first two decades of life. Involvement of the soft tissues surrounding the orbit and in the orbit is common, such that progressive unilateral *enophthalmos* occurs. Other findings include focal alopecia, loss of lashes and eyebrow hairs, linear scarring of the scalp (en coupe de sabre), exophthalmos, poliosis, ptosis, miosis, mydriasis, iris heterochromia, uveitis, motility disturbances, corneal opacities, refractive error, and optic nerve atrophy. The presence of subtle fundus abnormalities, including choroidal atrophy and retinal pigment epithelium changes, has been documented.[92] The most common neurologic complication is seizures, which may be generalized or focal in nature.[93] Other reported neurologic associations include hemiparesis, hemianesthesia, hemianopia, and aphasia. Chung and colleagues[94] reported a case of epilepsy with frontal lobe leptomeningeal sclerosis subjacent to forehead scleroderma. There is no treatment for this disorder, and reconstructive surgery is best delayed until progression ceases.

BILATERAL OR RECURRENT FACIAL NERVE PARESIS

Bilateral simultaneous facial nerve pareses present a special diagnostic and therapeutic challenge and may be a medical emergency. In our series, the onset of facial diplegia was acute in 12 cases, and the most common cause was the Guillain-Barré syndrome. Other causes of acute or chronic bilateral facial palsy include leukemia, meningeal carcinomatosis, idiopathic (Bell's) palsy, sarcoidosis, skull fracture, myasthenia gravis, polio, porphyria, Lyme disease, Möbius' syndrome, and myotonic dystrophy.

Recurrent facial paralysis has been noted to occur in an idiopathic form, the Melkersson-Rosenthal syndrome, and even with tumors.[95] The recurrence rate in our experience with idiopathic palsy was 12%. In contrast to recurrent facial paralysis on the same side, contralateral recurrence is almost always due to idiopathic palsy; alternating facial paralysis has been noted only rarely with other disorders.

Melkersson-Rosenthal syndrome (Fig. 8–20) is the most common example of a rare disorder that features recurrent alternating facial palsy; recurrent edema of the lips, face, and eyelids; cheilitis; and fissured tongue. Most authors agree that the presence of any two of these four manifestations permits the diagnosis.[96] It has been suggested that facial swelling is the most consistent finding in Melkersson-Rosenthal syndrome.[97] Perhaps

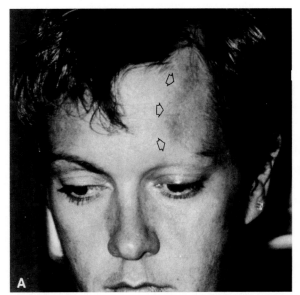
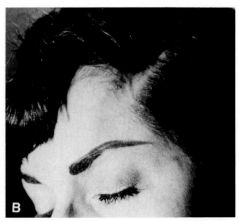

Fig. 8–19. Hemifacial atrophy (Parry-Romberg syndrome). **A.** Arrows outline depression of forehead due to loss of subcutaneous tissue; atrophy also extends to left cheek. Note loss of eyebrow hair and lashes from left upper lid. **B.** Spontaneous scalp creasing extending to forehead and upper brow (scleroderma en coupe de sabre). Lateral eyebrow is absent and lid lashes are false. Note slight left enophthalmos.

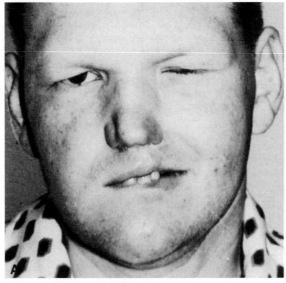
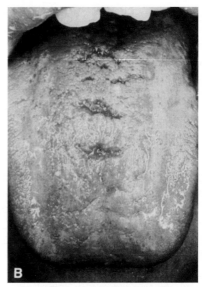

Fig. 8–20. Melkersson-Rosenthal syndrome. Patient with recurrent, alternating facial palsy. **A.** Facial swelling. **B.** Fissured tongue.

the diagnosis of this syndrome should be reserved for only those patients with the finding of facial edema, because there is recurrence in 12% of Bell's palsy patients and a fissured tongue can be seen in otherwise normal persons. The etiology of Melkersson-Rosenthal syndrome is unknown, although biopsy findings of buccal mucosa have shown noncaseating granulomas. Associated ophthalmic findings have included retrobulbar neuritis, lagophthalmos, corneal opacities, and keratoconjunctivitis sicca. Treatment has largely been unsuccessful and has included trials of antibiotics, antihistamines, irradiation, and steroids.[97]

FACIAL EMBRYOPATHIES AND CHILDHOOD PALSIES

Facial disorders in childhood constitute a special diagnostic category and should not be attributed so readily to the idiopathic category. The information presented here is based principally on the diagnosis and management of facial paralysis in 332 patients, newborn to 18 years. Although the causes of facial palsy in these children were generally similar to those in adults, the exceptions were neonatal paralysis and cases due to acute otitis media (Table 8–5). The principles of management of facial paralysis in children are similar to those in adults, with few exceptions.

The differential diagnosis and treatment of facial paralysis in the newborn have been reviewed by May and associates[98] and Harris and co-workers.[99] The two main differential diagnostic possibilities are developmental and traumatic (Table 8–6). Traumatic neonatal facial palsies are usually unilateral and may result from pressure on the infant's mastoid area from the maternal

sacral prominence.[100] Although Hepner[101] found the incidence of facial paralysis to be the same for natural and forceps deliveries, more recent studies implicate obstetric forceps as a risk factor for neonatal facial palsy. Among 44,292 babies delivered over a 5-year period,

TABLE 8–5. Causes of Facial Palsy in 332 Patients Newborn to 18 Years Old

Causes	No. of Patients	Percent
Bell's palsy	130	39
Herpes zoster cephalicus	13	4
Birth	61	18
Developmental (45)		
Traumatic (16)		
Trauma	56	17
Accidental (31)		
Iatrogenic (22)		
Surgical (3)		
Infection	38	11
Acute otitis media (27)		
Chronic otitis media (4)		
Cholesteatoma (1)		
Chickenpox (3)		
Mononucleosis (1)		
Mumps (1)		
Diphtheria (1)		
Tumor	15	5
Tumor suspect	3	1
Other	16	5
Melkersson-Rosenthal syndrome (4)		
Poliomyelitis (5)		
Guillain-Barré syndrome (3)		
Hypothyroidism (1)		
Sickle cell crisis (1)		
Myotonic dystrophy (1)		
Sarcoidosis (1)		
Total	332	

TABLE 8–6. Facial Palsy at Birth: Differential Diagnosis

	Developmental	Traumatic
History	No recovery after birth. Family history of facial and other anomalies.	Total paralysis at birth with some recovery noted subsequently
Physical	Other anomalies, bilateral palsy, lower lip or upper face palsy. Other cranial nerve deficits.	Hemotympanum, ecchymosis, synkinesis
Radiograph of temporal bone	Anomalous external, middle, or inner ear, or mandible; vertical segment of facial nerve	Fracture
Maximal stimulation/evoked electromyography	Response decreased or absent, without change on repeat testing	Normal at birth, then decreasing to possible loss of response
Electromyography	Reduced or absent response, no evidence of degeneration	Normal at birth, then loss of spontaneous motor units; 10 to 21 days later, appearance of fibrillation and giant motor unit potentials
Auditory brain stem response	Abnormality in cranial nerves III to V	Normal, provided hearing is normal

92 were found to have facial palsy.[102] Eighty-one of these palsies were believed to be related to birth trauma, most notably forceps use. The remaining 11 instances were developmental. Nearly 90% of the facial palsies related to birth trauma had complete spontaneous recovery by 1 year.[102]

The most common finding associated with developmental facial paralysis is the presence of one or more other congenital anomalies. Weakness of the lower lip has particular significance in that it may be associated with multiple congenital anomalies. In one study of asymmetric facies, noted especially during crying, associated congenital anomalies were found in the skeletal, genitourinary, respiratory, and cardiovascular systems.[103] Developmental bilateral facial palsy is often incomplete, with the lower portion of the face usually less affected than the upper part. This distinguishes it from facial palsy due to trauma, which is rarely bilateral and shows equal involvement of the lower and upper face. Bilateral immobility of the face may not be apparent at birth and may be manifested by incomplete eyelid closure when asleep, by a gaping mouth, and by an inability to suck.

Möbius' syndrome is a rare congenital disorder that usually includes bilateral hypoplasia of facial muscles, unilateral or bilateral horizontal gaze palsy, anomalies of the extremities, absence of chest muscles, and involvement of other cranial nerves, especially the hypoglossal. Many pathologic findings have been described in Möbius' syndrome, including nuclear aplasia and neuronal degeneration (Fig. 8–21) (see Chapter 13).[104]

There is no effective way to restore facial function in the newborn or young child with a facial paralysis due to a congenital anomaly. Management should be directed toward preventing complications and performing reanimation procedures as the patient approaches the teens.

Children with facial paralysis from birth usually do not have problems with keratitis and corneal scarring unless there is a poor Bell's phenomenon, decreased tearing, or entropion with irritation of the globe from eyelashes rubbing against the cornea. The child should undergo slit lamp evaluation periodically, and if there is any evidence of frank keratitis, medical and perhaps surgical measures should be considered to correct the deformities.

HYPERKINETIC FACIAL DISORDERS

A wide variety of spontaneous, anomalous facial movements occur with surprising frequency. These hyperkinesia syndromes include primary and secondary blepharospasm, hemifacial spasm, facial synkinesis following recovery of facial palsies, tonic contracture, and myokymias.

Blepharospasm

This condition is characterized by involuntary, bilateral spasmodic eye closure. Forceful contraction of the orbicularis oculi muscle is present, accompanied by tonic depression of the eyebrows (Fig. 8–22). Unlike hemifacial spasm, which is unilateral, blepharospasm tends not to involve the lower face or platysma. Secondary blepharospasm is the result of ocular irritation and may be seen in cases of keratitis, scleritis, or uveitis, or after the application of topical ocular medications. Once ocular irritation has been excluded, primary blepharospasm should be considered in a variety of extrapyramidal disorders, including Parkinson's disease, postencephalitic parkinsonism, Huntington's chorea, bilateral basal ganglia infarction,[105] and Meige's syndrome (blepharospasm and oral facial dystonia). It should also be consid-

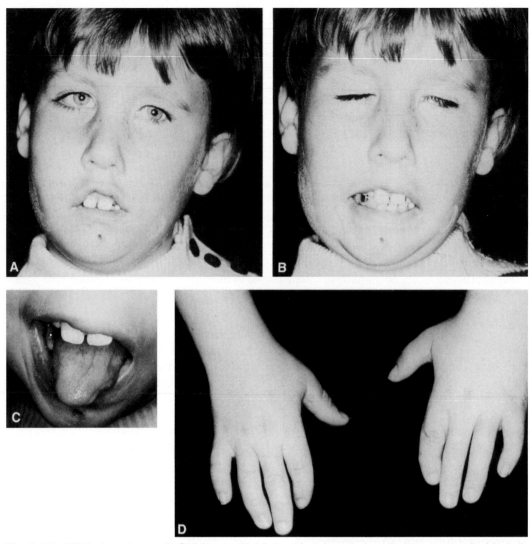

Fig. 8–21. Möbius' syndrome. **A.** Child born with bilateral facial weakness. **B.** Asymmetry of orbicularis function and relative sparing of lower face. This patient also showed horizontal gaze paresis. **C.** Moderate atrophy of the left side of the tongue, suggesting XII nerve involvement. **D.** Congenital finger anomalies, including webbed bases.

ered as a side effect of dopamine agonists and antagonists.[106] Most cases of blepharospasm are idiopathic, and medical therapy, for the most part, is often disappointing. Pharmacologic therapy with dopamine-depleting agents, neuroleptics, sedatives, centrally acting cholinergic drugs, and gamma-aminobutyric acid agonists has had variable success. Psychotherapy and biofeedback also have been helpful in a limited number of cases.[106] Surgical therapy is a last resort and has included procedures directed at weakening the facial nerve[107] or stripping the orbicularis oculi muscle.[108] These procedures are often limited by complications such as facial weakness, ectropion, and recurrent blepharospasm.

Botulinum, a presynaptic blocking agent injected subcutaneously into the orbicularis oculi muscles, is now the treatment of choice for blepharospasm.[109–113] Most patients enjoy a significant reduction in the facial spasm within a few days of the injection, and these effects last several months. Complications are usually mild and transient, including ptosis, exposure keratopathy, lower facial weakness, and ecchymosis around the injection sites. Recurrence of facial spasm occurs in almost all patients within several months, but repeated injections are well tolerated.

Hemifacial Spasm

Hemifacial spasm is the result of unilateral, hyperactive facial nerve dysfunction and is characterized by the spontaneous onset of unilateral intermittent spasms of the orbicularis oculi muscle. These spasms gradually increase in severity and frequency and spread downward to involve the muscles of facial expression, including the platysma (Fig. 8–23). Hemifacial spasm should be

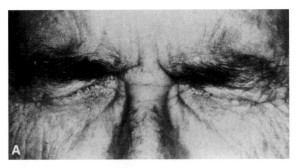

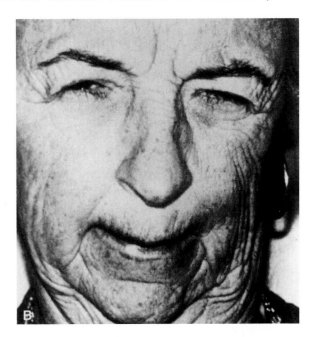

Fig. 8–22. Essential blepharospasm. **A.** Forceful spontaneous contraction of orbicularis oculi muscle. **B.** Meige's syndrome with blepharospasm and orofacial dystonia. (May M: The Facial Nerve. New York, Thieme Stratton, 1986)

distinguished from facial tics that begin in childhood and can be suppressed voluntarily for a period of time. Focal epilepsy involving the face can also be distinguished from hemifacial spasm by the presence of an abnormal electroencephalogram or the appearance of a postictal facial paralysis (Todd's paralysis). The spasms are usually brief, lasting only seconds, and may persist during sleep. Rarely is a specific cause of hemifacial spasm uncovered, but vascular compression of the facial nerve at its exit from the brain stem has been implicated.[114]

Although the underlying pathophysiology of this disorder is unknown, the concept of ephaptic transmission remains a dominant theory.[115,116] Ephaptic transmission refers to a lateral spreading of neural impulses by damaged axons that excite adjacent nerve fibers. This leads

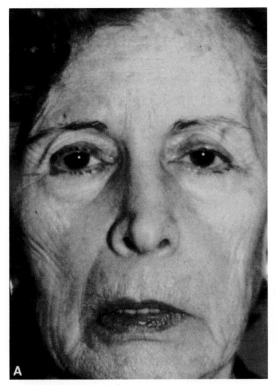

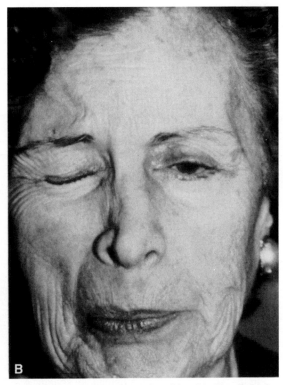

Fig. 8–23. Hemifacial spasm. **A.** At rest. **B.** During involuntary facial contraction.(May M: The Facial Nerve. New York, Thieme Stratton, 1986)

to the spontaneous and simultaneous contraction of adjacent facial muscles. Anomalous facial motor nucleus firing is an alternative theory. Ferguson[117] has suggested that damage to the facial nerve near its root entry zone, or in the brain stem, leads to deafferentation of the facial motor nucleus. This would result in augmented and automatic firing of the facial motor nucleus, presumably by disinhibition and reorganization of the central nuclear pool. Other cases are recorded after idiopathic palsy and with extramedullary compression by tumor.[118] Neuroradiologic imaging, especially MRI of the posterior fossa, should be performed to exclude compression of the facial nerve by tumor (Fig. 8–24). A recent study found magnetic resonance tomographic angiography to be the most sensitive test to detect vascular compression of the facial nerve at the root exit zone. Twenty-four of 37 (65%) patients had evidence of vascular compression of the seventh nerve at its exit zone, compared with 6% of control patients.[119]

Neurosurgical treatment is directed toward decompression of the facial trunk at its exit from the brain stem in proximity to a tortuous or dolichoectatic anteroinferior cerebellar, posteroinferior cerebellar, vertebral, or basilar artery (see Fig. 8–24).[9] The surgical approach is by way of a suboccipital craniotomy with placement of a sponge prosthesis between the facial nerve and the offending artery. In a series of 54 patients, Auger and colleagues[120] reported complete relief in 70% of patients who underwent microvascular decompression for hemifacial spasm; 11% had initial improvement followed by a recurrence of facial spasm within 2 years, whereas another 9% had improvement without total resolution. Only 9% of patients showed no benefit. The mean follow-up period was 3.9 years. Complications included unilateral hearing loss, transient and permanent facial weakness, facial numbness, and unsteady gait. In a recent series of 310 patients treated by microvascular decompression of the facial nerve, over 90% had complete relief of spasm with a late recurrence of only 1%.[121] Other surgical approaches include unilateral myectomy[122] and facial neurotomy.[107]

Medical therapy with carbamazepine[123] and baclofen[124] has also been successful in relieving hemifacial spasm in some patients. Injection of botulinum A toxin into the orbicularis oculi muscle has become standard treatment of hemifacial spasm.[111]

Facial Synkinesis

When a patient suffers a seventh nerve paresis, he or she may subsequently demonstrate ipsilateral involuntary narrowing of the palpebral fissure upon volitional contraction of the orbicularis oris and other facial muscles (*i.e.,* during pursing the lips, forceful opening of the mouth, smiling, or chewing with the mouth closed). In addition, lower facial muscles may contract during volitional eye closure. This phenomenon is due to aberrant regeneration of the seventh nerve with sprouting of axons to supply more than one muscle group. Frueh[125] used electromyography to show that the narrowing of the palpebral fissure was secondary to contraction of the ipsilateral orbicularis oculi muscles and not due to inhibition of the levator superioris. At present, there is no effective way to prevent intrafacial synkinetic phenomena. In one study, injections of botulinum toxin into the orbicularis oculi of several patients provided temporary relief.[111]

Facial synkinesis should be distinguished from the rare congenital inverse jaw-winking phenomenon, in which contraction of the trigeminal innervated pterygoid muscle induces narrowing of the ipsilateral palpe-

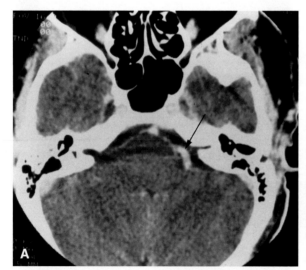
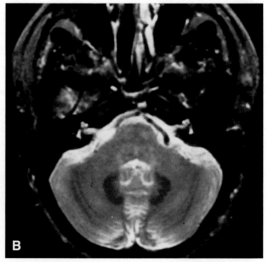

Fig. 8–24. Patient with left hemifacial spasm. **A.** CT with contrast shows dolichoectatic vertebrobasilar artery (*arrow*) abutting left facial nerve. **B.** Similar finding confirmed by axial T$_2$-weighted MRI scan.

bral fissure. In this condition, there is a mild ptosis at rest, which increases upon opening the mouth or with lateral deviation of the jaw. Electromyography has shown inhibition of the levator muscle without any change in the firing of the orbicularis oculi muscle.[126] This synkinesis has been attributed to abnormal central connections between the trigeminal and oculomotor nuclei, resulting in ipsilateral levator superioris inhibition.

Gustatory Tearing (Crocodile Tears)

Persons who have undergone a peripheral facial palsy may experience uncontrollable ipsilateral tearing while eating, or even in anticipation of a meal. This psychic or gustatory lacrimation phenomenon is the result of an aberrant resprouting of salivary fibers that gain access to the ipsilateral lacrimal glands. In such cases, the facial nerve is denervated at or above the level of the geniculate ganglion or along the course of the greater superficial petrosal nerve. This anomaly is known as "crocodile tears" and is reminiscent of the myth that crocodiles are said to tear while eating their prey.[127,128]

Gustatory Sweating

Unilateral profuse sweating in the preauricular area of the face while eating is known as gustatory sweating or Frey's syndrome.[129] This disorder usually occurs several months to years after injury to the facial nerve in the parotid gland.[130] Presumably, misdirected salivary fibers supply the sweat glands. This is a rare condition that often remits spontaneously. Drysol cream rubbed over the affected area every 3 days is a useful remedy for this disorder.

Facial Myokymia

Facial myokymia consists of fine fibrillary or undulating movement of the facial muscles. These contractions are unilateral, are intermittent, and may ripple across the face. This condition has been associated with several etiologies, including multiple sclerosis,[131] intrinsic brain stem tumors,[132] extramedullary compression,[133] brain stem infarction,[134] Guillain-Barré syndrome,[135] toxins,[136] anoxia,[137] and obstructive hydrocephalus.[124] This disorder may represent enhanced irritability of the facial motor unit, starting with the supranuclear pathways and ending at the neuromuscular junction of the facial nerve.[135] When facial myokymia is associated with ipsilateral tonic facial contracture and paresis (spastic-paretic facial contracture) (Fig. 8–25), the lesion is most likely to be within the pons.[138]

In a study of facial myokymia and multiple sclerosis, MRI demonstrated a high signal abnormality in the pontine tegmentum in the region of the postgenu segment of the facial nerve in 11 of 12 (90%) patients.[139]

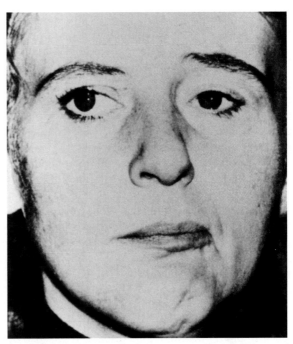

Fig. 8–25. Spastic-paretic facial contraction due to pontine glioma. Note constant spasm of left facial musculature. (May M: The Facial Nerve. New York, Thieme Stratton, 1986)

Facial myokymia should be distinguished from benign eyelid myokymia, a disorder that is transient and of no pathologic significance. Benign eyelid myokymia is seen in well persons and consists of fine twitching of the upper and lower eyelids on one side. Episodes last from several hours to several days or even weeks and are commonly associated with fatigue, anxiety, nicotine, or excessive caffeine.

DISORDERS OF EYELID OPENING

The hyperkinetic facial disorders that narrow or close the lid aperture are to be distinguished from mechanical or neural causes of ptosis (*e.g.*, senile or traumatic levator dehiscence, myasthenia, oculomotor palsy), and also from rather rare *supranuclear* defects of eyelid opening.

Apraxia of eyelid opening is a supranuclear disorder characterized by an inability to voluntarily open closed lids. This can be distinguished from blepharospasm by the absence of active orbicularis oculi and upper facial contractions, and it can be distinguished from bilateral cerebral ptosis by its intermittent nature. Lid opening can be triggered by backward head thrusts or extensive frontalis and brow elevation.[140] This defect of eyelid opening can be seen in patients with extrapyramidal dysfunction, including progressive supranuclear palsy, Parkinson's disease, the Shy-Drager syndrome, and Wilson's disease.[141] Lepore and Duvoisin[142] object to the term "apraxia" because of the associated extrapyramidal dysfunction seen in these patients. They prefer to regard the disorder as involuntary levator inhibition of supranuclear origin. It is now believed that apraxia of eyelid opening may result from a variable combination of involuntary levator inhibition and contraction of the pretarsal orbicularis oculi.[142a] Although technically difficult, electromyography may help distinguish the contribution of these two factors. Rarely, apraxia of eyelid opening is seen in patients with cortical lesions, particularly those involving the right hemisphere.[143] Two patients with isolated apraxia of eyelid opening had complete resolution of their eyelid dysfunction with the administration of levodopa.[144] Treatment of the condition is vexing, but botulinum injections can also be tried.

There is also a supranuclear disorder characterized by an inability to voluntarily close the lids. Such patients have intact reflex eye closure and sleep with the eyes closed. This condition should be distinguished from motor impersistence, in which the lids can be closed to command but eye closure is not maintained. Failure to maintain or initiate voluntary lid closure is most often seen with bilateral frontal lobe disease. It has also been

documented in several cases of Jakob-Creutzfeldt disease.[145] Lessell[146] believes that this disorder represents actual motor dysfunction rather than "apraxia" because there is no evidence for disconnection between the language and motor areas.

A study has been reported of bilateral *cerebral ptosis* occurring after acute right hemisphere damage.[147] All 13 patients showed a conjugate deviation of the eyes to the right and ptosis of at least 4 mm. Some cases had nearly complete ptosis. Asymmetric upper lid drooping was seen in 10 patients and may have resulted from associated left frontalis weakness. However, in 5 patients the ptosis was greater on the right side. This finding might imply the existence of unequal supranuclear innervation to the levator nuclear complex. Contralateral lower facial weakness was seen in 5 patients, and both upper and lower facial weakness was seen in the remaining 8 patients. One patient showed both bilateral cerebral ptosis and "apraxia" of eyelid opening. The predominance of bilateral cerebral ptosis with right hemisphere lesions implies functional or anatomic

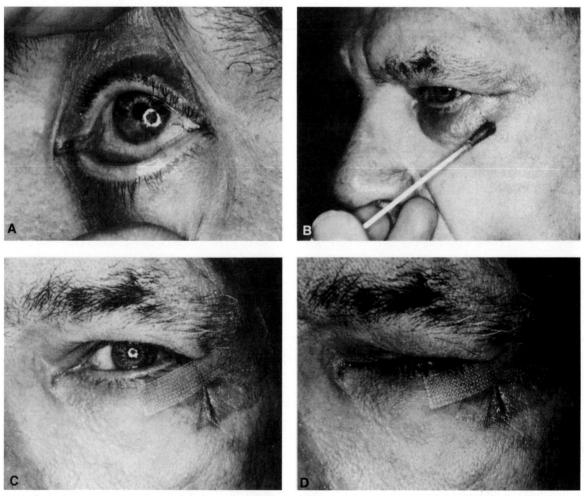

Fig. 8–26. Patient with Bell's palsy and BAD syndrome (inadequate *B*ell's phenomenon, *a*nesthesia of cornea, *d*ry eye). **A.** Corneal stain with fluorescein. **B.** Application of tincture of benzoin. **C.** Lower lid splinted with Transpore tape. **D.** Enhanced eye closure.

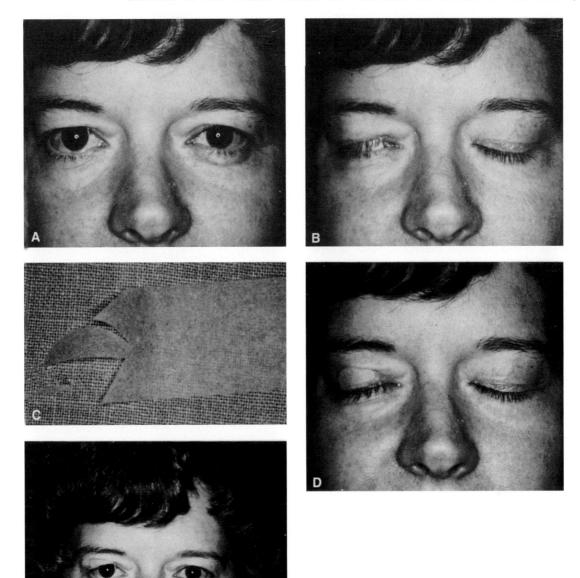

Fig. 8–27. Technique for improving upper lid position with tape. **A.** Note widened right palpebral fissure due to orbicularis weakness. **B.** Incomplete eyelid closure. **C.** Crescent of tape is cut. **D.** Tape is placed to override lid fold to assist lid closure. **E.** Appearance with eyes opened.

asymmetry in hemispheric control of eyelid opening. Also, bilateral "central" ptosis is reported in AIDS encephalopathy involving the periaqueductal midbrain.[148]

Recent experimental and clinical evidence supports a premotor eyelid control center that is dorsal to the oculomotor nucleus and is known as the supraoculomotor area or supra III. This area may be under the ultimate control of the nucleus of the posterior commissure. Le-

sions in this region have been implicated in cases of supranuclear ptosis and eyelid retraction and lag.[16,149]

MANAGEMENT OF FACIAL PALSY

Efforts should be directed toward keeping the eye moist to prevent exposure keratitis and corneal epithelial breakdown. The patient can manually close the eyelids on the involved side whenever the eye feels irritated or burns. In addition, artificial tears and a moisture chamber can be used during the day, and Lacri-Lube ointment and patching are used at night. If there is significant incomplete eyelid closure, the lower lid may need to be elevated to protect the cornea. Transpore tape works quite well for this purpose. The end of the tape is applied to the center of the lower lid with the upper edge about ¼ inch below the lashes. The tape is used like a pull-tab, with the tension directed up and laterally; it is secured laterally to the orbital rim (Fig. 8–26). In this fashion, the irritation to the palpebral conjunctiva, caused by ectropion, will be reduced. The palpebral aperture can be further narrowed by limiting the opening of the upper lid. A crescentic piece of tape resembling a half moon can be placed overriding the tarsal fold in the upper lid (Fig. 8–27).

When the eyelids are difficult to tape shut, temporary tarsorrhaphy using lid sutures or botulinum A toxin–induced ptosis may be preferable.[150] The latter technique involves injection of botulinum toxin into the levator palpebral muscle on the side of the facial paresis. This induced ptosis protects the cornea from further exposure and promotes healing of damaged epithelium for several weeks. These two techniques are reserved for those patients who are not responding to the methods already mentioned; they are the last resorts before considering more complicated surgical techniques. Surgery to reanimate the paralyzed eyelids should be considered if medical treatment is ineffective, especially for patients who lack *B*ell's phenomenon, have corneal *a*nesthesia, and have *d*ry eye—the BAD syndrome. A number of surgical procedures are available to achieve eyelid closure, including the use of a palpebral spring[151–153] or a gold weight[154,155] to correct upper lid lagophthalmos. The lower lid can also be elevated surgically to prevent corneal exposure. These techniques are preferable to permanent tarsorrhaphy, which may lead to a deformed lid configuration and a constricted visual field from a narrowed palpebral aperture. Finally, hypoglossal-facial anastomosis and temporalis muscle transposition[29] are useful procedures when lower facial movement is desired and direct anastomosis of the facial nerve cannot be performed within 30 days.

REFERENCES

1. Gasser RF: The development of the facial nerve in man. Ann Otol Rhinol Laryngol 76:37, 1967
2. Gasser RF: The development of the facial muscles in man. Am J Anat 120:357, 1967
3. Goycoolea MV, Paparell MM, Carpenter AM: Ganglia and ganglion cells in the middle ear. Arch Otolaryngol 108:276, 1982
4. Bischoff EPE: Microscopic analysis of anastomoses between the cranial nerves. In Sachs E, Valtin EW (eds): The Facial Nerve, pp 43–76. Hanover, NH, University Press of New England, 1977
5. Jahrsdoerfer RA: The facial nerve in congenital middle ear malformations. Laryngoscope 91:1217, 1981
6. Crosby EC, DeJonge BR: Experimental and clinical studies of the central connections and the central relations of the facial nerve. Ann Otol 72:735, 1963
7. Van Buskirk C: The seventh nerve complex. J Comp Neurol 82:303, 1945
8. Carpenter M: Core Text of Neuro-Anatomy, p 151. Baltimore, Williams & Wilkins, 1985
9. Martin RG, Grant JL, Peace D: Microsurgical relationship of the anterior inferior cerebellar artery and the facial-vestibulocochlear nerve complex. Neurosurgery 6:483, 1980
10. Guerrier Y: Surgical anatomy, particularly vascular supply of the facial nerve. In Fisch U (ed): Facial Nerve Surgery, pp 12–23. Birmingham, Aesculapius Publishing Co., 1977
11. Davis RA, Anson BJ, Puddinger JM, Kurth RE: Surgical anatomy of the facial nerve and parotid gland based upon a study of 350 cervical facial halves. Surg Gynecol Obstet 102:385, 1956
12. Nager GT, Nager N: The arteries of the human middle ear, with particular regard to the blood supply of the auditory ossicle. Ann Otol Rhinol Laryngol 62:923, 1953
13. Blunt MJ: The possible role of vascular changes in the etiology of Bell's palsy. J Laryngol 70:701, 1956
14. Donath T, Lengyel I: The vascular structure of the intrapetrosal section of the facial nerve, with special reference to peripheral facial palsy. Acta Med Acad Sci Hung 10:249, 1957
15. May M, Hardin WB: Facial palsy: interpretation of neurologic findings. Trans Am Acad Ophthalmol Otolaryngol 84:710, 1977
16. Schmidtke K, Büttner-Ennever JA: Nervous control of eyelid function. a review of clinical, experimental and pathologic data. Brain 115:227, 1992
17. Evinger C, Manning KA, Sibony PA: Eyelid movements. Mechanisms and normal data. Invest Ophthalmol Vis Sci 32:387, 1991
18. Francis IL, Loughhead JA: Bell's phenomenon. A study of 508 patients. Aust J Ophthalmol 12:15, 1984
19. Hauser WA, Karnes WE, Annis J: Incidence and prognosis of Bell's palsy in the population of Rochester, Minnesota. Mayo Clin Proc 46:258, 1971
20. Adour KK, Byl FM, Hilsinger RL: The true nature of Bell's palsy: analysis of 1000 consecutive patients. Laryngoscope 88:787, 1978
21. Peitersen E: The natural history of Bell's palsy. Am J Otol 4:107, 1982
22. Katusic SK, Beard CM, Wiederholt WC: Incidence, clinical features and prognosis in Bell's palsy. Ann Neurol 20:622, 1986
23. Park HW, Watkins AL: Facial paralysis: analysis of 500 cases. Arch Phys Med 30:749, 1949
24. Paolino E, Granieri E, Tola MR: Predisposing factor in Bell's palsy: a case control study. J Neurol 232:363, 1985
25. Pechet P, Schattner A: Concurrent Bell's palsy and diabetes mellitus: a diabetic mononeuropathy? J Neurol 232:363, 1985
26. Hilsinger RL, Aduor KK, Doty HE: Idiopathic facial paralysis, pregnancy and the menstrual cycle. Ann Otol Rhinol Laryngol 84:433, 1975
27. Alter M: Familial aggregation of Bell's palsy. Arch Neurol 8:557, 1963
28. Takahash A, Fujiwara R: Familial Bell's palsy. Report of seven families. Clin Neurol (Tokyo) 11:454, 1971
29. May M: Muscle transposition for facial reanimation. Indications and results. Arch Otolaryngol 110:184, 1984
30. Dumitru D, Walsh NE, Porter LD: Electrophysiologic evaluation of the facial nerve in Bell's palsy: a review. Am J Phys Med Rehabil 67:137, 1988
31. Morgan M, Nathwani D: Facial palsy and infection: the unfolding story. Clin Infect Dis 14:263, 1992
32. Adour KK: Medical management of idiopathic Bell's palsy. Otolaryngol Clin North Am 24:666, 1991
33. Hyden D, Roberg M, Forsberg P: Acute idiopathic peripheral facial palsy: clinical, serological, and cerebrospinal fluid findings and effects of corticosteroids. Am J Otolaryngol 14:179, 1993
33a. Murakami S, Mizobuchi M, Nakashiro Y et al: Bell palsy and herpes simplex virus: indentification of viral DNA in end neurial fluid and muscle. Ann Intern Med 124:27, 1996
34. Kohsyu H, Aoyagi M, Tojima H: Facial nerve enhancement in Gd-MRI in patients with Bell's palsy. Acta Otolaryngol 511(suppl):I65, 1994
35. May M, Klein SR, Taylor FH: Idiopathic (Bell's) facial palsy:

natural history defies steroid or surgical treatment. Laryngoscope 95:406, 1985

36. Stankiewicz JA: A review of the published data on steroids and idiopathic facial paralysis. Otolaryngol Head Neck Surg 97:481, 1987

36a. Adour KK, Ruboyianes JM, Von Doersten PG et al: Bell's treatment with acyclovir and prednisone compared with prednisone alone: A double-blind randomized controlled trial. Ann Otol Rhinol Laryngol 105:37, 1996

37. Hunt JR: On herpetic inflammations of the geniculate ganglion. A new syndrome and its implications. J Nerve Ment Dis 34:73, 1907

38. Hunt JR: A further contribution to herpetic inflammations of the geniculate ganglion. Am J Med Sci 136:226, 1916

39. Portenoy RK, Duma C, Foley KM: Acute herpetic and postherpetic neuralgia. Clinical review and current management. Ann Neurol 20:651, 1986

40. Stafford FW, Welch AR: The use of acyclovir in Ramsay Hunt syndrome. J Laryngol Otol 100:337, 1986

41. Inamura H, Aoyagi M, Tojima H, Koike Y: Effects of acyclovir in Ramsay Hunt syndrome. Acta Otolaryngol 446(suppl):111, 1988

42. Abramsky O, Webb C, Tietelbaum D: Cellular immune response to peripheral nerve basic protein in idiopathic facial paralysis (Bell's palsy). J Neurol Sci 26:13, 1975

43. Asbury AK: Diagnostic considerations in Guillain-Barré syndrome. Ann Neurol 9(suppl):1, 1981

44. Charous DI, Saxe BI: Landry-Guillain-Barré syndrome: report of an unusual case with a comment on Bell's palsy. N Engl J Med 267:1334, 1962

45. Clark JR, Carlson RD, Sasak CT: Facial paralysis in Lyme disease. Laryngoscope 95:1341, 1985

46. Markby DP: Lyme disease facial palsy: differentiation from Bell's palsy. Br Med J 299:605, 1989

47. Rawlings JA, Fournier PU, Teltow GJ: Isolation of *Borrelia* spirochetes from patients in Texas. J Clin Microbiol 25:1148, 1987

48. Hunter EF, Russel H, Farstly CE: Evaluation of sera from patients with Lyme disease in the fluorescent treponemal antibody–absorption test for syphilis. Sex Transm Dis 13:232, 1986

49. Kamitsuka M, Feldman R, Richardson M: Facial paralysis associated with otitis media. Pediatr Infect Dis 6:682, 1985

50. Gradenigo G: A special syndrome of endocranial otitic complications. Ann Otol Rhinol Laryngol 13:637, 1904

51. Kohut RF, Lindsay JR: Necrotizing (malignant) external otitis histopathologic processes. Ann Otol 88:714, 1979

52. Naldol JB: Histopathology of *Pseudomonas* osteomyelitis of the temporal bone starting as malignant external otitis. Am J Otolaryngol 115:359, 1980

53. McGove FH: Bilateral Bell's palsy. Laryngoscope 75:1070, 1965

54. Dreifus FE, Martin JD, Green RC: Brainstem encephalitis. Va Med Month 91:15, 1964

55. Yasui I, Miyasaki T: Case of poliomyelitis due to virus type I manifested only by right facial paralysis. J Jpn Assn Infect Dis 36:427, 1962

56. Sklar VEF, Patriarca PA, Onorato IM: Clinical findings and results of treatment in an outbreak of acute hemorrhagic conjunctivitis is southern Florida. Am J Ophthalmol 95:45, 1983

57. Bosher SK: Leprosy presenting as facial palsy. J Laryngol 76:827, 1962

58. Lucente FE, Tobias GW, Parisier SC: Tuberculous otitis media. Laryngoscope 88:1107, 1978

59. Bergstrom L, Hemenway WG, Barnhardt RA: Rhinocerebral and otologic mucormycosis. Ann Otol 79:70, 1970

60. Gussen R, Canalis RF: Mucormycosis of the temporal bone. Ann Otol 91:27, 1982

61. Verduijn PG, Bleeker JD: Secondary syphilis of the facial nerve. Arch Otolaryngol 48:675, 1939

62. Dastur FD, Shahani MT, Dastoor DH et al: Cephalic tetanus: demonstration of a dual lesion. J Neurol Neurosurg Psychiatry 40:782, 1977

63. Harrison TR: Principles of Internal Medicine, 12th ed, p 580. New York, McGraw-Hill, 1987

63a. Grant AC, Hunter S, Portin WC: A case of acute monocytic ehrlichiosis with prominent neurologic signs. Neurology 48:1619, 1997

64. Sahludovich S: Accidents due to antirabies vaccine: pseudoperitoneal syndrome followed by bilateral paralysis: case. Ed Dia Medico (Buenos Aires) 18:1454, 1946

65. Jappich G: Effects and side effects of oral poliomyelitis vaccinations. Monatsschr Kinderheilkd 112:112, 1964

66. Danforth HB: Familial Bell's palsy. Ann Otol 73:179, 1964

67. Lerond J: Ascending paralysis after tetanus antiserum's rapid regression in member lingering facial paralysis. Bull Mem Soc Med Hop Paris 50:1695, 1926

68. Wechsler AF, Ho DD: Bilateral Bell's palsy at the time of HIV seroconversion. Neurology 39:747, 1989

69. Wright RE: Blocking the main trunk of the facial nerve in cataract operations. Arch Ophthalmol 55:555, 1926

70. Lambert PR, Brackman DE: Facial paralysis in longitudinal temporal bone fractures: a review of 26 cases. Laryngoscope 94:1022, 1984

71. Cannon CR, Jahrsdoerfer RA: Temporal bone fractures: review of 90 cases. Arch Otolaryngol 109:285, 1983

72. Hitselberger WE, House WF: Tumors of the cerebellopontine angle. Arch Otolaryngol 80:720, 1964

73. Kettel K: Peripheral facial palsies due to tumors: pathology and clinical picture: review of the literature and a report of three cases of intratemporal tumors of the facial nerve. Arch Otolaryngol 69:276, 1959

74. Cawthorne T, Griffith A: Primary cholesteatoma of the temporal bone. Arch Otolaryngol 73:252, 1961

75. Koide C, Imai A, Nagaba A: Pathological findings of the facial nerve in a case of facial palsy associated with benign parotid tumor. Arch Otolaryngol Head Neck Surg 120:410, 1994

76. Pulec JL, House WF: Facial nerve involvement and testing in acoustic neuromas. Arch Otolaryngol 80:685, 1964

77. Lee SH, Rao K: Cranial Computed Tomography and MRI, 2nd ed. New York, McGraw-Hill, 1987

78. Harner SG, Daube JR, Beatty CW, Ebersold MJ: Intraoperative monitoring of the facial nerve. Laryngoscope 98:209, 1988

79. Uziel A, Benezech J, Frerebeau P: Intraoperative facial nerve monitoring in posterior fossa acoustic neuroma surgery. Otolaryngol Head Neck Surg 108:126, 1993

80. Pillsbury HE, Price HC, Gardner LH: Primary tumors of the facial nerve. Laryngoscope 93:1045, 1983

81. Wasserstorm WR, Glass PT, Posner JB: Diagnosis and treatment of leptomeningeal metastasis from solid tumors. Cancer 49:759, 1982

82. Olson ME, Chernik NC, Posner JB: Infiltration of the leptomeninges by systemic cancer. Arch Neurol 30:122, 1974

83. Cohen JP, Lachman LJ, Hammerschlag PE: Reversible facial paralysis in sarcoidosis. Confirmation by serum angiotensin-converting enzyme assay. Arch Otolaryngol 109:832, 1983

84. Stern BT, Krumholz A, Johns C: Sarcoidosis and its neurological manifestations. Arch Neurol 42:909, 1985

85. Lambert V, Richards SH: Facial palsy in Heerfordt's syndrome. J Laryngol 78:684, 1964

86. Lewis M, Kallenbach J, Hockman M: Otolaryngologic complications of acute prophyria. Laryngoscope 93:483, 1983

86a. Suarez JI, Cohen ML, Larkin J et al: Acute intermittent porphyria: Clinicopathologic correlation: report of a case and review of the literature. Neurology 48:1678, 1997

87. Ridley A: The neuropathy of acute intermittent porphyria. Q J Med 151:301, 1969

88. Osher RH, Griggs RC: Orbicularis fatigue: the "peek" sign of myasthenia gravis. Arch Ophthalmol 97:677, 1979

89. Milone M, Monaco ML, Evoli A: Ocular myasthenia: diagnostic value of single fiber EMG in the orbicularis oculi muscle. J Neurol Neurosurg Psychiatry 56:720, 1993

90. Shugar MA, Granich MS, Reardon EJ: The otolaryngologic presentation of botulism. Laryngoscope 91:121, 1981

91. Hanson PA, Rowland LP: Mo
bius' syndrome and facioscapulohumeral muscular dystrophy. Arch Neurol 24:31, 1971

92. Miller MT, Sloane H, Goldberg MF: Progressive hemifacial atrophy (Parry-Romberg disease). J Pediatr Ophthalmol Strabismus 24:27, 1987

93. Wolf SM, Verity MA: Neurological complications of progressive facial hematrophy. J Neurol Neurosurg Psychiatry 39:997, 1974

94. Chung MH, Sum J, Morrell MJ, Horoupian DS: Intracerebral involvement in scleroderma en coup de sabre: report of a case with neuropathologic findings. Ann Neurol 37:679, 1995
95. Saberman MN, Tenta LT: The Melkersson-Rosenthal syndrome. Arch Otolaryngol 84:292, 1966
96. Stevens H: Melkersson syndrome. Neurology 15:263, 1965
97. Minor MW, Fox RW, Bukantz SL: Melkersson-Rosenthal syndrome. J Allergy Clin Immunol 80:64, 1987
98. May M, Fria TJ, Blumenthal F: Facial paralysis in children: differential diagnosis. Otolaryngol Head Neck Surg 89:841, 1981
99. Harris JP, Davidson TM, May M: Evaluation and treatment of congenital facial paralysis. Arch Otolaryngol 109:145, 1983
100. McHugh HE: Facial paralysis in birth injury and skull fractures. Arch Otol 78:443, 1963
101. Hepner WR: Some observations on facial paresis in the newborn infant: etiology and incidence. Pediatrics 8:494, 1951
102. Falco NA, Eriksson E: Facial nerve palsy in the newborn: incidence and outcome. Plast Reconstr Surg 85:1, 1990
103. Pape KE, Pickering B: Asymmetric crying facies: an index of other congenital anomalies. J Pediatr 81:21, 1972
104. Towfighi T, Marks K, Palmer E: Möbius' syndrome: neuropath observations. Acta Neuropathol 48:11, 1979
105. Keane JR, Young JA: Blepharospasm with bilateral basal ganglia infarction. Arch Neurol 42:1206, 1985
106. Jankovic J, Havins WE, Wilkins RB: Blinking and blepharospasm: mechanism, diagnosis and management. JAMA 284:3160, 1982
107. Reynolds DH, Smith JL, Walsh TH: Differential sections of the facial nerve for blepharospasm. Trans Am Acad Ophthalmol Otolaryngol 71:656, 1967
108. Fox SA: Essential blepharospasm. Arch Ophthalmol 76:318, 1966
109. Savino PJ, Stern M, Hurtig H: Pharmacologic therapy versus botulinum in the treatment of blepharospasm: a preliminary report. Arch Neurol 16:125, 1984
110. Dutton JJ, Buckley E: Botulinum toxin in the management of blepharospasm. Arch Neurol 43:380, 1986
111. Biglan A, May M: Treatment of facial spasm with Oculinum. J Pediatr Ophthalmol Strabismus 23:216, 1986
112. Engstrom P, Arnoult J, Malow M: Effectiveness of botulinum toxin therapy for essential blepharospasm. Ophthalmology 94:971, 1987
113. Jordan DR, Patrinely JR, Anderson RL: Essential blepharospasm and related dystonias. Surv Ophthalmol 34:123, 1989
114. Jannetta PT, Abbasy M, Marion JC: Etiology and definitive microsurgical treatment of hemifacial spasm: operative techniques and results in 47 patients. J Neurosurg 47:321, 1977
115. Gardner WJ, Sava GA: Hemifacial spasm: a reversible pathophysiologic state. J Neurosurg 19:240, 1962
116. Nielsen VK: Pathophysiology of hemifacial spasm: a reversible pathophysiologic state. Neurology 34:418, 1984
117. Ferguson JH: Hemifacial spasm and the facial nucleus. Ann Neurol 4:97, 1978
118. Davis WE, Luterman BF, Pulliam MW: Hemifacial spasm caused by cholesteatoma. Am J Otol 2:272, 1981
119. Adler CH, Zimmerman RA, Savino PJ: Hemifacial spasm: evaluation by magnetic resonance imaging and magnetic resonance tomographic angiography. Ann Neurol 32:502, 1992
120. Auger R, Piepras D, Laws E: Hemifacial spasm: results in microvascular decompressions of the facial nerve in 54 patients. Mayo Clin Proc 61:650, 1986
121. Huang CI, Chen IH, Lee LS: Microvascular decompression of hemifacial spasm: analysis of operative findings and results in 310 patients. Neurosurgery 30:53, 1992
122. Garland PE, Patrinely JR, Andreson RI: Hemifacial spasm: results of unilateral myectomy. Ophthalmology 94:288, 1987
123. Alexander GE, Moses H: Carbamazepine for hemifacial spasm. Neurology 32:286, 1982
124. Sandyk R: Facial myokymia. J Neurosurg 59:1108, 1983
125. Frueh BR: Associated facial contracting after seventh nerve palsy mimicking jaw-winking. Ophthalmology 90:1105, 1983
126. Lubkin V: The inverse Marcus Gunn phenomenon. Arch Neurol 35:249, 1978
127. Chorobski J: Syndrome of crocodile tears. Arch Neurol Psychiatry 65:299, 1951
128. Axelsson A, Laage-Hellman JE: The gustolachrymal reflex: the syndrome of crocodile tears. Acta Otolaryngol 54:239, 1962
129. Frey L: Syndrome of auriculotemporal nerve. Rev Neurol 2:97, 1923
130. Laage-Hellman JE: Gustatory sweating and flushing. Aetiological implications of latent period and mode of development after parotidectomy. Acta Otolaryngol 49:366, 1958
131. Andermann F, Cosgrove JBR, Lloyd-Smith DL: Facial myokymia in multiple sclerosis. Brain 84:31, 1961
132. Tenser RB, Corbett JJ: Myokymia and facial contraction in brainstem glioma: an electrographic study. Arch Neurol 30:425, 1974
133. Espinosa RE, Lambert EH, Klass DW: Facial myokymia affecting the electroencephalogram. Mayo Clin Proc 42:258, 1967
134. Radu EW, Skorpil V, Raeser HE: Facial myokymia. Eur Neurol 13:499, 1975
135. Wasserstorm WR, Starr A: Facial myokymia in the Guillain-Barré syndrome. Arch Neurol 35:576, 1977
136. Feldman RG, Lessell S, Travers PM: Neuro-ophthalmologic and neuropsychological effect of trichloroethylene intoxication: 18 year follow-up. Neurology 34:242, 1984
137. Morris HH, Esters MC: Bilateral facial myokymia following cardiopulmonary arrest. Arch Neurol 38:393, 1981
138. Waybright EA, Gutman L, Chou SM: Facial myokymia. Pathological features. Arch Neurol 36:244, 1979
139. Jacobs L, Kaba S, Pullicino P: The lesion causing continuous facial myokymia in multiple sclerosis. Arch Neurol 51:1115, 1994
140. Goldstein JE, Cogan DG: Apraxia of lid opening. Arch Ophthalmol 73:155, 1965
141. Keane JR: Lid opening apraxia in Wilson's disease. J Clin Neuro-Ophthalmol 8:31, 1988
142. Lepore F, Duvoisin R: "Apraxia" of eyelid opening: an involuntary levator inhibition. Neurology 35:423, 1985
142a. Boghen D: Apraxia of lid opening: a review. Neurology 48:1491, 1997
143. Johnston J, Rosenbaum DM, Picone CM: Apraxia of eyelid opening secondary to right hemisphere infarction. Ann Neurol 25:622, 1989
144. Dewey RB, Maragonore DM: Isolated eyelid opening apraxia: report of a new levodopa-responsive syndrome. Neurology 44:752, 1994
145. Ross Russell RW: Supranuclear palsy of eyelid closure. Brain 103:71, 1980
146. Lessell S: Supranuclear paralysis of voluntary lid closure. Arch Ophthalmol 88:241, 1972
147. Lepore F: Bilateral cerebral ptosis. Neurology 37:1043, 1987
148. Barton JS: Bilateral central ptosis in acquired immunodeficiency syndrome. Can J Neurol Sci 22:52, 1995
149. Galetta SL, Gray LG, Raps EC, Schatz NJ: Pretectal eyelid retraction and lag. Ann Neurol 33:554, 1993
150. Adams GG, Kirkness JP: Botulinum toxin A induced protective ptosis. Eye 1:603, 1987
151. Morel-Fatio D, Lalardrie JP: Palliative surgical treatment of facial paralysis. The palpebral spring. Plast Reconstr Surg 33:446, 1964
152. Morel-Fatio D, Lalardrie JP: Le ressort palpebral: contribution a l'etude de la chirurgie plastique de la paralysie faciale. Neurochirurgia 11:303, 1965
153. Levine RE, House WF, Hitselberger WE: Ocular complications of seventh nerve paralysis and management with the palpebral spring. Am J Ophthalmol 73:219, 1972
154. Jobe RP: A technique for lid-loading in the management of lagophthalmos in facial palsy. Plast Reconstr Surg 53:29, 1974
155. Sansone V, Boyton J, Palenski C. Use of gold weights to correct lagophthalmos in neuromuscular disease. Neurology 48:1500, 1997

CHAPTER 9

Eye Movement Characteristics and Recording Techniques

Louis F. Dell'Osso and Robert B. Daroff

Physiologic Organization
Fast Eye Movements (Saccades)
  Plasticity
Slow Eye Movements
  Pursuit
  Fixation
  Vestibulo-ocular Reflex
  Optokinetic Reflex
  Visual-vestibulo-ocular Reflex
Internal Monitor (Efference Copy)
Corrective Movements
Vergence Eye Movements
Subsystem Synergism
The Near Triad
Micromovements of the Eye

Anatomic Architecture
  Unilateral and Bilateral Yoked Control
  Bilateral and Bilateral Yoked, Independent Control
Eye Movement Recording Techniques
  Afterimages
  Mechanical Transducers
  Photography
  Corneal Reflection
  Contact Lens
  Electro-oculography
  Photoelectric Oculography
  Electromagnetic Search Coil
  Video
  Ocular Electromyography

The muscles were of necessitie provided and given to the eye, so that it might move on every side: for if the eye stood fast, and immoveable, we should be constrained to turn our head and necke (being all of one peece) for to see: but by these muscles it now moveth it selfe with such swiftnes and nimblenes, without stirring of the head, as is almost incredible. . .

> Andreas Laurentius (1599) (du Laurens)
> *A Discourse of the Preservation of the Sight:*
> *Of Melancholike Diseases; Of Rheumes,*
> *and of Old Age. Facsimile Edition.*
> *Oxford University Press, London, 1938*

In foveate animals, the purpose of eye movements is to bring visual stimuli in the peripheral field of vision (peripheral retina) to the central point of best visual acuity (fovea) and to maintain foveal fixation of a moving object. The acquisition (gaze shifting) and securing (gaze holding) of stationary object images on the fovea and the stabilization of images on the fovea during head movement (gaze holding) or target movement (gaze shifting) constitute the basic functions of human eye movements. Although many specific types of eye movement abnormalities require sophisticated recording and analysis techniques, there are clinical tests that, when properly applied, can provide valuable information about diagnosis, pathophysiologic mechanism, or response to therapy.[1]

L. F. Dell'Osso: Departments of Neurology and Biomedical Engineering, Schools of Medicine and Engineering, Case Western Reserve University; and Ocular Motor Neurophysiology Laboratory, Veterans Administration Medical Center, Cleveland, Ohio

R. B. Daroff: Department of Neurology, Case Western Reserve University; and Medical Affairs, University Hospitals of Cleveland, Cleveland, Ohio

See Chapter 11 for Glossary.

PHYSIOLOGIC ORGANIZATION

The ocular motor system can be conceptualized as two independent major subsystems, version and vergence, acting synergistically (Fig. 9–1).[2] The version subsystem mediates all conjugate eye movements, whereas the vergence subsystem mediates all disjugate eye movements. Fixation and vestibulo-ocular inputs influence the version subsystem. At the most peripheral level, regardless of input, there are only three major categories of eye movement output: fast eye movements (FEM or

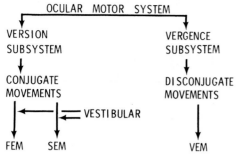

Fig. 9–1. Basic organization of ocular motor system emphasizing the division between vergence and dual-mode version subsystems. The three basic motor outputs are fast eye movements (*FEM*), slow eye movements (*SEM*), and vergence eye movements (VEM).

saccades) and slow eye movements (SEM) from the version subsystem, and vergence eye movements (VEM) from their own subsystem. All three outputs share a common neural pathway from the ocular motor neurons to the muscles (Fig. 9–2). In addition, the version subsystems share a common neural network that integrates (mathematically) velocity information into position signals. The fast mode of the version subsystem mediates all conjugate saccades (FEM), and the slow mode mediates all SEM. The latter includes, but is not limited to, the pursuit function. Without knowledge of the conditions that were used to elicit a particular response, one could not differentiate (1) the eye movement record of a voluntary saccade from a nystagmus fast phase or (2) the record made by pursuit of a slowly moving target from that of slow rotation of the subject while fixating a stationary target. The many terms used to describe eye movements generally specify the eliciting input, the functional subsystem, or the circumstance of occurrence, but the eye movements themselves consist of one or more of the three main outputs (FEM, SEM, VEM) of the ocular motor system (Table 9–1).

There is ample physiologic, anatomic, and clinical justification for regarding the subsystems as autonomous. However, the neurons within the oculomotor, trochlear, and abducens nuclei are not specific for types of eye movement. Rather, different firing patterns of homogeneous neuronal pools determine the type of eye movement.[3]

The simplified schema described above, which uses

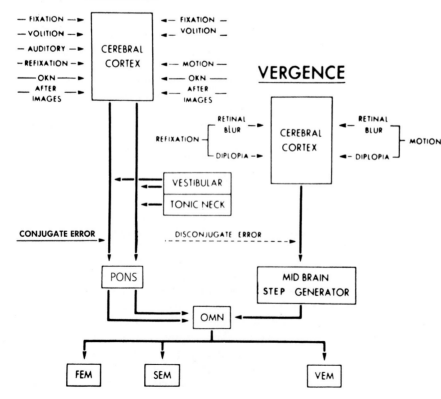

Fig. 9–2. The ocular motor control system is composed of the dual-mode version and the vergence subsystems. The output of the pons sums with that of the vergence neural pulse generator at the ocular motor nuclei (*OMN*) to produce the three basic types of eye movements: fast (*FEM*), slow (*SEM*), and vergence (*VEM*). *OKN*, optokinetic nystagmus. (Modified from Dell'Osso LF, Daroff RB: Functional organization of the ocular motor system. Aerospace Med 45:873, 1974)

TABLE 9–1. Eye Movement Classifications

Version		Vergence
Fast eye movements (FEM)	**Slow eye movements (SEM)**	**Vergence eye movements (VEM)**
Saccade: Refixation	Pursuit (tracking)	Refixation
Reflex		
Voluntary	Voluntary	Tracking (pursuit)
Microsaccade (flick)	Microdrift	Microdrift
Corrective saccade	Glissade	
Saccadic pursuit (cogwheel)	Compensatory	Voluntary
Fast phase of nystagmus (jerk)	Slow phase of nystagmus	
Saccadic intrusions		
Saccadic oscillations	Pendular nystagmus	
Afterimage induced	Afterimage induced	
Rapid eye movement (REM)	Slow sleep drifts	
Braking saccades	Imaginary tracking	Imaginary tracking
	Proprioceptive tracking	Proprioceptive tracking

the three unique ocular motor *outputs* as a basis for conceptualization of the ocular motor system, is used in this chapter for purely pedagogic reasons. If one used *inputs* as a basis, the ocular motor system could be divided into additional subsystems separated by phylogenetic origins and physiologic modes of action. From an evolutionary point of view, the vestibular subsystem probably developed first, closely followed by the optokinetic and saccadic subsystems; the latter are required to generate reflex fast (quick) phases associated with passive head movement and "afoveate" saccades for active head movement. With the development of a fovea came subsystems for fixation, pursuit, and voluntary saccades, and finally the vergence subsystem for binocular single vision and stereopsis. Because the neurophysiologic substrates and varied purposes of these subsystems result in specific properties and limitations, their origins and individual modes of action are key to a complete understanding of the ocular motor system and are especially important if one wishes to study them in situ or with the use of computer models. Observations indicate that a distinct subsystem may mediate the SEM of fixation in synergy with the saccadic and pursuit subsystems. Studies of the latter[4] and of human congenital nystagmus[5-7] have provided evidence in support of a separate fixation subsystem. Some of the quantitative characteristics of a fixation or "stabilization" subsystem have begun to be elucidated.[8-10] The different inputs, outputs, and components of these subsystems are discussed in the sections of this chapter dealing with the major output subsystem to which they belong (*i.e.,* FEM, SEM, or VEM).

FAST EYE MOVEMENTS (SACCADES)

Fast eye movements are rapid versional (conjugate) eye movements that are under both voluntary and reflex control. Examples of voluntary saccades are willed re-

fixations and those in response to command (*e.g.,* "Look to the right . . . Look up."). The sudden appearance of a peripheral visual object or an eccentric sound may evoke a reflex saccade in the direction of the stimulus. In the natural state, these saccades are usually accompanied by a head movement in the same direction. However, in clinical examinations and in most physiologic experiments, the head is stabilized.

The visual stimulus for FEM is target (object) displacement in space. After an instantaneous change in target position, the ocular motor system will respond with a FEM after a latency (delay) of 200 to 250 milliseconds. Both the peak velocity and the duration of FEM are dependent on the size (amplitude) of eye movement, which varies from 30°/second to 800°/second and 20 to 140 milliseconds, respectively, for movements from 0.5° to 40° in amplitude. FEM are conjugate and ballistic. The control system responsible for their generation is discrete. At discrete instants in time, control decisions are made based on the continuous inflow of visual information from the retina. In normal persons, these decisions are essentially irrevocable; once the eyes are in motion, their trajectory cannot be altered. The control signal is retinal error (disparity of image position from the fovea), which is automatically reduced to zero by the nature of negative feedback.

After the appropriate latency, the FEM response to target displacement (Fig. 9–3) consists of a period of acceleration to a peak velocity, and then deceleration of the eyes as they approach the new target position. The muscular activity in the agonist-antagonist pair of each globe is characterized by a burst of maximal facilitation in the agonist and total inhibition in the antagonist during the movement (Fig. 9–4). Electromyographic (EMG) recordings reveal that FEM deceleration is usually not consequent to active braking by the antagonist muscle. Rather, the two muscles merely assume the relative tensions necessary to hold the new target posi-

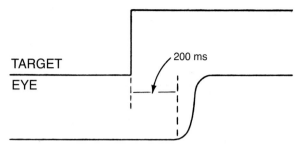

Fig. 9–3. FEM response to a rightward target displacement, illustrating the latency (200 milliseconds) and trajectory of the FEM (saccade).

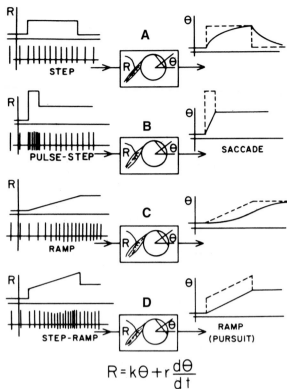

$$R = k\Theta + r\frac{d\Theta}{dt}$$

Fig. 9–5. Illustration of the FEM responses (**A** and **B**) and SEM responses (**C** and **D**) that would result from the neural innervation patterns depicted. The top left curves and the right dashed curves are plots of instantaneous firing rate versus time. The equation relates neural firing frequency (*R*) with eye position (*θ*) and velocity (*dθ/dt*). Note that the overdamped nature of muscle and eyeball plant dynamics produces sluggish responses to a simple step (**A**) or ramp (**C**) change in firing frequency. To generate a proper FEM (saccade), a pulse-step is required (**B**). To generate a proper SEM (pursuit), a step-ramp is required (**D**). (Robinson DA: Oculomotor control signals. In Lennerstrand G, Bach-y-Rita P (eds): Basic Mechanisms of Ocular Motility and Their Clinical Implications. New York, Pergamon Press, 1975)

tion. This is sufficient to accomplish the rapid deceleration because of the braking effect (damping) of the "ocular motor plant" (*i.e.,* globe, muscles, check ligaments, and fatty supporting tissue of the orbit). EMG recordings have identified active dynamic braking in the antagonist muscles for some saccades. The active braking seems to be associated more often with small saccades than with large saccades. Occasionally a saccade is of such magnitude that it overshoots the target and a saccade in the opposite direction follows it without latency; this is called a dynamic overshoot. There is also evidence that, with an unrestricted head, intersaccadic latencies may be reduced.[11]

The overdamped plant (mechanical resistance of orbital structures) requires that the neural signal necessary to achieve the rapid FEM acceleration must be a high-frequency burst of spikes, followed by the tonic spike frequency required to stop and then hold the eyes at the new position. This combination of phasic and tonic firing patterns is designated the "pulse-step" of neural innervation (Fig. 9–5). The eye movement in Figure 9–5A results from a step change in neural firing frequency and, reflecting the overdamped plant dynamics, is considerably slower than a normal FEM. A normal

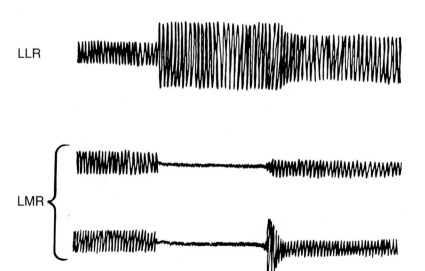

LLR

LMR

Fig. 9–4. Muscle activity of the agonistic left lateral rectus (*LLR*) and antagonistic left medial rectus (*LMR*) during FEM to the left. Note burst of LLR activity and total inhibition of LMR during the FEM and absence (*top*) or presence (*bottom*) of active braking activity in LMR.

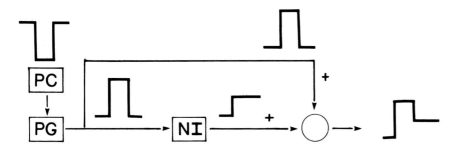

Fig. 9–6. Schematic drawing demonstrates how the pulse-step of neural innervation could be derived by summing the outputs of a neural pulse generator (*PG*) and a neural integrator (*NI*). The PG is triggered by a pause cell (*PC*) whose activity normally keeps the burst cells in the PG from firing.

FEM trajectory occurs only when a pulse precedes the step (see Fig. 9–5B). A neural "pulse generator" and "integrator" combine to form the required pulse-step of innervation (Fig. 9–6). The pulse generator consists of burst cells, whose activity is normally inhibited by pause cells (see Fig. 9–6). When the pause cells cease firing, the burst is turned on, and the duration of its high-frequency pulse of innervation is determined by a feedback circuit that contains a neural integrator. The *resettable* neural integrator, within the pulse generator, feeds back a signal that simultaneously turns off the burst cells and reactivates the pause cells. The neural integrator of the pulse generator is probably not the same as the *common* neural integrator used to generate the tonic innervation levels sent to the ocular motor nuclei. Because there are pathologic conditions (*e.g.,* gaze-evoked nystagmus) that affect the ability of the eyes to maintain gaze but do not alter the trajectory of saccades, two separate neural integrators seem to be required: a resettable integrator within the pulse generator that functions to set pulse width, and a second, common integrator that is responsible for generating the constant level of tonic innervation required to maintain gaze.[12,13] This hypothesis of normal saccade generation was supported by ocular motility studies of common human clinical conditions. Almost a decade passed before neurophysiologic studies in animals provided additional supportive evidence.[14] The pulse generator for horizontal eye movements is located within the pontine paramedian reticular formation (PPRF) at the level of the abducens nuclei, specifically, in the nucleus pontis caudalis centralis (see Chapter 10, Fig. 9–4).[15] Vertical burst neurons are located in the rostral interstitial nucleus of the medial longitudinal fasciculus (MLF). The horizontal common integrator may be located in the nucleus prepositus hypoglossi, the medial vestibular nucleus, and possibly other (cerebellum) locations. The vertical integrator is probably in the interstitial nucleus of Cajal.[16] The location of the summing junction for the pulse and step is uncertain but must be prenuclear with respect to the third cranial nerve, because MLF axons carry neural information that is already summated (pulse plus step).[17] Both burst neurons (pulse) and tonic neurons (step) project to an area of the nucleus of the abducens nerve, where intranuclear interneurons pro-

ject to the nucleus of the oculomotor nerve by way of the MLF. Thus, the summing junction is probably in the area of the nucleus of the abducens nerve.

Because saccades are not always accurate and their trajectories are not always normal, a scheme has been devised to describe both their metrics and their trajectories. The pulse-step of innervation necessary to make a saccade is used to define what is meant by orthometric, hypometric, or hypermetric eye movements. The final gaze position that the eye assumes (after the effects of both pulse and step) is used to measure saccadic accuracy. The step determines metrics, and the relationship between the pulse and step determines the trajectory (*i.e.,* the way in which the eye arrives at its final position). Saccades can be orthometric, hypometric, or hypermetric and can have numerous trajectory variations. The latter have been identified as normal, slow, overshoot, undershoot, dynamic overshoot, discrete decelerations, and multiple closely spaced saccades. A complete description of a particular saccade must include both metrics and trajectory; a refixation may include several saccades of varying metrics and trajectories. A thorough discussion of saccadic metrics along with a recursive shorthand notation for metrics and trajectories is found in the article by Schmidt et al.[18] All of the possible departures from the norm of the saccadic system were derived from and illustrated in Schmidt's article on myasthenia gravis.

Other factors may influence the speed of saccades; both attention and state of convergence can play a role. Saccades made under conditions of increased demand for accuracy are slower than normal.[19] This has been found to be associated with increased co-contraction of the extraocular muscles, presumably increasing the stiffness of the plant, both statically and dynamically.[20] The discovery of fibromuscular "pulleys," through which the extraocular muscles pass, provides a mechanism by which this can be accomplished.[21] These compliant pulleys are under active control and can change the effective moment arm of the muscles, thereby altering the dynamics of the resulting eye movement.

The closed-loop nature of the FEM mode of the version subsystem can be depicted in a block diagram (Fig. 9–7). The conjugate retinal error signal, representing a discrepancy between target and eye position, is sensed

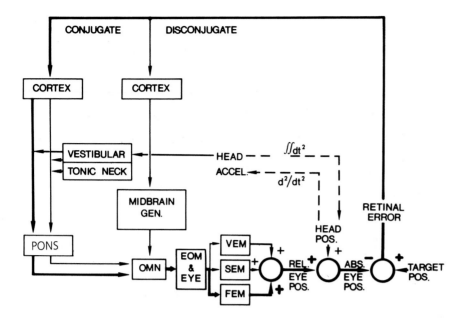

Fig. 9–7. Basic closed-loop block diagram of the FEM mode of the version subsystem (*heavy lines*) superimposed on the block diagram of the total ocular motor control system. The control signal, conjugate retinal error, is sent to the cortex, and the decision to reposition the eyes is forwarded to the paramedian reticular formation of the pons (*PONS*), where the motor commands are generated and passed on to the ocular motor nuclei (*OMN*). This innervation causes the extraocular muscles (*EOM*) to move the eye with FEM and thus change relative eye position (*REL. EYE POS.*). Assuming no change in head position, the relative position constitutes the absolute eye position (*ABS. EYE POS.*), which summates with the target position at the retina to produce zero retinal error.

in the cerebral cortex. Signals derived from this information are used in the brain stem to generate the neural command to the ocular motor neurons necessary for the FEM, which moves the eye to its new position, thereby reducing the retinal error to zero (foveal fixation).

The FEM subsystem can be modeled as a discontinuous or, more specifically, sampled-data control system in which visual information is used during sample intervals (intermittent sampling). Between samples, new visual information, although perceived, cannot be used to modify any eye movement decisions. The study of patients with pathologically slow saccades has revealed that under these conditions it is possible to modify a saccade in flight based on new visual information.[22] A detailed presentation of the control system analysis of the various types of eye movements is beyond the scope of this chapter.

Rapid eye movements (REM) of paradoxical sleep and the fast phases of evoked (vestibular, optokinetic) or pathologic nystagmus are also examples of saccadic eye movements. These saccades and those of refixation share the same physiologic characteristics.

During a saccade, the visual threshold is elevated about 0.5 log units (saccadic suppression). This phenomenon is controversial; some investigators postulate an active central inhibitory process,[23] whereas others[24] favor a retinal image "smear" mechanism. In either case, the relatively small visual threshold elevation cannot account entirely for the subjective sense of environmental stability during saccades. A mechanism designated "corollary discharge" or "efference copy," in which the visual system is "altered" centrally (by way of fronto-occipital connections) for forthcoming retinal image movement, probably serves to cancel conscious perception of environmental motion during a saccade.[25]

Plasticity

The saccadic system, as well as other ocular motor systems, is plastic (*i.e.*, its gain is under adaptive control based on feedback signals that monitor its performance). Although saccades are programmed in the brain stem, their size is controlled by means of cerebellar circuits, and it is these circuits that change saccadic gain in response to neurologic deficits. By alternately patching one eye in a patient with a third nerve palsy and studying the gain of the saccadic system as it varied with time, Abel et al[26] could document the plastic gain changes in the saccadic system and measure the time constants of this adaptation. The time constants were found to be on the order of 1 to 1.5 days; both the duration of the innervational pulse and the magnitude of the step were adjusted independently.

One of the ways in which the cerebellum is thought to make parametric adjustments in the saccadic system is by varying the amount of position information fed back to the input of the common neural integrator (Fig. 9–8). Because this neural integrator is an imperfect one (*i.e.*, it cannot hold its output without a decay in the signal, referred to as a "leak"), the gain (K_c) of the position feedback is adjusted to overcome its inherent leakiness. By using eye position feedback, the cerebellum evaluates the performance of the common neural integrator, and adjustments in K_c are made. Problems either in the neural integrator itself or in this parametric adjustment circuitry can cause various types of nystagmus. If K_c is too small, the inherent leakiness of the neural integrator will cause the eyes to gradually drift back toward primary position from any eccentric gaze position. If K_c is too high, the eyes will accelerate away from the desired gaze position with an ever-increasing velocity.

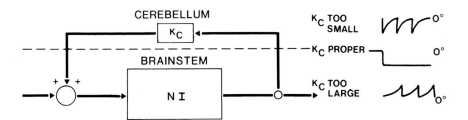

Fig. 9–8. Block diagram of the cerebellar positive feedback path with gain K_c around the leaky neural integrator (*NI*).

During evaluation of the ocular motility of a patient, the eye movements seen are a result of *both* the initial insult and the plastic adaptation that has resulted; if the insult is to the structures involved in system plasticity, either hypometric or hypermetric activity is possible.

SLOW EYE MOVEMENTS

Pursuit

The major stimulus for pursuit in foveate animals is a fixated target that moves; this evokes pursuit SEM after a latency of 125 milliseconds. The maximum sustained pursuit velocities are about 90°/second,[27] although higher values can be obtained for large-amplitude, full-field, or self-moved target motions.[28] The SEM of the vestibulo-ocular reflex (VOR) and of optokinetic nystagmus (OKN) or congenital nystagmus (CN) can be considerably faster. SEM are conjugate, smooth, and under a control system capable of *continuous* modification of motor output in response to visual input (in contrast to discrete FEM control). The input signal is retinal error ("slip") velocity, which is reduced to zero when eye velocity matches target velocity. The work of Yasui and Young[29] suggests that retinal slip velocity is used along with corollary discharge to recreate a target velocity signal, and it is this "perceived target velocity" that drives the SEM system. This would provide an explanation for many of the "pursuit" responses to non-moving targets (*e.g.,* afterimages). True pursuit is SEM in response to a *moving* target. There are many other ways to elicit SEM (see Table 9–1), and further study is required to uncover other mechanisms. Under normal conditions, a moving target is usually required for pursuit SEM; attempts to move the eyes smoothly without actual target motion result in a series of small saccades.[30]

When a foveated target suddenly moves at a constant velocity, the pursuit response begins after a 125-millisecond latency (Fig. 9–9). The initial movement is the same velocity as the target, but because of the latency, the eyes are behind the target and require a catch-up saccade for refoveation while continuing the tracking with pursuit SEM. The catch-up saccade follows the initiation of the pursuit movement because of the longer latency of the FEM subsystem. Plant dynamics do not permit a simple linear increase (ramp) in neural firing frequency to rapidly accelerate the eyes to the velocity of the moving

target (see Fig. 9–5C); a "step-ramp" of innervation is needed (see Fig. 9–5D). Thus, an instantaneous jump in firing frequency (the step) is followed by a linear increase in frequency (the ramp). It is commonly accepted that the same neural integrator used to generate the tonic firing level necessary for FEM is used for the step-ramp of SEM. Like FEM, the SEM subsystem is a closed loop with negative feedback (Fig. 9–10). The conjugate retinal error signal (slip velocity) is sensed at the visual cortex, and this information is used in the brain stem to generate the required pursuit SEM to reduce the retinal error velocity to zero. Target position, target velocity, and retinal slip velocity have all been related to the generation of smooth pursuit movements, but none of these alone adequately accounts for all of the observed characteristics of pursuit SEM. Efferent eye position, velocity information, or both are probably used in addition to the above stimuli. The role of target acceleration in smooth pursuit is in dispute.[31,32]

Because the FEM mode responds to target position errors and the SEM mode to target velocity errors (real or perceived), what would be the response to a sudden imposition of both types of error? Experiments using step-ramp stimuli (*i.e.,* the target simultaneously steps to a new position and assumes a constant velocity in the direction opposite its step of displacement) have shown that the pursuit SEM mode is independent of, but synergistic with, the FEM mode of the dual-mode version subsystem. Thus, the pursuit system will cause tracking in the direction of target motion at 125 milliseconds despite the target displacement in the opposite direction; that displacement will be corrected by a saccade at 200 milliseconds as tracking continues.

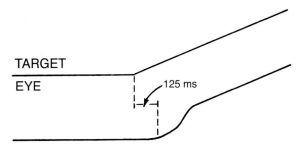

Fig. 9–9. SEM response to a target moving with a constant rightward velocity illustrating the latency (125 milliseconds) of the SEM as well as the catch-up FEM.

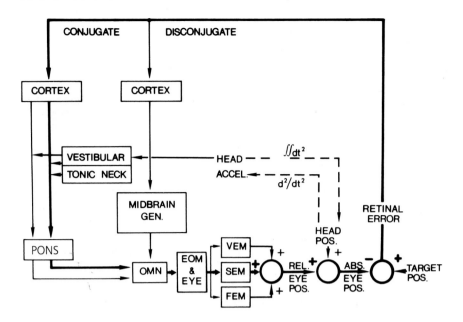

Fig. 9–10. Basic closed-loop diagram of the SEM mode of the version subsystem (*heavy lines*) superimposed on the block diagram of the total ocular motor control system. The pursuit control signal, conjugate retinal error velocity, is sent to the cortex, and the decision to move the eyes is forwarded to the pons, where the motor commands are generated and passed on to the ocular motor nuclei (*OMN*). This innervation causes the extraocular muscles (*EOM*) to move the eye with SEM and change relative eye velocity. Assuming no change in head position, this new absolute eye velocity summates with target velocity at the retina to produce zero retinal error velocity.

Fixation

Maintaining the image of a target of interest within the foveal area is the function of the fixation subsystem. Although it has been suggested that fixation is not active during smooth pursuit,[8] our studies of congenital nystagmus foveation suggest that fixation works synergistically to maintain target foveation during pursuit. Although it may not be true that fixation is pursuit at zero velocity, as Yarbus[30] suggested, we hypothesize that pursuit includes fixation at, or near, zero position (*i.e.,* when the pursuit and saccadic subsystems have positioned the target within the foveal area).

Current data suggest that maintenance of target foveation is accomplished by velocity control (similar to smooth pursuit).[9] However, we believe that some position control is also present to maintain the target in the center of the foveal area, where acuity is maximal. This would mimic the presence of position control during smooth pursuit.[33]

Vestibulo-ocular Reflex

Head movement is the stimulus for the VOR. The latency between the onset of sudden head movement and the resultant SEM can be as little as 15 milliseconds. The peak velocities of vestibulo-ocular SEM are also variable and may be as fast as 300° to 400°/second. The movements are conjugate and smooth, and the control system is continuous, but unlike the closed-loop saccadic and pursuit functions, the vestibulo-ocular system is an open loop (Figs. 9–11 and 9–12). The control signal is head acceleration transduced by the semicircular canals to a neural signal proportional to head velocity. The canals thus perform the mathematical step of integration

necessary to convert acceleration to velocity. The velocity information enters the vestibular nuclei, which project to the ocular motor neurons (see Fig. 9–11). The final step of mathematical integration that converts velocity data to the position signal may take place in the vestibular nuclei, nucleus prepositus hypoglossi, or both. In Figure 9–12, the open-loop vestibulo-ocular function is diagrammed as it would occur in darkness with no visual inputs. Final eye position is therefore equal to relative eye position plus head position.

The gain of the VOR (eye velocity/head velocity) is about 1 and does not vary much in the range of normal head movements (less than 7 Hz). Similarly, the phase shift is small, in the region of 0.01 to 7 Hz. In the dark, when doing mental arithmetic, a subject's VOR gain is about 0.65 at 0.3 Hz, but in the light, or when asked to look at an imaginary spot on the wall in total darkness, the gain rises to 1 and 0.95, respectively. Thus, to raise the natural gain of the VOR from 0.65, the subject must be attending to the environment. Unfortunately, below 0.01 Hz the gain and phase of the VOR change rapidly with frequency. Thus, for very slow movements, the VOR is not useful; low-frequency movements are discussed in the section on the optokinetic reflex (OKR). Because the time constant of the cupula is about 4 seconds, the low-frequency range of the VOR should not extend below 0.03 Hz. However, the fact that it does extend down to 0.01 Hz is due to a lengthening of the effective VOR time constant from the 4 seconds of the cupula to about 16 seconds. This is done in the vestibular nuclei, the cells of which exhibit the 16-second time constant rather than the cupula time constant.

With head-on-body movement, input from neck receptors summates with input from the vestibular end-

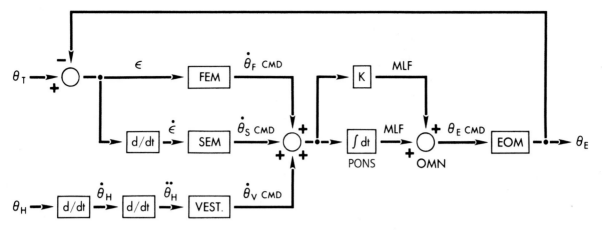

Fig. 9–11. Block diagram of the dual-mode version subsystems with vestibular input illustrates the difference between the closed-loop FEM and SEM mechanisms and the open-loop vestibulo-ocular apparatus (*VEST.*). The velocity commands of the FEM ($\dot{\theta}_F$ *CMD*), SEM ($\dot{\theta}_S$ *CMD*), and vestibular eye movements ($\dot{\theta}_V$ *CMD*) are shown summing and using the final common integrator ($\int$ dt) in the pons. Its output and the velocity outputs travel to the oculomotor nuclei (*OMN*) by way of the medial longitudinal fasciculus (*MLF*). The eye position command (θ_E *CMD*) is sent to the extraocular muscles (*EOM*) to effect the required eye position (θ_E). θ_T is the target position. In this way, the position error, $\varepsilon = \theta_T - \theta_E$, and the velocity error, $\dot{\varepsilon} = d/dt\,(\theta_T - \theta_E)$, are driven to zero; there is no feedback to the vestibular system, which responds to head acceleration ($\ddot{\theta}_H$). Head position (θ_H) and velocity ($\dot{\theta}_H$) are also shown along with their relationship to θ_H. *CMD*, command.

organ to produce compensatory eye movement.[34] For simplicity, we have not included this nuchal-ocular function in our block diagrams.

Optokinetic Reflex

The OKR is responsible for filling in where the VOR fails (*i.e.*, at the low end of the frequency spectrum of head and body movements). Proper excitation of the optokinetic system requires movement of the entire visual surround. This is most easily observed in afoveate

animals (such as the rabbit) that do not track small moving targets. Whereas in real life it is self-motion that stimulates the OKR, in the laboratory the OKR is more easily studied by placing the subject within a moving surround. When this surround begins to move, the eyes will begin to follow in the same direction after a latency of a little more than 100 milliseconds, and eye velocity will slowly build to a value equal to that of the surround. In humans, because of a well-developed pursuit system, this slow buildup of eye velocity is not seen, and the eyes quickly assume a velocity equal to

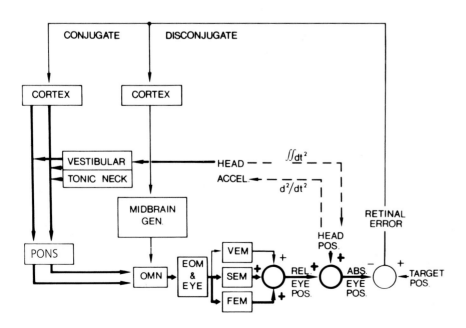

Fig. 9–12. Basic open-loop block diagram of the vestibulo-ocular mechanism (*heavy lines*) superimposed on the block diagram of the total ocular motor control system. The input is head acceleration, which is converted by the semicircular canals to a neural signal proportional to head velocity and sent to the vestibular nuclei. Here the motor commands are generated and passed on to the ocular motor nuclei (*OMN*). This innervation causes the extraocular muscles (*EOM*) to move the eyes with SEM in an attempt to match head velocity, and with FEM if eye position requires change consequent to an internal centering mechanism. Absolute eye position is the sum of relative eye position and the nonzero head position. The dashed lines show the mathematical relationships between head position and acceleration; they are *not* signal paths.

that of the surround. It is extremely difficult to study the isolated OKR in humans because of our well-developed pursuit system and the fact that the OKR reaches maximum velocity at a different velocity than the pursuit system. If one studies the eye movements that result in darkness after an optokinetic stimulus is removed (optokinetic after-nystagmus–OKAN), the effects of the pursuit system are removed and the basic OKR can be evaluated. Because of their complementary time constants (and, therefore, frequency responses), the OKR and VOR act synergistically during self-rotation to induce eye movements that are equal and opposite to motion of the surround. This joint activity is evidenced anatomically by the fact that the optokinetic signals (which are velocity commands) are mediated through the vestibular nuclei.

Visual-vestibulo-ocular Response

Because of their synergistic interaction as well as their virtual inseparability in normal head and body motions in a lighted environment, the VOR and OKR are usually combined as the visualvestibulo-ocular response. With the addition of vision (Fig. 9–13), a feedback loop is closed around the open-loop VOR, and what results is the visual-vestibulo-ocular response. The ability of the ocular motor system to relate eye position to target position in situations of head movement is thereby markedly enhanced for quick (high-frequency) movements of the head and for sustained rotation. Thus, the ocular motor system is able to accurately move the eyes opposite the moving environment.

INTERNAL MONITOR (EFFERENCE COPY)

Early studies of the saccadic system in normals,[35] as well as later studies of abnormalities in the saccadic system,[36] suggested that the FEM subsystem contained an internal monitor of efferent eye position commands that it used to generate subsequent saccades. By combining retinal error position with the internal copy of eye position, a reconstructed target position signal is used by the pulse generator to generate a saccade. The signals fed back by this internal monitor come from the output of the common neural integrator and enter the saccadic system at a point before the sampling that characterizes the saccadic system. This is not the feedback signal used in the actual generation of the pulse by the pulse generator (see discussion above). Similarly, studies of the pursuit system[29] have suggested that an internal monitor is used to feed back eye velocity commands. By this mechanism, the pursuit system would reconstruct target velocity and generate a velocity command to the eyes that was based on that signal rather than on retinal slip velocity. Figure 9–14 shows the internal monitor and its connections in both the FEM and SEM subsystems. The reconstructed target signals, both position (θ_T^r) and velocity ($\dot{\theta}_T^r$), are used to generate both position and velocity commands to the eyes.

CORRECTIVE MOVEMENTS

Large FEM (greater than 15°) are often inaccurate, necessitating corrective movements to bring the eyes on target. Inaccurate (dysmetric) conjugate refixation

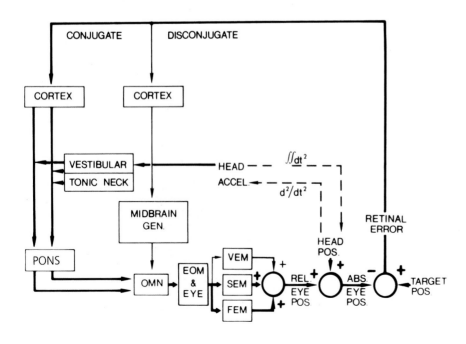

Fig. 9–13. Basic closed-loop diagram of the dual-mode version subsystem (*heavy lines*) with open-loop vestibular inputs (*heavy lines*) superimposed on the block diagram of the total ocular motor control system. The retinal error inputs combine with head acceleration and position inputs to create all version outputs (FEM, SEM, and FEM plus SEM). See Figures 9–7, 9–9, and 9–11 for explanations of the individual components of the version subsystem.

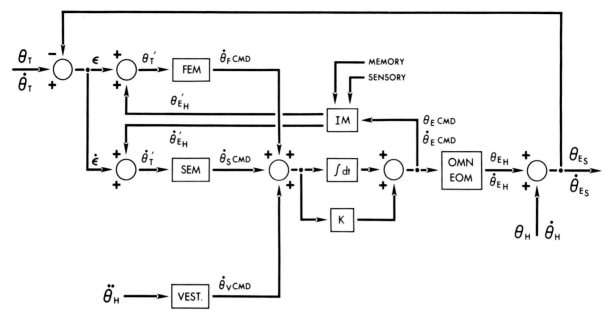

Fig. 9–14. Block diagram of the dual-mode version subsystem with vestibular input illustrates the use of an internal monitor (*IM*), which feeds back the eye position command (θ_E *CMD*) and eye velocity command ($\dot\theta_E$ *CMD*) to generate an efferent copy of eye position in the head (θ'_{E_H}) and eye velocity in the head ($\dot\theta'_{E_H}$). These signals sum with retinal error and retinal error velocity to produce an efferent copy of target position in space (θ'_T) and target velocity in space ($\dot\theta'_T$). Eye position and velocity in the head combine with head position and velocity, respectively, to produce eye position and velocity in space ($\theta_{E_H} + \theta_H = \theta_{E_S}$, and $\dot\theta_{E_H} + \dot\theta_H = \dot\theta_{E_S}$). The other symbols in this figure are identical to those in Figure 9–11.

saccades are followed by saccadic corrective movements after a latency of about 125 milliseconds. These are conjugate and occur even in darkness, thereby precluding any significant role of visual feedback information.[35] The exact mechanism responsible for these saccadic corrective movements is uncertain, but the internal monitor of eye position is probably involved. In addition, proprioceptive feedback remains a plausible explanation despite the ongoing controversy about the existence and importance of proprioception from the extraocular muscles.

Disjugate dysmetric refixation saccades usually involve one accurate eye, with the other either undershooting or overshooting. The dysmetric eye is brought to the target by a slow (usually less than 20°/second) movement, designated a "glissade."[35] The glissade results from a mismatch between the pulse and the step of the original saccade. Rather than a purposive corrective movement, a glissade is a passive drift dictated by the viscoelastic properties of the plant (orbit).

VERGENCE EYE MOVEMENTS

The stimulus for VEM is target displacement or motion along the visual Z-axis (toward or away from the observer). Vergence latency is about 160 milliseconds, maximum velocities are in the range of 20°/second, and the movements are disjugate and smooth. VEM control

is continuous, and the inputs are retinal blur (open-loop) or diplopia (closed-loop). The VEM subsystem is asymmetric (*i.e.,* convergence movements are faster than divergence movements) and is uniquely capable of generating a uniocular eye movement. The time course is similar to that depicted in Figure 9–5A for a step change in target position and in Figure 9–5C for a constant target velocity. Thus, VEM outputs simply reflect innervational signals on the overdamped plant dynamics. The VEM subsystem is a closed loop when diplopia is the error signal (Fig. 9–15). The step (of innervation) command from the midbrain generator to the ocular motor neurons results in appropriate VEM to reduce diplopia to zero.

SUBSYSTEM SYNERGISM

When eye movements are studied in the laboratory or evoked in clinical examinations, individual types are isolated by fixation of the head and/or provision of a simple appropriate stimulus. However, most naturally occurring eye movements are a combination of various versional movements admixed with VEM, reflecting the synergistic operation of all the subsystems (Fig. 9–16). Underactivity or overactivity in any subsystem may result in dynamic eye movement disturbances (Fig. 9–17). These constitute abnormal ocular oscillations, of which nystagmus is the most common.

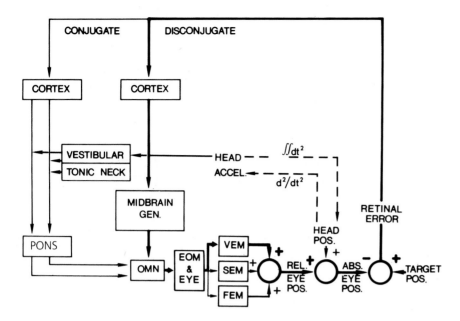

Fig. 9–15. Basic closed-loop block diagram of the vergence subsystem (*heavy lines*) superimposed on the block diagram of the total ocular motor control system. The control signal, disjugate retinal error (static diplopia), and/or error velocity (changing diplopia) is sensed by the cortex. The decision to move the eyes is forwarded to a midbrain generator where the motor commands are initiated and passed to the ocular motor nuclei (*OMN*). This innervation causes the extraocular muscles (*EOM*) to move the eyes with VEM and change relative eye position and/or velocity. Assuming no change in head position, this new absolute eye position and/or velocity sums with target position and/or velocity to produce zero disjugate retinal error(s).

THE NEAR TRIAD

Humans and other primates possess an intricate synergism linking accommodation, convergence, and pupillary constriction, an interrelationship variably termed "near response," "near reflex," "near-point triad," or "near synkinesis." The near triad can be elicited by electrical stimulation of the cerebral cortex at the junction of the occipital and temporal lobes (Brodmann area 19). Although abolition of any one of the functions does not interfere with the others, there is a definite causal relationship among the three phenomena. Pupillary constriction is directly dependent on both the convergence impulse and the accommodative impulse. As Figure

9–18 illustrates, the near triad is composed of three closed-loop subsystems, the signals of which are linked to their respective motor controllers. Thus, the accommodative signal also affects the pupillary and vergence motor controllers, and the vergence signal affects the accommodative and pupillary motor controllers. The net result is activity causing a response in each of the systems, whether the stimulus is image blur, light, disparity (diplopia), or any combination of the three. Because pupil diameter directly affects the depth of field of focal planes, a dotted feedback path has been included from the output of the pupillary system to the input of the accommodative system. Although the pupillary response to light is closed-loop, its function in the

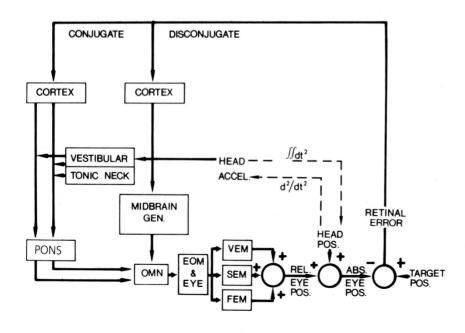

Fig. 9–16. Basic block diagram of the ocular motor system with vergence and dual-mode version subsystems. Explanations of the various components are provided in preceding figures.

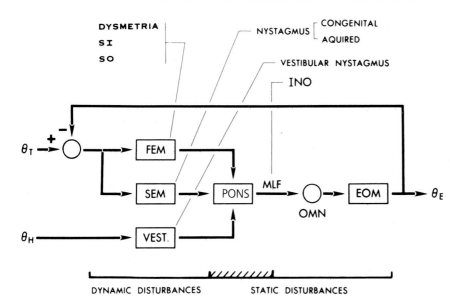

Fig. 9–17. Simplified block diagram of the dual-mode version subsystem and vestibular input with various ocular motor disorders related to disturbances in specific subsystems. θ_T is target position, θ_H is head position, and θ_E is eye position. *MLF*, medial longitudinal fasciculus; *EOM*, extraocular muscles; *OMN*, ocular motor nuclei; *SI*, saccadic intrusions; *SO*, saccadic oscillations; *INO*, internuclear ophthalmoplegia.

near response is essentially open-loop because of the small influences of blur and disparity on pupil diameter.[37]

MICROMOVEMENTS OF THE EYE

Sensitive recording techniques during fixation of a stationary target disclose three types of eye movements less than 1° in amplitude: microsaccades, microdrift, and microtremor.[30]

Microsaccades (flicks) are conjugate, although often of unequal amplitude in the two eyes. They range from 1 to 25 minutes (average of 6 minutes) of arc and demonstrate a velocity-amplitude relationship analogous to that of refixation saccades. The frequency of microsaccades is about 1 to 3 Hz. Microdrifts are disjugate and

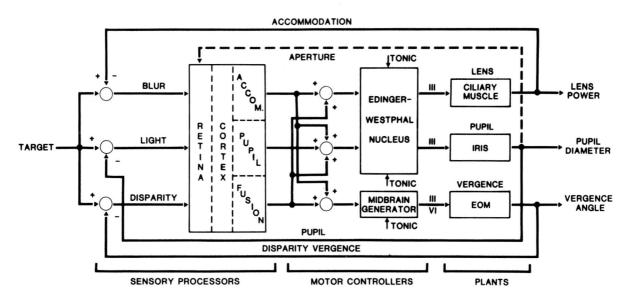

Fig. 9–18. The near triad. A block diagram shows the interrelationships among the accommodative, pupillary, and fusional subsystems that make up the near triad. When known, both functional and anatomic labels are provided. Each subsystem is a closed-loop negative feedback control system that is responsive to its own particular input as well as to the outputs of the other two systems as indicated. Both the accommodative and disparity version subsystems receive inputs from each other, and the pupillary subsystem receives inputs from both of the others. Because the aperture of the pupil directly affects the depth of field of the accommodative system, a dotted feedback pathway is shown.

TABLE 9–2. Eye Movement Characteristics

Type	Stimulus	Latency	Velocity	Amplitude	Conjugacy	Control system
FEM (saccade)	Volition, reflex	200 ms	30°–800°/s	<0.5°–90°	Conjugate	Sampled: finite width
SEM						
Pursuit	Target motion	125 ms	<90°/s	0°–90°	Conjugate	Continuous
Vestibulo-ocular	Head movement	<15 ms	<400°/s	0°–90°	Conjugate	Continuous
Optokinetic	Field motion	>100 ms	<60°/s	0°–90°	Conjugate	Continuous
VEM	Accommodative, fusional	160 ms	<20°/s	Age dependent	Disjugate	Continuous
Corrective saccade	Position error	125 ms	<150°/s	<4°	Conjugate	Refractory
Microsaccade	Fixation		3°–12°/s	1–25 min	Conjugate	Refractory
Microdrift	Fixation		0–30 min/s	<1°	Disjugate	
Tremor			50–100 Hz	5–30 s	Disjugate	Oscillatory

(Modified from Dell'Osso LF, Daroff RB: Functional organization of the ocular motor system. Aerospace Med 45:873, 1974)

slow, with speeds varying from 1 to 30 minutes of arc/second. Microtremor constitutes a disjugate, high-frequency vibration of the eyes ranging from 50 to 100 Hz, with amplitudes varying from 5 to 15 seconds of arc.

The significance of these micromovements is uncertain. It was originally believed that both microsaccades and drifts played a corrective role in fixation,[38] but later studies indicated that microsaccades probably do not occur naturally and are unique to eye movement recording conditions.[39]

Optical methods that stabilize retinal images completely, thereby eliminating the effect of micromovements, result in complete image fade-out after several seconds.[30] This implies that the small eye movements (especially tremor), by continuously sweeping images across several receptors, prevent cone saturation.

The characteristics of the various types of eye movements are summarized in Table 9–2.

ANATOMIC ARCHITECTURE

Most models of ocular motor control, including those in this chapter, are reduced to their simplest form. That is, they are unilateral in architecture with precise yoking presumed. Although such models are limited to simple, stereotyped responses, they are useful for many types of studies and for pedagogic purposes.

Unilateral and Bilateral Yoked Control

Unilateral yoked control (UYC) models contain both positive and negative signals despite the bilateral nature of brain stem organization and the positive-only nature of neuronal signals. UYC models have one eye and are essentially monocular representations of perfectly yoked eyes. As such, they cannot duplicate many of the properties of the physiologic system that are a function of internal interconnections. One basic tenet of control system theory is that behavior is a function of interconnections (feedback loops) and not the gains of individual

elements. Studies of the bilateral nature of ocular motor control required expansion (duplication) of the UYC models into bilateral yoked control (BYC). In these, perfect yoking is still assumed, but neuronal signals are positive, as are their physiologic counterparts. The "push-pull" interconnections across the midline can be modeled with BYC architecture.[40]

Bilateral and Bilateral Yoked, Independent Control

Studies of normal and, especially, abnormal eye movements of humans, and of dogs and humans with absent optic chiasms, suggest *independent* control of each eye. This directly implies independent control of each eye *muscle*,[41] which is due to the bilateral architecture of the brain stem. A bilateral independent control (BIC) model evolves from this data. A BIC model is necessary to model the ocular motor control of a chameleon, for instance. To include binocularity, yoking must be added to BIC, producing a bilateral, yoked, independent control (BYIC) model. Figure 9–19 shows such a model and includes the saccadic and pursuit subsystems; the addition of the four fixation, four VOR, four OKN, and vergence subsystems would greatly increase the complexity of a BYIC model, as can be seen by comparing Figure 9–19 with Figure 9–11 (minus the vestibular input).

EYE MOVEMENT RECORDING TECHNIQUES

Eye movement recording is required for quantitative information and as a permanent record in both basic research and clinical situations.

Afterimages

In one early technique of recording eye movements, a series of images was placed on the retina by regularly flashing lights. This necessitated subjective verbal re-

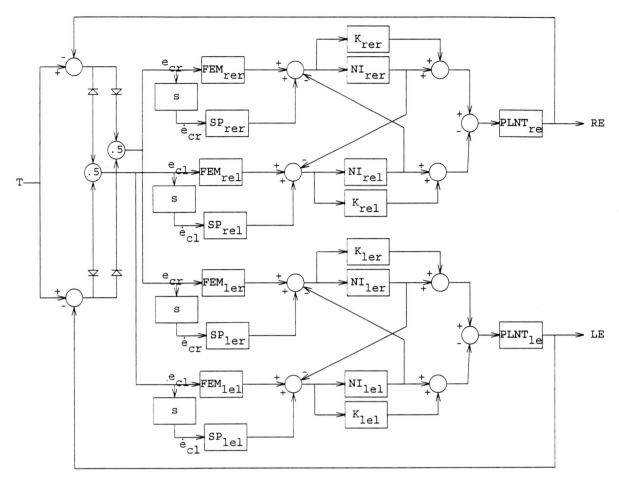

Fig. 9–19. A bilateral, yoked, independent control architecture in a model of both the fast eye movement (*FEM*) and smooth pursuit (*SP*) subsystems. *T*, target; *e*, retinal error position; *ė*, retinal error velocity; *NI*, common neural integrator; *PLNT*, ocular motor plant; *K*, proportional pathway; *E*, eye; *RE* or *re*, right eye; *LE* or *le*, left eye; *r*, right; *l*, left; *s*, Laplace notation for differentiation. (Dell'Osso LF: Evidence suggesting individual ocular motor control of each eye [muscle]. J Vestib Res 4:335, 1994)

ports, yielded no permanent record, and was replaced by mechanical recording devices.

Mechanical Transducers

Historically, mechanical transducers represented an improvement over the afterimage method in that a permanent record was obtained. They involved the attachment of instruments to the eye that interfered with normal eye movements. More sophisticated techniques are now used.

Photography

Motion picture recording of eye movements is an excellent, simple technique for gross clinical comparisons and teaching purposes. However, there are a number of compelling limitations in the use of photography for quantitative recordings. It is extremely time-consuming and requires careful frame-by-frame analy-

sis, large quantities of expensive film, and rigid head mounting.

Corneal Reflection

Corneal reflection is an offshoot of direct photography and involves photographing a light reflected on the cornea. The light beam is focused on a photographic film to provide permanent records. The use of photographic film prevents real-time monitoring of the data, but this limitation can be overcome by television scanning. The head must be rigidly stabilized for quantitative recording, because considerable error is introduced with slight head movement. The system is linear and accurate within a narrow range of amplitude and is suitable for quantitative recording of micromovements of the eye. Although not suitable for clinical purposes, it is an excellent technique for recording the scanning patterns of subjects viewing scenes or pictures.

Contact Lens

The contact lens method, which usually involves reflecting a beam of light from a mirror mounted on a corneal contact lens, is extremely sensitive and can measure eye movements of less than 10 seconds of arc, making it useful for the recording of micromovements.

Electro-oculography

Because of different metabolic rates, the cornea is about 1 mV positive with respect to the retina, a situation that creates an electrostatic field that rotates with eye movement. Skin electrodes placed around the eye can therefore record eye position. Although both eyes can be averaged with the use of bitemporal electrodes, this method does *not* result in correct eye position information about either eye and therefore can be very misleading. We recommend that each eye be measured separately with periorbital electrodes. Recording only one eye is preferable to bitemporal electrodes if only one channel is available; at least the movements of that eye will be recorded without the contamination that results from bitemporal electrode placement. Electro-oculography (EOG) is useful and convenient for recording eye movements from about 1° to 40°, but frequent calibration is essential because of nonlinearities and baseline drift.

Alternating-current-coupled EOG is a simple method of recording nystagmus and is used in electronystagmography. However, neither eye position nor slow pursuit can be recorded with the use of alternating-current amplification. For quantitative studies, direct-current oculography is essential. This introduces the problem of baseline drift, which can be overcome partially with strict attention to proper electrode and skin preparation and the use of modern, low-drift, direct-current amplifiers.

We recommend alternating-current-coupled EOG only for clinicians who want a recording of spontaneous and caloric-induced nystagmus and are *not* concerned with quantitative analysis.

Satisfactory recordings of vertical eye movements are difficult to perform with EOG because of muscle artifact and eyelid movement.

Photoelectric Oculography

Photoelectric oculography encompasses a variety of techniques, each involving the projection of light over the cornea and a photosensitive device that responds to the light reflected from the eye. The voltage output from the photosensors is a function of the angle of gaze. Infrared techniques yield a linear output to ±20° and are the most commonly used. As in EOG, both eyes can be recorded simultaneously in the horizontal direction.

Vertical eye movements can be measured accurately only if eyelid interference is eliminated; this usually restricts the range to ±10°. Compared with EOG, the system is virtually noise free, and its fast dynamic response is advantageous for the recording of saccades. It is useful for measuring eye movements during reading and is a preferred technique in research involving eye movements within 20° of primary position. Infrared photoelectric oculography is, in most respects, preferable to EOG for quantitative recording. Although it has a limited range when recording vertical eye movements, unlike EOG, the measurements are accurate. Because movement of the sensors relative to the eyes can produce artifacts in the eye signal, some systems measure the corneal reflection relative to either the pupil or fourth Purkinje image from the posterior surface of the lens. These systems have had limited success in eye movement monitoring.

Electromagnetic Search Coil

The scleral search coil is a wire coil embedded in a contact lens. The subject is placed in an alternating magnetic field, and eye position is recorded from the voltage induced in the coil. This scleral search coil is an accurate technique for both large and small movements.[42] Contact lens techniques now allow binocular tracings, because occlusion of the recorded eye is no longer required. Although the search coil is very sensitive (5 minutes of arc), has a large range (±90°), and can be used to record both horizontal and vertical eye movements simultaneously at bandwidths up to 500 Hz, the fact that it is an invasive technique makes it of limited clinical utility except in the hands of highly trained personnel. Despite this limitation, it is the most accurate and most versatile method available.

Video

With the advent of higher scan rate frequencies, digitization of video signals, and integrated software, eye movements can now be accurately measured and digitally stored by means of a video front end. Horizontal, vertical, and (in some systems) torsional eye movements can be simultaneously recorded by this noninvasive method. Linear ranges of ±40° horizontally and ±30° vertically are possible, with sampling rates of 120 Hz and noise of less than 0.1°. In comparison to the magnetic search coil, reliable horizontal and vertical position signals are provided, but the eye velocities are noisier.[43] Another advantage of the video signal is that the information necessary for pupillary diameter measurements is already present and can be extracted by the appropriate software.

The scanning laser ophthalmoscope (SLO) is a special device that makes use of video. The SLO provides a video record of the retina, on which the visual stimulus is superimposed. With appropriate video digitization and software, the SLO can also be used for quantitative analysis.

Ocular Electromyography

The methods described above measure eye position. Electromyography, in which concentric needle electrodes are inserted into the extraocular muscles, records muscle action potentials. The technique is difficult and provides little useful information to the pragmatic clinician. However, it is a research tool that has provided data about eye movement neurophysiology and explanations of clinical phenomena.

REFERENCES

1. Shaunak S, O'Sullivan E, Kennard C: Eye movements. J Neurol Neurosurg Psychiatry 59:115, 1995
2. Dell'Osso LF, Daroff RB: Functional organization of the ocular motor system. Aerospace Med 45:873, 1974
3. Keller EL, Robinson DA: Abducens unit behavior in the monkey during vergence movements. Vision Res 12:369, 1972
4. Robinson DA, Gordon JL, Gordon SE: A model of smooth pursuit eye movements. Biol Cybern 55:43, 1986
5. Dell'Osso LF: Fixation characteristics in hereditary congenital nystagmus. Am J Optom Arch Am Acad Optom 50:85, 1973
6. Dell'Osso LF, Van der Steen J, Steinman RM, Collewijn H: Foveation dynamics in congenital nystagmus I: fixation. Doc Ophthalmol 79:1, 1992
7. Dell'Osso LF, Van der Steen J, Steinman RM, Collewijn H: Foveation dynamics in congenital nystagmus II: smooth pursuit. Doc Ophthalmol 79:25, 1992
8. Luebke AE, Robinson DA: Transition dynamics between pursuit and fixation suggest different systems. Vision Res 28:941, 1988
9. Epelboim J, Kowler E: Slow control with eccentric targets: evidence against a position-corrective model. Vision Res 33:361, 1993
10. Tusa RJ, Zee DS, Hain TC, Simonsz HJ: Voluntary control of congenital nystagmus. Clin Vis Sci 7:195, 1992
11. Skavenski AA, Steinman RM: Free headed monkeys make saccades at very high frequencies in a novel laboratory environment. Invest Ophthalmol Vis Sci 36:S354, 1995
12. Dell'Osso LF, Daroff RB: Clinical disorders of ocular movement. In Zuber BL (ed): Models of Oculomotor Behavior and Control, p 233. West Palm Beach, CRC Press Inc, 1981
13. Abel LA, Dell'Osso LF, Daroff RB: Analog model for gaze-evoked nystagmus. IEEE Trans Biomed Eng BME-25:71, 1978
14. Scudder CA: A new local feedback model of the saccadic burst generator. J Neurophysiol 59:1455, 1988
15. Keller EL: Participation of medial pontine reticular formation in eye movement generation in monkey. J Neurophysiol 37:316, 1974
16. Fukushima K, Kaneko CRS, Fuchs AF: The neuronal substrate of integration in the oculomotor system. Prog Neurobiol 39:609, 1992
17. Pola J, Robinson DA: An explanation of eye movements seen in internuclear ophthalmoplegia. Arch Neurol 33:447, 1976
18. Schmidt D, Dell'Osso LF, Abel LA, Daroff RB: Myasthenia gravis: dynamic changes in saccadic waveform, gain and velocity. Exp Neurol 68:365, 1980
19. Hendriks AW, Enright JT: Eye movements become slower with increasing demand for accuracy. Invest Ophthalmol Vis Sci 36:S355, 1995
20. Enright JT, Hendriks AW: Cognitive influence on the relationship between peak velocity and amplitude of saccades. Invest Ophthalmol Vis Sci 36:S597, 1995
21. Demer JL, Miller JM, Poukens V et al: Evidence for fibromuscular pulleys of the recti extraocular muscles. Invest Ophthalmol Vis Sci 36:1125, 1995
22. Zee DS, Optican LM, Cook JD et al: Slow saccades in spinocerebellar degeneration. Arch Neurol 33:243, 1976
23. Chase R, Kalil RE: Suppression of visual evoked responses to flashes and pattern shift during voluntary saccades. Vision Res 12:215, 1972
24. Mitrani L, Mateef ST, Yakimoff N: Is saccadic suppression really saccadic? Vision Res 11:1157, 1971
25. Koerner F, Schiller PH: The optokinetic response under open and closed loop conditions in the monkey. Exp Brain Res 14:318, 1972
26. Abel LA, Schmidt D, Dell'Osso LF, Daroff RB: Saccadic system plasticity in humans. Ann Neurol 4:313, 1978
27. Meyer CH, Lasker AG, Robinson DA: The upper limit of human smooth pursuit velocity. Vision Res 25:561, 1985
28. Van Den Berg AV, Collewijn H: Human smooth pursuit: effects of stimulus extent and of spatial and temporal constraints of the pursuit trajectory. Vision Res 26:1209, 1986
29. Yasui S, Young LR: Perceived visual motion as effective stimulus to pursuit eye movement system. Science 190:906, 1975
30. Yarbus AL: Eye Movements and Vision, pp 1–222. New York, Plenum Press, 1967
31. Krauzlis RJ, Lisberger SG: A control systems model of smooth pursuit eye movements with realistic emergent properties. Neural Computation 1:116, 1989
32. Watamaniuk SNJ, Heinen SJ: Is the visual system's insensitivity to acceleration also evident in the smooth pursuit system? Invest Ophthalmol Vis Sci 36:S205, 1995
33. Pola J, Wyatt HJ: Target position and velocity: the stimuli for smooth pursuit eye movements. Vision Res 20:523, 1980
34. Rubin AM, Young JH, Milne AC et al: Vestibular-neck integration in the vestibular nuclei. Brain Res 96:99, 1975
35. Weber RB, Daroff RB: Corrective movements following refixation saccades: type and control system analysis. Vision Res 12:467, 1972
36. Dell'Osso LF, Troost BT, Daroff RB: Macro square wave jerks. Neurology 25:975, 1975
37. Hung GK, Semmlow JL, Ciuffreda KJ: The near response: modeling, instrumentation, and clinical applications. IEEE Trans Biomed Eng BME-31:910, 1984
38. St Cyr GJ, Fender DH: The interplay of drifts and flicks in binocular fixation. Vision Res 9:245, 1969
39. Steinman RM, Haddad GM, Skavenski AA, Wyman D: Miniature eye movement. Science 181:810, 1973
40. Doslak MJ, Dell'Osso LF, Daroff RB: A model of Alexander's law of vestibular nystagmus. Biol Cybern 34:181, 1979
41. Dell'Osso LF: Evidence suggesting individual ocular motor control of each eye (muscle). J Vestib Res 4:335, 1994
42. Robinson DA: A method of measuring eye movement using a scleral search coil in a magnetic field. IEEE Trans Biomed Electron BME 10:137, 1963
43. DiScenna AO, Das V, Zivotofsky AZ et al: Evaluation of a video tracking device for measurement of horizontal and vertical eye rotations during locomotion. J Neurosci Methods 58:89, 1995

CHAPTER 10

Supranuclear Disorders of Eye Movements

R. John Leigh, Robert B. Daroff, and B. Todd Troost

Brain Stem Control of Horizontal Gaze
  Effects of Lesions of the Pons and Medulla on
    Horizontal Gaze
**Brain Stem Connections for Vertical and Torsional
  Movements**
  Effects of Midbrain Lesions on Vertical and
    Torsional Gaze
  Sustained Vertical Deviations
  Dorsal Midbrain Syndrome
  Skew Deviation
  Progressive Supranuclear Palsy
**Brain Stem Control of Vergence Eye
  Movements**
  Disorders of Vergence
  Spasm of the Near Reflex
  Divergence Paresis or Paralysis
Cerebellar Influences on Eye Movements
  Effects of Cerebellar Lesions
  Common Vascular Syndromes of the
    Cerebellum

**Cerebral and Basal Ganglionic Control of Eye Move-
  ments**
  The Saccadic System
  Several Rules for Saccades
  Several Cortical Areas that Contribute to Saccade
    Generation
  Cortical Projections to Brain Stem Saccade
  Circuits
  The Superior Colliculus
  The Roles of Descending Parallel Projections
  Pursuit System
  Vestibulo-ocular System
  Gaze Holding
  Common Disturbances of Gaze with Unilateral
    Hemispheric Lesions
  Acute Bilateral Frontoparietal Lesions: Ocular Mo-
    tor Apraxia
  Parkinson Disease
  Huntington Disease
  Functional Disturbances of Gaze

> Doubt is not a pleasant condition but certainty is an
> absurd one.
>
> Voltaire

As a result of three decades of systematic research into the control of eye movements, it is now possible to provide a pathophysiologic explanation for most of the supranuclear disorders of gaze (see Chapter 9 for more detailed discussions of pathophysiology).[1] In applying this approach to the diagnosis of abnormal eye movements, the first important step is to use a system

of examination that tests each of the different functional classes of eye movements. Each functional class of eye movements has distinctive properties that suit it to its specific purposes; these were discussed in Chapter 9 but are recapitulated in Table 10–1. Knowledge of these purposes and properties helps guide the examination. The second step is to be familiar with the neural substrate that is important for each functional class of eye movements, because such knowledge helps with topologic diagnosis. Our approach in this chapter is "bottom-up," starting with the brain stem inputs to the ocular motoneurons that reside in the third, fourth, and sixth cranial nerve nuclei. Subsequently, the contributions of the cerebellum and cerebral hemispheres are reviewed. At each stage from ocular motoneuron to visual cortex, a summary of the relevant anatomy and physiology is followed by descriptions of the effects of discrete lesions and the characteristics of distinctive syndromes.

It is important to recognize that when the brain initiates any type of eye movement, it must take into account the properties of the eyeball, its suspensory ligaments, and the fascia. Although it is easy to take for granted

R. J. Leigh: Department of Neurology, Case Western Reserve University; and Neurology Service, Veterans Affairs Medical Center, Cleveland, Ohio

R. B. Daroff: Department of Neurology, Case Western Reserve University; and Medical Affairs, University Hospitals of Cleveland, Cleveland, Ohio

B. T. Troost: Department of Neurology, Wake Forest University School of Medicine; and Department of Neurology, North Carolina Baptist Hospital, Winston-Salem, North Carolina

See Chapter 11 for Glossary.

TABLE 10–1. Functional Classes of Eye Movements

Class of eye movement	Main function
Visual fixation	Holds the image of a stationary object on the fovea
Vestibulo-ocular reflex	Holds images of the seen world steady on the retina during brief head rotations
Optokinetic	Holds images of the seen world steady on the retina during sustained head rotations
Smooth pursuit	Holds the image of a moving target close to the fovea
Nystagmus quick phases	Reset the eyes during prolonged rotation, and direct gaze toward the on-coming visual scene
Saccades	Bring images of objects of interest onto the fovea
Vergence	Moves the eyes in opposite directions so that images of a single object are placed simultaneously on both foveas

(Adapted from Leigh RJ, Zee DS: The Neurology of Eye Movements, 3rd ed. New York, Oxford University Press, 1999)

that the brain will make adjustments, for example, when the eye is turned to look out of the corner or the orbit, such eccentric "gaze holding" demands an appropriate tonic contraction of the extraocular muscles. Otherwise, the eye would drift back toward the primary position. This gaze-holding function (sometimes referred to as the achievement of a "neural integrator") is really a separate functional property affecting all eye movements that also has its own identified neural substrate.

BRAIN STEM CONTROL OF HORIZONTAL GAZE

Motor Commands for Conjugate (Versional) Horizontal Movements

The *abducens nucleus* is of central importance in the control of horizontal gaze because it governs conjugate movements of both the ipsilateral lateral rectus *and* the contralateral medial rectus muscles. It houses two populations of neurons: (1) abducens motoneurons, which supply the lateral rectus muscle; and (2) abducens internuclear neurons, which project up the contralateral medial longitudinal fasciculus (MLF) to contact medial rectus motoneurons of the oculomotor nucleus (Fig. 10–1).[2,3] Thus, axons of the abducens nerve and axons of the abducens internuclear neurons that run in the MLF[4] together encode conjugate, horizontal eye movements. In other words, the mechanism for yoking of horizontal movements—Hering's law—has its neural basis in the abducens nucleus and its two populations of neurons. The abducens motoneurons and internuclear neurons are intermingled and show only minor morpho-

logic differences[5]; however, only the motoneurons contain acetylcholine.[6] Both types of abducens neurons receive the same afferent input. How do signals for each functional class of eye movements project to the abducens nucleus?

The abducens nucleus receives vestibular and optokinetic inputs from the vestibular nuclei.[7,8] Saccadic commands originate from burst neurons of the pontine and medullary reticular formation.[9,10] A descending smooth pursuit pathway probably projects to the abducens nucleus via the flocculus and cerebellar fastigial nuclei (see Pursuit System section).[1] The signals that are important for gaze-holding function reach the abducens nucleus from the nucleus prepositus hypoglossi and the medial vestibular nuclei.[11]

Effects of Lesions of the Pons and Medulla on Horizontal Gaze

Lesions of the abducens nucleus produce paralysis of both the ipsilateral lateral rectus and contralateral medial rectus for all conjugate eye movements,[12–14] but vergence movements are spared. Clinical lesions that affect only the abducens nucleus are rare, and there is usually involvement of adjacent structures as well, including the facial nerve fascicle, MLF, and paramedian pontine reticular formation (PPRF).

Lesions of the MLF produce *internuclear ophthalmoplegia* (INO), which is characterized by paresis of adduction, for conjugate movements, on the side of the lesion[15,16]; and "dissociated nystagmus," characterized by abduction overshoot of the eye contralateral to the lesion (see Chapter 11).[17] The MLF is paramedian in the pons and becomes slightly more lateral in the midbrain as it approaches the oculomotor nuclear complex. INO is often accompanied by skew deviation, probably as a result of disruption of the otolithic-ocular connections.[18] In addition, bilateral INO is usually associated with gaze-evoked vertical nystagmus, impaired vertical pursuit, and decreased vertical vestibular responses.[19] Small-amplitude saccadic intrusions may disrupt steady fixation.[20] The most frequent cause of INO in young adults, particularly when bilateral, is multiple sclerosis; other causes are summarized in Table 10–2.

Strictly speaking, the term internuclear ophthalmoplegia should refer to absolute adduction paralysis during horizontal versions, and the term internuclear ophthalmoparesis should be used to describe those cases where adduction past the midline is present, but with limitation of amplitude or decreased velocity. When INO is subtle, two maneuvers may be useful for demonstrating it: the optokinetic and ocular dysmetria signs,[21] which rely on demonstrating impairment of innervation of the medial rectus muscle compared with its yoke, the contralateral lateral rectus, during horizontal saccades. With the optokinetic tape moving to the side of the involved medial rectus muscle, the nystagmus response

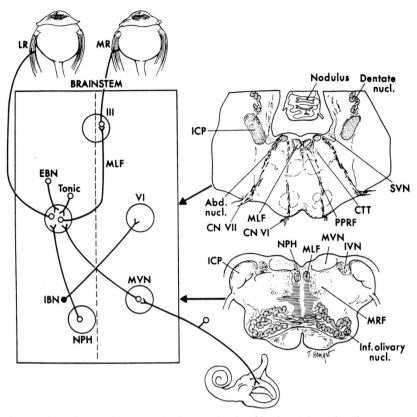

Fig. 10–1. Anatomic pathways important in the synthesis of horizontal versional eye movements. The abducens nucleus (*VI*) contains abducens motoneurons that innervate the ipsilateral lateral rectus muscle (*LR*), as well as abducens internuclear neurons with axons that ascend in the contralateral medial longitudinal fasciculus (*MLF*) to contact medial rectus (*MR*) motoneurons in the contralateral third nerve nucleus (*III*). From the horizontal semicircular canal, primary vestibular afferents project mainly to the medial vestibular nucleus (*MVN*), where they synapse and then send an excitatory connection to the contralateral abducens nucleus and an inhibitory projection to the ipsilateral abducens nucleus. Saccadic inputs reach the abducens nucleus from ipsilateral excitatory burst neurons (*EBN*) and contralateral inhibitory burst neurons (*IBN*). Eye position information (the output of the neural integrator) reaches the abducens nucleus from neurons within the nucleus prepositus hypoglossi (*NPH*) and adjacent MVN. The anatomic sections on the right correspond to the level of the arrow heads on the schematic on the left. *Abd. nucl.*, abducens nucleus; *CN VI*, abducens nerve; *CN VII*, facial nerve; *CTT*, central tegmental tract; *ICP*, inferior cerebellar peduncle; *IVN*, inferior vestibular nucleus; *Inf. olivary nucl.*, inferior olivary nucleus; *MVN*, medial vestibular nucleus; *MRF*, medullary reticular formation; *SVN*, superior vestibular nucleus. (Adapted from Leigh RJ, Zee DS: The Neurology of Eye Movements, 3rd ed. New York, Oxford University Press, 1999)

in that eye is reduced (especially the adduction saccade) compared with the opposite eye. The ocular dysmetria sign necessitates repetitive horizontal saccadic refixations that disclose slow, hypometric refixation of the adducting eye (medial rectus) and concomitant overshoot of the abducting eye (lateral rectus). Some care is required in interpreting these signs, since abducting saccades are faster in normal subjects[22]; quantitative comparison of the velocity of the two eyes may be required to make the diagnosis in subtle cases (see Chapter 9).

Most cases of INO are orthotropic (or exophoric) in primary position without symptomatic diplopia unless accompanied by skew deviation. Occasionally, patients with bilateral INO show exotropia, designated the WEBINO (wall-eyed bilateral INO) syndrome.[23] The explanation for this finding is unclear, since monkeys with lidocaine-induced INO show an *increased* accommodative vergence to accommodation ratio, indicating that the MLF actually carries signals that inhibit vergence.[24] Thus, the cause of exotropia in INO is uncertain, and it has been observed in patients with preserved convergence. Furthermore, the classification of INO into anterior and posterior types depending on the integrity of the convergence mechanism is not of localizing value in identifying the rostral-caudal location of the MLF lesion. The so-called posterior internuclear ophthalmoplegia of Lutz,[25] in which abduction (but not adduction) is impaired is rare. It has been difficult to conceptualize since the abducens contains neurons that

TABLE 10–2. Causes of Internuclear Ophthalmoplegia

1. Multiple sclerosis (commonly bilateral)
2. Brain stem infarction (commonly unilateral), including complication of arteriography and hemorrhage
3. Brain stem and fourth ventricular tumors
4. Arnold-Chiari malformation; associated hydrocephalus and syringobulbia
5. Infection: bacterial, viral, and other forms of meningoencephalitis; in association with AIDS
6. Hydrocephalus; subdural hematoma; supratentorial arteriovenous malformation
7. Nutritional disorders: Wernicke encephalography; pernicious anemia
8. Metabolic disorders: hepatic encephalography; maple syrup urine disease; abetalipoproteinemia; Fabry disease
9. Drug intoxications: phenothiazines, tricyclic antidepressants, narcotics, propranolol, lithium, barbiturates
10. Cancer: due to either carcinomatous infiltration or remote effect
11. Head trauma; cervical hyperextension or manipulation
12. Degenerative conditions: progressive supranuclear palsy
13. Syphilis
14. Pseudointernuclear ophthalmoplegia of myasthenia gravis; Fisher syndrome

(Adapted from Leigh RJ, Zee DS: The Neurology of Eye Movements, 3rd ed. New York, Oxford University Press, 1999)

innervate both lateral and medial rectus muscles for all conjugate eye movements.[26]

A combined lesion of one MLF and the adjacent abducens nucleus (or its inputs) produces paresis of all conjugate movements except for abduction of the eye contralateral to the side of the lesion—*"one-and-a-half" syndrome.*[27,28] This occurs with brain stem infarction, hemorrhage, multiple sclerosis and pontine glioma; rarer causes are brain stem arteriovenous malformation, basilar artery aneurysm, and posterior fossa tumor. When the lesion is acute, the patient may be profoundly exotropic.[29] The deviated eye may demonstrate marked nystagmus and is always on the side opposite that of the brain stem lesion.

Discrete *lesions of the PPRF,*[30,31] the PPRF mainly corresponding to the nucleus pontis centralis caudalis and containing saccadic burst neurons, cause loss of saccades and quick phases of nystagmus to the side of the lesion. Vertical saccades are misdirected obliquely away from the side of the lesion.[32] Selective impairment of horizontal saccades occurs in degenerative conditions, such as some variants of spinocerebellar atrophy. Other causes of slow or absent saccades are summarized in Table 10–3. Infarction of the paramedian pons usually also involves adjacent fibers conveying vestibular and pursuit inputs to the abducens nucleus.[33] Pontine disease may cause a unilateral defect of smooth pursuit by affecting the dorsolateral pontine nuclei and their projections to the cerebellum (see discussion below).[34,35] More

rostral brain stem lesions may cause ipsilateral smooth pursuit deficits, whereas caudal brain stem lesions tend to cause contralateral deficits (see discussion below).[36]

Bilateral, experimental *lesions of the nucleus prepositus hypoglossi and adjacent medial vestibular nucleus* abolish the gaze-holding mechanism for eye movements in the horizontal plane.[36] When healthy, the neural integrator generates the eye position command necessary to hold the eye steady in an eccentric orbital position. After damage to the neural integrator network (which includes connection with the vestibular cerebellum), however, the eye cannot be held in an eccentric position in the orbit and it drifts back to primary position. Corrective quick phases then produce gaze-evoked nystagmus. Thus, disease affecting the vestibular nuclei and nucleus prepositus hypoglossi cause vestibular imbalance—manifest as nystagmus or skew deviation—and impairment of gaze holding for all types of conjugate eye movement. This occurs with lateral medullary infarction (Wallenberg syndrome), in which the spontaneous nystagmus is usually horizontal or mixed horizontal-torsional, with the slow phases directed toward the side of the lesion; the nystagmus may reverse direction in eccentric positions, suggesting coexistent involvement of the gaze-holding mechanism. Skew deviation together with ipsilateral hypotropia, cyclodeviation (lower eye more extorted), and ipsilateral head tilt—the *ocular tilt reaction* (OTR)—reflects an imbalance of otolithic inputs.[37] In addition, patients with Wallenberg syndrome show a characteristic lateropulsion in which the eyes deviate conjugately toward the side of the lesion if the lids are closed, or with saccades.[38] A hypothetical explanation for lateropulsion has been proposed in which infarction of the inferior cerebellar peduncle leads to

TABLE 10–3. Causes of Slow Saccades

1. Olivopontocerebellar atrophy; spinocerebellar degenerations
2. Huntington disease
3. Progressive supranuclear palsy
4. Parkinson disease (advanced cases); diffuse Lewy body disease
5. Whipple diseases
6. Lipid storage diseases
7. Wilson disease
8. Drug intoxications: anticonvulsants, benzodiazepines
9. Tetanus
10. In dementia: Alzheimer disease (stimulus-dependent); in association with AIDS
11. Lesions of the paramedian pontine reticular formation
12. Internuclear ophthalmoplegia
13. Peripheral nerve palsy; diseases affecting the neuromuscular junction and extraocular muscle; restrictive ophthalmopathy

(Adapted from Leigh RJ and Zee DS: The Neurology of Eye Movements, 3rd ed. New York, Oxford University Press, 1999)

increased inhibition of the fastigial nucleus by the cerebellar vermis (see discussion below).

BRAIN STEM CONNECTIONS FOR VERTICAL AND TORSIONAL MOVEMENTS

The ocular motoneurons that control vertical and torsional eye movements lie in the oculomotor and trochlear nuclei. How do signals for each functional class of eye movements project to these motoneurons? To

epitomize, vertical and torsional saccadic commands and the vertical gaze-holding signal are synthesized in the midbrain, while vestibular and pursuit signals ascend to the midbrain from the lower brain stem.

In the prerubral fields of the mesencephalon, rostral to the tractus retroflexus and caudal to the mamillothalamic tract, lies a nucleus that is important for the generation of *vertical saccades* (Fig. 10–2). This structure has been variously termed the *rostral interstitial nucleus of the MLF (riMLF)*,[39] the nucleus of the prerubral fields,

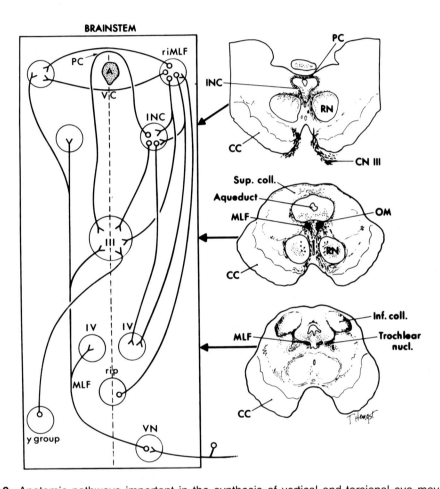

Fig. 10–2. Anatomic pathways important in the synthesis of vertical and torsional eye movements. Vestibular inputs from the vertical semicircular canals synapse in the vestibular nuclei (*VN*) and ascend in the medial longitudinal fasciculus (*MLF*) and brachium conjunctivum (not shown) to contact neurons in the trochlear nucleus (*IV*), oculomotor nucleus (*III*), interstitial nucleus of Cajal (*INC*), and rostral interstitial nucleus of the medial longitudinal fasciculus (*riMLF*). The riMLF, which lies in the prerubral fields, also receives an input from omnipause neurons of the nucleus raphe interpositus (*rip*), which lies in the pons. The riMLF contains saccadic burst cells that project ipsilaterally to the motoneurons of III and IV, and also send an axon collateral to INC. Connections between the right and left riMLF may pass in or near the posterior commissure (*PC*) and ventral commissure (*VC*). Cells in INC that may encode vertical eye position (contributing to the neural integrator) also project to III and IV: projections to the elevator subnuclei (innervating the superior rectus and inferior oblique muscles) pass above the aqueduct of Sylvius (*A*) in the posterior commissure; projections to the depressor subnuclei (innervating the inferior rectus and superior oblique) pass ventrally. Signals contributing to vertical smooth pursuit and eye-head tracking reach the III from the y-group via the brachium conjunctivum and a crossing ventral tegmental tract. The anatomic sections on the right correspond to the level of the arrowheads of the schematic on the left. *CC*, crus cerebri; *CN III*, oculomotor nerve; *RN*, red nucleus; *Sup. coll.*, superior colliculus; *Inf. coll.*, inferior colliculus; *OM*, oculomotor nucleus. (Adapted from Leigh RJ, Zee DS: The Neurology of Eye Movements, 2 ed. New York, Oxford University Press, 1999)

and the nucleus of the fields of Forel. It contains burst neurons for vertical saccades and quick phases and for torsional quick phases. Each riMLF contains neurons that burst for upward and downward eye movements; however, for torsional quick phases, they burst in only one direction. Thus, the right riMLF discharges for quick phases that are directed clockwise with respect to the subject.[40] In addition, each riMLF is connected to its counterpart by a commissure that lies ventral to the aqueduct. The riMLF appears to project to motoneurons innervating elevator muscles bilaterally, but to motoneurons innervating ipsilateral depressor muscles.[41,42] Furthermore, each burst neuron in the riMLF appears to send axon collaterals to motoneurons supplying yoke muscle pairs (*e.g.*, superior rectus, inferior oblique); this is the neural substrate for Hering's law (see Chapter 3) in the vertical plane.

The riMLF also projects to the *interstitial nucleus of Cajal* (INC), which has been shown to play an important role in vertical and torsional gaze-holding.[43] In addition, each INC also receives inputs from the vestibular nuclei and the contralateral INC.[44] The INC projects to motoneurons of the vertical ocular motor subnuclei.[45] The projections of the INC to the elevator ocular motor nuclei (superior rectus and inferior oblique) pass dorsally over the aqueduct in the posterior commissure, and this might explain why lesions of the posterior commissure limit mainly upward eye movements.[46] The INC also contains neurons that project to motoneurons of the neck and trunk muscles, and it appears to coordinate combined torsional-vertical movements of the eyes and head. The neural signals necessary for *vertical vestibular and smooth-pursuit eye movements* ascend from the cerebellum, medulla, and pons to the midbrain. The MLF is the most important route for these projections, but the brachium conjunctivum (superior cerebellar peduncle) and other pathways are also involved.[47]

Effects of Midbrain Lesions on Vertical and Torsional Gaze

Unilateral experimental *lesions of the riMLF* cause only a mild defect in vertical saccades, because each nucleus contains burst neurons for both upward and downward movements; however, unilateral riMLF lesions produce a specific defect of torsional quick phases.[48] For example, with a lesion of the right riMLF, torsional quick phases, clockwise from the point of view of the patient (*i.e.*, extorsion of the right eye and intorsion of the left eye), are lost. Vertical saccadic deficits with unilateral lesions of the riMLF in humans are rare and probably reflect involvement of the commissural pathways of the riMLF that make the lesion, in effect, bilateral.[49] In general, bilateral lesions are required to produce clinically apparent deficits of vertical eye movements.[50] Bilateral experimental lesions of the riMLF in monkeys cause a vertical saccadic deficit that may be more pronounced for downward eye movements[51]; vertical gaze-holding, vestibular eye movements, and possibly pursuit are preserved, as are horizontal saccades. Patients with discrete, bilateral infarction involving the riMLF show deficits of either downward or both upward and downward saccades.[52] Certain metabolic and degenerative disorders can lead to selective slowing or absence of vertical saccades (see Table 10–3).

Unilateral experimental *lesions of the INC* are reported to impair gaze-holding function in the vertical plane.[43] Skew deviation (ipsilateral hypertropia) extorsion of the contralateral eye, intorsion of the ipsilateral eye, and contralateral head tilt also occur. Stimulation of the INC in the monkey produces an OTR that consists of an ipsilateral head tilt and a synkinetic ocular reaction: depression and extorsion of the eye ipsilateral to the stimulation, and elevation and intorsion of the contralateral eye.[53] This OTR is similar to that produced by stimulation of the contralateral utricular nerve or an ipsilateral lesion of the vestibular nucleus (see discussion on Wallenberg syndrome). Bilateral lesions of the MLF (bilateral INO) impair vertical vestibular and smooth-pursuit movements but spare vertical saccades.[54] In addition, partial loss of the vertical eye position signal causes gaze-evoked nystagmus in the vertical plane.

Lesions of the posterior commissure cause loss of upward gaze.[46] All types of eye movements are usually affected, but the vestibulo-ocular reflex and Bell phenomenon are sometimes spared. Experimental inactivation of the posterior commissure with lidocaine impairs vertical gaze-holding function.[55] Other findings with posterior commissure lesions include slowing of vertical saccades below the horizontal meridian, disorders of convergence, "convergence-retraction nystagmus," light-near dissociation of the pupils, and eyelid retraction (see Dorsal Midbrain Syndrome section).

Sustained Vertical Deviations

A number of disparate conditions can lead to tonic upward or downward eye deviations. One dramatic example is the sustained upward deviation of oculogyric crisis (see Parkinson Disease section). Otherwise, tonic upgaze deviation is seen in unconscious patients, especially after hypoxic-ischemic brain injury, perhaps reflecting loss of cerebellar Purkinje cells that normally balance vestibular and gaze-holding mechanisms. This notion is supported by the observation that the few patients who survive such insults develop downbeating nystagmus.[56] Tonic downward deviation may occur transiently in neonates and does not necessarily indicate a neurologic abnormality. In comatose patients, sustained downward deviations, with small, unreactive pupils, usually indicate bilateral thalamic infarction or hemorrhage.[57] The setting-sun sign of infantile hydrocephalus is an analogous clinical phenomenon, with associated pathologic eyelid retraction. The reversibility of this

sign with ventricular decompression indicates a dynamic mechanism secondary to acutely increased intracranial pressure.[58] Tonic downward deviation may occur in metabolic encephalopathies.[59] Tonic convergent and downward deviation of the eyes in a patient with paralysis of upward gaze secondary to a large midbrain hematoma has been reported.[60] These downward deviations, which probably reflect pressure on or dysfunction of the posterior commissure, should be distinguished from "ocular bobbing," an oscillatory disorder consisting of an abrupt downward jerk followed by a slow, upward drift to midposition (see Chapter 11). Slow, spontaneously alternating skew deviations may occur with lesions of the dorsal midbrain.[61]

Dorsal Midbrain Syndrome

Dorsal lesions in the rostral midbrain produce a distinctive constellation of neuro-ophthalmologic signs involving supranuclear control of vertical gaze, eyelids, pupils, accommodation, and vergence. This entity encompasses many syndromes given eponymic and anatomic designations (e.g., Parinaud, sylvian aqueduct, pretectal, posterior commissural). Pineal area tumors[62,63] and midbrain infarction[49,52,64] are the most common causes. Other causes include congenital aqueductal stenosis, multiple sclerosis, syphilis, arteriovenous malformations, midbrain hemorrhage,[65,66] encephalitis, midbrain or third ventricle tumors, herniation of the uncus,[67] and lesions resulting from stereotactic surgery.[68] The lesions are usually large and involve one or more of the sites previously described as causing upgaze palsies. The pupils are usually large and demonstrate light-near dissociation; that is, the light reaction is smaller than the near response. Pathologic lid retraction (Collier sign) and lid lag are common findings. Paralysis of upward gaze is the hallmark sign. Upward saccades are affected initially, whereas pursuit is relatively spared. Both types of eye movements, as well as vestibulo-ocular responses and Bell phenomenon, may ultimately become paralyzed. Attempts at upward saccades evoke "convergence-retraction nystagmus," which persists as long as the refixation effort is maintained. The nystagmus is best elicited with down-going optokinetic targets providing a stimulus for repetitive upward saccades; each fast phase is replaced by a convergence or retraction movement. It is not truly nystagmus, but consists of opposed adducting saccades, followed by slow divergence movements (see Chapter 11).[69] This is in contrast to normal subjects, who show transient convergence during downward saccades and divergence during upward saccades.[70] Rarely, a divergence-retraction nystagmus may occur in patients with dorsal midbrain syndrome (see Chapter 12).

Cerebral hemispheric lesions associated with focal motor seizures may cause retraction nystagmus temporally associated with periodic lateralized epileptiform discharges on the electroencephalogram.[71]

Skew Deviation

Skew deviation may be defined as a vertical misalignment of the visual axes caused by a disturbance of prenuclear inputs. The hypertropia may be the same in all positions of gaze (concomitant), may vary with gaze position, or may even alternate (e.g., right hypertropia on right gaze, left hypertropia on left gaze).[72,73] When skew deviation is nonconcomitant, it should be differentiated from vertical extraocular muscle palsy by the coexistence of signs of central neurologic dysfunction and from trochlear nerve palsy by a negative head-tilt test. In some patients, skew deviation is accompanied by ocular torsion and head tilt (OTR)[18] (Fig. 10–3), which may be tonic (sustained)[74,75] or paroxysmal.[76,77] Such patients also show a deviation of the subjective vertical.[18] Rarely, skew deviation slowly alternates or varies in magnitude over the course of minutes.[61] These patients have midbrain lesions. The periodicity of the phenomena is reminiscent of periodic alternating nystagmus (see above), and the two phenomena may coexist.[78]

Skew deviation has been reported in association with a variety of disorders of the brain stem and cerebellum,[79,80] and as a reversible finding with raised intracranial pressure.[58] Current evidence suggests that skew deviation occurs whenever peripheral or central lesions cause an imbalance of otolithic inputs.[18] The characteristics of the OTR caused by lesions of the vestibular labyrinth, vestibular nuclei, MLF, and INC are summarized in Figure 10–3. When the skew deviation is paroxysmal, the mechanism is thought to be irritative. This interpretation is supported by observations in one patient: stimulation in the region of INC caused an OTR, with episodes of contralateral hypertropia and ipsilateral head tilt.[81]

Progressive Supranuclear Palsy

Progressive supranuclear palsy (PSP) is a degenerative disease of later life characterized by abnormal eye movements, axial rigidity, difficulties with swallowing and speech, and mental slowing. Disturbance of eye movements is usually present early in the course, but occasionally is noted late or not at all. The condition is usually fatal within 6 years of its onset; death is often the result of aspiration pneumonia or the consequence of falls (see Chapter 12).

Initially, the ocular motor deficit consists of impairment of vertical saccades and quick phases—either down or up, but usually down.[82–84] Saccades are slow at first and then small, eventually resulting in complete loss of voluntary vertical refixations. Smooth pursuit may be relatively preserved, and the vestibulo-ocular reflex (VOR) is intact until later on in the disease (although a characteristic nuchal rigidity may make the vertical doll's head maneuver difficult). Caloric stimulation induces tonic deviations without fast phases of nys-

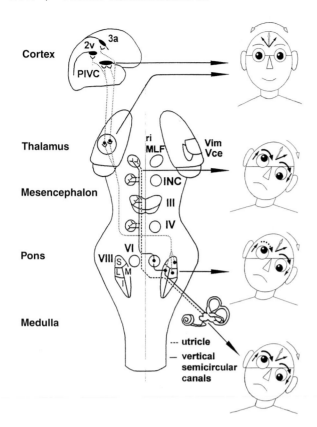

Fig. 10–3. Graviceptive pathways from the otoliths and vertical semicircular canals mediating the vestibular reactions in the roll plane. The projections from the otoliths and vertical semicircular canals to the ocular motor nuclei (trochlear nucleus *IV*, oculomotor nucleus *III*, abducens nucleus *VI*) and supranuclear centers of the interstitial nucleus of Cajal (*INC*), as well as the rostral interstitial nucleus of the medial longitudinal fasciculus (*riMLF*), are shown. They subserve the vestibulo-ocular reflex (VOR) in three planes. The VOR is part of a more complex vestibular reaction that also involves the vestibulospinal connections via the medial and lateral vestibulospinal tracts for head and body posture control. Furthermore, connections to the assumed vestibular cortex (areas *2v* and *3a* and the parietoinsular vestibular cortex, *PIVC*) via the vestibular nuclei of the thalamus (*Vim, Vce*) are depicted. Graviceptive vestibular pathways for the roll plane cross at the pontine level. The ocular tilt reaction (OTR) is depicted schematically on the right in relation to the level of the lesion (*i.e.*, ipsiversive OTR with peripheral and pontomedullary lesions, contraversive OTR with pontomesencephalic lesions). In vestibular thalamus lesions, the tilts of the subjective visual vertical may be contraversive or ipsiversive; in vestibular cortex lesions, they are preferably contraversive. OTR is not induced by supratentorial lesions above the level of INC. (Brandt T, Dieterich M: Vestibular syndromes in the roll plane: Topographic diagnosis from brainstem to cortex. Ann Neurol 36:337, 1994)

tagmus. Some patients have difficulty opening their eyes (eye-opening apraxia).[85] Horizontal eye movements also show characteristic changes: disruption of fixation by square-wave jerks, impaired smooth pursuit,[86] and saccades and quick phases that are small and eventually slow.[87] Patients show preserved ability to generate short-

latency ("express") saccades, but make errors on the antisaccade task; these findings suggest defects in frontal lobe function.[88] Although neuropathologic changes in these cases are mild, positron emission scanning indicates profound frontal lobe hypometabolism.[89] The ocular motor deficit may eventually progress to complete ophthalmoplegia. Administration of dopaminergic drugs may improve extremity rigidity and locomotion, but eye movements are not improved.

Pathologically, PSP is a diffuse disorder with neuronal loss, granulovascular degeneration, neurofibrillary tangles, and gliosis principally affecting the brain stem reticular formation, pontine, and ocular motor nuclei.[86,90] The midbrain often bears the brunt of the early pathology, accounting for the relative vulnerability of vertical saccades. Thus, slow vertical saccades reflect involvement of burst neurons in the riMLF, whereas the neck stiffness, often with dorsiflexion, might be due to involvement of the INC, which contributes to the control of eye-head movements.[91]

The differential diagnosis of PSP includes a similar syndrome due to multiple infarcts affecting the basal ganglia, internal capsule, and midbrain.[92,93] PSP should be differentiated from "cortical basal ganglionic degeneration," which may impair vertical and horizontal gaze, but causes focal dystonia and is pathologically distinct.[94] PSP should also be differentiated from Parkinson disease, since the former responds poorly to dopamine replacement. Although upward gaze may be limited in both PSP and Parkinson disease, impaired downward gaze and slow vertical saccades are more characteristic of PSP. Most important, PSP should be differentiated from Whipple disease, a rare multisystem disorder characterized by weight loss, diarrhea, arthritis, anemia, lymphadenopathy, and fever; sometimes this disease is confined to the nervous system.[95] It causes a defect of ocular motility that mimics PSP: initially vertical saccades are involved,[96] but eventually all eye movements may be lost.[97] A characteristic finding is pendular vergence oscillations and concurrent contractions of the masticatory muscles ("oculomasticatory myorhythmia").[98] Whipple disease can be treated with antibiotics.[99]

BRAIN STEM CONTROL OF VERGENCE EYE MOVEMENTS

Motor Commands for Vergence Movements

Neurophysiologic studies in monkeys have shown that almost all oculomotor neurons subserving the medial rectus and the majority of neurons in the abducens nucleus discharge for both conjugate (version) and disjunctive (vergence) eye movements, although there is evidence that different neurons play relatively smaller or larger roles in conjugate versus vergence eye movements.[100] Premotor signals for vergence have been found on neurons in the mesencephalic reticular formation, 1 to 2 mm dorsal and dorsolateral to the oculomotor nucleus.[101,102] Three main types of neurons can be found: those that discharge in relation to vergence angle, vergence velocity,[103] and both vergence angle and velocity. Recent evidence suggests that the nucleus reticularis tegmenti pontis (NRTP) houses neurons that are important for generating the vergence position signal (the "vergence integrator").[104,105] Abducens and oculomotor internuclear neurons (each of which has projections to the other nucleus via the MLF) contribute to the coordination of conjugate and vergence commands.[24]

Disorders of Vergence

Midbrain lesions may disrupt convergence, accommodation, and pupillary constriction—the near reflex. In addition, they produce vertical gaze disturbances and so-called convergence-retraction nystagmus (see Dorsal Midbrain Syndrome section). Convergence paralysis or paresis may be secondary to various organic processes, such as encephalitis, multiple sclerosis, and occlusive vascular disease involving the rostral midbrain. The distinction between organic and functional convergence palsy is based primarily on the assumption that accommodation and pupillary constrictions are provoked during attempted convergence in the former, but not in the latter. Senescence and lack of effort are the most common causes of poor convergence. Overall, the most common disorders of vergence are congenital, causing strabismus in childhood. In many such cases, abnormality of the accommodative-convergence synkinesis can be demonstrated. In adults, the most common disorders are spasm of the near reflex and divergence insufficiency (paresis).

Spasm of the Near Reflex

Spasm of the near reflex (accommodative or convergence spasm) is most commonly psychogenic. Affected patients may appear to have unilateral or bilateral abducens paresis[106]; however, the pupillary miosis accompanying failure of abduction is a diagnostic sign. Volitional excessive near effort is uncomfortable and rarely can be maintained for more than seconds to minutes. Symptoms include blurred vision, eye strain, dizziness, headache, and diplopia. Rarely, a tonic near reflex may occur in organic disease (e.g., during generalized seizures, after head trauma, in conditions including dorsal midbrain syndrome, craniocervical junction abnormalities, intoxications, and Wernicke encephalopathy).[107–110]

Divergence Paresis or Paralysis

Paresis (insufficiency) of divergence is a rare clinical syndrome characterized by orthophoria at near but relatively concomitant esotropia at distance, although abduction is normal. Diplopia while viewing distant objects is the principal complaint, although other vague symptoms may be emphasized. A prerequisite for the diagnosis of divergence paresis is the demonstration of normal abducting saccades, and this criteria has seldom been met. In many patients, the question of "decompensation" of a longstanding esophoria bias is usually raised, for example, in the setting of concussion or cervical hyperextension injury. Tests of vergence amplitudes and stereopsis may be equivocal, and the possibility of mild abduction defects remains. Mild abducens nerve dysfunction occurs after head trauma or raised intracranial pressure. The possibility of raised intracranial pressure must be excluded. Divergence insufficiency has been reported in PSP, seizure disorder, acute brain stem dysfunction, vascular disease, and after "viral" infections.[111,112] Most patients do well with base-out prisms incorporated in distant spectacle correction, and only rarely is ocular muscle surgery required.

CEREBELLAR INFLUENCES ON EYE MOVEMENTS

The cerebellum optimizes eye movements so that they can provide clear and stable vision. Two separate parts of the cerebellum play an important role in the control of eye movements: (1) the vestibulocerebellum (flocculus, paraflocculus, nodulus, and ventral uvula); and (2) the dorsal vermis of the posterior lobe, and the fastigial nuclei (Table 10–4).

The flocculi and ventral paraflocculi (tonsils) are paired structures that, in the human brain, lie ventral to the inferior cerebellar peduncle and next to the eighth cranial nerve. The flocculus receives bilateral inputs

---

TABLE 10–4. Ocular Motor Disorders Caused by Lesions of the Cerebellum

Vestibulocerebellum
Flocculus, paraflocculus, and ventral uvula:
1. Gaze-evoked nystagmus ("leaky neural integrator")
2. Impaired smooth pursuit (and eye-head tracking)
3. Downbeat nystagmus
4. Rebound nystagmus
5. "Uncalibrated" vestibulo-ocular reflex

Nodulus:
1. Prolongation of durations of vestibular nystagmus in response to rotational stimuli
2. Periodic alternating nystagmus (when in darkness)

Dorsal vermis, fastigial nucleus, and their projections
Dorsal vermis lesions: Saccadic dysmetria, with hypometria of contralateral saccades
Fastigial nucleus: Hypermetria of ipsilateral saccades, hypometria of contralateral saccades (ipsipulsion), and impairment of contralateral smooth pursuit
Uncinate fasciculus and superior cerebellar peduncle: Contralateral hypermetria (contrapulsion)

from the vestibular nuclei and nucleus prepositus hypoglossi, and inputs from the dorsal cap of the contralateral inferior olive.[113] The main efferent pathways of the flocculus are to the ipsilateral superior, medial, and y-group of vestibular nuclei.[114] The flocculus and ventral paraflocculus contain Purkinje cells that discharge during smooth pursuit and combined eye-head tracking to encode gaze velocity.[115] These floccular Purkinje cells may also contribute to vestibular eye movements during self-rotation.[116] The floccular Purkinje cells play an important role in the adaptive control of the VOR.[117]

The *nodulus,* which is the midline portion of the flocculonodular lobe lying immediately caudal to the inferior medullary velum, and the adjacent *ventral uvula* receive afferents from the vestibular nuclei and inferior olive.[118] The nodulus and uvula project to the vestibular nuclei and probably to other structures via the fastigial nucleus. Together, these structures affect the temporal response of the VOR, so that a sustained, constant-velocity rotation induces nystagmus that outlasts by two or three times the duration of displacement of the cupula of the labyrinthine semicircular canals (a process called "velocity storage").

Lobules IV to VII of the *vermis* (the culmen, folium, tuber, declive, and part of the pyramis) receive mossy fiber inputs from the PPRF, NRTP, dorsolateral pontine nuclei, vestibular nuclei and nucleus prepositus hypoglossi, and climbing fiber inputs from the inferior olive.[119] The projection from NRTP may relay information from the frontal eye fields necessary for the planning of saccades.[120] The dorsal vermis projects to the fastigial nucleus, which also receives inputs from the inferior olive.[121] The fastigial nucleus sends contralateral projections via the uncinate fasciculus (which runs in the dorsolateral border of the brachium conjunctivum) to the PPRF and riMLF. Purkinje cells in the dorsal vermis discharge before saccades. Stimulation of the vermis produces saccades, and with currents near threshold, a topographic organization is evident: upward saccades are evoked from the anterior part, downward saccades from the posterior part, and ipsilateral, horizontal saccades from the lateral part.[122] Neurons in the caudal fastigial nucleus show properties that suggest that they accelerate contralateral saccades and smooth pursuit.[123,124]

Effects of Cerebellar Lesions

Experimental lesions of the flocculus and paraflocculus in monkeys produce a syndrome[125] that is similar to that encountered clinically in patients with Arnold-Chiari malformation. This includes impaired smooth pursuit and eye-head tracking and impaired gaze holding. The gaze-holding deficit most probably reflects the contribution that the cerebellum makes to enhance the brain stem neural integrator, which lies in the medial vestibular nuclei and the nucleus prepositus hypoglossi. Another deficit caused by floccular lesions is loss of the ability to adapt the properties of the VOR in response to visual demands[117]; consequently, patients with disease involving the vestibular cerebellum may have vestibulo-ocular eye movements that are hypoactive or hyperactive, and they may complain of impaired vision and oscillopsia with head movements. Downbeat nystagmus is another common finding, and probably reflects an imbalance in central vestibular connections due to loss of floccular modulation of the vertical VOR (see Chapter 11).

Experimental lesions of the nodulus and uvula maximize the velocity storage effect[126]; maneuvers that would usually minimize the effect, such as pitching the head forward during postrotational nystagmus, are rendered ineffectual.[126] Similar effects are seen in patients with midline cerebellar tumors that involve the nodulus.[127] In addition, when monkeys that have nodular lesions are placed in darkness, they may develop periodic alternating nystagmus.[126] Patients with periodic alternating nystagmus often have lesions involving the nodulus and ventral uvula.[128]

Lesions of the dorsal vermis produce marked hypometria of ipsilateral saccades and mild hypometria of contralateral saccades. Experimental inactivation of the caudal fastigial nuclei with the GABA agonist muscimol causes hypermetria of ipsilateral saccades and hypometria of contralateral saccades.[129] It has been suggested that this mechanism of saccadic dysmetria may account for the ipsipulsion of saccades encountered in patients with Wallenberg syndrome; loss of inputs from an infarcted inferior cerebellar peduncle causes an increase in Purkinje cell activity that inhibits the ipsilateral fastigial nucleus.[130] Lesions that involve the fastigial nucleus in humans often produce a severe form of saccadic dysmetria in which the eye may repetitively overshoot a stationary target (so-called macrosaccadic oscillations; see Chapter 11). The posterior vermis also contributes to smooth pursuit; it has reciprocal connections with the dorsolateral pontine nuclei, and neurons encode target velocity during pursuit. Lesions of the posterior vermis impair smooth pursuit.[131] Unilateral lesions of the fastigial nucleus cause a defect of contralateral smooth pursuit, but bilateral lesions may leave smooth pursuit preserved, reflecting directional (acceleration-deceleration) influences of this nucleus on tracking.[132]

Common Vascular Syndromes of the Cerebellum

The cerebellum receives its blood supply from the three branches of the posterior circulation: the posterior-inferior cerebellar artery, anterior-inferior cerebellar artery, and superior cerebellar artery. Occlusion in these vessels often also produces brain stem infarction, making precise clinicopathologic correlation difficult.

Infarction in the distribution of the *distal posterior-inferior cerebellar artery* may cause acute vertigo and nystagmus that often simulates an acute peripheral vestibular lesion.[133] These symptoms probably reflect a central vestibular imbalance, created by asymmetric infarction in the vestibulocerebellum, which normally has a tonic inhibitory effect on the vestibular nuclei. Affected patients may have gaze-evoked nystagmus, which differentiates this cerebellar lesion from an acute peripheral vestibulopathy. The *anterior-inferior cerebellar artery* supplies portions of the vestibular nuclei, adjacent dorsolateral brain stem, and inferior lateral cerebellum (including the flocculus); it is also the origin of the labyrinthine artery in most persons. Consequently, ischemia in the anterior-inferior cerebellar artery distribution may cause vertigo, vomiting, hearing loss, facial palsy, and ipsilateral limb ataxia.[134] Infarction in the territory of the *superior cerebellar artery* causes ataxia of gait and limbs and vertigo.[135] A characteristic finding is saccadic *contrapulsion*. This consists of an overshooting of contralateral saccades and an undershooting of ipsilateral saccades; attempted vertical saccades are oblique, with a horizontal component away from the side of the lesion.[136-138] Thus, the saccadic disorder is the opposite of the saccadic ipsipulsion seen in Wallenberg syndrome and probably reflects interruption of crossed outputs from the fastigial nucleus running in the uncinate fasciculus adjacent to the superior cerebellar peduncle.

CEREBRAL AND BASAL GANGLIONIC CONTROL OF EYE MOVEMENTS

Our present notions of the cerebral hemispheric control of eye movements are founded on information from several lines of investigation, each with its own strengths and weaknesses. Thus, some caution is required, for example, in extrapolating the effects of discrete cortical lesions in monkeys to the effects of disease in humans, since the cortical architecture is significantly different.[139] Nonetheless, experimental studies in the Rhesus monkey have provided substantial insights into how neurons encode and program eye movements. Recent developments in imaging techniques (*e.g.*, proton emission tomography, functional magnetic resonance imaging) and transcranial magnetic stimulation have made it possible to identify similar cortical mechanisms in humans. Another advance has been the development of test paradigms to identify specific defects of eye movement control in patients with well-delineated cerebral lesions, such as infarcts. Thus, the following scheme should be viewed as a working hypothesis that future studies are likely to clarify and refine. Our approach is (1) to lay out the scheme and salient evidence to support it; and (2) to use it to account for the classic findings of cerebral disease.

The Saccadic System

Several Roles for Saccades

Fundamental to an understanding of how the cerebral hemispheres control saccadic movements is the recognition that rapid eye movements serve several distinct functions[1]:

1. At the lowest level are the fast phases of nystagmus, which reset the eyes following vestibular or optokinetic slow-phase movements.
2. Spontaneous saccades occur at a frequency of about 20 per minute and serve the purpose of repetitive scanning of the environment, although they also occur in darkness.
3. "Reflexive" (nonvolitional) saccades, characterized by short reaction times, occur in response to new visual, auditory, or tactile cues.
4. Voluntary (intentional or volitional) saccades carry the eyes to a predetermined location corresponding to the position of a visual target; they direct the fovea at a goal. Such voluntary saccades can also be made in a predictive fashion when the target is moving in a regular pattern: the eye movement anticipates the change in target position. Voluntary saccades can also be made toward imagined or remembered target locations, or in response to commands (*e.g.*, "Look right"). A special case of voluntary saccades is the "antisaccade," whereby a subject is required to respond to a visual stimulus by looking to the corresponding position in the opposite visual hemifield.
5. Saccades can be voluntarily suppressed when it is necessary to maintain steady foveal fixation.

Thus, saccades respond to the full range of sensory inputs (visual, vestibular, auditory, somato-sensory) and to internal cognitive factors. Each of these distinct functions of saccades depends on different cortical and subcortical areas. By examining each function, at the bedside or in the laboratory, it is possible to evaluate the separate neural substrates.

Several Cortical Areas That Contribute to Saccade Generation

It is now recognized that, in addition to the frontal and parietal eye fields, several other cortical areas contribute to the control of saccades, including the supplementary eye fields and the dorsolateral prefrontal cortex (Fig. 10–4). How do sensory and cognitive signals reach these areas? It is now established that different attributes of vision reaching striate cortex (Brodmann area 17, visual area V1), such as the fine features, color, spatial location, and motion of a viewed object, are mainly processed separately in different cortical areas.[140] Thus, striate cortex projects to many separate secondary

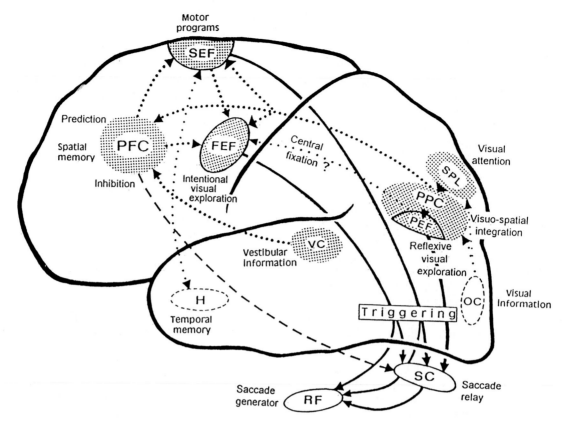

Fig. 10–4. A hypothetical scheme for the cortical control of saccades. The cortical relays of saccade pathways are represented by arrowheads. Note the presence of parallel descending pathways subserving the voluntary control of saccades. *FEF*, frontal eye fields; *H*, hippocampal formation; *OC*, occipital cortex; *PEF*, parietal eye fields; *PFC*, prefrontal cortex (area 46 of Brodmann); *PPC*, posterior parietal cortex; *RF*, reticular formation; *SC*, superior colliculus; *SEF*, supplementary eye fields; *SLP*, superior parietal lobule; *VC*, vestibular cortex. (Pierrot-Deseilligny C, Rivaud S, Gaymard B et al: Cortical control of saccades. Ann Neurol 37:557, 1995)

visual areas, each of which is mainly concerned with analysis of certain features of vision.

Important for the planning of saccades is the inferior parietal lobule. In monkeys, area 7a is important for localizing an object in space by taking into account the location of a stimulus within the visual field and the direction in which the eyes are pointing.[141] Neurons in this area discharge after saccades and seem more concerned with visuospatial integration than with eye movements per se. In humans, the homologue of area 7a is probably close to the intraparietal sulcus (posterior parietal cortex, PPC). In the posterior insula lies an area of "vestibular cortex" (VC) that may contribute information regarding head or body movements.[18] Together, this information is important for planning accurate saccadic eye movements and eye-head movements to objects in extrapersonal space. Also important for eye movements are the "middle temporal" (MT, or V5) and "medial superior temporal" (MST) visual areas,[140] which in humans probably lie at the junction of the temporal, parietal, and occipital lobes.[142] In monkeys, area MT contains neurons that encode the speed and

direction of moving visual targets; experimental lesions here cause a selective defect of motion vision.[143,144] Area MST, to which MT projects, contains neurons that combine visual motion information with eye movement and vestibular signals.[145] Areas MT and MST are important for generating smooth pursuit (see discussion below), and they also provide important information to cortical areas concerned with saccade generation, since we often make saccades toward moving targets.

The *parietal eye fields* in monkeys lie in the lateral intraparietal area (LIP), within the intraparietal sulcus. Neurons in this area discharge before saccades.[146] LIP projects to frontal eye fields and the superior colliculus, but not directly to the PPRF or riMLF.[147] Experimental lesions of LIP delay the onset of saccades made to visual stimuli.[148] In humans, the homologue of LIP probably lies in the superior part of the angular gyrus.[149] Parietal lesions in humans also cause an increase in the response time from presentation of a visual stimulus until the generation of a saccade ("increased saccadic latency"). Unilateral parietal disease may cause bilateral increases in saccadic latency, and the effect is more marked for right hemisphere lesions.[150,151] This defect in the initiation of saccades often coexists with disorders of hemivisual attention; however, the saccadic defect may occur alone, supporting the notion that the human homologue of LIP is distinct from areas concerned with directing visual attention, which may lie more superiorly.[149] Parietal lesions also cause an inability to make accurate saccades if a visual target is flashed just before the patient makes an eye movement.[152] In this "double-step" paradigm, the brain must take into account both the location in the visual field of the target flash before the eye movement and the size and direction of the eye movement that subsequently occurred; only if both pieces of information can be combined will it be possible to make an accurate saccade to the remembered location of the target flash. Thus, the parietal eye fields seem important for programming saccades concerned with reflexive exploration of the visual environment.

The *frontal eye fields* in monkeys lie along the posterior bank of the arcuate sulcus, corresponding to part of Brodmann area 8. They receive inputs from visual areas MT and MST, dorsolateral prefrontal cortex, parietal eye fields, supplementary eye fields, and intralaminar thalamic nuclei. In monkeys, neurons in the frontal eye fields discharge before volitional, but not reflexive, saccades. Furthermore, the frontal eye fields are important in suppressing saccades and maintaining steady fixation. The homologue of frontal eye fields in humans is not settled, but probably corresponds to confluent regions of Brodmann areas 8, 6, 4 and 9; this area includes the lateral part of the precentral sulcus, part of the posterior extremity of the middle frontal gyrus, and the adjacent precentral sulcus and gyrus, just anterior to the motor cortex.[149] The frontal eye fields project caudally to the superior colliculus, caudate nucleus, and brain stem reticular formation (see discussion below). Disease involving the frontal eye fields in humans causes increased latency of saccades to visual targets if the previous (fixation) target remains visible. If, however, the fixation target disappears before the new target is presented ("gap paradigm"), then there is no increase in the response time.[153] This evidence suggests that the frontal eye fields are important for "disengagement of fixation." In addition, unilateral lesions of the frontal eye fields cause increased saccadic latency to remembered target locations bilaterally.[154] Also impaired is the ability to generate predictive saccades and antisaccades that are directed into the visual hemifield opposite to that of the test stimulus.[153,155] Thus, the frontal eye fields are important for the programming of saccades concerned with intentional exploration of the visual environment.

In monkeys, the *supplementary eye fields* are located in the dorsomedial frontal lobes, in the anterior part of the supplementary motor area.[156] They receive inputs from the frontal eye fields, parietal cortex, and intralaminar thalamic nuclei, and project to the frontal eye fields, caudate nucleus, superior colliculus, and brain stem reticular formation.[157] In humans, the supplementary eye fields lie in the posteromedial portion of the superior frontal gyrus.[149] Disease affecting these fields in humans does not affect saccades to visual or remembered targets, but after patients are rotated to a new position, saccades are inaccurate.[154] Thus, one important difference between supplementary versus frontal eye fields is that only the former are important for generating saccades to specified spatial (rather than retinal) locations. Another function that is impaired by disease affecting the supplementary eye fields, especially on the left side, is the ability to make a sequence of saccades to several target lights that are turned and left on in a specified order.[158] It appears that the supplementary eye fields are aided by the hippocampus in remembering the chronologic sequence of target presentation.[159] Thus, the supplementary eye fields are important in programming saccades concerned with complex motor behaviors.

The *dorsolateral prefrontal cortex* (PFC, Brodmann area 46) is important for making accurate motor responses (including saccades) to the remembered spatial locations of targets.[157] Lesions of the PFC, including pharmacologic blockade of D1 dopamine receptors,[160] disrupt this "working memory" area, so that if a target is out of sight, it is also "out of mind."

Cortical Projections to Brain Stem Saccade Circuits

Parallel, descending pathways connect these cortical regions with brain stem and cerebellar structures concerned with the generation of saccades. No direct projection exists from cortical neurons to ocular motoneurons[161]; rather, several intermediate structures play important roles, including the caudate nucleus, substantia nigra, superior colliculus, and brain stem reticular formation. These are summarized in Figure 10–4.

Parietal area LIP projects to the superior colliculus and frontal eye fields, but not directly to the brain stem reticular formation concerned with saccade generation.[147] The projections of the frontal eye fields run in the internal capsule; clinical lesions involving the anterior portion of the internal capsule and adjacent deep frontal region are reported to increase saccadic latency.[151] Below the level of the internal capsule, several separate pathways can be discerned: one to the caudate nucleus, a second to the intralaminar thalamic nuclei and ipsilateral superior colliculus, and a third—the pedunculopontine pathway that runs in the most medial aspect of the cerebral peduncle and projects to the NRTP—to the cerebellum.[162-164] The PPRF and particularly the midline pontine raphe nuclei that house saccadic omnipause cells also receive projections from the frontal eye fields. A partial "saccadic decussation" may occur between the levels of the trochlear and abducens nuclei,[162] although its functional role requires clarification. The supplementary eye fields also project to the caudate nucleus, where convergence with frontal eye field projections occurs, as well as to the superior colliculus and pontine omnipause neurons.[165] The dorsolateral prefrontal cortex projects to the caudate nucleus and to the superior colliculus.[166] The *caudate nucleus* sends inhibitory projections to the non-dopaminergic *substantia nigra pars reticulata*, which, in turn, inhibits neurons in the superior colliculus. Thus, this basal ganglia system is composed of two serial, inhibitory links: a caudonigral inhibition that is only phasically active, and a nigrocollicular inhibition that is tonically active.[167,168] If the frontal cortex causes caudate neurons to fire, then the nigrocollicular inhibition is interrupted and the superior colliculus is able to activate a saccade. Disease affecting the caudate nucleus may impair the ability to make saccades to complex tasks; however, disease affecting the substantia nigra pars reticulata might disinhibit the superior colliculus, causing excessive, inappropriate saccades. Both deficits have been described in patients with disorders affecting the basal ganglia, such as Huntington disease.[169]

The Superior Colliculus

All three frontal areas as well as parietal area LIP project directly to the superior colliculus. Although the role of the superior colliculus in humans remains undefined, in monkeys it has been shown to be a crucial structure for generating saccades. The superior colliculus contains a "retinotopic" map in the cells of its superficial layers and a "motor" map in its intermediate layers.[170] Stimulation at any point on the motor map will produce a contralateral saccade of specific amplitude and direction; the smallest saccades are represented in the rostral superior colliculus and the largest in the caudal superior colliculus. The overall role of the superior colliculus in generating saccades was clarified by the demonstration that it is essential for programming saccades to visual stimuli made at short latency (so-called express saccades).[171] To produce such express saccades, the fixation light is turned off before the target light is illuminated (gap paradigm); this paradigm appears to facilitate the process of disengaging attention from one object and switching it to another.

The superior colliculus projects to the brain stem reticular formation, which contains saccade-generating burst neurons as well as omnipause neurons that tonically inhibit burst neurons except during saccades. Saccadic burst neurons project monosynaptically to ocular motoneurons. Unlike the superior colliculus, the burst neurons discharge as an ensemble and encode the characteristics of the saccade in terms of their temporal discharge; the total number of spikes in each burst of activity is proportional to the size of the saccade.[1] Recent studies on the superior colliculus have clarified how its saccadic command, which is encoded in terms of the location of active neurons within its maps, is transformed into the saccadic command on reticular burst neurons, which is encoded in terms of discharge frequency and duration.[172,173]

Three populations of cells within the intermediate layers of the superior colliculus contribute to saccade generation: fixation neurons and build-up neurons, which lie more ventrally; and collicular-burst neurons, which lie more dorsally.

Fixation neurons lie at the rostral pole of the superior colliculus and may suppress saccades via projections to omnipause neurons and by inhibiting collicular-burst neurons. Thus, cessation of activity of the fixation cells in superior colliculus plays a central role in the generation of express saccades. When a visual stimulus becomes the target for a saccade, *build-up neurons* start to discharge at a site on the motor map related to the size and direction of the upcoming saccade. Subsequently, the activity of fixation neurons begins to decline, and then *collicular-burst neurons* located at the appropriate part of the motor map (lying dorsal to the active build-up neurons) start to discharge. Although the location of discharging collicular-burst neurons for the saccade remains the same throughout the eye movement, there appears to be a rostral spread of activity of build-up neurons toward the fixation zone. This spread of activity may contribute to the spatial-temporal transformation of signals that is needed to provide the reticular burst neurons with the saccadic command. Furthermore, it appears that the collicular burst neurons encode motor error (the difference between desired eye position and instantaneous eye position during a saccade), which is the signal required to drive the saccadic burst neurons.[174]

In support of this scheme, selective inactivation of the rostral pole of the superior colliculus causes disruption of steady fixation by saccadic intrusions.[175] Pharmacologic inactivation of the caudal portions of the superior colliculus with muscimol, however, causes impaired initiation of saccades, which are hypometric and slow.[176]

The ability to perform express saccades depends on an intact superior colliculus and its cortical afferents.[177] Reported patients with disease restricted to the superior colliculus are rare, but in one patient with a unilateral lesion, contralateral saccades were produced at longer latency and were hypometric.[178] Involvement of the superior colliculus (and adjacent mesencephalic reticular formation) is an established feature of PSP,[90] and some patients show increased latency with the gap paradigm, as well as unstable fixation with multiple saccadic intrusions.[88] In summary, the great interest that the superior colliculus has received by basic scientists has produced a wealth of new information that stands ready to be applied to understanding the effects of midbrain disease in humans, specifically on the fixation system and saccadic precision. What is now required is application of the gap paradigm to patients with midbrain lesions, as well as systematic neuropathologic examination of the superior colliculus in patients with abnormal express saccades or prominent saccadic intrusions.

Ablation of the superior colliculus does not abolish saccades to visual targets,[177] so it seems likely that the frontal and parietal eye movements are also able to carry out the spatial-temporal translation in parallel. A direct pathway from the frontal eye fields to the PPRF is also able to initiate saccades (*e.g.*, after ablation of the superior colliculus; see discussion below). At present, however, the normal role of this rather small projection is unknown. The frontal eye fields project via the NRTP to the cerebellum. Although this pathway is probably important in optimizing saccadic metrics, it is not essential for the initiation of saccades, which persist even after total cerebellectomy.[179]

The Roles of Descending Parallel Projections

The relative importance of descending pathways for saccade generation has been elucidated by studies on the effects of restricted, experimental lesions. In monkeys, chronic lesions of the superior colliculus cause relatively minor deficits, such as an increase in saccadic latency.[177] Chronic lesions of the frontal eye fields in monkeys also cause minor deficits that affect saccades to remembered targets.[180] In contrast, combined lesions of the frontal eye fields and superior colliculi produce a severe and lasting deficit of eye movements, with a restricted range of movement.[181] Severe deficits of saccadic eye movements also follow combined, bilateral lesions of the parieto-occipital and frontal cortex in monkeys.[148] With unilateral, combined parietofrontal lesions, saccades to visual targets in contralateral hemispace are impaired[182]; with hemidecortication, the deficit is more severe and enduring.[183] In humans, combined lesions of the frontal and parietal cortex cause loss of ability to make voluntary saccades (ocular motor apraxia).[184]

Pursuit System

As indicated earlier, neurons in the secondary visual (MT) areas encode the speed and direction of a moving target.[142-144] MT projects to the adjacent visual area (MST), where neurons encode not only visual information, but also a corollary discharge (efference copy) of the eye movement command.[185] Adjacent parietal cortex also influences smooth pursuit, probably by enhancing attention to the moving target. The frontal eye fields also contribute to both the initiation and maintenance of smooth pursuit.[186] From MST, projections descend to

the dorsolateral pontine nuclei[187] and subsequently to the flocculus, paraflocculus, and vermis of the cerebellum.[188] The flocculus projects to the ipsilateral vestibular nuclei,[114] which, in turn, project to the ocular motor nuclei; the vermis projects to the underlying fastigial nucleus.

The effects of experimental or discrete clinical stimuli can be interpreted with reference to the above scheme (Fig. 10–5). Lesions of striate cortex abolish smooth pursuit of targets presented in the blind hemifield, but pursuit is normal in both directions in the seeing hemifield.[189] Lesions of MT do not cause a conventional visual field defect but produce a selective abnormality in target speed estimation; both saccades and smooth pursuit are consequently impaired.[190] Lesions of MST in monkeys cause a disturbance much like the ipsilateral pursuit deficit encountered with unilateral cortical lesions in humans (Fig. 10–6); horizontal pursuit is impaired for targets moving toward the side of the lesion.[190] Experimental lesions of the dorsolateral pontine nuclei cause a similar impairment of ipsilateral smooth pursuit.[191] Lesions of the cerebellar flocculus and dorsal vermis also impair ipsilateral smooth pursuit. Experimental or clinical lesions of the vestibular or fastigial nuclei, however, produce a defect of contralateral smooth pursuit.[35,192] Lesions of the PPRF that impair or abolish saccades do not necessarily affect smooth pursuit.[30,31] Therefore, the PPRF is not, as previously surmised, a major part of the pursuit pathway, although fibers may traverse it.

A large number of conditions *bilaterally* impair smooth-pursuit eye movements so that the eyes conse-

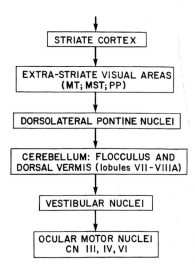

Fig. 10–5. A hypothetical scheme for smooth-pursuit eye movements, starting with striate cortex, which receives inputs from lateral geniculate nuclei (*uppermost arrow*). Not shown are projections from the frontal eye fields to the dorsolateral pontine nuclei. *MT*, middle temporal visual area; *MST*, medial superior visual area; *PP*, posterior parietal cortex.

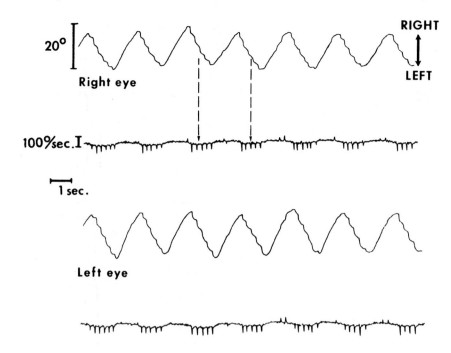

Fig. 10–6. Electro-oculography of unilateral saccadic (cogwheel) pursuit in a patient with left cerebral hemispherectomy. The upper two tracings represent position and velocity, respectively, from the right eye; the lower two tracings are from the left eye. Upward deflection represents rightward eye movement. The pursuit movement to the right (up-slope) is smooth, with only occasional interspersed saccades; pursuit toward the left (down-slope) is slower than the target and requires catch-up saccades to regain target foveation. The multiple saccades are particularly evident in the velocity tracings.

quently "fall behind" the moving target and require "catch-up" saccades to regain fixation. Such saccadic or cogwheel pursuit occurs with age, sedative drugs, inattention,[193] fatigue, and impaired consciousness, as well as in diffuse cerebral,[194] cerebellar, or brain stem disease.[195] A pursuit defect difficult to distinguish from that of inattention is reported in schizophrenia.[196]

Vestibulo-ocular System

The VOR is probably unaffected by cortical lesions during brief, natural head rotations[197]; only when vestibular responses are supplemented by pursuit eye movements—to enhance or suppress the response—may asymmetric deficits become evident. The posterior insula of the temporal lobe is the "area of vestibular sensation" in humans, and lesions in this area interfere with the ability to accurately detect earth-vertical.[18]

Gaze Holding

Gaze holding (sustaining the eyes conjugately in eccentric positions in the orbits) is dependent on vestibular nuclei, nucleus prepositus hypoglossi, and their cerebellar connections. The cerebral hemispheres, however, particularly the parietal lobes, do influence this ability

by encoding the location of a target in space. Thus, parietal neurons respond not simply to the location of a visual stimulus on the retina, but also to the direction of gaze.[141] Thus, unilateral parietal lobe lesions are manifest not only by hemispatial neglect, but also by a "gaze preference" ipsilateral to the side of the lesion.[183]

Common Disturbances of Gaze with Unilateral Hemispheric Lesions

With *acute* hemispheric lesions, the patient's eyes are often deviated conjugately toward the side of the lesion. Such deviations are more common after large strokes involving right post-Rolandic cortex[198]; visual hemineglect is a common accompaniment.[199] Conjugate deviation of patients' eyes away from the side of the lesion ("wrong-way deviation") occurs with subfrontal or thalamic lesions.[27]

Acutely, patients may not voluntarily direct their eyes toward the side of the intact hemisphere, but vestibular stimulation usually produces a full range of horizontal movement (with the slow phase) in contrast to gaze palsies associated with pontine lesions.[200] Sometimes, in addition to ipsiversive deviation of the eyes, there is a small-amplitude nystagmus with ipsilateral quick phases; the slow phases of this nystagmus may reflect unopposed pursuit drives directed away from the side of the lesion. Vertical saccades may be dysmetric with an inappropriate horizontal component toward the side of the lesion. Since both hemispheres are normally activated to elicit a purely vertical saccade, the loss of one hemisphere may be the cause of such oblique saccades.[201]

With *chronic* hemispheric lesions, there usually is no resting deviation of the eyes, and persistence of gaze deviation is associated with a prior lesion in the contralateral hemisphere.[202] Attempted forced eyelid closure may cause a contralateral "spastic" conjugate eye movement, the mechanism of which is not understood.[203] In primary position, a small-amplitude nystagmus may be observed (best seen during ophthalmoscopy), with slow phases directed toward the side of the intact hemisphere[204]; it may represent an imbalance in smooth pursuit tone. Horizontal pursuit is relatively impaired for tracking of targets moving toward the side of the lesion; a convenient way to demonstrate this asymmetry of pursuit is with a hand-held optokinetic drum or tape.[205] The response is decreased when the stripes are moved toward the side of the hemispheric lesion. At the bedside, this "optokinetic" response is usually judged by the frequency and amplitude of quick phases of nystagmus. A variety of defects in the control of saccades can be brought out by special testing, as outlined earlier. When prolongation of saccadic reaction time is evident at the bedside, however, it may reflect defects in visual detection, visual attention, or abnormal programming of saccades.

Acute Bilateral Frontoparietal Lesions: Ocular Motor Apraxia

Large bihemispheric lesions cause a disturbance of ocular motility that has been called acquired ocular motor apraxia. It is characterized by loss of voluntary control of eye movements, with preservation of reflex movements, including the VOR and quick phases of nystagmus. Acquired ocular motor apraxia has been associated with volitional difficulty in eyelid opening (lid apraxia).[206] Acquired apraxia limited to the vertical plane is reported with bilateral lesions at the mesencephalic-diencephalic junction.[207,208]

The eponym Balint syndrome has been used to describe acquired ocular motor apraxia associated with acute optic ataxia and disturbance of visual attention.[184,209] Voluntary movements of the eyes are restricted in the horizontal and vertical planes. Gaze shifts are usually achieved by combined movements of the eyes and head.[184] Both slow and quick phases of vestibular nystagmus are largely preserved, indicating that the brain stem mechanisms are intact. The defect of voluntary eye movements probably reflects disruption of descending pathways from both the frontal and the parietal

eye fields, so that the superior colliculus and brain stem reticular formation lack their supranuclear inputs; similar results have been produced experimentally in monkeys.[181]

Sometimes the term "spasm of fixation" is applied to such patients who have difficulty voluntarily shifting gaze. Holmes[210] described a group of such patients and noted that voluntary eye movements became possible when the visual scene was a homogenous white screen. As reviewed above, one effect of frontal eye fields is difficulties in "disengagement of fixation." Thus, it appears that spasm of fixation might have a real physiologic basis; however, before applying the term to patients, it would seem necessary to demonstrate differences in saccadic latency between trials in which the fixation stimulus disappeared before the new visual stimulus appeared ("gap stimulus") and trials in which the fixation stimulus remained visible.[211] Certainly, brain stem disorders that affect the saccade-generating reticular formation should be not be included in this category. Another factor in evaluating such patients is the nature and size of the visual stimulus. We have seen a patient with extreme difficulty making saccades to command who did so only after prolonged tight eye closure. There was slightly less difficulty with small refixation targets; with larger targets, the saccades were initiated with more ease until, finally, normal command saccades occurred as he alternately refixated between two closely spaced faces.

Congenital oculomotor apraxia is characterized by absence of horizontal saccadic refixations and smooth pursuit movement, although some patients show normal smooth pursuit. During childhood, fast phases of nystagmus are absent during either optokinetic or caloric stimulation. This implicates a basic saccadic rather than apraxic disorder, and the condition is better designated *congenital saccadic palsy* or *congenital gaze palsy,* depending on the integrity of smooth-pursuit eye movements. The most striking feature of this syndrome is head thrusts used to accomplish ocular refixations. The head thrust may not be present in early infancy, but it develops between 4 and 8 months of age.[212] Children with inadequate head control may never develop the thrusts.[213] These head movements are more exaggerated than those in patients with acquired saccadic palsy. The head moves toward the position of the eccentric new target, and the eyes, responding to the active vestibulo-ocular system, rotate conjugately in the opposite direction (Fig. 10–7). The eyelids close at the onset of the head movement as if to lower the gain of the vestibulo-ocular reflex and thus reduce the amount of head thrust. Head rotation overshoots the intended target, enabling the contraversively deviated eyes to fixate the target. While maintaining fixation, the head slowly moves back until the eyes are straight forward. With

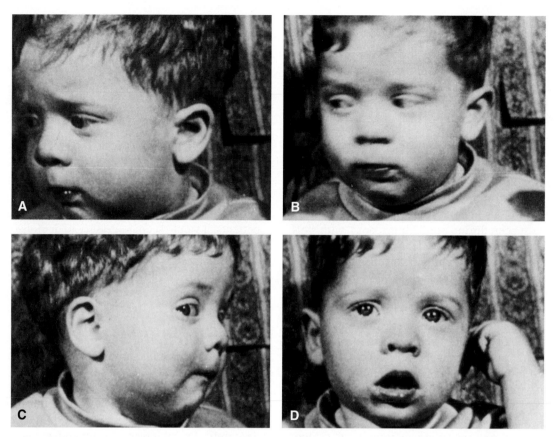

Fig. 10–7. Congenital ocular motor apraxia. **A.** Patient looking to the right. **B.** The child's attention is drawn to the camera, the head turning to the left, with contraversion of the eyes. **C.** Overshoot of the head with extreme contraversion of the eyes. **D.** Fixation and realignment of the head and eyes. (Felker GV, Ide CH, Hart WM: Congenital ocular motor apraxia. EENT Monthly, March 1973)

advancing age, the head thrust becomes less prominent, and saccadic eye movements, albeit abnormal, may emerge.[214] Only one patient has been followed longitudinally to adult life, and head thrusts were noted only rarely.[215] This syndrome may be familial, and significant developmental central nervous system defects, such as hypoplasia of the corpus callosum and cerebrum, may be associated with it.[212,216] Infrequently, a brain stem neoplasm may mimic the condition.[76] Rarely, the apraxia may be primarily in the vertical direction.[217]

Parkinson Disease

Most patients with Parkinson disease show only minor changes on clinical examination: disruption of steady fixation by square wave jerks, mild hypometria of saccades, and impairment ("cog-wheeling") of smooth pursuit.[218,219] Upward gaze is often moderately restricted,[220] but this is a frequent finding in normal, elderly persons.[221] Vertical saccades are usually of normal velocity in Parkinson disease, helping differentiate this condition from PSP.

Saccades in Parkinson disease become hypometric when patients are asked to perform rapid, self-paced refixations between two stationary targets. During such a test, which allows a predictive strategy, intersaccadic intervals increase above values during nonpredictable tracking.[222,223] In contrast, saccades made "reflexively" to novel visual stimuli are of normal amplitude.[224] Thus, during saccadic tracking, parkinsonian patients often lack a predictive strategy.[225]

Smooth-pursuit eye movements of a target moving in a predictable, sinusoidal pattern are impaired, necessitating catch-up saccades.[226,227] Despite the impairment of smooth-pursuit gain, the phase relationship between eye and target movement during periodic (sinusoidal) tracking is normal, indicating a normal, predictable strategy.[225]

Although caloric vestibular responses in darkness may be hypoactive,[220] head rotations at natural frequencies made during visual fixation produce normal vestibular responses, which accounts for the lack of complaint of oscillopsia among patients with Parkinson disease.[221] Patients with multisystem (striatonigral) degeneration have eye movements similar to those of classic Parkinson disease,[228] whereas patients with "diffuse Lewy body disease" may show more severe deficits, with loss of vertical or horizontal gaze.[229]

In general, levodopa treatment for Parkinson disease does not seem to improve the ocular motor deficits[220] except for improving saccadic accuracy (*i.e.*, saccades become larger).[226] Some newly diagnosed patients with idiopathic Parkinson disease have been reported to show improved smooth pursuit after the institution of dopaminergic therapy.[226] In patients with parkinsonism due to 1-methyl-4-phenyl-1,2,3,6-tetrahydropyridine (MTPT) toxicity from "synthetic heroin," saccadic latency was shortened and saccadic accuracy improved by dopaminergic agents; in addition, reflex blepharospasm in these patients was improved.[230]

Oculogyric crisis, first encountered as a feature of postencephalitic parkinsonism, now usually occurs as a side effect of drugs, particularly the neuroleptic agents.[231] A typical attack is heralded by an obsessive thought. The eyes typically deviate upward, sometimes laterally, and rarely downward. During the period of upward deviation, movement of the eyes in the upper field of gaze appears nearly normal. Affected patients have great difficulty looking down, except by combining a blink and downward saccade. Thus, the ocular disorder may reflect an imbalance of the vertical gaze-holding mechanism. Anticholinergic drugs promptly terminate both the thought disorder and the ocular deviation, a finding suggesting that the disorders of thought and eye movements are linked by a pharmacologic imbalance common to both.[231] Oculogyric crises are distinct from brief upward ocular deviations that occur in some patients with tardive dyskinesia.[232]

Huntington Disease

A variety of abnormalities of saccades have been described in Huntington disease that probably reflect involvement of the caudate–substantia nigra–superior colliculus pathway.[168,232–235] Thus, in some patients, the prominent defect involves fixation (*i.e.*, difficulty suppressing saccades toward new visual stimuli). Paradoxically, the same patients may have difficulties in initiating saccades with increased reaction time or even inability to initiate a saccade without an associated head movement or blink. In other patients, the most prominent defect is slowing of saccades, particularly in the vertical direction; the issue as to whether such slowing reflects involvement of the saccadic burst neurons or inputs to them remains unsettled.[236] Smooth pursuit has low gain, but the VOR is normal.

Functional Disturbances of Gaze

Spasm of the near reflex (convergence spasm), which may mimic a lateral rectus paresis, has been discussed earlier. In rare cases, patients may present with a psychogenic paralysis of horizontal gaze. Pursuit and saccades are usually symmetrically restricted. Sophisticated neuro-ophthalmologic testing using passive head rotations, optokinetic stimuli, and pursuit stimulation with the large "mirror test" should demonstrate the ability of these patients to make fast and slow eye movements and uncover the psychogenic nature of the disturbance.[237] In the mirror test, the patient is asked to look into a large hand-held mirror that is then tilted right and left or up and down. The patient's eyes are observed readily to follow the moving reflection of the visual environment.

REFERENCES

1. Leigh RJ, Zee DS: The Neurology of Eye Movements, 3rd ed. New York, Oxford University Press, 1999
2. Highstein SM, Baker R: Excitatory termination of abducens internuclear neurons on medial rectus motoneurons: relationship to syndrome of internuclear ophthalmoplegia. J Neurophysiol 41:1647, 1978
3. Maciewicz RJ, Spencer RF: Oculomotor and abducens internuclear pathways in the cat. In Baker R, Berthoz A (eds): Control of Gaze by Brain Stem Neurons, p 99. New York, Elsevier, 1977
4. King WM, Lisberger SG, Fuchs AF: Responses of fibers in medial longitudinal fasciculus (MLF) of alert monkeys during horizontal and vertical conjugate eye movements evoked by vestibular or visual stimuli. J Neurophysiol 39:1135, 1976
5. McCrea RA, Strassman A, Highstein SM: Morphology and physiology of abducens motoneurons and internuclear neurons intracellularly injected with horseradish peroxidase in alert squirrel monkeys. J Comp Neurol 243:291, 1986
6. Spencer RF, Baker R: Histochemical localization of acetylcholinesterase in relation to motor neurons and internuclear neurons of the cat abducens nucleus. J Neurocytology 15:137, 1986
7. McCrea RA, Strassman A, May E, Highstein SM: Anatomical and physiological characteristics of vestibular neurons mediating the horizontal vestibulo-ocular reflex of the squirrel monkey. J Comp Neurol 264:547, 1987
8. Langer T, Kaneko CRS, Scudder CA, Fuchs AF: Afferents to the abducens nucleus in the monkey and cat. J Comp Neurol 245:379, 1986
9. Strassman A, Highstein SM, McCrea RA: Anatomy and physiology of saccadic burst neurons in the alert squirrel monkey: I. Excitatory burst neurons. J Comp Neurol 249:337, 1986
10. Strassman A, Highstein SM, McCrea RA: Anatomy and physiology of saccadic burst neurons in the alert squirrel monkey: II. Inhibitory burst neurons. J Comp Neurol 249:358, 1986
11. Belknap DB, McCrea RA: Anatomical connections of the prepositus and abducens nuclei in the squirrel monkey. J Comp Neurol 268:13, 1988
12. Pierrot-Deseilligny C, Goasguen J: Isolated abducens nucleus damage due to histiocytosis X. Brain 107:1019, 1984
13. Meienberg O, Buttner-Ennever JA, Kraus-Ruppert R: Unilateral paralysis of conjugate gaze due to lesion of the abducens nucleus: Clinico-pathological case report. Neuroophthalmology 2:47, 1981
14. Bronstein AM, Morris J, Du Boulay G et al: Abnormalities of horizontal gaze: clinical, oculographic and magnetic resonance imaging findings: I. Abducens palsy. J Neurol Neurosurg Psychiatry 53:194, 1990
15. Kommerell G: Unilateral internuclear ophthalmoplegia: the lack of inhibitory involvement in medial rectus muscle activity. Invest Ophthalmol Vis Sci 21:592, 1981
16. Baloh RW, Yee RD, Honrubia V: Internuclear ophthalmoplegia: I. Saccades and dissociated nystagmus. Arch Neurol 35:484, 1978
17. Zee DS, Hain TC, Carl JR: Abduction nystagmus in internuclear ophthalmoplegia. Ann Neurol 21:383, 1987
18. Brandt T, Dieterich M: Vestibular syndromes in the roll plane: topographic diagnosis from brainstem to cortex. Ann Neurol 36:337, 1994

19. Ranalli PJ, Sharpe JA: Vertical vestibulo-ocular reflex, smooth pursuit and eye-head tracking dysfunction in internuclear ophthalmoplegia. Brain 111:1299, 1988
20. Herishanu YO, Sharpe JA: Saccadic intrusions in internuclear ophthalmoplegia. Ann Neurol 14:67, 1983
21. Smith JL, David NJ: Internuclear ophthalmoplegia: two new clinical signs. Neurology 14:307, 1964
22. Collewijn H, Erkelens CJ, Steinman RM: Binocular co-ordination of human horizontal saccadic eye movements. J Physiol (Lond) 40:157, 1988
23. McGettrick P, Eustace P: The w.e.b.i.n.o. syndrome. Neuro-ophthalmology 5:109, 1985
24. Gamlin PDR, Gnadt JW, Mays LE: Lidocaine-induced unilateral internuclear ophthalmoplegia: effects on convergence and conjugate eye movements. J Neurophysiol 62:82, 1989
25. Lutz A: Ueber die Bahnen der Blickwendung und deren Dissozierung. Klin Monatsbl Augenheilkd 70:213, 1923
26. Bogousslavsky J, Regli F, Ostinelli B, Rabinowicz T: Paresis of lateral gaze alternating with so-called posterior internuclear ophthalmoplegia: a partial paramedian pontine reticular formation—abducens nucleus syndrome. J Neurol 232:38, 1985
27. Fisher CM: Some neuro-ophthalmological observations. J Neurol Neurosurg Psychiatry 30:383, 1967
28. Pierrot-Deseilligny C, Chain F, Serdaru M et al: The "one-and-a-half" syndrome: electro-oculographic analyses of five cases with deductions about the physiological mechanisms of lateral gaze. Brain 104:665, 1981
29. Sharpe JA, Rosenberg MA, Hoyt WF, Daroff RB: Paralytic pontine exotropia: a sign of acute unilateral pontine gaze palsy and internuclear ophthalmoplegia. Neurology 24:1076, 1974
30. Hanson MR, Hamid MA, Tomsak RL et al: Selective saccadic palsy caused by pontine lesions: clinical, physiological, and pathological correlations. Ann Neurol 20:209, 1986
31. Henn V, Lang W, Hepp K, Reisine H: Experimental gaze palsies in monkeys and their relation to human pathology. Brain 107:619, 1984
32. Johnston JL, Sharpe JA, Ranalli PJ, Morrow MJ: Oblique misdirection and slowing of vertical saccades after unilateral lesions of the pontine tegmentum. Neurology 43:2238, 1993
33. Pierrot-Deseilligny C, Goasguen J, Chain F, Lapresle J: Pontine metastasis with dissociated bilateral horizontal gaze paralysis. J Neurol Neurosurg Psychiatry 47:159, 1984
34. Thier P, Bachor A, Faiss J et al: Selective impairment of smooth-pursuit eye movements due to an ischemic lesion of the basal pons. Ann Neurol 29:443, 1991
35. Johnston JL, Sharpe JA, Morrow MJ: Paresis of contralateral smooth pursuit and normal vestibular smooth eye movements after unilateral brainstem lesions. Ann Neurol 31:495, 1992
36. Cannon SC, Robinson DA: Loss of the neural integrator of the oculomotor system from brain stem lesions in monkey. J Neurophysiol 57:1383, 1987
37. Dieterich M, Brandt T: Wallenberg's syndrome: lateropulsion, cyclorotation and subjective visual vertical in 36 patients. Ann Neurol 31:399, 1992
38. Kirkham TH, Guitton D, Gans M: Task dependent variations of ocular lateropulsion in Wallenberg's syndrome. Can J Neurol Sci 8:21, 1981
39. Büttner-Ennever JA, Büttner U: A cell group associated with vertical eye movements in the rostral mesencephalic reticular formation of the monkey. Brain Res 151:31, 1978
40. Vilis T, Hepp K, Schwartz U, Henn V: On the generation of vertical and torsional rapid eye movements in the monkey. Exp Brain Res 77:1, 1989
41. Moschovakis AK, Scudder CA, Highstein SM: Structure of the primate oculomotor burst generator: I. Median-lead burst neurons with upward on-directions. J Neurophysiol 65:203, 1991
42. Moschovakis AK, Scudder CA, highstein SM: Structure of the primate oculomotor burst generator: II. Median-lead burst neurons with downward on-directions. J Neurophysiol 65:218, 1991
43. Crawford JD, Cadera W, Vilis T: Generation of torsional and vertical eye position signals by the interstitial nucleus of Cajal. Science 252:1551, 1991
44. King WM, Precht W, Dieringer N: Synaptic organization of frontal eye field and vestibular afferents to the interstitial nucleus of Cajal in cat. J Neurophysiol 43:912, 1980
45. Carpenter MB, Harbison JW, Peter P: Accessory oculomotor nuclei in the monkey: projections and effects of discrete lesions. J Comp Neurol 140:131, 1970
46. Pasik P, Pasik T, Bender MB: The pretectal syndrome in monkeys: I. Disturbances of gaze and body posture. Brain 92:521, 1969
47. McCrea RA, Strassman A, Highstein SM: Anatomical and physiological characteristics of vestibular neurons mediating the vertical vestibulo-ocular reflexes of the squirrel monkey. J Comp Neurol 264:571, 1987
48. Henn V, Hepp K, Vilis T: Rapid eye movement generation in the primate: physiology, pathophysiology, and clinical implications. Rev Neurol (Paris) 145:540, 1989
49. Ranalli PJ, Sharpe JA, Fletcher WA: Palsy of upward and downward saccadic, pursuit, and vestibular movements with a unilateral midbrain lesion: pathophysiologic correlations. Neurology 38:114, 1988
50. Bender MB: Brain control of conjugate horizontal and vertical eye movements: a survey of the structural and functional correlates. Brain 103:23, 1980
51. Kompf D, Pasik T, Pasik P, Bender MB: Downward gaze in monkeys: stimulation and lesion studies. Brain 102:527, 1979
52. Büttner-Ennever JA, Büttner U, Cohen B, Baumgartner G: Vertical gaze paralysis and the rostral interstitial nucleus of the medial longitudinal fasciculus. Brain 105:125, 1982
53. Westheimer G, Blair SM: The ocular tilt reaction: a brainstem oculomotor routine. Invest Ophthalmol 14:833, 1975
54. Evinger LC, Fuchs AF, Baker R: Bilateral lesions of the medial longitudinal fasciculus in monkeys: effects on the horizontal and vertical components of voluntary and vestibular induced eye movements. Exp Brain Res 28:1, 1977
55. Partsalis AM, Highstein SM, Moschovakis AK: Lesions of the posterior commissure disable the vertical neural integrator of the primate oculomotor system. J Neurophysiol 71:2582, 1994
56. Keane JR: Sustained upgaze in coma. Ann Neurol 9:409, 1981
57. Fisher CM: The pathologic and clinical aspects of thalamic hemorrhage. Trans Am Neurol Assoc 84:56, 1959
58. Frohman LP, Kupersmith MJ: Reversible vertical ocular deviations associated with raised intracranial pressure. J Clin Neuro Ophthalmol 5:158, 1985
59. Keane JR, Rawlinson DG, Lu AT: Sustained downgaze deviation: two cases without structural pretectal lesions. Neurology 26:594, 1976
60. Lapresle J, Said G: Deviation forcée des yeux ver le bas et en dedans et mouvements oculaires periodiques au cours d'une hemorrhagie aneurysmale de la calotte mesencephalique. Rev Neurol 133:497, 1977
61. Corbett JJ, Schatz NJ, Shults WT et al: Slowly alternating skew deviation: description of a pretectal syndrome in three patients. Ann Neurol 10:540, 1981
62. Wray SH: The neuro-ophthalmic and neurologic manifestations of pinealomas. In Schmider HH (ed): Pineal Tumors, pp 21–59. New York, Masson, 1977
63. Büttner-Ennever JA, Acheson JF, Büttner U et al: Ptosis and supranuclear downgaze paralysis. Neurology 39:385, 1989
64. Tatu L, Moulin T, Bogousslavsky J, Duvernoy H: Arterial territories of human brain: brain stem and cerebellum. Neurology 47:1125, 1996
65. Weisberg LA: Mesencephalic hemorrhages: clinical and computed tomographic correlations. Neurology 36:713, 1986
66. Sand JJ, Biller J, Corbett JJ et al: Partial dorsal mesencephalic hemorrhages: report of three cases. Neurology 36:529, 1986
67. Keane JR: Bilateral ocular motor signs after tentorial herniation in 25 patients. Arch Neurol 43:806, 1986
68. Seaber JH, Nashold BS: Comparison of ocular motor effects of unilateral stereotactic midbrain lesions in man. Neuro-ophthalmology 1:95, 1990
69. Ochs AL, Stark L, Hoyt WF, D'Amico D: Opposed adducting saccades in convergence-retraction nystagmus: a patient with sylvian aqueduct syndrome. Brain 102:497, 1979
70. Zee DS, Fitzgibbon EJ, Optican LM: Saccade-vergence interactions in humans. J Neurophysiol 68: 1624, 1992

71. Brenner RP, Carlow TJ: PLEDS and nystagmus retractorius. Ann Neurol 5:403, 1979

72. Keane JR: Alternating skew deviation: 47 patients. Neurology 35:725, 1985

73. Moster ML, Schatz NJ, Savino PJ et al: Alternating skew on lateral gaze (bilateral abducting hypertropia). Ann Neurol 23:190, 1988

74. Brandt T, Dieterich M: Pathological eye-head coordination in roll: tonic ocular tilt reaction in mesencephalic and medullary lesions. Brain 110:649, 1987

75. Halmagyi GM, Brandt T, Dieterich M et al: Tonic contraversive ocular tilt reaction due to unilateral mesodiencephalic lesion. Neurology 40:1503, 1990

76. Rabinovitch HE, Sharpe JA, Sylvester TO: The ocular tilt reaction: a paroxysmal dyskinesia associated with elliptical nystagmus. Arch Ophthalmol 95:1395, 1977

77. Hedges TR III, Hoyt WE: Ocular tilt reaction due to an upper brainstem lesion: paroxysmal skew deviation, torsion, and oscillation of the eyes with head tilt. Ann Neurol 11:537, 1982

78. Lewis JM, Kline LB: Periodic alternating nystagmus associated with periodic alternating skew deviation. J Clin Neuro Ophthalmol 3:115, 1983

79. Keane JR: Ocular skew deviation: analysis of 100 cases. Arch Neurol 32:185, 1975

80. Zee DS: Considerations on the mechanisms of alternating skew deviations in patients with cerebellar lesions. J Vestib Res 6:395, 1996

81. Lueck CJ, Hamlyn P, Crawford TJ et al: A case of ocular tilt reaction and torsional nystagmus due to direct stimulation of the midbrain in man. Brain 114:2069, 1991

82. Steele JC, Richardson JC, Olszewski J: Progressive supranuclear palsy: a heterogeneous degeneration involving the brain stem, basal ganglia and cerebellum with vertical gaze and pseudobulbar palsy, nuchal dystonia and dementia. Arch Neurol 10:333, 1964

83. Leigh RJ, Newman SA, King WM: Vertical gaze disorders. In Lennerstrand G, Zee DS, Keller EL (eds): Functional basis of ocular motility disorders, pp 257–266. Oxford, Pergamon, 1982

84. Tanyeri S, Lueck CJ, Crawford TJ, Kennard C: Vertical and horizontal saccadic eye movements in Parkinson's disease. Neuro-ophthalmology 9:165, 1989

85. Dehaene I: Apraxia of eyelid opening in progressive supranuclear palsy. Ann Neurol 15:115, 1984

86. Malessa S, Gaymard B, Rivaud S et al: Role of pontine nuclei damage in smooth pursuit impairment of progressive supranuclear palsy: a clinico-pathological study. Neurology 44:716, 1994

87. Troost BT, Daroff RB: The ocular motor defects in progressive supranuclear palsy. Ann Neurol 2:397, 1977

88. Pierrot-Deseilligny C, Rivaud S, Pillon B et al: Lateral visually-guided saccades in progressive supranuclear palsy. Brain 112:471, 1989

89. Goffinet AM, De Volder AG, Gillian C et al: Positron tomography demonstrates frontal lobe hypometabolism in progressive supranuclear palsy. Ann Neurol 25:131, 1989

90. Collins SJ, Ahlskog JE, Parsi JE, Maraganore DM: Progressive supranuclear palsy: neuropathologically based diagnostic clinical criteria. J Neurol Neurosurg Psychiatry 58:167, 1995

91. Fukushima-Kudo J, Fukushima K, Tashiro K: Rigidity and dorsiflexion of the neck in progressive supranuclear palsy and the interstitial nucleus of Cajal. J Neurol Neurosurg Psychiatry 50:1197, 1987

92. Dubinsky RM, Jankovic J: Progressive supranuclear palsy and a multi-infarct state. Neurology 37:570, 1987

93. Moses H III, Zee D: Multiinfarct PSP. Neurology 37:1819, 1987

94. Lang AE, Riley DE, Bergeron C: Cortical-basal ganglionic degeneration. In Calne DB (ed): Neurodegenerative Diseases, pp 877–894. Philadelphia, WB Saunders, 1994

95. Adams M, Rhyner PA, Day J et al: Whipple's disease confined to the central nervous system. Ann Neurol 21:104, 1987

96. Finelli PF, McEntee WJ, Lessell S et al: Whipple's disease with predominantly neuroophthalmic manifestations. Ann Neurol 1:247, 1977

97. Knox DL, Bayless TM, Pittman FE: Neurologic disease in patients with treated Whipple's disease. Medicine 55:467, 1976

98. Schwartz MA, Selhorst JB, Ochs AL et al: Oculomasticatory myorhythmia: a unique movement disorder occurring in Whipple's disease. Ann Neurol 20:677, 1986

99. Fleming JL, Wiesner RH, Shorter RG: Whipple's disease: clinical, biochemical, and histopathologic features and assessment of treatment in 29 patients. Mayo Clin Proc 63:539, 1988

100. Mays LE, Porter JD: Neural control of vergence eye movements: activity of abducens and oculomotor neurons. J Neurophysiol 52:743, 1984

101. Mays LE: Neural control of vergence eye movements: convergence and divergence neurons in midbrain. J Neurophysiol 51:1091, 1984

102. Judge SJ, Cumming BG: Neurons in the monkey midbrain with activity related to vergence eye movement and accommodation. J Neurophysiol 55:915, 1986

103. Mays LE, Porter JD, Gamlin PDR, Tello CA: Neural control of vergence eye movements: neurons encoding vergence velocity. J Neurophysiol 56:1007, 1986

104. Gamlin PD, Clarke RJ: Single-unit activity in the primate nucleus reticularis tegmenti pontis related to vergence and ocular accommodation. J Neurophysiol 73:2115, 1995

105. Gamlin PDR, Mitchell KR: Reversible lesions of nucleus reticularis tegmenti pontis affect convergence and ocular accommodation (abstr). Soc Neurosci Abstr 19:346, 1993

106. Keane JR: Neuro-ophthalmologic signs and symptoms of hysteria. Neurology 32:757, 1982

107. Hermans P: Convergence spasms. Mt Sinai J Med 44:510, 1977

108. Guiloff RJ, Whiteley A, Kelly RE: Organic convergence spasm. Acta Neurol Scand 61:252, 1980

109. Coria F, Rebollo M, Quintana F et al: Occipitoatlantal instability and vertebrobasilar ischemia: case report. Neurology 32:303, 1982

110. Rabinowitz L, Chrousos GA, Cogan DG: Spasm of the near reflex associated with organic disease. Am J Ophthalmol 103:582, 1987

111. Krohel GB, Tobin DR, Hartnett ME et al: Divergence paralysis. Am J Ophthalmol 94:506, 1982

112. Roper-Hall G, Burde RM: Diagnosis and management of divergence paralysis. Am Orthoptic J 37:113, 1987

113. Langer T, Fuchs AF, Scudder CA, Chubb MC: Afferents to the flocculus of the cerebellum in the Rhesus macaque as revealed by retrograde transport of horseradish peroxidase. J Comp Neurol 235:1, 1985

114. Langer T, Fuchs AF, Chubb MC et al: Floccular efferents in the Rhesus macaque as revealed by autoradiography and horseradish peroxidase. J Comp Neurol 235:26, 1985

115. Lisberger SG, Fuchs AF: Role of primate flocculus during rapid behavioral modification of vestibulo-ocular reflex: I. Purkinje cell activity during visually guided horizontal smooth-pursuit eye movements and passive head rotation. J Neurophysiol 41:733, 1978

116. Waespe W, Henn V: Visual-vestibular interaction in the flocculus of the alert monkey: II. Purkinje cell activity. Exp Brain Res 43:349, 1981

117. Lisberger SG, Miles FA, Zee DS: Signals used to compute errors in monkey vestibuloocular reflex: possible role of flocculus. J Neurophysiol 52:1140, 1984

118. Walberg F, Dietrichs E: The interconnection between the vestibular nuclei and the nodulus: a study of reciprocity. Brain Res 449:47, 1988

119. Yamada J, Noda H: Afferent and efferent connections of the oculomotor cerebellar vermis in the macaque monkey. J Comp Neurol 265:224, 1987

120. Leichnetz GR, Smith DJ, Spencer R: Cortical projections to the paramedian tegmental and basilar pons in the monkey. J Comp Neurol 228:388, 1984

121. Ikeda Y, Noda H, Sugita S: Olivocerebellar and cerebelloolivary connections of the oculomotor region of the fastigial nucleus in the macaque monkey. J Comp Neurol 284:463, 1989

122. Noda H, Fujikado T: Topography of the oculomotor area of the

cerebellar vermis in macaques as determined by microstimulation. J Neurophysiol 58:359, 1987

123. Fuchs AF, Robinson FR, Straube A: Role of caudal fastigial nucleus in saccade generation: I. Neuronal discharge patterns. J Neurophysiol 70:1723, 1993

124. Fuchs AF, Robinson FR, Straube A: Participation of the caudal fastigial nucleus in smooth-pursuit eye movements: I. Neuronal activity. J Neurophysiol 72: 2714, 1994

125. Zee DS, Yamazaki A, Butler PH, Gucer G: Effects of ablation of flocculus and paraflocculus on eye movements in primate. J Neurophysiol 46:878, 1981

126. Waespe W, Cohen B, Raphan T: Dynamic modification of the vestibulo-ocular reflex by nodulus and uvula. Science 228:199, 1985

127. Hain TC, Zee DS, Maria BL: Tilt suppression of vestibulo-ocular reflex in patients with cerebellar lesions. Acta Otolaryngol (Stockh) 105:13, 1988

128. Furman JMR, Wall III C, Pang D: Vestibular function in periodic alternating nystagmus. Brain 113:1425, 1990

129. Sato H, Noda H: Saccadic dysmetria induced by transient functional decortication of the cerebellar vermis. Exp Brain Res 88:455, 1992

130. Robinson FR, Straube A, Fuchs AF: Role of caudal fastigial nucleus in saccade generation: II. Effects of muscimol inactivation. J Neurophysiol 70:1741, 1993

131. Pierrot-Deseilligny C, Amarenco P, Roullet E, Marteau R: Vermal infarct with pursuit eye movement disorders. J Neurol Neurosurg Psychiatry 53:519 1990

132. Büttner U, Straube A, Spuler A: Saccadic dysmetria and "intact" smooth pursuit eye movements after bilateral deep cerebellar nuclei lesions. J Neurol Neurosurg Psychiatry 57:832, 1994

133. Duncan GW, Parker SW, Fisher CM: Acute cerebellar infarction in the PICA territory. Arch Neurol 32:364, 1975

134. Grad A, Baloh RW: Vertigo of vascular origin: clinical and electronystagmographic features in 84 cases. Arch Neurol 46:281, 1989

135. Kase CS, White JL, Joslyn JN et al: Cerebellar infarction in the superior cerebellar artery distribution. Neurology 35:705, 1985

136. Ranalli PJ, Sharpe JA: Contrapulsion of saccades and ipsilateral ataxia: a unilateral disorder of the rostral cerebellum. Ann Neurol 20:311, 1986

137. Benjamin EE, Zimmerman CF, Troost BT: Lateropulsion and upbeat nystagmus are manifestations of central vestibular dysfunction. Arch Neurol 43:962, 1986

138. Uno A, Mukuno K, Sekiya H et al: Lateropulsion in Wallenberg's syndrome and contrapulsion in the proximal type of the superior cerebellar artery syndrome. Neuro-ophthalmology 9:75, 1989

139. Andersen RA, Gnadt JW: Posterior parietal cortex. In Wurtz, RH, Goldberg ME (eds): Reviews in Oculomotor Research, Vol 3, The Neurobiology of Saccadic Eye movements, pp 315–335. Amsterdam, Elsevier, 1989

140. Zeki S: A Vision of the Brain. Oxford, Blackwell, 1993

141. Andersen RA, Bracewell RM, Barach S et al: Eye position effects on visual, memory, and saccade-related activity in areas LIP and 7a of macaque monkey. J Neurosci 10:1176, 1990

142. Zeki S, Watson JDG, Lueck CJ et al: A direct demonstration of functional specialization in human visual cortex. J Neurosci 11:641, 1991

143. Newsome WT, Wurtz RH, Dürsteler MR, Mikami A: Deficits in visual motion processing following ibotenic acid lesions of the middle temporal visual area of the macaque monkey. J Neurosci 5:825, 1985

144. Newsome WT, Paré EB: A selective impairment of motion perception following lesions of the middle temporal visual area (MT). J Neurosci 8:2201, 1988

145. Thier P, Erickson RG: Vestibular inputs to visual-tracking neurons in area MST of awake Rhesus monkeys. Ann New York Acad Sci 656:960, 1992

146. Barash S, Bracewell RM, Fogassi L et al: Saccade-related activity in the lateral intraparietal area: I. Temporal properties; comparison with area 7a. J Neurophysiol 66:1095, 1991

147. Lynch JC, Graybiel AM, Lobeck LJ: The differential projection of two cytoarchitectonic subregions of the inferior parietal lobule

148. Lynch JC: Saccade initiation and latency deficits after combined lesions of the frontal and posterior eye fields in monkeys. J Neurophysiol 68:1913, 1992

149. Pierrot-Deseilligny C, Rivaud S, Gaymard B et al: Cortical control of saccades. Ann Neurol 37:557, 1995

150. Pierrot-Deseilligny C, Rivaud S, Gaymard B, Agid Y: Cortical control of reflexive visually guided saccades in man. Brain 114:1473, 1991

151. Pierrot-Deseilligny C, Rivaud S, Penet C, Rigolet M-H: Latencies of visually guided saccades in unilateral hemispheric cerebral lesions. Ann Neurol 21:138, 1987

152. Heide W, Blankenburg M, Zimmermann E, Kömpf D: Cortical control of double-step saccades: Implications for spatial orientation. Ann Neurol 38:739, 1995

153. Rivaud S, Müri RM, Gaymard B et al: Eye movement disorders after frontal eye field lesions in humans. Exp Brain Res 102:110, 1994

154. Pierrot-Deseilligny C, Israël I, Berthoz A et al: Role of the different frontal lobe areas in the control of the horizontal component of memory-guided saccades in man. Exp Brain Res 95:166, 1993

155. Guitton D, Buchtel HW, Douglas RM: Frontal lobe lesions in man cause difficulties in suppressing reflexive glances and in generating goal-directed saccades. Exp Brain Res 58:455, 1985

156. Schlag J, Schlag-Rey M: Evidence for a supplementary eye field. J Neurophysiol 57:179, 1987

157. Goldman-Rakic PS: Circuitry of primate prefrontal cortex and regulation of behavior by representational memory. In Plum F (ed): Handbook of Physiology, Sect 1, Vol V, The Nervous System, pp 373–417. Bethesda, MD, American Physiological System, 1987

158. Gaymard B, Rivaud S, Pierrot-Deseilligny C: Role of the left and right supplementary motor areas in memory-saccades sequences. Ann Neurol 34:404, 1993

159. Müri RM, Rivaud S, Timsit S et al: The role of the right medial temporal lobe in the control of memory-guided saccades. Exp Brain Res 101:165, 1994

160. Sawaguchi T, Goldman-Racik PS: D1 dopamine receptors in prefrontal cortex: involvement in working memory. Science 251:947, 1991

161. Iwatsubo T, Kuzuhara S, Kanemitsu A et al: Corticofugal projections to the motor nuclei of the brainstem and spinal cord in humans. Neurology 40:309, 1990

162. Leichnetz GR: The prefrontal cortico-oculomotor trajectories in the monkey: a possible explanation for the effects of stimulation/lesion experiments on eye movement. J Neurol Sci 49:387, 1981

163. Stanton GB, Goldberg ME, Bruce CJ: Frontal eye field efferents in the macaque monkey: I. Subcortical pathways and topography of striatal and thalamic terminal fields. J Comp Neurol 271:473, 1988

164. Stanton GB, Goldberg ME, Bruce CJ: Frontal eye field efferents in the macaque monkey: II. Topography of terminal fields in midbrain and pons. J Comp Neurol 271:493, 1988

165. Huerta MF, Kaas JH: Supplementary eye fields as defined by intracortical microstimulation: connections in macaques. J Comp Neurol 293:299, 1990

166. Selemon LD, Goldman-Rakic PS: Common cortical and subcortical targets of the dorsolateral prefrontal and posterior parietal cortices in the Rhesus monkey: evidence for a distributed neural network subserving spatially guided behavior. J Neurosci 8:4049, 1988

167. Hikosaka O, Sakamoto M, Usui S: Functional properties of monkey caudate neurons: I. Activities related to saccadic eye movements. J Neurophysiol 61:780, 1989

168. Hikosaka O, Wurtz RH: The basal ganglia. In Wurtz RH, Goldberg ME (eds): The neurobiology of saccadic eye movements, Chap 6, pp 257–281. Amsterdam, Elsevier, 1989

169. Lasker AG, Zee DS, Hain TC et al: Saccades in Huntington's disease: initiation defects and distractability. Neurology 37:364, 1987

170. Sparks DL, Hartwich-Young R: The deep layers of the superior colliculus. In Wurtz RH, Goldberg ME (eds): The Neurobiology

of macaque upon the deep layers of the superior colliculus. J Comp Neurol 235:241, 1985

of Saccadic Eye Movements, Chap 5, pp 213–255. Amsterdam, Elsevier, 1989

171. Fischer B, Weber H: Express saccades and visual attention. Behav Brain Sci 16:553, 1993

172. Munoz DP, Wurtz RH: Saccade-related activity in monkey superior colliculus: I. Characteristics of burst and buildup cells. J Neurophysiol 73:2313, 1995

173. Munoz DP, Wurtz RH: Saccade-related activity in monkey superior colliculus: II. Spread of activity during saccades. J Neurophysiol 73:2334, 1995

174. Waitzman DM, Ma TP, Optican LM, Wurtz RH: Superior colliculus neurons mediate the dynamic characteristics of saccade. J Neurophysiology 66:1716, 1991

175. Munoz DP, Wurtz RH: Fixation cells in monkey superior colliculus: II. Reversible activation and deactivation. J Neurophysiology 70:576, 1993

176. Hikosaka O, Wurtz RH: Modification of saccadic eye movements by GABA-related substances: I. Effect of muscimol and bicuculline in monkey superior colliculus. J Neurophysiol 53:266, 1985

177. Schiller PH, Sandell JH, Maunsell JHR: The effect of frontal eye field and superior colliculus lesions on saccadic latencies in the Rhesus monkey. J Neurophysiol 57:1033, 1987

178. Pierrot-Deseilligny C, Rosa A, Masmoudi K et al: Saccade deficits after a unilateral lesion affecting the superior colliculus. J Neurol Neurosurg Psychiatry 54:1106, 1991

179. Westheimer G, Blair SM: Oculomotor defects in cerebellectomized monkeys. Invest Ophthalmol 12:618, 1973

180. Deng S-Y, Goldberg ME, Segraves MA et al: The effect of unilateral ablation of the frontal eye fields on saccadic performance in the monkey. In Keller EL, Zee DS (eds): Adaptive Processes in Visual and Oculomotor Systems, pp 201–208. Oxford, Pergamon, 1986

181. Schiller PH, True SD, Conway JL: Deficits in eye movements following frontal eye-field and superior colliculus ablations. J Neurophysiol 44:1175, 1980

182. Lynch JC, McLaren JW: Deficits of visual attention and saccadic eye movements after lesions of parietoocipital cortex in monkeys. J Neurophysiol 61:74, 1989

183. Tusa RJ, Zee DS, Herdman SJ: Effect of unilateral cerebral cortical lesions on ocular motor behavior in monkeys: saccades and quick phases. J Neurophysiol 56:1590, 1986

184. Pierrot-Deseilligny C, Gautier J-C, Loron P: Acquired ocular motor apraxia due to bilateral fronto-parietal infarcts. Ann Neurol 23:199, 1988

185. Newsome WT, Wurtz RH, Komatsu H: Relation of cortical areas MT and MST to pursuit eye movements: II. Differentiation of retinal from extraretinal inputs. J Neurophysiol 60:604, 1988

186. Gottlieb JP, Macavoy MG, Bruce CJ: Neural responses to smooth-pursuit eye movements and their correspondence with electrically elicited smooth eye movements in the primate frontal eye field. J Neurophysiol 72:1634, 1995

187. Glickstein M, Cohen JL, Dixon B et al: Corticopontine visual projections in macaque monkeys. J Comp Neurol 190:209, 1980

188. Suzuki DA, Noda H, Kase M: Visual and pursuit eye movement-related activity in posterior vermis of monkey cerebellum. J Neurophysiol 46:1120, 1981

189. Segraves MA, Goldberg ME, Deng S-Y et al: The role of striate cortex in the guidance of eye movements in the monkey. J Neurosci 7:3040, 1987

190. Dürsteler MR, Wurtz RH: Pursuit and optokinetic deficits following chemical lesions of cortical areas MT and MST. J Neurophysiol 60:940, 1988

191. May JG, Keller EL, Suzuki DA: Smooth-pursuit eye movement deficits with chemical lesions in the dorsolateral pontine nucleus of the monkey. J Neurophysiol 59:952, 1988

192. Büttner U, Straube A: The effect of cerebellar midline lesions on eye movements. Neuro-Ophthalmology 15:75, 1995

193. Kaufman SR, Abel LA: The effects of distraction on smooth pursuit in normal subjects. Acta Otolaryngol (Stockh) 102:57, 1986

194. Leigh RJ, Tusa RJ: Disturbance of smooth pursuit caused by infarction of occipitoparietal cortex. Ann Neurol 17:185, 1985

195. Osorio I, Daroff RB: Absence of REM and altered NREM sleep in patients with spinocerebellar degeneration and slow saccades. Ann Neurol 7:277, 1980

196. Levin S, Luebke A, Zee DS et al: Smooth pursuit eye movements in schizophrenics: quantitative measurements with the search-coil technique. J Psychiatr Res 22:195, 1989

197. Huebner WP, Leigh RJ, Seidman SH, Billian C: An Investigation of horizontal combined eye-head tracking in patients with abnormal vestibular and smooth pursuit eye movements. J Neurol Sci 116:152, 1993

198. De Renzi E, Colombo A, Faglioni P, Gibertoni M: Conjugate gaze paresis in stroke patients with unilateral damage. Arch Neurol 39:482, 1982

199. Kompf D, Gmeiner H-J: Gaze palsy and visual hemineglect in acute hemisphere lesions. Neuro-ophthalmology 9:49, 1989

200. Daroff RB, Hoyt WF: Supranuclear disorders of ocular control systems in man: Clinical, anatomical and physiological correlations—1969. In Bach-y-Rita P, Collins CC, Hyde JE (eds): The Control of Eye Movements, pp 175–235. New York, Academic Press, 1971

201. Fletcher WA, Gellman RS: Saccades in humans with lesions of frontal eye fields (FEF) (abstr). Soc Neurosci Abstr 15:1203, 1989

202. Steiner I, Melamed E: Conjugate eye deviation after acute hemispheric stroke: delayed recovery after previous contralateral frontal lobe damage. Ann Neurol 16:509, 1984

203. Sullivan HC, Kaminski HJ, Maas EF et al: Lateral deviation of the eyes on forced lid closure in patients with cerebral lesions. Arch Neurol 48:310, 1991

204. Sharpe JA, Lo AW, Rabinovitch HE: Control of the saccadic and smooth pursuit systems after cerebral hemidecortication. Brain 102:387, 1979

205. Cogan DG, Loeb DR: Optokinetic response and intracranial lesions. Arch Neurol Psychiatry 61:183, 1949

206. Monaco F, Pirisi A, Sechi GP, Cossu G: Acquired ocular-motor and right-sided cortical angioma. Cortex 16:159, 1980

207. Mills RP, Swanson PD: Vertical oculomotor apraxia and memory loss. Ann Neurol 4:149, 1978

208. Ebner R, Lopez L, Ochoa S, Crovetto L: Vertical ocular motor apraxia. Neurology 40: 712, 1990

209. Husain M, Stein J: Rezso Balint and his most celebrated case. Arch Neurol 45:89, 1988

210. Holmes G: Spasm of fixation. Trans Ophthalmol Soc UK 50:253, 1930

211. Johnston JL, Sharpe JA, Morrow MJ: Spasm of fixation: a quantitative study. J Neurol Sci 107:166, 1992

212. Fielder AR, Gresty MA, Dodd KL et al: Congenital ocular motor apraxia. Trans Ophthalmol Soc UK 105:589, 1986

213. Rosenberg ML, Wilson E: Congenital ocular motor apraxia without head thrusts. J Clin Neuro Opthalmol 7:26, 1987

214. Zee DS, Yee RD, Singer HS: Congenital ocular motor apraxia, Brain 100:581, 1977

215. Cogan DG, Chu FC, Reingold D et al: A longterm follow-up of congenital ocular motor apraxia: case report. Neuro-ophthalmology 1:145, 1980

216. Borchert MS, Sadun AA, Sommers JD et al: Congenital ocular motor apraxia in twins: findings with magnetic resonance imaging. J Clin Neuro Ophthalmol 7:104, 1987

217. Zaret CR, Behrens MM, Eggers HM: Congenital ocular motor apraxia and brainstem tumor. Arch Ophthalmol 98:328, 1980

218. Kennard C, Lueck CJ: Oculomotor abnormalities in diseases of the basal ganglia. Rev Neurol (Paris) 145:587, 1989

219. Huaman AG, Sharpe JA: Vertical saccades in senescence. Invest Ophthalmol Vis Sci 34:2588, 1993

220. Crawford T, Goodrich S, Henderson L, Kennard C: Predictive responses in Parkinson's disease: manual keypresses and saccadic eye movements to regular stimulus events. J Neurol Neurosurg Psychiatry 52:1033, 1989

221. Kennard C, Crawford TJ, Henderson L: A pathophysiological approach to saccadic eye movements in neurological and psychiatric disease. J Neurol Neurosurg Psychiatry 57:881, 1994

222. Crawford TJ, Henderson L, Kennard C: Abnormalities of nonvisually-guided eye movements in Parkinson's disease. Brain 112:1573, 1989

223. Bronstein AM, Kennard C: Predictive ocular motor control in Parkinson's disease. Brain 108:925, 1985

224. Gibson JM, Pimlott R, Kennard C: Ocular motor and manual tracking in Parkinson's disease and the effect of treatment. J Neurol Neurosurg Psychiatry 50:853, 1987

225. White OB, Saint-Cyr JA, Tomlinson RD, Sharpe JA: Ocular motor deficits in Parkinson's disease: II. Control of the saccadic and smooth pursuit systems. Brain 106:571, 1983

226. Reichert WH, Doolittle J, McDowell FH: Vestibular dysfunction in Parkinson disease. Neurology 32:1133, 1982

227. White OB, Saint-Cyr JA, Sharpe JA: Ocular motor deficits in Parkinson's disease: I. The horizontal vestibulo-ocular reflex and its regulation. Brain 106:555, 1983

228. Vidailhet M, Rivaud S, Gouider-Khouja N et al: Eye movements in parkinsonian syndromes. Ann Neurol 35:420, 1994

229. Fearnley JM, Revesz T, Brooks DJ et al: Diffuse Lewy body disease presenting with a supranuclear gaze palsy. J Neurol Neurosurg Psychiatry 54:159, 1991

230. Hotson JR, Langston EB, Langston JW: Saccade responses to dopamine in human MPTP-induced parkinsonism. Ann Neurol 20:456, 1986

231. Leigh RJ, Foley JM, Remler BF, Civil RH: Oculogyric crisis: A syndrome of thought disorder and ocular deviation. Ann Neurol 22:13, 1987

232. Fitzgerald P, Jankovic J: Tardive oculogyric crises. Neurology 39:1434, 1989

233. Leigh RJ, Newman SA, Folstein SE et al: Abnormal ocular motor control in Huntington's disease. Neurology 33:1268, 1983

234. Collewljn H, Went LN, Tamminga EP et al: Oculomotor defects in patients with Huntington's disease and their offspring. J Neurol Sci 86:307, 1988

235. Lasker AG, Zee DS, Hain TC et al: Saccades in Huntington's disease: slowing and dysmetria. Neurology 38:427, 1988

236. Leigh RJ, Parhad IM, Clark AW et al: Brainstem findings in Huntington's disease. J Neurol Sci 71:247, 1985

237. Troost BT, Troost EG: Functional paralysis of horizontal gaze. Neurology 29:82, 1979

CHAPTER 11

Nystagmus and Saccadic Intrusions and Oscillations

Louis F. Dell'Osso and Robert B. Daroff

Nystagmus
   Nystagmus in Infancy
      Congenital
      Latent/Manifest Latent
      Nystagmus Blockage Syndrome
      Acquired
         Secondary to Visual Loss
         Spasmus Nutans
   Acquired Pendular Nystagmus (Adults)
   Acquired Horizontal Jerk Nystagmus
      Vestibular
      Gaze-Evoked (Gaze-Paretic) Nystagmus
   Special Nystagmus Types
      Physiologic (End-Point)
      Dissociated
      Torsional
      See-Saw
      Convergence/Convergence-Evoked
      Periodic Alternating
      Downbeat
      Upbeat
      Rebound
      Circular, Elliptic, and Oblique
      Cervical
      Muscle-Paretic (Myasthenic)
      Lid
      Epileptic

Induced Nystagmus
   Caloric
   Rotational
   Positional
   Optokinetic
   Drug- and Toxin-Induced
Special Anatomic Categories
   Acoustic Neuroma
   Lateral Medullary Syndrome
   Albinism and Achiasma
   Cerebellum
Saccadic Intrusions and Oscillations
   Square-Wave Jerks/Oscillations
   Square-Wave Pulses
   Macro-Saccadic Oscillations
   Saccadic Pulses/Pulse Trains
   Double Saccadic Pulses
   Dysmetria
   Flutter
   Flutter Dysmetria
   Opsoclonus
   Myoclonus
   Superior Oblique Myokymia
   Bobbing/Dipping
   Voluntary "Nystagmus"

The day of the last hypothesis would also be the day of the last observation. . . . An hypothesis which becomes dispossessed by new facts dies an honorable death; and if it has called up for examination those truths by which it is annihilated, it deserves a moment of gratitude.

Jacob Henle (1809–1885)

L. F. Dell'Osso: Departments of Neurology and Biomedical Engineering, Schools of Medicine and Engineering, Case Western Reserve University; and Ocular Motor Neurophysiology Laboratory, Veterans Administration Medical Center, Cleveland, Ohio
R. B. Daroff: Department of Neurology, Case Western Reserve University; Medical Affairs, University Hospitals of Cleveland, Cleveland, Ohio

See Chapter 11 for Glossary.

NYSTAGMUS

Nystagmus, the rhythmic to-and-fro oscillation of the eyes, has been regarded as enigmatic. In fact, the distinguished neuro-ophthalmologist Wilbrand once advised, "Never write on nystagmus, it will lead you nowhere."[1]

Although technologic advances have permitted quantitative insights into nystagmus analysis, the clinician should not be daunted. Many useful, often diagnostic, observations can be made by physical examination alone. Figures 11–1 and 11–2 are examples of one convenient method of diagramming nystagmus. Also, nystagmus can be further described when the globes are inspected under slit-lamp magnification, or when the fundus is viewed.

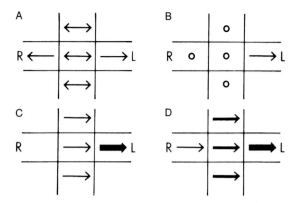

Fig. 11–1. Simple diagrammatic method for depicting nystagmus. The velocity of the nystagmus phases (*two arrowheads*) are equal (*i.e.,* pendular). Jerk nystagmus (*single arrowhead*) points in direction of fast phase. *Heavy lines* indicate more intense nystagmus. **A.** Pendular nystagmus in primary position and up or down, converting to jerk on lateral gaze. **B.** First-degree jerk nystagmus present only on left lateral gaze. **C.** Second-degree jerk nystagmus beating leftward in primary position and increasing on left gaze. **D.** Third-degree leftward jerk nystagmus.

This chapter is a coalescence of the traditional neuro-ophthalmologic approach to nystagmus diagnosis and the impact of the newer capabilities of electronic eye movement recording and mathematical "biomodeling."

Eye movement recordings have allowed definition of 47 types of nystagmus (Table 11–1) and new insights into their pathophysiology. For precise analysis, special recording techniques are necessary, such as infrared, magnetic search-coil, or video recording systems, which can faithfully reproduce the eye-movement trajectories and provide accurate information on eye position without drift or noise. For quantitative purposes, all systems should record by way of direct current, with a bandwidth of 100 Hz. The eyes should be recorded separately in horizontal, vertical, and (if possible) torsional directions, with the tracing analogs written on rectilinear graph paper. Recording should be performed during fixation of visible targets and sometimes in the dark with eyes open (see Chapter 9). For detailed quantitative analysis, the data should be digitized at 200 Hz or higher.

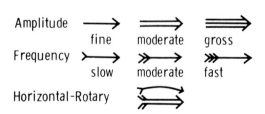

Fig. 11–2. Nystagmus diagrams can be detailed and complex if one uses these symbols.

Nystagmus has traditionally been divided into two types on the basis of the clinical impression of the waveform. Thus, if the eyes appeared to oscillate with "equal speed" in either direction, it was called "pendular" nystagmus; if movement in one direction was faster than in the other, it was called "jerk" nystagmus. True pendular nystagmus is sinusoidal, whereas jerk nystagmus has a slow phase away from the object of regard, followed by a fast (saccadic) phase toward the target. The direction of the fast component, by convention, defines the nystagmus direction. These criteria can often be assessed only by accurate recordings. Nystagmus should be described not only by its waveform and direction but also by its amplitude (A) and frequency (F), the product of which is intensity (I). The examiner should also note the positions of gaze in which the nystagmus occurs and whether the intensity changes with gaze direction. Jerk nystagmus is usually accentuated in amplitude upon gaze in the direction of the fast component, a characteristic referred to as Alexander's law.[2]

The field of gaze in which nystagmus intensity is minimal is termed the "null zone" (see Fig. 11–12). The "neutral zone" is that eye position in which a reversal of direction of jerk nystagmus occurs and in which no nystagmus, any of several bidirectional waveforms, or pendular nystagmus is present. The null and neutral zones usually overlap; however, several cases have been recorded where they do not.

Based on quantitative eye-movement recordings, we have identified three underlying defects in the slow eye movement (SEM) subsystem (see Chapter 9) that produce nystagmus:

1. *High gain instability.* In some persons, because of abnormally high gain in the SEM subsystem, a runaway (increasing velocity) movement or a pendular oscillation is evoked. In this chapter, the term *high gain* can also imply excessive delay for the gain present (*i.e.,* the control loop may have a normal gain, but an increased delay). Control theory suggests how particular changes in gain can result in either a pendular or a jerk nystagmus. Pendular nystagmus can be congenital or acquired, whereas horizontal jerk nystagmus with slow phases of increasing velocity usually is associated with congenital nystagmus; however, the latter may result from an Arnold-Chiari malformation.[3] Vertical nystagmus with an exponential slow phase of increasing velocity may be secondary to acquired cerebellar disease.[4]

2. *Vestibular tone imbalance.* The nystagmus of vestibular tone imbalance results from the imposition of asymmetric vestibular input on an inherently normal horizontal gaze generator. This asymmetric input occurs if one vestibular apparatus (labyrinths, nerve, and brain stem nuclei) functions abnormally or if both sides are asymmetrically defective. The nystag-

TABLE 11–1. Forty-seven Types of Nystagmus*

Acquired	Gaze-evoked	Pseudospontaneous
"Fixation"	Deviational	Induced
Anticipatory	Gaze-paretic	Rebound
Induced	"Neurasthenic"	Reflex
Arthrokinetic	"Seducible"	Baer's
Induced	"Setting-in"	See-saw
Somatosensory	Horizontal	Somatosensory
Associated	Induced	Induced
Induced	Provoked	Spontaneous
Stransky's	Intermittent vertical	Stepping around
Audiokinetic	Jerk	Apparent/real
Induced	Latent/manifest latent	Induced
Bartels'	Monocular "fixation"	Somatosensory
Induced	Unimacular	Torsional
Bruns'	Lateral medullary	Rotary
Centripetal	Lid	Uniocular
Cervical	Miner's†	Upbeat
Neck torsion	Occupational	Vertical
Vertebrobasilar artery insufficiency	Muscle-paretic	Vestibular
Circular/elliptic/oblique	Myasthenic	A(po)geotropic/geotropic
Alternating windmill	Optokinetic	Alternating current
Circumduction	Induced	Bechterew's
Diagonal	"Kinetic"	Caloric/caloric-after
Elliptic	"Optic"	Compensatory
Gyratory	Optomotor	Electrical/faradic/galvanic
Oblique	Panoramic	Head-shaking
Radiary	"Railway"	Induced
Congenital	Sigma	L-
"Fixation"	"Train"	Labyrinthine
Hereditary	Optokinetic after-	Perverted
Convergence	Induced	Pneumatic/compression
Convergence-evoked	Postoptokinetic	Positional/alcohol
Dissociated	Reverse postoptokinetic	Positioning
Disjunctive	Pendular	Postrotational
Downbeat	Talantropia	Pseudocaloric
Drug-induced	Periodic/aperiodic alternating	Rotational/perrotary
Barbiturate	Alternans	Secondary phase
Bow tie	Physiologic	
Induced	End-point	
Epileptic	Fatigue	
Ictal	Pursuit after-	
Flash-induced	Induced	
Flicker-induced	Pursuit-defect†	
Induced		

* Synonyms and other terms indented under either the preferred or the more inclusive designation; some nystagmus types may be acquired or congenital; quoted terms are erroneous or nonspecific.
    † May not exist.

mus recording always shows a linear (straight line) slow phase, reflecting a persistent tone to drive the eyes toward the side of the relatively damaged vestibular apparatus. The slow-phase amplitude is reduced by fixation and enhanced by darkness, Frenzel (high-plus) lenses, or closing the eyes. Fixation inhibition may be related to an opposing smooth-pursuit force and requires the integrity of the cerebellar flocculus.

3. *Integrator leak.* Nystagmus caused by a "leaky integrator" occurs only in an eccentric gaze position; thus, it is gaze-evoked. The eyes are unable to maintain the eccentric position and drift back to the primary position with a decreasing velocity, reflecting

a passive movement resisted by the viscous forces of orbital soft tissues. The defect may reside in the brain stem "neural integrator" or its connections (such as in the cerebellum), which mediate eye deviation. This form of gaze-evoked nystagmus is called "gaze-paretic" nystagmus (see Fig. 9–8 for an illustration of the gaze-paretic waveform).

One means of classification of nystagmus is based on whether it is a "gazed-evoked" or "gaze-modulated" type; the former category requires that there be no primary-position nystagmus. Two benign types of nystagmus (congenital and latent), physiologic types (vestibular), and symptomatic types (vestibular) fall in the gaze-modulated category. Some physiologic types (endpoint) and symptomatic types (gaze-paretic) are gaze evoked. Although these concepts of a control mechanism represent useful approaches toward a more meaningful classification of nystagmus, they are far from inclusive. For practical reasons, an empirical nystagmus classification is presented that will aid the clinician in bedside and office evaluation, without the use of sophisticated recording instrumentation. This classification continues to change as our understanding of nystagmus advances.

The localizing significance of nystagmus is often a mere indication of dysfunction somewhere in the posterior fossa (*i.e.*, vestibular end-organ, brain stem, or cerebellum). However, certain nystagmus patterns are quite specific and permit reasonably accurate neuroanatomic diagnosis. When possible, the specific and nonspecific forms are separated on the basis of clinical appearance and associated signs and symptoms.

Nystagmus in Infancy

There are several types of benign nystagmus usually seen in infancy. Congenital nystagmus (CN) is the most common infantile nystagmus. Others are latent/manifest latent nystagmus (LMLN) and the pendular nystagmus of spasmus nutans.

Congenital

Congenital nystagmus is usually present at birth or noted in early infancy at the time of development of visual fixation, and it persists throughout life. Rarely, CN becomes manifest later in life,[5] so the term *congenital* should be thought of as a congenital predisposition for this particular type of ocular motor instability rather than taken literally. This form of nystagmus may accompany primary visual defects, which has led to the assumption that the nystagmus is secondary to poor vision, and that both "sensory defect" and "motor defect" types of CN exist. In fact, recordings have shown that all CN is the same with regard to waveforms and underlying mechanism, regardless of the coincidental existence of a sensory deficit. CN is the *direct* result of an ocular motor control instability that may develop with or without an accompanying sensory deficit. Thus, for those cases in which a sensory deficit exists, it can only be a subordinate factor in the development of CN, perhaps interfering with the normal calibration of a key ocular motor subsystem and thereby precipitating its instability. The common association of "pendular" CN with a sensory defect and the "jerk" form with a primary motor abnormality is both simplistic and erroneous. Studies of infants with CN show no difference in waveforms associated with the presence or absence of sensory defi-

cits; the infants exhibited the same CN waveforms that have been recorded in children and adults.[6] Specifically, the development of foveation periods in CN waveforms begins early in infancy as acuity and fixation develop. This is clearly seen in infrared recordings of infants when they are attending to a visual task.

When oculography has been used in systematic investigations, no consistent association between wave type and the presence (or absence) of primary visual loss has been found.[7] The relationship of the visual defect to the nystagmus possibly represents simple genetic association. Although the visual problem may not be causal, it can contribute to the intensity of the nystagmus. CN represents a high-gain instability in a SEM subsystem,[8] and fixation attempt (the effort to see) is its main driving force. Poor vision will increase fixation effort and increase the intensity of the nystagmus. Moreover, a subclinical motor instability may become manifest by this exaggerated visual effort. Although the exact location of the source of the instability present in CN is unknown, we hypothesize that CN is due to a gain/delay problem in an internal (brain stem) feedback loop in the pursuit subsystem.[8] The much greater incidence of horizontal CN, compared with vertical or diagonal CN, probably reflects inherent differences in the stability of the respective pursuit subsystems (*i.e.*, the horizontal is more unstable than the vertical). Another factor in support for this hypothesis is that no oscillopsia is perceived from oscillations in pursuit velocity, not in normals and not in those with CN. Thus, no additional mechanism need be proposed to account for the absence of oscillopsia in CN; it is suppressed by the same mechanism by which normals suppress it during pursuit. The common neural integrator is *not* the site of the CN instability.[9] Several models have been proposed that attempt to explain the genesis of CN.[10–12] While each can generate some CN characteristics, they exhibit behaviors inconsistent with data from individuals with CN. Because CN appears to be activated and intensified by fixation attempt, the deficit may also be linked to the fixation subsystem (see Chapter 9). The co-existence of a high-frequency pendular oscillation with a low-frequency jerk CN (causing a dual-jerk waveform) in some subjects, and with LMLN in others, suggests that the high-frequency pendular oscillation is due to an instability at a different site. It has also been suggested that CN is caused by oscillations at two frequencies whose interactions may produce some of the known CN waveforms.[13]

Distinguishing the lower frequency pendular nystagmus from jerk nystagmus may be difficult clinically, particularly in CN. Certain forms of jerk nystagmus are invariably mislabeled as pendular, or the direction is misidentified. Even with oculographic recordings, the direction of the fast phase may be misinterpreted unless velocity tracings are obtained.[14] In the absence of oculography, clinicians should describe the nystagmus carefully or use diagrammatic methods (Fig. 11–3; see Figs. 11–1 and 11–2). A diagonal nystagmus whose horizontal component initially looked like latent nystagmus slow phases (see below) and then developed to resemble CN slow phases was induced in monkeys by monocular visual deprivation. This deprivation took place from birth to 25 days and was followed by monocular deprivation of the other eye.[15]

Congenital nystagmus usually damps significantly with convergence. Although the exact mechanism responsible for this damping in unknown, we have long felt that it might result from an effective increase in the stiffness of the ocular motor plant brought about by the increased innervation to the antagonist medial recti. Because convergence results in a change in the muscle pulley system,[16] that may be the mechanism by which the stiffness is increased. The observations of convergence-induced damping of other types of nystagmus support this "peripheral" mechanism in preference to one relaying on an inherent property of CN. As previously mentioned, the intensity of CN is related to the fixation attempt, which probably explains why it sometimes persists with eyes open in darkness (when the subject will probably attempt to "see") and damps behind closed lids (when the subject will, unless instructed to the contrary, reduce any attempt to "see").[14] The defining criterion is fixation attempt, *not* retinal illumination or lid position. Therefore, reports of the presence or absence of CN with lid closure or darkness that lack a description of the instructions to the subject provide no useful information.

The recognition of CN is of extreme importance, particularly in the adult patient, and may obviate unnecessary neurodiagnostic procedures. The characteristics of CN are listed in Table 11–2. CN is almost always binocular and never shows more than minor amplitude dissociation between the two eyes. Clinically, the nystagmus usu-

TABLE 11–2. Characteristics of Congenital Nystagmus

Binocular with similar amplitude in both eyes
Provoked or increased by fixation attempt
Gaze-modulated, not gaze-evoked
Diminished (damped) by gaze or convergence
Usually horizontal and torsional (vertical rare)
Increasing velocity slow phases
Distinctive waveforms (foveation periods and braking saccades)
Superimposition of latent component possible
"Inversion" of the optokinetic reflex (actually, CN reversal)
Associated head oscillation or turn
No oscillopsia
Aperiodic alternation possible (Baclofen ineffective)
Abolished in sleep or inattention to visual tasks

ally appears uniplanar. Like vestibular end-organ nystagmus, horizontal nystagmus remains horizontal when the eyes are deviated vertically and does not convert to vertical nystagmus. Using new, sensitive techniques for recording torsional eye movements, we have found small but significant torsional components in the CN of subjects previously thought to have purely horizontal CN. Because the prominent horizontal movement masks the usually smaller torsional component, the latter appears to be a common characteristic of "horizontal" CN. In most patients, rightward movements were accompanied by clockwise torsion and leftward movements by counterclockwise torsion.[17] The superimposition of a latent component on an ongoing CN is discussed below.

Eye movement recordings of CN occasionally show a pure pendular waveform (sinusoidal) or a saw-toothed waveform (equiamplitude linear slow phase with foveating saccade) (see Fig. 11–8) typically seen in vestibular nystagmus. These pure forms are neither frequent nor pathognomonic for CN. More often, CN manifests distinctive waveforms that have not been reported in acquired nystagmus. These waveforms are an expression of the attempts by the ocular motor control system to increase foveation time imposed on inherently unstable slow control. The CN waveforms shown in Figures 11–4 through 11–7 (other than pure pendular or jerk) have never been recorded in acquired horizontal nystagmus.[7,18] The target position is indicated by a dashed line. For pendular waveforms, the target is foveated at the peaks that are more flattened, indicating extended foveation. Extended foveation in an adult with lifelong nystagmus secondary to a congenital brain stem hamartoma, and in an adult given gabapentin for treatment of nystagmus secondary to an arteriovenous malformation,[19] supports the hypothesis that extended foveation periods in CN represent the action of a normal fixation system on the underlying CN oscillation. Figures 11–8 and 11–9 demonstrate how these waveforms serve to increase the time of foveal imaging.

The pure pendular (P) and jerk (J) waveforms in Figure 11–8 are not conducive to good acuity because

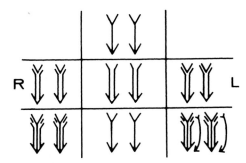

Fig. 11–3. A typical nystagmus is maximum in frequency and amplitude on eccentric and downward gaze. The nystagmus is absent during up and left gaze and up and right gaze; it is minimal during straight up or straight down gaze. In primary position the down-beating nystagmus is moderate in amplitude and slow in frequency. The frequency but not the amplitude increases on gaze right and left. On oblique downward gaze both amplitude and frequency increase, and on down and left gaze the eyes have a mixed pattern combining vertical and rotary components.

of the extremely short foveation time (instants 0 and 2 on the time axis). Although these are common acquired waveforms, when afflicted with CN, the developing nervous system "modifies" pendular and jerk nystagmus; therefore, foveation time (and thus acuity) is increased. Examples of some resultant waveforms are shown in Fig. 11–9. In pendular nystagmus with a foveating saccade waveform (P_{FS}), there is usually a substantial period of time when the target is imaged on the fovea and the eye is motionless (instant 3 on the time axis). In jerk-right nystagmus with extended foveation (JR_{EF}), the position from time 0 to 1 is when foveation takes place, and in the bidirectional jerk-left (BDJL) waveform, the position from instants 4 to 5 is conducive to good acuity. Waveform, gaze angle nulls, and convergence nulls are affected by heredity.[20] Members of the same family show higher incidences of specific combinations of waveforms or of either waveform, having only a convergence null or no convergence null (*i.e.*, having only a gaze angle null), than do members of the general CN population. Our experience has shown greater damping of CN with convergence than with gaze angle, in patients who exhibited both types of null, and this translated into acuity increases.[21] Comparison of the results of the Anderson-Kestenbaum and artificial divergence procedures also favored the artificial divergence.[22]

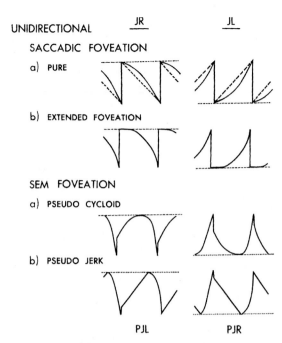

Fig. 11–5. Unidirectional types of jerk nystagmus including two with saccadic foveation (*pure* jerk and jerk with *extended foveation*) and two with slow eye movement (*SEM*) foveation (*pseudocycloid* and *pseudojerk*). For the pure jerk waveform, the more common increasing velocity slow phases are shown *solid,* and the rarer linear slow phases are shown *dashed.* Note small and variable saccadic amplitude in pseudocycloid waveform and further reduction in pseudojerk waveform.

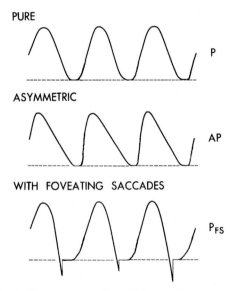

Fig. 11–4. Three types of pendular nystagmus: pure (*P*), asymmetric (*AP*), and pendular with foveating saccades (P_{FS}). Note that although foveating saccades vary in amplitude, they all return the eyes to same point (the target). Foveation takes place at the peaks that are more flattened; here shown as the leftmost peaks. In this and Figs. 11–5 through 11–7 and Fig. 11–13, *dashed lines* indicate target position (see text).

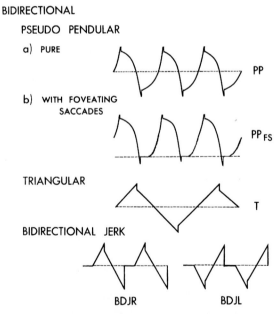

Fig. 11–6. Four types of bidirectional jerk nystagmus: pseudopendular (*PP*), pseudopendular with foveating saccades (PP_{FS}), triangular (*T*), and bidirectional jerk (*BDJ*). All saccades are in a corrective direction (*i.e.*, toward target). Foveating saccades of PP_{FS} vary in amplitude, but all achieve foveation, indicated by the flattened portions of the slow phases.

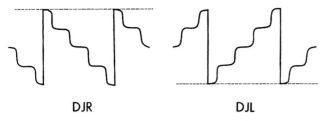

Fig. 11–7. Dual-jerk nystagmus showing sinusoidal modulation of slow eye movement off target. *DJR,* dual-jerk right; *DJL,* dual-jerk left.

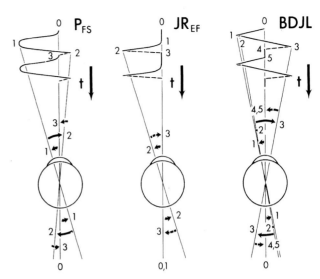

Fig. 11–9. Foveation "strategy" used during pendular nystagmus with foveating saccades (P_{FS}), jerk right with extended foveation (JR_{EF}) nystagmus, and bidirectional jerk left (*BDJL*) nystagmus. The longer the target is foveated, the better will be the good acuity. *t,* time scale.

Increased foveation time is *the most effective* determinant of increased acuity.[23-26] In most CN subjects, the best waveform (*i.e.,* most foveation time per cycle) is in the null region associated with a particular gaze or convergence angle, but in other subjects it is not; these latter subjects prefer the gaze or convergence angle that yields the best waveform, even if it is not the waveform with the least amplitude. We have hypothesized and tested a new type of surgery that shows promise in damping the CN of subjects that do not have either a gaze-angle or a convergence null, have a primary-position null, or do not have a static null [*i.e.,* they have asymmetric (a)periodic alternating CN].[27] The surgery consists of a simple tenotomy, dissection, and suture of the involved extraocular muscles in place, with neither recession nor resection. The various therapies available for CN, based on the presence or absence of gaze and convergence nulls, are summarized in Table 11–3. Note that for patients with both convergence and gaze-angle nulls, exploitation of the former (surgically or with

vergence prisms) usually damps the CN and increases acuity most; it is necessary to add −1.00 S [both eyes (OU)] to vergence prisms for pre-presbyopic patients. As indicated in Table 11–3, afferent stimulation can be used in all patients, regardless of the presence of nulls, who exhibit CN damping with active stimulation (see below).

Despite a nulling of the CN, a subject may not show an increase in acuity with convergence if the resulting waveform has little foveation time per cycle, or if acuity is limited by a primary visual deficit. The fixation system of a subject with CN is able to repeatedly foveate a target within minutes of arc, almost

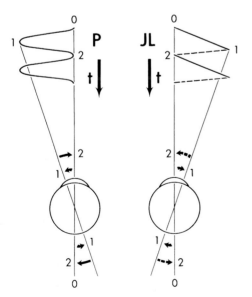

Fig. 11–8. Foveation "strategy" employed during pendular (*P*) and jerk (jerk left, [*JL*]) nystagmus. The target is only briefly foveated at points 0, 2, and so forth. *t,* time scale.

TABLE 11–3. Therapies for Congenital Nystagmus

If the CN nulls ONLY with gaze
  Resection and recession (OU)
  Version prisms
  Afferent stimulation (passive or active)
If the CN nulls ONLY with convergence
  Bimedial recession (artificial divergence)
  Vergence prisms with −1.00 S (OU)
  Afferent stimulation (passive or active)
If the CN nulls with BOTH gaze and convergence
  Bimedial recession alone or combined with resection and
    recession
  Vergence or composite prisms with −1.00 S (OU)
  Afferent stimulation (passive or active)
If the CN nulls with NEITHER gaze nor convergence or is
  asymmetric aperiodic alternating CN
  Tenotomy, dissection, and suture* (OU)
  Maximal recession (OU)
  Afferent stimulation (passive or active)

* This surgery is presently experimental.

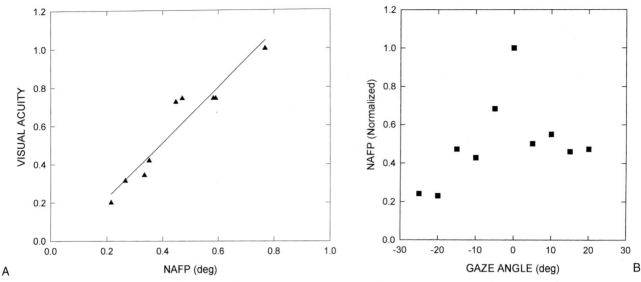

Fig. 11–10. A. The nystagmus acuity function (*NAFP*) vs. visual acuity for nine subjects with congenital nystagmus. **B.** A normalized NAFP vs. gaze angle for a subject with achiasma. (**A,** from ref. 31)

as accurately as a normal person.[21,24,28] The use of "phase-plane" analysis allows definition of a "foveation window" ($\pm 0.5°$ by $\pm 4.0°$/second) for the study of fixation, smooth pursuit, and the vestibulo-ocular reflex (VOR).[21,29,30] These studies demonstrate the extremely accurate fixation, pursuit, and VOR possible in subjects with CN.

The "nystagmus acuity function" (NAF) provides an objective determination of potential visual acuity from measurements of the key characteristics of the CN waveform: foveation time and the standard deviations of foveation position and velocity means (for NAF) or position mean alone (NAFP).[31] Plots of the NAF or NAFP vs. visual acuity reveal a linear relationship that allows intersubject prediction of potential visual acuity (Fig. 11–10A). The NAFs can be used both to compare potential acuity across subjects with different types of nystagmus (CN or LMLN), and to predict the acuity increase due to therapeutic intervention in a given subject. The latter is accomplished by plotting either of the NAFs vs. gaze or convergence angle. Finally, for those subjects whose foveation ability is not well developed (*i.e.*, the target image always falls within the above foveation window), the window used for its calculation can be expanded, and the expanded NAF plotted vs. gaze or convergence angle. Figure 11–10B is a plot of NAFP (normalized to the highest value) from a subject with achiasma, first seen at the Amsterdam Medical Center (see Albinism and Achiasma, below).[32] As the NAFP clearly shows, conditions for highest visual acuity occurred during gaze in primary position. Software that calculates the NAF (or expanded NAF) from eye-movement data provides a quantitative method for evaluating

different therapies for their effect on potential visual acuity.

The so-called inversion of the optokinetic reflex seems to occur only with CN.[33] When optokinetic stimuli are presented to a patient with CN, a peculiar phenomenon may occur: the resulting nystagmus may be opposite in direction from what would be anticipated if the evoked optokinetic nystagmus (OKN) simply summated with the ongoing nystagmus. For example, in the presence of left-beating CN, the response to right-going optokinetic targets (a leftward fast phase) should add to the congenital left-beating nystagmus to produce enhancement of the nystagmus intensity. Instead, the nystagmus may either damp or be converted to right-beating CN. If right-going targets are presented at a gaze angle at which the nystagmus is either absent or pendular, a right-beating CN may result. Inversion of the optokinetic reflex is present in 67% of CN patients. The observation of optokinetic inversion establishes the nystagmus as CN. The phenomenon is, in reality, merely a reversal of the CN direction due to a null shift; it is not a true inversion of the optokinetic response (see discussion of "reversed pursuit," below). The basic function of the optokinetic system is to stabilize slowly moving retinal images, but this function may be interfered with by the rapidly moving retina of a CN patient. It is not surprising that the optokinetic response appears suppressed in some patients; however, the perceived circularvection is in the proper direction, and OKN dynamics appear to be normal in individuals with CN.

The head oscillations that often accompany CN increase with visual intent and have traditionally been regarded as compensatory. For compensation to be achieved, head movements would have to be equal in amplitude and opposite in direction to the eye movements. For such a mechanism to work, the VOR would have to be totally inhibited (gain reduced to 0). Accurate objective observations of the head movements in patients with CN do not support that hypothesis.[34] Rather, the head oscillation is merely an extension of the motor instability, and the VOR functions normally to cancel the effects of head oscillation during the periods of target foveation normally present in the CN waveform.[30] The head tremor in CN can be distinguished from that in acquired disease; it is easily suppressed voluntarily in the former but not in the latter.

> Point out the head tremor to the patient. If it stops, the nystagmus is CN; if it persists, both are acquired.

Patients with CN usually do not experience an illusory oscillatory movement of their environment (oscillopsia). This lack of oscillopsia in CN, and also in LMLN, suggests that both oscillations occur within an efference copy feedback loop that serves to nullify the effects of retinal-image oscillation induced by either of these instabilities.[35] Like most ocular oscillations (myoclonus being the exception), CN disappears in sleep. In two patients with CN plus an acquired nystagmus, their acquired oscillopsia seemed to be related to an inability to maintain repeatable periods of good foveation in a particular plane.[36,37] However, that inability was an epiphenomenon caused by the addition of a transitory acquired nystagmus to the ever-present CN.[35] Oscillopsia suppression in CN and other types of nystagmus appears to be accomplished by efference copy of the nystagmus signal.[35,38–41]

During fixation of stationary targets, many patients with CN have a permanent null region representing the gaze angle at which the intensity of the nystagmus is the lowest (Fig. 11–11). They often turn their heads to permit straight-ahead viewing with the eyes in the null region. Such patients benefit from appropriate prism spectacles that alleviate the necessity for the head turn and the resulting increased fixation attempt.[14,23]

Some CN patients may exhibit a "superimposed latent" component that induces null shifts toward an eye that is covered (Fig. 11–12).[42] Demonstration of such a shift and maintenance of any of the CN waveforms establish the nystagmus as congenital rather than latent (see below). Rarely, a null shift is toward the viewing eye.[14]

Some studies of CN and smooth pursuit have led to confusion between the reversal of CN direction that may occur during pursuit and "reversed pursuit." This confusion is similar to that discussed earlier for the optokinetic response. Accurate eye-movement recordings show that neither subsystem responds in a reversed manner, as should be obvious both by the ab-

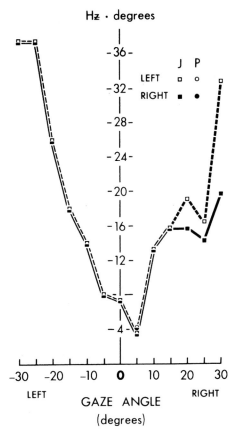

Fig. 11–11. Binocular intensity function for both pendular (P) and jerk (J) nystagmus. The null angle is at 5° right gaze.

sence of any symptoms of such a grave deficit and the normal abilities of CN patients in sports. Also, their perceptions of both the direction and magnitude of movements in the periphery and on the fovea are equal to those of normals. Just as the CN waveform is distorted by SEM (creating periods of extended foveation) during fixation of a stationary target, the pursuit system is able to generate pursuit movements with a direction and velocity that match those of a moving target during these same periods of the CN waveform.[29,38,43] This ensures extended foveation of the moving target and results in accurate smooth pursuit during the periods when the target image is on the fovea. Pursuit during foveation is all that is necessary for good acuity; the same conditions are met during smooth pursuit as are met during fixation of a stationary target. It has been documented that during smooth pursuit (or during optokinetic or VOR stimuli) the gaze angle at which the CN null region occurs shifts in the direction opposite to the pursuit (optokinetic grating or VOR-induced eye motion).[29,30] The amount of null shift is related to the pursuit or VOR velocity. It is this shift in the CN null angle that causes the CN reversal that has been mistakenly equated

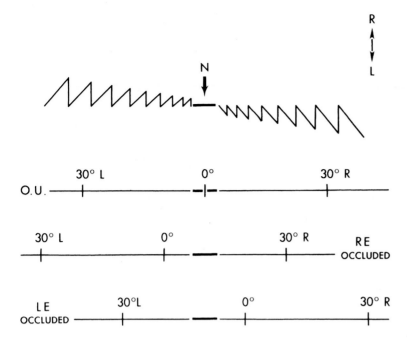

Fig. 11–12. Depiction of shifts of neutral zone or null (*N*) in congenital nystagmus. Tracing demonstrates an idealized nystagmus pattern with both eyes open (*O.U.*). Neutral zone extends over several degrees on either side of 0°. When gaze is directed laterally, nystagmus of increasing amplitude develops with fast phase in direction of gaze. Occlusion of right eye (*RE*) shifts zone to the right; at 0° there is left-beating nystagmus. Occlusion of left eye (*LE*) shifts zone to the left; at 0° there is right-beating nystagmus.

with "reversed" responses of both the optokinetic and pursuit subsystems.

In many subjects with CN, afferent stimulation of the ophthalmic division of the trigeminal nerve or of the neck may damp the nystagmus, allowing increased visual acuity.[31,44] Neck or forehead vibration prolonged foveation periods, yielding higher values of the NAF and improved visual acuity in 9 of 13 patients with CN.[31] This non-invasive and benign therapy (active afferent stimulation) may prove useful in both CN and acquired nystagmus. The use of soft contact lenses to improve the acuity of individuals with CN takes advantage of the damping effect on CN of (passive) afferent stimulation.[45–48]

> Soft contact lenses are not contraindicated in CN and can provide better acuity than spectacles in patients whose CN damps with afferent stimulation. Plano soft contact lenses can be used if no refractive correction is required.

Relatives of patients with CN may have *saccadic* instabilities,[49] and carriers of blue-cone monochromatism may have vertical (upbeat and downbeat) nystagmus and LMLN.[50]

Latent/Manifest Latent

Latent/manifest latent nystagmus (LMLN) is a jerk nystagmus with either a linear or decreasing-velocity exponential slow phase identical to that of gaze-paretic nystagmus. Occasionally, when both eyes are closed, a jerk nystagmus with a linear slow phase is present.

Classically, "pure" or "true" latent nystagmus (LN) occurs only with uniocular fixation. There is no nystagmus with both eyes viewing, but when one eye is occluded, nystagmus develops in both eyes, with the fast phase toward the uncovered eye (Fig. 11–13). LN is always congenital. However, several cases of manifest latent nystagmus (MLN) associated with retrolental fibroplasia have been recorded.[51]

Early theories postulated that a unilateral retinal stimulus was the necessary condition for LN, but this concept was discounted by observations of LN in monocular fixation with a blind eye or with an acoustic stimulus in complete darkness. Similarly, the hypothesis that LN is caused by nasal-temporal asymmetries in the optokinetic reflex is not supported by evidence that subjects with LMLN are able to use retinal slip information to adapt motion-detection sensitivities[52] and are able to pursue symmetrically.[53] Also, because nasal-temporal asymmetries exist in individuals with strabismus but not LMLN,[52] this cannot be the primary causal factor in the genesis of LMLN. Asymmetries in the monocular optokinetic response of monkeys deprived of binocular input early in life may result from, rather than cause, their LN. In normal monkeys, each nucleus of the optic tract (NOT) is driven binocularly; in these monkeys, they are driven by the contralateral eye.[54] Although the resulting imbalance may provide the tonic signal that produces the LMLN slow phases (inactivation of the NOT with muscimol abolishes the LMLN), the cause of the imbalance appears to lie in higher centers.

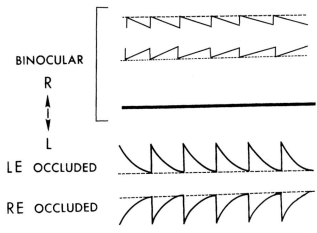

Fig. 11–13. Latent/manifest latent nystagmus. With both eyes open there is either low-amplitude manifest latent nystagmus (when only one eye is fixating) or, rarely, no nystagmus (when both eyes are fixating). Closure of either eye results in jerk nystagmus with fast phases toward the viewing (unoccluded) eye. When both eyes are open, the nystagmus fast phases are toward the fixating eye. Slow phases may be either linear (usually when both eyes are open) or decreasing-velocity exponentials (usually upon occlusion of one eye), unlike those of CN. Note that the fast phases may be foveating (for low-amplitude LMLN with linear slow phases) or defoveating (for the higher amplitude LMLN with decreasing velocity slow phases).

Our own observations have led us to relate LMLN to the cortical switching that must occur in the calculation of egocentric direction when going from binocular to monocular viewing.[51] Under binocular conditions, the gaze angle of each eye is summed with the other and divided by two to obtain the egocentric direction, referenced to the "cyclopean eye." However, with monocular viewing, egocentric direction depends only on the viewing eye, and the cortical operation of summing and dividing by two must be altered to process unchanged information from the viewing eye. The shift in egocentric direction toward the nonviewing eye causes the slow drift of the eyes in that direction. Both eyes are then corrected by a saccade in the direction of the viewing eye, which brings the eyes to the target (or, in darkness, to the intended gaze angle). This contention is supported by unilateral strabismus surgery causing central effects on egocentric localization.[55] Thus, LMLN can be generated by this inability to properly alter the cortical mathematical operation normally used to define egocentric direction.

The shift to monocular egocentric localization can also produce a mode whereby the saccadic system is used to produce defoveating saccades that momentarily carry the fixating eye past the target in a temporal direc-tion, followed by a decelerating-velocity nasal drift back toward the target.[56] This would be equivalent to generating a pulse, but not a step, of innervation to drive the fast phases of the LMLN. Presumably, the common neural integrator is kept from integrating these defoveating pulses by the signal representing the correct eye position vis-à-vis the target.

MLN occurs in patients with strabismus who, although viewing with both eyes open, are fixing monocularly. The slow phases are of the expected decreasing exponential form, and the fast phases are always in the direction of the viewing eye.[51] The nystagmus of patients with strabismus, alternating fixation, and MLN has fast phases always in the direction of the fixating eye. Such patients are usually misdiagnosed as having CN, because the nystagmus is present with both eyes open. Recordings are required to document the decreasing exponential slow phase that delineates LMLN from CN, which has an increasing exponential slow phase. LMLN may be part of a syndrome with strabismus, alternating hyperphoria, and pendular torsional nystagmus in primary position.

Strabismus is a necessary (but not sufficient) condition for LMLN.[57] That is, all patients with LMLN have strabismus, consisting of a phoria under cover and a tropia with both eyes open, if LN or MLN is present under these respective conditions. Conversely, LMLN is not significantly associated with early-onset strabismus.[58] Rarely, on occlusion of a preferred eye, during which fixation with an amblyopic eye is forced, both eyes drift in the direction of the covered eye without corrections by fast phases. This is called "latent deviation." Early surgical correction of infantile strabismus may convert MLN to LN,[59] thereby supporting a previous hypothesis.[57]

Because the good acuity of CN patients is related to the long, postsaccadic foveation periods of many waveforms, it is difficult to explain the equally good acuity of LMLN patients, given the absence of such periods. Accurate studies of LMLN foveation have revealed a dual strategy.[56] During low-amplitude, linear-slow-phase LMLN, the saccadic fast phases foveate the target, and the low-velocity slow phases take the eye away from the target with little effect on acuity. During the higher amplitude, decreasing-velocity slow-phase MLN, the saccadic fast phases defoveate the target, allowing foveation during the low-velocity, tail ends of the slow phases (see Fig. 11–13); this ensures the best acuity possible.

Although most patients have either CN or LMLN, some have both; three unambiguous patient groups have been identified: CN, LMLN, and CN + LMLN.[20] The three groups exhibit different clinical signs and relations to strabismus; most CN patients do not have strabismus, but all LMLN patients do. Thus, CN and

LMLN are specific, easily differentiated disorders and do not, as has been suggested,[60] represent a unitary disorder with a broad spectrum of expression. Because no acquired, time-independent, primary-position jerk nystagmus reverses direction with alternate eye cover, a simple reverse-cover test can be a powerful clinical tool.

> To distinguish among benign, infantile, primary-position, jerk nystagmus, and that which is acquired and symptomatic, first verify that there is no periodic alternation in direction and then perform a reverse-cover test. If the cover test causes a reversal in the nystagmus direction consistent with LMLN, the nystagmus is benign (LMLN or CN with a latent component). If not, rule out CN (history, clinical signs (see Table 11–2), waveforms).

Nystagmus Blockage Syndrome

The nystagmus blockage syndrome (NBS) is both a poorly understood and an overdiagnosed phenomenon related to CN. As the name suggests, the nystagmus of these patients diminishes or disappears with the act of *willed esotropia* while fixating a distant target. This should not be confused with the damping of CN during convergence on a near target. There are two mechanisms by which blockage of the ongoing nystagmus can be accomplished.[61] During the willed esotropia, some CN merely damps or stops, in much the same way as with true convergence. In the second type of NBS, the CN converts to MLN with the onset of the strabismus. Normally, the substitution of the MLN slow phases for the CN waveforms that allow for better foveation would not be advantageous. However, in these few patients, the small MLN amplitude results in better acuity than the larger CN amplitude. NBS is often misdiagnosed in MLN patients with a strong Alexander's law variation of their nystagmus, which causes them to fixate with their adducting eye.[61]

Acquired

Secondary to Visual Loss

Nystagmus occurring in early childhood consequent to progressive bilateral visual loss should not be classified as CN unless CN waveforms are documented. The conceptual problems in the classification were discussed above. Usually, nystagmus secondary to visual loss cannot be distinguished from CN in a patient with coexisting primary visual abnormalities.

The nystagmus associated with rod monochromacy (complete congenital achromatopsia) is said to be distinguishable from other forms of CN on the basis of slow buildup of the slow component velocity of OKN. This occurs during monocular stimulation and directional asymmetry of OKN when the temporal-to-nasal direction is compared with the nasal-to-temporal direction.[62] Patients with blindness from birth and nystagmus may have an impaired VOR and an inability to initiate saccades voluntarily, despite the presence of quick phases of nystagmus.[63] Adults with "eye movements of the blind" exhibit features similar to those of patients with cerebellar disease.[63] Cats reared from birth in stroboscopic illumination develop low-amplitude nystagmus; this is believed to be an animal model for nystagmus secondary to visual loss.[64]

Monocular visual loss may produce monocular nystagmus, usually vertical, at any age from birth through adult life. The fact that the nystagmus is monocular and usually vertical makes it distinguishable from CN, but it may mimic spasmus nutans, particularly if there is associated head nodding.

Spasmus Nutans

Spasmus nutans is a rare constellation of ocular oscillation, head nodding, and torticollis that begins in infancy (usually between 4 and 18 months of age) and disappears in childhood (usually before 3 years of age). The nystagmus is generally bilateral (but can differ in each eye and may even be strictly monocular), and it oscillates in horizontal, torsional, or vertical directions. An instance of spasmus nutans presenting with monocular nystagmus in monozygous twins has been reported.[65] Spasmus nutans may sometimes be mimicked by tumors of the optic nerve, chiasm, or third ventricle[66]; therefore, any child with suspected spasmus nutans should have brain imaging. Retinal disease has been reported to mimic the clinical signs of spasms nutans,[67] as has a case of opsoclonus-myoclonus.[68]

The nystagmus tends to be asymmetric in the two eyes, to vary in different directions of gaze, and to be rapid and of small amplitude. The head nodding is inconstant and irregular and can be horizontal or vertical, or both. The average duration of spasmus nutans is 12 to 24 months; rarely, it lasts a number of years. Studies of quantitative head- and eye-movement recordings indicate that the head movement may, using the normal VOR, actually serve to abolish the eye movements.[69] In some patients, it may be only compensatory with suppression of the VOR.

The pendular oscillation of spasmus nutans is characterized by a variable phase difference between the oscillations of each eye.[70] These phase differences can appear from minute to minute and during the child's development. The dissociated nystagmus is usually of a higher frequency than CN, and the result can be disconjugate, conjugate, or uniocular. We hypothesize that spasmus nutans is a yoking abnormality, perhaps due to delayed development. Recordings show that, in some cases, spasmus nutans may not disappear completely but may recede to a subclinical level; CN and LMLN do not disappear with age.

Acquired Pendular Nystagmus (Adults)

Acquired pendular nystagmus may reflect brain stem or cerebellar dysfunction, or both. It occurs in patients with vascular or demyelinating disease. In the latter, it has been regarded as a sign of cerebellar nuclear lesions. The nystagmus is multivectorial (i.e., horizontal, vertical, diagonal, elliptic, or circular) and usually is associated with a head tremor. Marked dissociation between the two eyes often exists and may not correlate with differences in visual acuity from co-existing optic neuropathy.[71] Despite the dissociation, the oscillations of the two eyes are phase-locked, even when there is a difference in their frequencies.[72] Acquired pendular nystagmus has also been found in autosomal peroxisomal disorder.[73] Gabapentin was found to be effective in treating some forms of acquired pendular nystagmus.[73,74]

Rarely, acquired pendular nystagmus in the adult becomes manifest with acquired amblyopia, as mentioned above. Scopolamine has been reported to be an effective treatment,[75] but botulinum toxin is of limited efficacy in treating acquired pendular nystagmus.[76] A review of current therapeutic approaches to various types of nystagmus and saccadic oscillations, based on known physiology and pharmacology, points out the need for more precise, double-blind studies.[77]

Miner's nystagmus is a rarity limited presumably to mine workers in the United Kingdom. It is described as a small-amplitude, horizontal, and vertical nystagmus that is often more pronounced in upward gaze. The pathogenesis of this putative dysfunction is uncertain, but functional contamination with voluntary "nystagmus" is suspected; a secondary gain setting is usually present.

Except for the dissociation between the two eyes, acquired pendular nystagmus may be similar to pendular CN; both can have associated head tremor and characteristically damp with eyelid closure. Studies into the pathogenesis of acquired pendular nystagmus have ruled out delayed visual feedback and increased gain in the visually enhanced VOR as causal factors.[78]

Acquired Horizontal Jerk Nystagmus

Vestibular

We generally delimit vestibular nystagmus as being consequent to dysfunction of the vestibular end-organ, nerve, or nuclear complex within the brain stem. It is a horizontal-torsional or purely horizontal, primary-position jerk nystagmus with a linear slow phase. The nystagmus intensity increases with gaze toward the fast phase (obeying Alexander's law); it decreases and, with central lesions, may reverse directions upon gaze toward the direction of the slow phase. The symptom of vertigo usually co-exists. As might be expected, acute lesions of the cerebellar flocculus (the vestibulocerebellum) can produce a similar nystagmus (see Chapter 10). Cases of discrete cerebellar infarction are quite rare. Nystagmus may accompany episodic attacks of ataxia.[79] Evidence has been presented supporting a specific chromosomal abnormality in some cases[80] and brain stem lesions in others.[81] For practical clinical purposes, the responsible lesion in vestibular nystagmus is located in either the end-organ, nerve, or brain stem. Such localization requires an appreciation of the manifestations of end-organ dysfunction. In normal subjects, some degree of nystagmus and vertigo develops when the labyrinth (end-organ) is stimulated with warm or cold water applied to the tympanic membrane. The direction of the resulting nystagmus, in terms of the fast (jerk) phase, can be remembered by the mnemonic "COWS" (cold, opposite; warm, same). Cold water in the left ear (or warm water in the right) induces a right-beating nystagmus; cold water in the right ear (or warm water in the left) induces a left-beating nystagmus. In addition, the subject experiences vertigo and, with eye closure, past-points with an outstretched arm and falls in a consistent direction on Romberg testing. The apparent direction of the vertiginous movement, whether of the environment or self, is always in the direction of the fast phase of the nystagmus. The past-pointing and Romberg fall are always in the direction of the slow phase. For example, with cold water placed in the external canal of the left ear, the subject develops a right-beating jerk nystagmus and experiences environmental or bodily movement to the right (paradoxically appearing to move continuously in one direction).[82] With the eyes closed, the patient's attempts at pointing an outstretched finger at a target in front of him result in past-pointing to the left; on standing there is a tendency to fall to the left (in the direction of the slow phase of the nystagmus). This Romberg fall can be directionally altered by head turning: with the head turned to the left, the slow phase is directed toward the rear and the fall is backward; with the head turned to the right, the fall is forward.[83]

These manifestations of cold-water irrigation mimic the effects of a destructive lesion of the vestibular end-organ; warm-water irrigation mimics an irritative lesion. Clinically, most diseases of the end-organ create destructive effects. Irritative phenomena occur but are transient, often subclinical, and usually of interest only to the electronystagmographer. During an attack of Meniere's disease, there may be ipsilateral (jerk toward the affected side) nystagmus. Perhaps the most common cause of ipsilateral nystagmus secondary to end-organ disease is "recovery nystagmus."[84] Here, spontaneous nystagmus that occurs after a unilateral labyrinthine lesion may transiently reverse direction as some function is restored in the damaged end-organ. This probably reflects the compensatory "central rebalancing" of the vestibular nuclei. This compensation can also change a primary-position vestibular nystagmus (of peripheral or central etiology) to a paroxysmal positional nystagmus.[85]

A patient with unidirectional jerk nystagmus, vertigo in the direction of the fast-phase component, and past-pointing and Romberg fall in the direction of the slow component is suffering acute dysfunction of the vestibular end-organ on the side of the nystagmus *slow phase*. When the pattern of direction for the nystagmus, vertigo, past-pointing, and Romberg fall is not as just described but varies in some aspect, the symptom complex represents an abnormality of the central vestibular nuclei. Thus, in central vestibular disease, the vertigo may be in the direction of the slow phase of the nystagmus, and the past-pointing or Romberg fall may be toward the fast phase.

Other factors distinguish peripheral from central vestibular nystagmus. Pure vertical or pure torsional nystagmus is never peripheral and always represents central dysfunction. Similarly, pure horizontal nystagmus without a torsional component is suggestive of central disease.[82] Nystagmus that is reduced in intensity by visual fixation is peripheral, whereas nystagmus due to central lesions is usually not reduced, and may even be enhanced, by fixation. Peripheral vestibular nystagmus is best visualized clinically behind Frenzel lenses (+20 diopters), which eliminate the inhibiting effects of visual fixation and magnify the eyes.[86] A marked bidirectionality to the nystagmus (left-beating on left gaze, and a similarly severe right-beating nystagmus on right gaze) is almost always central. Table 11–4 presents the differential features of peripheral and central vestibular nystagmus.

Gaze-Evoked (Gaze-Paretic) Nystagmus

Gaze-evoked nystagmus is elicited by the attempt to maintain an eccentric eye position, and it is the most common form of nystagmus encountered in clinical practice. Patients recovering from a central gaze palsy show a phase in which lateral gaze movement is possible but cannot be maintained in the deviated position; that is, the eyes drift back slowly toward primary position (see Chapter 10). A corrective saccade repositions the eyes eccentrically, and repetition

TABLE 11–4. Vestibular Nystagmus

Symptom or sign	Peripheral (end-organ)	Central (nuclear)
Direction of nystagmus	Unidirectional, fast phase opposite lesion	Bidirectional or unidirectional
Pure horizontal nystagmus without torsional component	Uncommon	Common
Vertical or purely torsional nystagmus	Never present	May be present
Visual fixation	Inhibits nystagmus and vertigo	No inhibition
Severity of vertigo	Marked	Mild
Direction of spin	Toward slow phase	Variable
Direction of past-pointing	Toward slow phase	Variable
Direction of Romberg fall	Toward slow phase	Variable
Effect of head turning	Changes Romberg fall	No effect
Duration of symptoms	Finite (minutes, days, weeks) but recurrent	May be chronic
Tinnitus and/or deafness	Often present	Usually absent
Common causes	Infection (labyrinthitis), Meniere's disease, neuronitis, vascular, trauma, toxicity	Vascular, demyelinating, and neoplastic disorders

of this pattern produces nystagmus, aptly designated "gaze-paretic." This was a clinical description that was not based on oculographic findings. Information about the role of the brain stem neural integrators (see Chapter 9) led to the presumption that a defective integrator would result in the inability of the eyes to maintain an eccentric position, causing them to drift toward the center with a decreasing-velocity exponential waveform. This is indeed the waveform that defines the gaze-paretic subtype of gaze-evoked nystagmus, which is particularly prevalent in patients with cerebellar disease that especially involves the flocculus (see Chapter 10). It has been postulated that there is an inherent "leakiness" of the brain stem neural integrators, namely, a tendency to drift from a given firing level. The cerebellar flocculus normally corrects for this drift. With a floccular lesion, the leakiness and drift are unchecked, and gaze-paretic nystagmus develops. If the integrator leak is small and the time-constant long, a gaze-paretic nystagmus could have a slow phase that is linear rather than a decreasing-velocity exponential. Such nystagmus cannot be designated as gaze-paretic with any degree of certainty and may only be described as gaze-evoked.

In summary, the term *gaze-paretic nystagmus* is restricted to a subgroup of gaze-evoked nystagmus with a decreasing-velocity exponential slow phase. It is "integrator nystagmus" with a defect in the step function of neural firing frequency constituting the pathophysiologic mechanism. The same integrators are probably responsible for smooth-pursuit eye movements, which seem to be invariably abnormal in patients with gaze-paretic nystagmus.

The most common cause of pathologic, bidirectional, gaze-evoked nystagmus is sedative or anticonvulsant medication. The nystagmus fast phase is always in the direction of gaze (toward the right on right gaze, left-beating on left gaze, and upbeating on upward gaze; down gaze is usually without nystagmus). In the absence of drugs, horizontal gaze-evoked nystagmus with linear slow phases can be localized only enough to indicate brain stem or, if unilateral, labyrinthine dysfunction. Analysis of the associated neurologic signs and symptoms would be required for more precise localization.

Gaze-evoked vertical nystagmus almost always coexists with the horizontal variety. Primary-position vertical jerk nystagmus (upbeat and downbeat) is discussed below.

Special Nystagmus Types

Physiologic (End-Point)

There are three basic types of nystagmus that are regarded as normal (physiologic) phenomena:[87]

Fatigue nystagmus begins during extended maintenance of an extreme gaze position and has been found in up to 60% of normals when horizontal gaze is maximally deviated for a time exceeding 30 seconds. It may become increasingly torsional with prolonged deviation effort and may be greater in the adducting eye. Fatigue nystagmus is not a clinically important phenomenon, because routine examinations do not include the maintenance of far eccentric gaze.

Unsustained end-point nystagmus is certainly the most frequently encountered physiologic nystagmus. Its incidence and characteristics have never been studied quantitatively. All experienced clinicians recognize that a few beats of nystagmus are within perfectly normal limits at gaze deviations of 30° or more.

Sustained end-point nystagmus begins immediately upon, or within several seconds of, reaching an eccentric lateral-gaze position. It has been found in more than 60% of normal subjects with horizontal-gaze maintenance greater than 40°. Quantitative oculography reveals that physiologic nystagmus can begin with only a 20° deviation[87] and is almost universal at deviations of 40° or more.[88] The slow phase is linear, except with an extreme 40° to 50° deviation, in which a decreasing-velocity exponential may develop. The nystagmus may be different in the two eyes, but it is symmetric in the two lateral directions. The amplitude of physiologic nystagmus does not exceed 3°.[87] Thus, small-amplitude gaze-evoked nystagmus may be a normal phenomenon, provided the slow phase, with gaze angles up to 40°, is linear. The onset of end-point nystagmus is related to slow drift velocity,[89] and the reduction of drift velocity during fixation (probably by the fixation subsystem) inhibits the nystagmus. Gaze-evoked nystagmus is by necessity "pathologic" if any of three features are present: (1) asymmetry in the two directions, (2) amplitude of 4° or more, or (3) exponential slow phase within a gaze angle of less than 40°.

Dissociated

Nystagmus in which the two eyes show a significant asymmetry in either amplitude or direction is considered "dissociated." The most common type of dissociation is that observed in internuclear ophthalmoplegias; it is most marked in the abducting eye (see Chapter 10). Abduction "nystagmus," which is sometimes designated by the confusing term *ataxic nystagmus*, is not really a nystagmus. This saccadic oscillation is secondary to lesions of the medial longitudinal fasciculus, and is discussed under Saccadic Pulses/Pulse Trains later in this chapter and in Chapter 10.

The pendular nystagmus in patients with multiple sclerosis is usually dissociated. A variety of nystagmus dissociations with diverse lesions of the posterior fossa have been described (*e.g.,* asymmetric vertical nystagmus greater in one eye on looking up and in the other eye on looking down in a young girl with a recurrent cerebellar medulloblastoma).

Torsional

Torsional nystagmus describes a torsional movement of the globe about its anteroposterior axis; the term *rotary nystagmus* is used interchangeably. Most nystagmus consequent to vestibular end-organ dysfunction has a torsional component admixed with a major horizontal or vertical nystagmus. A purely torsional nystagmus never occurs with vestibular end-organ disease. When of small amplitude, torsional nystagmus may reflect a medullary lesion. Larger-amplitude torsional nystagmus may be congenital, but when it is acquired it often indicates diencephalic (thalamic) involvement, in which case it is the underlying pattern in see-saw nystagmus. Torsional nystagmus can be classified into two groups.[90] In group I the nystagmus is in primary position, and in group II it is gaze-evoked. The etiologies of both groups are either demyelinating, vascular, or neoplastic.

For consistency, nystagmus in the torsional plane should be defined with respect to the subject, *not* the observer. When a subject's nystagmus beats to his or her right, it is called jerk-right nystagmus; if it beats toward his or her forehead, it is upbeat (even if the subject is in the head-hanging position). Therefore, when the nystagmus fast phases bring the top of the eye toward the subject's right shoulder, it is *clockwise* nystagmus. Clinical descriptions of torsional nystagmus, made from the observer's point of view, deviate from the accepted convention that applies to both horizontal and vertical movements. Maintaining the subject-based directions reduces confusion, eases understanding of anatomic substrates, and anchors the subject's perception of oscillopsia to the direction of his nystagmus. Just as leftward horizontal slow phases cause rightward perceived world motion, clockwise torsional slow phases cause counterclockwise perceived world motion (see Circular, Elliptic, and Oblique, below).

See-Saw

See-saw nystagmus is characterized by conjugate, pendular, torsional oscillation with a superimposed disjunctive vertical vector. The intorting eye rises and the opposite, extorting eye falls. Repetition of this sequence in the alternate direction provides the see-saw effect. The torsional movements predominate in all fields of gaze, but the see-saw feature may be restricted to the primary position or, more commonly, to downward or lateral gaze. See-saw nystagmus can be of the jerk type (with one phase being slow and the other fast) with unilateral meso-diencephalic lesions.[91] Most patients with acquired see-saw nystagmus have bitemporal hemianopias consequent to large parasellar tumors expanding within the third ventricle. It is occasionally evoked transiently after blinks or saccades.[92] Upper brain stem vascular disease and severe head trauma are the next most common etiologies. Post-traumatic see-saw may be temporarily abolished by ingestion of alcohol.[93] Rarely, the nystagmus is associated with septo-optic dysplasia, an Arnold-Chiari malformation,[94] multiple sclerosis,[95] or loss of vision alone.[96] See-saw nystagmus probably reflects diencephalic (thalamic) dysfunction possibly of a pathway or pathways from the zona incerta to the interstitial nucleus of Cajal. A study of visual-vestibular interaction concluded that see-saw nystagmus resulted from a loss of retinal error signals secondary to disruption of chiasmal crossing fibers.[97]

Congenital see-saw nystagmus manifests either in constant vertical disconjugacies without a significant torsional component or in conjugate torsional nystagmus with a vertical component that can be opposite to that of the acquired variety; that is, the intorting eye falls while the extorting eye rises. Congenital see-saw nystagmus is also seen in canine and human achiasma (see Albinism and Achiasma, below). An unusual instance of congenital see-saw nystagmus in two mentally retarded adult siblings, associated with retinitis pigmentosa, had the typical vertical/torsional relationship associated with acquired see-saw.[98]

The ocular tilt reaction, described in Chapter 10, is actually one-half of a see-saw cycle.

Convergence/Convergence-Evoked

The act of convergence usually damps nystagmus, particularly the congenital type.[99] Convergence can also damp[99] or evoke[100] lid nystagmus and may damp or enhance downbeat nystagmus.[101] Upbeat nystagmus may change to downbeat with convergence.[102]

Repetitive divergence is a term describing a slow divergence movement followed by a rapid convergence to the primary position. The movements occur at irregular intervals, distinguishing this from nystagmus.[103] In the single reported instance of this phenomenon in a patient with hepatic encephalopathy, an entire cycle lasted from 4 to 10 seconds, and the interval between cycles was 1 to 15 seconds.

Nystagmus evoked by convergence must be distinguished from "convergence nystagmus." Convergence-retraction "nystagmus" as a manifestation of the dorsal midbrain syndrome is discussed in Chapter 10; here, the initiating convergence movements are saccadic,[104] and thus not a true nystagmus. Fast divergent movements, followed by a slow convergence, associated with epileptic electroencephalographic activity, occurred in a neonate with an intraventricular hemorrhage.[105]

With the exception of pure convergence nystagmus in infants with spasmus nutans, true pendular convergence nystagmus is uncommon. It was observed in a patient with presumed progressive supranuclear palsy who had paralysis of all volitional eye movements. In retrospect, however, it is probable that the patient had central nervous system Whipple's disease, perhaps the most common cause of pendular convergence nystagmus (see Chapter 10). A study of three patients with convergence nystagmus revealed phase shifts of about 180° in both the horizontal and torsional planes with conjugate nystagmus in the vertical plane.[106] Convergence increased the nystagmus in two of the patients. The waveforms were either sinusiodal or complex sums of sinusoids, and in one patient they were cycloidal. Unlike the pseudocycloid waveform of CN, there were no initiating saccades to these cycloidal movements. Low-frequency convergence nystagmus was hypothesized to result from a visually mediated vergence instability, whereas high-frequency forms might have arisen from an instability in internal brain stem connections associated with vergence.

Nystagmus evoked by convergence is unusual and may be either conjugate or disconjugate, congenital or acquired.[107] In two cases reported, no definite clinical correlation could be made with a specific lesion. The neuropathologic examination revealed no morphologic explanation for nystagmus in the patient with congenital convergence-evoked nystagmus; the patient with the acquired form had demyelinating disease with a spastic paraparesis and no cranial nerve abnormality other than the ocular motor findings.[107] Horizontal pendular nystagmus rarely is evoked by accommodative vergence.[108] This is to be distinguished from the so-called voluntary nystagmus (discussed below), which is often best accomplished when the eyes are slightly converged.

Periodic Alternating

Periodic alternating nystagmus (PAN) is an extraordinary ocular motor phenomenon in which a persisting horizontal jerk nystagmus periodically changes directions. PAN may be congenital or acquired. The congenital variety, which may be associated with albinism,[109,110] has the slow-phase waveform of an increasing-velocity exponential and usually lacks the well-defined stereotyped periodicity seen in acquired PAN (i.e., it is asym-

metric aperiodic alternating nystagmus). The periodicity of the congenital PAN is markedly influenced by changes in gaze position, supporting the hypothesis that the PAN is a result of a temporal shift in the null zone (Fig. 11–14).[42]

> Patients with CN and a varying head turn should be examined for PAN.

The usual sequence in acquired PAN consists of about 90 seconds of nystagmus beating in one direction, 10 seconds of a neutral phase in which the eyes stop or beat downward irregularly, and 90 seconds of beating in the opposite direction. This periodicity is continuous during waking hours and may prevail during sleep. Some patients demonstrate asymmetries in the timing of the two major phases, but the basic pattern for each patient is usually invariable.

In a detailed clinical and control-system study, Leigh and colleagues[111] proposed that PAN arises from (1) a defect in the brain stem neural networks that generates slow phases of vestibular and optokinetic nystagmus; (2) the action of an adaptive network that normally acts to null prolonged, inappropriate nystagmus; and (3) an inability to use retinal-error velocity information. They proposed a control system model that denied access of

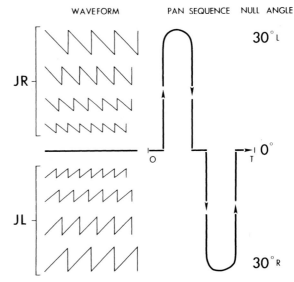

Fig. 11–14. Periodic alternating nystagmus (*PAN*) sequence is depicted in relation to waveform and null angle. Sequence reflects one PAN period (from *O* to *T*). Period begins in a neutral phase; null is at 0°. As null shifts to the left, jerk-right (*JR*) nystagmus develops and gradually increases in amplitude to maximum when null is at extreme left (*e.g.,* 30°L). Null then shifts back toward 0° and *JR* nystagmus decreases, finally stopping and forming the next neutral phase when null reaches 0°. The same sequence of null shifting to right and back accounts for jerk left (*JL*) phase. The diagram is idealized and does not reflect the asymmetries of the true clinical state. (From ref. 42.)

visual signals to the OKN-vestibular system. This model is particularly appealing because of the occasional relationship between impaired vision and PAN. Support for their hypothesis of impairment in the velocity storage element was presented by Furman and colleagues,[112] who studied four patients with PAN. PAN has been described after bilateral vitreous hemorrhages (associated with a massive subarachnoid hemorrhage) and after cataracts. It disappeared after bilateral vitrectomy and after cataract surgery. Ablation of the nodulus and ventral uvula of the cerebellum in monkeys produces PAN.[113]

Although numerous conditions have been associated with PAN, including CN, head trauma, vascular insufficiency, encephalitis, syphilis, multiple sclerosis, spinocerebellar degenerations, and posterior fossa tumors, particular attention should be directed to an abnormality of the craniocervical junction. The possibility of a lesion should be investigated with magnetic resonance imaging. PAN may coexist with downbeat nystagmus, which also suggests an abnormality in the same location.

PAN has been described as secondary to phenytoin intoxication in a patient with alcoholic cerebellar degeneration.[114] The antispasticity drug baclofen abolishes acquired PAN but has no effect on the congenital variety.[115] The drug abolished experimentally created PAN in the monkey,[113] as well as a single case of aperiodic alternating nystagmus in a patient with vertebrobasilar insufficiency.[116]

PAN may be associated with a periodic alternating skew deviation.[117] Periodic alternating gaze deviations, with and without associated alternating nystagmus or alternating head turning, are rare, related phenomena.[118] PAN should not be confused with the nystagmus occurring in the enigmatic, usually familial, acetazolamide-responsive, paroxysmal ataxia syndrome.[119]

Downbeat

Downbeat nystagmus is defined as nystagmus in primary gaze position, with the fast phase beating in a downward direction. Patients with brain stem disease or drug intoxications usually lack gaze-evoked downward nystagmus despite nystagmus in all other fields of gaze. Thus, nystagmus beating downward in the primary position is a striking phenomenon and is highly suggestive of a disorder of the craniocervical junction, such as Arnold-Chiari malformations.[120,121] Downbeat nystagmus is usually of sufficient amplitude in primary position to cause oscillopsia, and, contrary to Alexander's law,[2] it is not maximal at the extreme of downward gaze. Rather, it is usually of maximum intensity when the eyes are deviated laterally and slightly below the horizontal[121]; the nystagmus may be intermittent.

The other major cause of downbeat nystagmus is spinocerebellar degeneration. Indeed, it is difficult to ascertain from the literature whether an Arnold-Chiari malformation or spinocerebellar degeneration is the most common cause. However, because the latter is correctable, a defect of the craniocervical junction must be carefully considered in all patients with downbeat nystagmus. Downbeat nystagmus may co-exist with PAN, another type of nystagmus suggestive of an abnormality of the craniocervical junction. A variety of miscellaneous conditions have also been reported to produce downbeat nystagmus.[101,121] These include anticonvulsant, alcohol, and lithium intoxication; magnesium deficiency; B_{12} deficiency; brain stem encephalitis; alcoholic cerebellar degeneration; dolichoectasia of the ventral artery; and vertebral artery occlusion.[122] Rarely, downbeat nystagmus is secondary to upper brain stem or supratentorial disease, or it may appear as a form of congenital nystagmus. (See Schmidt[123] for an excellent clinical review of downbeat nystagmus.)

Downbeat nystagmus was regarded as the prototype of nystagmus secondary to a "pursuit defect," but studies have cast serious doubt as to whether a unidirectional pursuit defect has been established as a cause of any form of nystagmus.[120] The slow-phase waveform of downbeat nystagmus can vary from a linear, to an increasing-velocity, to a decreasing-velocity exponential in the same patient, presumably reflecting short-term gain changes by cerebellar compensation for leaky brain stem neural integrators.[4] One patient with a pseudocycloid waveform damped with convergence; this prompted treatment with base-out prism spectacles.[101] This has subsequently proved superior to retinal image stabilization as a means of reducing oscillopsia.[124] Downbeat is usually increased in intensity with head-hanging[120] as well as linear acceleration, and occasionally convergence. The mechanism of downbeat is postulated to be disruption of central vestibular pathways,[120] possibly involving specific connections from the otoliths or an asymmetry of the vertical semicircular canal gains.[125] It is associated with lesions of the caudal midline cerebellum, as opposed to the central medulla with upbeat nystagmus.[126–128]

Upbeat

Primary-position nystagmus with the fast phase beating upward rarely reflects drug intoxication. Most often, the nystagmus is acquired and indicates structural disease, usually of the brain stem.[129–131] The location of the lesions in patients with upbeat nystagmus after meningitis, Wernicke's encephalopathy, or organophosphate poisoning is uncertain. The localizing value of upbeat and other types of nystagmus has been found to be specific in some cases but not in others.[132] Cyclosporin A therapy has also been identified as a possible cause of upbeat nystagmus.[133] With convergence, upbeat may enhance[130] or convert to downbeat.[102] The slow-phase waveform is usually linear but may be an increasing-velocity exponential.

Upbeat nystagmus has been regarded as "pursuit defect" nystagmus, but for the reasons given above in the discussion of downbeat nystagmus, a pursuit defect has not been established as an etiology. Upbeat may be enhanced[130] or suppressed[134] by head tilt. Therefore, it is conceptualized hypothetically as secondary to a disruption of central otolithic pathways; the effects of convergence on the nystagmus are presumed to reflect vergence effects on these pathways. Tobacco smoking causes upbeat nystagmus in normal human subjects in darkness, but the nystagmus is suppressed by visual fixation.[135] The mechanism is presumed to be the excitatory effects of nicotine on central vestibular pathways.

Rebound

Rebound nystagmus is either the diminution and direction change of gaze-evoked horizontal nystagmus during sustained ocular deviation or a horizontal gaze-evoked nystagmus that, on refixation to primary position, transiently beats in the opposite direction. The sign is often present in patients with cerebellar disease.[136] Rebound nystagmus is conceptualized as a smooth eye movement bias generated to oppose gaze-evoked centripetal drift of the eyes. Normal subjects may demonstrate rebound nystagmus after prolonged far lateral gaze if the lights are shut off the moment the eyes are returned to primary position; rebound nystagmus may even occur in normals during fixation in a fully lit room.[88] Rebound and centripetal nystagmus have been reported in Creutzfeldt-Jakob disease.[137]

Circular, Elliptic, and Oblique

Circular nystagmus, sometimes confusingly mislabeled as "rotary," is a form of pendular nystagmus in which the globe oscillates continuously in a fine, rapid, circular path. Unlike torsional nystagmus, in which the 12 o'clock meridian of the limbus torts laterally, this point maintains its position in circular nystagmus. The nystagmus represents the summation of simultaneous, equal-amplitude, horizontal, and vertical pendular oscillations that are 90° out of phase. Elliptic nystagmus is produced when the horizontal and vertical oscillations are 90° out of phase but are of unequal amplitude. Analysis of the vertical and horizontal pendular nystagmus movements, which summate to form circular and elliptic

nystagmus, indicates that a true circular pattern is rarely sustained. More often, the nystagmus varies between elliptic and circular. This type of nystagmus is often congenital and identical in the two eyes, and the patient is otherwise free of neurologic signs. Acquired circular-elliptic nystagmus occurs in multiple sclerosis, is often dissociated in the two eyes, and almost always co-exists with truncal or extremity ataxia. Drug treatment with isoniazid may be effective.[138]

Oblique or diagonal nystagmus results when simultaneous pendular, horizontal, and vertical vectors are either in phase or 180° out of phase. The angle of the diagonal vector depends on the relative amplitudes of the horizontal and vertical components. This type is more often acquired than congenital and has the same significance as acquired circular-elliptic nystagmus. Unlike all other types of nystagmus, the oscillopsia induced by elliptical nystagmus is in the *same* direction as the slow phases.[138] Thus, if the subject's eye moves in a clockwise, circular-elliptic manner (from the subject's point of view), the direction of perceived world motion will also be clockwise.

Cervical

The literature on cervical (cord) nystagmus contains numerous examples of spontaneous or positional nystagmus allegedly secondary to lesions of the cervical spinal cord or roots.[139-141] Although this form of positional nystagmus occurs only rarely, it is claimed to support the legitimacy of dizziness in patients who have sustained whiplash injuries and are involved in litigation. For that reason, the entire concept of cervical nystagmus has become highly suspect.[140,141] We have not seen a patient with convincing cervical nystagmus.

Muscle-Paretic (Myasthenic)

A paretic eye muscle, from whatever cause, can fatigue quickly during contraction, and muscle-paretic nystagmus can be observed. This is often evident as gaze-evoked nystagmus in myasthenia gravis, in which there is usually asymmetry between the two eyes.[142] Another form of oscillation in myasthenia is "nystagmus" of the abducting eye (may be saccadic pulse trains, discussed below), co-existing with paresis of adduction; this mimics an internuclear ophthalmoplegia. Here the oscillation is not due to lateral rectus paresis, but rather to excessive innervation by increased central gain, the result of paresis of the contralateral yoke medial rectus. Cessation of both muscle-paretic and contralateral yoke nystagmus in myasthenia usually follows administration of anticholinesterase medication.

Lid

Lid nystagmus is a rhythmic, upward jerking of the upper eyelids that usually consists of the normally coordinated movements of the lids and eyes during vertical ocular nystagmus. Several types of pathologic lid nystagmus are recognized. Type I, with no specific localizing value, co-exists synchronously with vertical ocular nystagmus, but the amplitude of the lid movements exceeds significantly that of the eyes. Type II is evoked by lateral gaze and is characterized by rapid phasic twitches of the lids that are synchronous with the fast phases of horizontal ocular nystagmus. This second type may be a sign of the lateral medullary syndrome and can be inhibited by near-effort.[99] Type III lid nystagmus is provoked by ocular convergence.[100,143] In a patient with this type of nystagmus studied pathologically, a large area of subacute demyelinization in the rostral medulla was found. Lid nystagmus has been identified as a sign of midbrain disease in a subject with an astrocytoma.[144]

Epileptic

Nystagmus associated with epileptic activity includes retraction, pendular, torsional, and divergent-convergent forms.[105] At times, the pupils may constrict and dilate synchronously with the nystagmus.[145] The usual form of epileptic nystagmus is horizontal jerk with the fast phase contralateral to a posterior parietal focus, but a vertical nystagmus may be present.[146] The eyes may tonically deviate toward or away from the side of the epileptic focus.[147] The decreasing-velocity slow phases suggest that a gaze-holding failure[148] causes the slow phases, and the relationship of the ictal activity suggests activation of the saccadic system (see Chapter 10).[149]

Induced Nystagmus

Caloric

The characteristics of caloric-induced vestibular nystagmus were described above. With unilateral irrigation, the nystagmus is either horizontal, torsional, or oblique, depending on the position of the head. Bilateral simultaneous caloric stimulation produces vertical nystagmus; the direction of the fast (jerk) phase can be remembered by the mnemonic "CUWD" (pronounced "cud" and designating cold, up; warm, down).

Traditionally, caloric nystagmus was regarded as being evoked entirely by thermal convection of the endolymph. However, the fact that such nystagmus exists in the zero-gravity conditions of outer space indicates the necessity of an alternative mechanism.[150] Indeed, investigations have revealed two mechanisms responsible for the induction of caloric nystagmus.[151] In addition to the convection mechanism, a direct temperature effect on the canal's sensory apparatus was identified that was independent of head orientation. A review of the technique of quantitative bithermal caloric testing for evaluating vestibular function is provided elsewhere. Caloric and head rotation (doll's) are useful tests in the evaluation of comatose patients.[152]

Rotational

Rotating or accelerating head movements induce motion of endolymph in the semicircular canals, with a resultant jerk nystagmus. If the axis of rotation passes through the upright head, as happens with the Bárány chair, the nystagmus fast phase is in the same direction as head (or chair) rotation. After cessation of the rotation, the postrotary nystagmus is in the opposite direction. Rotational nystagmus is used in evaluating the ocular motor system in infants (see Fig. 3–2), but its primary use in recent years has been to evaluate vestibulo-ocular gain and other aspects (visual suppression of the VOR) of the vestibular system.

Positional

In patients complaining of vertigo related to shifts in position of the head or body, the possibility of positional nystagmus should be investigated. The test is performed by observing for nystagmus produced when the patient rapidly reclines from a sitting to a supine position, with the head either turned alternately to one side and then the other, or hyperextended (hanging). Two types of nystagmus, peripheral and central, can be differentiated (Table 11–5).

Peripheral positional nystagmus is associated with marked vertigo, which begins after a delay of 2 to 20 seconds. The nystagmus and vertigo eventually fatigue, usually within 1 minute. A rapid return to the sitting position causes another brief burst of nystagmus and vertigo ("rebound"). Repositioning in the provocative supine posture again induces nystagmus and vertigo, but to a lesser extent. Repetition of the shifts of posture

TABLE 11–5. Positional Nystagmus

Features	Peripheral	Central
Latency	3–40 s	None; nystagmus begins immediately
Fatigability	Yes	No
Rebound	Yes	No
Habituation	Yes	No
Intensity of vertigo	Severe	Mild
Reproducibility	Poor	Good
Directionality and waveforms	Stereotyped	Variable

ultimately results in diminution and disappearance of the nystagmus and vertigo. Characteristic of the peripheral variety is variable reproducibility: the nystagmus and vertigo may not be present every time the offending position is attained. Whereas latency, fatigability, and habituation have traditionally been regarded as the major features distinguishing peripheral from central positional nystagmus, Baloh et al[153] emphasize that the nystagmus vector is the critical determinant. Positional nystagmus with a torsional-vertical vector, with the torsional component greater in the undermost eye and the vertical component (upbeating) greater in the uppermost eye, is always peripheral, irrespective of the nature of latency, fatigability, and habituation. The torsional component increases when gaze is directed toward the down eye, and the upbeating component increases with gaze directed toward the upper eye.[153] With head-hanging (extended), a downbeating nystagmus (fast phase beating toward the chin) probably has the same significance as downbeating nystagmus with the patient upright.

Central positional nystagmus, which is invariably reproducible, begins immediately on movement to the provoking position; the nystagmus neither fatigues nor habituates, and the vertigo is usually mild. Positional nystagmus that changes direction while the head position remains fixed has been regarded as a central sign. However, direction-changing positional nystagmus occurs with peripheral disease and even in normal subjects.[154]

The peripheral variety, designated "benign paroxysmal positional vertigo" (BPPV), is indicative of labyrinthine disease, and neuroradiologic procedures are rarely indicated. The most common specific etiology is head trauma. However, no cause is found in most cases. The malady increases in prevalence with age. The traditional presumption has been that the provoking position occurred with the diseased ear undermost, and that the fast phase of nystagmus beat toward that ear. The direction of the nystagmus and the lateralization of the labyrinthopathy have been challenged.[153] Nystagmus, identical to the benign peripheral variety, may result from the slow drift produced by central vestibular compensation consequent to either peripheral or central vestibular dysfunction.[85]

The most reasonable etiology of BPPV is "canalolithiasis." The hypothesis is that otoconia detach from a utricle, congeal to form a "plug," and float freely in the endolymph of a posterior semicircular canal. Because the plug is of greater specific gravity than the endolymph, the canal becomes a gravity receptor and symptoms and signs are produced when the head is in a particular position. This concept has led to a form of "physical therapy" in which repetitive movement, or a single provocative movement, dislodges the displaced otoconia.[155] Most patients with the disorder recover spontaneously after several weeks. However, if a person has persistent symptoms and the attacks are consistently evoked with the head in the offending position, a liberatory maneuver is performed. With BPPV, in addition to positional vertigo, patients develop symptoms on arising, bending over, leaning forward, and with head movements while upright.

The central type of positional nystagmus is often associated with neoplastic, vascular, demyelinating, or degenerative disorders involving the brain stem or cerebellum.[156] Intermediate forms of positional nystagmus, such as those that fatigue and habituate but have no noticeable latency, should raise suspicions of central disease.

Testing for positional nystagmus is fairly standardized and does not require electronystagmography. We prefer self-illuminated Frenzel glasses (highly convex lenses, +20 D, which blur vision), but testing can also be performed in a completely darkened room, with the examiner periodically observing the eyes with a dim light. Routine testing for positional nystagmus in patients without the specific symptom of positional vertigo does not generally yield useful results.

The BPPV just mentioned is due to dysfunction of the posterior semicircular canals. Some patients have horizontal BPPV[157] for which a liberatory maneuver has also been described.[158] The term *positional nystagmus* is often used interchangeably with *positional vertigo* in designating a syndrome, and *positional* and *positioning* are used interchangeably to describe nystagmus.

Optokinetic

The localizing value of OKN with cerebral hemispheric lesions is discussed in Chapter 10. OKN is used for several other important functions in clinical neuro-ophthalmology. It provides evidence of at least gross levels of visual function in infants or patients with functional visual loss. As mentioned in Chapter 10, OKN in the downward direction is used to induce convergence-retraction "nystagmus," and horizontal OKN is used to demonstrate the adduction insufficiency in internuclear ophthalmoparesis. "Inversion" of OKN is diagnostic of CN. OKN can be used to diagnose oculomotor nerve misdirection, and, finally, it may be quite useful as a diagnostic test in myasthenia gravis, because the velocity of the fast phase is significantly increased after the standard edrophonium chloride (Tensilon) test.

Drug- and Toxin-Induced

Drug-induced nystagmus is a common sequela of barbiturate, tranquilizer, phenothiazine, and anticonvulsant therapy.[159] The nystagmus is generally regarded as gaze-evoked and is usually horizontal or horizontal-torsional in direction. Vertical nystagmus is often present on upward gaze and only rarely on downward gaze. At times the nystagmus may be dissociated in the two eyes despite the lack of structural disease to account for the asymmetry. Although primary-position nystagmus is usually indicative of severe drug intoxication, it may appear 10 hours after the oral ingestion of only 100 mg of secobarbital.[85] In addition, this amount of secobarbital can produce positional nystagmus. As mentioned, lithium can produce downbeat nystagmus,[160,161] tobacco can induce upbeat nystagmus,[135] and severe alcohol intoxication can produce downbeat nystagmus that abates during sobriety.[162]

Unfortunately, the fact that alcohol can produce horizontal gaze-evoked nystagmus has led to a roadside sobriety test conducted by law-enforcement officers.[163] Nystagmus as an indicator of alcohol intoxication is fraught with extraordinary pitfalls: many normal individuals have physiologic end-point nystagmus; small doses of tranquilizers that wouldn't interfere with driving ability can produce nystagmus; nystagmus may be congenital or consequent to structural neurologic disease; and often a sophisticated neuro-ophthalmologist or oculographer is required to determine whether nystagmus is pathologic. It seems unreasonable that such judgments should be the domain of cursorily trained law officers, no matter how intelligent, perceptive, and well meaning they might be. As noted, meticulous history taking and drug-screening blood studies are often essential in evaluating patients with nystagmus. Toluene (glue-sniffing) can induce pendular nystagmus with both horizontal and vertical components.[164]

Special Anatomic Categories

Acoustic Neuroma

Schwannomas of the eighth nerve grow so slowly that adaptive mechanisms often obscure clinical vestibular manifestations. Vestibular nystagmus beating contralateral to the lesion may be present, particularly if fixation is eliminated. As the tumor expands to compress the brain stem, a slow, gaze-evoked ipsilateral nystagmus is often added. The combination of a small-amplitude, rapid primary-position jerk nystagmus beating contralateral to the lesion, and a slower, larger-amplitude, gaze-evoked (Bruns') nystagmus ipsilateral to the lesion also occurs with other extra-axial masses, including cerebellar tumors, compressing the brain stem. Rarely, Bruns' nystagmus is inverted.[165]

Lateral Medullary Syndrome

The lateral medullary syndrome (Wallenberg) is a distinctive constellation of signs. The nystagmus in this syndrome tends to be stereotyped. With the eyes open there is horizontal-torsional jerk nystagmus beating con-

tralateral to the lesion; when recorded with the eyes closed, the nystagmus beats ipsilateral to the lesion. Other rare manifestations, confined to single cases, are gaze-evoked eyelid and ocular nystagmus inhibited by the near reflex[99] and horizontal gaze-evoked monocular downbeat nystagmus.

An extraordinarily dramatic eye-movement abnormality, saccadic lateropulsion, may occur with lateral medullary infarction. Eye movements as well as body and limb movements are biased toward the side of the lesion (ipsipulsion). The ocular motor abnormality is most striking during shifts of fixation; all ipsilateral saccades are too large (hypermetric), whereas those to the opposite side are too small (hypometric). Spontaneous drifts to the side of the lesion are gaze-dependent and may reflect disruptions of the gaze-holding mechanism.[166] There is also reduced capability to adjust saccadic gain in response to the dysmetria,[167] significant tilt in the subjective vertical, with ipsilateral excyclotropia,[168] and torsional nystagmus and torsipulsion.[169,170] Upward or downward refixations veer ipsilaterally along an oblique rather than a vertical line. Lateropulsion away from the side of the lesion (contrapulsion) has been described with a unilateral disorder of the rostral cerebellum.[171] Both types of lateropulsion are regarded as saccadic instabilities (Table 11–6). The gaze deviation may reflect increased inhibition of the ipsilateral vestibular nucleus, and ipsipulsion may reflect decreased excitation of contralateral premotor areas in the pontine paramedian reticular formation.[172]

Albinism and Achiasma

Ocular albinism is associated with anomalous visual projections that result in a variety of eye movement disturbances, with considerable intersubject variability. These individuals may have pendular or jerk nystagmus, absent OKN, "inverted" pursuit, or "defective" pursuit (see section on CN) when targets are projected onto the temporal half-retina.[173] Periodic alternating nystagmus may also occur.[109,110] Albinism may also exist in the *absence* of any nystagmus.[174,175]

Achiasma is a very rare condition, first recognized in dogs (circa 1974) and then in humans (circa 1992). It is associated with the combination of CN and see-saw nystagmus, the latter diagnosed from videotape (in dogs in 1991 and in a human in 1993) and subsequently studied using eye-movement recordings.[32,176–181] In achiasma, all retinal fibers remain ipsilateral, passing to the ipsilateral lateral geniculates and visual cortexes. Thus, each visual cortex has a representation of the entire visual field, but stereopsis is impossible. There is no bitemporal hemianopia in achiasma. Figure 11–15 shows both the horizontal CN and the vertical component of the see-saw nystagmus in an achiasmatic canine (Fig. 11–15A) and an achiasmatic human (Fig. 11–15B). The hori-

TABLE 11–6. Saccadic Intrusions and Oscillations*

Bobbing/dipping	Saccadic lateropulsion
Inverse bobbing	Ipsipulsion
Reverse bobbing	Contrapulsion
Convergence-retraction "nystagmus"	Saccadic pulses/pulse trains
"Nystagmus" retractoris	Abduction "nystagmus"
Double saccadic pulses (single/multiple)	Ataxic "nystagmus"
Saccadic intrusions/oscillations	Saccadic intrusions/oscillations
Dynamic overshoot	Stepless saccades
"Quiver"	Square-wave jerks/oscillations
Dysmetria	Gegenrucke
Flutter	Hopping "nystagmus"
Flutter dysmetria	"Lightning eye movements"
Macrosaccadic oscillations	Myoclonus
Myoclonus	Saccadic intrusions/oscillations
Laryngeal "nystagmus"	Zickzakbewegungen
"Lightning eye movements"	Square-wave pulses (bursts/single)
Pharyngeal "nystagmus"	"Macro square-wave jerks"
Opsoclonus	Kippdeviationen/"Kippnystagmus"
"Dancing eyes"	"Pendular macro-oscillations"
"Lightning eye movements"	Saccadic "nystagmus"
Saccadomania	Saccadic oscillations/intrusions
Psychogenic flutter	Superior oblique myokymia
Hysterical flutter	
Hysterical "nystagmus"	
"Ocular fibrillation"	
"Ocular shuddering"	
Psychological "nystagmus"	
Voluntary flutter	
Voluntary "nystagmus"	

* Synonyms and other terms are indented under either the preferred or the more inclusive designation; quoted terms are erroneous or misleading.

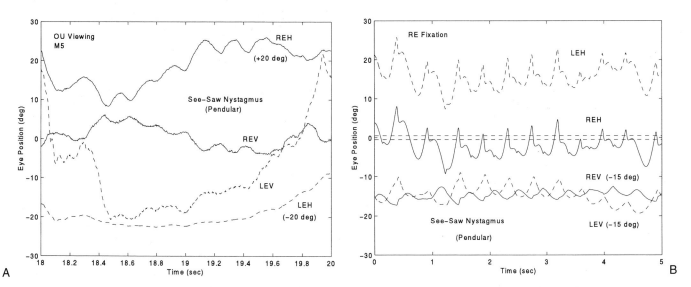

Fig. 11–15. The horizontal congenital nystagmus and vertical component of see-saw nystagmus in an achiasmatic Belgian sheepdog during binocular (*OU*) viewing **(A)** and an achiasmatic human during right-eye fixation **(B).** Note that the left eye in (B) was approximately 15° esotropic. When indicated, traces were shifted for clarity. *Dashed lines* in (B) define the foveal extent. *REH*, right eye horizontal; *LEH*, left eye horizontal; *REV*, right eye vertical; *LEV*, left eye vertical. Upward deflections indicate rightward or upward eye movements.

zontal and vertical waveforms of the canine's nystagmus and the human's vertical nystagmus were pendular, whereas the human's horizontal waveforms were pendular with foveating saccades (P_{FS}) or pseudopendular with foveating saccades (PP_{FS}). Since the achiasmatic human subject was not always able to achieve well-developed foveation, as shown by her inability to repeatedly foveate the target with her fixating right eye, the expanded NAF would be required to assess the best potential visual acuity in this segment. Unlike CN, which may or may not be associated with a particular sensory deficit, the see-saw nystagmus appears to be directly associated with achiasma in both species. In achiasma, there is no lesion, indeed no chiasm, and disruption of thalamic inputs to the nucleus of Cajal, postulated as the cause of acquired see-saw nystagmus, cannot be causal. In *hemichiasma*, abnormalities at the chiasm prevent decussation of the retinal fibers from one eye, the other decussating normally.[182] Whereas achiasma appears to be sufficient for SSN, hemichiasma is not. Because of the rarity of congenital see-saw nystagmus and its identification in both canines and humans with achiasma and in one of two canines with hemichiasma, we regard its presence in infants as a diagnostic sign of possible achiasma or hemichiasma.[183]

> The presence of SSN in an infant is a strong indication for imaging of the optic chiasm to rule out achiasma or structural abnormalities conducive to hemichiasma.

Tenotomy of the vertical and oblique muscles can damp SSN.[27]

Cerebellum

Some of the various eye signs seen with cerebellar system disease are discussed above and in Chapter 10. Descriptions of others will follow.

SACCADIC INTRUSIONS AND OSCILLATIONS

Non-nystagmic (*i.e.*, saccadic) ocular oscillations and intrusions represent specific and classifiable eye movement anomalies (Table 11–6). Many reflect cerebellar dysfunction. In Table 11–6, 16 types of saccadic intrusions and oscillations are identified, the most important of which are discussed below.

Square-Wave Jerks/Oscillations

Square-wave jerks (SWJs), so named because of their rectangular appearance on eye movement records (Fig. 11–16), are usually small-amplitude (0.5° to 5°), conjugate saccadic eye movements that spontaneously move the eyes away from, and back to, a fixational point. Between the two saccades that constitute this saccadic intrusion is a latent period of about 200 msec (the visual

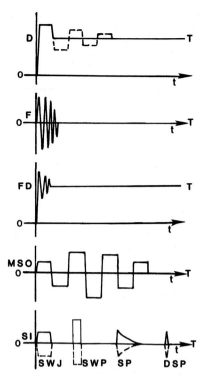

Fig. 11–16. Schematic illustrations of dysmetria (*D*), flutter (*F*), flutter dysmetria (*FD*), macro-saccadic oscillations (*MSO*), and the saccadic intrusions (*SI*): square-wave jerks (*SWJ*), square-wave pulses (*SWP*), saccadic pulses (*SP*), and double saccadic pulses (*DSP*). *T*, target; *O*, primary position; *t*, time.

reaction time). SWJs have a maximum frequency of about 2 Hz and occur in normals on closure of eyelids. However, when they are prominent during fixation, they must be considered abnormal, although lacking diagnostic specificity, much like saccadic pursuit. SWJs are a subtle disturbance that is easily missed clinically. However, they are obvious with eye-movement recordings, which also allow other types of saccadic intrusions to be identified.[184] Clinically, they are often best identified during slit-lamp biomicroscopy or funduscopy, but they may be difficult to distinguish among other intrusions.

The occurrence of SWJs is significantly greater in the elderly population than in young subjects. Their appearance at a rate greater than 9/minute in young patients is considered abnormal. SWJs also are found in 70% of patients with acute or chronic focal cerebral lesions and are the rule in progressive supranuclear palsy and Parkinson's disease. Schizophrenic patients and their parents[185] have been found to exhibit SWJs, which are also present during smooth pursuit and have been mistaken for a deficit in the pursuit system.

Square-wave oscillations (SWOs) are continuously occurring SWJs and have been recorded in patients with a variety of neurologic deficits. The characteristics are identical to those of SWJs (Table 11–7). In a patient with progressive supranuclear palsy, SWOs appeared to

TABLE 11–7. Characteristics of Saccadic Instabilities

	Square-wave jerks	Square-wave oscillations	Square-wave pulses*	Macro-saccadic oscillations
Amplitude	0.5°–5°†	0.5°–5°†	4°–30°	1°–30°
	Constant	Constant	Variable	Increasing then decreasing
Time course	Sporadic/bursts	Bursts	Bursts/sporadic	Bursts
Latency	200 msec	200 msec	50–150 msec	200 msec
Foveation	Yes	Yes	Yes	No
Presence in darkness	Yes	Yes	Yes	No

* Previously designated macro–square-wave jerks.
† Occasionally up to 10°.

be part of a continuum with SWJs; at times, single or several SWJs occurred, and at other times there were long runs of SWJs that were identified as SWOs.[186]

Square-Wave Pulses

Square-wave pulses (SWPs), originally called "macro square-wave jerks," are usually larger in amplitude than SWJs, are related to fixation, and have a frequency of about 2 Hz.[187] They generally occur in bursts but may appear as a single saccadic intrusion. Both eyes suddenly and conjugately move off target with a saccade, and after a latent period of only about 80 msec, a nonvisually evoked reflex saccade brings them back on target (see Fig. 11–16). SWPs are not merely large SWJs; the characteristics of both are summarized in Table 11–7. SWPs usually occur in patients with marked extremity ataxia suggestive of cerebellar outflow disease, especially when the patient has demyelinating lesions.[187] A unique variety of SWP, present with binocular fixation at distance but stopping when either eye was closed, prompted the designation "inverse latent SWP."[188]

Macro-Saccadic Oscillations

Macro saccadic oscillations (MSOs) increase and then damp in amplitude, bypassing the fixation angle with each saccade (see Fig. 11–16).[189] Unlike SWJs, SWOs, and SWPs, MSOs are not present in darkness and have a longer latency for the return saccade than do SWPs. In a patient with suspected multiple sclerosis, MSOs were recorded as part of a constellation of saccadic intrusions and oscillations including SWJs, saccadic pulses (SPs), double saccadic pulses (DSPs), flutter, and flutter dysmetria (FD)[184] (see below for descriptions of these latter eye signs). A case has been reported in which SWP and MSO appeared to have a vertical component.[190] Administration of several sedative drugs caused these oscillations to disappear.

A comparison of the features of the four saccadic instabilities described above (SWJ, SWO, SWP, and MSO) appears in Table 11–7.

Saccadic Pulses/Pulse Trains

Saccadic pulses are intrusions on fixation caused by a spurious pulse of innervation, provided by the burst cells without the usual accompanying step; they were originally called "stepless saccades." The resultant eye movement is a saccade off-target followed immediately by a glissadic drift back to the target (see Fig. 11–16). The glissadic drift in SP represents failure of the neural integrator to produce a step of innervation from the burst producing the SP. This difference from SWJ suggests dysfunction in the pause cell/burst cell circuitry for SP and a more central dysfunction for SWJ.

Saccadic pulse trains (SPTs) are continuous runs of SPs that are often confused with nystagmus. Even on good eye-movement records, SPTs cannot be distinguished from jerk nystagmus with decreasing-velocity slow phases, unless both eye position and target position are known. The initiation of an SP is a saccade off-target, whereas jerk nystagmus is initiated by the slow phase off-target, with the saccadic fast phase bringing the eye back to the target. The so-called abduction nystagmus of internuclear ophthalmoplegia is SPT.[191] Recordings of several patients with congenital achromatopsia and thought to have CN have been recorded; however, their oscillations did not contain any of the known CN waveforms and were most consistent with SPT. The waveforms mimicked those of LMLN, but there were no evident effects of monocular fixation.

Double Saccadic Pulses

Double saccadic pulses (DSPs) are intrusions on fixation, consisting of two back-to-back saccades without latency between them (see Fig. 11–16).[184] Small DSPs are common in normals and also occur occasionally in some CN patients. Multiple DSPs (mDSPs) are runs of

DSPs.[184] There is a continuum between the saccadic intrusion DSP, mDSP, and the saccadic oscillation, flutter.[186]

Dysmetria

Strictly speaking, dysmetria refers to any inaccurate saccadic eye movement. With small saccades, normal subjects may undershoot or overshoot; with large saccades, small undershooting is the rule. Consistent overshooting during small refixations (10° or less), or more than occasional overshooting during refixations greater than 30°, is abnormal and indicative of cerebellar dysfunction (see Fig. 11–16).[192] The term *ocular dysmetria* is used to denote pathologic hypermetria. In experimental animals with cerebellar lesions, dysmetria may be unequal in the two eyes.[193] The components of the oscillation are usually flat at the peaks, indicating an intersaccadic latency,[192] but they may also be triangular or sinusoidal in appearance; the latter are probably cycles of flutter dysmetria (FD) (see below).

Quantitative studies can differentiate normal from pathologic saccadic dysmetria,[194] especially for saccades of 20° or more. Saccadic dysmetria with preserved smooth pursuit has been reported to be caused by midline lesions of cerebellar structures.[195] This occurs despite the known involvement of these areas with control of smooth pursuit. Dorsal cerebellar vermis angioma has produced dysmetria of all types of saccades (visually guided and visually, vestibularly, and cervically remembered)[196]; the observation that final eye position was normal in the memory-guided saccades suggests that this area is involved in the neural integration of the saccadic pulse for such saccades.

Flutter

Ocular flutter was originally defined clinically as any brief, intermittent, binocular, horizontal ocular oscillation occurring spontaneously during straight-ahead fixation. It differs from the oscillation of dysmetria, which always follows a saccadic refixation. In eye-movement recordings, flutter is triangular or sinusoidal in appearance, consisting of several back-to-back saccades (see Fig. 11–16).

Flutter represents a disturbance of the pause cells in the pontine paramedian reticular formation subserving horizontal eye movements.[197] Inappropriate inhibition of the pause cells leads to the burst cell activity that produces the flutter. Rarely, a blink will initiate a large-amplitude ocular flutter in patients with neurologic disease, and short bursts of low-amplitude flutter in normal subjects.[198] A microflutter ("microsaccadic" flutter) has been described in five patients with no identifiable neurologic disorders.[199] It was attributed to malfunction of the omnipause neurons. Flutter has also been reported

with the AIDS-related complex[200] and in association with opsoclonus and myoclonus in patients with anti-Ri antibodies.[201]

Flutter and opsoclonus represent a continuum of ocular motor instability. Patients recovering from opsoclonus often develop a picture of flutter in which opsoclonus emerges, especially during upward gaze. As with opsoclonus, flutter may be a manifestation of a paraneoplastic syndrome,[202] and it may remit spontaneously even before the neoplasm is diagnosed.[203]

Flutter Dysmetria

Flutter dysmetria (FD) is the occurrence of flutter immediately after a saccade (see Fig. 11–16).[197] Although it superficially resembles dysmetria, eye-movement recordings reveal that FD is an oscillation about the intended fixation angle and consists of back-to-back saccades with no intersaccadic latencies. This contrasts with dysmetria in which the saccadic oscillation has normal intersaccadic latencies. FD is seen in a setting of cerebellar disease.

Opsoclonus

Opsoclonus is a bizarre ocular motor oscillation consisting of rapid, involuntary, chaotic, repetitive, unpredictable, conjugate saccadic eye movements in all directions and persisting during sleep. The movements are usually continuous except during patient recovery and in mild forms, during which brief paroxysms interrupt stable fixation. In this instance, the continuum between opsoclonus and ocular flutter, mentioned earlier, is readily apparent. Some paroxysms have characteristic oblique or half-circle vectors,[204] whereas others are entirely horizontal and indistinguishable from flutter.

Opsoclonus, usually associated with extremity myoclonus and ataxia, occurs in a number of clinical settings. In children, opsoclonus and generalized limb myoclonus may continue enigmatically for years, except when suppressed by adrenocorticotropic hormone (ACTH) therapy, which seems to be considerably more effective than corticosteroids. Opsoclonus and acute cerebellar ataxia may represent the sole manifestations of occult neuroblastoma, and the eye movements usually, but not always, remit after tumor removal. This variety of opsoclonus may also respond to ACTH. Opsoclonus only on eye closure was reported in two brothers with hereditary cerebellar ataxia.[205]

Rarely, opsoclonus is a self-limiting phenomenon that occurs in otherwise normal neonates. The so-called ocular tics seen in children usually occur with other types of tics, may be imitated on request, and may be associated with stress.[206] They appear to be bursts of opsoclonus when recorded.[207] In adults, opsoclonus can be secondary to a postinfectious syndrome (which has an excellent prognosis for a complete recovery); brain stem encephalitis; toxicity due to amitriptyline, lithium, haloperidol, chlordecone, thallium, toluene, chlorophenothane, phenytoin, or diazepam; hyperosmolar nonketotic coma; and degenerative diseases.[208,209] It also occurs as a nonmetastatic, paraneoplastic complication of visceral carcinoma; some of these patients have anticerebellar antibodies in the serum and cerebrospinal fluid,[210,211] and their manifestations may improve with steroid[201,212] or immunoadsorption[213] therapy. Brain stem pause cell dysfunction is the presumed etiology, but these cells are normal pathologically in this syndrome.[214] Radiologic and pathologic correlation in a patient suggests involvement of both cerebellum and brain stem.[215] Electrophysiologic data suggest brain stem and cerebellar circuits are involved in idiopathic opsoclonus-myoclonus.[216] Extensive reviews of the literature are available.[217,218]

Myoclonus

Ocular myoclonus is a pendular oscillation that conforms to our definition of nystagmus and is indeed regarded as nystagmus by European writers. However, the eye movement is usually classified separately as myoclonus because of associated rhythmic movements of nonocular muscles in synchrony with the eyes. The soft palate is most commonly involved, but the tongue, facial muscles, pharynx, larynx, and diaphragm may also participate.

The term *myoclonus* is used, often confusingly, to describe several movement disorders. It may refer to spontaneous, episodic, single or multiple jerks of the extremities that constitute a form of seizure particularly prevalent in infants. The same movement provoked by a loud noise is termed *startle myoclonus* and occurs in adults with specific types of cerebral dysfunction, such as anoxic encephalopathy or Creutzfeldt-Jakob disease. Similar movements occur in normal subjects before falling asleep and represent a physiologic phenomenon, probably of spinal origin. Myoclonus also describes the arrhythmic, asymmetric, sudden, brief, involuntary jerks of one or more muscles of the extremities, often reflecting a metabolic derangement or degenerative central nervous system disease with cerebellar involvement.

Ocular myoclonus is a form of segmental myoclonus and is characterized by continuous, rhythmic, to-and-fro pendular oscillation, usually in the vertical plane, with a rate of 1.5 to 5 beats per second. Only the coexisting movements of other structures, such as the palate, distinguish ocular myoclonus from pendular nystagmus. Actually, isolated palatal myoclonus (symptomatic or essential)[219] is more common than the oculopalatal variety and may be a benign, self-limited process that variably responds to anticonvulsants. At times the eye movements have an oblique and rotary vector.[220]

Oculopalatal myoclonus has a rather specific pathologic correlate—hypertrophy of the inferior olivary nucleus in the medulla. The myoclonic triangle involves three structures: the red nucleus in the midbrain, the ipsilateral inferior olive in the medulla, and the contralateral dentate nucleus of the cerebellum. The connecting pathways are the central tegmental tract, the inferior cerebellar peduncle, and the superior cerebellar peduncle. Pathologic involvement of the central tegmental tract produces hypertrophy of the ipsilateral inferior olive after a latency of 2 to 49 months, with a mean at about 10.5 months.[221] Damage to a dentate nucleus results in contralateral olivary hypertrophy after a similar latency. Oculopalatal myoclonus develops as a consequence of the olivary hypertrophy and, therefore, is not a manifestation of acute lesions. The mechanism for the hypertrophy is believed to be denervation supersensitivity[221] related to transneuronal degeneration.[222] Once established, myoclonus ordinarily persists, even during sleep, as a chronic sign until the death of the patient.[223] Occasionally, isolated palatal myoclonus disappears during sleep.[224] A single case of ocular myoclonus responded dramatically to valproic acid[225] and another to chronic one-eye patching.[226] Trihexyphenidyl seems to be the most effective therapy.[227]

Superior Oblique Myokymia

Superior oblique myokymia is an intermittent, small-amplitude, monocular, torsional eye movement ("microtremor") evoking oscillopsia, which appears spontaneously in otherwise healthy adults and only rarely, perhaps even coincidentally, with other neurologic disease.[228] The oscillation is rapid in rate (12 to 15 per second) and reflects phasic contraction of the superior oblique muscle.[229] The movement is detected most readily during ophthalmoscopy or by use of the slit lamp. Eye movement recordings reveal either slow, sustained tonic intorsion and depression, or a phasic intorsion with superimposed high-frequency oscillations in both the vertical and torsional planes; each intorsion is followed by a decreasing-velocity return.[230,231] The spectrum of the oscillations includes low-amplitude components up to 50 Hz and high-amplitude components from 1 to 6 Hz.

Recognition of the entity and reassurance of the patient are essential. Rosenberg and Glaser[232] have presented an extensive longitudinal study of patients and emphasize that the disorder may have varying clinical manifestations and that spontaneous remissions and relapses occur. Treatment with carbamazepine provides short-term benefit to most patients.[232] There is disagreement as to the appropriateness of the term *myokymia*,[233] but the usual benignity of the condition can no longer remain unquestioned.[230] The source of the oscillation is uncertain.[234,235] A review of the history and results of treatment is available.[236]

Bobbing/Dipping

Ocular bobbing is a distinctive spontaneous eye-movement disturbance, readily distinguished from downbeat nystagmus and ocular myoclonus. Bobbing refers to fast downward jerks of both eyes followed by a slow drift to midposition. The downward jerks may be disconjugate in the two eyes, and often the eyes remain deviated for several seconds before returning to midposition. Bobbing usually occurs in comatose patients with extensive destruction of the pons, but extrapontine compressions, obstructive hydrocephalus, metabolic encephalopathy, and encephalitis occasionally are causative.[237]

Bobbing can be divided into three types. Typical bobbing involves both eyes and appears in patients with paralysis of horizontal conjugate eye movements. A monocular type reflects co-existing contralateral third-nerve paresis. The third category, atypical bobbing, includes downward bobbing with convergence movements, asymmetric bobbing without an associated oculomotor palsy, and bobbing with intact spontaneous or reflex horizontal eye movements; the latter variety suggests diffuse encephalopathy, hydrocephalus, or organophosphate poisoning, rather than severe intrinsic pontine disease. The pathophysiology of all forms of ocular bobbing is uncertain, but imaginative hypotheses abound. In two cases, a pontine lesion plus an oculomotor lesion resulted in uniocular bobbing,[238] but in another, no explanation could be found.[239]

In addition to these three types of bobbing (typical, monocular, and atypical), we described a phenomenon designated "reverse bobbing," in which the eyes jerked upward with a fast movement and then slowly returned to the horizontal; the patients were deeply comatose as a result of metabolic encephalopathy. Reverse bobbing may co-exist with typical bobbing with lesions of the dorsal median portion of the pontine tegmentum.[240]

In 1981 there were two reports of comatose patients who demonstrated a slow downward eye movement, followed, after a variable delay, by a quick saccade up to midposition. This disorder was called "inverse bobbing" in one report[241] and "ocular dipping" in the other.[242] The latter term, *dipping,* seems to have achieved favor.[243,244] The upward jerking of the eyes is occasionally associated with contraction of the orbicularis oculi.[245] The phenomenon is regarded as mechanistically similar to the sustained down-gaze deviation seen occasionally in comatose patients. This sign occurred in a patient with a pinealoblastoma[246]; a depressed level of consciousness is not a prerequisite for its appearance. Some patients in coma may demonstrate all three types of spontaneous vertical movements: ocular bobbing, ocular dipping, and reverse bobbing.[247]

Voluntary "Nystagmus"

Voluntary "nystagmus" consists of bursts of an extremely rapid, conjugate, horizontal oscillation that appears pendular but actually consists of back-to-back saccades.[248] As shown in Table 11–6, it is equivalent to flutter.[197] It may be used as a party trick or as a conscious attempt to feign illness. The oscillation is readily identified by the extreme rapidity (approximately 20 Hz, with a range of 8 to 23 Hz) and brevity of each burst (maximum duration usually less than 30 seconds). Most subjects do not sustain the oscillation for more than 10 seconds, and manifest facial distortions with eyelid closure to "rest" their eyes in preparation for another outburst. The ability to perform this stunt may be hereditary, and is present in about 5% of the population.[249] Rarely, voluntary "nystagmus" is in the vertical plane[250] or is multidirectional, mimicking opsoclonus.[251]

REFERENCES

1. Wartenberg R: Diagnostic Tests in Neurology. A Selection for Office Use. Chicago, Yearbook, 1953
2. Doslak MJ, Dell'Osso LF, Daroff RB: Alexander's law: a model and resulting study. Ann Otol Rhinol Laryngol 91:316, 1982
3. Barton JJS, Sharpe JA: Oscillopsia and horizontal nystagmus with accelerating slow phases following lumbar puncture in the Arnold-Chiari malformation. Ann Neurol 33:418, 1993
4. Abel LA, Traccis S, Dell'Osso LF et al: Variable waveforms in downbeat nystagmus imply short-term gain changes. Ann Neurol 13:616, 1983
5. Gresty MA, Bronstein AM, Page NG et al: Congenital-type nystagmus emerging in later life. Neurology 41:653, 1991
6. Hertle RW, Dell'Osso LF: Clinical and ocular motor analysis of congenital nystagmus in infancy. J Am Pediatr Ophthalmol Strab 3:70, 1999
7. Dell'Osso LF, Daroff RB: Congenital nystagmus waveforms and foveation strategy. Doc Ophthalmol 39:155, 1975
8. Dell'Osso LF, Gauthier G, Liberman G et al: Eye movement recordings as a diagnostic tool in a case of congenital nystagmus. Am J Optom Arch Am Acad Optom 49:3, 1972
9. Dell'Osso LF, Weissman BM, Leigh RJ et al: Hereditary congenital nystagmus and gaze-holding failure: the role of the neural integrator. Neurology 43:1741, 1993
10. Optican LM, Zee DS: A hypothetical explanation of congenital nystagmus. Biol Cyber 50:119, 1984
11. Tusa RJ, Zee DS, Hain TC et al: Voluntary control of congenital nystagmus. Clin Vis Sci 7:195, 1992
12. Harris CM: Problems in modelling congenital nystagmus: towards a new model. In Findlay JM, Walker R, Kentridge RW (eds): Eye Movement Research: Mechanisms, Processes and Applications, p 239. Amsterdam, Elsevier, 1995
13. Goldstein HP: Extended slow phase analysis of foveation, waveform and null zone in infantile nystagmus. Invest Ophthalmol Vis Sci 36:S174, 1995
14. Dell'Osso LF, Flynn JT, Daroff RB: Hereditary congenital nystagmus: an intrafamilial study. Arch Ophthalmol 92:366, 1974
15. Tusa RJ, Smith CB, Herdman SJ: The development of nystagmus in infant monkeys following visual deprivation. Soc Neurosci Abstr 13:172, 1987
16. Demer JL, Poukens V, Micevych P: Nitroxidergic and catecholaminergic innervation of the smooth muscle of the medial rectus pulley in humans. Invest Ophthalmol Vis Sci 36:S959, 1995

17. Bedell HE, White JM: The torsional component of idiopathic congenital nystagmus. Invest Ophthalmol Vis Sci 36:S174, 1995

18. Abadi RV, Dickinson CM: Waveform characteristics in congenital nystagmus. Doc Ophthalmol 64:153, 1986

19. Stahl JS, Rottach KG, Averbuch-Heller L et al: A pilot study of gabapentin as treatment for acquired nystagmus. Neuro-ophthalmology 16:107, 1996

20. Dell'Osso LF: Congenital, latent and manifest latent nystagmus—similarities, differences and relation to strabismus. Jpn J Ophthalmol 29:351, 1985

21. Dell'Osso LF, Van der Steen J, Steinman RM et al: Foveation dynamics in congenital nystagmus I: fixation. Doc Ophthalmol 79:1, 1992

22. Zubcov AA, Stärk N, Weber A et al: Improvement of visual acuity after surgery for nystagmus. Ophthalmology 100:1488, 1993

23. Dell'Osso LF: Fixation characteristics in hereditary congenital nystagmus. Am J Optom Arch Am Acad Optom 50:85, 1973

24. Bedell HE, White JM, Abplanalp PL: Variability of foveations in congenital nystagmus. Clin Vision Sci 4:247, 1989

25. Abadi RV, Worfolk R: Retinal slip velocities in congenital nystagmus. Vision Res 29:195, 1989

26. Guo S, Reinecke RD, Goldstein HP: Visual acuity determinants in infantile nystagmus. Invest Ophthalmol Vis Sci 31:83, 1990

27. Dell'Osso LF, Hertle RW, Williams RW, Jacobs JB: A new surgery for congenital nystagmus: effects of tenotomy on an achiasmatic canine and the role of extraocular proprioception. J Am Acad Pediatr Ophthalmol Strab 3:166, 1999

28. Abadi RV, Pascal E, Whittle J et al: Retinal fixation behavior in human albinos. Optom Vis Sci 66:276, 1989

29. Dell'Osso LF, Van der Steen J, Steinman RM et al: Foveation dynamics in congenital nystagmus II: smooth pursuit. Doc Ophthalmol 79:25, 1992

30. Dell'Osso LF, Van der Steen J, Steinman RM et al: Foveation dynamics in congenital nystagmus III: vestibulo-ocular reflex. Doc Ophthalmol 79:51, 1992

31. Sheth NV, Dell'Osso LF, Leigh RJ et al: The effects of afferent stimulation on congenital nystagmus foveation periods. Vision Res 35:2371, 1995

32. Dell'Osso LF: See-saw nystagmus in dogs and humans: an international, across-discipline, serendipitous collaboration. Neurology 47:1372, 1996

33. Halmagyi GM, Gresty MA, Leech J: Reversed optokinetic nystagmus (OKN): mechanism and clinical significance. Ann Neurol 7:429, 1980

34. Gresty MA, Halmagyi GM, Leech J: The relationship between head and eye movement in congenital nystagmus with head shaking: objective recordings of a single case. Br J Ophthalmol 62:533, 1978

35. Dell'Osso LF, Leigh RJ: Oscillopsia suppression: efference copy or foveation periods? Invest Ophthalmol Vis Sci 36:S174, 1995

36. Dell'Osso LF, Leigh RJ: Foveation period stability and oscillopsia suppression in congenital nystagmus. An hypothesis. Neuro-ophthalmology 12:169, 1992

37. Dell'Osso LF, Leigh RJ: Ocular motor stability of foveation periods. Required conditions for suppression of oscillopsia. Neuro-ophthalmology 12:303, 1992

38. Dell'Osso LF: Evaluation of smooth pursuit in the presence of congenital nystagmus. Neuro-ophthalmology 6:383, 1986

39. Leigh RJ, Dell'Osso LF, Yaniglos SS et al: Oscillopsia, retinal image stabilization and congenital nystagmus. Invest Ophthalmol Vis Sci 29:279, 1988

40. Goldstein HP, Gottlob I, Fendick MG: Visual remapping in infantile nystagmus. Vision Res 32:1115, 1992

41. Bedell HE, Currie DC: Extraretinal signals for congenital nystagmus. Invest Ophthalmol Vis Sci 34:2325, 1993

42. Daroff RB, Dell'Osso LF: Periodic alternating nystagmus and the shifting null. Can J Otolaryngol 3:367, 1974

43. Kurzan R, Büttner U: Smooth pursuit mechanisms in congenital nystagmus. Neuro-ophthalmology 9:313, 1989

44. Dell'Osso LF, Leigh RJ, Daroff RB: Suppression of congenital nystagmus by cutaneous stimulation. Neuro-ophthalmology 11:173, 1991

45. Abadi RV: Visual performance with contact lenses and congenital idiopathic nystagmus. Br J Physiol Optics 33:32, 1979

46. Allen ED, Davies PD: Role of contact lenses in the management of congenital nystagmus. Br J Ophthalmol 67:834, 1983

47. Dell'Osso LF, Traccis S, Abel LA et al: Contact lenses and congenital nystagmus. Clin Vision Sci 3:229, 1988

48. Matsubayashi K, Fukushima M, Tabuchi A: Application of soft contact lenses for children with congenital nystagmus. Neuro-ophthalmology 12:47, 1992

49. Shallo-Hoffmann J, Watermeier D, Petersen J et al: Fast-phase instabilities in normally sighted relatives of congenital nystagmus patients—autosomal dominant and x-chromosome recessive modes of inheritance. Neurosurg Rev 11:151, 1988

50. Gottlob I: Eye movement abnormalities in carriers of blue-one monochromatism. Invest Ophthalmol Vis Sci 35:3556, 1994

51. Dell'Osso LF, Schmidt D, Daroff RB: Latent, manifest latent and congenital nystagmus. Arch Ophthalmol 97:1877, 1979

52. Shallo-Hoffman J, Faldon ME, Acheson JF et al: Temporally directed deficits for the detection of visual motion in latent nystagmus: evidence for adaptive processing. Neuro-ophthalmology 16:343, 1996

53. Dickinson CM, Abadi RV: Pursuit and optokinetic responses in latent/manifest latent nystagmus. Invest Ophthalmol Vis Sci 31:1599, 1990

54. Fuchs AF, Mustari MJ: The optokinetic response in primates and its possible neuronal substrate. In Wallman J, Miles FA (eds): Reviews of Oculomotor Research, Vol 5, Visual Motion and its Role in Stabilization of the Gaze, p 343. Amsterdam, Elsevier, 1993

55. Steinbach MJ, Smith D, Crawford JS: Egocentric localization changes following unilateral strabismus surgery. J Pediatr Ophthalmol Strab 25:115, 1988

56. Dell'Osso LF, Leigh RJ, Sheth NV et al: Two types of foveation strategy in 'latent' nystagmus. Fixation, visual acuity and stability. Neuro-ophthalmology 15:167, 1995

57. Dell'Osso LF, Traccis S, Abel LA: Strabismus—a necessary condition for latent and manifest latent nystagmus. Neuro-ophthalmology 3:247, 1983

58. Schor CM, Wilson N, Fusaro R: Prediction of early onset esotropia from components of the infantile squint syndrome. Invest Ophthalmol Vis Sci 36:S645, 1995

59. Zubcov AA, Reinecke RD, Gottlob I et al: Treatment of manifest latent nystagmus. Am J Ophthalmol 110:160, 1990

60. Gresty MA, Metcalfe T, Timms C et al: Neurology of latent nystagmus. Brain 115:1303, 1992

61. Dell'Osso LF, Ellenberger C Jr, Abel LA et al: The nystagmus blockage syndrome: congenital nystagmus, manifest latent nystagmus or both? Invest Ophthalmol Vis Sci 24:1580, 1983

62. Yee RD, Baloh RW, Honrubia V: Eye movement abnormalities in rod monochromacy. Ophthalmology 88:1010, 1981

63. Leigh RJ, Zee DS: Eye movements of the blind. Invest Ophthalmol Vis Sci 19:328, 1980

64. Melvill Jones G, Mandl G, Cynader M et al: Eye oscillations in strobe reared cats. Brain Res 209:47, 1981

65. Hoyt CS, Aicardi E: Acquired monocular nystagmus in monozygous twins. J Pediatr Ophthalmol Strab 16:115, 1979

66. Lavery MA, O'Neill JF, Chu FC et al: Acquired nystagmus in early childhood: a presenting sign of intracranial tumor. Ophthalmology 91:425, 1984

67. Lambert SR, Newman NJ: Retinal disease masquerading as spasmus nutans. Neurology 43:1607, 1993

68. Allarakhia IN: Opsoclonus-myoclonus presenting with features of spasmus nutans. J Child Neurol 10:67, 1995

69. Gresty MA, Leech J, Sanders MD et al: A study of head and eye movement in spasmus nutans. Br J Ophthalmol 160:652, 1976

70. Weismann BM, Dell'Osso LF, Abel LA et al: Spasmus nutans: a quantitative prospective study. Arch Ophthalmol 105:525, 1987

71. Barton JJS, Cox TA: Acquired pendular nystagmus: its characteristics, localizing value and pathophysiology. J Neurol Neurosurg Psychiatry 56:262, 1993

72. Barton JJS: Is acquired pendular nystagmus always phase locked? J Neurol Neurosurg Psychiatry 57:1263, 1994

73. Kori AA, Robin NH, Jacobs JB et al: Pendular nystagmus in autosomal peroxisomal disorder. Arch Neurol 55:554, 1998
74. Averbuch-Heller L, Tusa RJ, Fuhry L et al: A double-blind controlled study of gabapentin and baclofen as treatment for acquired nystagmus. Ann Neurol 41:818, 1997
75. Barton JS, Huaman AG, Sharpe JA: Muscarinic antagonists in the treatment of acquired pendular and downbeat nystagmus: a double-blind, randomized trial of three intravenous drugs. Ann Neurol 35:319, 1994
76. Tomsak RL, Remler BF, Averbuch-Heller L et al: Unsatisfactory treatment of acquired nystagmus with retrobulbar injection of botulinum toxin. Am J Ophthalmol 119:489, 1995
77. Averbuch-Heller L, Remler B: Opsoclonus. Semin Neurol 16:21, 1996
78. Averbuch-Heller L, Zivotofsky AZ, Das VE et al: Investigations of the pathogenesis of acquired pendular nystagmus. Brain 118:369, 1995
79. Baloh RW, Winder A: Acetazolamide-responsive vestibulocere-bellar syndrome: clinical and oculographic features. Neurology 41:429, 1991
80. Kramer PL, Yue Q, Gancher ST et al: A locus for the nystagmus-associated form of episodic ataxia maps to an 11 cM region on chromosome 19p. Am J Hum Genet 57:182, 1995
81. Lawden MC, Bronstein AM, Kennard C: Repetitive paroxysmal nystagmus and vertigo. Neurology 45:276, 1995
82. Brandt T, Daroff RB: The multisensory physiological and pathological vertigo syndromes. Ann Neurol 7:195, 1980
83. Holtmann S, Clarke A, Scherer H: Cervical receptors and the direction of body sway. Arch Otorhinolaryngol 246:61, 1989
84. Zee DS, Preziosi TJ, Proctor LR: Bechterew's phenomenon in a human patient. Ann Neurol 12:495, 1982
85. Dayal VS, Farkashidy J, Mai M et al: Vestibular compensation and nystagmus. Acta Otolaryngol Suppl (Stockh) 406:105, 1984
86. Reker U: Peripheral-vestibular spontaneous nystagmus. Analysis of reproducibility and methodologies. Arch Otorhinolaryngol 226:225, 1980
87. Abel LA, Parker L, Daroff RB et al: Endpoint nystagmus. Invest Ophthalmol Vis Sci 17:539, 1978
88. Shallo-Hoffmann J, Schwarze H, Simonsz HJ et al: A reexamination of end-point and rebound nystagmus in normals. Invest Ophthalmol Vis Sci 31:388, 1990
89. Eizenman M, Cheng P, Sharpe JA et al: End-point nystagmus and ocular drift: an experimental and theoretical study. Vision Res 30:863, 1990
90. Lopez L, Bronstein AM, Gresty MA et al: Torsional nystagmus. A neuro-otological and MRI study of thirty-five cases. Brain 115:1107, 1992
91. Halmagyi GM, Aw ST, Dehaene I et al: Jerk-waveform see-saw nystagmus due to unilateral mesodiencephalic lesion. Brain 117:789, 1994
92. Barton JJS: Blink- and saccade-induced seesaw nystagmus. Neurology 45:831, 1995
93. Frisén L, Wikkelsø C: Posttraumatic seesaw nystagmus abolished by ethanol ingestion. Neurology 36:841, 1986
94. Zimmerman CF, Roach ES, Troost BT: See-saw nystagmus associated with Chiari malformation. Arch Neurol 43:299, 1986
95. Samkoff LM, Smith CR: See-saw nystagmus in a patient with clinically definite MS. Eur Neurol 34:228, 1994
96. May EF, Truxal AR: Loss of vision may result in seesaw nystagmus. J Neuro-ophthalmol 17:84, 1997
97. Nakada T, Kwee IL: Seesaw nystagmus. Role of visuovestibular interaction in its pathogenesis. J Clin Neuro-ophthalmol 8:171, 1988
98. Bergin DJ, Halpern J: Congenital see-saw nystagmus associated with retinitis pigmentosa. Ann Ophthalmol 18:346, 1986
99. Daroff RB, Hoyt WF, Sanders MD et al: Gaze-evoked eyelid and ocular nystagmus inhibited lby the near reflex: unusual ocular motor phenomena in a lateral medullary syndrome. J Neurol Neurosurg Psychiatry 31:362, 1968
100. Safran AB, Berney J, Safran E: Convergence-evoked eyelid nystagmus. Am J Ophthalmol 93:48, 1982
101. Lavin PJM, Traccis S, Dell'Osso LF et al: Downbeat nystagmus with a pseudocycloid waveform: improvement with base-out prisms. Ann Neurol 13:621, 1983
102. Cox TA, Corbett JJ, Thompson HS et al: Upbeat nystagmus changing to downbeat nystagmus with convergence. Neurology 31:891, 1981
103. Noda S, Ide K, Umezaki H et al: Repetitive divergence. Ann Neurol 21:109, 1987
104. Oohira A, Goto K, Ozawa T: Convergence nystagmus. Neuro-ophthalmology 6:313, 1986
105. Nelson KR, Brenner RP, Carlow TJ: Divergent-convergent eye movements and transient eyelid opening associated with an EEG burst-suppression pattern. Neuro-ophthalmology 6:43, 1986
106. Averbuch-Heller L, Zivotofsky AZ, Remler BF et al: Convergent-divergent pendular nystagmus: possible role of the vergence system. Neurology 45:509, 1995
107. Sharpe JA, Hoyt WF, Rosenberg MA: Convergence-evoked nystagmus: congenital and acquired forms. Arch Neurol 32:191, 1975
108. Hara T, Kawazawa S, Abe Y et al: Conjugate pendular nystagmus evoked by accommodative vergence. Eur Neurol 25:369, 1986
109. Guyer DR, Lessell S: Periodic alternating nystagmus associated with albinism. J Clin Neuro-ophthalmol 6:82, 1986
110. Abadi RV, Pascal E: Periodic alternating nystagmus in humans with albinism. Invest Ophthalmol Vis Sci 35:4080, 1994
111. Leigh RJ, Robinson DA, Zee DS: A hypothetical explanation for periodic alternating nystagmus: instability in the optokinetic-vestibular system. Ann NY Acad Sci 374:619, 1981
112. Furman JMR, Wall C III, Pang D: Vestibular function in periodic alternating nystagmus. Brain 113:1425, 1990
113. Waespe W, Cohen B, Raphan T: Dynamic modification of the vestibulo-ocular reflex by the nodulus and uvula. Science 228:199, 1985
114. Campbell WW Jr: Periodic alternating nystagmus in phenytoin intoxication. Arch Neurol 37:178, 1980
115. Halmagyi GM, Rudge P, Gresty MA et al: Treatment of periodic alternating nystagmus. Ann Neurol 8:609, 1980
116. Nuti D, Ciacci G, Giannini F et al: Aperiodic alternating nystagmus: report of two cases and treatment by baclofen. Ital J Neurol Sci 7:453, 1986
117. Lewis JM, Kline LB: Periodic alternating nystagmus associated with periodic alternating skew deviation. J Clin Neuro-ophthalmol 3:115, 1983
118. Kennard C, Barger G, Hoyt WF: The association of periodic alternating nystagmus with periodic alternating gaze. J Clin Neuro-ophthalmol 1:191, 1981
119. Vighetto A, Froment JC, Trillet M et al: Magnetic resonance imaging in familial paroxysmal ataxia. Arch Neurol 45:547, 1988
120. Baloh RW, Spooner JW: Downbeat nystagmus: a type of central vestibular nystagmus. Neurology 31:304, 1981
121. Halmagyi GM, Rudge P, Gresty MA et al: Downbeating nystagmus. A review of 62 cases. Arch Neurol 40:777, 1983
122. Rosengart A, Hedges TR III, Teal PA et al: Intermittent downbeat nystagmus due to vertebral artery compression. Neurology 43:216, 1993
123. Schmidt D: Downbeat nystagmus. A clinical review. Neuro-ophthalmology 11:247, 1991
124. Egan DJ: Optical treatment of downbeat nystagmus induced oscillopsia. Invest Ophthalmol Vis Sci 36:S351, 1995
125. Gresty MA, Barratt H, Rudge P et al: Analysis of downbeat nystagmus. Arch Neurol 43:52, 1986
126. Baloh RW, Yee RD: Spontaneous vertical nystagmus. Rev Neurol 145:527, 1989
127. Rousseaux M, Dupard T, Lesoin F et al: Upbeat and downbeat nystagmus occurring successively in a patient with posterior medullary hemorrhage. J Neurol Neurosurg Psychiatry 54:367, 1991
128. Tokumasu K, Fujino A, Yoshio S et al: Upbeat nystagmus in primary eye position. Acta Otolaryngol (Stockh) 481:366, 1991
129. Ranalli PJ, Sharpe JA: Upbeat nystagmus and the ventral tegmental pathway of the upward vestibuloocular reflex. Neurology 38:1329, 1988
130. Fisher A, Gresty MA, Chambers B et al: Primary position upbeating nystagmus: a variety of central positional nystagmus. Brain 106:949, 1983
131. Keane JR, Itabashi HH: Upbeat nystagmus: clinicopathologic study of two patients. Neurology 37:491, 1987
132. Büttner U, Helmchen Ch, Büttner-ennever JA: The localizing

value of nystagmus in brainstem disorders. Neuro-ophthalmology 15:283, 1995

133. Albera R, Luda E, Machetta G et al: Cyclosporine A as a possible cause of upbeating nystagmus. Neuro-ophthalmology 17:163, 1997

134. Kattah JC, Dagi TF: Compensatory head tilt in upbeating nystagmus. J Clin Neuro-ophthalmol 10:27, 1990

135. Sibony PA, Evinger C, Manning KA: Tobacco-induced primary-position upbeat nystagmus. Ann Neurol 21:53, 1987

136. Bondar RL, Sharpe JA, Lewis AJ: Rebound nystagmus in olivo-cerebellar atrophy: a clinicopathological correlation. Ann Neurol 15:474, 1984

137. Helmchen Ch, Büttner U: Centripetal nystagmus in a case of Creutzfeldt-Jakob disease. Neuro-ophthalmology 15:187, 1995

138. Traccis S, Rosati G, Monaco MF et al: Successful treatment of acquired pendular elliptical nystagmus in multiple sclerosis with isoniazid and base-out prisms. Neurology 40:492, 1990

139. De Jong JMBV, Bless W, Bovenkerk G: Nystagmus, gaze shift, and self-motion perception during sinusoidal head and neck rotation. Ann NY Acad Sci 374:590, 1981

140. Hamann KF: Kritische Anmerkungen zum sogenannten zerviko-genen Schwindel. Laryngol Rhinol Otol 64:156, 1985

141. Norre ME, Stevens A: Diagnostic and semiological problem with special emphasis upon "cervical nystagmus." Acta Otorhino-laryngol Belg 41:436, 1987

142. Schmidt D, Dell'Osso LF, Abel LA et al: Myasthenia gravis: dynamic changes in saccadic waveform, gain and velocity. Exp Neurol 68:365, 1980

143. Howard RS: A case of convergence evoked eyelid nystagmus. J Clin Neuro-ophthalmol 6:169, 1986

144. Brodsky MC, Boop FA: Lid nystagmus as a sign of intrinsic midbrain disease. J Neuro-ophthalmol 15:236, 1995

145. Lavin PJM: Pupillary oscillations synchronous with ictal nystagmus. Neuro-ophthalmology 6:113, 1986

146. Kaplan PW, Lesser RP: Vertical and horizontal epileptic gaze deviation and nystagmus. Neurology 39:1391, 1989

147. Tusa RJ, Kaplan PW, Hain TC et al: Ipsiversive eye deviation and epileptic nystagmus. Neurology 40:662, 1989

148. Thurston SE, Leigh RJ, Osorio I: Epileptic gaze deviation and nystagmus. Neurology 35:1518, 1985

149. Kaplan PW, Tusa RJ: Neurophysiologic and clinical correlations of epileptic nystagmus. Neurology 43:2508, 1993

150. Von Baumgarten R, Benson A, Brand U et al: Effects of recti-linear acceleration and optokinetic and caloric stimulations in space. Science 225:208, 1984

151. Paige GD: Caloric responses after horizontal canal inactivation. Acta Otolaryngol (Stockh) 100:321, 1985

152. Buettner UW, Zee DS: Vestibular testing in comatose patients. Arch Neurol 46:561, 1989

153. Baloh RW, Honrubia V, Jacobson K: Benign positional vertigo: clinical and oculographic features in 240 cases. Neurology 37:371, 1987

154. Lin J, Elidan J, Baloh RW et al: direction-changing positional nystagmus. Am J Otolaryngol 7:306, 1986

155. Brandt T, Steddin S, Daroff RB: Therapy for benign paroxysmal positioning vertigo, revisited. Neurology 44:796, 1994

156. Kattah JC, Kolsky MP, Luessenhop AJ: Positional vertigo and the cerebellar vermis. Neurology 34:527, 1984

157. Baloh RW, Jacobson K, Honrubia V: Horizontal semicircular canal variant of benign positional vertigo. Neurology 43:2542, 1993

158. Lempert T: Horizontal benign positional vertigo. Neurology 44:2213, 1994

159. Esser J, Brandt T: Pharmakologisch verursachte Augenbewe-gungsstörungen—Differentialdiagnose und Wirkungsmechanis-men. Fortschr Neurol Psychiatr 51:41, 1983

160. Coppeto JR, Monteiro MLR, Lessel S et al: Downbeat nystagmus. Arch Neurol 40:754, 1983

161. Corbett JJ, Jacobson DM, Thompson HS et al: Downbeating nystagmus and other ocular motor defects caused by lithium toxicity. Neurology 39:481, 1989

162. Rosenberg ML: Reversible downbeat nystagmus secondary to excessive alcohol intake. J Clin Neuro-ophthalmol 7:23, 1987

163. Kattah JC, Schilling R, Liu S-J et al: Oculomotor manifestations of acute alcohol intoxication. In Smith JL, Katz RS (eds): Neuro-Ophthalmology Enters the Nineties, p 233. Miami, Dutton Press, 1988

164. Maas EF, Ashe J, Spiegel BA et al: Acquired pendular nystagmus in toluene addiction. Neurology 41:282, 1991

165. Yokota J-I, Imai H, Okuda O et al: Inverted Bruns' nystagmus in arachnoid cysts of the cerebellopontine angle. Eur Neurol 33:62, 1993

166. Waespe W, Wichmann W: Oculomotor disturbances during visual-vestibular interaction in Wallenberg's lateral medullary syndrome. Brain 113:821, 1990

167. Waespe W, Baumgartner R: Enduring dysmetria and impaired gain adaptivity of saccadic eye movements in Wallenberg's lateral medullary syndrome. Brain 115:1125, 1992

168. Dieterich M, Brandt T: Wallenberg's syndrome: lateropulsion, cyclorotation, and subjective visual vertical in thirty-six patients. Ann Neurol 31:399, 1992

169. Morrow MJ, Sharpe JA: Torsional nystagmus in the lateral medullary syndrome. Ann Neurol 24:390, 1988

170. Brazis PW: Ocular motor abnormalities in Wallenberg's lateral medullary syndrome. Mayo Clin Proc 67:365, 1992

171. Ranailli PJ, Sharpe JA: Contrapulsion of saccades and ipsilateral ataxia: a unilateral disorder of the rostral cerebellum. Ann Neurol 20:311, 1986

172. Solomon D, Galetta SL, Grant TL: Possible mechanisms for horizontal gaze deviation and lateropulsion in the lateral medullary syndrome. J Neuro-ophthalmol 15:26, 1995

173. Collewijn H, Apkarian P, Spekreijse H: The oculomotor behaviour of human albinos. Brain 108:1, 1985

174. Apkarian P, Shallo-Hoffmann J: VEP projections in congenital nystagmus; VEP asymmetry in albinism: a comparison study. Invest Ophthalmol Vis Sci 32:2653, 1991

175. Cheong PYY, King RA, Bateman JB: Oculocutaneous albinism: variable expressivity of nystagmus in a sibship. J Pediatr Ophthalmol Strabismus 29:185, 1992

176. McCarty JW, Demer JL, Hovis LA et al: Ocular motility anomalies in developmental misdirection of the optic chiasm. Am J Ophthalmol 113:86, 1992

177. Williams RW, Hogan D, Garraghty PE: Target recognition and visual maps in the thalamus of achiasmatic mutant dogs. Nature 367:637, 1994

178. Apkarian P, Dell'Osso LF, Ferraresi A, Van derSteen J: Ocular motor abnormalities in human achiasmatic syndrome. Invest Ophthalmol Vis Sci 35:1410, 1994

179. Dell'Osso LF: Evidence suggesting individual ocular motor control of each eye (muscle). J Vestib Res 4:335, 1994

180. Dell'Osso LF, Williams RW: Ocular motor abnormalities in achiasmatic mutant Belgian sheepdogs: unyoked eye movements in a mammal. Vision Res 35:109, 1995

181. Dell'Osso LF, Williams RW, Jacobs JB et al: The congenital and see-saw nystagmus in the prototypical achiasma of canines: comparison to the human achiasmatic prototype. Vision Res 38:1629, 1998

182. Dell'Osso LF, Williams RW, Hogan D: Eye movements in canine hemichiasma. Invest Ophthalmol Vis Sci 38:S1144, 1997

183. Dell'Osso LF, Daroff RB: Two additional scenarios for see-saw nystagmus: achiasma and hemichiasma. J Neuro-ophthalmol 18:112, 1998

184. Doslak MJ, Dell'Osso LF, Daroff RB: Multiple double saccadic pulses occurring with other saccadic intrusions and oscillations. Neuro-ophthalmology 3:109, 1983

185. Whicker L, Abel LA, Dell'Osso LF: Smooth pursuit and fixation in the parents of schizophrenics. Soc Neurosci Abstr 9:70, 1983

186. Abel LA, Traccis S, Dell'Osso LF et al: Square wave oscillation. The relationship of saccadic intrusions and oscillations. Neuro-ophthalmology 4:21, 1984

187. Dell'Osso LF, Troost BT, Daroff RB: Macro square wave jerks. Neurology 25:975, 1975

188. Dell'Osso LF, Abel LA, Daroff RB: "Inverse latent" macro square wave jerks and macro saccadic oscillations. Ann Neurol 2:57, 1977

189. Selhorst JB, Stark L, Ochs AL et al: Disorders in cerebellar ocular motor control. II. Macro saccadic oscillation: an oculo-

graphic, control system and clinico-anatomical analysis. Brain 99:509, 1976

190. Fukazawa T, Tashiro K, Hamada T et al: Multisystem degeneration: drugs and square wave jerks. Neurology 36:1230, 1986

191. Herishanu YO, Sharpe JA: Saccadic intrusions in internuclear ophthalmoplegia. Ann Neurol 14:67, 1983

192. Selhorst JB, Stark L, Ochs AL et al: Disorders in cerebellar ocular motor control. I. Saccadic overshoot dysmetria: an oculographic, control system and clinico-anatomical analysis. Brain 99:497, 1976

193. Vilis T, Snow R, Hore J: Cerebellar saccadic dysmetria is not equal in the two eyes. Exp Brain Res 51:343, 1983

194. Bötzel K, Rottach K, Büttner U: Normal and pathological saccadic dysmetria. Brain 116:337, 1993

195. Büttner U, Straube A, Spuler A: Saccadic dysmetria and "intact" smooth pursuit eye movements after bilateral deep cerebellar nuclei lesions. J Neurol Neurosurg Psychiatry 57:832, 1994

196. Kanayama R, Bronstein AM, Shallo-Hoffmann J et al: Visually and memory guided saccades in a case of cerebellar saccadic dysmetria. J Neurol Neurosurg Psychiatry 57:1081, 1994

197. Zee DS, Robinson DA: a hypothetical explanation of saccadic oscillations. Ann Neurol 5:405, 1979

198. Hain TC, Zee DS, Mordes M: Blink induced saccadic oscillations. Ann Neurol 19:299, 1986

199. Ashe J, Hain TC, Zee DS et al: Microsaccadic flutter. Brain 114:461, 1991

200. Kaminski HJ, Zee DS, Leigh RJ et al: Ocular flutter and ataxia associated with AIDS-related complex. Neuro-ophthalmology 11:163, 1991

201. Dropcho EJ, Kline LB, Riser J: Antineuronal (anti-Ri) antibodies in a patient with steroid-responsive opsoclonus-myoclonus. Neurology 43:207, 1993

202. Prier S, Larmande P, Dairou R et al: Oscillations macro-saccadiques au cours d'un cas d'encéphalopathie myoclonique paranéoplasique. Rev Neurol 135:339, 1979

203. Furman JMR, Eidelman BH, Fromm GH: Spontaneous remission of paraneoplastic ocular flutter and saccadic intrusions. Neurology 38:499, 1988

204. Gresty MA, Findley LJ, Wade P: Mechanism of rotatory eye movements in opsoclonus. Br J Ophthalmol 64:923, 1980

205. Hattori T, Takaya Y, Tsuboi Y et al: Opsoclonus showing only during eye closure in hereditary cerebellar ataxia. J Neurol Neurosurg Psychiatry 56:1036, 1993

206. Binyon S, Prendergast M: Eye-movement tics in children. Dev Med Child Neurol 33:343, 1991

207. Shawket F, Harris CM, Jacobs M et al: Eye movement tics. Br J Ophthalmol 76:697, 1992

208. Hunter S, Kooistra C: Neuropathologic findings in idiopathic opsoclonus and myoclonus. Their similarity to those in paraneoplastic cerebellar cortical degeneration. J Clin Neuro-ophthalmol 6:236, 1986

209. Dehaene I, Van Vleymen B: Opsoclonus induced by phenytoin and diazepam. Ann Neurol 21:216, 1987

210. Greenlee JE, Lipton HL: Anticerebellar antibodies in serum and cerebrospinal fluid of a patient with oat cell carcinoma of the lung and paraneoplastic cerebellar degeneration. Ann Neurol 19: 82, 1986

211. Anderson NE, Corinna CB, Budde-Steffen C: Opsoclonus, myoclonus, ataxia, and encephalopathy in adults with cancer: a distinct paraneoplastic syndrome. Medicine 67:100, 1988

212. Herishanu Y, Apte R, Kuperman O: Immunological abnormalities in opsoclonus cerebellopathy. Neuro-ophthalmology 5:271, 1985

213. Nitschke M, Hochberg F, Dropcho E: Improvement in paraneoplastic opsoclonus-myoclonus after protein A column therapy. N Engl J Med 332:192, 1995

214. Ridley A, Kennard C, Scholtz CL et al: Omnipause neurons in two cases of opsoclonus associated with oat cell carcinoma of the lung. Brain 110:1699, 1987

215. Tuchman RF, Alvarez LA, Kantrowitz AB et al: Opsoclonus-myoclonus syndrome: correlation of radiographic and pathological observations. Neuroradiology 31:250, 1989

216. Gwinn KA, Caviness JN: Electrophysiological observations in idiopathic opsoclonus-myoclonus syndrome. Mov Disord 12:438, 1997

217. Borodic GE, Miller DC, Bienfang DC: Opsoclonus: three cases and literature review. In Smith JL, Katz RS (eds): Neuro-Ophthalmology Enters the Nineties, p 213. Miami, Dutton Press, 1988

218. Caviness JN, Forsyth PA, Layton DD et al: The movement disorder of adult opsoclonus. Mov Disord 10:22, 1995

219. Deuschl G, Mischke G, Schenck E, et al: Symptomatic and essential rhythmic palatal myoclonus. Brain 113:1645, 1990

220. Nakada T, Kwee IL: Oculopalatal myoclonus. Brain 109:431, 1986

221. Matsuo F, Ajax ET: Palatal myoclonus and denervation supersensitivity in the central nervous system. Ann Neurol 5:72, 1979

222. Koeppen AH, Barron KD, Dentinger MP: Olivary hypertrophy: histochemical demonstration of hydrolytic enzymes. Neurology 30:471, 1980

223. Keane JR: Acute vertical ocular myoclonus. Neurology 36:86, 1986

224. Jacobs L, Newman RP, Bozian D: Disappearing palatal myoclonus. Neurology 31:748, 1981

225. Carlow TJ: Medical treatment of nystagmus and ocular motor disorders. In Beck RW, Smith CH (eds): Neuroophthalmology, p 251. Boston, Little, Brown, 1986

226. Herishanu YO, Zigoulinski R: The effect of chronic one-eye patching on ocular myoclonus. J Clin Neuro-ophthalmol 11:166, 1991

227. Jabbari B, Rosenberg M, Scherokman B et al: Effectiveness of trihexyphenidyl against pendular nystagmus and palatal myoclonus: evidence of cholinergic dysfunction. Mov Disord 2:93, 1987

228. Neetens A, Martin JJ: Superior oblique myokymia in a case of adrenoleukodystrophy and in a case of lead intoxication. Neuro-ophthalmology 3:103, 1983

229. Kommerell G, Schaubele G: Superior oblique myokymia. An electromyographical analysis. Trans Ophthalmol Soc UK 100:504, 1980

230. Morrow MJ, Sharpe JA, Ranalli PJ: Superior oblique myokymia associated with a posterior fossa tumor: oculographic correlation with an idiopathic case. Neurology 40:367, 1990

231. Leigh RJ, Tomsak RL, Seidman SH et al: Superior oblique myokymia: quantitative characteristics of the eye movements in three patients. Arch Ophthalmol 109:1710, 1991

232. Rosenberg ML, Glaser JS: Superior oblique myokymia. Ann Neurol 13:667, 1983

233. Breen LA, Gutmann L, Riggs JE: Superior oblique myokymia. A misnomer. J Clin Neuro-ophthalmol 3:131, 1983

234. Thurston SE, Saul RF: Superior oblique myokymia: quantitative description of the eye movement. Neurology 41:1679, 1991

235. Komai K, Mimura O, Uyama J et al: Neuro-ophthalmological evaluation of superior oblique myokymia. Neuro-ophthalmology 12:135, 1992

236. Brazis PW, Miller NR, Henderer JD et al: The natural history and results of treatment of superior oblique myokymia. Arch Ophthalmol 112:1063, 1994

237. Rudick R, Satran R, Eskin T: Ocular bobbing in encephalitis. J Neurol Neurosurg Psychiatry 44:441, 1981

238. Dehaene I, Lammens M, Marchau M: Paretic ocular bobbing. Neuro-ophthalmology 13:143, 1993

239. Gaymard B: Disconjugate ocular bobbing. Neurology 43:2151, 1993

240. Brusa A, Firpo MP, Massa S et al: Typical and reverse bobbing: a case with localizing value. Eur Neurol 23:151, 1984

241. Knobler RL, Somasundaram M, Schutta HS: Inverse ocular bobbing. Ann Neurol 9:194, 1981

242. Ropper AH: Ocular dipping in anoxic coma. Arch Neurol 38:297, 1981

243. Van Weerden TW, Van Woerkom TCAM: Ocular dipping. Clin Neurol Neurosurg 84:221, 1982

244. Stark SR, Masucci EF, Kurtzke JF: Ocular dipping. Neurology 34:391, 1984
245. Safran AB, Berney J: Synchronism of inverse ocular bobbing and blinking. Am J Ophthalmol 95:401, 1983
246. Toshniwal P, Yadava R, Goldbarg H: Presentation of pineal-oblastoma with ocular dipping and deafness. J Clin Neuro-ophthalmol 6:128, 1986
247. Rosenberg ML: Spontaneous vertical eye movements in coma. Ann Neurol 20:635, 1986
248. Shults WT, Stark L, Hoyt WF et al: Normal saccadic struc-ture and voluntary nystagmus. Arch Ophthalmol 95:1399, 1977
249. Nagle M, Bridgeman B, Stark L: Voluntary nystagmus, saccadic suppression, and stabilization of the visual world. Vision Res 20:717, 1980
250. Krohel G, Griffin JF: Voluntary vertical nystagmus. Neurology 29:1153, 1979
251. Yee RD, Spiegel PH, Yamada T et al: Voluntary saccadic oscil-lations, resembling ocular flutter and opsoclonus. J Neuro-ophthalmol 14:95, 1994

Glossary for Chapters 9 through 11

Amplitude   The size of an eye movement (measured in angular degrees), either horizontal or vertical excursion (e.g., "The amplitude of the saccades was 20°").

Ballistic   Having characteristics similar to the trajectory or path of motion of a projectile after it is launched. Implies lack of any ongoing control or guidance. Used in reference to fast eye movements (saccades), the course of which is regarded as ballistic.

Bandwidth   Range of input signal frequencies processed without major distortion by a given piece of electronic equipment or by a given physiologic system.

Closed-loop system   In control-systems theory, a system that has feedback by the way of some connection, such as a neural pathway. In such systems the output signal is monitored and fed back to the input signal; it can be either added to or subtracted from the input signal. In the control of eye movements, the output (eye movement) may be fed back by measurement of the retinal error to determine accuracy. If there is a retinal error, a corrective eye movement may be made (see also Fig. 9–7).

Continuous   Uninterrupted in time. In eye-movement control, this refers to a system that is continuously monitoring eye position or velocity (e.g., the pursuit system performs accurate tracking of a moving target by continuously recognizing differences between velocities [rates of change] of the target and of the eye).

Control system   A mechanism that functions to maintain its output at a given level dependent upon an input reference signal. In eye movements, a system that functions to bring images from the peripheral retina to the fovea and/or to maintain foveation, as during pursuit of a moving target. The output is the eye movement; the input reference signal is the position or velocity of the retinal image.

Cyclopean eye   A reference eye theoretically located midway between, and in the same place as, the two anatomic eyes.

Damp (damping, damped)   To retard the energy or reduce the amplitude of a movement (e.g., convergence may damp the oscillation of the eyes in congenital nystagmus).

Differentiation   A mathematical operation that yields a measure of the rate of change of a variable (e.g., the slope of a straight line). Differentiation of eye position with respect to time will define velocity at a given instant.

Discontinuous   Interrupted in time. In eye-movement control, this refers to a system that samples eye and target positions at discrete intervals (e.g., the saccadic system intermittently samples differences between target and eye positions).

Discrete   Consisting of separate, individual parts or date points. In eye-movement control, this refers to a system that is monitoring eye position or velocity at or during finite intervals (e.g., the saccadic eye-movement system).

Displacement   The total distance that a target, retinal image, or eye has moved.

Exponential   A mathematically defined motion with a constantly increasing or decreasing rate of change. Graphically seen as a curving rather than a straight line.

Feedback   Return of portions or entire output signal information to influence the input signal (e.g., continuous return of eye-movement data [output] to the system controlling eye movements). See **Closed-loop system.**

Feedback (negative)   Subtracting portions of a system's output from its input (e.g., subtracting a new retinal image position closer to the fovea from a prior image position further in the periphery in an attempt to reduce the eccentric image position [retinal error] to zero and produce foveation).

Feedback (positive)   Adding portions of a system's output to its input. In eye-movement control, such addition causes greater retinal error.

Foveate (foveation, refoveation)   To bring a peripheral retinal image onto the fovea (by way of a saccade) or to maintain the image on the fovea during target movement (by way of pursuit).

Frequency   Number of oscillations per second or cycles per second, measured in Hertz (Hz) (e.g., a nystagmus cycle [slow and fast phase] that is completed five times per second has a frequency of 5 Hz).

Gain   The ratio of a system's output to its input (e.g., when the eyes move 20° [output] in response to a retinal-image position error of 20° [input], the gain of the eye-movement system is output/input: $20°/20°=1$).

Generator   The source of a signal. The pontine reticular formation is regarded as the final prenuclear source or generator (pulse generator) of the neural signal for horizontal eye movements.

Hertz (Hz)   See **Frequency**.

Input   The information signal upon which a system operates (e.g., retinal-position error [image not on fovea] that elicits voluntary ocular refixation to new target positions [with image on fovea]).

Integrator (integral, integrate)   A mathematical function/operation analogous to summation. The inverse operation is differentiation (e.g., in eye movements the integral of the velocity yields eye position). A brainstem neural integrator processes information to produce a signal proportional to eye position. If the integrator is imperfect or leaky, the neural signal tends to change and the eye drifts from an eccentric gaze position toward primary position, resulting in nystagmus (see also Fig. 9–8).

Latency Reaction time after a specific stimulus (*e.g.*, with a shift in target position, there is a 200-millisecond interval before eye movements begin [see Fig. 9–3]).

Linear (nonlinear) Can (cannot) be described by a simple straight-line relation.

Neutral zone That eye position (region of gaze angles) in which a reversal of direction of jerk nystagmus occurs and in which any of several bidirectional waveforms, pendular nystagmus or no nystagmus, may be present.

Null Field of gaze in which nystagmus intensity is minimal (see Fig. 11–12).

Open loop A control system with no feedback from output to input (*e.g.*, the vestibulo-ocular system is open loop, since there is no feedback from the output [compensatory eye movement] to the input [acceleration stimulating the semicircular canals]).

Output The outgoing signal resulting from a system's response to an input signal or signals (*e.g.*, a saccadic eye movement [output] in response to a peripheral retinal image or target displacement [input]).

Plant (plant dynamics) The globe, muscles, check ligaments, fascia, and fatty supporting tissues of the orbit have physical properties described as viscoelastic (including inertia); these characteristics can be defined mathematically. In general, the orbital plant dynamics have a braking (damping) effect on eye movement.

Position error Discrepancy between position of eccentric retinal image and the fovea. Represented in space by the difference between target position and visual direction of the eye. Position error is the stimulus for foveation and is an example of a feedback signal.

Pulse A high-frequency burst of neural firing beginning and ending at well-defined times (see Fig. 9–5B).

Pulse-step A high-frequency burst followed by a constant frequency of neural firing beginning and ending at a well-defined time. It is pulse-step of neural firing

that brings about a saccade or rapid change in eye position (see Fig. 9–5B).

Ramp A linearly increasing frequency of neural firing beginning at a well-defined time (see Fig. 9–5C).

Rectilinear In a recording system, this refers to pen motion perpendicular to paper motion.

Retinal error Distance on the retina between eccentric image and fovea. See **Position error.**

Retinal-slip velocity Rate of change of retinal error.

Saccade A fast eye movement, voluntary or reflex, usually accomplishing foveal fixation.

Sampled data System operating on information gathered at separate time intervals, as opposed to continuous data analysis (*e.g.*, the saccadic eye-movement control system has been considered a sampled-data system).

Signal An electrical or neural analog to a physical quantity (*e.g.*, input and output signals).

Sinusoidal A mathematical function that describes the motion of a pendulum. Ordinary house current is sinusoidal. In pendular nystagmus the eyes oscillate in a sinusoidal fashion.

Step A constant frequency of neural firing beginning at some well-defined time (see Fig. 9–5A).

Step-ramp A constant frequency added to a linearly increasing frequency of neural firing beginning at a well-defined time (see Fig. 9–5D).

Target An object of regard. Stimulus for foveation and fixation.

Time constant A measure of the response time of a system to a transient input (*e.g.*, the response of a system to a step change in input is usually considered to be the interval given by 3 to 5 time constants).

Trajectory The motion of a target or eye in time and space.

Transfer function The mathematical function that is the ratio of a system's output to its input, the magnitude of which is the gain of the system.

Velocity error The rate of change of position error (*e.g.*, the difference between the velocity of the tracking eye and of the target).

CHAPTER 12

Infranuclear Disorders of Eye Movement

Joel S. Glaser and R. Michael Siatkowski

Neuroanatomy
Abducens Palsies
Etiology
Isolated Abducens Palsy
Trochlear Palsies
Oculomotor Palsies
Nuclear Lesions
Fascicular Lesions
Interpeduncular Lesions
   Cavernous Sinus Lesions
   Orbital Lesions
Ischemic ("Diabetic") Oculomotor Palsy
Oculomotor Synkinesis
Herpes Zoster
Acute Infectious Polyneuropathy
Ophthalmoplegic Migraine
Oculomotor Palsies of Childhood
Cyclic Oculomotor Palsy

Combined Oculomotor Palsies and Painful
   Ophthalmoplegias
Orbital Lesions
Tolosa-Hunt Syndrome
Parasellar Syndromes
Other Ocular Polyneuropathies
Disorders of the Neuromuscular Junction and
     Ocular Myopathies
   Myasthenia
   Myasthenia-Like Syndromes
   Thyroid-Related Myopathy (Graves' Disease)
   Progressive (Chronic) External Ophthalmoplegia
Conditions Simulating Progressive External
     Ophthalmoplegia
Myotonic Dystrophy
Ocular Neuromyotonia
Dorsal Midbrain Syndrome
Diplopia after Ocular Surgery
Miscellaneous Ocular Muscle Conditions

Not only the novice but also many well-trained and experienced oculists consider motor anomalies to be hte most difficult field in ophthalmology because of the great variety of signs and symptoms which frequently cannot be reconciled with one another . . . In examining and treating motor anomalies, one never loses an uneasy feeling of incompetence until one has become familiar with the physiologic fundamentals . . .

Alfred Bielschowsky, 1938
Lectures on Motor Anomalies

NEUROANATOMY

The supranuclear control of eye movements is discussed in detail in Chapters 9 and 10. However, for purposes of review it should be recalled that supranuclear ocular motor pathways descend from the cerebral hemispheres, decussate in the caudal midbrain, and terminate in the pontine horizontal gaze complex (Fig. 12–1). From here,

J. S. Glaser: Departments of Neurology and Ophthalmology, Bascom Palmer Eye Institute, University of Miami School of Medicine, Miami; and Neuro-ophthalmology, Cleveland Clinic Florida, Ft. Lauderdale, Florida

R. M. Siatkowski: Department of Ophthalmology, Dean A. McGee Eye Institute, University of Oklahoma, Oklahoma City, Oklahoma

the motor nuclei of the ocular muscles are integrated by way of the medial longitudinal fasciculus.

The nuclear complex of the third (oculomotor) nerve lies beneath the aqueductal gray matter of the rostral midbrain at the level of the superior colliculus (Fig. 12–2). The medial longitudinal fasciculus (MLF) passes just lateral to the oculomotor nuclei, and the fourth (trochlear) cranial nerve nucleus is contiguous caudally. The organization of the oculomotor nuclear complex into distinct motor cell pools subserving individual extraocular muscles was investigated by Warwick,[1] from whose schema (Fig. 12–3) the following points are especially noteworthy: (1) both lid levators are served by a single dorsal-caudal midline nucleus; (2) the motor cell pool of the superior rectus muscle sends fibers across to the contralateral oculomotor nerve; (3) a nucleus for convergence (Perlia) has not been consistently demonstrated in primates, including humans; and (4) at the caudal aspect of the oculomotor complex is the trochlear nucleus, whose axons turn dorsally to cross in the anterior medullary velum and innervate the contralateral superior oblique. Therefore, the nuclear motor pools of the superior rectus and superior oblique muscles are contralateral to the eye that they move. Warwick proposed that each muscle (intrinsic and extrinsic) inner-

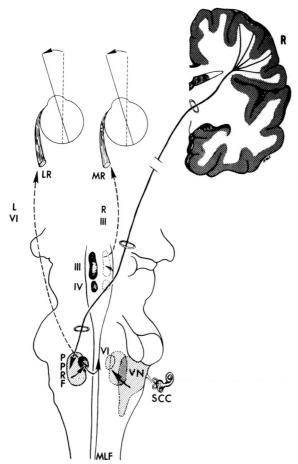

Fig. 12–1. Supranuclear oculomotor system. Conjugate horizontal gaze to left originates in right frontal optomotor cortex (*R*). Pathway descends in area of internal capsule, decussates at level of trochlear nucleus (*IV*) to synapse in left pontine paramedian reticular formation (*PPRF*). Via direct connection to abducens nucleus (*VI*; labeled on right side), left lateral rectus (*LR*) is innervated. From abducens nucleus via contralateral medial longitudinal fasciculus (*MLF*) impulse is directed to contralateral oculomotor nuclear complex (*III*; labeled on left side), then to right medial rectus (*MR*). (*VN*, vestibular nuclear complex; *SCC*, semicircular canals)

ate the median mesencephalon in the interpeduncular space.

The sixth (abducens) nucleus is situated in the caudal portion of the paramedian pontine tegmentum, beneath the floor of the fourth ventricle (see Fig. 12–2). Facial nerve fibers loop around the abducens nucleus before exiting in the cerebellopontine angle. This intimate relationship accounts for frequent concurrent damage seen clinically. Although lateral to the third nuclear complex in the rostral mesencephalon, the MLF passes medial to the abducens nucleus. There are two populations of neurons with cell bodies within the abducens nucleus.[5,6] One group forms the sixth nerve; these abducens fibers pass ventrally to exit at the pontomedullary junction. The other internuclear neurons send fibers to join the contralateral MLF, with projection to the medial rectus subnucleus. Therefore, lesions involving the sixth nucleus produce an ipsilateral conjugate gaze palsy (*i.e.*, ipsilateral lateral rectus and contralateral medial rectus).[7]

The abducens, trochlear, and oculomotor nuclei are integrated via the MLF, which also has major connections with the vestibular nuclear complex (see Fig. 12–1). Lesions involving the MLF typically result in *internuclear ophthalmoplegia* (see Chapter 10), which consists of faulty adduction of the ipsilateral eye (observed especially with attempted saccades) and dissociated nystagmus greater in the abducting eye on attempted lateral horizontal gaze (Fig. 12–4). In addition, some degree of vertical nystagmus in upward gaze is often present, and skew deviation may account for vertical diplopia.[8] Internuclear ophthalmoplegia, usually bilateral, is by far the most common ocular motor disturbance of demyelinative origin. As a rule, unilateral ophthalmoplegia is usually due to a vascular incident, but bilateral involvement should not be considered rare in brain stem infarction.[9]

The peripheral course of the third nerve is as follows (Fig. 12–5): as the nerve exits ventrally from the midbrain into the interpeduncular space, it passes beneath the origin of the posterior cerebral artery and lies parallel and lateral to the posterior communicating artery. Klintworth[10] pointed out that, in instances where the basilar artery bifurcates at a low level, the oculomotor nerve may be angled downward at the point where the posterior cerebral artery crosses the nerve, and vascular grooving of the superior aspect of the nerve is present in approximately one third of normal brains. The nerve runs between the free edge of the tentorium and the lateral aspect of the posterior clinoid, where it pierces the dura to enter the cavernous sinus. The oculomotor trunk occupies the superior aspect of the cavernous sinus (see ahead to Fig. 12–17) and separates into superior and inferior divisions at 4 to 5 mm before the superior orbital fissure. Fiber count of the superior division is about one-third that of the inferior,[11] and it has been

vated by the oculomotor nerve is subserved by a single, circumscribed mass of cells called a *subnucleus*. Modern tracer techniques have, to date, confirmed this concept for all the extrinsic muscles except the medial rectus, which has three definable subnuclei[2,3]; there are also afferent fibers to the ipsilateral trigeminal ganglion. Results of elegant axonal tracer studies mapping the intricate connections of the visceral nuclei of the oculomotor complex have been summarized by Burde.[4]

From the oculomotor complex the efferent fibers exit ventrally and pass through the red nucleus and medial aspect of the cerebral peduncles. The fascicles emerge in the interpeduncular space anterior to the midbrain as the paired oculomotor nerves. The oculomotor nuclei obtain their vascular supply from the terminal bifurcation of the basilar artery. Multiple arteries perfor-

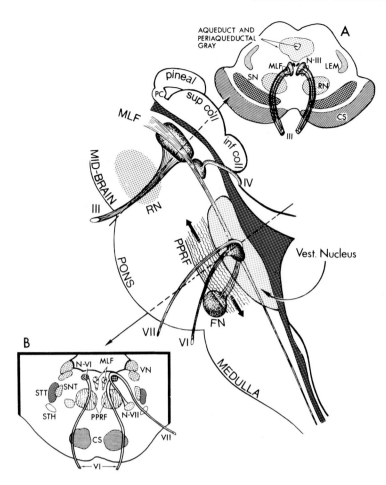

Fig. 12–2. Diagrammatic section of brain stem. **A.** Cross-section at level of superior colliculus. (*N-III*, oculomotor nucleus; *MLF*, medial longitudinal fasciculus; *LEM*, medial lemniscus; *RN*, red nucleus; *SN*, substantia nigra; *CS*, corticospinal tract) **B.** Cross-section at level of abducens nucleus (*N-VI*). (*PPRF*, pontine paramedian reticular formation [note that reticular formation continues rostrally and caudally (*arrows*)]; *N-VII* [*FN*], facial nucleus; *VN*, vestibular nuclear complex; *SNT*, spinal nucleus of trigeminal; *STT*, spinal tract of trigeminal; *STH*, spinothalamic tract)

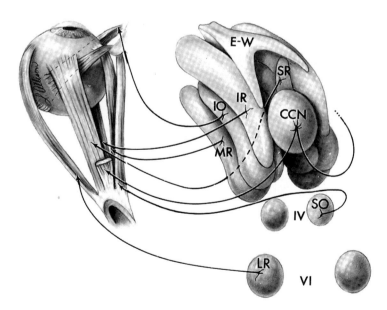

Fig. 12–3. Organization of oculomotor nuclear complex viewed from above, left posterior. *E-W*, Edinger-Westphal parasympathetic subnucleus; subnuclei *IR*, inferior rectus; *IO*, inferior oblique; *MR*, medial rectus. Note that *SR*, superior rectus motor pool, is crossed, as is *SO*, superior oblique; *CCN*, caudal nucleus to both lid levators; *LR*, abducens nucleus for lateral rectus (Adapted Warwick R: Representation of the extra-ocular muscles in the oculomotor complex. J Comp Neurol 98:449, 1953)

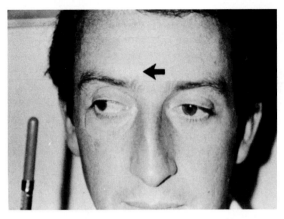

Fig. 12–4. Left internuclear ophthalmoplegia. On attempted right gaze, the left eye fails to adduct due to lesion of left medial longitudinal fasciculus.

suggested that relative pupil sparing in cavernous sinus or orbital apex lesions may reflect preservation of the inferior branch. The inferior branch supplies the medial and inferior recti, inferior oblique, and parasympathetic root to the ciliary ganglion (pupil sphincter); the superior branch innervates the superior rectus and levator palpebrae.

According to Kerr,[12] the pupillomotor fibers are superficial in the oculomotor nerve trunk, lying just internal to the epineurium. It is thought that this superficial position makes the pupillomotor fibers especially vulnerable to compression. In more anterior segments (*e.g.*, cavernous sinus), however, pupillomotor fibers may be preferentially spared even in the presence of total oculomotor palsy. It is likely that involvement or "sparing" of the pupil reflects the nature and acuteness of the

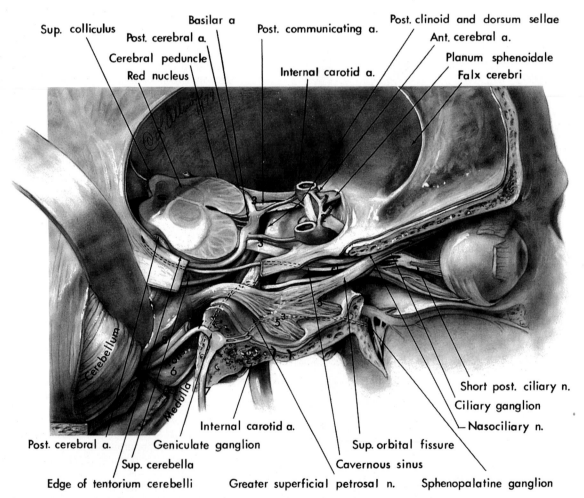

Sup. colliculus
Post. cerebral a.
Cerebral peduncle
Red nucleus
Basilar a
Post. communicating a.
Internal carotid a.
Post. clinoid and dorsum sellae
Ant. cerebral a.
Planum sphenoidale
Falx cerebri
Short post. ciliary n.
Ciliary ganglion
Nasociliary n.
Post. cerebral a.
Geniculate ganglion
Sup. cerebella
Internal carotid a.
Sup. orbital fissure
Cavernous sinus
Edge of tentorium cerebelli
Greater superficial petrosal n.
Sphenopalatine ganglion

Fig. 12–5. Representation of cranial nerves and related basal structures in the area of the midbrain, middle fossa, cavernous sinus, and orbital apex. The roof of the right orbit, sphenoid wing, floor of middle fossa, and petrous ridge have been sectioned; a section of the tentorial edge is removed to demonstrate the course of trochlear nerve (*4*). The cerebellum is retracted to show structures in the posterior fossa. Cross-section of the midbrain is at level of superior colliculi and red nuclei. (*2*, optic nerves and chiasm; *3*, oculomotor nerves [note relationship to posterior cerebral and posterior communicating arteries]; *4*, trochlear nerve in edge of tentorium; *5*, trigeminal nerve [*5¹*, ophthalmic division; *5²*, maxillary division; *5³*, mandibular division]; *6*, abducens nerve [note course up clivus and passage under petroclinoid ligament into posterior aspect of cavernous sinus]; *7*, facial nerve; *8*, acoustic nerve)

lesion, rather than which specific segment of the oculomotor trunk is compromised.

The trochlear fascicles pass dorsally, lateral to the aqueduct, and the nerve exits the midbrain and crosses the contralateral fourth nerve in the anterior medullary velum, just caudal to the inferior colliculi. The fourth nerve is the only cranial nerve to exit the brain stem dorsally. The nerve continues laterally around the midbrain tectum, crosses the superior cerebellar artery, and reaches the free edge of the tentorium, where it enters the dura and runs forward into the cavernous sinus (see Fig. 12–5). The fourth nerve enters the orbit through the superior orbital fissure, but above the annulus formed by the origin of the recti muscles, and innervates only the superior oblique muscle.

The abducens nerve emerges from the brain stem at the lower border of the pons in the pontomedullary sulcus, approximately 1 cm from the midline. The nerve ascends the ventral face of the pons for a short distance, is crossed by the anterior inferior cerebellar artery, and pierces the dura of the clivus approximately 2 cm below the posterior clinoids (see Fig. 12–5). The sixth nerve traverses or passes above the inferior petrosal sinus, runs beneath the petroclinoid ligament (Gruber), and enters the cavernous sinus. The sixth nerve lies freely within the body of the cavernous sinus, unlike the oculomotor and trochlear nerves that are supported in the lateral wall of the sinus. Some sympathetic fibers are briefly attached to the abducens, passing onward to the ophthalmic trigeminal.[13] From the cavernous sinus, the nerve passes through the annular segment of the superior orbital fissure and innervates only the lateral rectus.

Milisavljević and associates[14] demonstrated penetration of oculomotor trunks by circumflex mesencephalic arteries or branches of the posterior cerebral perforating vessels, but clinical implications of such anatomic anomalies are not clear.

According to the anatomic review by Lapresle and Lasjaunias,[15] there are three arterial "systems" that vascularize the cranial nerves: the inferolateral trunk arises from the intracavernous siphon of the internal carotid artery and nourishes cranial nerves III, IV, VI, and V-1; the middle meningeal system supplies nerves VII and V-2,3; and the ascending pharyngeal system supplies nerves IX through XII. The oculomotor nerve is also vascularized by the basilar artery system in the region of the posterior perforated substance, and in the supracavernous region by the artery of the free tentorial margin (Bernasconi). The clinical correlation of ischemic cranial neuropathies with these arterial territories is not entirely clear.

ABDUCENS PALSIES

It is not proper to equate all lateral rectus malfunction with "sixth nerve palsy": to do so confuses the issue and leads to inappropriate diagnostic procedures. For example, myasthenia, Graves' (dysthyroid) myopathy, or orbital inflammation may all produce deficits of abduction, none of which is due to sixth nerve lesions. The "neural" etiology of lateral rectus weakness must be established or, at least, other causes excluded when possible (Table 12–1). Along with details provided by a thorough medical history, special diagnostic techniques should always be employed, including intravenous edrophonium (Tensilon), forced duction (see Fig. 3–6), and forced generation tests. Until local orbital diseases have been excluded, it is premature for the ophthalmologist to refer a patient for a "neurologic workup."

ETIOLOGY

The causes of actual sixth nerve palsy are legion (Table 12–2). As noted previously, the peripheral course of the abducens nerve is a lengthy one that predisposes this cranial nerve to involvement at all levels, from the brain stem and base of the skull, through the

TABLE 12–1. Causes of Abduction Deficits

Sixth nerve palsies
Graves' myopathy (fibrotic medial rectus)
Myasthenia gravis
Orbital pseudotumor/myositis
Orbital trauma (medial rectus entrapment)
Congenital defects (Duane, Möbius syndromes)
"Convergence spasm" (spasm of the near reflex)

TABLE 12–2. Causes of Sixth Nerve Palsies

Nonlocalizing
Increased intracranial pressure
Intracranial hypotension
Head trauma
Lumbar puncture or spinal anesthesia
Vascular, hypertension
Diabetes/microvascular
Parainfectious processes (postviral; middle ear infections in children)
Basal meningitis

Localizing
Pontine syndromes (infarction, demyelination, tumor); contralateral hemiplegia; ipsilateral facial palsy, ipsilateral horizontal gaze palsy ($\pm$ ipsilateral internuclear ophthalmoplegia); ipsilateral facial analgesia
Cerebellopontine angle lesions (acoustic neuroma, meningioma): in combination with disorders of the eighth, seventh, and ophthalmic-trigeminal nerves (especially corneal hypoesthesia), nystagmus, and cerebellar signs
Clivus lesions (nasopharyngeal carcinoma, clivus chordoma)
Middle fossa disorders (tumor, inflammation of medial aspect of petrous): facial pain/numbness, $\pm$ facial palsy
Cavernous sinus or superior orbital fissure (tumor, inflammation, aneurysm): in combination with disorders of the third, fourth, and ophthalmic-trigeminal nerves (pain/numbness)
Carotid-cavernous or dural arteriovenous fistula

petrous tip and cavernous sinus, to the superior orbital fissure and orbit.

Lesions in the area of the abducens nucleus produce an ipsilateral horizontal gaze paresis, since both the internuclear neurons and the motor neurons of the sixth nerve originate in this nucleus. Although it is not certain whether the horizontal gaze palsy that occurs from damage to the abducens nucleus is always symmetric, it is clear that isolated lateral rectus pareses should never be considered nuclear in origin.

The fascicular (intrapontine) portion of the abducens nerve may be involved along with adjacent structures (see Fig. 12–2) to produce (1) ipsilateral paralysis of abduction (ipsilateral gaze palsy if sixth nucleus and/or pontine paramedian reticular formation [PPRF] is affected); (2) ipsilateral facial palsy; (3) ipsilateral Horner syndrome; (4) ipsilateral facial analgesia; (5) ipsilateral peripheral deafness; and (6) contralateral hemiparesis. These signs constitute the dorsolateral and ventral pontine syndromes (Foville, Millard-Gubler) at the level of the abducens fasciculus in the distribution of the anterior inferior cerebellar artery or its paramedian perforating arteries.

As the sixth nerve ascends the clivus in the subarachnoid space it is vulnerable to various insults, including neoplasms in the prepontine basal cistern (e.g., clivus chordoma, intraforaminal extension of nasopharyngeal carcinoma), compression by downward or forward movement of the brain stem (e.g., transtentorial herniation from supratentorial space-occupying lesions, head trauma, posterior fossa masses or structural anomalies, intracranial hypotension from cerebrospinal fluid leaks), and meningitis. It is here also that the nerve is probably affected by changes in intracranial pressure. Unilateral or bilateral abducens palsies can develop in association with pseudotumor cerebri or the syndrome of spontaneous intracranial hypotension,[16] as well as after the following procedures: lumbar puncture, shunting for hydrocephalus, contrast myelography, spinal anesthesia,[17] and treatment of cervical fractures.[18]

Before entering the cavernous sinus, the abducens nerve lies in relationship to the medial aspect of the petrous bone. Inflammation of the petrous bone and its dura may occur secondary to middle-ear infections, with involvement of the facial nerve (facial palsy), the trigeminal ganglion (pain in the eye or face), and the abducens nerve (lateral rectus palsy). These signs and symptoms constitute the now rare Gradenigo syndrome. The combination of sixth and seventh nerve palsies, even bilateral, is not uncommon in closed-head trauma, especially when the skull is compressed in its horizontal diameter (Fig. 12–6); this results in transverse fractures of the temporal bone. Leakage of blood or spinal fluid from the external ear canal, hemotympanum, or mastoid ecchymosis (Battle's sign) may be further evidence of basal fracture.

In the cavernous sinus, the abducens nerve may be involved in combination with the ophthalmic-trigeminal, third, or fourth nerves. Abducens monoparesis is frequent with cavernous sinus lesions, perhaps related to the nerve's location within the sinus, inferolateral to the carotid artery and unsupported by the dural wall of the sinus.[19,20] Isolated abducens palsy occurs with carotid-cavernous fistulas (especially with spontaneous dural shunts[21]) and intracavernous aneurysms[20] (Fig. 12–7), and is the earliest indication of contralateral spread of cavernous sinus thrombosis. Sixth nerve palsy accompanied only by ipsilateral Horner's syndrome also points to the cavernous sinus, since the ocular sympathetics from the carotid plexus may be simultaneously involved.[22]

Lesions involving abducens nerve function at the superior orbital fissure or orbital apex regularly involve other motor nerves to the eye, or produce proptosis and/or visual compromise.

Keane[23] provided an analysis of 125 cases of *bilateral* sixth nerve palsies. Unlike the many isolated, unilateral abducens palsies that wander in the limbo of "vascular disease," more accurate pathoanatomic diagnoses were made where bilateral palsies existed. One fourth of the

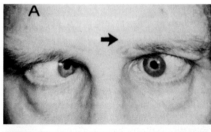
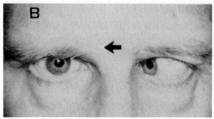
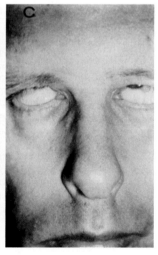

Fig. 12–6. Bilateral sixth and seventh nerve palsies due to basal skull fracture. **A.** Left gaze. **B.** Right gaze. **C.** Attempted lid closure demonstrates intact Bell's phenomenon and lagophthalmos.

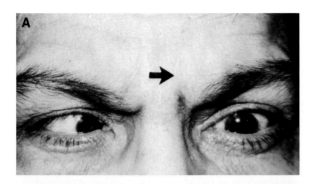

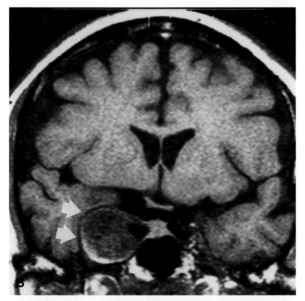

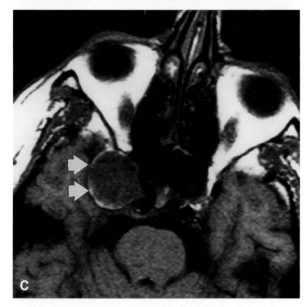

Fig. 12–7. A. Chronic isolated sixth nerve palsy. Coronal **(B)** and axial **(C)** MRI sections showing large intracavernous internal carotid aneurysm (*arrows*).

patients in this series demonstrated deficits of other cranial nerves, and many had additional neurologic signs and symptoms, as well as spinal fluid abnormalities.

ISOLATED ABDUCENS PALSY

As noted previously, all patients with abduction defects do not have sixth nerve lesions per se, and additional diagnostic techniques such as forced ductions/generations and intravenous Tensilon tests are mandatory. If the onset of diplopia is associated with acute eye, orbital, or head pain, then neither Graves' disease nor myasthenia is a likely cause. In addition to the ocular motor (III, IV, VI) nerves, the function of cranial nerves V (especially corneal sensation), VII, and VIII should be examined.

The question now arises as to how one should proceed in the workup of the patient with a truly isolated sixth nerve palsy. In the elderly, as well as in younger adults (see later discussion), vascular disease (hypertensive or otherwise) has been considered a cause of sixth nerve palsies, and remitting abducens palsies are regularly encountered in the adult diabetic population. Therefore, a history of hypertension or diabetes should be sought. Considering the latter, a fasting and 2-hour postprandial glucose level or glycosylated hemoglobin should be obtained. There is no correlation between severity of glucose metabolism defect and occurrence of cranial nerve palsies; thus, an isolated sixth, fourth, or pupil-sparing third nerve palsy may signal the presence of otherwise occult diabetes. Diabetic retinopathy is frequently absent in these cases.

Although it would be rather extraordinary for cranial arteritis to present as an isolated sixth nerve palsy, an erythrocyte sedimentation rate is a reasonable laboratory study in patients 65 years of age or older. Of the neurologic complications of systemic lupus erythematosus, both sixth and third nerve palsies, and brain stem motility disorders, are recognized.[24] Because of the propensity for nasopharyngeal carcinoma to spread through the extradural space via basal skull foramina, basisphenoidal sections should be included in gadolinium-enhanced magnetic resonance imaging (MRI) (Table 12–3).

When associated orbital and cranial signs and symptoms are absent, and when laboratory and appropriate radiologic studies are normal, the most prudent and practical course to follow is continued observation. An examination by a neurologist is comforting, but even Tensilon testing may be postponed. In this specific clinical situation, neuroimaging is infrequently productive, and its application in the elucidation of acute or subacute isolated sixth nerve palsies is moot. However, further radiologic evaluation must be undertaken if pain persists or develops, if other cranial nerves become involved, or if the palsy does not begin to improve over

TABLE 12–3. Diagnostic Studies for Isolated Abduction Palsy

Tensilon test
Forced ductions/forced generations
Serum glucose: fasting or after glucose load, or
  glycosylated hemoglobin
Erythrocyte sedimentation rate
Imaging studies*
  Contrast-enhanced CT: axial and coronal views, espe-
  cially of orbital apex, cavernous sinus, sella, and clivus
  Contrast-enhanced MRI: cavernous sinus, clivus

* Pain or mild ocular discomfort may occur with onset of
ischemic-diabetic abducens palsy. If pain persists or worsens,
imaging studies should be performed.

a 3- to 4-month period. Although it is true that some isolated "chronic" sixth nerve pareses last longer than 6 months, yet follow a completely benign course,[25] others are indeed caused by potentially treatable basal tumors.[26] Volpe and Lessell[27] reported seven patients with relapsing or remitting sixth nerve palsies, which were ultimately identified to be secondary to extramedullary compression of the abducens nerve by skull-based tumors. No patients had diabetes or vascular disease, and all recovered completely at least once (and in one case in five separate episodes) without surgical intervention, radiotherapy, or chemotherapy before a definitive diagnosis was made. Lesions included chordomas (Fig. 12–8), chondrosarcomas, and presumed meningiomas.

When pain persists and all radiologic and orbital investigations are unrevealing, a trial of corticosteroids (e.g., 60 mg prednisone orally for 5 days) may result in prompt and dramatic relief, in which case a tentative diagnosis of nonspecific inflammation of the superior orbital fissure or cavernous sinus may be made. However, the "response to steroid trial" may produce relief of pain with neoplasms as well as inflammation (see below, Combined Ocular Motor Palsies and Painful Ophthalmoplegia). Certainly, unrelenting eye or orbital or facial pain is an indication for exquisite visualization of the cavernous sinus and parasellar area by thin-section MRI scanning and either magnetic resonance or conventional angiography, if vascular abnormalities are suspected.

Isolated sixth nerve palsies in children often resolve spontaneously. Newborns may rarely manifest a transient lateral rectus weakness, with resolution occurring by 6 weeks.[28] Knox and colleagues[29] called attention to transient isolated abducens palsy of presumed postviral origin developing in children 1 to 3 weeks after nonspecific febrile or respiratory illness. The age range of the patients reviewed was 18 months to the early teens; recovery of abducens function occurred within 10 weeks (one case continued for 9 months). A similar pattern may be seen with specific viral illnesses such as varicella,[30] after immunization,[31] or in association with Ep-

stein-Barr viremia.[32] A spate of reports indicates that some patients have multiple recurrences of these isolated "benign" sixth nerve palsies and that these recurrences have no serious implications.[31,33–36] A 35-year-old with cluster headaches also experienced three consecutive right lateral rectus palsies, on each occasion beginning a day or two after onset of pain, with recovery within 2 weeks[37]; radiologic studies were unremarkable, suggesting the possibility of migrainous abducens palsy.

Robertson and co-workers[38] found a high incidence of brain tumor in his Mayo Clinic series of children with sixth nerve paresis. Although referred to as cases of "isolated" sixth nerve paresis, this definition signifies only that no other ocular motor nerves were defective. Indeed, of the children with neoplasms, one-third had papilledema and one-half demonstrated nystagmus at the time of initial examination. Of the patients with tumor who truly presented with only isolated abducens palsy, additional signs appeared within a few weeks or, rarely, within 2 to 3 months. Harley,[39] in his series of children with sixth nerve palsies of all causes, whether isolated or not, noted that approximately one third had suffered trauma and one fourth had underlying tumors; the total clinical picture in these cases is not described.

In the child with an isolated sixth nerve palsy without other neurologic signs, including papilledema, headaches, or ataxia, the following approach is suggested: (1) rule out middle-ear infection; and (2) obtain a peripheral blood count (lymphocytosis may be considered an indication of recent viral infection). The child must be reexamined at regular intervals until the paresis clears, and the parents must be advised to observe for new signs or symptoms. If the paresis persists or worsens, MRI is mandated. A persistent sixth nerve paresis

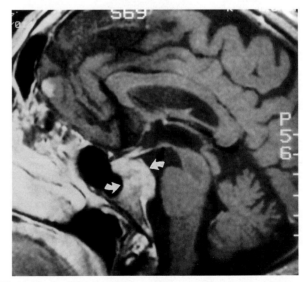

Fig. 12–8. MRI sagittal section, gadolinium enhanced, shows clivus chordoma (*arrows*). Patient presented with chronic bilateral sixth nerve palsies.

in childhood may be the first clinical sign of a pontine astrocytoma or other posterior fossa mass lesion.

In a 10-year series of 49 "younger adults" (age range, 15 to 50 years) with isolated sixth nerve palsy, Moster and colleagues[40] reported that about one third had diabetes and/or hypertension; 8 had basal tumors; 6 had isolated abducens palsies as the initial sign of multiple sclerosis (all with subsequent clinical or spinal fluid abnormalities), usually with spontaneous resolution; and 11 had no specific etiology disclosed, but did have a sanguine outcome. This series excluded patients with a positive Tensilon test, abnormal forced ductions, other known neurologic disease, or with bilateral palsies.

Larger series of sixth nerve palsies reported[41–43] are helpful in reviewing the causes, although these patients were somewhat preselected. The largest number of cases fell into the nonspecific "vascular" category (37%, 7%, and 18%, respectively) and the "undetermined" category (24%, 21%, and 29%, respectively). All three series included a modest number of patients with multiple sclerosis (13%, 7%, and 4%, respectively; also 12% in the Moster[40] series), but abducens palsy in demyelinative disease has been exceedingly rare in our personal experience. Nevertheless, with the advent of MRI, acute sixth nerve palsies with multiple sclerosis may be more frequently discovered, with abnormal signals in the pons.[44]

Minimal abduction paresis may herald increased intracranial pressure, such that the patient complains of horizontal diplopia when viewing distant objects. Clinically, these symptoms and findings may mimic divergence insufficiency. Kirkham and co-workers,[45] using electro-oculographic techniques, have demonstrated reduced abduction saccadic velocities, which suggest bilateral minimal sixth nerve dysfunction. Although neurons that discharge with divergence (and convergence) have been found in the mesencephalic reticular formation of the monkey,[46] the existence of a "divergence center" in the brain stem still remains controversial.

Symptomatic treatment of an acute sixth nerve palsy includes the use of Fresnel prisms, or alternate patching to avoid diplopia and possible medial rectus contracture. The injection of botulinum toxin type A (Botox) into the ipsilateral medial rectus is quite effective at preventing muscle contracture and improving fusion in the primary position of gaze. However, this procedure carries the disadvantage of significant crossed diplopia (exotropia) in contralateral gaze. Definitive surgical correction of a sixth nerve paresis should be employed when the deviation has been stable for at least 6 months. The primary consideration in these cases is the amount of residual abducting power of the lateral rectus, since moderate to good abduction is associated with successful ipsilateral recess/resect procedures (perhaps combined with contralateral medial rectus recession). However, if residual abduction is poor or absent, ipsilateral medial rectus recession may be combined with either a full- or partial-thickness tendon transplant procedure of the superior and inferior recti, or a Jensen procedure. The latter may have a decreased risk of anterior segment ischemia in susceptible patients.

Divergence paralysis is characterized by acute comitant esotropia at distance, normal fusion at near, and full ocular ductions. Of 11 patients with nontraumatic cause, Krohel and associates[47] found 3 with neurologic disease and other findings. Otherwise, there was no tendency to late evolution of neurologic sequelae. Stern and Tomsak[48] reported a young adult with a lower pontine lesion and also provided a useful overview of "divergence paralysis." Divergence paralysis has been reported in association with the Arnold-Chiari malformation; in some cases, fusion returns to normal after neurosurgical correction.[49] In general, however, the process is idiopathic and benign, and neuroimaging is neither useful nor necessary. When surgical correction is indicated in these cases, lateral rectus resection, without medial rectus recession, effectively eliminates diplopia.

TROCHLEAR PALSIES

Palsy of the superior oblique, as in the case of isolated lateral rectus weakness, may be due to local orbital processes that should be distinguished from a neurogenic lesion per se. As always, myasthenia and Graves' myopathy (an especially frequent cause of incomitant vertical strabismus) must be suspected and appropriate tests performed. The pattern of muscle imbalance and ocular versions can be quite similar in ipsilateral inferior rectus fibrosis (e.g., in Graves' disease) and contralateral superior oblique paresis[50]; however, worsening of the vertical deviation in upgaze is seen in inferior rectus fibrosis, and in downgaze in superior oblique palsy. Also, intraocular pressure may increase in attempted upgaze in restrictive (Graves') disease. Excyclodeviations are more prominent in superior oblique paresis than in thyroid myopathy, which may show significant excyclotorsion only in abduction.

Superior oblique palsies may present spontaneously in late childhood and possibly represent "decompensated" congenital fourth nerve palsies. This diagnostic concept (i.e., that fusional mechanisms decompensate in later life) has also been applied to otherwise healthy adults with spontaneously acquired, unremitting superior oblique palsies of unknown origin (Fig. 12–9). A similar, often transient, occurrence of superior oblique palsy has been reported during pregnancy.[51] These adults complain of reading difficulties, principally momentary diplopia, and show all of the attributes of superior oblique palsy. Old photographs may document tilting of the head, and further inquiry may uncover a forgotten history of childhood squint. Patients with congenital trochlear palsies commonly show increased am-

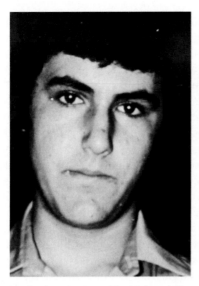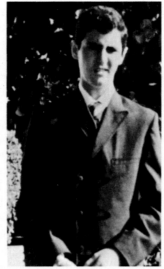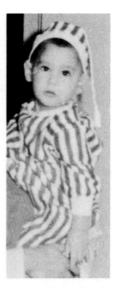

Fig. 12–9. An 18-year-old with head tilt complained of intermittent diplopia for several months. Muscle balance measured 8Δ of right hypertropia in primary position and 16Δ in left gaze. Snapshots at ages 12 and 2 demonstrate habitual head tilt consistent with right superior oblique palsy.

plitudes of vertical vergence.[52] Normally, only 2 to 4 prism diopters (pd) of vertical fusional amplitude are found, but patients with congenital superior oblique pareses may be able to fuse a 10-pd or even a 30-pd deviation. However, the presence of large vertical fusional amplitudes does not necessarily imply a congenital etiology, because vertical fusional vergence may increase in adults within weeks or months after an acquired vertical strabismus.

The cause of most congenital superior oblique palsies is unknown; however, agenesis of the trochlear nucleus has been described in association with agenesis of other cranial-nerve nuclei,[53] but never in the situation of an isolated congenital fourth nerve palsy. Dysplasia (aplasia) of cranial nuclei may occur after perinatal peripheral injuries to nerves, with secondary "dying back." Also, axonal death, with selective elimination and preservation, is an established phenomenon during neurogenesis of all cranial nerves.[54] Absence of the superior oblique tendon has been observed during surgery to correct putative isolated congenital superior oblique palsies. This phenomenon may be more common in patients with craniofacial dysostoses.[55] Indeed, Helveston et al[56] reported congenital absence of the superior oblique tendon in 18% of patients with congenital superior oblique palsy, in whom a tuck of the superior oblique had been contemplated, and in another subgroup of patients with congenital superior oblique pareses, abnormally lax superior oblique tendons have been described. Bilateral congenital superior oblique palsies (particularly asymmetric pareses), as with bilateral acquired superior oblique palsies, may initially appear to be unilateral until corrective surgery "unmasks" the contralateral palsy.

Other than in the context of trauma, acquired isolated fourth nerve palsy occurs far less frequently than abducens or oculomotor palsies. In a retrospective study of 412 patients,[57] third and sixth nerve palsies were seven times more common than fourth nerve palsy. As with isolated abducens palsy, many spontaneous trochlear palsies are classified as "unknown" or "vascular." In the older age group, isolated fourth nerve palsy is frequently associated with diabetes. Keane[58] provided an excellent overview of fourth nerve palsy among 215 patients, with head trauma representing the cause in more than 50%; no tumors showed isolated palsies, but were accompanied by other defects related to lesions in the cavernous sinus. In comparison, 149 patients with ocular myasthenia did not show isolated superior oblique palsies. Bilateral fourth palsies occurred in 19%; again, the majority of these cases were due to head trauma. Herpes zoster ophthalmicus may be associated with isolated trochlear palsy,[59] with variable recovery, but meningitis produces other signs and symptoms.[58] Although extremely rare, intracranial aneurysms (*e.g.*, superior cerebellar artery) have been documented to cause superior oblique palsy as well.[60] Autosomal-dominant inheritance of superior oblique palsy, some bilateral, is also documented.[61] The causes of fourth nerve palsies are listed in Table 12–4.

Susceptibility of the trochlear nerve to injury in closed head traumas has been attributed to the position of the nerves with respect to the tentorial edge. According to Lindenberg,[62] the tectum of the midbrain is subject to contrecoup contusion at the tentorial notch when the forehead or skull vertex strikes a stationary object, with the impact force directed toward the tentorium. The fourth nerves may be injured as they sweep laterally around the midbrain or dorsally in the anterior medul-

TABLE 12-4. Causes of Superior Oblique Paresis

Fourth nerve palsy
   Traumatic (may be bilateral)
   Vascular mononeuropathy
   Diabetic
   Decompensated congenital paresis
   Posterior fossa tumor (rare)
   Cavernous sinus/superior orbital fissure syndromes
   Neurosurgical procedures
   Herpes zoster
Myasthenia gravis
Graves' myopathy (fibrotic inferior oblique, superior rectus)*
Orbital inflammatory pseudotumor
Orbital injury to trochlea

_____

   * Note that a fibrotic inferior rectus may mimic a *contralateral* superior oblique palsy.

lary velum, or in the substance of the lower midbrain. In these situations, bilateral fourth nerve palsies are common. Lindenberg also pointed out that, in blows to the base of the occiput or even in falls on the buttocks, forces are transmitted such that the cerebellum is thrust against the tentorium from below. In contrast to Lindenberg's neuropathologic material, fourth nerve palsies may result from minimal, if not insignificant, trauma. Radiographic documentation of the site of damage to the fourth nerve is unusual after trauma, but MRI of the posterior fossa has greatly increased the possibility of identifying minor intra- and extra-axial lesions in these cases.

As a rule, the diagnosis of an acute superior oblique palsy is not difficult (Fig. 12–10). Many patients rapidly learn to tilt the head toward the side opposite the defective eye. Such head tilting is not an exclusive sign of trochlear palsy, but it is seen more consistently here than with other vertical muscle pareses.[63] Nevertheless, it must be cautioned that a number of patients will have no consistent head tilt, or may even show a tilt toward the palsied side, possibly to achieve greater subjective image separation so that the more peripheral image can be ignored.

According to the data accumulated by Khawam et al,[63] all patients with unilateral superior oblique palsies show vertical deviation in the primary position, with an increase in deviation on adduction of the involved eye. A common pattern wherein the vertical deviation is greatest in adduction and elevation is seen with secondary inferior oblique overaction. With time, the vertical deviation often becomes comitant. In patients with bilateral palsies, almost all due to head trauma, the vertical deviation in primary position tends to be smaller. Anomalous head positions were present in half of the unilateral palsies and 70% of the bilateral palsies, but more than 90% of all patients demonstrated greater vertical deviation with the head tilted toward the side of the paretic muscle (*i.e.*, a positive Bielschowsky forced head-tilt test; see Fig. 12–10). Sydnor and colleagues[64] concurred that unilateral fourth nerve palsies have large hypertropias and more vertical than torsional diplopia, whereas bilateral palsies show small hypertropias in primary gaze, large V-pattern esotropias, a compensating chin-down position that permits fusion in upgaze, and excyclotorsion greater than 10° to 12°. Lee and Flynn[65] noted that bilateral superior oblique palsies should be suspected when the Bielschowsky test is positive with head tilt in both directions, especially after a relatively severe head trauma.

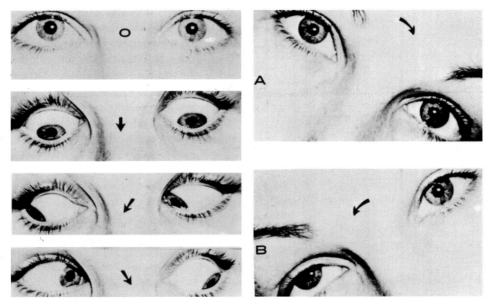

Fig. 12–10. Ocular deviation with right superior oblique palsy. **Left**. Defective duction of right eye on gaze down and left. **Right**. Bielschowsky head-tilt test: (*A*) Tilt to left; (*B*) Tilt to right (note increased right hyperdeviation).

In the clinical dilemma of acquired verticle deviations, Trobe[66] provided practical data regarding cyclotorsional defects: excyclodeviation occurred in 30 of 33 patients with trochlear palsies, 8 of 15 patients with Graves' ophthalmopathy, and 1 of 13 patients with myasthenia, but did not occur in any case of skew deviation. Keane[67] provided an excellent summary of the vertical diplopia syndromes seen during a 15-year inpatient hospital experience, including oculomotor palsy (579 cases), trochlear palsy (133 cases), skew deviation (434 cases), myasthenia (94 cases), and others, such as Guillain-Barré syndrome, orbital floor fracture, and Graves' ophthalmopathy.

In the patient with an isolated superior oblique palsy, without antecedent trauma and with a negative Tensilon test, forced duction, and serum glucose tests, observation is the rule. Radiologic studies are of minimal value, but schwannoma of the trochlea nerve has been reported.[68] If the deviation is stable, prisms can be incorporated into spectacles, but this may fail because of torsional defects or persistent incomitance. After measurements remain stable for at least 6 months, surgical correction may be undertaken with a high rate of success. In general, ductional defects when present should be addressed: for example, if the superior oblique is underactive, a tendon-tucking procedure is preferred; with significant inferior oblique overaction, inferior oblique myectomy or recession is quite effective. Depending on the degree and pattern of the vertical misalignment, recessions of the ipsilateral superior rectus and/or contralateral inferior rectus using the adjustable suture technique may be employed. These procedures have worked well in cases of congenital absence of the superior oblique tendon or in cases of bilateral superior oblique palsies. For bilateral cases, surgery should be commensurate with the relative degree of symmetry between the two eyes. In cases of persistent V-pattern esotropia and excyclodeviation, after bilateral superior oblique tucks, bilateral inferior rectus recessions often yield significant improvement.[69] Finally, in cases where there is minimal vertical deviation but excyclodiplopia is the chief complaint, advancement of the anterior superior oblique tendon fibers (Harada-Ito procedure) may improve the torsional diplopia without disturbing vertical ocular alignment.

Acting as a pseudopalsy of the inferior oblique, Brown's syndrome refers to an anomalous articulation between the trochlea and superior oblique tendon sheath, resulting in a restrictive strabismus showing lack of elevation in adduction. This is most often a congenital disorder, in which diplopia is infrequent and good fusion is the rule. Many patients enjoy spontaneous improvement by late childhood or early adulthood.[70] When surgery is required for large hypotropia in the primary position, or for disfiguring chin-up posture in order to promote fusion, superior oblique tenectomy with or without ipsilateral inferior oblique weakening is the most commonly employed procedure. Other surgical techniques include introduction of a silicone tendon expander and superior oblique and trochlear luxation.[71] A form of secondary Brown's syndrome may also be acquired after orbital trauma[72] or with orbital metastasis.[73] It has been described in association with systemic collagen vascular disease, such as juvenile rheumatoid arthritis,[74] systemic lupus erythematosus,[75] and hypogammaglobulinemia. Such cases typically respond well to oral steroids or nonsteroidal agents. Local injection of depot steroids in the region of the trochlea can produce improvement as well, but may cause secondary scarring and fibrosis. Brown's syndrome has also been described as a transient phenomenon in the postpartum period.[76]

Superior oblique myokymia (see also Chapter 11) consists of spasms of cyclotorsional and vertical eye movements. These are often difficult to appreciate on gross examination, but are easily seen with the slit lamp or ophthalmoscope. There is an initial intorsion and depression of the affected eye, followed by irregular torsional oscillations of minor amplitude. This phenomenon is strictly unilateral, and generally occurs in the absence of neurologic disease. Brazis et al[77] have reported a long-term follow-up of 16 patients. Therapeutic options include carbamazepine or propranolol. If medical treatment is ineffective or intolerable, superior oblique tenectomy combined with inferior oblique myectomy to avoid iatrogenic trochlear paresis has been documented to be an effective treatment.

OCULOMOTOR PALSIES

Oculomotor nerve function may be affected at a nuclear level, in the fascicular portion within the midbrain, in the interpeduncular space, in its course forward alongside the posterior communicating artery, at its entrance into the dura lateral and anterior to the dorsum sellae, in the cavernous sinus, in the superior orbital fissure, and in the orbit itself. The combination of oculomotor palsy with other cranial nerve (II, IV, VI, V) deficits, or with corticospinal or cerebellar-system signs, permits accurate localizing diagnoses (Table 12–5).

NUCLEAR LESIONS

Disorders of the oculomotor nerve at its nuclear source may be encountered in rare instances. Based on Warwick's anatomic configuration of the third nerve nuclear complex (see Fig. 12–3), the following clinical rules are applicable:

1. Conditions that cannot represent nuclear lesions
   a. Unilateral external ophthalmoplegia (with or without pupil involvement) associated with normal contralateral superior rectus function

b. Unilateral internal ophthalmoplegia

c. Unilateral ptosis

2. Conditions that may be nuclear
   a. Bilateral total third nerve palsy
   b. Bilateral ptosis
   c. Bilateral internal ophthalmoplegia
   d. Bilateral medial rectus palsy
   e. Isolated single muscle involvement (except levator and superior rectus)

3. Obligatory nuclear lesions
   a. Unilateral third nerve palsy with contralateral superior rectus and bilateral partial ptosis
   b. Bilateral third nerve palsy (with or without internal ophthalmoplegia) associated with spared levator function

Because ocular myasthenia, and in some instances, Graves' myopathy, may mimic various patterns of oculomotor nerve dysfunction, Tensilon testing and forced ductions should be considered in cases of painless ophthalmoplegia where pupils are normal. Supranuclear lesions involving midbrain structures near the third nerve nucleus may closely simulate direct damage to the nucleus. If ocular motility improves with vestibular stimulation (oculocephalic reflex, calorics) or with Bell's phe-

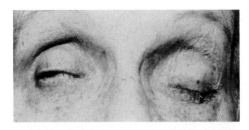
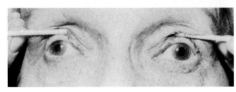

Fig. 12–11. Bilateral oculomotor palsies (nuclear?) associated with abrupt onset of vertigo and mild left hemiparesis. Patient could not be imaged.

nomenon, a supranuclear lesion is present. Failure of ocular motility to improve with any of these stimuli indicates the presence of a nuclear or infranuclear lesion, but does not exclude additional supranuclear abnormalities.

Several clinicopathologic studies have supported Warwick's schema. There are documented instances of isolated bilateral ptosis, with discrete foci in the nuclear complex of the third nerve, in the midline at the level of the central caudal nucleus.[78] Keane et al[79] described a case of unilateral oculomotor palsy, complete except for near-normal levator function; at autopsy, a solitary midbrain metastasis was seen involving the rostral ipsilateral third nerve nucleus, but sparing the central caudal levator nucleus. The MRI findings in two instances of levator-sparing nuclear oculomotor palsies, with contralateral elevator palsy, defined focal rostral midbrain infarcts.[80] In several patients, isolated extraocular muscle palsies (*e.g.*, isolated inferior rectus palsy) have been ascribed on clinical grounds to small lesions of the oculomotor nuclear complex.[81]

Acquired bi-nuclear total ophthalmoplegia is occasionally seen (Fig. 12–11), as reported by Masucci.[82] These findings are the result of thrombotic or embolic processes at the level of the basilar bifurcation, with occlusion of the median mesencephalic perforating arteries. Congenital bilateral total ophthalmoplegia with or without levator and pupil sparing has been reported and may be associated with dysplasia of the corpus callosum.[83]

FASCICULAR LESIONS

Deficits of the oculomotor fasciculus are usually identified by the accompanying brain stem signs. Oculomotor palsy with contralateral hemiplegia (Weber syndrome) indicates involvement of the corticospinal tracts. Contralateral ataxia and intention tremor (Benedikt

---

TABLE 12–5. Causes of Oculomotor Palsies

Nuclear
Infarction
Demyelination
Metastatic tumor

Fascicular
Infarction
Demyelination (rare)
Tumor

Interpeduncular
Aneurysm
Trauma
Meningitis

Cavernous sinus
Carotid-cavernous fistula
Granulomatous inflammation (Tolosa-Hunt syndrome)
Intracavernous aneurysm
Extrasellar extension of pituitary tumor
Meningioma
Sphenoid sinus carcinoma
Metastatic tumor
Mucormycosis (other fungus)
Herpes zoster

Orbit
Nonspecific inflammation (pseudotumor)
Trauma
Tumor

Ischemic (diabetic) ophthalmoplegia

Miscellaneous
Polyneuritis (Guillain-Barré-Fisher syndrome)
Cyclic oculomotor palsy (Bielschowsky)
Migraine
Arteritis

syndrome) indicates involvement of the red nucleus (see Fig. 12–2). Nothnagel syndrome is an eponym given when signs of both Weber and Benedikt syndromes are present. Midbrain vascular accidents account for most fascicular defects.

Ksiazek[84] shed some light on the fascicular arrangement of the oculomotor nerve based on two patients with partial oculomotor paresis, each with pupillary mydriasis, significant inferior rectus paresis, and medial rectus paresis. Neuroimaging revealed a lesion in the fascicular portion of the nerve, thus indicating the proximity of these fibers in the fasciculus. Monocular elevator paresis (superior rectus and inferior oblique) in mass compression of the oculomotor fasciculus has also been reported.[85] In this regard, Castro and associates[86] proposed the mediolateral somatotopy of the oculomotor fascicular fibers within the mesencephalon with the inferior oblique and superior rectus muscles being most lateral, and the pupilloconstrictor fibers and inferior rectus being most medial. The levator palpebrae fascicles are in an intermediate location between the superior rectus and medial rectus fascicles.

INTERPEDUNCULAR LESIONS

Basal lesions, including the rare rostral basilar artery aneurysm, may encroach on the oculomotor nerves as they exit in the interpeduncular space. Such slow-growing aneurysms, either saccular or fusiform, may present as partial oculomotor palsies with or without involvement of pyramidal tracts, and without subarachnoid hemorrhage.[87] Aneurysms of the posterior communicating artery, on the other hand, are probably the most common lesions causing acute spontaneous oculomotor palsies (Fig. 12–12). According to Hyland and Barnett,[88] the oculomotor palsy that occurs with posterior communicating aneurysm is not necessarily due to mass effect per se, but rather is attributed to hemorrhage that suddenly enlarges the aneurysmal sac to which the oculomotor nerve is adherent, or to hemorrhage into the substance of the nerve itself. Most patients present, therefore, with an intensely painful, complete unilateral oculomotor palsy in association with other signs and symptoms of subarachnoid hemorrhage. Few patients with symptomatic posterior communicating aneurysms are found in office waiting rooms: they are usually obtunded or comatose in emergency rooms.

Involvement of pupillary fibers is such a consistent finding in third nerve palsies due to bleeding aneurysms that most clinicians concur in this useful dictum: a pupil-sparing, but otherwise complete, third nerve palsy is very unlikely to be due to posterior communicating aneurysms. Careful pupil evaluation may disclose subtle abnormalities in "apparent pupil-sparing," especially in cases of aberrant regeneration or with chronic cavernous sinus lesions. Generally, in patients at least 50 years

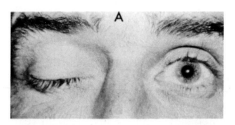
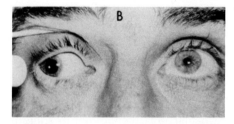
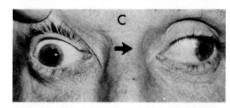
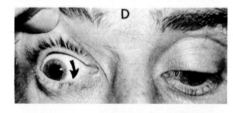
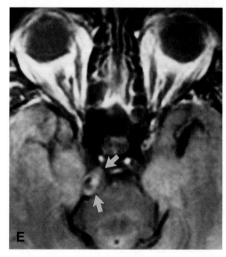

Fig. 12–12. Sudden total right ophthalmoplegia accompanied by orbital pain, due to posterior communicating artery aneurysm. **A.** Complete right ptosis. **B.** Right eye in abducted position, with dilated pupil, fixed to light. **C.** Failure of adduction on left gaze. **D.** Right eye intorts (*arrow*) on downward gaze, indicating retained function of fourth nerve. **E.** Contrast-enhanced T-1 weighted MRI axial section shows aneurysm (*arrows*). Confirmed by angiography.

of age or older, an acute, isolated, painful oculomotor palsy that spares the pupil is caused by intraneural ischemia; nevertheless, these patients must be carefully observed for further evolution. In our opinion, an acute complete oculomotor palsy with moderate to major mydriasis, even when diabetes is present, is an indication for cerebral arteriography. It should be emphasized that magnetic resonance angiography may not detect aneurysms smaller than 3 to 4 mm.[89]

The clinical management of patients with relative pupil-sparing third nerve palsies remains in debate. Observation alone arguably is appropriate management of such patients; however, since practically every conceivable combination of partial ophthalmoplegia and pupillary abnormality has been reported in aneurysmal compression of the third nerve, it is better to err on the side of caution and perform angiography more frequently. It is incumbent upon the physician to evaluate carefully the proportion of ophthalmoplegia and ptosis in relation to the degree of pupillary abnormality when deciding appropriate workup of these patients. Again, the increasing sensitivity of magnetic resonance angiography has not yet entirely replaced formal angiography. Certainly, neurosurgical intervention requires conventional cerebral arteriography before surgical treatment. Capó and colleagues[90] pointed out that the interval from onset to maximal ophthalmoplegia does not differentiate between microvascular (3.3 days) and aneurysm (3 days), but that failure to recover within 4 to 8 weeks requires further evaluation.

Other partial oculomotor palsies occur regularly with cavernous sinus masses and parasellar syndromes (see below), accompanied by variable pupillary findings. Furthermore, both acute and chronic lesions may produce incomplete palsy of the superior division (supplying levator palpebrae and superior rectus muscles) or of the inferior division (medial and inferior recti, inferior oblique and pupillomotor fibers). If pain or first trigeminal division numbness are absent, and if the pupil is uninvolved, such fractional oculomotor pareses are regularly misinterpreted as myasthenia or local orbital inflammations. Guy et al[91] described five patients with isolated ptosis and elevator paresis in abduction, consistent with selective "superior division" involvement. They also discussed five previously reported cases with the following respective diagnoses: (1) intracavernous aneurysm (usually with associated Horner's syndrome) and basilar artery aneurysm; (2) diabetic ophthalmoplegia; (3) meningitis; (4) dural lymphoma; and (5) postsurgical manipulation of parasellar structures. In essence, there was little anatomic correlation with the physical separation into superior and inferior oculomotor trunks that occurs in the cavernous sinus. Moreover, two patients sustained superior division palsies during surgical manipulation of the subarachnoidal portion of the oculomotor nerve trunk. A number of cases of infe-

rior rectus paresis, isolated or in combination with ipsilateral or contralateral superior rectus paresis, have been construed as focal lesions involving the rostral portion of the oculomotor nuclear complex.[80–82]

Oculomotor palsy following head trauma is not rare, but probably occurs less frequently than traumatic fourth nerve palsies. As a rule, such closed-head injury causes loss of consciousness and is accompanied by skull fracture, but this is not invariable. Injury to the ocular motor nerves in road accidents was studied by Heinze,[92] who dissected the cadavers of 21 fatal cases. He found that the relationship of frontal or temporal fractures to neural damage was unpredictable. In fact, intact nerves were encountered adjacent to gross fracture sites. The oculomotor nerve was damaged at three locations: (1) avulsion of the rootlets at their ventral exit from the brain stem; (2) contusion necrosis of the most proximal portion of the nerve trunk; and (3) intraneural and perineural hemorrhage of the nerve trunks at the level of the superior orbital fissure. Of great interest are Heinze's findings of focal hemorrhages in extraocular muscles, usually associated with fractured orbital bones.

Eyster et al[93] reported three patients with large basicranial tumors, who presented with oculomotor palsies precipitated by mild blows to the head that were insufficient to cause fracture or loss of consciousness. The oculomotor nerves were encased and stretched by tumor, which apparently rendered these tethered nerves vulnerable when innocent head blows abruptly shifted the brain. The authors pointed out that such atypical presentations of intracranial tumors may further mimic aneurysms, since subarachnoid hemorrhage does occasionally occur with tumors. Neetens[94] reported an additional three cases of oculomotor nerve palsies after minor trauma in the presence of basal intracranial tumors; the trochlear nerve was involved in all three cases, and in two cases the oculomotor nerve was partially affected. Walter et al[95] reported two instances of minor head trauma resulting in complete third nerve palsies attributed to occult posterior communicating artery aneurysms. We have seen a 45-year-old school teacher who experienced an immediate right abducens palsy when playfully slapped on the back of the head; within weeks, other cranial nerve palsies announced the presence of diffuse meningeal spread of carcinoma.

In the United States, basilar meningitis is rare, but was formerly encountered with tuberculosis and syphilis. When the third nerve is involved in such cases, progressive defects are the rule and other cranial nerve palsies are commonly found. Oculomotor palsy may especially occur with meningitides in infants, including instances of viral and bacterial (e.g., *Streptococcus pneumoniae, Haemophilus influenzae*) infections.[96]

Oculomotor nerve compression by the proximal segment of the posterior cerebral artery, or by the uncus against the petroclinoid ligament, can be seen with increasing cerebral edema or with an ipsilateral expanding supratentorial mass, and it is often heralded by unilateral pupillary dilation (Hutchinson pupil). Progression rapidly leads to complete ocular motor nerve palsy. Keane[97] reviewed the ocular motor signs of tentorial herniation, which include anisocoria and parasympathetic pupillary abnormalities, unilateral or bilateral ptosis, internuclear ophthalmoplegia, vertical gaze paresis, and partial third nerve palsies.

Cavernous Sinus Lesions

The oculomotor nerve may be involved by inflammatory disease, tumor, aneurysm, arteriovenous fistula, or thrombosis at the level of the cavernous sinus. The third nerve is usually involved in combination with the fourth, sixth, and ophthalmictrigeminal nerves, and accompanying sympathetic paresis may minimize pupillary dilation. The syndrome of the cavernous sinus, therefore, includes multiple ocular motor nerve palsies and pain or numbness in the first trigeminal division. In practice, lesions involving primarily the superior orbital fissure produce signs and symptoms that, with the possible exception of proptosis, cannot be distinguished from those of the anterior cavernous sinus. In particular, dural carotid cavernous fistulas that drain primarily into the inferior petrosal sinus may cause third nerve pareses without significant orbital congestion.[98]

Third nerve palsies due to lesions in the cavernous sinus tend to be partial in that all muscles innervated by the oculomotor branches need not be involved. This is especially true of pupillomotor fibers, such that the pupil may be normal or minimally involved. This "pupil-sparing" is offhandedly attributed to the superimposition of sympathetic paresis (Horner syndrome), but appropriate pharmacologic tests rarely substantiate this explanation (see below, Parasellar Syndrome). More likely, slowly expanding masses (*e.g.*, infraclinoid aneurysm, meningioma) functionally spare the pupilloconstrictor fibers in the intracavernous portion of the oculomotor nerve. In addition, the levator, superior, inferior, and medial recti may be involved in unequal degrees, but progressive paresis evolves. (Once again, myasthenia must be suspected in any nonpainful, pupil-sparing, nonproptotic ophthalmoplegia, with or without ptosis.) Cavernous sinus lesions are further discussed below.

Primary neurinoma of the oculomotor nerve is a relatively rare lesion that should be considered in children or young adults with insidious third nerve palsy. These may occur in the cavernous or interpeduncular portion of the nerve (Fig. 12–13), as with the trochlear nerve.[68,99,100]

Orbital Lesions

Oculomotor nerve palsies with orbital lesions are usually accompanied by abducens weakness and proptosis. In the absence of proptosis, anterior cavernous sinus

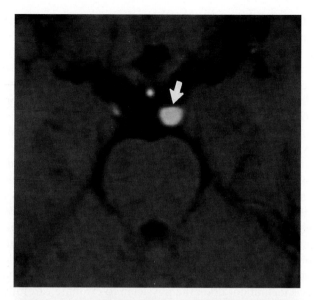

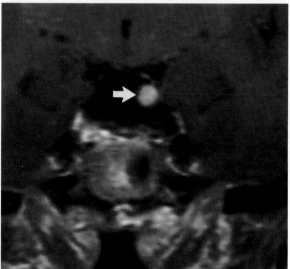

Fig. 12–13. Insidiously progressive third nerve palsy due to oculomotor neurinoma (*arrows*) in 16-year-old girl. MRI T-1, enhanced axial (**top**) and coronal (**bottom**) sections.

lesions may not be distinguishable from those involving the superior orbital fissure or orbital apex. Nonspecific inflammations of orbital tissues (orbital pseudotumor) may produce palsies of extraocular muscles in variable combinations, but other manifestations (*e.g.*, pain, chemosis, ocular inflammation, proptosis) are usually present. Orbital trauma, unless overlooked or forgotten, usually presents no difficulty in diagnosis. Forced duction testing and orbital ultrasonography and/or enhanced CT imaging are indicated.

ISCHEMIC ("DIABETIC") OCULOMOTOR PALSY

As noted in the discussion of fourth and sixth nerve palsies, self-limited vasculopathic extraocular muscle pareses may be associated with diabetes, although the incidence of ophthalmoplegia in diabetes is relatively rare. Jacobson et al[101] reported that diabetes and left ventricular hypertrophy are associated risk factors, but often enough the patient is an adult with latent diabetes first brought to light during the evaluation of the acute ophthalmoplegia. Surprisingly, very few of these patients have significant diabetic retinopathy at the time of their ophthalmoplegia. Although recurrences, on either the same or opposite side and involving either the same or other nerves (III, IV, VI), are not infrequent, simultaneous involvement of two or more ocular motor nerves is a rare occurrence in diabetes and should be viewed with caution.[102] We may enunciate a useful clinical dictum: a patient with diabetes is permitted one cranial neuropathy at a time; exceptions to this rule, that is, either more than one motor nerve per eye, or simultaneous bilateral cranial palsies, make investigation mandatory. Nevertheless, Eshbaugh et al[103] reported three patients with multiple simultaneous bilateral cranial neuropathies secondary to diabetes mellitus, all of which spontaneously resolved without sequelae. Their paper also reviewed the literature regarding reports of such patients, as well as those with multiple recurrent episodes.

Clinically, patients with ischemic oculomotor palsy present with acute pain in and about the involved eye. The pain may precede actual ophthalmoplegia and can be so severe as to suggest a bleeding aneurysm (but without neck stiffness, photophobia, obtundation, etc.), or it may accompany the onset of ptosis or diplopia as a mild brow pain or headache. The pupil is almost always spared, in contradistinction to posterior communicating artery aneurysm (see above). Iridoplegia, when present, is moderate. Ophthalmoplegia may be partial, with some muscles spared entirely (Fig. 12–14). Recovery is predictable, occurring after several weeks and usually before 4 months.

Studies by Weber et al[104] and Asbury et al[105] have indicated the following: (1) the lesion is primarily a focal demyelinization with minimal axonal degeneration; (2) remyelinization is thought to be responsible for recovery without aberrant regeneration; and (3) ischemia due to closure of intraneural arterioles is thought to cause the demyelinative lesion, which may occur in the intracavernous[105] or subarachnoid[104] segment of the third nerve. However, the advent of MRI has clearly demonstrated that intraparenchymal midbrain lesions may be responsible for pupil-sparing ophthalmoplegia.[106,107]

The key to diagnosis is threefold: a high level of suspicion should be entertained when a middle-aged or elderly person (1) presents with a pupil-sparing ophthalmoplegia involving all or most of the ocular muscles innervated by the third nerve only (with or without accompanying pain); (2) has elevated serum glucose levels either during fasting or after a measured glucose load; most recently, the American Diabetes Association

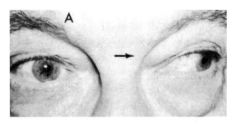
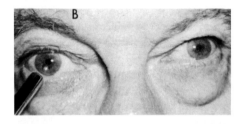
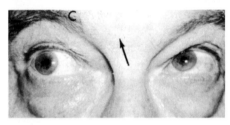
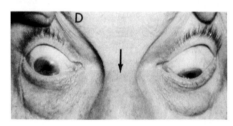

Fig. 12–14. Ischemic (diabetic) right oculomotor ophthalmoplegia of mild degree. **A.** Note failure of adduction on left gaze and unusual lack of ptosis. **B.** Pupil is spared, with intact light reaction. **C.** Superior rectus weakness. **D.** Inferior rectus weakness. Mild pain accompanied onset of diplopia, with complete resolution in 3 weeks. This was the second episode in a 62-year-old patient with known diabetes.

has recommended[108] a more reliable assay of hyperglycemia, namely, glycosylated hemoglobin (GHb or hemoglobin A1c), reflecting mean glycemia over the preceding 2 to 3 months; and (3) has a documented recovery within 3 to 4 months. The significant proportion of cranial nerve pareses due to diabetes or another microvascular disease cannot be overemphasized. The Mayo Clinic has reviewed more than 4000 cases of third, fourth, or sixth cranial nerve palsy.[43] The order of frequency was as follows: abducens pareses (43.9%), oculomotor pareses (28%), trochlear pareses (15%), and multiple simultaneous oculomotor pareses (13.1%). Slightly more than 15% of all cranial neuropathies were attributed to vascular causes (*e.g.*, diabetes, hypertension, atherosclerosis, vasculitis). Note, however, that these figures pertain to adults only: microvascular cranial neuropathies do not occur in the pediatric population.

OCULOMOTOR SYNKINESIS

Since the era of Ramon y Cajal, it has been appreciated that, following trauma, regenerating axons of peripheral motor nerves may randomly access structures other than those originally innervated. This neurophysiologic phenomenon accounts for intrafacial dyskinesias following seventh nerve palsies, or for paradoxic gustatory facial sweating (Frey syndrome) and gustatory tearing ("crocodile tears") with misdirection of regenerated autonomic axons. Since the oculomotor nerve innervates multiple extraocular muscles, the levator palpebrae, and the pupil sphincter, aberrant innervation patterns may be produced by misdirected axonal sprouting after injury, producing variable patterns of dyskinetic ocular movement.

The precise mechanism whereby oculomotor synkinesis occurs is controversial and unsettled. Sibony et al[109] reviewed the various hypotheses proposed to explain oculomotor synkinesis. Random misdirection of regenerating motor axons within an injured oculomotor nerve trunk, with erroneous muscle re-innervation, is the traditional explanation for oculomotor synkinesis, and indeed histopathologic, clinical, and experimental evidence may be cited in support of this hypothesis.[110] But transient oculomotor synkinesis,[111-113] spontaneous "primary" oculomotor synkinesis,[111,114-117] and synkinesis involving superior and inferior divisions of the third nerve after damage to only the superior division[112] have been observed and are difficult, but not impossible,[109] to explain by the hypothesis of indiscriminate axonal regeneration. Such clinical oddities prompted Lepore and Glaser[111] to challenge the concept that misdirection of regenerating oculomotor fibers is responsible for *all* oculomotor synkinesis, and to invoke two alternative mechanisms: ephaptic transmission (axo-axonal "cross-talk"), and synaptic reorganization of the oculomotor nucleus following retrograde axonal degeneration.

After acute ophthalmoplegia, clinical signs of dyskinesia begin at about 8 to 10 weeks, accompanying variable degrees of recovered function (Fig. 12–15). When recovery begins earlier, synkinesia is less frequent—and, of course, when there is no recovery, there is no synkinesia. Several paradoxic patterns may evolve: elevation of the upper lid on attempted use of the inferior (pseudo–von Graefe sign) or medial rectus muscles ("reverse Duane" syndrome) (see Fig. 12–13); adduction or retraction of the globe on attempted downward or upward gaze; and a light-near (or lateral gaze) pupillary dissociation with constriction of a larger than normal pupil occurring on attempted adduction. According to Hepler and Cantu,[118] of 25 patients with aberrant oculomotor regeneration after posterior communicating artery aneurysms, 20 demonstrated the pseudo–von Graefe phenomenon of lid elevation on attempted downgaze. This critical sign is best appreciated by direct-

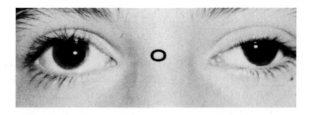
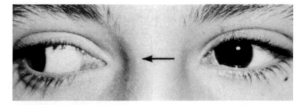
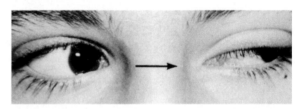
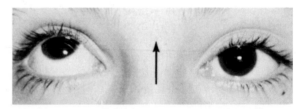
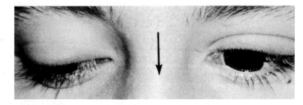

Fig. 12–15. Aberrant regeneration of left oculomotor nerve following head trauma. Note modest limitation of medial rectus function and marked deficit of superior rectus. On attempted downward gaze (inferior rectus) the left lid elevates, that is, the pseudo-Graefe phenomenon.

ing the patient's gaze first downward, and then slowly from side to side. Czarnecki and Thompson[119] reported other pupillary anomalies, including asynchronous sectoral contractions with both light stimulation and eye movement.

Oculomotor synkinesis is frequently observed in congenital third nerve palsies.[39,120–122] The spontaneous and progressive development of oculomotor synkinesis in patients with no prior acute oculomotor palsy[111,114–117] is seen most commonly with slowly growing lesions in the cavernous sinus, usually meningiomas or aneurysms, and has been termed primary oculomotor synkinesis. Varma and Miller[123] pointed out that although aneurysms typically present with acute, painful oculomotor pareses, they may produce painless third nerve palsies with primary aberrant regeneration. Secondary oculomotor synkinesis, that is, synkinesis following recognized acquired oculomotor palsy, most commonly occurs in association with trauma or aneurysms, but may rarely be seen with neoplasia or even ophthalmoplegic migraine.[124] Misdirection has not been documented after ischemic (diabetic) ophthalmoplegia or demyelinative syndromes.

Bilateral misdirection produces the extraordinary picture of gaze-dependent (adduction and/or depression) alternating lid retraction: that is, right lid retraction on left gaze, and left lid retraction on right gaze. An instance of apparent combined oculomotor-abducens synkinesis has been reported[125] in one unusual case of posttraumatic "total ophthalmoplegia": on attempted adduction, the right eye slightly abducted, but adducted upon attempted abduction; in addition, attempted abduction produced pupillary constriction. An extraordinary case of trigeminal-abducens synkinesis has been reported[126] following head trauma. In a 29 year old woman, left eye abduction was enhanced by 30° when accompanied by tight jaw closure, attributed to misdirection of mandibular division motor fibers accessing the abducens sheath at the petrous bone.

Pallini and colleagues,[127] in their work in adult guinea pigs, noted frequent aberrant regeneration following oculomotor nerve repair after transection proximally at the tentorial edge, versus full recovery without aberrant phenomena when the nerve was severed distally at the orbital fissure. The presence of aberrant regeneration correlated inversely with reestablishment of normal topographic bias in the regenerated nerves.

HERPES ZOSTER

Ocular motor nerve palsies are frequently enough encountered in herpes zoster ophthalmicus, but their presence neither reflects special severity nor predicts a complicated outcome. Since lid swelling with complete ptosis is so common a finding, many instances of ocular motor deficits may be muted. Of such deficits, partial or complete oculomotor palsy is the most common (Fig. 12–16), but isolated internal ophthalmoplegia, independent of iritis, is also frequent. Pupillary involvement, with or without oculomotor palsy, may resolve as a "pseudo–Argyll Robertson pupil" (i.e., a mid-dilated pupil with defective light reaction, but constriction on near effort). Marsh et al[128] reviewed 58 patients with herpes zoster pareses: 34 had involvement ipsilateral to the cutaneous eruption (16 oculomotor, 11 abducens) and 9 had contralateral involvement (2 oculomotor, 8 abducens); 6 had evolving contralateral paresis; 5 had bilateral involvement; and 4 had complete ophthalmoplegia. Prognosis for full recovery of motor function is excellent, although an interval of several months may be required. The mechanism whereby other cranial

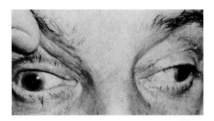
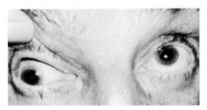

Fig. 12–16. Herpes zoster ophthalmicus with right oculomotor palsy. Double vision was noted when lid swelling abated and patient held up lid. Pupil is dilated and fixed.

nerves are involved in herpes zoster ophthalmicus is not known, but in ipsilateral cases it is likely that inflammation extends from the trigeminal ganglion to the ocular motor nerves as they traverse the cavernous sinus and superior orbital fissure (see also Trochlear Palsies). Other cranial neuropathies include those of the facial, glossopharyngeal, and vagus nerves.

ACUTE INFECTIOUS POLYNEUROPATHY

The bulbar variant of the Guillain-Barré syndrome (Landry ascending paralysis) often presents as a painless, rapidly progressive bilateral ophthalmoplegia. As it evolves, this cranial polyneuropathy may mimic unilateral or bilateral oculomotor palsies, but it usually progresses to a more or less total symmetric ophthalmoplegia that may include the pupils and accommodation. Lid elevators can be normal or minimally involved. The presence of acute or subacute facial diplegia confirms the diagnosis and practically excludes other considerations (Fig. 12–17).

Commonly, the disorder follows a febrile or "viral" illnesses, or is seen in association with infectious mononucleosis. Although the well-known cerebrospinal fluid protein elevation, in the absence of cellular response, is a *sine qua non* of this disorder, by no means is this dissociation a constant finding. Detailed nerve conduction studies in one patient with generalized Guillain-Barré syndrome[129] revealed that demyelination occurred first in the most distal nerve and progressed to the spinal root; during recovery, remyelination occurred initially at the spinal root level. This sequence may explain the typical interval of days to weeks between onset of symptoms and rise in cerebrospinal fluid protein, which probably increases only when the spinal roots become involved.

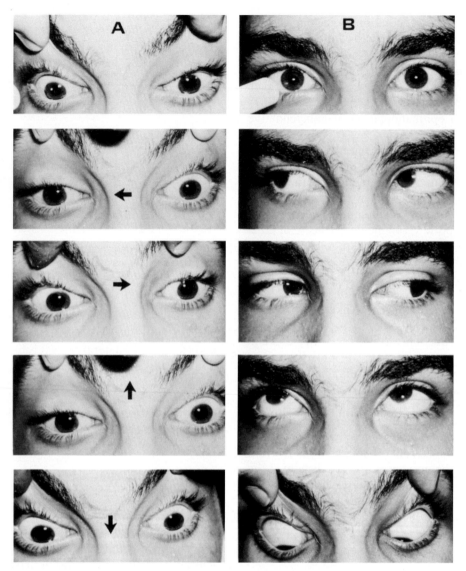

Fig. 12–17. Bulbar polyneuritis (Fisher syndrome) in a 16-year-old boy with rapidly progressive facial diplegia and total ophthalmoplegia, including pupillary and accommodative paresis. **A.** Acute phase. **B.** Complete resolution 3 months later.

In 1956, Fisher[130] documented the ophthalmoplegic variant of acute idiopathic polyneuritis, characterized by oculomotor palsies, areflexia, and ataxia. Pathologic material published by Asbury et al[131] demonstrated inflammatory infiltration of nerve roots, including peripheral and cranial nerves; these authors proposed that their findings suggest that the polyneuritis syndrome is related to a lymphocyte-mediated autoimmune reaction. The patient studied by Grunnet and Lubow,[132] however, showed central chromatolysis in the nuclei of the third, fourth, fifth, and twelfth nerves, and of the anterior horn cells, with only sparse lymphocytic infiltration. Additional clinical evidence that Fisher's syndrome can indeed affect the central nervous system (CNS) includes the following: loss of voluntary saccades with preservation of pursuit; upgaze paresis with intact Bell's phenomenon; internuclear ophthalmoplegia; cerebellar ataxia;

hemiparesis; extrapyramidal signs; and disorders of consciousness, including obtundation and electroencephalographic abnormalities.[133] Radiologic abnormalities include enhancing midbrain tegmental lesions and enhancement of trochlear, abducens, and oculomotor nerves, likely reflecting in inflammation and demyelination.[134]

Although it is estimated that ophthalmoplegia occurs in 15% of patients with Guillain-Barré syndrome,[135] nonetheless, on the basis of both clinical and neuropathologic findings, Fisher's syndrome (ophthalmoplegia, ataxia, areflexia) may not always represent a variant of the Guillain-Barré syndrome, but could represent several disease states. In fact, ophthalmoplegia may accompany a third type of idiopathic demyelinative polyneuropathy characterized by a prolonged course of symmetric sensory and motor limb symptoms.[136] Acute ophthalmoparesis may be associated with high serum IgG antibody to GQ$_{1b}$ ganglioside, with or without ataxia.[137] (See also Other Ocular Polyneuropathies, below).

In an extensive review of patients with Fisher's syndrome, Berlit and Rakicky[133] provided the following data:

Male : female ratio: 2 : 1
Mean age of onset: 43.6 years
Percentage with a preceding viral prodrome: 72%, with a 10-day interval
Symptoms: diplopia (39%), ataxia (21%), and areflexia (82%)
Non-ocular nerve involvement included: seventh (46%), ninth and tenth (40%), and twelfth (13%) nerves
Percentage with elevated CSF protein: 64%

Prognosis was considered good, with a mean recovery time of 10 weeks, but residual symptoms were present in 33% of cases. Therapy with corticosteroids or plasmaphoresis seemed without benefit.

OPHTHALMOPLEGIC MIGRAINE

Although rarely encountered, migrainous ophthalmoplegia is a distinct clinical entity; at times it is confused with carotid aneurysm, even though the victims are usually in the pediatric age group (Fig. 12–18). Migraine in its various forms occurs in *at least* 5% of school-age children, but may actually begin in infancy. In the early years, head pain is less frequent than cyclic vomiting or vertigo, and the typical episode in infancy is characterized by crying, irritability, photophobia, pallor, and vomiting, followed by sleep. In older children, cyclic vomiting may be the only sign of migraine, but more frequently the child experiences either classic recurrent migraine or "cluster" episodes. A family history of migraine is obtained in nearly 90% of the childhood cases of migraine (see also Chapter 16). Many clinicians believe that childhood "motion sickness" is also a migraine variant.

Friedman et al[138] analyzed eight cases of ophthalmoplegic migraine culled from 5000 migraine patients. Ages at onset of the first ophthalmoplegic episode were as follows: 2, 2, 3, 3, 5, 8, 17, and 30 years; that is, six of eight patients experienced ocular palsy at age 8 years or younger. All patients had oculomotor nerve involvement, the majority of which involved the pupil. A typical episode consisted of pain in and about the involved eye, nausea, and vomiting. With the onset of ophthalmoplegia, the head pain often resolved. As a rule, paresis clears completely within 1 month, but residua may persist (see Fig. 12–16D). Although patients can suffer multiple attacks, many years may intervene.

The mechanism of ophthalmoplegic migraine is ob-

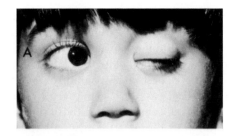
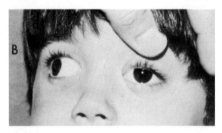
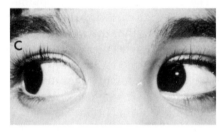
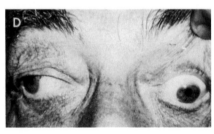

Fig. 12–18. Ophthalmoplegic migraine. This 3-year-old experienced an episode of nausea, vomiting, and headache of several hours' duration. After 12 hours of sleep, child awoke with left ptosis but felt absolutely well. **A** and **B.** Examination revealed complete left oculomotor palsy. The pupil was slightly dilated but reactive. **C.** Five weeks later all deficits had cleared. No diagnostic studies beyond skull x-rays were performed. One year later a second episode occurred exactly duplicating the first. **D.** A 60-year-old man with history of multiple episodes of left hemicrania in childhood, relieved by onset of left ptosis. At age 18 years, the left oculomotor palsy became fixed following typical attack. Residua include mild ptosis, left exotropia, elevation deficit, and small nonreactive pupil (fixed to all pharmacologic agents except strong mydriatics).

scure, but surely is peripheral in nature. Vijayan[139] observed sparing of the pupil in a single patient during three episodes of ophthalmoplegic migraine and, on reviewing the literature, reiterated that pupil sparing is not uncommon in this entity. He argued that this makes compressive neuropathy an unlikely mechanism, but proposed instead that "swelling of the walls of the carotid or basilar arteries leads to occlusion of the smaller vessels which supply the involved cranial nerves." However, MRI has shown enhancement of the oculomotor nerve in acute ophthalmoplegic migraine, with normal appearance on repeat imaging after the attack.[140–142]

The question of cerebral angiography is an important one. In the typical case of a young child with nausea, vomiting, and headache followed by third nerve palsy upon resolution of the premonitory symptoms, as well as a positive family history of migraine, perhaps no angiography is indicated. It is extremely unlikely than an intracranial tumor would present as a sudden painful third nerve palsy in a child, and aneurysms are quite rare among pediatric patients. A small perimesencephalic vascular anomaly was found angiographically in a 31-year-old patient with a partial oculomotor palsy and a 25-year history of recurrent ophthalmoplegic migraine.[143] The point that migrainous ophthalmoplegia and Tolosa-Hunt syndrome (see below) share many features is well taken,[141,144] but the argument that steroids should be used seems superfluous given the rapid resolution of pain and spontaneous recovery.

Osuntokun and Osuntokun[145] reported an extraordinarily high incidence of ophthalmoplegic migraine in Nigerians. Of practical importance is their finding of concurrent hemoglobin AS, and they suggested that hemoglobin electrophoresis be obtained in any black patient presenting with complicated migraine, including the ophthalmoplegic form.

OCULOMOTOR PALSIES OF CHILDHOOD

Isolated, nontraumatic oculomotor palsy is a rare event in childhood, but as noted above, ophthalmoplegic migraine occurs almost exclusively in the first decade of life, and may be suspected as a cause of recurrent, benign oculomotor palsies in this age group. Miller[120] reviewed 30 cases of isolated third nerve palsy occurring in childhood (23 patients younger than 10 years of age). Thirteen children (43%) had congenital palsies, but in only 4 was the palsy associated with birth trauma or forceps delivery. Aberrant regeneration was a common sequela, and cyclic phenomena developed in 3 patients (see below). Six patients had palsies secondary to trauma, most commonly orbital fractures, and 4 had palsies secondary to established or presumed (possibly viral) meningitis. Only 3 cases of tumor-related palsies were recorded: 1 case each of leptomeningeal sarcoma, leptomeningeal lymphoma, and orbital apex tumor. Migraine ophthalmoplegia occurred in 2 children, ages 3 and 6. Posterior communicating artery aneurysms occurred in 2 adolescents, ages 16 and 17, both with signs and symptoms of subarachnoid hemorrhage. Likewise, Ing et al[96] reviewed 54 cases of childhood third nerve palsy, 31 of which were related to trauma, and 11 were evident at birth; of the remaining cases, 4 were associated with meningitis, 3 were "viral," 2 were migrainous, and only 1 brain stem glioma (late in the course with accompanying sixth and seventh nerve palsies), and 1 due to an orbital hemangioma.

Balkan and Hoyt[122] cautioned that congenital third nerve palsies may not be monosymptomatic. Of their 10 patients with congenital third nerve palsies, 4 had associated focal neurologic deficits and 2 had generalized developmental delay. In children, isolated third nerve palsy may follow viral illness[123,146] or immunization,[147] but seems to occur much less frequently in this setting than sixth nerve palsy. Recall also that "cryptogenic," progressive oculomotor pareses may be secondary to a neurinoma of the peripheral nerve or masses in the cavernous sinus, for which thin-section MRI is required.

Harley[123] provided a useful overview of "paralytic strabismus" in children, a retrospective analysis of the Wills Eye Hospital experience of 121 patients ranging in age from birth to 16 years. The common causes of isolated oculomotor palsy included 15 congenital cases (including 4 with double elevator palsies), frequently showing aberrant regeneration signs; 4 traumatic cases; and 3 migrainous cases. Of the abducens palsy cases, 21 were traumatic; 17 were associated with neoplasms, including brain stem gliomas, and posterior fossa astrocytomas and medulloblastomas. Although no further clinical data are supplied, in the tumor group surely other neurologic signs and symptoms were present, although the abducens may have been the predominant malfunctioning motor nerve to the eye. Of 18 trochlear palsy cases, 12 were congenital (including 5 bilateral cases) and 5 were the result of head trauma. Other patients in this series showed eye movement defects that were due to local orbital inflammation or tumor, but not strictly due to focal ocular motor palsies per se.

In the situation of nontraumatic, acquired, isolated oculomotor palsy in childhood, where the diagnosis is in doubt, it is reasonable to proceed with MRI scanning of basal structures including the orbits. In cases where meningitis or intracranial hemorrhage is suspected, cerebrospinal fluid examination is also mandatory.

CYCLIC OCULOMOTOR PALSY

Alternating paresis and spasm of the extraocular and intraocular muscles supplied by the oculomotor nerve is an extraordinary cyclical phenomenon that usually occurs in early childhood or may be noted at birth. With few exceptions, once the cycles begin, they persist throughout life. The relationship to birth trauma is unsettled, and other mechanistic concepts are speculative. Loewenfeld and Thompson[148] reviewed 57 cases, and their analysis is authoritative. During the paretic phase, the eyelid is ptotic, the pupil is dilated but not necessarily fixed to light, accommodation is impaired, and the eye is usually in an exotropic position with paresis of abduction and vertical movement. The shorter spastic phase may be initiated by attempts at adduction and begins with lid twitching, which progresses to lid elevation. The pupil constricts, accommodation increases, and the globe may turn to the midline or beyond. As a rule, cycles continue during sleep but may be abolished during deep anesthesia.

One extraordinary case[149] showed involvement of the pupil and accommodation only, with no evidence of levator or extraocular muscle involvement. In another unusual case,[150] cyclic oculomotor palsy accompanied by oculomotor synkinesis was presumably caused by a supraclinoid aneurysm in an elderly woman.

COMBINED OCULAR MOTOR PALSIES AND PAINFUL OPHTHALMOPLEGIAS

It is imperative to distinguish simultaneous palsies of the oculomotor, trochlear, and abducens nerves (Table 12–6) from oculoparesis due to diffuse orbital inflammatory disease (Graves ophthalmopathy, myositis), slowly progressive myopathy (chronic progressive external ophthalmoplegia), and ocular myasthenia.

Combined ocular neural palsies are most commonly unilateral because lesions involve the superior orbital fissure or cavernous sinus. Orbital diseases producing oculoparesis usually also result in some degree of proptosis and congestion of the lids and conjunctiva. Minimal proptosis (2 to 3 mm) has been attributed to lack of tone of the extraocular muscle cone in the presence of profound oculomotor nerve palsy, but with such "neurogenic proptosis," the globe may be easily retropulsed into the orbit by applying firm digital pressure through the closed lids. In the presence of an orbital mass lesion or Graves disease, increased orbital resistance prevents retropulsion of the globe.

Bilateral combined palsies may be seen in a variety of etiologic settings (see Table 12–6), including the following: acute infectious polyneuropathy (Fisher syndrome), enterovirus 70 infections, brain stem toxoplasmosis, infiltrative brain stem tumors, basicranial extension of nasopharyngeal carcinoma, basal sarcoidosis, carcinomatous seeding of basal arachnoid, clivus chordoma, extrasellar extension of pituitary tumor into both cavernous sinuses (may occur acutely with hemorrhage [i.e., "pituitary apoplexy"]), sphenoid carcinoma, cavernous sinus thrombosis, or arteriovenous fistula. In a review of 4278 cases of ocular palsies encountered at the Mayo Clinic,[108] the abducens nerve was affected in 1918, oculomotor in 1225, trochlear in 657, and multiple cranial nerve palsies in 573. According to this series, in patients with simultaneous multiple ocular cranial neuropathies, neoplasm was by far the most common cause (35.3%). However, 4.1% of such patients had microvascular disease as the underlying etiology. These diverse clinical situations are usually differentiated by temporal course, associated signs and symptoms (including involvement of other cranial nerves), examination of the cerebrospinal fluid, and neuroimaging techniques that include CT, arteriography, and MRI, all performed with special regard to orbital and basicranial areas.

The combination of single or multiple ocular motor nerve palsies with pain in and about the eye, usually unilateral, constitutes the syndrome of painful ophthalmoplegia. This syndrome has a wide variety of underlying pathophysiologic mechanisms, ranging from benign ischemic oculomotor palsy to carcinoma involving the cavernous sinus (Table 12–7).

ORBITAL LESIONS

In the orbit (also see Chapter 14), acute painful ophthalmoplegia may be associated with inflammation in the adjacent sinuses, in children[151] as well as adults.

TABLE 12–6. Combined Oculopareses

	Graves' ophthalmopathy	Myasthenia	Ocular myopathy	Combined III, IV, VI
Course*	Chronic/rarely acute; ± history of dysthyroidism	Acute/chronic; intermittent	Chronic	Acute/chronic
Bilateral	Usually	Usually; may alternate	Always	Rarely
Pain	± Foreign body sensation	No	No	Variable
Pupils	Normal	Normal	Normal	Variable
Tensilon test	Negative	Positive	Negative	Negative
Forced duction†	Positive	Negative	Variable	Negative
Other signs	Lid retraction, scleral injection, proptosis, lid edema; classic echographic, CT or MRI changes	Ptosis, lid fatigability, orbicularis weakness, Cogan's lid twitch	Ptosis, orbicularis weakness, ± temporalis wasting	± Trigeminal hypoesthesia

* Regardless of etiology, diplopia is considered acute by most patients.
† Any chronic oculoparesis may show positive forced ductions.

TABLE 12–7. Painful Ophthalmoplegia Syndromes

Orbit
Inflammatory pseudotumor
Contiguous sinusitis
Mucormycosis or other fungal infections
Metastatic tumor
Lymphoma

Superior orbital fissure/anterior cavernous sinus
Nonspecific granulomatous inflammation (Tolosa-Hunt syndrome)
Metastatic tumor
Nasopharyngeal carcinoma
Lymphoma
Herpes zoster
Carotid-cavernous fistula
Cavernous sinus thrombosis

Parasellar area
Pituitary adenoma
Intracavernous aneurysm
Metastatic tumor
Nasopharyngeal carcinoma
Sphenoid sinus mucocele
Meningioma, chordoma
Petrositis (Gradenigo's syndrome)

Posterior fossa
Posterior communicating artery aneurysm
Basilar artery aneurysm (rare)

Miscellaneous
Diabetic ophthalmoplegia
Migrainous ophthalmoplegia
Cranial arteritis

Orbital cellulitis per se is not a requisite, but thrombosis of orbital veins, demonstrable by echography, may account for congestive signs and symptoms. Bergin and Wright[152] found abnormal sinuses radiographically in 61% of 49 cases of orbital cellulitis, with an average age presentation of 31 years. Some degree of proptosis and lid swelling is invariably present, but fever is more common in infants and children.

Of great clinical importance is the early recognition of an acute orbital inflammatory syndrome in the diabetic patient, which should immediately suggest an opportunistic fungal infection such as mucormycosis (phycomycosis). Contrary to popular opinion, uncontrolled acidosis need not be present, and in fact, orbitocerebral phycomycosis can occur in otherwise healthy patients.[153] Although the exception, mucormycosis may run a subacute or even chronic course. Retinal artery occlusion is highly suggestive, and classically a progressive and often fatal picture of cavernous sinus thrombosis rapidly evolves.

The basic pathophysiologic process by which mucormycosis produces orbital signs and symptoms is ischemic necrosis due to arterial thrombosis. All orbital structures may be involved, and there may also be occlusion of the cavernous sinus, other cerebral venous sinuses, the arterial circle, internal carotid artery, and central retinal artery. Rarely, orbital disease is minimal, but more commonly a full-blown orbital apex syndrome is observed. Premorbid diagnosis is dependent on a high index of suspicion and immediate sinus exploration with mucosal biopsy. Survival depends on the combined effort of the ophthalmologist, rhinologist, mycologist, and internist. Amphotericin B is the drug of choice, but adequate therapy also requires surgical débridement of necrotic tissue.

A major review by Yohai et al[154] analyzed survival factors in mucormycosis. Criteria related to a lower survival rate included delayed diagnosis and treatment, the presence of hemiparesis or hemiplegia, bilateral sinus involvement, leukemia, renal disease, and prior treatment with deferoxamine. Facial necrosis also played an important role in the clinical prognosis of these patients. Newer adjunctive therapies include local irrigation with amphotericin B and alteration of immunosuppressive regimens in patients being treated for transplants or malignancies. In addition, hyperbaric oxygen therapy had a favorable effect on prognosis.

Inflammatory orbital pseudotumor is a distinct, if somewhat difficult to define, clinical entity that may run an acute or indolent course. Usually associated with proptosis, orbital pseudotumor is a source of variable degrees of ophthalmoplegia and pain, but visual loss is infrequent. It occurs in all age groups; recurrences are common, and both orbits may be involved.[155] Orbital pseudotumor is an infrequent manifestation of the collagen vasculitides,[156] and in rare cases may be part of a syndrome of multifocal idiopathic fibrosclerosis.[157]

Rootman and Nugent,[158] in their series of 17 patients with acute orbital pseudotumor, described five patterns determined by clinical and CT criteria: anterior, diffuse, posterior, lacrimal, and myositic. Of particular interest here is the myositis form of orbital pseudotumor (orbital myositis). This entity, like other forms of orbital pseudotumor, is characterized by inflammation of unknown etiology; may be associated with systemic collagen vascular disease; may be recurrent or chronic; occurs in all age groups; and shows a dramatic response to steroids. The patient typically presents with symptoms of acute periorbital pain, eyelid swelling, and diplopia with proptosis. Ocular echography and CT or MRI quickly exclude a number of diagnostic possibilities, such as carotid-cavernous fistula, infectious cellulitis, metastatic neoplasm, and cavernous sinus thrombosis.

Siatkowski et al[159] performed a large retrospective review of 75 patients (age range, 9 to 84 years) with orbital myositis. Female patients were affected more than twice as frequently as male patients; 68% of patients had single muscle involvement, the lateral and medial recti being affected most commonly. In almost half of these patients, affected muscles functioned normally, but in the other patients muscle function was equally distributed between paretic or restrictive, or combined "paretic-restrictive" myopathies. Early treatment with systemic corticosteroids was advocated to avoid permanent restrictive myopathies. Interestingly, in 9% of patients with typical unimuscular orbital myositis, classic thyroid eye disease later developed. Usually, the clinical distinction between these two entities is straightforward: myositis presents with pain, muscle enlargement, and involvement of the tendon insertion on CT or orbital echography, with low muscle reflectivity seen on standardized A-scan; thyroid myopathy is typically painless and spares the tendon, with notably high reflectivity echographically.

On relatively infrequent occasions, the clinical symptoms of cranial arteritis include defects of ocular motility. The incidence of subjective diplopia is uncertain, but it is estimated at 10% to 17%.[160] Ophthalmoplegia of any degree, however, may be obscured by the more dramatic symptoms of visual loss. In the only complete pathologic study of ophthalmoplegia occurring in cranial arteritis,[161] the ocular motor system was unremarkable except for the extraocular muscles, which showed variable degrees of ischemic necrosis. It is also possible that some instances of diplopia may be due to cranial nerve infarctions, but pathologic confirmation of this mechanism is lacking.

Slowly progressive ophthalmoplegia, usually without pain, may occur rarely in amyloidosis, and intraductal (sclerosing) breast carcinoma produces a syndrome of insidious fibrous fixation (desmoplasia) of orbital soft tissues with atrophy and enophthalmos, despite infiltrative metastases.[162]

Combined unilateral palsies of the third, sixth, or fourth nerves, or involvement of the trigeminal nerve (producing pain or hypoesthesia), suggest a lesion at the skull base, especially in the cavernous sinus or parasellar area. Keane[163] reviewed case material accrued at the Los Angeles County Medical Center and documented that 30% of such cases were due to tumors, two thirds of which were malignant.

TOLOSA-HUNT SYNDROME

It is probable that the same nonspecific inflammatory reaction that characterizes orbital pseudotumor also accounts for acute inflammatory syndromes that involve the superior orbital fissure or anterior cavernous sinus (i.e., the so-called Tolosa-Hunt syndrome, or "painful ophthalmoplegia"). In 1954, Tolosa[164] described a 47-year-old man with recurrent orbital pain and ophthalmoplegia, who died after exploratory craniotomy. At autopsy, the intracavernous carotid was surrounded by granulomatous tissue that invested cranial nerves and partially filled the cavernous sinus. In 1961, Hunt et al[165] described six similar clinical cases and concluded that the process was self-limited and responded to corticosteroid therapy, and that Tolosa's case did not represent

an actual arteritis. The use of corticosteroids as a "diagnostic test," often with dramatic therapeutic response, should be viewed with caution because both spontaneous and steroid-induced remissions of symptoms and signs, in both tumorous and nontumorous lesions, have been recorded.[166] Therefore, prompt clinical response to corticosteroid therapy does not confirm the nature of the disease process.[167]

The lesions responsible for the Tolosa-Hunt form of painful ophthalmoplegia have been pathologically confirmed in very few instances; these descriptions include nonspecific granulation tissue in the cavernous sinus[164] and pachymeningitis of the superior orbital fissure. Kline[168] provided a subject review with additional cases cited, and a patient with necrotizing inflammation of the intracavernous and intracranial portions of the internal carotid artery is documented.[169]

The following criteria are suggested for the diagnosis of the Tolosa-Hunt (painful ophthalmoplegia) syndrome:

1. The patient has steady, boring pain in and about the eye (ophthalmic division of the trigeminal nerve).
2. There is ophthalmoplegia with partial or total palsy of the extraocular muscles innervated by nerves III, IV, or VI, in any combination.
3. The pupil may be partially dilated and sluggish, dilated and fixed, spared entirely, or small (because of involvement of the sympathetic nerves).
4. Sensory defects may be found in the distribution of the ophthalmic-trigeminal nerve (rarely the second division).
5. The optic nerve may rarely be involved.
6. Symptoms are acute or subacute and respond dramatically to large doses of corticosteroids (e.g., 60 to 100 mg prednisone).
7. Spontaneous remissions may occur with complete or partial regression of deficits.
8. Episodes may recur at intervals of months or years.
9. Diagnostic studies (CT, MRI, arteriography, rhinologic examination) show no evidence of involvement of structures outside of the cavernous sinus).

Radiologic findings may be relatively meager, but include soft tissue densities (Fig. 12–19) in the cavernous sinus,[170,171] some with resolution following corticosteroid therapy; sellar erosion,[172] and, in a patient with painful ophthalmoplegia associated with diabetes and hypoadrenalism, enlargement of the hypophysis and infundibulum[173], biopsy of which demonstrated chronic inflammation. Other various mechanisms that mimic Tolosa-Hunt include dural arteriovenous fistula,[174] ophthalmoplegic migraine with enhanced oculomotor nerves,[141,142] and lymphoma.[175]

The clinician should be mindful that a diagnosis of Tolosa-Hunt syndrome is one made by default when exhaustive examination has seemingly ruled out other

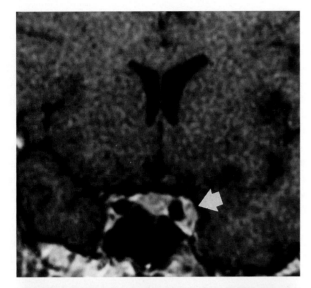
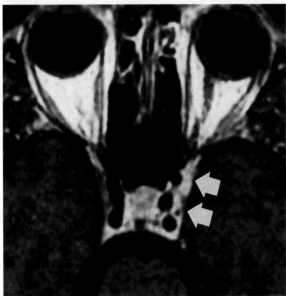

Fig. 12–19. A 42-year-old woman presented with severe pain in left orbit and brow, and diplopia due to partial oculomotor paresis. MRI with enhancement showed soft tissue densities (*arrows*) in left cavernous sinus. Coronal **(top)** and axial **(bottom)** sections. All laboratory studies and CSF results were normal. There was complete clinical resolution with corticosteroid therapy. Follow-up neuroimages were declined.

causes of painful ophthalmoplegia (see Table 12–7). More specific underlying processes may surface with the passage of time, and radiologic studies may bear repeating. If the preceding criteria are met, it is reasonable to begin corticosteroid therapy to alleviate severe pain while radiologic studies are being completed. If mucormycosis or other fungal infection is suspected, the use of corticosteroids is strictly contraindicated, and may indeed cause or hasten a fatal course.

The relationship between nonspecific inflammation involving the cavernous sinus or superior orbital fissure and idiopathic orbital pseudotumor is of interest. One may consider that these syndromes are indeed caused by the same process, in different locations. It is speculated that, on the basis of antineutrophil cytoplasmic antibodies, Tolosa-Hunt may represent a limited form of Wegener granulomatosis[176] in some instances. Also, idiopathic cranial pachymeningitis or fibrosclerosis may be related.[177] Concurrent autoimmune diseases such as Hashimoto's thyroiditis may be likewise incriminated.[178]

PARASELLAR SYNDROMES

Lesions in and about the sella turcica may involve the ocular motor nerves in their course through the cavernous sinus (Figs. 12–20 and 12–21). Pituitary tumors, or even supposedly normal glands, may suddenly enlarge and expand laterally into the cavernous sinus. Such extrasellar extension produces a clinical picture of multiple ocular motor palsies (often bilateral), severe headache, and variable disturbances of vision, including abrupt bilateral blindness. This constellation is highly suggestive of spontaneous infarction of a pituitary adenoma (*i.e.*, so-called "pituitary apoplexy"). An enlarged sella confirms the diagnosis, and enhanced CT or MRI can discriminate among densities related to blood, infarction, and necrosis. Chronically progressive cavernous sinus syndromes due to pituitary tumors are relatively rare; rather, an acute or rapidly progressive ophthalmoplegia is the rule. Bills et al[179] noted oculomotor pareses in 78% of patients with pituitary apoplexy, and Vidal et al[180] in 67%. As Weinberger et al[181] noted, pituitary tumors that produce visual symptoms due to insidious chiasmal compression do not, as a rule, cause ophthalmoplegias. They quoted Schaeffer's observation that anatomic variations in the size of the aperture in the diaphragma sellae, and the strength of the diaphragma itself, may influence the growth pattern and actually determine the direction of extrasellar extension of pituitary adenomas. Pituitary apoplexy is further considered in Chapter 6.

Intracavernous aneurysms (see Fig. 12–7B and C) constitute only 2% to 3% of all intracranial aneurysms, but they may represent up to 15% of symptomatic unruptured aneurysms,[19] and 20% to 25% of lesions producing a cavernous sinus syndrome.[166] The only other entities that are as frequently responsible for this syndrome are nasopharyngeal and metastatic neoplasms.[163,166,182] As Meadows[183] noted, intracavernous aneurysms "behave differently from aneurysms arising elsewhere in the skull by virtue of their position . . . and [they] tend to present themselves to ophthalmologists on account of ocular features." Although Meadows wrote that "rupture may certainly occur," with subsequent formation of an intracavernous arteriovenous fistula, this complication must be exceedingly rare. Fatal subarachnoid hemorrhage

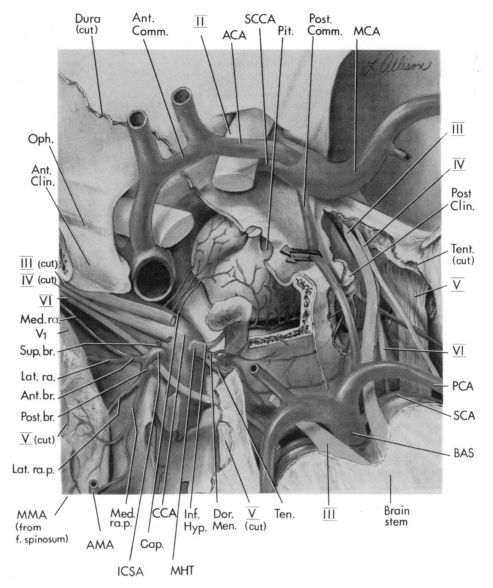

Fig. 12–20. An exposed view of the cavernous sinus. The neurovascular anatomy of the cavernous sinus is shown in detail. [*BAS,* basilar artery; *SCA,* superior cerebellar artery; *PCA,* posterior cerebral artery; *Tent. (cut),* tentorium cut to demonstrate underlying arteries and nerves; *Post Clin.,* posterior clinoid; *MCA,* middle cerebral artery; *Post. Comm.,* posterior communicating artery; *Pit.,* pituitary gland; *SCCA,* supraclinoid carotid artery; *ACA,* anterior cerebral artery; *Ant. Comm.,* anterior communicating artery; *Dura (cut),* dura cut for exposure of cavernous sinus; *Oph.,* ophthalmic artery; *Ant. Clin.,* anterior clinoid; *MMA (from f. spinosum),* middle meningeal arterial branch coming from foramen spinosum; *AMA,* accessory meningeal artery at level of foramen ovale; *ICSA,* artery to the inferior cavernous sinus; *Sup. br.,* superior branch of ICSA; *Ant. br.,* anterior branch of ICSA; *Med. ra.,* medial ramus of anterior branch of ICSA; *Lat. ra.,* lateral ramus of anterior branch of medial ICSA; *Post. br.,* posterior branch of ICSA; *Med. ra.p.,* medial ramus of posterior branch of ICSA, *Cap.,* capsular arteries; *CCA,* cavernous carotid artery; *MHT,* meningohypophyseal trunk; *Inf. Hyp.,* inferior hypophyseal artery of MHT; *Brain stem,* anterior portion of mesencephalon exposed; *II,* optic nerve; *III (cut),* oculomotor nerve cut to allow visualization of intracavernous carotid artery and its branches; *IV (cut),* trochlear nerve cut; *VI,* abducens nerve cut; *V₁,* first division of fifth cranial nerve ophthalmic; *III,* oculomotor nerve seen posteriorly and anteriorly (not cut) on reader's right; *V,* fifth cranial nerve seen (not cut) on reader's right. *V (cut)* on left. *Dor. Men.,* dorsal meningeal artery; *Ten,* tentorial artery.]

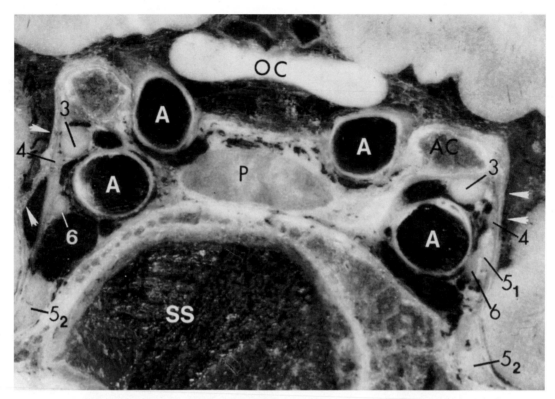

Fig. 12–21. Microtomic preparation, coronal section through cavernous sinuses. *SS*, sphenoid sinus; *P*, pituitary gland; *AC*, anterior clinoids; *OC*, optic chiasm; *3, 4, 6, 5₁* (ophthalmic), and *5₂* (maxillary, cranial nerves). Siphons of intracavernous carotid arteries (*A*) cut in cross-section. White arrowheads indicate dura of lateral wall of cavernous sinuses. (Courtesy of Dr. David Daniels, Medical College of Wisconsin, Milwaukee)

has been reported.[184] On occasion, uncontrollable nasal bleeding may be caused by erosion into the sphenoid sinus, but this phenomenon pertains to the post-traumatic, acquired intracavernous aneurysm.[185]

The clinical features of intracavernous aneurysms may be summarized as follows:[186]

1. There is usually slowly progressive diplopia first noted on eccentric gaze, due to variable involvement of the ocular motor nerves.

2. There is usually an abduction defect (abducens palsy) coupled with partial oculomotor palsy; pure abduction defects have been reported.[186,187]

3. Less frequently, patients present with an abrupt and simultaneous onset of diplopia, unilateral ptosis, and severe ipsilateral periocular pain or trigeminal dysesthesia; however, pain may be minimal or absent, even in the presence of profound ocular motor palsies.

4. Ptosis may be minimal to complete.

5. The pupil may show sympathoparesis, parasympathoparesis, or (rarely) a combination that renders the pupil smaller (pharmacologic testing for Horner syndrome confirms the presence of sympathoparesis, whereas sluggish light reaction suggests parasympathoparesis).

6. "Primary misdirection" (see above) may be observed.

7. There is an unexplained higher frequency of these aneurysms in middle-aged and elderly women (Fig. 12–22).

8. Involvement of the optic nerve (visual loss and optic atrophy) is rare, and indicates encroachment of the aneurysm superiorly toward the ipsilateral anterior clinoid.

9. Thin-section, enhanced CT scanning of basicranial structures, or MRI, demonstrates the lesion, which may be confirmed by angiography or radionuclide dynamic flow studies.

10. Longstanding, unruptured aneurysms are compatible with long life, and indications for surgical intervention are indistinct, although intervention would seem reasonable to treat intractable trigeminal pain.

11. Cardiovascular disease, including hypertension, is commonly associated with these aneurysms.

Of 59 cavernous aneurysms reported with ocular motor involvement,[188] 17 involved the sixth nerve only, 5 involved the third nerve, and 37 involved multiple nerves, including 13 with complete unilateral ophthalmoplegia. The onset of oculomotor involvement was painful in all but three patients, and the conditions of all nine patients

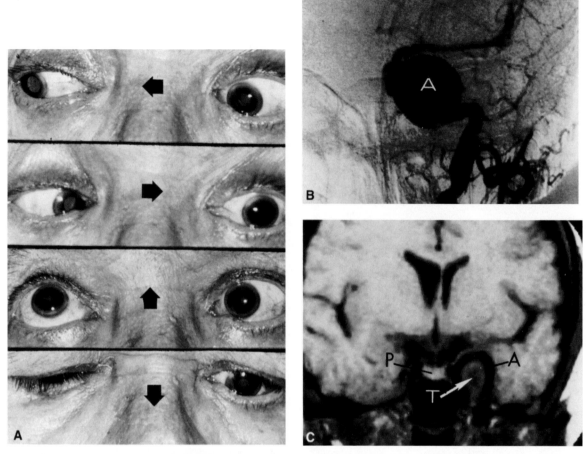

Fig. 12–22. A. A 72-year-old man with slowly progressive left ophthalmoplegia. Note paresis of left medial, lateral, superior, and inferior recti. Left pupil showed inextensive motor function. Left lid retraction on downward gaze (pseudo-vonGraefe phenomenon) indicates oculomotor "misdirection." **B.** Left carotid arteriogram demonstrates large intracavernous aneurysm (*A*). **C.** Similar left intracavernous aneurysm (*A*) displayed on coronal MRI; note partial thrombosis (*T*) surrounded by signal void. (*P*, pituitary gland)

with sudden ophthalmoplegia improved spontaneously within 6 weeks.[188]

Barr et al[19] documented the pathologic changes of intracavernous aneurysms, including the disposition of the ocular motor nerves displaced on the medial convexity of the aneurysmal sac.

It is clinically valid to separate from the general category of middle fossa or sphenoid ridge meningiomas, a distinctive type whose center of growth, symptomatically and radiologically, is the cavernous sinus. Although meningiomas represent 15% to 20% of intracranial tumors, origin in the dura of the cavernous sinus is not acknowledged in most comprehensive series.[189] In all probability, these tumors derive from the meninges covering the floor of the middle fossa, but they are clinically unlike the tumors designated as "middle fossa meningiomas." Typical middle fossa tumors, which constitute 2% to 15% of meningiomas, evidently originate at some

distance lateral to the cavernous sinus, for they produce headaches, seizures, memory disturbances, hemiparesis, homonymous hemianopia, and papilledema before producing ophthalmoplegia. Meningiomas of the more medial sphenoid ridge frequently produce ophthalmoplegia, proptosis, and possible compromise of the optic nerve.

As with intracavernous aneurysms, "intracavernous" meningiomas may masquerade for years as slowly progressive unilateral ophthalmoplegia without pain, but commonly with proptosis, moderate ptosis, and occasionally primary aberrant regeneration phenomena.[186] Pupillary abnormality is usually of the parasympathoparetic type (*i.e.*, somewhat dilated and with a sluggish light reflex). CT or MRI of the sellar area is typical, if not pathognomonic (Fig. 12–23).

Aside from histopathologic confirmation, surgery generally affords no relief of diplopia; the effectiveness

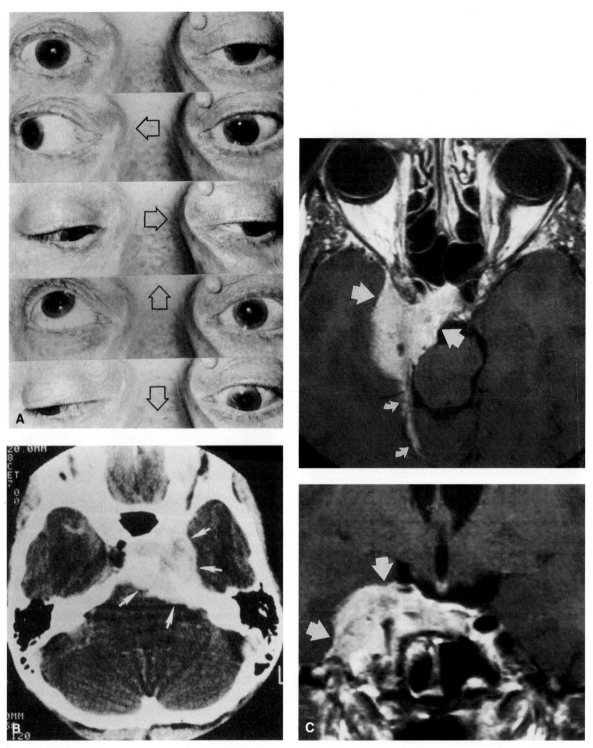

Fig. 12–23. A. A 68-year-old man with progressive left ptosis and diplopia. Left pupil slightly larger than right, with sluggish light reaction. Note pseudo-vonGraefe lid retraction in downgaze. **B.** CT shows enhancing soft tissue mass involving left cavernous sinus, petrous ridge, dorsum, and sella, compatible with meningioma. **C.** Enhanced T-1 weighted MRI. Axial **(top)** and coronal **(bottom)** sections show medial sphenoidal ("cavernous") meningioma (*large arrows*). Note tentorial extension (*small arrows*).

of fractionated or stereotactic radiation therapy is moot.[190]

In the Thomas and Yoss[166] series of 102 patients with parasellar syndrome, nasopharyngeal carcinoma was the most common cause, accounting for approximately 1 in every 5 patients. Also, according to Godtfredsen and Lederman,[182] 20% of nasopharyngeal tumors present as a cavernous sinus syndrome and, conversely, 20% of cavernous sinus syndromes are due to malignant nasopharyngeal tumors. Although nasopharyngeal tumors may occur at any age, they most frequently do so in the seventh and eight decades and occur more frequently in males. Tumorous growth usually begins in the roof of the nasopharynx or in the lateral region about the ostium of the eustachian tube. Therefore, symptoms of tubal occlusion, including recurrent serous otitis, may be the initial sign of a nasopharyngeal tumor. Tumor extension commonly involves the basal foramina of the middle cranial fossa such that trigeminal involvement, especially maxillary division (*e.g.*, pain or numbness in the cheek or side of the face), is common. According to Godtfredsen and Lederman,[182] among patients with neuro-ophthalmic signs of nasopharyngeal tumors, the following frequencies of involvement are found: in 70%, neuralgias of the first and second trigeminal divisions; in 65%, ophthalmoplegia (most often affecting the abducens, then the oculomotor and trochlear nerves); in 17%, exophthalmos; in 12%, optic nerve defect; and in 16%, Horner syndrome. Although strictly ocular signs occurred alone in 25% of the patients, they were associated either with first- or second-division trigeminal defects or with varying lower cranial nerve palsies in 50% of the patients.

Because of the high rate of ophthalmologic signs and symptoms in nasopharyngeal tumors, and the large percentage of cavernous sinus syndromes due to such lesions, competent nasopharyngeal examination is mandatory in multiple ocular motor palsies or painful ophthalmoplegia. Since subtle submucosal extension of tumor occurs, "blind" nasopharyngeal biopsy may be positive in the absence of visible tumor mass, but CT and MRI studies of the paranasal sinuses often disclose evidence of soft tissue masses or bone erosion, in which case biopsy is performed at the indicated site.

Although associated with a more chronic variety of frontal and periocular headaches, sphenoidal sinus mucoceles (pyoceles) may also produce ophthalmoplegia. The review by Nugent et al[191] indicates that approximately one in three patients with a sphenoidal mucocele evidences palsy of the oculomotor or abducens nerves. However, in the series by Valvassori and Putterman,[192] no patient showed oculoparesis. One or both optic nerves are commonly involved, with a picture of chronically progressive visual loss and optic atrophy, but visual loss may be abrupt.[193] Occasionally, patients demonstrate chiasmal defects, usually with severe visual loss

in one eye and a temporal hemianopic field defect in the other. It should be recalled that the sphenoidal sinus shares a common bony wall with the optic canal, tuberculum sellae, cavernous sinus, and superior orbital fissure (see Figs. 4–5 and 5–32). With large expansion, exophthalmos may occur, as well as disc edema.[194]

Patients harboring sphenoidal mucoceles may have a history of otolaryngologic disease, but many do not. The diagnosis rests on typical radiologic features best seen by CT scanning, and recovery of visual and ocular motor function is dependent on chronicity of symptoms.

Metastatic tumors to the cavernous sinus comprised 23% of the 102 parasellar lesions reviewed by Thomas and Yoss,[166] and 33% of all neoplastic disease. Other than the nasopharynx, common primary sites include lung, breast, prostate, and systemic lymphomas. In the series of 17 patients with cavernous sinus metastases reported by Post et al,[195] unilateral, rather severe periorbital pain was the initial symptom in 12; 9 patients, including most of those with pain, had decreased sensation in trigeminal distribution, the ophthalmic division alone or with the maxillary in six cases, with the mandibular division in two cases, and isolated maxillary division in one case; four patients also had ipsilateral optic nerve involvement. High-resolution, contrast CT scanning demonstrated an enhancing soft tissue mass that bulged the wall of the cavernous sinus laterally, and secondary bone invasion was often present (see also Kline et al[196]). In 6 of 17 patients, the cavernous sinus syndrome was the initial presentation of occult malignancy, and it represented the first sign of metastases in 5 patients with known disease. Median survival was 4.5 months from onset of parasellar symptoms, but focal radiation therapy was useful in pain control.

Skin carcinoma, especially squamous cell, may spread centripetally from the face or neck via perineural routes to the orbital apex or superior fissure, and may present years after dermatologic excisions.[197] Patients may present with diplopia due to minimal ocular duction deficits with few orbital signs and can also have trigeminal hypoesthesia or pain, or facial neuropathies.[198] tenHove et al[199] documented nine such patients, noting that enhanced MRI of infraorbital and orbital nerves was helpful for confirmatory biopsy; in addition, radiation therapy may stabilize the diplopia in these patients, allowing for the possibility of strabismus surgery. Contiguous perineural and endoneural extension may also lead to meningeal carcinomatosis.[200]

Identification of specific pathologic entities causing the cavernous sinus syndrome is rarely possible by clinical criteria alone. The mode of onset, frequency of remissions, rate of progression, presence or absence of pain, pattern of neurologic deficit, and response to steroid therapy cannot reliably predict the precise nature of a cavernous sinus lesion. Nonetheless, it is often possible, on the basis of history, physical findings, radiography, and other clinical factors, at least to limit etiologic considerations and manage accordingly. Although it is true that ultimate diagnosis rests with biopsy, either transnasal or transcranial, in some instances even without histologic confirmation radiation therapy may be a better choice than craniotomy, especially if abnormal tissue is not encountered outside of the cavernous sinus. Surgery indeed may further jeopardize visual function or intensify general morbidity.

OTHER OCULAR POLYNEUROPATHIES

Diffuse or multifocal seeding of the leptomeninges by carcinoma, so-called meningeal carcinomatosis, often presents as simultaneous or rapidly sequential cranial nerve disorders, with or without headache, altered mentation, or signs of meningeal irritation. Although such neurologic complications are usually a late manifestation of systemic cancer, on occasion these signs may be the first evidence of occult carcinoma. According to the reviews by Olson et al,[201] Little et al,[202] and Wasserstrom et al,[203] ophthalmoplegia due to oculomotor and/or abducens involvement is strikingly common; also frequently involved are the facial, trigeminal, and acoustic nerves. Cerebrospinal fluid findings variably include raised pressure, elevated protein, depressed glucose, lymphocytic pleocytosis, and atypical (malignant) cells on cytologic preparations. Filling defects of the basal cisterns, subarachnoid space, and enhancement of leptomeninges, fissures, and cerebral sulci are best seen with gadolinium-MRI studies; hydrocephalus may be an indirect sign.[204]

Although the nervous system is involved relatively infrequently in patients with systemic sarcoidosis, multiple cranial neuropathies, aseptic meningitis, hydrocephalus, disease of CNS parenchyma, peripheral neuropathies, and myopathies may all occur with neurosarcoidosis. Of cranial palsies, peripheral facial nerve weakness is most frequent,[205] but the ocular motor nerves may also be involved as well as the optic nerves and chiasm (see Chapter 5). Of 50 cases of neurosarcoidosis, Oksamen[206] found that the angiotensin-converting enzyme (ACE) level in the cerebrospinal fluid was elevated in 18 of 31 patients.

Ocular motor nerve palsies may be the initial presenting sign of CNS toxoplasmosis, a potentially treatable disorder. *Toxoplasma gondii* is an opportunistic, neurotropic organism that usually causes multifocal CNS lesions and frequently involves the thalamus and brain stem.[207] We have observed several immunodeficient or immunosuppressed patients who presented with ptosis or diplopia due to toxoplasmosis involving the brain stem. Asymptomatic lesions are often found elsewhere in the brain. Other cranial nerve and brain stem functions may become progressively involved.

The acquired immunodeficiency syndrome (AIDS)

provides the clinical substrate for cranial neuropathies secondary to infections and lymphomas (Table 12–8). Third and sixth nerve palsies may herald CNS infection with cryptococcosis and toxoplasmosis,[207] as well as with large cell lymphoma.[208] Other ocular motility disorders include conjugate gaze palsies and internuclear ophthalmoplegia.[209]

Another infectious agent, enterovirus 70, causes acute hemorrhagic conjunctivitis that, in a number of cases, is associated with dysfunction of any of the spinal cord and/or cranial motor nerves.[210,211] One series[211] yielded the following results: 50% of the patients showed cranial nerve disturbances; sole involvement of the seventh or fifth cranial nerves was most common, and when multiple cranial nerves were involved, these same two nerves were again most frequently affected; prognosis was related to both severity and type of cranial nerve dysfunction; and patients with mild initial weakness and involvement of cranial nerves VII, IX, and X showed complete

TABLE 12–8. The Potential Etiologies of Cranial Nerve Palsies with HIV Infection

Infectious meningitis
Fungal
   Cryptococcus
   Histoplasmosis
   Mucormycosis
Bacterial
   Mycobacteria tuberculosis
   Listeria monocytogenes
   Treponema pallidum
Viral
   Herpes zoster/varicella
   Cytomegalovirus
   HIV meningitis

Neoplastic meningitis
Lymphoma
Other malignancies

Compression from intracranial mass lesions
Neoplastic
   Brain lymphoma
   Other malignancies
Infectious
   Toxoplasmosis
   Cryptococcoma
   Tuberculomas and tuberculous abscess

Vasculitis complicating HIV infection

Inflammatory
Guillain-Barré syndrome
Chronic inflammatory polyradiculoneuropathy

Miscellaneous
Malignant otitis externa
Idiopathic Bell's palsy
Other

(Berger JR, Flaster M, Schatz N et al: Cranial neuropathy heralding otherwise occult AIDS-related large cell lymphoma. J Clin Neuro Ophthalmol 13:113, 1993)

recovery, whereas patients with severe weakness or involvement of nerves III, IV, VI, and V did not show significant improvement.

The spirochete *Borrelia burgdorferi* produces Lyme disease, which may manifest a variety of acute, subacute, and chronic ocular and neurologic symptoms, including conjunctivitis, scleritis, uveitis, panophthalmitis, neuroretinitis, fluctuating meningoencephalitis, peripheral radiculopathies, and cranial nerve palsies.[212] By far, the facial nerve is most commonly affected, but other cranial nerve involvement, including the third, sixth, or optic nerve, is relatively rare even in endemic areas. Elevated serum IgM or IgG antibody titers are variably present, but false-negative results are common. The Western blot is a helpful confirmatory test, but cases of seronegative neuroborreliosis are well documented in the literature. Lyme disease is also a common cause of false-positive FTA-absorbed tests. Polymerase chain reaction may provide a sensitive tool for organism detection to complement immunologic techniques. The circular cutaneous lesion of erythema chronicum migrans is pathognomonic, as is the characteristic tick bite, but these phenomena may be unnoticed by the patient. The optimal treatment regimen for Lyme disease has not been defined, but a course of ceftriaxone (2 g/day) or cefotaxime (6 g/day) for 3 to 4 weeks is commonly prescribed. Intravenous penicillin and oral doxycycline (200 mg/day) for 2 weeks have been used successfully to treat Lyme meningitis, but these results require confirmation.

DISORDERS OF THE NEUROMUSCULAR JUNCTION AND OCULAR MYOPATHIES

Although of diverse nosology, disorders that primarily involve the neuromuscular junction of the extraocular muscles, or the muscles themselves, will be considered together in this section. Myasthenia and related myasthenic syndromes represent neuromuscular conduction defects. Graves' ocular myopathy represents a more or less specific immunologically mediated inflammatory reaction, especially of the extraocular muscles. What constitutes a primary ocular muscle dystrophy versus a neural abiotrophy is not precisely understood, but the presentation here nonetheless provides a useful clinical classification (Table 12–9).

Myasthenia

The diagnosis of myasthenia is at times simple and straightforward, and on other occasions frustrating and elusive. Despite the well-publicized ocular signs, myasthenia ranks high on the list of "missed diagnoses," simply because many physicians are unaware of the variations in presentation, do not know how to examine for subtle signs, and often do not think of this possibility, at any rate. Any puzzling acquired ocular motility distur-

TABLE 12–9. Disorders of the Neuromuscular Junction and Ocular Muscles

Myasthenia
Myasthenia-like syndromes
  Eaton-Lambert syndrome (distant effect of neoplasia)
  Drug-induced myopathies
Thyroid-related myopathy (Graves' disease)
Progressive external ophthalmoplegia
  Congenital
  Mitochondrial cytopathies
    Isolated ocular
    Oculofacial
    With pigmentary retinopathy
    Kearns-Sayre syndrome
  Oculopharyngeal (oculofacial-pharyngeal, oculo-pharyngodistal)
  Familial ophthalmoplegia with intestinal pseudo-obstruction
  Associated with neurodegenerative disorders
    Spinocerebellar degenerations, heredoataxias
    Juvenile spinal muscular atrophy (Wohlfart-Kugelberg-Welander syndrome)
    Infantile spinal muscular atrophy (Werdnig-Hoffman syndrome)
    Abetalipoproteinemia (Bassen-Kornzweig syndrome)
Myotonic dystrophy
Ocular neuromyotonia
Conditions simulating progressive external ophthalmoplegia
  Progressive supranuclear (bulbar) palsy (Steele-Richardson-Olszewsky)
  Parkinsonism
  Rostral-dorsal midbrain syndrome

bance—with or without ptosis, but with clinically normal pupils—should raise the question of myasthenia.

Myasthenia may be characterized as follows: weakness without other signs of neurologic deficit (no reflex changes, sensory loss, or muscle atrophy); variability of muscle function within minutes, hours or weeks; remissions and exacerbations (sometimes triggered by infection, fever, or trauma); and tendency to affect extraocular, facial, and oropharyngeal muscles. In addition, there is usually reversal or improvement of muscle function with cholinergic drugs. The onset of myasthenia may occur at any age, but before age 40, the disease is more common in women. Neonatal forms are rarely encountered, and the clinical course in children and infants differs from adults, demonstrating a wider spectrum of myasthenic syndromes.[213] (See also Chapter 13.) The association with thymoma is well known (approximately 10% of myasthenia patients), and in such patients morbidity tends to be more severe and mortality rates are higher. In addition, dysthyroidism is found in approximately 5% of myasthenic patients, such that ocular signs may be admixed (*e.g.*, exophthalmos and ptosis, paretic and restrictive motility defects). There is also a distinct relationship between collagen vascular disorders, thymoma, and myasthenia, and a familial incidence of myasthenia has been reported.

Myasthenia gravis is an autoimmune disorder characterized by a reduction of available postsynaptic acetylcholine receptors on the end plates of the neuromuscular junctions of skeletal muscle. Antibody-receptor interactions block neuromuscular transmission and subsequently destroy the receptor complex. The humoral immune response (*e.g.*, polyclonal IgG produced by B lymphocytes) apparently plays a critical role in producing this disease. Antiacetylcholine receptor antibody is said to be present in 85% to 90% of patients with generalized myasthenia gravis (GMG) but less in patients with myasthenia "restricted" to ocular muscles (OMG).[214] Indeed, given the "embryonic" type of acetylcholine receptor in ocular muscles, there is evidence for considerable immunologic heterogeneity between GMG and OMG.[215] This phenomenon may partially account for cases of "sero-negative" OMG. Although actual antibody titers correlate poorly with the severity of the disease, Drachman et al[216] demonstrated that the antibodies do accelerate degradation of acetylcholine receptors and increase the extent of receptor blockade. In turn, increased receptor degradation and blockade correspond closely with clinical status, and thus confirm the relevance of antiacetylcholine receptor antibodies in the pathogenesis of myasthenia. Thus, the concept of a "safety margin" is important in the pathophysiology of myasthenia. Normally, both acetylcholine receptors and acetylcholine molecules at the neuromuscular junction are in significant excess. Any aberration that decreases the likelihood of molecular interaction between these two entities reduces this safety margin and produces clinical symptoms. The cause of the autoimmune attack on acetylcholine receptors is not known, but the thymus regularly shows prominent germinal centers (presumably the source of antibody-forming cells), if not actual tumoral growth. Epithelial ("myoid") cells normally present in the thymus do indeed histologically resemble skeletal muscle, complete with acetylcholine receptors; these cells may become antigenic.

Ocular muscle involvement eventually occurs in 90% of all myasthenia and accounts for the initial complaint in approximately 75%.[217] In a study involving 1487 patients,[218] more than 50% presented with manifestations limited solely to extraocular muscles and levator palpebrae; of those patients with strictly ocular involvement during the first month after onset, 34% continued to have clinically "ocular" myasthenia over a four-decade follow-up period. That is, in 14% of this series, clinical manifestations were limited to the ocular muscles during the entire observation interval (mean, 17 years). Generalized myasthenia evolved in 68% of the initially "ocular" group, 78% of whom had clinical evidence within 12 months. Bever et al,[219] in a similar study, reported that 49% of "ocular" myasthenia remains "ocular," and that 82% of those patients who later developed generalized myasthenia did so within 2 years.

Since muscle fatigability and remissions are the hallmarks of the disease, it is not surprising that ocular signs may vary, lasting from a period of hours to a course of weeks or months. Although some degree of ptosis is almost invariable, it may at first be unilateral and noted only as the day or the fatigue progresses, or the ptosis

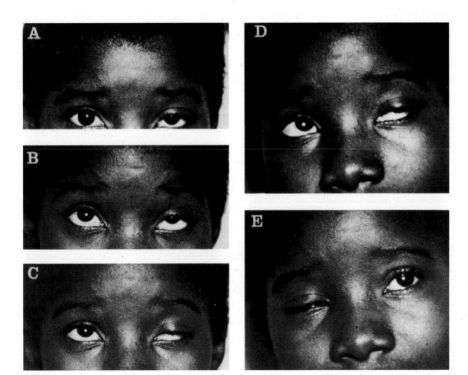

Fig. 12–24. **A.** Ocular myasthenia presenting as unilateral ptosis in an 8-year-old child. **B.** Levator can be fatigued by sustained upward gaze. **C.** Increasing ptosis. **D.** With ptosis accentuated, intravenous edrophonium (Tensilon) relieves fatigued left lid. **E.** Paradoxically, right lid is paralyzed.

may "shift" from eye to eye. Clinically, ptosis may be made more apparent by repeated eyelid closure or during sustained upward gaze (Fig. 12–24). In cases of unilateral ptosis, the contralateral upper lid may be retracted, but will assume a normal position if the eye with ptosis is occluded or if the ptotic lid is lifted with a finger ("curtaining" sign or "enhanced ptosis"). This represents an example of Hering's law of equivalent innervation to the lid levators, the intact lid responding to increased innervation evoked by the effort to raise the ptotic lid. Cogan[220] described a "lid twitch" sign that is elicited by having the patient rapidly redirect gaze from the downward to the primary position. The lid will be seen to twitch upward and then resettle to its original ptotic position. Occasionally, fine fluttering vibrations of the lash margins are observed in myasthenic lids. Although this is not a pathognomonic sign, Cogan's lid twitch is only rarely associated with other causes of ptosis.

Authoritative consensus dictates that pupillary and accommodative musculature is clinically uninvolved by myasthenia, sporadic reports and laboratory data to the contrary, notwithstanding.[217,221] If pupillary signs are present, another diagnosis must be entertained.

Extraocular muscle involvement does not follow any set pattern, although some have suggested that upward movements may be involved earliest. In our experience, medial rectus weakness is quite common, but essentially any ocular movement pattern may develop, such that isolated muscle palsies, or even total external ophthalmoplegia, may evolve. The motility pattern can mimic central gaze palsies or even internuclear ophthalmoplegia, complete with nystagmoid movements in the abducting eye (Fig. 12–25).[222] Myasthenic "nystagmus" has been otherwise documented.[223] Eye movement recordings may be helpful in the diagnosis of myasthenia, which tends to demonstrate hypometric large saccades, hypermetric smaller saccades, and intrasaccadic fatigue (resolved with edrophonium).[224] Intersaccadic fatigue may result in the appearance of a bimodal saccade or very rapid small saccades ("lightning eye movements") terminating in an apparent, small "quiver." These movements are quite characteristic and may be observed clinically. That is, supernormal saccadic velocities are the rule in myasthenia, even when significant ductional defects are present. Weakness of the orbicularis oculi is a very consistent sign in ocular myasthenia (Fig. 12–26) and serves as a further clue in diagnosis. Rarely does corneal exposure occur, but lower lid ectropion is occasionally seen. The "peek" sign results from orbicularis fatigue during eyelid closure, resulting in one or both eyes slightly opening spontaneously as the patient appears to peek at the examiner.[225]

Although it is true that the diagnosis of myasthenia is made on the basis of history and careful physical observations, one of the most helpful and dramatic (if

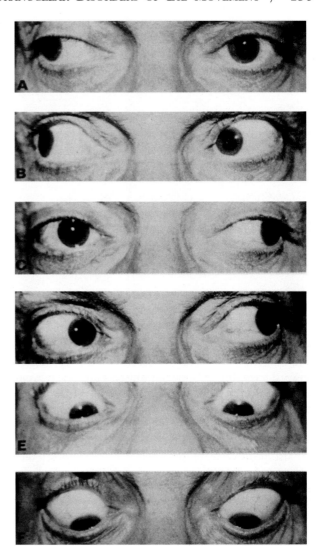

Fig. 12–25. Ocular myasthenia with motility pattern mimicking bilateral internuclear ophthalmoplegia. Lag of adducting eye on right (**A**) and left (**C**) gaze, relieved with edrophonium (Tensilon) (**B** and **D**). Convergence before (**E**) and after (**F**) edrophonium administration. Note relief of ptosis (**B** and **D**). (Glaser JS: Myasthenic pseudointernuclear ophthalmoplegia. Arch Ophthalmol 75:363, 1966. Copyright © 1966, American Medical Association)

positive) tests in medicine is the Tensilon test (edrophonium infusion). However, Tensilon testing is complicated by the problem of interpretation of response. When deficits in lid elevation or ocular motility are moderate or marked, evaluation of response to anticholinesterase drugs is usually a simple matter. However, when signs are minimal or inconstant, edrophonium or neostigmine (Prostigmin) response is more difficult to assess. The patient's interpretation of change in diplopia pattern may be made easier by placing a red filter before one eye, but this technique shares the inadequacies of all subjective examinations. In fact, patients have reported "improvement" after intravenous saline placebo. Such artificial reactions may indicate a functional disorder,

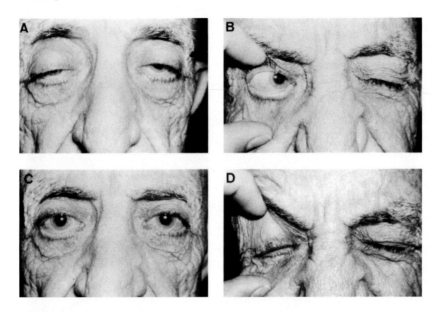

Fig. 12–26. A. Ocular myasthenia with ptosis. **B.** Marked orbicularis weakness. **C.** After administration of edrophonium, ptosis is relieved. **D.** Orbicularis strength increased.

or "neurasthenia." Before edrophonium is administered, lid weakness may be accentuated by prolonged upward gaze, but extraocular muscles are rarely weakened by exercise, with uncommon exceptions such as fatigue of sustained lateral gaze.[226] The orbicularis strength should also be noted before and after administration of edrophonium (see Fig. 12–26).

False-positive reactions occur with both neostigmine and edrophonium, but are fortunately infrequent. False-negative tests are not uncommon. This is in part due to the physician's often rough evaluation of subtle and inconstant oculoparesis and ptosis, dependency on the patient's subjective impressions, day-to-day variability of signs, and inadequate observations of "end points." Paradoxical edrophonium responses are recognized, including producing paresis of previously nonparetic muscles in myasthenics. Retzlaff et al[227] believe such paradoxical reactions to be present in half of myasthenics subjected to Tensilon testing, using red-green glasses for diplopia assessment.

In the chronic or "fixed" form, ocular myasthenia may be confused with chronic progressive external ophthalmoplegia (CPEO), because either entity can demonstrate symmetric total external ophthalmoplegia, ptosis, facial weakness, edrophonium resistance, and pharyngeal symptoms. A slow, progressive symmetric course, without fluctuations or remissions and little or no complaints of diplopia, speaks strongly in favor of CPEO, as does familial incidence. The "fixed" type of chronic ocular myasthenia may also show mechanical resistance to attempted forced duction testing.

For the most part, intravenous edrophonium has replaced neostigmine in diagnostic testing for myasthenia, although neostigmine is useful in children or in adults with poor intravenous access. The Tensilon test is performed in the following manner: (1) ptosis and motility

defects are evaluated as objectively as possible; (2) 1 mL (10 mg) edrophonium is drawn into a tuberculin or other small syringe and, after venipuncture, 0.2 mL of test dose is injected, but the needle is left in the vein; (3) tearing and fasciculations in the lids are indicators of cholinergic effect; and (4) if lid or extraocular muscle function is not improved within 30 to 60 seconds, the remaining 0.8 mL is slowly injected over similar intervals until a positive test result is observed, systemic effects (e.g., lid myokymia, tearing) occur, or the entire vial is injected, and the lid positions and eye movements assessed again.[228] We have had no problem with the use of intravenous edrophonium, even in children. The effect of edrophonium is short lived, and all evaluations must be completed within 5 minutes. Many myasthenics show improvement within 30 to 45 seconds after doses as low as 0.3 mL. Rarely is the entire vial necessary to provoke a response, and in fact, large doses of edrophonium may paradoxically cause worsening of ocular motility in myasthenia.

The Hess diplopia screen (red-green glasses and matching projector lights) combined with intravenous edrophonium was used to test 10 normal control subjects, 12 nonmyasthenic patients with acquired strabismus, and 10 patients with acquired strabismus caused by OMG. A positive response to the edrophonium-Hess screen test was defined as a 50% or greater reduction in the strabismic deviation at the fixation point associated with maximum deviation within 1 minute of edrophonium infusion. All myasthenic patients had a 50% or greater reduction in the initial deviation within 1 minute of edrophonium infusion. Myasthenic patients had a statistically significant reduction in the average deviation up to 150 seconds after edrophonium infusion. In contrast, with or without edrophonium infusion, control subjects had a purely horizontal fluctuation in binocular alignment of less than or equal to 2° for the entire 4-minute period after edrophonium infusion. None of the 12 nonmyasthenic patients tested positive to the edrophonium-Hess screen test. These results suggest that clearly defined endpoint criteria make the edrophonium-Hess screen test a sensitive and specific quantitative study.[229]

Siatkowski et al[230] performed Tensilon tests on 30 normal subjects and 14 patients with nonmyasthenic strabismus. There were no clinically significant changes in muscle balance after Tensilon injection in any of the subjects, although the normal subjects had a slight *increase* in their near exophorias (mean, 2 prism diopters). The strabismic patients tended to have a slight change in their vertical deviation (mean change, 1.7 prism diopters; maximum change, <5 prism diopters) which was neither clinically nor statistically significant. The mean dose of edrophonium required for systemic response was 7.1 mg.

Just as the Tensilon test may on occasion be positive when the Prostigmin test is negative, the Prostigmin test may be positive when the Tensilon test is negative. Miller et al[231] suggested that neostigmine be used in patients whose signs are minimal, particularly in those with diplopia but no ptosis. Arguably, the longer duration of neostigmine's effect allows more time for quantitative measurements of ocular motility. Such patients are usually pretreated with intramuscular atropine (approximately 0.6 mg) before receiving intramuscular injection of neostigmine (approximately 1.5 mg). Ocular motility is reassessed 30 to 45 minutes thereafter.

It should be emphasized that *neurasthenia* may masquerade as myasthenia, especially where the chronically fatigued or tired patient shows no real eye muscle involvement, the so-called findings being limited to variable limb weakness. A placebo injection of, for example, physiologic saline that produces increased muscle strength and/or rapid alleviation of fatigue will quickly provide a useful diagnostic distinction. A small pediatric scalp-vein needle permits alternate connection of syringes first with saline and then with edrophonium.

Diagnostic procedures that complement Tensilon and Prostigmin testing, particularly in generalized myasthenia, include (1) electromyography (EMG) of muscle action potentials evoked by repetitive supramaximal nerve stimulation (approximately 3 to 5 Hz), and for the presence of the jitter phenomenon on single muscle fiber studies; and (2) antiacetylcholine receptor antibody titer (see above). In OMG, testing of the orbicularis muscles may be helpful. The relative importance of several methods—stimulated single fiber EMG (stimulated SFEMG), repetitive nerve stimulation test (RNS) of orbicularis oculi muscle, and infrared reflection oculography (IROG)—was investigated.[232] Based on the results of the three neurophysiologic tests, the patients can be divided into three groups:

Group 1: Those with an abnormal stimulated SFEMG, abnormal RNS, and/or abnormal IROG
Group 2: Those with only a slightly abnormal stimulated SFEMG
Group 3: Those with normal results in all three tests

The clinical diagnosis of OMG was made in all 11 patients in the first group; in 6 of 7 patients (86%) in the second group; and in 1 of 14 patients (7%) in the third group. This study emphasizes that the orbicularis oculi muscle is a suitable muscle for stimulated SFEMG in patients with suspected OMG. A seemingly simple "sleep test" was proposed,[233] based on the phenomenon of myasthenic symptoms and signs improving after rest: patients are kept in a quiet room in a restful state for 30 minutes, and levator and extraocular muscle function is assessed before and after rest. In this series, the sleep test was positive in cases of known OMG.

A diagnosis or firm suspicion of myasthenia on the part of the ophthalmologist is an indication for thorough examination by a neurologist. Thin-section, contrast-enhanced CT scan or MRI of the mediastinum should be performed to search for occult thymoma, but in a significant number of patients with only hyperplastic or normal thymus glands,[234] CT scan may suggest thymoma. Ideally, tests to determine thyroid function and the presence of collagen vascular disease should be performed.

The pharmacologic treatment of myasthenia, ocular or otherwise, is beyond the purlieu of even the interested ophthalmologist and is strictly the domain of an experienced neurologist, who would be more familiar with the response of myasthenics to medications, with the minor and major complications of the primary disorder, and with the difficulties of dose variations and medication schedules. The ophthalmologist should collaborate by reevaluating ocular motility and using press-on prisms and lid crutches when indicated. Large, variable, or incomitant deviations are best treated with an opaque lens. Ptosis surgery is dangerous because defective ocular motility can lead to problems of corneal exposure.

Therapy for myasthenia at present is somewhat individualized,[235] but is based on one of the following options: (1) increasing the amount of acetylcholine available with cholinesterase inhibitors such as pyridostigmine (Mestinon); or (2) blunting the autoimmune response with corticosteroids, especially for the often-resistant ocular symptoms, or less frequently with immunosuppressive agents (*e.g.*, azathioprine, cyclosporine), plasmapheresis, and/or thymectomy. Gamma-globulin therapy and plasmapheresis are rarely, if ever, indicated for purely ocular myasthenia. Other pharmacologic agents include ambenonium, a biquaternary compound that binds irreversibly to acetylcholinesterase, with a duration of approximately 8 hours.

Thymectomy is rarely used in OMG but often used in GMG. Remission postoperatively is well documented, although the benefit of surgery may be delayed from 1 to 3 years. For OMG, we have found that a combination of pyridostigmine bromide and oral corticosteroid provides salutary results, but some authors have reported improvement with the use of steroids alone.[236]

Myasthenia-Like Syndromes

The Eaton-Lambert syndrome is a paraneoplastic disorder of the neuromuscular junction that produces proximal limb weakness and fatigability resembling myasthenia in some aspects. In contrast to true myasthenia, ocular, facial, and oropharyngeal musculature is preferentially spared, a temporary increase in muscle power is seen after brief exercise, and deep tendon reflexes are diminished or absent.[237] EMG diagnosis entails demonstrating a characteristic *incremental response* to repetitive nerve stimulation, which is precisely the opposite of myasthenia. Although patients with this disorder are sensitive to small doses of curare, as in true myasthenia the weakness is due to a presynaptic mechanism that causes impaired release of acetylcholine[238] at both nicotinic and muscarinic nerve terminals. Specifically, antibodies to voltage-gated calcium channels in motor and autonomic nerve terminals disrupt calcium influx and reduce acetylcholine release. Approximately 70% of patients with Eaton-Lambert syndrome harbor malignant neoplasms, usually small-cell bronchogenic carcinoma; other instances are associated with autoimmune disorders, such as Sjögren's syndrome or discoid lupus,[239] but in some cases no other primary disease can be discovered.

Ocular involvement is distinctly rare and, if present (particularly if there is *isolated* ocular involvement), practically excludes the diagnosis of Eaton-Lambert syndrome. Patients have been reported with ptosis and/or ocular motility disorders,[240] as well as with documented abnormal eye movement recordings.[241] Breen et al[242] reported transient improvement of ptosis after sustained upgaze as a clinically useful sign in distinguishing Eaton-Lambert syndrome from myasthenia gravis. Grisold et al[243] provided a general review of paraneoplastic neurologic syndromes in which detection of autoantibodies directed against central and peripheral nervous system structures has suggested an autoimmune etiology. The therapeutic results of 258 patients with paraneoplastic neurologic disease (*e.g.*, paraneoplastic encephalomyelitis, sensory neuronopathy, cerebellar degeneration, motor neuron disease, stiff-man syndrome) were summarized. The results showed that in some entities, such as Lambert-Eaton syndrome, successful treatment can be expected. In other syndromes, such as subacute sensory neuronopathy or paraneoplastic cerebellar degeneration, therapeutic success varies from 5% to 10%.

Some pharmacologic agents may induce a clinical picture closely mimicking myasthenia. For example, D-penicillamine, given for rheumatoid arthritis, can produce isolated ocular signs and symptoms or generalized muscle involvement, and affected patients have elevated antiacetylcholine receptor antibodies, along with the same HLA antigens seen in true myasthenia.[244] A number of antibiotics, including the polypeptides (Colistin, polymyxin B) and aminoglycosides (neomycin, streptomycin, kanamycin, azithromycin) can also induce weakness resembling myasthenia gravis.[245] Diplopia, accommodative insufficiency, and bulbar muscle weakness may be encountered. The antineoplastic agents vincristine and vinblastine have special neurotoxic propensity, including ocular signs such as ptosis, external ophthalmoplegia, isolated muscle paresis, facial palsy, and lagophthalmos.[246]

Numerous other pharmacologic agents can decrease transmission at the neuromuscular junction,[247] such as neuromuscular blockers, anticholinesterase agents, antiarrhythmics (procainamide and quinidine), anticonvulsants (phenytoin), β-blockers (propranolol, timolol), corticosteroids, cisplatin, lithium, and magnesium. Obviously, great care must be taken when patients with myasthenia or other disorders of neuromuscular transmission are exposed to or treated with these agents. Corticosteroids, for example, are commonly used to treat myasthenia and may exacerbate muscle weakness, in some instances to the point where respiratory support is necessary.

Toxins elaborated by scorpions, ticks, wasps, spiders, and bacteria (*Clostridium botulinum, Clostridium tetani*) also affect the neuromuscular junction. Botulinum toxin acts presynaptically to prevent release of acetylcholine and also destroys nerve endings, which require several months for regeneration. Ophthalmologic findings in botulism include ptosis, ophthalmoparesis, and dilated, poorly reactive pupils.[248,249] Of course, botulinum toxin is commonly used therapeutically to produce isolated transient paresis of the extraocular muscles and of the facial and neck muscles in treating strabismus, blepharospasm, hemifacial spasm (including Meige's syndrome) and torticollis.

Thyroid-Related Myopathy (Graves' Disease)

Restricted eye movement caused by pathologic changes in extraocular muscles commonly, but not exclusively, associated with dysthyroidism is an extraordinarily frequent cause of diplopia. Encountered in all age groups (but rarely occurring in those less than 20 years old), thyroid-related restrictive myopathy (TRM) is *the most common cause of spontaneous double vision in middle age and early senescence*. Like myasthenia, TRM ranks high on the list of frequently missed diagnoses; patients are constantly subjected to inappropriate, invasive, and expensive radiodiagnostic studies. The ophthalmologist and neurologist should learn well the subtle ocular signs that usually accompany TRM and should know how to perform the single most important office maneuver, the forced duction test, to establish the presence of mechanical resistance (see Fig. 3–6). Comments here are limited to those aspects of TRM pertinent to neuro-ophthalmology: that is, those findings that permit a clinical diagnosis and obviate further uncomfortable and costly studies.

In subtle cases of TRM, the striking clinical signs of congestive proptosis are absent, but spontaneous lid retraction (stare) or lag on downward gaze is observable (see Fig. 3–11; Fig. 14–4). These lid signs may be elicited by having the patient perform pursuit eye movements while fixating some object moved vertically at a moderately fast speed. As the eyes turn downward, one or both lids are noted to lag (or "hang up"). A peculiar "jelly roll" edema is often evident in the upper or lower lids, but at times is difficult to distinguish from the redundancy of lid tissue that accompanies aging.

Careful inspection of the globe itself may reveal the conjunctival vessels overlying the anterior aspect of the horizontal recti muscles to be dilated and tortuous. The hypertrophied extraocular muscles themselves are occasionally visible (Fig. 12–27).

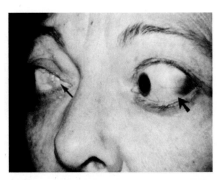

Fig. 12–27. Graves' disease. Note chemotic caruncle (*small arrow*) in right eye and clearly visible insertion of hypertrophied left lateral rectus (*large arrow*). The overlying conjunctival vessels are engorged.

The single most common ocular motility abnormality encountered in TRM is unilateral "elevator palsy" (Fig. 12–28), or a hypodeviation that increases on upward gaze. While mimicking a superior rectus palsy, the actual problem is fibrotic shortening of the inferior rectus, which restricts upward rotations. That the globe is tethered by a taut muscle is established by the palpable resistance to mechanical elevation (*i.e.*, a positive forced duction test). If both inferior recti are involved, the patient shows an upward gaze palsy somewhat mimicking midbrain syndromes (Fig. 12–29). Similar fibrotic

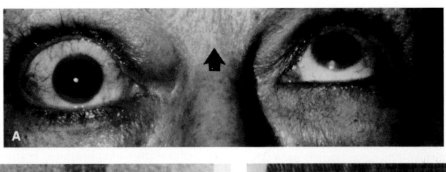
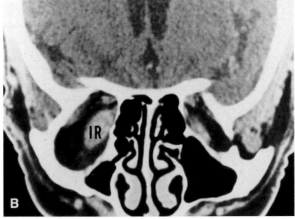
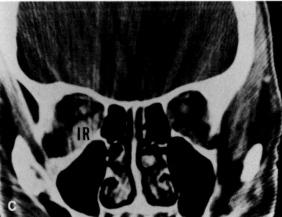

Fig. 12–28. Graves' disease. Typical uniocular elevator palsy (**A**) due to enlarged inferior rectus (see also Fig. 12–30). Off-axial (**B**) and coronal (**C**) CT sections show selective enlargement of right inferior rectus muscle (*IR*).

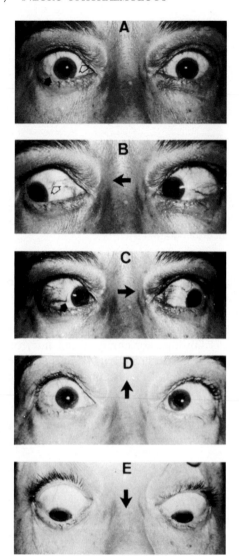

Fig. 12-29. Graves' disease. Marked lid retraction (**A**) is evident. Small solid arrow marks vessel loop that indicates intorsion when right eye adducts (**C**). Small open arrow marks vessel loop that indicates extorsion when right eye abducts (**B**). Note that abducting eye (**B** and **C**) depresses in lateral gaze (? tight inferior rectus). Attempted upward gaze (**D**) results in minimal convergence and increased lid retraction. Full downgaze (**E**) is achieved. A misdiagnosis of pinealoma had been made.

contraction of the medial rectus produces an abduction deficit that mimics a sixth nerve palsy, but the globe resists outward rotation when the insertion of the medical rectus is grasped. Downward gaze is limited when restrictive fibrosis of the superior rectus occurs. Isolated lateral rectus involvement, with abduction deficits, is uncommon, but all gaze functions may be reduced. In addition to the myopathy itself, impaired orbital venous outflow may play a role in the exophthalmos and strabismus of this disorder.[250]

Commonly, torsional movements of the globe are observed on attempted horizontal or vertical versions (see Fig. 12-29A and B). For example, on attempted right

gaze, the right eye abducts incompletely and extorts slightly as it reaches the position of maximum abduction. This excyclotorsion is seen especially in the company of elevation deficits (tight inferior rectus).

In the early stages of the disease, an affected muscle may in rare cases appear paretic rather than restricted. Hermann[251] reported on two patients with diplopia with negative forced ductions, but with saccadic velocities consistent with inferior rectus paresis. We also have observed a patient with obvious Graves disease who presented with an inferior rectus paresis, including a positive three-step test and negative forced ductions; echography revealed a greatly enlarged inferior rectus muscle. Several months later the hypertropia converted to a hypotropia, as a typical restrictive pattern evolved. Such paresis is distinctly unusual, and may represent thyroid "myositis" as a precursor to muscle fibrosis. However, mechanical restriction by the involved muscle with positive forced duction testing is the rule.

An additional clue to the restrictive nature of TRM is the finding of elevation of intraocular pressure on attempted upward gaze.[252] This phenomenon, attributed to a fibrotic and taut inferior rectus muscle, may aid in establishing the cause of otherwise puzzling spontaneously acquired diplopia.

The diagnosis of TRM is not so difficult a task on clinical grounds, if the physician bears in mind the characteristic lid and orbital congestive signs, the typical patterns of motility disturbance, and the use of the forced duction test. Increase in extraocular muscle bulk, the hallmark of Graves orbitopathy, may be assessed by standardized A-scan ultrasonography,[253] CT scanning, or MRI (Fig. 12-30). Usually multiple muscles in both orbits are enlarged, but asymmetry may be striking. To affirm the diagnosis in terms of biochemical tests of thyroid function is another problem altogether. Ocular manifestations may antedate laboratory or clinical evidence of dysthyroidism, but many patients present with ophthalmologic complications occurring months to years after surgery or radioactive iodine therapy for hyperthyroid states. At the time of ocular diagnosis, many of these patients are euthyroid by all parameters of multiple laboratory tests of thyroid function. However, hypothyroidism with elevated thyrotropin (thyroid-stimulating hormone, TSH) levels after radioactive iodine treatment appears to be an important adverse risk factor for development or exacerbation of ophthalmopathy.[254] In addition to a history and physical examination, laboratory procedures to determine triiodothyronine (T_3), thyroxine (T_4), TSH, and T_3 resin uptake have assumed a fundamental role. T_4 and T_3 are the major circulating hormones produced by the thyroid. By increasing the sensitivity of analysis, radioimmunoassay (RIA) techniques have dramatically simplified thyroid hormone assessment. Furthermore, T_3 (RIA) and T_4 (RIA) levels are not influenced by inorganic iodine contamination from outside sources. Hence, the administra-

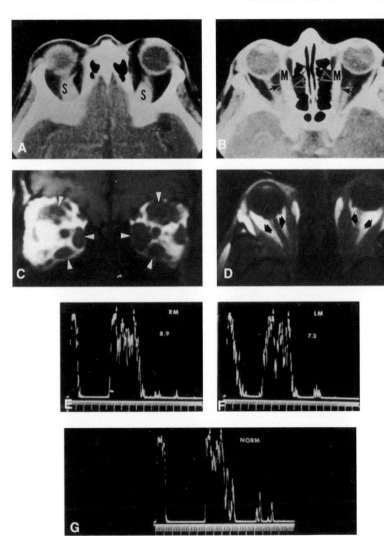

Fig. 12-30. Graves' ophthalmopathy. **A.** CT axial section through superior aspect of orbits shows symmetrically enlarged superior rectus muscles (*S*). **B.** Midorbital plane shows enlarged medial rectus muscles (*M*, and *arrows*). **C.** Coronal MRI shows hypertrophied ocular muscles (*arrowheads*) in both orbits. **D.** Axial section of MRI reveals enlarged medial and horizontal recti (*arrows*). **E.** Orbital ultrasonography (A-scan) provides sensitive measurement of muscle belly diameters. Enlarged right medial rectus shows interspike interval (*small arrows*) corresponding to 8.9 mm. **F.** Left medial rectus, 7.3 mm. **G.** Normal muscle diameter, 4.5 mm.

tion of iodinated radiologic contrast dye does not confound the evaluation of thyroid function when RIA methods are employed. Both the T_4 (RIA) and the previously widely used T_4 measurement by the Murphy-Pattee competitive protein-binding assay require simultaneous T_3 resin uptake determination. The T_3 resin uptake analyzes the unbound thyroxine-binding globulin. Numerous conditions (*e.g.*, pregnancy, hepatitis, recent surgery, renal failure) and pharmacologic agents (*e.g.*, estrogens, corticosteroids, phenytoin) may alter thyroxine-binding globulin affinity; therefore a computed value, the free T_4 index, is often used to estimate the amount of free thyroid hormone available to the tissues. The free T_4 index is calculated from the serum T_4 concentration and the T_3 resin uptake.

Although T_3 thyrotoxicosis is well recognized by internists and endocrinologists as a distinct clinical entity, ophthalmologists must be aware that T_4 determination alone does not completely evaluate peripheral blood thyroid hormone status. In addition, T_3 is often elevated out of proportion to T_4 in Graves' disease. Long-acting thyroid stimulation determinations, although still avail-

able, have no currently recognized value in diagnosis or patient care.

Since approximately two thirds of patients with euthyroid Graves' disease demonstrate an autonomously functioning pituitary-thyroid axis, this homeostatic system must be evaluated. An autonomous pituitary-thyroid axis indicates that the thyroid gland has escaped the normal feedback, regulatory control of circulating TSH; it is thus known as the *autonomous* thyroid gland. For many years, the Werner suppression test was employed to assess any "escape" of the thyroid from normal TSH control. This test involved the administration of oral T_3 (Cytomel) for 7 days with prior and follow-up determination of radioactive iodine uptake detected over the thyroid gland. With disruption of the pituitary-thyroid balance, the administration of oral T_3 fails to suppress radioactive iodine uptake below 50% of the initial level, thereby indicating autonomous thyroid activity (provided that the initial uptake is at least 15%).

The intravenous thyrotropin-releasing hormone (TRH) test has now virtually supplanted the more cumbersome, time-consuming, and costly Werner suppression test. TRH is the hypothalamic regulatory factor controlling the release of TSH from the anterior pituitary gland. Normally, intravenous administration of TRH causes a four- to five-fold peak rise in blood TSH level within 20 to 30 minutes after injection. The TSH response to TRH is fairly constant, except in patients with Cushing's syndrome from either endogenous or exogenous excess corticosteroids. In addition, patients with an autonomous pituitary-thyroid axis will fail to show the expected increase in TSH response. A blunted or absent pituitary TSH response to TRH injection signifies a positive test, as found in approximately 50% of patients with Graves ophthalmopathy considered "euthyroid" by conventional testing.[255] A normal TRH test is therefore seen in the remaining 50% of these patients and designates them truly euthyroid by currently available laboratory criteria.

Autoimmune abnormalities, such as thyroid-stimulating antibodies and thyroid-displacing activity, may be used in conjunction with the TRH test to detect occult thyroid disease. The collaboration of a competent endocrinologist is of obvious advantage. In addition, elevated serum IgE[256] and anti–eye-muscle antibodies[257] have been reported in patients with thyroid-related myopathy.

For the internist, a medical approach to therapy should be tempered by knowledge that thyroid-related orbitopathy is more or less a self-limited disease, and that emphasis should be placed on the prevention of serious ocular complications. It seems reasonable that rendering hyperthyroid patients euthyroid, and preventing them from becoming hypothyroid, is advantageous. If the euthyroid state is preferable, then no specific medical manipulation of euthyroid ophthalmopathic patients is indicated.[255]

Treatment of optic neuropathy in Graves' disease is considered in Chapter 5. The strabismus in acute and subacute orbitopathy has been demonstrated to improve with both corticosteroid and radiation therapy,[258–260] but definitive surgical treatment should be postponed until deviations have been stable for a minimum of 6 months. Because of the incomitance of the strabismus, prisms are often inadequate to control patients' symptoms, necessitating extraocular muscle surgery. As a general rule, muscle resections should not be employed in this disease, because such procedures do not address the underlying mechanism of the restrictive strabismus and may, in fact, worsen it. Long-term results of rectus muscle recessions employing the adjustable suture technique are quite favorable,[261] and adjustable suspensions of the lower eyelid retractors may be employed concurrently to minimize lower eyelid retraction after inferior rectus surgery.[262] The surgeon should attempt initially to undercorrect the deviation, since late overcorrections are common in Graves' ophthalmopa-

thy.[263] Botulinum toxin has a limited role, if any, in Graves' ophthalmopathy, but may be used in those rare patients with extraocular muscle paresis in order to minimize or delay contracture of the antagonist muscle.

Progressive (Chronic) External Ophthalmoplegia

There is considerable controversy regarding the precise nosologic classification of the "muscular dystrophies," including the chronic external ophthalmoplegias (i.e., those not involving the internal ocular muscles of the pupil). Although they were once traditionally considered primary myopathies, later contributions have challenged this etiologic concept and have argued strongly in favor of another: primary neurogenic disorders or abnormal proliferation of mitochondria are believed to cause "ragged-red fibers" (so called because of their dark red color on modified Gomori trichrome stain), which are a hallmark of the severe biochemical defects in oxidative phosphorylation characteristic of many mitochondrial encephalomyopathies.[264] Recent literature has focused on the importance of diffuse, systemic mitochondrial abnormalities (Table 12–10). In patients with progressive external ophthalmoplegia (PEO) or CPEO, light microscopic examination of extraocular muscle, orbicularis oculi, and at times other

TABLE 12–10. Manifestations of the Kearns-Sayre-Daroff Syndrome ("Ophthalmoplegia Plus")

Cardinal manifestations
External ophthalmoplegia with onset in childhood
Retinal pigmentary degeneration
Cardiac conduction defects
Elevated cerebrospinal fluid protein
Abnormal muscle mitochondria
Spongiform encephalopathy, including brain stem
Negative family history

Associated manifestations
Short stature
Neurologic
  Deafness
  Cerebellar ataxia
  Mild corticospinal tract signs
  "Descending" myopathy of face and limbs
  Subnormal intelligence
  Slowed electroencephalogram
  Aseptic meningitis (by history)
  Demyelinating radiculopathy
  Decreased ventilatory drive
  Hyperglycemic acidotic coma/death
Endocrine
  Diabetes mellitus
  Hypogonadism
  Hypoparathyroidism
  Growth hormone deficiency
  Adrenal dysfunction
Skeletal and dental anomalies
Corneal edema

skeletal muscle reveals ragged-red muscle fibers admixed within a population of relatively normal muscle fibers. On electron microscopic examination, these same ragged-red fibers demonstrate strikingly abnormal mitochondria. Ragged-red fibers may be found in other diseases, and small numbers are indeed seen in the orbicularis and extraocular muscles of normal persons, but not in their limb muscles. Also, mitochondria are morphologically abnormal in skeletal muscle biopsies from PEO patients with or without ragged-red fibers.[265] In the Kearns-Sayre variant, such abnormal mitochondria have also been observed in liver cells, sweat glands, and granular and Purkinje cells of the cerebellum.[266] All recent studies have suggested that mitochondrial dysfunction plays an essential role in producing the multisystem involvement in many PEO patients. Mitochondrial dysfunction is associated with a variety of genetic defects due to nucleotide mutations.[264,267,268] Muscle mitochondrial DNA (mtDNA) deletions may be detected, localized, and quantitated by Southern blot analysis of transfer RNA (tRNA) genes in the mtDNA (+RNA leucine, glutamine, isoleucine, and formylmethionine).[269] Such techniques confirm the high frequency of mtDNA deletions or point mutations in PEO. At the onset of the disease, no clinical, morphologic, or molecular features can predict whether PEO will remain isolated or become part of a more severe multisystem disease. However, patients with mtDNA deletions are characterized by more severe ophthalmoplegia of earlier onset. Muscle alterations are roughly parallel in severity to the proportion of deleted mtDNA molecules in muscle. There are sporadic cases of patients with multitissue disease and mtDNA deletions; their clinical presentation usually closely resembles Kearns-Sayre syndrome.

Clinically, PEO is characterized by insidiously progressive, symmetric immobility of the eyes, which are fixed to oculocephalic or caloric stimulation. There is no pain and the pupils are spared, but the lids typically are ptotic and the orbicularis oculi weak (Figs. 12–31 and 12–32). Unlike Graves' ophthalmopathy, there is no lid retraction, proptosis, or congestive conjunctival signs. In longstanding PEO, however, fibrotic changes in extraocular muscles may produce mechanical resistance and a positive forced duction test. Chronic or "fixed" ocular myasthenia may be confused with PEO, because both disorders tend to demonstrate the following: symmetric total or subtotal external ophthalmoplegia; ptosis; normal pupils; orbicularis oculi, facial, and bulbar weakness; and resistance to Tensilon or other cholinergic agents. A slowly progressive symmetric ophthalmoplegia, without fluctuations or remissions, speaks strongly in favor of PEO (see below, hereditary form). Otherwise, electrophysiologic testing and muscle biopsy may be required to distinguish between chronic myasthenia and PEO.

Although not always an easy task, it is usually possible clinically to distinguish ophthalmoplegia due to CNS lesions from the PEO syndromes. Patients with PEO, however, do not demonstrate an increase in ocular motility when the doll's head maneuver is employed. On the other hand, cerebral gaze palsies are acute, usually asymmetric, and show retention of reflex eye movements, including oculocephalic deviations. Pontine gaze palsies are usually asymmetric and accompanied by other neurologic deficits, such as hemiparesis, hyperreflexia, and other ipsilateral cranial nerve palsies. Supranuclear gaze palsies that otherwise may simulate PEO (e.g., progressive supranuclear bulbar palsy, parkinsonism) are discussed in the next section.

Depending on the associated signs and symptoms, PEO may be classified into several subgroups (see Table

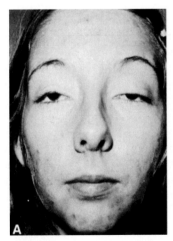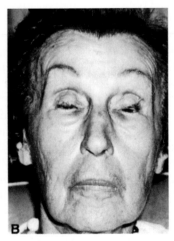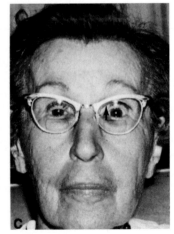

Fig. 12–31. Progressive external ophthalmoplegia. **A.** Marked ptosis and facial wasting in 18-year-old woman (see motility and fundus in the same patient, Fig. 12–32). **B.** Adult-onset familial oculopharyngeal dystrophy. Note marked temporalis wasting. **C.** Patient with lid crutches attached to glass frames (*arrow*). The bifocal segments are useless.

12–9). Accompanying the Kearns-Sayre form of PEO, a mild to moderate "salt and pepper" disturbance of peripheral retinal pigment epithelium has been described (see Fig. 12–32B), especially in adolescents.[270] Unlike retinitis pigmentosa, as a rule there is neither optic atrophy, arteriolar attenuation, nor visual disturbance to any real degree. Visual fields are grossly full, and electroretinography may be surprisingly normal. The major manifestations of Kearns-Sayre syndrome are as follows: childhood onset of PEO without family history; retinal pigmentary degeneration; cardiac conduction defects, often leading to complete heart block and Stokes-Adams attacks; ragged-red muscle fibers on skeletal muscle biopsy; elevated cerebrospinal fluid protein; and marked vacuolization (status spongiosus) of the cerebrum and brain stem.

A number of other findings are frequently, but not invariably, associated with this syndrome. Whether or not the Kearns-Sayre symptom complex represents an atypical ("slow") viral, toxic, or multisystem genetic mitochondrial disturbance is currently unknown. Rowland[271] reviewed a number of reports of familial occurrence and found that "among the 70 cases, there has been only one family in which more than one person had the entire syndrome." Administration of coenzyme Q-10, a component of the mitochondrial electron transport system, has been observed to normalize serum pyruvate and lactate levels and improve both atrioventricular block and ocular movements in a patient with Kearns-Sayre syndrome.[272]

Oculopharyngeal dystrophy of Victor is a rather benign hereditary condition, usually autosomal dominant, which has an onset in the fifth and sixth decades and involves the bulbar musculature. Temporalis wasting may be striking (see Fig. 12–31). Pathologically, ragged-red fibers with abnormal mitochondria are not described in this condition. Rather, there is marked reduction in the number of muscle fibers, and those fibers that remain show significant degenerative changes and characteristic nuclear inclusions.[273] A large number of French Canadians are affected with this variety of PEO, which is traceable to a common ancestor from a Quebec isolate. Other variations, which may occur either sporadically or in an heredofamilial form, include involvement of muscles of the neck and upper extremities. Autopsy of one such case showed no pathologic changes in either the peripheral or the central nervous system.[274] Some patients have ptosis and pharyngeal symptoms with relative sparing of ocular motility, and we have seen one case of profound ophthalmoplegia and pharyngeal involvement, but without ptosis.

Ionescu et al[275] described the association between inherited ophthalmoplegia and intestinal pseudo-obstruction due to decreased motility of the stomach and small bowel. Ptosis and ophthalmoplegia begin in childhood, and gastrointestinal symptoms appear in adolescence;

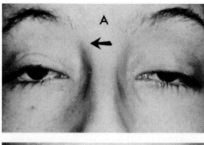
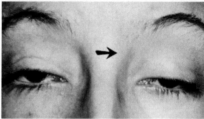
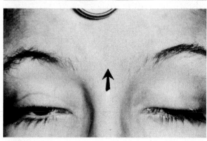
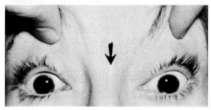

Fig. 12–32. A. Progressive external ophthalmoplegia. Almost complete absence of eye movements in all fields of gaze.

there is progressively worsening malnutrition, and death occurs before age 30 regardless of medical treatment. Abnormal synthesis of contractile proteins in muscle cells was demonstrated in the one case studied.

Mitochondrial myopathy, encephalopathy with lactic acidosis, and strokelike episodes (MELAS) syndrome is one of the mitochondrial encephalomyopathies that has distinct clinical features, including strokelike episodes with migrainous headache, nausea, vomiting, encephalopathy, and lactic acidosis.[276] For example: A 27-year-old woman presented with a history of partial seizure, strokelike episodes including hemiparesis, hemianopia and hemihypesthesia, sensorineural hearing loss, migrainelike headache, and lactic acidosis. A brain CT scan showed encephalomalacia in the right parieto-occipital area and hypodensity in the left temporoparieto-occipital area with cortical atrophy. Muscle biopsy revealed ragged-red fibers and paracrystalline inclusions in the mitochondria. Genetic study revealed an A to

B

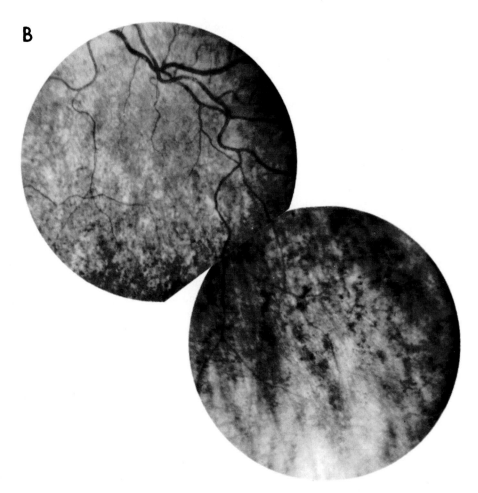

Fig. 12–32. (*continued*) **B.** Peripheral fundus of patient shows mottled degeneration of retinal pigment epithelium with minimal pigment clumping.

G point mutation at nucleotide position (np) 3243 of mtDNA. External ophthalmoplegia and ptosis were also found during two exaggerated episodes in this patient. Therefore, the overlapping syndrome of CPEO in the MELAS syndrome was considered. This patient was also found to have a carnitine deficiency, and she responded to steroid therapy. Muscle biopsy revealed excessive lipid-droplet deposits. It was concluded that a carnitine deficiency may occur in MELAS syndrome with the A to G point mutation at np 3243, and it was recommended that patients with MELAS syndrome and carnitine deficiency be started on steroid or carnitine supplement therapy.[276]

Hereditary abetalipoproteinemia (Bassen-Kornzweig syndrome) refers to the association of PEO, pigmentary retinopathy, ataxia, and intestinal fat malabsorption. The laboratory assessment of patients with potential mitochondrial disease is extensive, as outlined by Johns[264] (Table 12–11).

Regarding therapy, there is no pharmacologic relief for the weak muscles, including systemic or locally injected corticosteroids; in fact, in Kearns-Sayre syndrome systemic corticosteroids may precipitate hyperglycemic

TABLE 12–11 Possible Laboratory Findings in Patients with Mitochondrial Diseases

Ragged-red fibers in skeletal muscle–biopsy specimens
Elevated lactate concentrations in serum and cerebrospinal fluid
Myopathic potentials on electromyography
Axonal and demyelinating peripheral neuropathy on nerve-conduction studies
Sensorineural hearing loss on audiography
Cardiac conduction defects
Basal-ganglia calcification or focal signal abnormalities on magnetic resonance imaging
Abnormalities on phosphorus-31 nuclear-magnetic-resonance spectroscopy
Defective oxidative phosphorylation on biochemical studies
Molecular genetic evidence of mitochondrial-DNA mutation

(Johns DR: Mitochondrial DNA and disease. N Engl J Med 333:638, 1995)

acidotic coma and death.[277] If exotropia or diplopia develop, standard extraocular muscle surgery may be performed. However, these patients rarely complain of diplopia, perhaps in part because of slow onset of the disease, symmetry of the ophthalmoplegia, and comitancy of the strabismus. Surgical repair of ptotic lids should be approached with caution because, in the presence of poor ocular motility (specifically minimal upward movement), patients may experience severe complications of corneal exposure after lid-lifting procedures. Lid crutches are an excellent alternative (see Fig. 12–31C). In patients with an early onset, cardiac evaluation is mandatory to rule out complete heart block. A cardiac pacemaker is often indicated and may be lifesaving, although sudden neurologic deterioration and death can occur in Kearns-Sayre patients despite a functioning cardiac pacemaker.[278]

CONDITIONS SIMULATING PROGRESSIVE EXTERNAL OPHTHALMOPLEGIA

There are a number of other disorders that may simulate PEO because of deficits in conjugate eye movements.

Progressive supranuclear palsy is a slowly progressive degenerative disease of the CNS affecting persons in the fifth to seventh decades; it is characterized by supranuclear ophthalmoplegia involving primarily vertical gaze, at least in the early stages. Downward gaze is most affected, and victims complain of difficulty with the following: seeing food or table utensils, walking downstairs, using bifocals, reading, and other visual tasks dependent on vertical eye movements. Manifestations also include postural instability with frequent falls, bradykinesia, dystonic rigidity of neck and trunk, masked face, dysesthesia, hyperreflexia, and insidious dementia.[279] Blepharospasm[280] and apraxia of lid opening[281] may also be seen.

The ophthalmoplegia in progressive supranuclear palsy first affects volitional vertical gaze, especially downward. That the lesion is at first supranuclear can be demonstrated by full vertical deviations with oculocephalic (doll's head) maneuvers (Fig. 12–33). Pursuit movements may be preserved, such that optokinetic testing "draws" the eyes tonically in the direction of stimulus movement. Eventually, horizontal gaze is involved, with both saccadic and pursuit palsies. Although oculocephalic deviations may be demonstrable even late

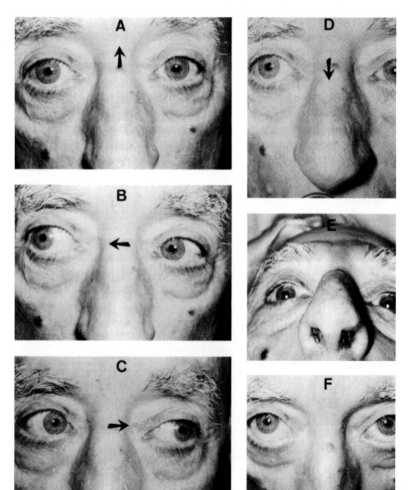

Fig. 12–33. Progressive supranuclear palsy. **A.** Volitional up-gaze absent. **B** and **C.** Horizontal gaze relatively spared. **D.** Volitional down-gaze absent. Oculocephalic (doll's head) maneuvers roll eyes downward (head back) (**E**) and upward (chin down) (**F**).

in the disease, marked neck dystonia makes doll's head maneuvers difficult to assess. Cold calorics show slow tonic deviation. Finally, all eye movements, including reflex movements, may be lost.

Therapy in these patients is generally directed at education and instruction regarding appropriate head movements; however, the use of idazoxan has proved useful in some patients.[282] Interestingly, although progressive supranuclear palsy is considered a supranuclear disorder, mitochondrial adenosine triphosphate production in the extraocular muscles has also been shown to be defective in these patients.[283]

Progressive supranuclear palsy is distinguished from Parkinson's disease by the pattern of ophthalmoplegia, lack of tremor, presence of pyramidal tract signs, dementia, and death, which usually ensues within 10 years. MRI is also helpful in distinguishing these two entities. In progressive supranuclear palsy, definitive atrophy of the midbrain and the region around the third ventricle is seen in more than 50% of cases. In Parkinson's disease, alterations in the pars compacta of the substantial nigra may be encountered.[284] Levodopa does not alter eye movement but may alleviate rigidity.[280] Since ocular symptomatology is marked, the ophthalmologist should be aware that defective vertical gaze movement may explain these patients' difficulty seeing objects in the inferior visual field. Bifocals are unsuitable, but single-vision reading glasses are indicated.

Patients with Parkinson's disease demonstrate a relative deficiency in spontaneous eye movements, which in association with infrequent blinking, produce a rather typical parkinsonian stare. As with progressive supranuclear palsy patients, blepharospasm and apraxia of lid opening may be seen. Upward gaze is more commonly initially involved and, along with convergence, may be weak or absent, even more so than those deficits associated with aging alone. Rapid volitional eye movements are fragmented into multiple saccades, and slow pursuit is accomplished similarly by a series of small amplitude saccades ("cogwheel" eye movements). Ophthalmoplegia in Parkinson's disease may well mimic progressive supranuclear palsy.[285]

Knox et al[286] reviewed Whipple's disease, a rare cause of supranuclear ophthalmoplegia, dementia, and facial myoclonia, but not necessarily gastrointestinal symptoms of diarrhea. Pathological confirmation is provided by jejunal biopsy for periodic acid-Schiff–positive, foam-filled macrophages containing microorganisms.

A number of spontaneous and heredodegenerative CNS disorders characterized chiefly by *ataxia* tend to produce uncompensated small-angle heterotropias, with momentary diplopia, or frank ophthalmoplegia. These disorders include Friedreich's ataxia, cerebellar and spinocerebellar degenerations, familial or sporadic olivopontocerebellar atrophies, multisystem atrophy, and spastic or myoclonic ataxias.[287]

MYOTONIC DYSTROPHY

Myotonic dystrophy is a rare but especially interesting cause of symmetric external ophthalmoplegia. Myotonic dystrophy is an adult form of muscular dystrophy affecting approximately 1 in 8000 people in most populations. Although common symptoms include progressive muscle weakness and stiffness, it is characterized by a heterogeneous clinical picture. Despite this variation in both the nature and severity of the symptoms seen in affected persons, myotonic dystrophy is genetically homogeneous, segregating as a single locus on the proximal long arm of human chromosome 19.[288] There is a molecular mutation event within the gene in which it lies: the expansion of a trinucleotide repeat (CTG) at the 3′ end of a gene encoding a member of the cyclic adenosine monophosphate-dependent protein kinase family. This has diagnostic implications because an easy, reliable, and predictive test can now be offered to persons with a family history of myotonic dystrophy. In addition, the striking similarity between findings at the DNA level in myotonic dystrophy and those in fragile X syndrome and spinal and bulbar muscular atrophy suggests that the mechanism leading to the increase in copy number of trinucleotide repeats at particular loci may be responsible for a number of other genetic diseases.

Lessell et al[289] reviewed myotonic ophthalmoplegia and presented reports on two men with ptosis; PEO; face, neck, and limb myopathy with atrophy; testicular atrophy; polychromatophilic cataracts (*i.e.* with multicolored, iridescent opacities); and baldness. They discussed the oculomotor signs of myotonic dystrophy and noted that ophthalmoplegia may be either minimal or profound. We have seen a patient demonstrating full range of eye movement, slowly performed, with myotonia of upward gaze and convergence: that is, when extreme upgaze or convergence was sustained, downward gaze and divergence were accomplished slowly (Fig. 12–34).

Burian and Burns[290] examined 25 myotonic patients and catalogued the ocular changes, including macular and peripheral retinal pigment epithelial dystrophy (Table 12–12). Thompson et al[291] documented sluggishly reacting, miotic pupils, which also dilated poorly with mydriatics, in myotonic patients. Some patients with myotonic dystrophy have neovascular tufts on the iris that leak on fluorescein angiography and may bleed spontaneously. Short, depigmented ciliary processes have been described and may contribute to the low intraocular pressure seen in these patients.[292] Pryse-Phillips et al[293] examined 133 members of an affected family and found a number of subjects with incomplete manifestations of the disease. Twenty-seven of the subjects lacked clinical or EMG evidence of myotonia; the most common signs in this group were upper facial weakness, brachial hyporeflexia, ocular hypotension, and lens changes.

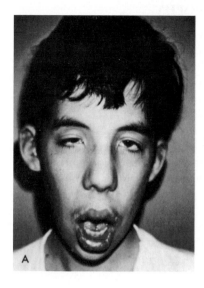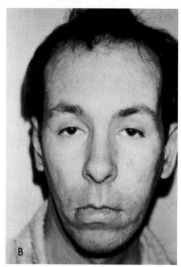

Fig. 12–34. Myotonic dystrophy, **A.** Narrow "hatchet" face, slack-jaw, and ptosis in young boy. **B.** Older male with frontal balding and ptosis. After sustained upward gaze this patient demonstrated inability to lower eyes for several seconds.

Electro-oculography of *horizontal saccades* and *smooth-pursuit eye movements* studied in 26 patients with myotonic dystrophy showed a significant decrease of the maximum velocity of the visually guided saccades in 83% of the patients.[294] Smooth-pursuit eye movements were not significantly different from age-matched controls. Visual evoked potential latencies (P100) were significantly prolonged compared with controls in 64% of the patients. The saccadic latency of the visually guided saccades was correlated with the prolonged visual evoked potential latencies, indicating that lesions in the primary visual pathways probably contribute to the oculomotor dysfunction. The isolated decrease of the maximum velocity of the saccades in combination with EMG findings favors a peripheral (dystrophic) pathophysiologic mechanism. Additionally, neuronal loss in the medullary reticular formation is also documented.[295]

TABLE 12–12. Ocular Signs of Myotonic Dystrophy

Lids: ptosis, myotonic lag, blepharitis
Extraocular movements: symmetric external ophthalmoplegia, pursuit decomposition (? cerebral), Bell's and convergence myotonia, intermittent horizontal tropias
Orbicularis: weakness, myotonic closure
Cornea: keratitis sicca (diminished tears, infrequent blink)
Orbit: enophthalmos
Pupils: miotic, sluggish to light and near
Intraocular pressure: hypotonia (average 10 mmHg)
Lens: subcapsular polychromasia, "snowballs," posterior cortex star figure, posterior subcapsular plaques
Retina: macular and peripheral pigmentary degeneration, diminished electroretinogram, elevated dark-adapt threshold
Fields: usually normal; generalized constriction

OCULAR NEUROMYOTONIA

Ocular neuromyotonia is an uncommon disorder characterized by episodic, sustained contractions of ocular muscles due to involuntary firing of ocular motor nerves. Schults et al[296] reported on six patients, four of whom showed involvement of muscles innervated by the oculomotor nerve, and one patient each with superior oblique or lateral rectus defects, implying abnormal spontaneous discharge in the third, fourth, and sixth cranial nerves. Four patients had received prior radiation therapy for invasive pituitary adenomas, suggesting that compression and irradiation of motor axons were the inciting events. Lessell et al[297] recorded four additional patients and provided a useful discussion on the question of radiation-induced cranial neuropathy. Other reports of radiation-induced neuromyotonia include one case of the lateral rectus after radiation therapy for a sinonasal carcinoma,[298] and another of episodic exotropia from lateral rectus neuromyotonia after radiation for a thalamic glioma in a 7-year-old boy.[299] Frohman and Zee[300] provided an inclusive review, and documented a case of unilateral oculomotor nerve myotonia in a 71-year-old man without a history of prior radiation therapy. Indeed, typical myotonia has been reported to be due to internal carotid artery aneurysm.[301] Membrane-stabilizing agents (*e.g.*, phenytoin, carbamazepine) may be useful in these cases.[300]

DORSAL MIDBRAIN SYNDROME

The dorsal midbrain (*e.g.*, Parinaud or sylvian aqueduct) syndrome is discussed briefly here to clarify clinical points that distinguish it from disorders of peripheral neuromuscular mechanisms, including Graves' restrictive myopathy, which may show a somewhat similar motility pattern. Unlike the forms of ophthalmoplegia considered in the preceding section, the internal neuromuscular mechanism of the eye is involved, with both hypertonicity and paresis of pupillary constriction and accommodation.

Upward gaze is typically affected, with preservation of downward movement (Fig. 12–35). The vertical palsy is supranuclear, and doll's head maneuver or Bell's phenomenon should elevate the eyes; however, eventually all upward gaze mechanisms fail. Skew deviation may be present, accounting for vertical diplopia. Attempts at upward saccades produce variable degrees of retraction-convergence nystagmus, in bursts or sustained. Retraction of the globe is especially evoked by downward rotation of optokinetic targets (saccadic phase upward). Accommodative spasms also occur on attempted upward gaze, and these episodes of momentary myopia may presage other signs and symptoms. Ultimately, accommodative paresis ensues, and pupils become mid-

dilated and show light-near dissociation[302] (see Fig. 12–35). There may be spasms or paralysis of convergence and "pseudoabducens palsy": that is, slower movement of the abducting eye than the adducting eye during horizontal saccades can also be observed.

Pinealomas are the most common lesion producing the "Parinaud-plus" syndrome (Fig. 12–36). Mass lesions involving the periaqueductal gray matter may arise in the posterior third ventricle, quadrigeminal plate (tectum), supracollicular subarachnoid space, or falco-tentorium. As the aqueduct becomes obstructed, internal hydrocephalus develops, and headache and papilledema appear. In addition to neoplasms, vascular occlusions, trauma, extra-axial and intra-axial arteriovenous malformations, demyelination, giant aneurysms of the posterior fossa, infections, trauma, stereotactic surgery for pain, and hydrocephalus from various causes have all been associated with the dorsal midbrain syndrome. Paralysis of upgaze can be an early sign of malfunctioning

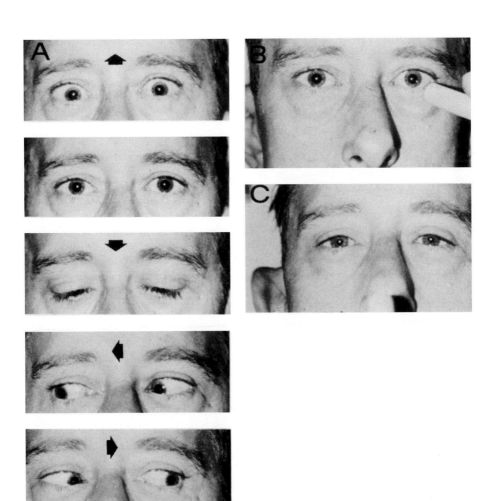

Fig. 12–35. Dorsal midbrain (Parinaud) syndrome. Upgaze palsy (**A**) with normal downgaze and horizontal movement. Pupils mid-dilated and fixed to light (**B**) but react to near-effort (**C**).

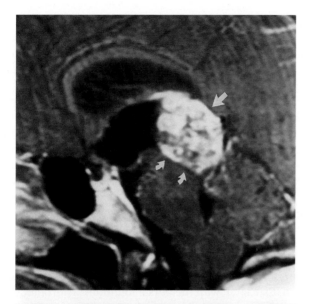

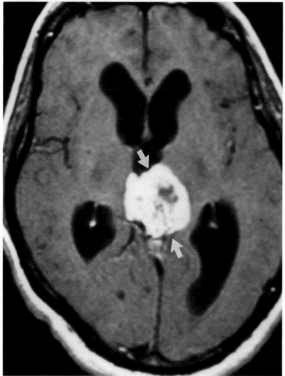

Fig. 12–36. Large, partially calcified pineal tumor (*arrows*) causing dorsal midbrain (Parinaud) syndrome. Gadolinium-enhanced T-1 weighted MRI. Saggital (**top**) and axial (**bottom**) sections. Note compression deformation (*small arrows*) of rostral midbrain, and obstructive dilation of ventricular system.

of a shunt placed to treat hydrocephalus, and it is reversible with repair or replacement of the shunt. Also, a reversible dorsal midbrain syndrome has been observed after jejunoileal bypass for obesity.[303] CNS toxoplasmosis in AIDS patients has now become an important cause of Parinaud syndrome as well.[304] A single case of Pari-

naud syndrome has been described in association with Leber's hereditary optic neuropathy.[305]

Vertical supranuclear ophthalmoplegia has been associated with metabolic disorders, including certain lipid storage diseases such as Niemann-Pick type C,[306,307] which may present in adults as dementia and ataxia.[308] The Niemann-Pick variant is characterized by sea-blue histiocytes in the bone marrow and visceromegaly. Ocular motor abnormalities include loss of voluntary vertical saccades, especially downward; loss of the fast phase of optokinetic nystagmus; defective convergence; and substitute "head-thrusting." Pathologically, lipid storage has been demonstrated in numerous ocular tissues, but ophthalmologic changes are observed only in later life, when the optic nerves appear pale and the perimacular areas show gray discoloration.[309] Final clinicopathologic correlation is lacking, but clinical features suggest diffuse involvement of cortical gray matter, basal ganglia, cerebellum, and upper midbrain, where corticobulbar ocular motor fibers may be preferentially involved in the subthalamic and pretectal regions.

Other forms of ophthalmoplegia are present in Wilson's disease,[310] kernicterus,[311] and barbiturate overdose.[312]

DIPLOPIA AFTER OCULAR SURGERY

Strabismus following cataract surgery has recently drawn much attention. The profile of more or less immediate postsurgical diplopia and a careful motility examination generally confirm the diagnosis. Inferior rectus contracture/fibrosis is arguably the most common type,[313,314] although the inferior oblique[315] and superior rectus muscles may be involved as well. Most evidence points to anesthetic myotoxicity, "with or without direct muscle trauma," as the etiologic agent. These patients typically demonstrate an increase in strabismus in gaze opposite the affected muscles, and forced ductions show restriction. However, isolated overaction of the affected muscle with deviation increasing in its field of action has also been described.[316] As bridle sutures become less commonly used, superior rectus paresis from needle or suture trauma is now infrequent. Capó et al[317] showed that both the inferior and superior recti can be injured with retrobulbar injections, although peribulbar injections were more likely to damage the inferior rectus. The left eye was involved twice as often as the right, perhaps reflecting the handedness of the person administering the block.

Postoperative strabismus is not peculiar to cataract surgery alone, and it is well known to occur after scleral buckling procedures, as well as after implantation of aqueous drainage devices in glaucoma.[318,319] In these cases, a restrictive strabismus results from the presence of foreign objects in Tenon's space and around the extraocular muscles.

Patients with strabismus after ocular surgery now constitute an increasing proportion of adults with diplopia. Many smaller deviations resolve spontaneously, or become comitant with time, lending themselves to prism therapy. Most cases, however, eventually require strabismus surgery and demonstrate excellent results with conventional techniques and the use of adjustable sutures.[317]

MISCELLANEOUS OCULAR MUSCLE CONDITIONS

Granulomas within the extraocular muscles have been described in sarcoidosis.[320,321] Such ocular deviations typically respond well to corticosteroid therapy. Patients with spontaneous hemorrhage within a rectus muscle present with painful proptosis and ophthalmoplegia, usually with uncomplicated resolution.[322] Orbital myositis has been reported as a paraneoplastic effect of non-Hodgkin's lymphoma,[323] and in association with giant cell myocarditis.[324] Serum antibodies reacting to eye muscle membrane antigens have been demonstrated in patients with typical and atypical orbital inflammation and myositis.[325]

REFERENCES

1. Warwick R: Representation of the extra-ocular muscles in the oculomotor complex. J Comp Neurol 98:449, 1953
2. Buttner-Ennever JA, Grob P, Akert K: A transsynaptic autoradiographic study of the pathways controlling the extraocular muscles using [125l]B-IIb tetanus toxin fragment. Ann NY Acad Sci 374:157, 1981
3. Porter JD, Guthrie BL, Sparks DL: Innervation of monkey extraocular muscles: localization of the sensory and motor neurons by retrograde transport of horseradish peroxidase. J Comp Neurol 218:208, 1983
4. Burde RM: The visceral nuclei of the oculomotor complex. Trans Am Ophthalmol Soc 81:533, 1983
5. Highstein SM, Baker R: Excitatory termination of abducens internuclear neurons on medial rectus motoneurons: relationship to syndrome of internuclear ophthalmoplegia. J Neurophysiol 41:1647, 1978
6. Destombes J, Horcholle-Bossavit G, Rouviere A: Données récentes concernant le noyau oculomoteur externe: centre du mouvement oculaire horizontal. J Fr Ophthalmol 6:605, 1983
7. Henn V, Lang W, Hepp K, Reisine H: Experimental gaze palsies in monkeys and their relation to human pathology. Brain 107:619, 1984
8. Crane TB, Yee RD, Baloh RW, Hepler RS: Analysis of characteristic eye movement abnormalities in internuclear ophthalmoplegia. Arch Ophthalmol 101:206, 1983
9. Gonyea EF: Bilateral internuclear ophthalmoplegia: association with occlusive cerebrovascular disease. Arch Neurol 31:168, 1974
10. Klintworth GK: The neuro-ophthalmic manifestations of transtentorial herniation. In Smith JL (ed): Neuro-Ophthalmology: Symposium of the University of Miami and the Bascom Palmer Eye Institute, Vol 4, pp 113–131. St. Louis, CV Mosby, 1972
11. Ishikawa H, Inagaki M, Kitano S: The oculomotor nerve in the cavernous sinus and orbit. Orbit 5:91, 1986
12. Kerr FW: The pupil: functional anatomy and clinical correlation. In Smith JL (ed): Neuro-Ophthalmology: Symposium of the University of Miami and the Bascom Palmer Eye Institute, Vol 4, pp 49–80. St. Louis, CV Mosby, 1968
13. Parkinson D, Johnston J, Chaudhuri A: Sympathetic connections of the fifth and sixth cranial nerves. Anat Record 191:221, 1978

14. Milisavljević M, Marinković S, Lolić-Draganić V, Kovacević M: Oculomotor, trochlear, and abducens nerves penetrated by cerebral vessels: microanatomy and possible clinical significance. Arch Neurol 43:58, 1986
15. Lapresle J, Lasjaunias P: Cranial nerve ischaemic arterial syndromes: a review. Brain 109:207, 1986
16. Horton JC, Fishman RA: Neurovisual findings in the syndrome of spontaneous intracranial hypotension from dural cerebrospinal fluid leak. Ophthalmology 101:244, 1994
17. Perlman EM, Barry D: Bilateral sixth-nerve palsy after water-soluble contrast myelography. Arch Ophthalmol 102:1968, 1984
18. Nabors MW, McCrory ME, Fischer BA et al: Delayed abducens nerve palsies associated with cervical spine fractures. Neurology 37:1565, 1987
19. Barr HWK, Blackwood W, Meadows SP: Intracavernous carotid aneurysms: a clinical-pathological report. Brain 94:607, 1971
20. O'Connor PS, Glaser JS: Intracavernous aneurysms and isolated sixth nerve palsy. In Smith JL (ed): Neuro-Ophthalmology Focus, pp 155–159. New York, Masson, 1982
21. Newton TH, Hoyt WF: Dural arteriovenous shunts in the region of the cavernous sinus. Neuroradiology 1:71, 1970
22. Gutman I, Levartovski S, Goldhammer Y et al: Sixth nerve palsy and unilateral Horner's syndrome. Ophthalmology 93:913, 1986
23. Keane JR: Bilateral sixth nerve palsy. Arch Neurol 33: 681, 1976
24. Keane JR: Eye movement abnormalities in systemic lupus erythematosus. Arch Neurol 52:1145, 1995
25. Savino PJ, Hiliker JK, Casell GH, Schatz NJ: Chronic sixth nerve palsies: are they really harbingers of serious disease? Arch Ophthalmol 100:1442, 1982
26. Currie J, Lubin JH, Lessell S: Chronic isolated abducens paresis from tumors at the base of the brain. Arch Neurol 40:226, 1983
27. Volpe NJ, Lessell S: Remitting sixth nerve palsy in skull base tumors. Arch Ophthalmol 3:1391, 1993
28. Reisner SH, Perlman M, Ben-Tovim N et al: Transient lateral rectus muscle paresis in the newborn infant. J Pediatr 78:461, 1971
29. Knox DL, Clark DB, Schuster FF: Benign VI nerve palsies in children. Pediatrics 40:560, 1967
30. Nemet P, Ehrlich D, Lazar M: Benign abducens palsy in varicella. Am J Ophthalmol 78:859, 1984
31. Werner DB, Savino PJ, Schatz NJ: Benign recurrent sixth nerve palsies in childhood: secondary to immunization or viral illness. Arch Ophthalmol 101:607, 1983
32. Straussberg R, Cohen AH, Amir J, Versano I: Benign abducens palsy associated with EBV infection. J Pediatr Ophthalmol Strabismus 30:60, 1993
33. Bixenman WW, von Noorden GK: Benign recurrent VI nerve palsy in childhood. J Pediatr Ophthalmol Strabismus 18:29, 1981
34. Reinecke RD, Thompson WE: Childhood recurrent idiopathic paralysis of the lateral rectus. Ann Ophthalmol 13:1037, 1981
35. Boger WP III, Puliofito CA, Magoon EH et al: Recurrent isolated sixth nerve palsy in children. Ann Ophthalmol 16:237, 1984
36. Sullivan SC: Benign recurrent isolated VI nerve palsy of childhood. Clin Pediatr 24:160, 1985
37. Peatfield RC: Recurrent VI palsy in cluster headache. Headache 25:225, 1985
38. Robertson DM, Hines JD, Rucker CW: Acquired sixth-nerve paresis in children. Arch Ophthalmol 83:574, 1970
39. Harley RD: Paralytic strabismus in children: etiologic incidence and management of the third, fourth and sixth nerve palsies. Ophthalmology 87:24, 1980
40. Moster ML, Savino PJ, Sergott RC et al: Isolated sixth-nerve palsies in younger adults. Arch Ophthalmol 102:1328, 1984
41. Shrader EC, Schlezinger NS: Neuro-ophthalmologic evaluation of abducens nerve paralysis. Arch Ophthalmol 63:84, 1960
42. Rucker CW: The causes of paralysis of the third, fourth and sixth cranial nerves. Am J Ophthalmol 61:1294, 1966
43. Richards BW, Jones FR, Younge BR: Causes and prognosis in 4,278 cases of paralysis of the oculomotor, trochlear, and abducens cranial nerves. Am J Ophthalmol 113:489, 1992
44. Rose JW, Digre KB, Lynch SG, Marnsberger RH: Acute VIth cranial nerve dysfunction in multiple sclerosis. J Clin Neuro Ophthalmol 12:17, 1992
45. Kirkham TH, Bird AC, Sanders MD: Divergence paralysis with

raised intracranial pressure: an electro-oculographic study. Br J Ophthalmol 56:776, 1972

46. Mays LE: Neural control of vergence eye movements: convergence and divergence neurons in the midbrain. J Neurophysiol 51:1091, 1984

47. Krohel GB, Tobin DR, Hartnett ME, Barrows NA: Divergence paralysis. Am J Ophthalmol 94:506, 1982

48. Stern RM, Tomsak RL: Magnetic resonance images in a case of "divergence paralysis." Surv Ophthalmol 30:397, 1986

49. Lewis AR, Kline LB, Sharpe JA: Acquired esotropia due to Arnold-Chiari I malformation. J Neuro Ophthalmol 16:49, 1996

50. Moster ML, Bosley TM, Slavin ML, Rubin SE: Thyroid ophthalmopathy presenting as superior oblique paresis. J Clin Neuro Ophthalmol 12:94, 1992

51. Jacobson DM: Superior oblique palsy manifested during pregnancy. Ophthalmology 98:1874, 1991

52. Astle WF, Rosenblum AL: Familial congenital fourth cranial nerve palsy. Arch Ophthalmol 103:552, 1985

53. Aleksic S, Fudzilovich G, Choy A et al: Congenital ophthalmoplegia in oculoauriculovertebral dysplasia-hemifacial microsomia (Goldenhar-Gorlin syndrome): a clinicopathologic study and review of the literature. Neurology 26:638, 1976

54. Cowan WM, Fawcett JW, O'Leary DDM et al: Regressive events in neurogenesis. Science 225:1258, 1984

55. Pinchoff BS, Sandall G: Congenital absence of the superior oblique tendon in craniofacial dysostosis. Ophthalmic Surg 16:375, 1985

56. Helveston EM, Krach D, Plager DA, Ellis FD: A new classification of superior oblique palsy based on congenital variations in the tendon. Ophthalmology 99:1609, 1992

57. Berlit P: Isolated and combined pareses of cranial nerves III, IV and VI: a retrospective study of 412 patients. J Neurol Sci 103:10, 1991

58. Keane JR: Fourth nerve palsy: historical review and study of 215 patients. Neurology 43:2439, 1993

59. Grimson BS, Glaser JS: Isolated trochlear nerve palsies in herpes zoster ophthalmicus. Arch Ophthalmol 96:1233, 1978

60. Agostinis C, Caverni L, Moschini L et al: Paralysis of fourth cranial nerve due to superior cerebellar artery aneurysm. Neurology 42:457, 1992

61. Botelho PJ, Giangiacomo JG: Autosomal-dominant inheritance of congenital superior oblique palsy. Ophthalmology 103:1508, 1996

62. Lindenberg R: Significance of the tentorium in head injuries from blunt forces. Clin Neurosurg 12:129, 1966

63. Khawam E, Scott AB, Jampolsky A: Acquired superior oblique palsy. Arch Ophthalmol 77:761, 1967

64. Sydnor CF, Seaber JH, Buckley EG: Traumatic superior oblique palsies. Ophthalmology 89:134, 1982

65. Lee J, Flynn JT: Bilateral superior oblique palsies. Br J Ophthalmol 69:508, 1985

66. Trobe JD: Cyclodeviation in acquired vertical strabismus. Arch Ophthalmol 102:717, 1984

67. Keane JR: Vertical diplopia. Semin Neurol 6:147, 1986

68. Feinberg AS, Newman NJ: Schwannoma in patients with isolated unilateral trochlear nerve palsy. Am J Ophthalmol 127:183, 1999

69. Kushner BJ: 'V' esotropia and excyclotropia after surgery for bilateral fourth nerve palsy. Arch Ophthalmol 110:1419, 1992

70. Gregersen E, Rindziunski E: Brown's syndrome: a longitudinal long-term study of spontaneous course. Acta Ophthalmol 71:371, 1993

71. Mombaerts I, Koornneef L et al: Superior oblique luxation and trochlear luxation as new concepts in superior oblique muscle weakening surgery. Am J Ophthalmol 120:83, 1995

72. Clarke WN, Noel LP, Agapitos PJ: Traumatic Brown's syndrome. Am Orthoptic J 37:100, 1987

73. Booth-Mason S, Kyle GM, Rossor M, Bradbury P: Acquired Brown's syndrome: an unusual cause. Br J Ophthalmol 69:791, 1985

74. Hickling P, Beck M: Brown's syndrome: an unusual ocular complication of rheumatoid arthritis. Ann Rheum Dis 50:66, 1991

75. Alonso-Valdivielso JL, Alvarez Lario B et al: Acquired Brown's syndrome in a patient with systemic lupus erythematosus. Ann Rheum Dis 52:63, 1993

76. Christiansen SP, Thomas AH: Postpartum Brown's syndrome. Arch Ophthalmol 112:23, 1994

77. Brazis PW, Miller NR, Henderer JD, Lee AG: The natural history and results of treatment of superior oblique myokymia. Arch Ophthalmol 112:1063, 1994

78. Martin TJ, Corbett JJ, Babikian PV et al: Bilateral ptosis due to mesencephalic lesions with relative preservation of ocular motility. J Neuro Ophthalmol 16:258, 1996

79. Keane JR, Zaias B, Itabashi HH: Levator-sparing oculomotor nerve palsy caused by a solitary midbrain metastases. Arch Neurol 14:210, 1984

80. Bryan JS, Hamed LM: Levator-sparing nuclear oculomotor palsy: clinical and magnetic resonance imaging findings. J Clin Neuro Ophthalmol 12:26, 1992

81. Van Dalen JTW, Van Mourek-Noordenbos AM: Isolated inferior rectus paresis: a report of six cases. Neuro Ophthalmology 4:89, 1984

82. Masucci EF: Bilateral ophthalmoplegia in basilar-vertebral artery disease. Brain 88:97, 1965

83. Acers TE: Oculomotor-corpus callosum dysplasia. Trans Am Ophthalmol Soc 80:172, 1982

84. Ksiazek SM, Slamovits TL, Rosen CE et al: Fascicular arrangement in partial oculomotor paresis. J Ophthalmol 118:97, 1994

85. Gauntt CD, Kashii S, Nagata I: Monocular elevation paresis caused by an oculomotor fascicular impairment. J Neuro Ophthalmol 15:11, 1995

86. Castro O, Johnson LN, Mamourian AC: Isolated inferior oblique paresis from brain-stem infarction: perspective on oculomotor fascicular organization in the ventral midbrain tegmentum. Arch Neurol 47:235, 1990

87. Trobe JD, Glaser JS, Quencer RC: Isolated oculomotor paralysis. Arch Ophthalmol 96:1236, 1978

88. Hyland HH, Barnett HJM: The pathogenesis of cranial nerve palsies associated with intracranial aneurysms. Proc R Soc Med 47:141, 1956

89. Ross JS, Masaryk TJ, Modic MT et al: Intracranial aneurysms: evaluation by MR angiography. AJNR 11:449, 1990

90. Capó H, Warren F, Kupersmith MJ: Evolution of oculomotor nerve palsies. J Clin Neuro Ophthalmol 12:21, 1992

91. Guy J, Savino PJ, Schatz NJ et al: Superior division paresis of the oculomotor nerve. Ophthalmology 92:777, 1985

92. Heinze J: Cranial nerve avulsion and other neural injuries in road accidents. Med J Aust 2:1246, 1969

93. Eyster EF, Hoyt WF, Wilson CB: Oculomotor palsy from minor head trauma: an initial sign of basal intracranial tumor. JAMA 220:1083, 1972

94. Neetens A: Extraocular muscle palsy from minor head trauma: initial sign of intracranial tumor. Neuro Ophthalmology 3:43, 1983

95. Walter KA, Newman NJ, Lessell S: Oculomotor palsy from minor head trauma: initial sign of intracranial aneurysm. Neurology 44:148, 1994

96. Ing EB, Sullivan TJ, Clarke MP, Buncic JR: Oculomotor nerve palsies in children. J Pediatr Ophthalmol Strabismus 29:331, 1992

97. Keane JR: Bilateral ocular motor signs after tentorial herniation in 25 patients. Arch Neurol 43:806, 1986

98. Acierno MD, Trobe JD, Cornblath WT, Gebarski SS: Painful oculomotor palsy caused by posterior-draining dural carotid cavernous fistulas. Arch Ophthalmol 113:1045, 1995

99. Schultheiss R, Kristol R, Schramm J: Complete removal of an oculomotor nerve neurinoma without permanent functional deficits. Ger J Ophthalmol 2:228, 1993

100. Kaye-Wilson LG, Gibson R, Bell JE et al: Oculomotor nerve neurinoma. Neuro-ophthalmology 14:37, 1994

101. Jacobson DM, McCanna TD, Layde PM: Risk factors for ischemic ocular motor palsies. Arch Ophthalmol 112:961, 1994

102. Sergott RC, Glaser JS, Buerger LJ: Simultaneous, bilateral diabetic ophthalmoplegia: report of two cases and discussion of differential diagnosis. Ophthalmology 91:18, 1984

103. Eshbaugh CG, Siatkowski RM, Smith JL, Kline LB: Simultaneous multiple cranial neuropathies in diabetes mellitus. J Neuro Ophthalmol 15:219, 1995

104. Weber RB, Daroff RB, Mackey EA: Pathology of oculomotor nerve palsy in diabetics. Neurology 20:835, 1970

105. Asbury AK, Aldredge H, Hershberg R et al: Oculomotor palsy in diabetes mellitus: a clinicopathological study. Brain 93:555, 1970

106. Breen LA, Hopf HC, Farris BK et al: Pupil-sparing oculomotor nerve palsy due to midbrain infarction. Arch Neurol 48:105, 1991

107. Pratt DV, Orengo-Nania S, Horowitz BL, Oram O: Magnetic resonance imaging findings in a patient with nuclear oculomotor palsy. Arch Ophthalmol 113:141, 1995

108. Position Statement: Tests of glycemia in diabetes. American Diabetes Association: Clinical practice recommendations. Diabetes Care, ADA, 1:S18, 1997

109. Sibony PA, Lessell S, Gittenger JW Jr: Acquired oculomotor synkinesis. Surv Ophthalmol 28:382, 1984

110. Sibony PA, Evinger C, Lessell S: Retrograde horseradish peroxidase transport after oculomotor nerve injury. Invest Ophthalmol Vis Sci 27:975, 1986

111. Lepore FE, Glaser JS: Misdirected revisited: a critical appraisal of acquired oculomotor nerve synkinesis. Arch Ophthalmol 98:2206, 1980

112. Wartenberg R: Associated movements in the oculomotor and facial muscles. Arch Neurol Psychiatry 55:439, 1946

113. Sibony PA, Lessell S: Transient oculomotor synkinesis in temporal arteritis. Arch Neurol 41:87, 1984

114. Schatz NJ, Savino PJ, Corbett JC: Primary aberrant oculomotor regeneration: A sign of intracavernous meningioma. Arch Neurol 34:29, 1977

115. Trobe JD, Glaser JS, Post JD: Meningiomas and aneurysms of the cavernous sinus: neuro-ophthalmologic features. Arch Ophthalmol 96:457, 1978

116. Cox TA, Wurster JB, Godfrey WA: Primary aberrant oculomotor regeneration due to intracranial aneurysm. Arch Neurol 36:570, 1979

117. Boghen D, Chartrand JP, LaFlamme P et al: Primary aberrant third nerve regeneration. Ann Neurol 6:415, 1979

118. Hepler RS, Cantu RC: Aneurysms and third nerve palsies: ocular status of survivors. Arch Ophthalmol 77:604, 1967

119. Czarnecki JSC, Thompson HS: The iris sphincter in aberrant regeneration of the third nerve. Arch Ophthalmol 96:1606, 1978

120. Miller NR: Solitary oculomotor nerve palsy in childhood. Am J Ophthalmol 83:106, 1977

121. Victor DI: The diagnosis of congenital unilateral third nerve palsy. Brain 99:711, 1976

122. Balkan R, Hoyt CS: Associated neurologic abnormalities in congenital third nerve palsies. Am J Ophthalmol 97:315, 1984

123. Varma R, Miller NR: Primary oculomotor nerve synkinesis caused by an extracavernous intradural aneurysm. Am J Ophthalmol 118:83, 1994

124. O'Day J, Billson F, King J: Ophthalmoplegic migraine and aberrant regeneration of the oculomotor nerve. Br J Ophthalmol 64:534, 1980

125. Packer AJ, Bienfang DC: Aberrant regeneration involving the oculomotor and abducens nerves. Ophthalmologica 189:80, 1984

126. Krzizok T, Gräf M: Acquired trigemino-abducens synkinesia. Proposed mechanisms and consequences for eye muscle surgery. Klin Monatsbl Augenheilkd 205:33, 1994

127. Pallini R, Fernandez E et al: Experimental repair of the oculomotor nerve: the anatomical paradigms of functional regeneration. J Neurosurg 77:768, 1992

128. Marsh RJ, Dulley B, Kelly V: External ocular motor palsies in ophthalmic zoster: a review. Br J Ophthalmol 61:677, 1977

129. Wexler I: Sequence of demyelination-remyelination in Guillain-Barré disease. J Neurol Neurosurg Psychiatry 46:168, 1983

130. Fisher CM: An unusual variant of acute idiopathic polyneuritis (syndrome of ophthalmoplegia, ataxia and areflexia). N Engl J Med 255:57, 1956

131. Asbury AK, Arnason BG, Adams R: The inflammatory lesion in idiopathic polyneuritis. Medicine 48:173, 1969

132. Grunnet ML, Lubow M: Ascending polyneuritis and ophthalmoplegia. Am J Ophthalmol 74:1155, 1972

133. Berlit P, Rakicky J: The Miller Fisher syndrome. J Clin Neuro Ophthalmol 12:59, 1992

134. Hideaki T, Nobuhiro Y, Koichi H: Trochlear nerve enhancement on three-dimensional magnetic resonance imaging in Fisher syndrome. Am J Ophthalmol 126:322, 1998

135. Ropper AH: The Guillain-Barré syndrome. N Engl J Med 326:1130, 1992

136. Chalmers AC, Miller RG: Chronic inflammatory polyradiculoneuropathy with ophthalmoplegia. J Clin Neuro Ophthalmol 6:166, 1986

137. Yuki N: Acute paresis of extraocular muscles associated with IgG anti-GQ$_{1b}$ antibody. Ann Neurol 39:668, 1995

138. Friedman AP, Harter DH, Merritt HH: Ophthalmoplegic migraine. Arch Neurol 7:320, 1962

139. Vijayan N: Ophthalmoplegic migraine: ischemic or compressive neuropathy? Headache 20:300, 1980

140. Stigmal EW, Ward TN, Harris RD: MRI findings in a case of ophthalmoplegic migraine. Headache 33:234, 1993

141. Straub A, Bondman O, Butter U, Schmidt H: A contrast enhances lesion of the III nerve on MR of a patient with ophthalmoplegic migraine as evidence for a Tolosa-Hunt syndrome. Headache 33:446, 1993

142. Østergaard JR, Moller HU, Christensen T: Recurrent ophthalmoplegia in childhood: diagnostic and etiologic considerations. Cephalgia 16:276, 1996

143. Imes RK, Monteiro MLR, Hoyt WF: Ophthalmoplegic migraine with proximal posterior cerebral artery vascular anomaly. J Clin Neuro Ophthalmol 4:221, 1984

144. Kandt RS, Goldstein GW: Steroid-responsive ophthalmoplegia in a child: diagnostic considerations. Arch Neurol 42:589, 1985

145. Osuntokun O, Osuntokun BO: Ophthalmoplegic migraine and hemoglobinopathy in Nigerians. Am J Ophthalmol 74:451, 1972

146. Sharf B, Hyams S: Oculomotor palsy following varicella. J Pediatr Ophthalmol 9:245, 1972

147. Chan CC, Sogg RL, Steinman L: Isolated oculomotor palsy after measles immunization. Am J Ophthalmol 89:446, 1980

148. Loewenfeld IE, Thompson HS: Oculomotor paresis with cyclic spasms: a critical review of the literature and a new case. Surv Ophthalmol 20:81, 1975

149. Bourgon P, LaFlamme P: Cited by Thompson HS: 13th Pupil Colloquium. Am J Ophthalmol 96:100, 1983

150. Bateman DE, Saunders M: Cyclic oculomotor palsy: description of a case and hypothesis of the mechanism. J Neurol Neurosurg Psychiatry 46:451, 1983

151. Dudim A, Othman A: Acute orbital swelling: evaluation and protocol. Pediatr Emerg Care 12:16, 1996

152. Bergin DJ, Wright JE: Orbital cellulitis. Br J Ophthalmol 70:174, 1986

153. Del Valle ZA, Suarez RA, Encinas PM et al: Mucormycosis of the sphenoid sinus in an otherwise health patient: case report and literature review. J Laryngol Otol 110:471, 1996

154. Yohai RA, Bullock JD, Aziz AA, Mirkert RJ: Survival factors in rhino-orbital cerebral mucormycosis. Surv Ophthalmol 39:3, 1994

155. Kennerdell JS, Dresner SC: The nonspecific orbital inflammatory syndromes. Surv Ophthalmol 29:93, 1984

156. Grimson BS, Simmons KB: Orbital inflammation, myositis and systemic lupus erythematosus. Arch Ophthalmol 101:36, 1983

157. Schonder AA, Clift RC, Brophy JW, Dane LW: Bilateral recurrent orbital inflammation associated with retroperitoneal fibrosclerosis. Br J Ophthalmol 69:783, 1985

158. Rootman J, Nugent R: The classification and management of acute orbital pseudotumors. Ophthalmology 89:1040, 1982

159. Siatkowski RM, Capó H, Byrne SF et al: Clinical and echographic findings in idiopathic orbital myositis. Am J Ophthalmol 118:343, 1994

160. Koorey DJ: Cranial arteritis: a twenty-year review of cases. Aust NZ J Med 14:143, 1984

161. Baricks ME, Traviesa DB, Glaser JS, Levy IS: Ophthalmoplegia in cranial arteritis. Brain 100:209, 1977

162. Cline RA, Rootman J: Enophthalmos: a clinical review. Ophthalmology 91:229, 1984

163. Keane JR: Cavernous sinus syndrome: analysis of 151 cases. Arch Neurol 53:967, 1996

164. Tolosa EJ: Periarteritic lesions of the carotid siphon with clinical features of carotid infraclinoid aneurysms. J Neurol Neurosurg Psychiatry 17:300, 1954

165. Hunt WE, Meagher JN, Lefever HE, Zeman W: Painful ophthal-

moplegia: its relation to indolent inflammation of the cavernous sinus. Neurology 11:56, 1961

166. Thomas JE, Yoss RE: The parasellar syndrome: problems in determining etiology. Mayo Clin Proc 45:617, 1970

167. Spector RH, Fiandaca MS: The "sinister" Tolosa-Hunt syndrome. Neurology 36:198, 1986

168. Kline LB: The Tolosa-Hunt syndrome. Surv Ophthalmol 27:79, 1982

169. Campbell RJ, Okazaki H: Painful ophthalmoplegia (Tolosa-Hunt variant): autopsy findings in a patient with necrotizing intracavernous carotid vasculitis and inflammatory disease of the orbit. Mayo Clin Proc 62:520, 1987

170. Aktan S, Aykut C, Erzen C: Computed tomography and magnetic resonance imaging in three patients with Tolosa-Hunt syndrome. Eur Neurol 33:393, 1993

171. Takahashi Y, Abe T, Kojima K et al: Tolosa-Hunt syndrome with atypical intrasellar and juxtasellar lesions. Two case reports. Kurume Med J 43:165, 1996

172. Drevelengas A, Kalaitzoglou I, Tsolaki M: Tolosa-Hunt syndrome with sellar erosion: case report. Neuroradiology 35:451, 1993

173. Hama S, Arita K, Kurisu K et al: Parasellar chronic inflammatory disease presenting as Tolosa-Hunt syndrome, hypopituitarism and diabetes insipidus: a case report. Endocr J 43:503, 1996

174. Brazis PW, Capobianco DJ et al: Low flow dural arteriovenous shunt: another cause of "sinister" Tolosa-Hunt syndrome. Headache 34:523, 1994

175. Sanchez Pina C, Pascual-Castroviejo I et al: Burkitt's lymphoma presenting as Tolosa-Hunt syndrome. Pediatr Neurol 9:157, 1993

176. Montecucco C, Caporali R, Pacchetti C, Turla M: Is Tolosa-Hunt syndrome a limited form of Wegener's granulomatosis?: report of two cases with anti-neutrophil cytoplasmic antibodies. Br J Rheumatol 32:640, 1993

177. Masson C, Henin D, Hauw JJ et al: Cranial pachymeningitis of unknown origin: a study of seven cases. Neurology 17:1329, 1993

178. Vailati A, Marena C et al: Hashimoto's thyroiditis in association with Tolosa-Hunt syndrome: a case report. Thyroid 3:125, 1993

179. Bills DC, Meyer FB et al: A retrospective analysis of pituitary apoplexy. Neurosurgery 33:602, 1993

180. Vidal E, Cevallos R et al: Twelve cases of pituitary apoplexy. Arch Intern Med 152:1893, 1992

181. Weinberger LM, Adler FH, Grant FC: Primary pituitary adenoma and the syndrome of the cavernous sinus. Arch Ophthalmol 24:1197, 1940

182. Godtfredsen E, Lederman M: Diagnostic and prognostic roles of ophthalmoneurologic signs and symptoms in malignant nasopharyngeal tumors. Am J Ophthalmol 59:1063, 1965

183. Meadows SP: Intracavernous aneurysms of the carotid artery. Arch Ophthalmol 62:566, 1959

184. Lee AG, Mawad ME, Baskin DS: Fatal subarachnoid hemorrhage from the rupture of a totally intracavernous carotid artery aneurysm: case report. Neurosurgery 38:596, 1996

185. Keane JR, Talalla A: Post traumatic intracavernous aneurysm: epistaxis with monocular blindness preceded by chromatopsia. Arch Ophthalmol 87:701, 1972

186. Trobe JD, Glaser JS, Post JD: Meningiomas and aneurysms of the cavernous sinus: neuro-ophthalmologic features. Arch Ophthalmol 96:457, 1978

187. Rapport R, Murtagh FR: Ophthalmoplegia due to spontaneous thrombosis in a patient with bilateral cavernous carotid aneurysms. J Clin Neuro Ophthalmol 1:225, 1981

188. Kupersmith MJ, Hurst R, Berenstein A et al: The benign course of cavernous carotid artery aneurysms. J Neurosurg 77:690, 1992

189. Cushing H, Eisenhardt L: Meningiomas: Their Classification, Regional Behavior, Life History and Surgical End Results. New York, Hofner, 1962

190. Ojemann RG, Thornton AF, Harsh GR: Management of anterior cranial base and cavernous sinus neoplasms with conservative surgery alone or in combination with fractionated photon or stereotactic proton radiotherapy. Clin Neurosurg 42:71, 1995

191. Nugent GR, Sprinkle P, Bloor BM: Sphenoid sinus mucoceles. J Neurosurg 32:443, 1970

192. Valvassori GE, Putterman AM: Ophthalmological and radiologi-

cal findings in sphenoidal mucoceles. Trans Am Acad Ophthalmol Otolaryngol 77:703, 1973

193. Casteels I, DeLoof E, Brock P et al: Sudden blindness in a child: presenting symptoms of sphenoid sinus mucocele. Br J Ophthalmol 76:502, 1992

194. El-Fiki ME, Abdel-Fattah HM, el-Deeb AK: Sphenoid sinus mucopyocele with marked intracranial extension. Surg Neurol 39:115, 1993

195. Post MJD, Mendez DR, Kline LB et al: Metastatic disease to the cavernous sinus: clinical syndrome and CT diagnosis. J Comput Assist Tomogr 9:115, 1985

196. Kline LB, Acker JD, Post JDM: Computed tomographic evaluation of the cavernous sinus. Ophthalmology 89:374, 1982

197. Moore CE, Hoyt WF, North JB: Painful ophthalmoplegia following treated squamous carcinoma of the forehead: orbital apex involvement from centripetal spread via the supraorbital nerve. Med J Aust 1:657, 1976

198. Catalano PJ, Sen C, Biller HF: Cranial neuropathy secondary to perineural spread of cutaneous malignancies. Am J Otol 16:772, 1995

199. ten Hove MW, Glaser JS, Schatz NJ: Occult perineural tumor infiltration of the trigeminal nerve. Diagnostic considerations. J Neuro Ophthalmol 17:170, 1997

200. Hayat G, Ehsan T, Selhorst JB, Manepali A: Magnetic resonance evidence of perineural metastasis. J Neuroimaging 5:122, 1995

201. Olson ME, Cornice NL, Posner JB: Infiltration of the leptomeninges by systemic cancer: a clinical and pathologic study. Arch Neurol 30:122, 1974

202. Little JR, Dale AJD, Okazaki H: Meningeal carcinomatosis: clinical manifestations. Arch Neurol 30:138, 1974

203. Wasserstrom WR, Glass JP, Posner JB: Diagnosis and treatment of leptomeningeal metastases from solid tumors: experience with 90 patients. Cancer 49:759, 1982

204. Watanabe M, Tanaka R, Takeda N: Correlation of MRI and clinical features in meningeal carcinomatosis. Neuroradiology 35:512, 1993

205. Stern BJ, Krumholz A, Johns C et al: Sarcoidosis and its neurological manifestations. Arch Neurol 49:909, 1985

206. Oksamen V: Neurosarcoidosis: clinical presentations and course in 50 patients. Acta Neurol Scand 73:283, 1986

207. Post MJD, Chan JC, Hensley GT et al: Toxoplasma encephalitis in Haitian adults with acquired immunodeficiency syndrome: a clinical-pathologic-CT correlation. Am J Neuroradiol 4:155, 1983

208. Berger JR, Flaster M, Schatz N et al: Cranial neuropathy heralding otherwise occult AIDS-related large cell lymphoma. J Clin Neuro Ophthalmol 13:113, 1993

209. Hamed LM, Schatz, NJ, Galetta SL: Brainstem ocular motility defects and AIDS. Am J Ophthalmol 106:437, 1988

210. Wadia NH, Wadia PN, Katrak SM, Misra VP: A study of the neurological disorder associated with acute hemorrhagic conjunctivitis due to enterovirus 70. J Neurol Neurosurg Psychiatry 46:559, 1983

211. Katiyar BC, Misra S, Singh RB et al: Adult polio-like syndrome following enterovirus 70 conjunctivitis (natural history of the disease). Acta Neurol Scand 67:263, 1983

212. Lesser RL: Ocular manifestations of Lyme disease. Am J Med 98:60, 1995

213. Rodriguez M, Gomez MR, Howard FM, Taylor WF: Myasthenia in children: long-term follow-up. Ann Neurol 13:504, 1983

214. Vincent A, Newsom-Davis J: Acetylcholine receptor antibody characteristics in myasthenia gravis: I. Patients with generalized myasthenia or disease restricted to ocular muscles. Clin Exp Immunol 49:257, 1982

215. Zimmerman CW, Eblen F: Repertoires of autoantibodies against homologous eye muscle in ocular and generalized myasthenia gravis. Clin Invest 71:445, 1993

216. Drachman DB, Adams RN, Josifek LF, Self SG: Functional activities of autoantibodies to acetylcholine receptors and the clinical severity of myasthenia gravis. N Engl J Med 307:769, 1982

217. Weinberg DA, Lesser RL, Vollmer TL: Ocular myasthenia: a protean disorder. Surv Ophthalmol 39:169, 1994

218. Grob D, Arsura EL, Brunner NG, Namba T: The course of

myasthenia gravis, and therapies affecting outcome. Ann NY Acad Sci 505:472, 1987

219. Bever CT, Aquino AV, Penn AS et al: Prognosis of ocular myasthenia. Ann Neurol 14:526, 1983

220. Cogan DG: Myasthenia gravis: A review of the disease and a description of lid twitch as a characteristic sign. Arch Ophthalmol 74:217, 1965

221. Dutton GN, Garson JA, Richardson RB: Pupillary fatigue in myasthenia gravis. Trans Ophthalmol Soc UK 102:510, 1982

222. Glaser JS: Myasthenic pseudo-internuclear ophthalmoplegia. Arch Ophthalmol 75:363, 1966

223. Keane JR, Hoyt WF: Myasthenic (vertical) nystagmus: verification by edrophonium tonography. JAMA 212:1209, 1970

224. Barton JJS, Jama A, Sharpe JA: Saccadic duration and intrasaccadic fatigue in myasthenic and nonmyasthenic ocular palsies. Neurology 45:2065, 1995

225. Osher RH, Griggs RC: Orbicularis fatigue: the "peek" sign of myasthenia gravis. Arch Ophthalmol 97:677, 1979

226. Osher RH, Glaser JS: Myasthenic sustained gaze fatigue. Am J Ophthalmol 89:443, 1980

227. Retzlaff JA, Kearns TP, Howard FM Jr et al: Lancaster red-green test in evaluation of edrophonium effect in myasthenia gravis. Am J Ophthalmol 67:13, 1969

228. Seybold ME, Daroff RB: The office Tensilon test for ocular myasthenia. Arch Neurol 43:842, 1986

229. Coll GE, Demer JL: The edrophonium-Hess screen test in the diagnosis of ocular myasthenia gravis. Am J Ophthalmol 114:489, 1992

230. Siatkowski RM, Shah L, Feuer WJ: The effect of edrophonium chloride on muscle balance in normal subjects and those with nonmyasthenic strabismus. J Neuro Ophthalmol 17:7, 1997

231. Miller NR, Morris JE, Maguire M: Combined use of neostigmine and ocular motility measurements in the diagnosis of myasthenia gravis. Arch Ophthalmol 100:761, 1982

232. Oey PL, Wieneke GM, Hoogenraad TU, van Hofgelen AC: Ocular myasthenia gravis: the diagnostic yield of repetitive nerve stimulating and stimulated single fiber EMG of orbicularis oculi muscle and infrared reflection oculography. Muscle Nerve 16:142, 1993

233. Odel J, Winterkorn J, Behrens M: The sleep test for myasthenia gravis: a safe alternative. J Clin Ophthalmol 11:288, 1991

234. Janssen RS, Kaye AD, Lisak RP et al: Radiologic evaluation of the mediastinum in myasthenia gravis. Neurology 33:534, 1983

235. Sanders DB, Howard JF: Disorders of neuromuscular transmission. In Bradley WG, Daroff RB, Fenichel GM, Marsden CD (eds): Neurology in Clinical Practice, Chap 83, p 1983. Boston, Butterworth-Heinemann, 1996

236. Kupersmith MJ, Moster M, Bhuiyan S et al: Beneficial effects of corticosteroids on ocular myasthenia gravis. Arch Neurol 53:802, 1996

237. McEvoy KM: Diagnosis and treatment of Lambert-Eaton myasthenic syndrome. Neurol Clin 12:387, 1994

238. Molenaar PC, Newson-Davis J, Polak RL, Vincent A: Eaton-Lambert syndrome: acetylcholine and choline acetyltransferase in skeletal muscle. Neurology 32:1062, 1982

239. Tsuchiya N, Sato M et al: Lambert-Eaton myasthenic syndrome associated with Sjögren's syndrome and discoid lupus erythematosus. Scand J Rheumatol 22:302, 1993

240. Cruciger MP, Brown B, Denys EH et al: Clinical and subclinical oculomotor findings in the Eaton-Lambert syndrome. J Clin Neuro Ophthalmol 3:19, 1983

241. Dell'Osso LF, Ayyar DR, Daroff RB, Abel LA: Edrophonium test in Eaton-Lambert syndrome: quantitative oculography. Neurology 33:1157, 1983

242. Breen LA, Gutmann L, Birck JF, Riggs JR: Paradoxical lid elevation with sustained upgaze: a sign of Lambert-Eaton syndrome. Muscle Nerve 14:863, 1991

243. Grisold W, Drlicek M, Liszka-Setinek U, Wondrusch E: Antitumour therapy in paraneoplastic neurological disease. Clin Neurol Neurosurg 97:106, 1995

244. Katz LJ, Lesser RL, Merikangas JR, Silverman JP: Ocular myasthenia gravis after D-penicillamine administration. Br J Ophthalmol 73:1015, 1989

245. McQuillen MP, Cantor HE, O'Rourke JR: Myasthenic syndromes associated with antibiotics. Arch Neurol 18:402, 1968

246. Albert DM, Wong VG, Henderson ES: Ocular complications of vincristine therapy. Arch Ophthalmol 78:709, 1967

247. Blanton CL, Sawyer RA: Myasthenia gravis by another name: an elusive impostor [clinical conference]. Surv Ophthalmol 38:219, 1993

248. Hedges TR III, Jones A, Stark L, Hoyt WF: Botulin ophthalmoplegia: clinical and oculographic observations. Arch Ophthalmol 101:211, 1983

249. Schubart P, Kasperski S, Schroder P: Ocular involvement in botulism. Klin Monatsbl Augenheilkd 187:142, 1985

250. Hudson HL, Levin L, Feldon SE: Graves exophthalmos unrelated to extraocular muscle enlargement. Ophthalmology 98:1495, 1991

251. Hermann JS: Paretic thyroid myopathy. Ophthalmology 89:473, 1982

252. Gamblin FT, Galentine PG, Eil C: Intraocular pressure and thyroid disease. In Gorman CA, Waller RR, Dyer JA (eds): The Eye and Orbit in Thyroid Disease, pp 155–166. New York, Raven Press, 1984

253. Byrne SF, Glaser JS: Orbital tissue differentiation with standardized echography. Ophthalmology 90:1071, 1983

254. Kung AW, Yau CC, Cheng A: The incidence of ophthalmopathy after radioiodine therapy for Graves' disease: prognostic factors and the role of methimazole. J Clin Endocrinol Metabol 79:542, 1994

255. Gorman CA, Waller RR, Dyer JA: The Eye and Orbit in Thyroid Eye Disease. New York, Raven Press, 1984

256. Raikow RB, Tyutyunikov A et al: Correlation of serum immunoglobulin E elevations with clinical states of dysthyroid orbitopathy. Ophthalmology 99:361, 1992

257. Khuteta A, Mishra YC et al: Mesenchymal chondrosarcoma of orbit with intracranial extension (a rare case). Ind J Ophthalmol 40:92, 1992

258. Prummel MF, Mourits MP et al: Randomized double-blind trial of prednisone versus radiotherapy in Graves' ophthalmopathy. Lancet 342:949, 1993

259. Wilson WB, Prochoda M: Radiotherapy for thyroid orbitopathy. Arch Ophthalmol 113:1420, 1995

260. Shine CSK, Kendler DL et al: Radiotherapy in the management of thyroid orbitopathy. Arch Ophthalmol 111:819, 1993

261. Lueder GT, Scott WE, Kutschke PJ, Keech RV: Long-term results of adjustable suture surgery for strabismus secondary to thyroid ophthalmopathy. Ophthalmology 99:993, 1992

262. Kushner BJ: A surgical procedure to minimize lower-eyelid retraction with inferior rectus recession. Arch Ophthalmol 110:1011, 1992

263. Hudson HL, Feldon SE: Late overcorrection of hypotropia in Graves ophthalmopathy. Ophthalmology 99:356, 1992

264. Johns DR: Mitochondrial DNA and disease. N Engl J Med 333:638, 1995

265. Mitsumoto H, Aprille JR, Wray SH et al: Chronic progressive external ophthalmoplegia (CPEO): clinical, morphologic and biochemical studies. Neurology 33:452, 1983

266. Hyman BN, Patten BM, Dodson RF: Mitochondrial abnormalities in progressive external ophthalmoplegia. Am J Ophthalmol 83:362, 1987

267. Seibel P, Lauber J et al: Chronic progressive external ophthalmoplegia is associated with a novel mutation in the mitochondrial tRNA (Asn) gene. Biochem Biophys Res Commun 204:482, 1994

268. Hattori Y, Goto Y et al: Point mutations in mitochondrial tRNA genes: sequence analysis of chronic progressive external ophthalmoplegia (CPEO). J Neurol Sci 125:50, 1994

269. Laforet P, Lombes A, Eymard B et al: Chronic progressive external ophthalmoplegia with ragged-red fibers: clinical, morphological and genetic investigations in 43 patients. Neuromuscul Disord 5:399, 1995

270. Mullie MA, Harding AE, Petty RKH et al: Retinal manifestations of mitochondrial myopathy: a study of 22 cases. Arch Ophthalmol 103:1825, 1985

271. Rowland LP: Molecular genetics, pseudogenetics, and clinical neurology. Neurology 33:1179, 1983

272. Ogasahara S, Yorifuji S, Nishikawa Y et al: Improvement of

abnormal pyruvate metabolism and cardiac conduction defect with coenzyme Q10 in Kearns-Sayre syndrome. Neurology 35:372, 1985

273. Coquet M, Vallat JM, Vital C et al: Nuclear inclusions in oculopharyngeal dystrophy: an ultrastructural study of six cases. J Neurol Sci 60:151, 1983

274. Satoyoshi E, Kinoshita M: Oculopharyngodistal myopathy: report of four families. Arch Neurol 34:89, 1977

275. Ionescu V, Thompson SH, Ionescu R et al: Inherited ophthalmoplegia with intestinal pseudo-obstruction. J Neurol Sci 59:215, 1983

276. Hsu CC, Chuang YH, Tsai JL et al: CPEO and carnitine deficiency overlapping in MELAS syndrome. Acta Neurol Scand 92:252, 1995

277. Flynn JT, Bachynski BN, Rodrigues MM et al: Hyperglycemic acidotic coma and death in Kearns-Sayre syndrome. Trans Am Ophthalmol Soc 83:131, 1985

278. Coulter DL, Allen RJ: Abrupt neurological deterioration in children with Kearns-Sayre syndrome. Arch Neurol 38:247, 1981

279. Litvan I, Agid Y, Caine D et al: Clinical research criteria for the diagnosis of progressive supranuclear palsy (Steele-Richardson-Olszewski syndrome). Neurology 47:1, 1996

280. Jackson JA, Jankovic J, Ford J: Progressive supranuclear palsy: clinical features and response to treatment in 16 patients. Ann Neurol 13:273, 1983

281. Dehaene J: Apraxia of lid opening in progressive supranuclear palsy. Ann Neurol 15:115, 1984

282. Cole DG, Growdon JH: Therapy for progressive supranuclear palsy: past and future. J Neural Transm 42(suppl):283, 1994

283. DiMonte DA, Harati Y et al: Muscle mitochondrial ATP production in progressive supranuclear palsy. J Neurochem 62:1631, 1994

284. Savoiardo M, Girotti F, Strada L, Ciceri E: Magnetic resonance imaging in progressive supranuclear palsy and other parkinsonian disorders. J Neural Transm 42(suppl):93, 1994

285. Calabrese VP, Hadfield MG: Parkinsonism and extraocular motor abnormalities with unusual neuropathological findings. Mov Disord 6:257, 1991

286. Knox DL, Green WR, Troncoso JC et al: Cerebral ocular Whipple's disease: a 62-year odyssey from death to diagnosis. Neurology 45:617, 1995

287. Rabiah PK, Bateman JB, Demer JL, Perlman S: Ophthalmologic findings in patients with ataxia. Am J Ophthalmol 123:108, 1997

288. Shelbourne P, Johnson K: Myotonic dystrophy: another case of too many repeats? Hum Mutat 1:183, 1992

289. Lessell S, Coppeto J, Samet S: Ophthalmoplegia in myotonic dystrophy. Am J Ophthalmol 71:1231, 1971

290. Burian HM, Burns CA: Ocular changes in myotonic dystrophy. Am J Ophthalmol 63:22, 1967

291. Thompson HS, Van Allen MW, von Noorden GK: The pupil in myotonic dystrophy. Invest Ophthalmol 3:325, 1964

292. Hayasaka S, Kiyosawa M, Katsumata S et al: Ciliary and retinal changes in myotonic dystrophy. Arch Ophthalmol 102:88, 1984

293. Pryse-Phillips W, Johnson GJ, Larsen B: Incomplete manifestations of myotonic dystrophy in a large kinship in Labrador. Ann Neurol 11:582, 1982

294. Ter Bruggen JP, Bastiaensen LA, Tyssen CC, Gielen G: Disorders of eye movement in myotonic dystrophy. Brain 113(pt 2):463, 1990

295. Ono S, Kanda F, Takahashi K et al: Neuronal loss in the medullary reticular formation in myotonic dystrophy: a clinicopathological study. Neurology 46:228, 1996

296. Schults WT, Hoyt WF, Behrens M et al: Ocular neuromyotonia: a clinical description of six patients. Arch Ophthalmol 104:1028, 1986

297. Lessell S, Lessell IM, Rizzo JF: Ocular neuromyotonia after radiation therapy. Am J Ophthalmol 102:766, 1986

298. Newman SA: Gaze-induced strabismus (clinical conference). Surv Ophthalmol 38:303, 1993

299. Barroso L, Hoyt WF: Episodic exotropia from lateral rectus neuromyotonia: appearance and remission after radiation therapy for a thalamic glioma. J Pediatr Ophthalmol Strabismus 30:56, 1993

300. Frohman EM, Zee DS: Ocular neuromyotonia clinical features, physiological mechanisms, and response to therapy. Ann Neurol 37:620, 1995

301. Ezra E, Spalton D, Sanders MD et al: Ocular neuromyotonia. Br J Ophthalmol 80:350, 1996

302. Seybold ME, Yoss RE, Hollenhorst RW, Moyer NJ: Pupillary abnormalities associated with tumors of the pineal region. Neurology 21:232, 1971

303. Gressel MG, Hanson MR, Tomsak RL: Reversible Sylvian aqueduct syndrome following jejunoileal bypass. In Smith JL (ed): Neuro-ophthalmology Focus, pp 231–233. New York, Masson, 1981

304. Daras M, Koppel BS, Samkoff L, Marc J: Brain stem toxoplasmosis in patients with acquired immunodeficiency syndrome. J Neuroimaging 4:85, 1994

305. Paulus W, Straube A, Bauer W, Harding AE: Central nervous system involvement in Leber's optic neuropathy. J Neurol 240:251, 1993

306. Neville BGR, Lake BD, Stephens R, Sanders MD: A neurovisceral storage disease with vertical supranuclear ophthalmoplegia, and its relationship to Niemann-Pick disease: a report of nine patients. Brain 96:97, 1973

307. Yan-Go FL, Yanagihara T, Pierre RV, Goldstein NP: A progressive neurologic disorder with supranuclear vertical gaze paresis and distinctive bone marrow cells. Mayo Clin Proc 59:404, 1984

308. Shulman LM, David NJ, Weiner WJ: Psychosis as the initial manifestation of adult-onset Niemann-Pick disease type C. Neurology 45:1739, 1995

309. Palmer M, Green WR, Maumenee IH et al: Niemann-Pick disease—type C. Arch Ophthalmol 103:817, 1985

310. Kirkham TH, Kamin DF: Slow saccadic eye movements in Wilson's disease. J Neurol Neurosurg Psychiatry 37:191, 1974

311. Hoyt CS, Bilson FA, Alpins N: The supranuclear disturbances of gaze in kernicterus. Ann Ophthalmol 10:1487, 1978

312. Edis RH, Mastaglia FL: Vertical gaze palsy in barbiturate intoxication. Br Med J 1:144, 1977

313. Hamed LM, Mancuso A: Inferior rectus muscle contracture syndrome after retrobulbar anesthesia. Ophthalmology 98:1506, 1991

314. Hamilton SM, Elsas FJ, Dawson TL: A cluster of patients with inferior rectus restriction following local anesthesia for cataract surgery. J Pediatr Ophthalmol Strabismus 30:288, 1993

315. Hunter DG, Lam GC, Guyton DL: Inferior oblique muscle injury from local anesthesia for cataract surgery. Ophthalmology 102:501, 1995

316. Muñoz M: Letter to the Editor: Inferior rectus muscle overaction after cataract extraction. Am J Ophthalmol 118:664, 1994

317. Capó H, Roth E, Johnson T et al: Vertical strabismus after cataract surgery. Ophthalmology 103:918, 1996

318. Muñoz M, Parrish RK II: Strabismus following implantation of Baerveldt drainage devices. Arch Ophthalmol 111:1096, 1993

319. Smith SL, Starita RJ, Fellman RL, Lynn JR: Early clinical experience with the Baerveldt 350-mm² glaucoma implant and associated extraocular muscle imbalance. Ophthalmology 100:914, 1993

320. Cornblath WT, Elner V, Rolfe M: Extraocular muscle involvement in sarcoidosis. Ophthalmology 100:501, 1993

321. Patel AS, Kelman SE, Duncan GW, Rismondo V: Painless diplopia caused by extraocular muscle sarcoid. Arch Ophthalmol 112:879, 1994

322. Hakin KN, McNab AA, Sullivan TJ: Spontaneous hemorrhage within the rectus muscle. Ophthalmology 101:1631, 1994

323. Harris GJ, Murphy ML et al: Orbital myositis as a paraneoplastic syndrome. Arch Ophthalmol 112:380, 1994

324. Leib ML, Odel JG, Cooney MJ: Orbital polymyositis and giant cell myocarditis. Ophthalmology 101:950, 1994

325. Atabay C, Tyutyunikov A et al: Serum antibodies reactive with eye muscle membrane antigens are detected in patients with nonspecific orbital inflammation. Ophthalmology 102:145, 1995

CHAPTER 13

Pediatric Neuro-ophthalmology: General Considerations and Congenital Motor and Sensory Anomalies

R. Michael Siatkowski and Joel S. Glaser

The Patient Encounter
Visual Development
The Blind Infant
Acquired Visual Loss in Childhood
Congenital Motor Anomalies
  Anomalies of Innervation
    Duane Retraction Syndrome
    Möbius Syndrome (Congenital Bulbar Palsies)
    Elevator Deficiencies
    Vertical Retraction Syndrome
    Synergistic Divergence
    Marcus Gunn Jaw-Winking Synkineses
  Restrictive Syndromes
    Brown Tendon Sheath Syndrome
    Congenital Familial Fibrosis Syndrome
Nystagmus and Related Disorders
  Congenital Nystagmus
  Latent Nystagmus
  Periodic Alternating Nystagmus
  Heimann-Bielschowsky Phenomenon
  Congenital Ocular Motor Apraxia

  Spasmus Nutans
  Ocular Flutter/Opsoclonus
Dyslexia
Headache in Children
  Pediatric Migraine
  Pediatric Pseudotumor Cerebri
Ocular Motor Cranial Neuropathies
Symptomatic Sensory and Strabismic Abnormalities
  Failure of Fusional Mechanisms
    Acquired Central Defects
    Congenital Anomalies
    Acquired Visual Loss
  Special Forms of Acquired Esotropia
    Acute Comitant Esotropia
    Cyclic Esotropia
    Progressive Esotropia with Myopia
  Problems at Near
    Convergence Insufficiencies
    Accommodative Effort Syndrome
Ocular Torticollis

The question as to the origin of squint has been discussed for more than two centuries. Innumerable theories have been published, not one of them applicable to all the different kinds of strabismus.

Lectures on the Motor Anomalies
Alfred Bielschowsky, 1938

Neuro-ophthalmologic problems of congenital origin or childhood onset may come to diagnostic attention in

R. M. Siatkowski: Department of Ophthalmology, Dean A. McGee Eye Institute, University of Oklahoma, Oklahoma City, Oklahoma

J. S. Glaser: Departments of Neurology and Ophthalmology, Bascom Palmer Eye Institute, University of Miami School of Medicine, Miami; and Neuro-ophthalmology, Cleveland Clinic Florida, Ft. Lauderdale, Florida

infancy (the blind baby), later in childhood (the grade school child with migraine), or in some cases, not until adulthood, when a congenital motor or sensory defect may be attributed to an acquired abnormality. For example, Duane retraction syndrome may be confused with a sixth nerve palsy, or anisometropic amblyopia may be interpreted as an acquired optic neuropathy. This chapter reviews and summarizes many of the important entities that fall into these potentially confounding categories.

THE PATIENT ENCOUNTER

Children are not "little adults" and infants are not even "little children." Accordingly, the neuroophthal-

TABLE 13–1. Neurodevelopmental Milestones

Behavioral event	Age
Sucking, rooting, and swallowing reflexes	Neonatal period
Lifts head in sitting position	4 mo
Rolls over	6 mo
Sits up	9–10 mo
Crawls	10–11 mo
Walks unassisted	12–15 mo
Walks up and down stairs holding on	18 mo
Can stand on one foot	3 yr

mologic history in infancy and childhood must be selectively focused; inquiries must often be directed toward the details of the pregnancy and postpartum period, including the gestational age, maternal illnesses, medications used during pregnancy, infant birth weight, Apgar scores, and use of perinatal oxygen. A detailed family history of ocular, neurologic, or musculoskeletal problems, as well as parental consanguinity must be explored. Neuro-developmental milestones (Table 13–1) should be documented when indicated; height, weight, and head circumference should be charted on standard nomograms.

Because the attention span of infants and children is quite limited, the physical examination must be conducted in a relatively brief time period. Simple inspection may allow the examiner to assess skull, facial, and other physical anomalies; note the presence of lid malposition or globe displacement; evaluate spontaneous ductional eye movements or the presence of nystagmus; and assess cognitive and, to some extent, visual function.

Vision in infants is evaluated by noting response to light or hand-motion threat, the accuracy of the fixation reflex toward a hand-light or other attractive object, and the capacity of each eye to follow during contralateral occlusion. In many cases, an infant's gross objection to occlusion of one eye, by crying or avoiding or pushing away the occluder, will provide the first clue that vision in the uncovered eye is significantly impaired. Elicitation of optokinetic nystagmus assesses a visual sensory, as well as a motor, response.

The measurement of grating acuity by forced preferential looking tests (Teller acuity cards) is arguably the most useful method of obtaining reliable, reproducible, quantifiable information on visual acuity in infants and nonverbal children (Fig. 13–1).[1-3] However, some have questioned the definition of "normal limits." Kushner et al[4] noted the often poor correlation between Teller (grating) acuity and Snellen (optotype recognition) acuity, the former yielding significantly better results, particularly when Snellen acuity is less than 20/70. It has been suggested that Teller acuity card testing results are imprecise and should not be used by social service agencies to determine legal blindness.[5] Vernier acuity may also be measured in infants and children using preferential looking techniques.[6] This may be more sensitive than grating acuity in detecting visual changes due to amblyopia. Clinical strategies for measuring visual acuity in children are summarized in Table 13–2.

Infants and children present particular challenges for successful visual evoked potential (VEP) recording, including their sleep-wake status, often poor postural positioning of the patient, and the inability to control and monitor ocular fixation and accommodation. Overestimation of acuity by VEP, particularly in amblyopia, may occur[7]; thus, for each laboratory, normative data for age group must be established. In many centers, VEP testing

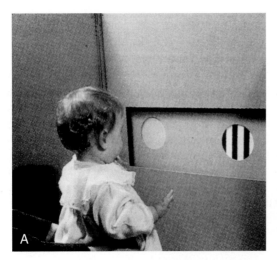
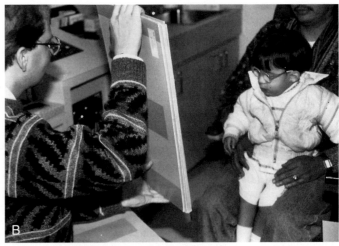

Fig. 13–1. A. The examiner, masked to orientation of the stripes in the cards, evaluates visually directed eye movements during Teller acuity card testing. **B.** Cards may be presented at closer distances for children with low vision; vertical presentation is particularly helpful for patients with horizontal nystagamus.

TABLE 13–2. Clinical Applications of Vision Testing in Children

Neonatal
Phototropism (turning toward light)
Avoidance of bright light

Infancy
Fixation and following behavior
Optokinetic responses
Forced preferential looking test (Teller acuity cards)
Pattern visual evoked potential

Childhood
Allen pictures
Snellen "E"
Landolt "C"
H-O-T-V letter game
Snellen acuity

for the purpose of measuring acuity is unrewarding and inaccurate. However, in standardized laboratories with experienced personnel who are comfortable and familiar with administering the test, the visual evoked response, particularly *pattern* VEP, may be useful for monitoring visual development in both preterm and full-term infants.[8]

The visual field in infants may be assessed by gross confrontation mechanisms, such as visually evoked eye movements or withdrawal or fright to threatening maneuvers (see Figs. 2–13 through 2–15). Hemifield defects are easily detected when a child regularly fails to look at an object of interest (such as a toy) held in the nonseeing field. The patient's response to simultaneous presentation of objects in both hemifields can be assessed. Visually elicited eye movements are quite easily noted by the examiner. By 3 years of age, children are able to comply with finger-mimicking tests. An experienced examiner is frequently able to perform simple kinetic perimetry in children older than 5 years, and many children aged 7 years and older are able to perform suprathreshold automated static perimetric testing, which may be presented as a "video-game" with rewards for "good scores."

VISUAL DEVELOPMENT

Visual and ocular developmental milestones are summarized in Table 13–3. The "critical period" of visual development refers to the period early in infancy when the visual system is sensitive to deprivation. It is believed that two different types of visual processing occur. *Magnocellular* (M) pathways deal with perception of motion, whereas *parvocellular* (P) neurons are more attuned to image shape and color (see Chapter 4). These two pathways are separated at the retinal ganglion cell level through to the lateral geniculate nucleus, and are represented in different areas in layer V-1 of the striate cortex.

The parieto-occipital extrastriate cortex deals more with motion perception, whereas the temporo-occipital region is concerned with image shape and color. There is direct neural communication between these two areas. Maldevelopment of the magnocellular system occurs with infantile esotropia, latent and congenital nystagmus, impairment of gross stereopsis, and motion VEP deficits. Maldevelopment of the P system is associated with anisometropic and strabismic amblyopia, deficits in fine stereopsis, and spatial sweep VEP deficits.[9]

Although normal binocular vision requires aligned eyes with intact sensory and motor fusion mechanisms, in the first few months of life some children have intermittent or constant ocular deviations, most commonly exotropia. Nevertheless, in normal infants, at about 3 months of age, there is a relatively rapid maturation of binocularity, including fusional convergence and sensory fusion (stereopsis). It has been hypothesized that refinement of cortical circuits, particularly those in the ocular dominance columns, occurs during this period of instability.[10] It is well documented that children with esotropia, amblyopia, or early visual deprivation have asymmetric monocular pursuit noted on optokinetic

TABLE 13–3. Visual and Ocular Developmental Milestones

Event	Age
Pupilllary light reaction	30 wks' gestation
Lid closure and response to bright light	30 wks' gestation
Visual fixation	Birth
Blink response to visual threat	2–5 mo
Well-developed fixation	6–9 wk
Visual following well developed	3 mo
Accommodation well developed	4 mo
Visual acuity potential at adult level by visual evoked potential	6–12 mo
Grating preferential (Teller) acuity at adult level	3 yr
Snellen acuity at adult level	2–5 yr
End of critical period for monocular visual deprivation	8–12 yr
Conjugate horizontal gaze well developed	Birth
Conjugate vertical gaze well developed	2 mo
Ocular alignment stable	1–3 mo
Fusional convergence well developed	6 mo
Stereopsis well developed	6 mo
Stereoacuity at adult level	7 yr
Foveal maturation completed	4 mo
Myelination of optic nerve completed	7–24 mo
Iris stromal pigmentation well developed	6 mo

(Modified from Greenwald MJ: Pediatr Clin North Am 30:977, 1983)

nystagmus testing, favoring targets moving in a temporal-to-nasal direction; however, the presence of normal stereoacuity and binocular function is not necessarily sufficient to prevent this bias.[11] The relationship among binocularity, fusion, visual deprivation, and monocular optokinetic nystagmus asymmetry is complex and not precisely understood.

Visual development in infants with severe ocular disorders (*e.g.*, retinal dystrophies, congenital optic nerve anomalies) may show delayed improvement of assessable visual function later in childhood, even up to several years.[12] Continuing posterior visual pathway maturation may be the mechanism responsible for late visual improvement in some cases. Of course, significant improvement in visual acuity as a result of amblyopia therapy may also occur in patients with either unilateral or bilateral, asymmetric structural abnormalities.[13] It is imperative that the clinician exercise restraint when attempting to predict final levels of visual function in such children.

THE BLIND INFANT

Assessment of the infant with subnormal or absent visual responses usually distinguishes between two major groups: those with and those without *congenital nystagmus*. Congenital nystagmus (see below) may appear as a jerk or pendular horizontal, uniplanar eye movement disorder, which frequently diminishes on convergence and is absent during sleep. In the past, congenital nystagmus has been divided into "sensory" and "motor" types. Although these concepts may be helpful clinically, they do not accurately reflect the underlying pathophysiology or the complex foveation strategies that the ocular motor system employs. It should be noted that a variety of other clinical features may be encountered in congenital nystagmus, including inversion of the optokinetic response and vertical or torsional movements (see Chapter 11).

Congenital nystagmus occurs in 1 in 1000 to 6550 births, and it is frequently associated with bilateral visual loss of prechiasmal or chiasmal origin.[14] When occurring in the presence of bilateral corneal or lens opacities, optic nerve disorders, or macular disease, the diagnosis is straightforward. In the infant population, Gelbart and Hoyt[15] demonstrated anterior visual pathway disease in 119 of 152 patients with congenital nystagmus, including diagnoses of bilateral optic nerve hypoplasia, Leber's congenital amaurosis, and ocular or oculocutaneous albinism. Likewise, Cibis and Fitzgerald[16] noted bilateral retinal disease in 56% of patients with congenital nystagmus. Unilateral anomalies, however, allow development of normal foveation in the sound eye and, with rare exception, are not associated with congenital nystagmus. Typically, congenital nystagmus does not present until the third or fourth month of life, when central, steady fixation and foveation should be established in normal infants.

In an infant with poor vision and nystagmus, but with an apparently otherwise normal eye examination, electroretinography (ERG) should be performed. Lambert et al[17] reviewed this clinical scenario. *Leber's congenital amaurosis* is an autosomal-recessive retinal rod/cone disorder that causes poor vision from birth. Although initial fundus examination may be unremarkable, pigmentary retinopathy, vessel attenuation, and optic atrophy occur over time. ERG shows nonrecordable or grossly attenuated electrical potentials of both rods and cones ("flat ERG") (Fig. 13–2). Although initial acuity is quite poor, it is unlikely to deteriorate substantially over the course of the patient's life.[18] No treatment is available. *Achromatopsia* (rod monochromatism) is an autosomal-recessive or X-linked disease characterized by a partial or complete absence of retinal cone function. Acuity is generally better than in Leber's amaurosis and frequently exceeds 20/200. In this condition, the rod ERG is normal while the cone ERG is significantly impaired (Fig. 13–3). Photophobia, which may be marked, is quite common, and these children show marked preference for dim lighting. Other hereditary retinal disorders may be seen in *Joubert syndrome* (cerebellar vermis hypoplasia), *congenital stationary night-blindness*, *Refsum's disease*, *neonatal adrenoleukodystrophy*, *neuronal ceroid lipofuscinosis*, *Jeune syndrome*, and *osteopetrosis*. Patients with *albinism* and *aniridia*, both of which may be associated with foveal (and optic nerve) hypoplasia, may present with congenital nystagmus. Anomalous (excessive) chiasmal crossing defects and cortical miswiring[19] have been reported in ocular albinism. Note that the nystagmus in association with disorders of bilateral anterior visual pathway disease should not be confused with the bilateral "manifest latent nystagmus" seen in patients with monocular decreased vision, which acts as an occluder, thus manifesting what otherwise would have been truly latent nystagmus (see Chapter 11).[20]

Optic nerve hypoplasia, unless subtle, is usually diagnosed on fundus examination. If bilateral, this condition may be associated with congenital nystagmus. *De Morsier syndrome* (septo-optic dysplasia) refers to the constellation of bilateral optic nerve hypoplasia, absence of the septum pellucidum, thinning or absence of the corpus callosum, dysplasia of the anterior third ventricle, and pituitary dysfunction (see Fig. 5–9). Brodsky and Glasier[21] broadened the spectrum of this condition. In a study of 40 children, some optic nerve anomalies were isolated, but in other children, midline craniofacial defects, hemispheric gray matter dystrophic anomalies, and posterior pituitary ectopia were noted. Of 21 cases of optic nerve hypoplasia described by Zeki et al,[22] there were midline central nervous system defects in 6 and endocrine deficiencies in 9. In the series of 35 patients

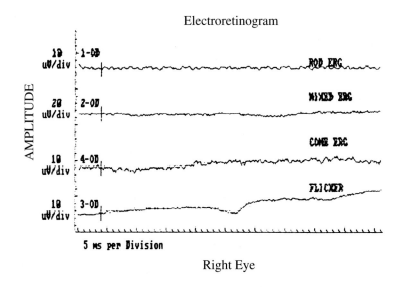

Fig. 13–2. ERG from patient with Leber's congenital amaurosis demonstrates absent rod and cone responses.

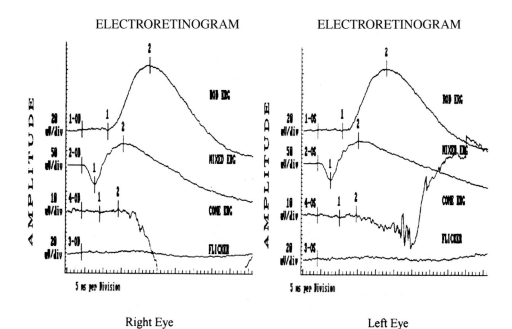

	Amplitude (uV) RE / LE	Timing (ms) RE / LE
ROD ERG		
b-wave	326.6.0 / 311.0	93.5 / 94.0
MIXED ERG		
b-wave	515.9 / 499.4	57.0 / 55.5
a-wave	209.1 / 245.7	17.5 / 18.0
CONE ERG		
single flash b-wave	14.2 / 12.3	50.5 / 53.0
30 Hz flicker	-- / --	-- / --

Fig. 13–3. ERG from a patient with achromatopsia. Rod (**top**) and mixed (**second**) tracings are normal, but the cone flash and flicker responses (**bottom** two tracings) are severely reduced or absent.

with bilateral optic nerve hypoplasia described by Siatkowski et al,[23] neuroradiographic abnormalities were seen in 46% and endocrinopathies in 27%. Growth hormone deficiency was the most common endocrine abnormality. The visual spectrum ranged from 20/20 in one case to no light perception in 34% of patients; 80% were legally blind (20/200 or less in both eyes). Absence of the septum pellucidum and corpus callosum, with panhypopituitarism, occurred in only 11.5% of all patients with bilateral optic nerve hypoplasia.

Optic disc colobomata (Fig. 13–4), if bilateral, may be seen in association with congenital nystagmus. Of greater import, however, is the association of colobomas or other dysplastic optic discs with basal encephaloceles, particularly in conjunction with hypertelorism, midfacial anomalies, or tongue-shaped retinochoroidal pigmentary disturbances.[24] The morning glory disc syndrome, although typically unilateral, does not present in association with nystagmus, but may rarely be seen with midline central nervous system defects and endocrinopathies as well.[25]

The infant with poor vision and no nystagmus is likely to have visual impairment on an occipital basis. Good et al[26] extensively reviewed this entity. These patients have normal pupillary light reaction, unremarkable fundi, and absence of nystagmus; however, they do have various neurobehavioral signs of cortical visual impairment:

1. They have a preference for brightly colored objects and stare at bright lights (although up to one third may have photophobia).
2. They adopt peculiar head turns when attempting to look at or reach for an object of interest, because peripheral visual field, rather than central vision, is used.
3. They may use extrageniculate vision, or "blindsight," in some cases enabling them to localize targets or

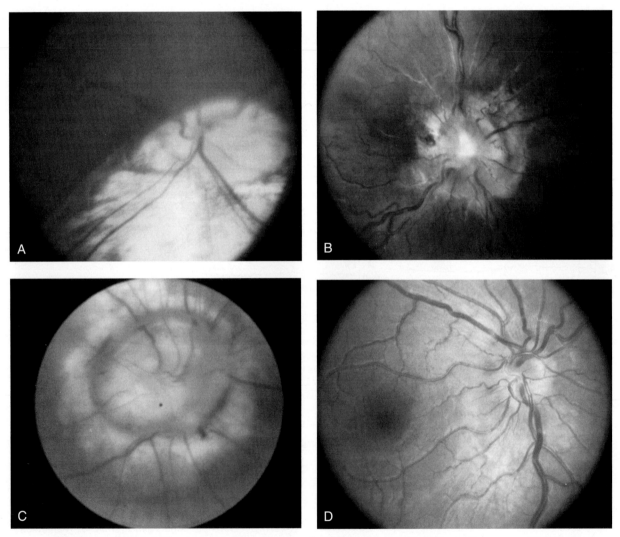

Fig. 13–4. Spectrum of congenital disc anamolies. **A.** Large coloboma involving optic nerve and inferior retina. **B.** Dysplastic disc, central cup filled with fibroglial tissue. **C.** Morning glory disc anamoly. **D.** Markedly hypoplastic optic nerve.

to see colors. This concept remains much in debate however, and many instances of "blindsight" may, in fact, be due to preservation of some portions of visual cortex.

4. They exhibit varying degrees of alertness and employ idiosyncratic visual "strategies" to use patches of visual field remnants.

Prognosis for recovery depends on etiology, age of onset, and severity of brain damage. Although such children remain visually handicapped, dramatic recovery may occasionally ensue.[26] Cortical visual loss from perinatal hypoxia/ischemia has a particularly poor prognosis if congenital, but up to a 70% recovery rate if acquired.[27]

Delayed maturation of vision is a diagnosis of exclusion and retrospection.[28] This pertains to visually impaired infants with normal ocular examinations, normal neuroimaging and ERG, and no nystagmus. The exact etiology is unknown. Delayed myelination of the posterior visual pathways has been implicated, but in most cases, magnetic resonance imaging (MRI) shows age-appropriate myelination. Another hypothesis is that eye movement abnormalities (apraxia) may be misinterpreted as poor vision. This retrospective diagnosis should be made only when visual function indeed spontaneously improves to normal or near-normal levels, as best ascertainable by the end of the first year of life.

Children with unilateral hemianopic defects may adopt a head turn toward the side of the field defect so that the eyes are rotated toward the objects of visual interest. In addition, many of these children develop an exotropia,[29,30] possibly to increase the panoramic visual field in compensation for the underlying hemianopic defect. It has been suggested that strabismus surgery in these children should, therefore, be avoided.

ACQUIRED VISUAL LOSS IN CHILDHOOD

Hereditary optic atrophies, neuroretinitis, optic nerve tumors, and trauma are discussed in Chapter 5 of this text. A few statements, however, are in order regarding several entities.

Optic neuritis has somewhat different characteristics in the pediatric population than in adults. Various authors have reviewed this entity.[31-34] Childhood optic neuritis commonly presents as simultaneous bilateral papillitis (see Fig. 5–22). Antecedent viral illnesses, ranging from upper respiratory infections to varicella, mumps, and mononucleosis, may precede visual loss by 2 to 6 weeks. Initial visual acuity is typically poor, 20/200 or less, in many instances. Cerebrospinal fluid pleocytosis and elevated protein are common, but the eventual association with multiple sclerosis appears less frequent in children than in adults. Prompt responses (within days)

to systemic corticosteroids in doses ranging from 1 mg/kg prednisone to high-dose intravenous methylprednisolone are the rule. Steroid taper over several weeks is recommended to reduce rebound inflammation. Although MRI may in some cases demonstrate optic nerve enhancement or cortical white matter lesions, the results of the Optic Neuritis Treatment Trial (see Chapter 5) are not applicable to children.

Leber's hereditary optic neuropathy commonly presents in the second decade of life,[35] but several cases occurring within the first decade have also been reported.[36-38] There is some evidence that those patients with the mtDNA 14484 mutation presenting in the second decade may show a higher incidence of spontaneous visual recovery, generally within 12 to 18 months of the initial visual loss.[35]

Anterior visual pathway gliomas account for the bulk of intrinsic optic nerve tumors in childhood. Although they are true neoplasms, malignant features are extraordinarily rare in the pediatric population (see Chapter 5). Dutton[39] provided a thorough review of this subject. When the glioma is initially confined to the optic nerve alone, the mortality rate is 5%. However, when the hypothalamus is involved, survival is less than 50% in some series. With a typically indolent course, these tumors can generally be managed conservatively, especially when confined to the optic nerve. Hoffman et al[40] reviewed 62 cases of optic pathway/hypothalamic gliomas over a 14-year period, with 48 of these exhibiting relative stability with only visual defects: 6 patients had significant neurologic abnormalities, and 8 died. Spontaneous regression and visual improvement has also been reported[41,42]; this phenomenon may be more likely in those patients with neurofibromatosis.

Tumors abutting the visual system that may cause progressive visual loss by extrinsic compression, including craniopharyngiomas, are discussed in Chapter 5.

Other causes of *progressive* visual loss in childhood are those syndromes associated with retinal pigmentary abiotrophies (tapetoretinal degenerations). These have a later onset than the congenital photoreceptor dystrophies, which profoundly affect vision at birth, and are generally stable. Included among these progressive retinal degenerations are the Bardet-Biedl syndrome (an autosomal-recessive disorder of polydactyly, obesity, hypogenitalism, renal disease, and tapetoretinal degeneration); Refsum's disease; Bassen-Kornzweig syndrome (abetalipoproteinemia with intestinal malabsorption); and Kearns-Sayre syndrome (progressive external ophthalmoplegia [see Chapter 12]).

Aicardi's syndrome consists of agenesis of the corpus callosum, chorioretinal lacunae (Fig. 13–5), and infantile spasms with seizures. The condition is limited to females and, with one exception, is lethal in males. Additional ocular features may include microphthalmia, optic nerve colobomas, and peripapillary glial tissue.[43,44]

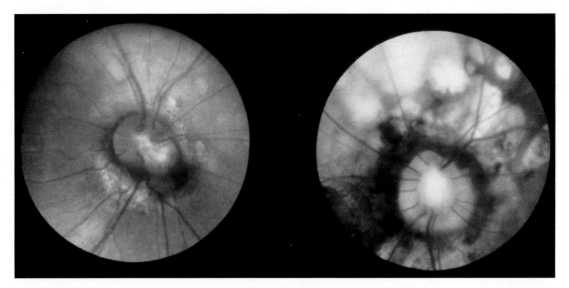

Fig. 13–5. Fundus of a 3-year-old girl with Aicardi's syndrome. Note dysplastic optic discs surrounded by hypopigmented retinal lacunae. (Courtesy of John T. Flynn, MD)

CONGENITAL MOTOR ANOMALIES

Anomalies of Innervation

For many decades, clinical descriptions of eye movements, coupled with gross observations made during surgery, have generated a preoccupation with malformations of extraocular muscles, fascial connections, tendon sheaths, or check ligaments. In addition, the phenomena of "overacting" and "underacting" single ocular muscles are invoked by way of "explanations" of defective motor patterns. Currently, electromyography (EMG) provides a technique whereby the electrical activity of extraocular muscles may be sampled. Thus, an interest in the neural basis of paradoxical ocular motor defects has been renewed.

Hoyt and Nachtigaller[45] reviewed the evidence for peripheral anomalies in the number and distribution of human ocular motor nerves, and have catalogued examples of omission, substitution, and duplication. In the dissection room, absence of the abducens nerve(s) has been documented, as well as agenesis of the sixth nerve nucleus, despite the presence of normal lateral rectus muscles. The lateral rectus may indeed be aggrandized by the oculomotor nerve in the absence of an abducens nerve, or it may receive a dual innervation from both the abducens and oculomotor nerve.[45] In 1919, Magath[46] reported the finding of a superior rectus muscle innervated by a branch of the abducens nerve as well as by a branch of the superior division of the oculomotor nerve. In none of the foregoing anatomic studies was clinical information available, and the incidence of such anomalies of innervation cannot be assessed. Phillips et al[47] reported pathologic correlation in a 5-year-old girl with bilateral abducens palsy, who died during surgical correction of convergent strabis-

mus; neither abducens nerve was present, and the corresponding nuclei were diminutive. Rarely is such clinico-anatomic correlation possible, but sufficient material has accrued to validate the concept of "congenital miswiring," including both failure of innervation and anomalous annexation of extraocular muscles by inappropriate nerve branches.

Simultaneous electrical activity in agonist-antagonist pairs of extraocular muscles (co-firing, co-contraction) has been documented on EMG, further substantiating the role of anomalous innervation in the production of paradoxical eye movements. For example, since the early work of Blodi,[48] such paradoxical innervation of one of the horizontal rectus muscles is the most outstanding and consistent feature of Duane retraction syndrome.

Although birth trauma is often invoked to explain congenital ocular motor defects, their association with other congenital neural and musculoskeletal defects, as well as their occurrence in members of the same family, make this explanation rarely tenable.

Duane Retraction Syndrome

This syndrome is so named because of retraction of the globe and narrowing of the lid fissure, which occur on attempted adduction (Fig. 13–6). Huber[49] classified three patterns as follows:

Type I: Palsy of abduction with retraction on adduction
Type II: Palsy of adduction with retraction, and intact abduction
Type III: Palsy of adduction and abduction, with retraction on attempted adduction

According to both Blodi[48] and Huber,[49] EMG evi-

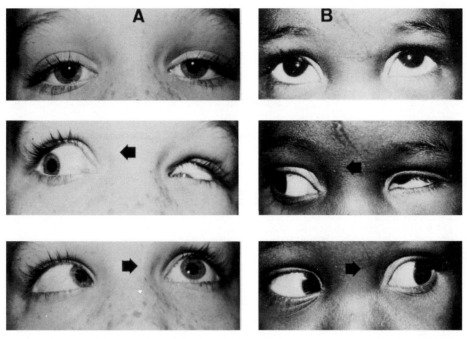

Fig. 13–6. Duane retraction syndrome. **A.** Type I. Forward gaze, eyes straight with slightly narrowed left fissure. Right gaze, retraction of left globe with downward oblique deviation. Left gaze, failure of abduction. **B.** Type II. Forward gaze, slight exotropia. Right gaze, retraction of left globe with upward oblique deviation. Left gaze, normal abduction.

dence of paradoxical innervation is incontrovertible: that is, electrical activity increases in a seemingly "paretic" muscle (Fig. 13–7). It is conceivable that Duane types I and II represent dual innervation of the lateral rectus by both the abducens and oculomotor nerves, whereas type III represents innervation of the medial and lateral recti by the oculomotor nerve. At any rate, retraction of the globe is caused by synchronous contraction (co-contraction) of the horizontal recti, and not for strictly mechanical reasons. Additionally, it is likely that orbital mechanical factors play a role in the globe retraction seen in Duane syndrome.[50]

There are several reported autopsies of patients with clinically assessed Duane syndrome. Matteucci[51] reported a case of unilateral Duane syndrome with a normal medial rectus, but a hypoplastic lateral rectus and hypoplastic abducens nucleus and nerve. In a patient with bilateral Duane syndrome, Hotchkiss et al[52] found bilateral absence of abducens nuclei and nerves; both lateral recti were partially innervated by branches from the inferior division of the oculomotor nerve and appeared histologically normal in innervated areas, but fibrotic in areas not innervated. Miller et al,[53] in a Duane type I patient who had had eye-movement recordings before death, demonstrated that the left abducens nerve was absent and, as in the previous case, the lateral rectus was innervated by branches from the inferior division of the third nerve, with fibrosis in areas not innervated, but normal in innervated areas. These studies provide elegant support for the hypothesis derived from previ-

ous EMG studies. Hickey and Wagoner[54] presented a pathologic study of bilaterally absent abducens, and argued that Möbius and Duane syndromes, as well as congenital horizontal gaze paralysis, represent different degrees of severity in the spectrum of developmental abnormalities that involve a small area of pontine tegmentum, which in all cases is found to be disorganized and hypoplastic.

Documentation of other brain stem abnormalities has been inconclusive. Jay and Hoyt[55] found brain stem auditory-evoked potential abnormalities in 9 of 14 patients with Duane syndrome (increased latency of wave III), but other authors[56,57] could not confirm this finding. Gourdeau et al[58] reported somewhat slowed adduction saccades in the sound eye, and asymmetric vestibulo-ocular reflex, optokinetic nystagmus, and after-nystagmus in five cases; they concluded that premotor brain stem structures (vestibular nuclei, medial longitudinal fasciculus, and paramedian pontine reticular formation) were abnormal in these patients. Metz,[59] however, found normal saccadic velocities in the sound eye of Duane syndrome patients. Hedera and Friedland[60] reported on a 36-year-old man with Duane syndrome and a giant aneurysm at the vertebral-basilar junction, providing support for an embryologic vascular etiology. Additionally, Saad and Lee[61] demonstrated paradoxical medial rectus EMG activity in patients with Duane syndrome type I, further lending support to the presence of a brain stem anomaly.

In all types of Duane syndrome, vertical deviations

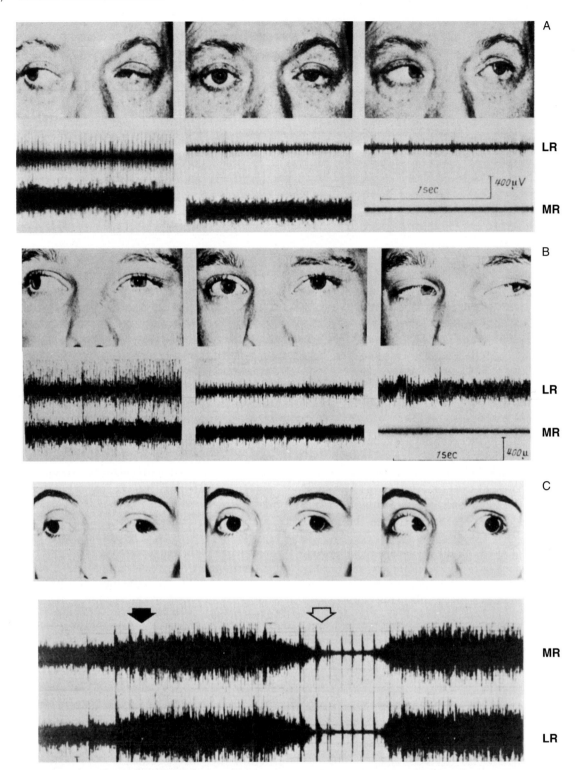

Fig. 13–7. Electromyography in Duane retraction syndrome. Simultaneous recordings of left lateral rectus (*LR*) and medial rectus (*MR*). **A.** Type I. Peak innervation of lateral rectus on right gaze (paradoxic innervation) and minimal innervation on left gaze. Normal electrical behavior of medial rectus throughout. **B.** Type II. Lateral rectus innervation on both right and left gaze. Normal electrical behavior of medial rectus throughout. **C.** Type III. Synchronous and strikingly similar electrical activity in both recti, with intense firing in right gaze (*black arrow*) and marked inhibition in left gaze (*open arrow*). (Huber A: Electrophysiology of the retraction syndromes. Br J Ophthalmol 58:293, 1974)

of the adducting eye may take the form of "upshoots and downshoots" (see Fig. 13–6). Scott and Wong[62] recorded increased activity in both the inferior oblique and superior rectus muscles during upshoot in adduction, most consistently in the superior rectus. However, a tightly fibrosed lateral rectus insertion may also act as a mechanical leash, causing dynamic vertical "overaction."[63]

According to Raab[64] and others, Duane syndrome occurs more commonly in women (about 2 : 1 over men), and the left eye is involved perhaps three times more commonly than the right eye. Approximately 10% to 18% of cases are bilateral. Approximately 75% of cases are type I; type II cases are much rarer. In bilateral cases, types I and II may coincide. Familial cases are not uncommon, and bilateral retraction has been reported in monozygotic twins.[65] Duane syndrome has also been reported in association with abnormalities on chromosomes 4q[66] and 22.[67]

Patients with Duane syndrome may demonstrate a peculiar sensory adaptation, with excellent binocular function in directions of gaze where visual axes are aligned, and suppression without diplopia in the field of the affected lateral rectus (i.e., a facultative suppression scotoma, as is employed in intermittent exotropia). Occasionally, mild amblyopia may be present in the involved eye, but the reported incidence of amblyopia varies greatly, as does the incidence of anisometropia.[68] A few patients who as children became accustomed to avoiding the diplopic field, may present as adults complaining of an "acute" onset of diplopia. However, microtropia or larger angles of strabismus may be present, convergence is often poor, and sensory adaptations are complex and sometimes tenuous in any case. Age-related deterioration in fusion ability and in convergence can produce symptoms of diplopia and asthenopia.

Certainly surgery on the adult Duane syndrome patient can upset a delicate sensory balance. As a rule, surgery should be considered only when patients have cosmetically unacceptable strabismus in the primary position or significantly anomalous head positions. Some suggest splitting the lateral rectus into a "Y" configuration, to diminish the "leashing" effect of a taut lateral rectus muscle.[69] Pressman and Scott[63] recommended using the adjustable suture technique for recession of the appropriate horizontal rectus muscle. Additionally, surgery on the normal eye may in some cases be the best approach for producing the widest range of postoperative fusion. Full-tendon transpositions of the superior or inferior recti to the lateral rectus (Type I) or the medial rectus (Type II), with or without posterior fixation sutures, may also yield excellent alignment and even afford some degree of abduction or adduction.

Pfaffenbach et al[70] reviewed 186 cases of Duane retraction syndrome and noted the association with congenital malformations of the face, ear, and upper verte-bral column. Numerous congenital ocular, skeletal, and neural anomalies have been seen in Duane syndrome, including (1) congenital gustolacrimal reflex[71] ("crocodile tears") ipsilateral to a Duane syndrome type I, but without facial palsy; and (2) Marcus Gunn jaw-winking phenomenon[72] (see below). Both represent "miswiring" phenomena. These associations again provide substantial evidence of a central pathophysiologic basis for Duane syndrome.

Duane retraction may accompany other syndrome complexes encompassing ear and cervical spine anomalies, including (1) Wildervanck cervico-oculoacoustic triad of Klippel-Feil spine deformity, sensorineural deafness, and Duane syndrome; and (2) Goldenhar variant of hemifacial microsomia.[73]

Retraction of the globe somewhat mimicking Duane syndrome may be seen with acquired orbital lesions that cause mechanical restriction. The chronic fibrotic changes of extraocular muscles in Graves' disease may cause a leash effect, most typically observed on abduction attempts, but possible on gaze opposite the field(s) of action of any involved muscle(s). The tethering also prevents full ductional range, and forced-duction testing (see Chapter 12) confirms the restrictive process. Proptosis and other orbital congestive signs are generally present. Similarly, infiltration of muscles by granulomatous inflammation (orbital pseudotumor) or by carcinoma may cause restrictive contraction, but rarely to the degree observed in Duane syndrome.[74] Medial orbital wall fractures can entrap the medial rectus muscle, with variable abduction limitation and globe retraction,[75] and retraction also has been reported with muscle fixations due to orbital metastases.[76] For more detailed information, the reader is referred to the comprehensive review by DeRespinis et al.[77]

Möbius Syndrome (Congenital Bulbar Palsies)

The discovery in 1888 of the condition of facial diplegia of variable degree associated with paralysis of lateral gaze, and usually esotropia, is attributed to Möbius. Although traditionally considered simply as palsies of the facial and abducens nerves, EMG and neuropathologic evidence indicates a more complex situation, as does involvement of other body systems. Variable associations include tongue hemiatrophy; head and extremity deformities; abnormalities of lower cranial nerves, producing hearing, speech, and swallowing difficulties; chest malformations; congenital heart defects; mental retardation; and Kallmann syndrome (hypogonadism and anosmia).[73,78,79] Although generally considered a static neonatal disorder, there have been reports of progressive, increasing motor deficits during later life.

Clinically, children present with feeding problems because of their inability to suck, and their lack of facial expression is noted especially when crying (Fig. 13–8). Because vertical gaze and convergence are typically preserved, the ocular motor anomaly mimics bilateral abducens palsy, usually with convergent squint. Convergence is used as a substitution phenomenon to "cross-fixate" (*i.e.*, the left eye adducts to look rightward, and the right eye adducts to look leftward). Vertical gaze is typically preserved, but total ophthalmoplegia may be present. Möbius syndrome is infrequently familial, with evidence of autosomal transmission, but many involved members show only facial palsies with intact eye movement, possibly a *forme fruste* of Möbius syndrome. In rare instances, thalidomide use during pregnancy has been implicated.[80]

The mechanism of Möbius syndrome is not precisely known. Blodi[48] previously used EMG to demonstrate simultaneous activity (co-contraction) of the horizontal recti, but bilateral aplasia of medial and lateral recti, with replacement by fibrous bands, has been reported.[81] A complete autopsy conducted by Pitner et al[82] revealed the following: almost total absence of facial musculature, but normal eyes and extraocular muscles; normal intracranial nerves and nuclei; decreased bulk of right side of tongue; hypoplasia of right cerebellar hemisphere and left inferior olivary nucleus; and hypoplasia of right brachium conjunctivum and central pontine tegmental tract. They concluded that Möbius syndrome could result from multiple causes involving the brain stem and/or musculature derived from branchial arches, and they noted the similarity to arthrogryposis, which can involve the spinal cord and/or musculature derived from the somites.

Towfighi et al[83] reported autopsy findings in one instance of Möbius syndrome, and reviewed 14 other such cases in the literature. They distinguished four groups according to the neuropathologic appearance of the brain stem nuclei:

Group 1: Atrophy or hypoplasia of the cranial nerve nuclei
Group 2: Atrophy plus neuronal degeneration
Group 3: Atrophy plus frank focal necrosis
Group 4: No lesions in the cranial nerve nuclei

It was proposed that group 4 represents primarily a myopathic disorder, and that cases of Möbius syndrome with facioscapulohumeral muscular dystrophy clinically fall within this type. In one case, computed tomography revealed a greatly enlarged cisterna magna, small dysplastic cerebellum and brain stem, and a deformed fourth ventricle.[84]

These varied associated anomalies and pathologic findings suggest a multiplicity of syndrome complexes that include more or less characteristic eye-movement deficiencies. Based on pathologic information, D'Cruz et al[85] suggested vascular-induced necrosis as the etiology of Möbius syndrome. McDermot et al[86] studied the phenomenon of familial transmission of this syndrome, noting that those with sixth and seventh nerve paralysis along with skeletal defects have a low (2%) transmission risk; the presence of deafness, complete ophthalmoplegia, and digital contracture increased the transmission risk rate to 25% to 30%.

The clinician should also be aware of central respiratory dysfunction and sleep disorder in infants with Möbius syndrome.[87,88] Additionally, these children may have a higher incidence of psychological and emotional difficulties as a result of their inability to smile and communicate their affect noticeably.[89]

Elevator Deficiencies

Congenital vertical eye movement anomalies are the result of supranuclear, nuclear, or cranial nerve defects,

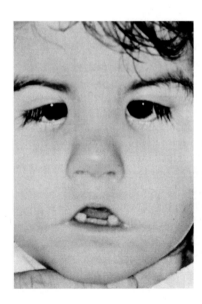
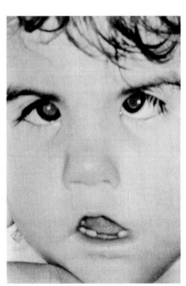

Fig. 13–8. Möbius syndrome. Esotropic deviation with bilateral deficit of horizontal gaze. Vertical gaze is intact. Note facial diplegia.

mechanical restrictions of the globe itself, or variable combinations of these factors. Ziffer et al[90] delineated three such groups of patients: (1) those with primary inferior rectus restriction; (2) those with primary superior rectus paresis; and (3) those with supranuclear elevation deficiency. Monocular elevation deficiency usually takes the form of a *double elevator palsy*: that is, an apparent weakness of superior rectus and inferior oblique muscles. The involved eye may be without deviation in the primary position or may be hypotropic, but diplopia is generally absent and the pupil categorically is uninvolved. Mild to moderate homolateral ptosis is frequently observed.

Metz[91] showed positive forced-ductions and normal upward saccadic velocity, indicating intact superior rectus function. In fact, in most such cases of double elevator palsy, upward gaze is improved by surgical relief of inferior restrictions. In some proportion of cases, preservation of Bell's phenomenon (Fig. 13–9) indicates a supranuclear lesion. Indeed, Jampel and Fells[92] reported on cases of diplopia with acquired monocular elevation paresis of sudden onset, clearly not due to a peripheral disorder such as restrictive dysthyroid myopathy or myasthenia. Forced duction tests were negative,

and they believed that these cases were examples of unilateral, discrete vascular lesions involving the *contralateral* pretectal, supranuclear fibers destined for the superior rectus subnucleus in the oculomotor nuclear complex. Ford et al,[93] however, reported on a case of acquired monocular elevation paresis due to a tumor metastatic to the *ipsilateral* dorsal mesodiencephalic junction. Muñoz and Page[94] reported a progressive monocular double elevator palsy in an 8-year-old girl complaining of diplopia. MRI disclosed a pineocytoma, and her strabismus and ocular motility improved postoperatively.

Surgery for double elevator palsy is indicated when there is a large hypotropia in the primary position or significant chin-up posture in order to maintain fusion. If forced ductions are positive, recession of the inferior rectus should be performed. Otherwise, vertical transposition of the horizontal recti (Knapp procedure) offers good, long-lasting effects.

That the anatomic pathways for the control of vertical eye movements are not completely understood should be evident (see Chapter 10). For acquired monocular elevation paresis, consensus dictates that the lesion must lie immediately adjacent to the oculomotor nucleus on

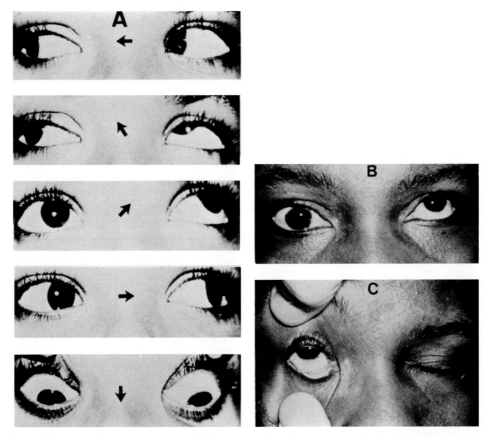

Fig. 13–9. Double elevator palsy. **A.** Defective elevation of the right eye is demonstrated in abduction and adduction. **B.** In similar situation right eye does not elevate in volitional upward gaze. **C.** Upward deviation of right eye on forced lid closure (Bell's phenomenon) indicates supranuclear nature of defect.

the *opposite* side, because the motor fibers to the superior rectus muscle arise in the *contralateral* superior rectus subnucleus. Such cases have been documented with unequal, large pupils showing light-near dissociation,[95] and with miotic, Argyll Robertson–type pupils also with light-near dissociation.[96]

Monocular depressor deficiency is quite rare, and it has been recorded as a congenital defect.[97] Acquired forms occur with restrictive orbital lesions and "inferior rectus"-type oculomotor palsies (see Chapter 12: Oculomotor Palsies), or with skew deviation (see Chapter 10).

Acquired bilateral downgaze palsies are the result of bilateral lesions located dorsomedial to the red nuclei, with variable rostral and caudal extension, and involving the rostral interstitial nucleus of the medial longitudinal fasciculus. Jacobs et al[98] reported an unusual cause of bilateral downgaze palsy (*i.e.*, a bilateral lesion of the dorsolateral mesencephalic periaqueductal gray matter), remote from the rostral interstitial nucleus of the medial longitudinal fasciculus.

Vertical Retraction Syndrome

Vertical retraction syndrome, comparable to horizontal retraction seen with Duane syndrome, is rarely encountered. One sporadic unilateral case,[99] as well as familial bilateral cases,[100] have been reported. Typically, there is limited elevation or depression associated with retraction of the globe and narrowing of the lid fissure on either upward or downward gaze. There may be an associated esotropia or exotropia more marked in the direction of the restricted field of vertical movement. Forced duction test was positive, but EMG data are not available.

In an atypical case, there was poor abduction and elevation of the right eye associated with retraction of the right globe on leftward, upward, and downward gaze.[101] EMG showed co-firing of the right vertical recti in three gaze directions; eye movement recordings also suggested anomalous innervation involving fibers to the right vertical recti and right lateral rectus.

Synergistic Divergence

Synergistic divergence produces the picture of monocular medial rectus palsy with paradoxical abduction in the field of action of the paretic medial rectus (*i.e.*, the motility pattern consists of exotropia, with *both* eyes abducting synchronously on attempted lateral gaze). There have been 14 reported cases, of which only 2 were bilateral.[102] In the case presented by Jimura et al,[103] the patient also had ipsilateral congenital Horner's syndrome. EMG has been performed in two cases. Wilcox et al[104] proposed, on the basis of clinical and EMG findings in their case, that the major portion of the oculomotor nerve branch intended to innervate the medial rectus instead anomalously innervated the lateral rectus, and that there was minimal or absent innervation of the lateral rectus by the abducens nerve; simultaneous innervation of the horizontal recti without retraction of the globe was observed on adduction. In analyzing this innervational pattern, they suggested that congenital adduction palsy with synergistic divergence is a variant of Duane syndrome.

Marcus Gunn Jaw-Winking Synkineses

Synkinesis is defined as a simultaneous movement or a coordinated sequence of movements of muscles supplied by different nerves or by separate peripheral branches of the same nerve. Normally occurring cranial nerve synkineses are exemplified by sucking, chewing, conjugate eye movements, or Bell's phenomenon, all of which are mediated by supranuclear pathways.

Abnormal cranial nerve synkineses may be either acquired or congenital. Intrafacial dyskinesia may follow peripheral facial nerve palsies (the "inverted" Marcus Gunn phenomenon, or syndrome of Marin Amat[105] [see Chapter 8]), and aberrant oculomotor misdirection is commonly a sequel to trauma (see Chapter 12). Marcus Gunn jaw-winking (trigemino-oculomotor synkinesis) and indeed the Duane retraction syndrome (see above) are examples of pathologic congenital synkineses. There are also a number of peculiar yet physiologically associated movements, including the coupling of volitional horizontal gaze shift with involuntary ear wiggle (oculoaural) or brow elevation (oculofrontal).[106]

Using EMG in normal subjects, Sano[107] demonstrated distinct *co-firing* of the extraocular muscles innervated by the oculomotor nerve, and of the muscles of mastication innervated by the trigeminal nerve. Sano believes that such findings support Wartenberg's hypothesis of "release phenomena": that is, synkineses result from damage to cranial nerve nuclei incurred secondary to peripheral nerve injury (*réaction á distance*), and that the secondary nuclear lesion "releases phylogenetically older [neural] mechanisms with their tendency toward associated movements."[108] Therefore, release phenomena represent *failure of inhibition of primitive reflexes*, as exemplified by palmomental, suck, snout, and primitive grasp-feeding reflexes, and by the dysraphic "mirror movements" seen occasionally in Duane syndrome or in the lid-facial-oral dyskinesia of Meige's syndrome.

Although not necessarily associated with disturbances of ocular motility, the congenital trigemino-oculomotor synkineses involving the jaw muscles and the lid levator are included here as examples of anomalous innervational patterns. Originally described by Gunn in 1883, this extraordinary phenomenon presents as unilateral ptosis of variable degree, usually noted shortly after birth. As the infant nurses, the ptotic lid rhythmically jerks upward. In a series of nearly 1500 cases of congenital ptosis,[109] 80 patients (5%) displayed the Marcus Gunn phenomenon. Although the left side is said to be involved more frequently, in this large group there were 42 right eyes and 35 left eyes; and three patients had bilateral Marcus Gunn phenomenon. There was no gender preponderance, and only two cases were familial. Amblyopia was present in 54%, anisometropia in 26%, and some degree of strabismus in 56%, including 19 cases each of superior rectus palsy and "double elevator palsy" and 2 cases of Duane syndrome. The question of spontaneous amelioration with aging was not clarified. Other authors have commented that the synkinesia does become less conspicuous, but it is possible that adults learn to minimize lid excursions consciously.[110]

Sano[107] extensively reviewed the subject of trigemino-oculomotor synkinesis. Two major groups are classified: (1) external pterygoid-levator synkinesis (i.e., elevation when jaw is thrust to opposite side [homolateral external pterygoid], when jaw is projected forward [bilateral external pterygoid], or when mouth is opened widely); and (2) internal pterygoid-levator synkinesis (i.e., lid elevation on teeth clenching). The first group is by far the more common. Regarding pathogenesis, Sano presented EMG evidence that the jaw-winking phenomenon is an exaggeration of a normally existing, but barely detectable, physiologic co-contraction (associated movement), which a congenital brain stem lesion has "released" from higher central control. Sano also demonstrated that direct stimulation of the pterygoid muscle results in lid retraction; however, damage to the trigeminal motor fibers relieves the lid activity. Mrabet et al[111] described two families with Marcus Gunn jaw-winking, demonstrating an autosomal-dominant type of inherited pattern with incomplete penetrance.

The surgical management of Marcus Gunn jaw-winking phenomenon is complex, and the reader is referred elsewhere for discussions of the various proposed surgical approaches.[110,112,113]

A rare condition in which the lid *falls* as the mouth opens has been dubbed the "inverse Marcus Gunn phenomenon." Lubkin[114] used EMG to demonstrate inhibition of the affected levator palpebrae superioris concurrent with external pterygoid contraction, but no associated activity of the orbicularis oculi. Therefore, in this condition, trigeminal innervation to the pterygoids is associated with *inhibition* of the oculomotor branch to the levator, whereas in the true Marcus Gunn phenomenon it is associated with *excitation* of the oculomotor branch to the levator.

A peculiar case of torsional diplopia associated with the initiation of swallowing (i.e., deglutition-trochlear synkinesis) has been reported,[115] incriminating a dyskinesia that couples the fourth cranial nerve with bulbar musculature, which is innervated by the trigeminal, facial, or hypoglossal nerves. The cases of two sisters, each

with monocular lid retraction on adduction or downward gaze, have also been reported.[116]

Restrictive Syndromes

The term "restrictive" refers to mechanical tethering of the globe due to congenital anomalies of the extraocular muscles and/or fascial attachments, rather than to supranuclear or infranuclear synkinesias or peripheral neural miswiring patterns. The mechanical nature of the motor defect is proved by resistance to passive (forced) duction of the eye when the conjunctiva or muscle insertions are used in attempts to rotate the globe (see Chapter 12 and Fig. 3–6).

Brown Tendon Sheath Syndrome

In 1950, Brown[117] described patients with apparent congenital paresis of the inferior oblique muscle, with restricted elevation upon forced duction testing when the globe was in the adducted position (see Chapter 12). At surgery, thickening of the superior oblique tendon sheath was observed, and passive movement was restored after the sheath was stripped. The positive forced duction test clearly distinguishes this disorder from inferior oblique palsy; however, other common features can be observed, including increasing exotropia in upgaze (V-pattern), downward displacement of the eye on attempted adduction ("superior oblique overaction"), and occasional widening of the palpebral fissure in adduction. Most patients enjoy good binocular function with or without compensatory head position, and amblyopia is uncommon. The syndrome may be bilateral, is rarely familial, and has been documented with mirror symmetry in monozygotic twins.[118]

Catford and Dean-Hart[119] demonstrated normal reciprocal firing patterns in the oblique muscles of three patients with tendon sheath syndrome, and concluded that the syndrome was due strictly to a local mechanical defect rather than to paradoxical innervation with co-firing, which Papst and Stein[120] had previously thought to be the case. Sevel[121] provided a useful review of etiologic considerations and added the suggestion, derived from this investigation of the trochlear region in embryonic life, that there may be persistent fine trabeculae between the superior oblique tendon and the cartilaginous trochlea.

Although the majority of patients with congenital Brown syndrome do not require surgery, correction should be considered when the eye is significantly hypotropic in the primary position, or a disfiguring or otherwise unsatisfactory head position is present. A superior oblique weakening procedure (tenotomy, tenectomy, or silicone tendon expander) is preferred. Although these maneuvers effectively free the mechanical restriction so that the globe can elevate in adduction, additional surgery may be necessary to correct *an induced* superior oblique palsy (*e.g.*, inferior oblique recession).

Restriction of elevation in adduction may be due to acquired lesions localized to the superior oblique muscle or the trochlea itself. This acquired form of tendon sheath syndrome can be a rare complication of rheumatoid arthritis (adult or juvenile form),[122–124] orbital trauma,[125] sinusitis, sinus surgery,[126] encircling scleral buckles, blepharoplasty,[127] and superior oblique tuck procedures, or may occur as an idiopathic form of painful tenosynovitis.[128] An isolated metastasis to the superior oblique muscle has also been reported.[129] Several authors have advocated administering a trial of local steroid injection when acute tenderness and swelling in the region of the trochlea indicate an inflammatory cause.[122,124,128] However, both oral nonsteroidal and steroidal anti-inflammatory drugs often afford relief as well.

Both congenital and acquired forms of tendon sheath syndrome may be momentarily intermittent, and numerous instances of audible "clicks" or "snaps" have been reported at the instant of restoration of full elevation.

Congenital Familial Fibrosis Syndrome

Replacement of extraocular muscles by fibrous tissue is a relatively rare form of fixed congenital ophthalmoplegia. Variable motility restrictions are dependent on the number and location of involved muscles. Rarely, all of the extraocular muscles and lid levator may be fibrosed. These conditions are frequently familial and are clinically characterized by downward or inward fixation of both eyes, moderate to marked ptosis, and jerky convergent movements on attempted upgaze. The head is thrown backward to compensate for fixed downward gaze. Astigmatism, amblyopia, and less frequently, some degree of enophthalmos are present. Strictly unilateral

cases are recognized, and may be seen in association with ptosis and enophthalmos.[130] Gillies et al[131] described a new syndrome of dominantly inherited fibrosis of the vertical-acting extraocular muscles, with normal horizontal excursions. Harley et al[132] provided a thorough review of these infrequent fibrosis syndromes.

A discussion of anomalies of muscle and tendon malformations is beyond the scope of this section, and the reader is referred to the publications of Francois (Table 13–4) and Duke-Elder and Wybar.[133]

NYSTAGMUS AND RELATED DISORDERS

Although the following entities are discussed in Chapter 11, they are reviewed here with particular attention to the pediatric population.

Congenital Nystagmus

Congenital nystagmus is frequently seen in association with bilateral anterior visual pathway disease, although it may be isolated as well and occur in patients with normal vision. The waveforms are typical and have been well described, consisting of a velocity-increasing slow phase (see Chapter 11). The clinical findings and eye movement recordings of congenital nystagmus are identical in cases with and without visual loss. The nystagmus is usually horizontal and uniplanar, although small vertical or torsional movements may occur. Congenital nystagmus presents typically at 3 to 4 months of life, and may diminish somewhat in amplitude and frequency in adulthood. Although many consider congenital nystagmus to be the result of a primary fixation defect, Dell'Osso et al[134] have demonstrated accurate and maintained target-foveation in patients with congenital nystagmus. Furthermore, they demonstrated

---

TABLE 13–4. Congenital Ocular Motor Anomalies

Anomalous innervation patterns	Absent muscles*
Duane retraction syndrome	Inferior rectus (most common)
Double elevator palsy	Medial rectus
Double depressor palsy	Superior rectus
Möbius syndrome	Superior oblique
Medial rectus palsy and lateral rectus	Lateral rectus
contraction	Inferior rectus and superior rectus
Fibrotic muscle and sheath defects	Inferior rectus, superior rectus, and superior oblique
Duane retraction syndrome	Inferior rectus and lateral rectus
Brown tendon-sheath syndrome	Muscle malformations*
Crawford fibrosis syndrome	Medial rectus bifurcation
Strabismus fixus	Lateral rectus bifurcation
Vertical retraction	Superior rectus bifurcation
Nonprogressive external ophthalmoplegia	Oblique reduplication
moplegia	Inferior rectus reduplication
Anomalous muscle insertions*	Supernumerary muscles

*See Francois J: Congenital ophthalmoplegias. In Brunette JR, Barbeau A (eds): Progress in Neuro-Ophthalmology, pp 387–421. Amsterdam, Excerpta Medica, 1969.

that eye velocity matched target velocity during foveation intervals and concluded that the smooth-pursuit mechanisms in patients with congenital nystagmus were relatively normal.[135]

Most investigators now believe that congenital nystagmus is due to an instability of the brain stem neural integrator responsible for gaze-holding, although apparently normal gaze-holding mechanisms have been demonstrated in at least some congenital nystagmus patients.[136] Oscillopsia is not a typical feature in cases of congenital nystagmus, but it has been described by Abel et al,[137] who postulated that suppression of oscillopsia is operable only within certain limits of foveation stability: when nystagmus exceeds these, oscillopsia will result. Additionally, Gresty et al[138] described six patients who had eye-movement recordings characteristic of congenital nystagmus, but who presented in adulthood with symptoms of oscillopsia; no etiology was uncovered, and the process was believed to be benign.

Various therapeutic modalities have been attempted in congenital nystagmus. Contact lenses are well known to dampen nystagmus, although worsening (rebound phenomena) may occur after their removal.[139] In those patients with a null point and consequent anomalous head position, Anderson-Kestenbaum strabismus surgery yields improvement in head position as well as visual acuity.[140] Alternatively, for patients without a null point, Helveston[141] reported improvement in nystagmus and near visual acuity after large retroequatorial recessions of all four horizontal recti. In our experience, eye muscle surgery in cases of congenital nystagmus is most beneficial when a significant anomalous head posture is present or the nystagmus is of very high amplitude. Underlying structural ocular anomalies and/or amblyopia often precludes significant improvement in visual acuity. However, in infants with bilateral congenital cataracts, early surgery may reduce or resolve the nystagmus.

Latent Nystagmus

Clinically, latent nystagmus is defined as nystagmus that appears when one eye is covered, the fast component (jerk phase) occurring away from the covered eye. This form is common in children with congenital strabismus, particularly with esotropia. It is *not* an acquired condition and *does not require* extensive neurologic investigation. Latent nystagmus may become manifest if visual acuity is decreased in one eye (*e.g.*, because of injury or amblyopia), which effectively acts as an "occluder" over that eye. On eye movement recordings, latent nystagmus demonstrates linear or exponentially decreasing slow phase velocity. Although conventional wisdom holds that a nasotemporal optokinetic imbalance occurs with congenital strabismus and latent nystagmus, because of failure to develop binocular vision,

Gresty et al[142] believe that both latent and congenital nystagmus arise from a genetic or acquired embryologic disorder. Kommerell and Zee[143] described two patients who were able to release or suppress latent nystagmus at will, presumably on the basis of voluntary control of visual input contributed by the amblyopic eye. Most patients with latent nystagmus are asymptomatic and do not require treatment, but in patients with cosmetically bothersome oscillations, strabismus surgery or injection with botulinum toxin type A (BOTOX) may be helpful.[144] The primary clinical importance of latent nystagmus is that its presence always signifies a congenital or infantile abnormality of the ocular motor and binocular fusion systems.

Periodic Alternating Nystagmus

Periodic alternating nystagmus is a conjugate horizontal jerk oscillation, during which there are regular reversals of the direction of the fast phase, separated by brief, quiet intervals. The time period of each cycle is variable, ranging from 1 to 5 minutes, and may be asymmetric. During the beating phases, the amplitude, frequency, and velocity progressively change. For the most part, this is an acquired condition after caudal brain stem or cerebellar disease. However, there have been a few reports of congenital periodic alternating nystagmus, particularly in patients with albinism.[145] Some cases respond well to oral lioresal (Baclofen Tablets).

Heimann-Bielschowsky Phenomenon

The Heimann-Bielschowsky phenomenon is an unusual motility pattern that develops after monocular visual loss, potentially many years later, and therefore is frequently incorrectly interpreted as a sign of acquired neurologic disease. The phenomenon consists of strictly monocular, coarse, pendular, primarily vertical oscillations occurring only in the poorly seeing eye. It is more prominent at distance and is inhibited by convergence or fixation. The oscillations vary from 1 to 5 cycles/second, and vertical amplitude from a few to more than 25 degrees.[146] It has been suggested that there is a correlation among the amplitude, oscillations, and duration of visual loss.[147] As with latent nystagmus, the presence of these movements does not require neuroimaging or further laboratory investigation unless the cause of the visual loss remains unclear.

Congenital Ocular Motor Apraxia

Originally described by Cogan in 1952, congenital ocular motor apraxia is characterized by a deficiency in the generation of voluntary horizontal saccadic eye movements despite the presence of spontaneous saccades (see Chapter 10). Vertical saccades are unaffected, and are completely normal. Affected infants may present with delayed visual and/or psychomotor development, or may even appear to be blind. During the later half of the first year, compensatory head thrust movements become apparent. The ocular motor abnormalities tend to improve with increasing age, and there is a clear tendency for natural resolution between the first and second decades of life,[148] but often subclinical abnormalities of the horizontal saccades are noted on careful examination or eye movement recordings. The cause of congenital ocular motor apraxia is unknown. Acquired ocular motor apraxia may occur in ataxia-telangiectasia[149] or Leigh's syndrome.[150] In adults, infarcts or demyelinating disease may produce a similar clinical picture. Familial incidence is unusual.[148]

Spasmus Nutans

Spasmus nutans is a triad of asymmetric nystagmus, head nodding, and torticollis, usually in infants, but without a known neural substrate. The syndrome is noted clinically in infancy or during the first several years of life and is often self-limited, resolving by the mid to late first decade. Young et al[151] emphasized that spasmus nutans is a condition occurring during stages of visual development ("amblyogenic period"), and is associated with strabismus and amblyopia, in the eye with the greater amplitude of nystagmus. Gottlob et al[152] showed that, in some cases, the head nodding in spasmus nutans is a compensatory mechanism oscillating at the same amplitude in phase and 180° out of phase to the head movements, as a result of a normal compensatory vestibulo-ocular reflex. Long-term follow-up reveals that good acuity is expected in these patients, and one-third have normal binocular function. However, subclinical nystagmus persists until at least the second decade.[153] Retinal diseases, particularly congenital stationary night blindness, and optic nerve or chiasmal gliomas, may produce an identical eye movement abnormality. Therefore, all patients with spasmus nutans require appropriate neuro-imaging.[154,155]

Ocular Flutter/Opsoclonus

These eye-movement disorders consist of bursts of conjugate saccades with no intersaccadic intervals, ocular flutter being horizontal and opsoclonus being multidirectional. Smooth pursuit and optokinetic mechanisms are generally normal, but ocular dysmetria, primarily consisting of saccadic overshoots, is quite common; this suggests that these abnormal eye movements are of cerebellar origin. Shawkat et al,[156] however, believe that the cerebellar flocculus is spared, as evidenced by the persistence of normal smooth pursuit and absence of gaze-paretic, downbeat, or rebound nystagmus; they proposed the origin to be in the cerebellar fastigial nuclei. In children, this entity may be seen after acute encephalitis[157] or as a paraneoplastic syndrome,[158] particularly in association with neuroblastoma.[159] Anti-Hu antibodies have been present in some cases.[160] Opsoclonus-myoclonus syndrome has also been described in association with Beckwith-Wiedemann syndrome and hepatoblastoma.[161] Treatment with intravenous corticotropic hormone (ACTH) is often helpful; indeed, antibodies to ACTH have been shown in patients with opsoclonus and myoclonus.[162] Additionally, volitional control of saccadic oscillations that resemble ocular flutter or myoclonus has been described in apparently otherwise normal individuals.[163]

DYSLEXIA

Dyslexia is used to describe a variety of learning disorders presenting as difficulty with reading in persons with otherwise normal intelligence. The cause is unknown, and the clinical spectrum is quite variable, resulting in the absence of a universally accepted definition, even by those who routinely diagnose and treat this disorder. Although anatomic abnormalities in dyslexics have been reported to occur in the magnocellular layer of the lateral geniculate nucleus, the region of the planum sphenoidale, and on various chromosomes, no definitive etiology has been established. MRI of brain morphology, specifically surface area of planum temporale and temporal lobe volume, has disclosed no significant differences between dyslexics and nonimpaired children.[164]

In the 1980s, the use of Irlen lenses was propagated based on the assumption that many of these children suffer from a condition called "scotopic sensitivity syndrome."[165] A large cohort study by Menacker et al,[166] however, showed no correlation between the use of tinted lenses and the reading performance of dyslexic children. The hazards of endorsing such therapies for this condition without having preliminary information from well-controlled clinical trials are obvious. The duty of the ophthalmologist is to perform a careful clinical examination on these children, treating refractive errors, anisometropia, muscle imbalance, and fusional deficits to the greatest extent possible. A joint statement by the American Academies of Ophthalmology and Pediatrics in 1993 reiterated this approach and did not support the use of any optical or pharmaceutical therapy for this condition. Until the etiology of dyslexia is better understood, therapy for this condition should rest with professional teachers and educational psychologists. The clinician should also recommend baseline auditory evaluation in these children, because hearing difficulty may contribute to or exacerbate a variety of types of learning disorders.

HEADACHE IN CHILDREN

Pediatric Migraine

The International Headache Society has developed criteria for the diagnosis of pediatric migraine.[167] In addition to the common and classic forms in the adult, patients with pediatric migraine may present with gastrointestinal distress alone (*i.e.*, without cephalgia)[168] or with somnambulism[169]; pediatric migraine may also be associated with transient oculosympathetic paresis.[170] Motion sickness may be a *forme fruste* of migraine as well, particularly in the pediatric population. Complicated migraines, such as those resulting in ophthalmoplegia (Chapter 12) or hemiplegia (Chapter 16), are discussed elsewhere. Treatment strategies have included the use of tinted lenses,[171] systemic trazodone,[172] and subcutaneous sumatriptan.[173] In the authors' experience, when attacks are frequent or severe enough to warrant prophylaxis, the use of cyproheptadine (Periactin) 2 to 4 mg nightly has been quite effective. Additionally, the comorbidity of migraine and epilepsy has been recognized in recent years[174] and should not be overlooked because of the frequent clinical overlap of these disorders.

Pediatric Pseudotumor Cerebri

Lessell[175] presented an excellent review of pediatric pseudotumor cerebri; its etiology, associated conditions, and treatment are discussed elsewhere (see Chapter 5). Important points in assessing children with idiopathic intracranial hypertension include the often rather minimal headache in this condition. Infants and youngsters are more likely to present with irritability, apathy, somnolence, dizziness, or ataxia. Some children present with visual loss due to papilledema, discovered during routine examination. Unlike the adult form, pediatric pseudotumor cerebri does not occur predominantly in females and is often not associated with obesity. This condition is more frequent in children around the age of menarche and early adolescence, suggesting an endocrine connection. Importantly, in children, mastoiditis with lateral dural sinus thrombosis must be considered (see Color Plate 5–4D). Cases have been reported to be associated with both oral and topical tetracycline, vitamin A use, and malnutrition. Management strategies are similar to those in adults.

OCULAR MOTOR CRANIAL NEUROPATHIES

Kodsi and Younge[176] reported on 160 pediatric patients with third, fourth, or sixth nerve palsies, as follows: there were 88 isolated sixth nerve palsies, 35 oculomotor palsies, 19 trochlear palsies, and 18 multiple cranial neuropathies. Trauma accounted for 40% of cases of oculomotor palsies; 17.1% of cases were idiopathic, 14.3% were due to neoplasm. Ophthalmoplegic migraine was responsible for 8.6% of cases. No aneurysms were encountered in their series. Trauma and congenital causes comprise the largest group of fourth nerve palsies; trauma and intracranial neoplasms were responsible for the bulk of isolated abducens and of multiple cranial neuropathies. No microvascular lesions were encountered in this series.

Hamed[177] reported 14 patients with congenital third nerve palsies, noting the frequent phenomenon of pupillary miosis as a result of aberrant regeneration. Ing et al[178] studied 54 children with oculomotor nerve palsy, the majority of whom had acquired lesions as a result of trauma or bacterial meningitis, rather than congenital cases. Although aneurysms causing oculomotor palsy are rare in children, Wolin and Saunders[179] and Branley et al[180] reported two such cases, in an 11-year-old boy and a 7-year-old girl, respectively.

Although not a cranial neuropathy per se, Hamed et al[181] noted the high frequency of A-pattern strabismus and superior oblique overaction in children with neurologic diseases such as hydrocephalus or cerebral palsy. They speculated that superior oblique overaction may be a clinical marker for associated neurologic dysfunction and may represent a form of skew deviation in some cases. In their companion paper,[182] with seven children who had alternating skew on lateral gaze, all subjects had tumors involving the level of the cervicomedullary junction and/or cerebellum.

SYMPTOMATIC SENSORY AND STRABISMIC ABNORMALITIES

The business of the ocular sensory and motor systems is to provide a clear, stable image precisely at the foveas of the two eyes. Binocular sensory input from the retinas is aligned by higher cortical centers that determine a "fusional reflex," providing a single panoramic view (cyclopean) with the advantage of depth perception (stereoacuity, stereopsis). The neural pathways for binocular visual coordination are only poorly understood, but are partially under volitional control. Moreover, most persons harbor a constant tendency toward imprecise ocular muscle balance, and if fusion is insufficient, the eyes may momentarily diverge (*i.e.*, an *exophoria* bias becomes a frank *exotropic* deviation); converge (*i.e.*, an *esophoria* bias becomes a frank *esotropic* deviation); or engage in vertical slippage (*i.e.*, a *hyperphoria* bias becomes a frank *hypertropia* deviation, "hyper-" referring to the higher eye).

The fusional reflex holds these tendencies toward muscular imbalance "in check" to a greater or lesser degree: strongly in childhood and adolescence, and progressively less firmly with increasing age. That is not to say that many persons are actually troubled by symptomatic diplopia due to failure of fusional mechanisms.

Double vision is itself the greatest stimulation for the fusional mechanism to correct the intolerable sensory situation of simultaneous perception of two dissimilar images. In infancy, when one eye receives a defective image by virtue of, for example, an uncorrected refractive error, the less clear image is suppressed and, if uncorrected, the eye becomes *amblyopic*, with variable degrees of reduction in acuity. Alternately, a muscular imbalance that would produce diplopia *in adults* leads to a failure of neuronal maturation in the deviating eye—a state of *strabismic amblyopia*. Thus, the cortical mechanism of "suppression" rids the infantile brain of diplopia, but at the expense of permanent failure of visual maturation of one eye and, hence, absence of normal binocularity.

The adult is much less likely to employ suppression of a deviated image, and thus symptomatic diplopia heralds the onset of acquired ocular imbalance or, less frequently, of spontaneous "decompensation" of central fusional reflexes, or of fusional deficiencies evoked by fatigue, sedatives, even small amounts of alcohol, or seemingly trivial head trauma. However, in adults with acquired ocular deviations of large magnitude, the two images may be sufficiently separated such that it is possible for the subject to "suppress" or otherwise ignore the more peripheral image. Typically, even if paretic, the dominant eye is preferred for fixation, and the *secondary deviation* of the nonfixing eye carries the second image toward the periphery of visual space. In long-standing monocular visual deprivation (*e.g.*, with monocular cataract or corneal opacity), when vision is restored, the adult fusional mechanism may be insufficient to reestablish binocularity (*i.e.*, a single fused image) despite full ocular ductions.

The term *sensory correspondence* (normal retinal correspondence) implies that corresponding retinal points (*e.g.*, the two foveas) have a common visual direction in space, and that an object in space is appreciated as a single image so long as corresponding retinal points are simultaneously stimulated. Any disparity in image location on the retina results in diplopia, itself a strong sensory stimulus for fusion. Motor fusion is a combination of both saccadic and *vergence* eye movements (see Chapter 10), the first being conjugate and the latter being *disjugate* or disjunctive (*i.e.*, the eyes move in opposite directions, either toward or away from one another). Although retinal image disparity at the fovea is the principle stimulus for fusion (particularly stereopsis), the retinal periphery also plays a role (*e.g.*, extrafoveal correspondence).

Fusion of retinal images is an essential characteristic of overlapping visual fields. The uncrossed (temporal) retinal fiber projection is a relatively recent phylogenetic innovation, and the segregation of afferent fibers in the chiasm was the logical adaptation for successful fusion of a binocular panorama (see Chapter 4). Of the more

central cortical and interhemispheric neural mechanisms for vergence and fusion, very little is known. The putative supranuclear defects of fusion, aside from surgically created stereotactic lesions of the midbrain that affect principally convergence,[183] are not precisely localized. We may infer empirically that major or minor lesions of the midbrain disrupt neural substrates for convergence (and divergence) that will result in loss of fusional amplitudes. Nevertheless, the vast majority of patients with disruption of convergence and divergence show little evidence of brain stem dysfunction, and a benign course is the rule.

Convergence and divergence amplitudes may be measured by determining the amount of base-out prism (provoking convergence) and base-in prism (provoking divergence) that the patient's versional system can overcome by re-aligning and fusing the prismatically separated images. Vertical vergence may be similarly evaluated. But when there is central loss of fusion, even prismatic correction of image malposition (either due to cranial nerve palsy or to vergence deficiency) fails to gain image superimposition, except briefly and intermittently.

The variety of tests that assess fusion, stereopsis, and other features of binocularity are beyond the scope of this presentation; the reader is referred to works dealing principally with the theory and management of strabismus, especially the excellent text of von Noorden.[97]

Failure of Fusional Mechanisms

Acquired Central Defects

Acquired central disruption of fusion is most commonly associated with moderate to severe closed head trauma. Indeed, with nonparalytic heterotropia, convergence and/or accommodative insufficiency should be suspected after head trauma.[184] The patient displays loss of fusional convergence and divergence and an inability to sustain superimposition of images. Ocular ductions are *generally* normal, but even when existing ocular nerve palsies are compensated by prismatic balance (*e.g.*, a left abducens palsy is corrected by appropriate strength base-out prism), fusion is absent or incomplete. At best there is a single distance at which fleeting, unsustainable fusion occurs, resulting in rather constant diplopia that requires occlusion of an eye. Pratt-Johnson and Tillson[185] pointed out that *bilateral* trochlear palsies especially, which cause considerable excyclotorsional diplopia, may mimic central disruption of fusion, but such patients can indeed hold fusion when any vertical, horizontal, and torsional defects are neutralized on, for example, the synoptophore (amblyoscope).

Central disruption of fusional amplitude has also been reported in association with cerebrovascular accidents and brain tumors, and after neurosurgical procedures.[186]

Given that vergence movements and accommodation are linked and under volitional control, it is a difficult task to distinguish the dissembler from the unfortunate patient with true fusional deficiencies. In fact, spontaneous recovery is so infrequent[185,187] that improvement in symptoms after legal settlements often suggests a functional, nonstructural cause.

Kushner[188] noted the phenomenon of unexpected cyclotropia (*e.g.*, in association with prior ocular surgery, corneal scarring, or longstanding strabismus) simulating disruption of fusion. In these patients, diplopia could not be eliminated by prisms, but fusion was restored after appropriate eye muscle surgery for the cyclodeviation. Miller and Guyton[189] hypothesized that loss of fusion, particularly "sensory torsion," predisposes patients to the development of A or V patterns in strabismus. Of 21 patients with consecutive esotropia after surgery for intermittent exotropia, 43% had an A or V pattern, versus only 5% of bifoveating patients after similar surgery. Indeed, continuing clinical observations have shed light on the complex mechanism of fusion, and many dogmatic concepts are being challenged. Of 24 patients with strabismus in the first 2 years of life (13 in the first 6 months of life), 50% (two thirds in the congenital group) achieved stereopsis of 200 seconds of arc or better after undergoing strabismus surgery in adulthood.[190] Kushner and Morton[191] reported development of binocularity as measured with the Bagolini lens test in 86% of 359 adults who underwent surgery for longstanding strabismus. Obviously, a great deal of plasticity must exist in the visual cortex; the reader is directed to Daw's[192] 1994 Friedenwald Lecture for further details in this regard.

Congenital Anomalies

Rarely, congenital (or infantile) lack of fusional amplitudes may be the cause of long-standing, but intermittent, diplopia in children or adults. Failure of fusion, whether "primary" (central) or "secondary" to muscle imbalance, excessive accommodation, or visual malfunction of an eye, usually results in infantile esotropia. That is, as a rule, anomalies of fusion produce manifest eye deviations (heterotropias), regardless of a "central" versus "peripheral," or a "motor" versus "sensory" cause. Such patients, however, are *free of diplopia*, possibly as a result of suppression (see above) or because of other sensory anomalies (*e.g.*, anomalous retinal correspondence). *Microtropia (monofixation syndrome)* represents one of these anomalous states, characterized by amblyopia (often minor) and a very small angle (less than 8 prism diopters) of manifest deviation. Thus, "visual loss of unknown cause" *may* become the clinical dilemma. The finding of eccentric (nonfoveal) fixation is essential. Although some authors comment that microtropia is symptomless, this is clearly not always the

case for adults with microtropia.[97,193] The use of the 4-diopter base-out prism test[194] is quite helpful in identifying these patients. In a normal person, when a 4-diopter base-out prism is placed over one eye, both eyes will deviate toward the side of the eye without the prism (the prism-covered eye because of displacement of the visual image, and the fellow eye because of Hering's law), followed by a secondary refusional movement of the fellow eye only *toward the prism-covered eye*. In a patient with microtropia or monofixation syndrome, only one eye foveates at a time, and there is a central suppression scotoma in the fellow eye. If the prism is placed over the preferred (foveating) eye, both eyes will deviate toward the eye without the prism, but no refixation movement of the other eye will be noted; if, however, the prism is placed over the eye with the suppression scotoma, no movement will occur in either eye. Although the monofixation syndrome is almost always congenital in origin, it may be acquired in, for example, patients with a very small macular lesion. Competence of the fusion reflex appears to deteriorate with time in these patients, their underlying phorias become manifest, and symptoms may appear in the teenage years or later in life; diplopia is often initially intermittent. Treatment is directed toward restoring the original microtropic state, with either prisms or surgery; only very rarely, if ever, can bifoveal fixation be established.

Although neither congenital nor infantile in presentation, *convergence insufficiency* is a constitutional disorder that represents a commonly symptomatic form of defective fusional amplitudes, noted intermittently during prolonged reading or other near-effort tasks. This clinical entity is probably the most significant cause of asthenopia associated with reading, and even enthusiastic students may fall asleep. More frequent episodes of frank diplopia occur, corrected by momentary eye closure or cessation of reading. The demands of unaccustomed schoolwork, aggravated by late hours and apprehension, impose an additional burden on weak fusional mechanisms. The near point of convergence may be remote, but the hallmark finding is decreased fusional convergence at near, as determined by base-out prism testing (see below).

Acquired Visual Loss

Because binocular sensory input is so vital, being a requisite for coordinated ocular muscle balance, it is surprising how infrequently loss of central visual acuity produces diplopia. In some patients with macular diseases that distort retinal topography (*e.g.*, epiretinal membrane), foveal photoreceptors will be shifted to a noncorresponding point, with good levels of acuity but with diplopia. This situation is not to be confused with monocular diplopia, which is detailed in Chapter 1. Burgess et al[195] suggested that such patients (*e.g.*, those with subretinal neovascular membranes) acquire a form of "rivalry" between central and peripheral fusional mechanisms. Small vertical deviations are regularly present, and prisms can correct this form of fusional disturbance.[196] In other situations where visual acuity is reduced in one or both eyes, peripheral retinal fusional capacity may be insufficient to control ocular motor balance, with resultant diplopia of peripheral visual space. We have seen patients with dense unilateral (after optic neuritis) or bilateral (ethambutol optic neuropathy) central scotomas with severe diplopia who required monocular occlusion.

Other patterns of visual loss may be associated with nonparetic forms of diplopia. With chiasmal interference and bitemporal field loss, the remaining nasal field sectors may be insufficiently overlapped by depressed temporal hemifield function, leading to defective fusion and a *hemifield slide phenomenon* (see Chapter 6). Usually acuity is also depressed in one or both eyes. Latent deviations (phorias) then permit the "free-floating" nasal hemifields to slip horizontally and/or vertically.

Special Forms of Acquired Esotropia

Acute Comitant Esotropia

The sudden onset of laterally comitant esotropia in patients with no prior history or evidence of strabismus demands that a new paretic cause be excluded. In children more commonly than adults, otherwise benign strabismus may follow febrile illnesses or even incidental short-term patching; sometimes no obvious inciting cause is uncovered.[197] Preverbal children will not complain of diplopia, nor will a head-turn suffice, but usually one eye is habitually closed. An accommodative anomaly may be present, and fusional reserves are often deficient.[198] After cataract or other ocular surgery in adults, comitant esodeviation or, more frequently, exodeviation may constitute an insuperable form of diplopia likely related to minimal fusional reserves, although this phenomenon is not nearly as common as diplopia secondary to injury of extraocular muscles from local anesthetic agents (see Chapter 12).

Two additional groups of adults may develop sudden, nonparetic diplopia: those with accommodative esotropia who stop wearing the corrective lenses as teen-agers, and patients with microtropia-monofixation syndrome (see above). Microtropia that "decompensates" by manifesting a large-angle esotropia (unlike the situation described earlier, where the original ability to fuse is lost) can be corrected by prisms or surgery. Although abnormal fusion generally ensues, these patients are nonetheless free of diplopia.

Cyclic Esotropia

This rare *circadian* form of strabismus usually occurs in children 2 to 4 years old, but it has also been reported in adults.[199] It should not be confused with sixth nerve palsy. Usually a temporal rhythm occurs, during which a 24-hour period of 30 to 50 prism diopter esotropia is followed by a 24-hour period of normal binocular vision. Other rhythms of 72- and 96-hour cycles have been reported, however. Generally, the condition occurs spontaneously, but has followed surgery for intermittent exotropia and for retinal detachment.[200] Treatment consists of surgery to correct the maximum deviation; the cycles stop after surgery. Although Friendly et al[201] could find no associated cyclic phenomena after monitoring numerous psychologic and physiologic functions, Roper-Hall and Yapp[202] reported cyclic changes in behavior, frequency of micturition, and electroencephalographic abnormalities. Troost et al[200] recorded normal eye movements in both eyes when straight and also when esotropic. Therefore, recurrent cranial nerve dysfunction is extremely unlikely, and the mechanism of cyclic esotropia remains unknown. Most strabismologists recommend bimedial rectus recession for these cases; surprisingly, postoperative exotropia is rarely seen. It is intriguing that other cyclic heterotropias do occur: the cyclic oculomotor palsy of Bielschowsky and a rare case of cyclic superior oblique paresis following trochlear trauma.[203]

Progressive Esotropia with Myopia

The gradual onset of esotropia in adults with significant myopia of -7.00 to -35.00 diopters has been documented.[204] The esotropia progresses until the eyes are markedly adducted, often with positive forced ductions found in the later stages. Surprisingly (as in chronic progressive external ophthalmoplegia), diplopia is not usually disturbing to these patients. Instead, the presenting complaint is of cosmetically unacceptable, large-angle esotropia; thus, the early stages of this syndrome are not well described. No underlying disease is found, and muscle surgery is required.

Problems at Near

Convergence Insufficiencies

As noted briefly above (see Congenital Anomalies), symptomatic convergence insufficiency occurs when fusional convergence is poor, but accommodation is normal. The patient is often a young adult in good general health, but with the complaint of "eyestrain" and other asthenopic symptoms, or even frank diplopia at near. Examination reveals the following: (1) normal near point of accommodation; (2) remote near point of convergence; (3) exophoria at near, made worse by $+3.00$ lenses; and (4) poor convergence (base-out prism) amplitudes. Such patients respond well to orthoptic exercises aimed at improving fusional vergence amplitudes.

Prisms or surgery are rarely necessary, and often yield less than dramatic results. However, patients with a manifest exotropia of smaller magnitude at distance often do well with horizontal recess-resect procedures, with proportionately more surgical displacement of the medial than the lateral rectus. Unfortunately, for patients who do not have significant distance deviation, the long-term results of bimedial rectus resection are poor.

Convergence insufficiency may also be accompanied by a remote near point of accommodation, especially in the following patients: myopes, patients accustomed to presbyopic corrections, generally debilitated patients, patients taking any of a variety of psychoactive medications (see Chapter 15), or patients with an accompanying condition (*e.g.*, neurologic disease, endocrine disease, head trauma,[184] systemic infections, decompression sickness in divers).[205]

Accommodative Effort Syndrome

Accommodative effort syndrome is a less common problem that also causes asthenopia and diplopia at near. As with convergence insufficiency, the patient is often young and in good health. Examination reveals: (1) normal near point of accommodation; (2) normal near point of convergence; (3) esophoria at near lessened by +3.00 lenses; and (4) poor divergence amplitudes. Treatment includes plus lenses (and/or phospholine iodide) as well as orthoptic exercises, as in other cases of increased accommodative convergence-accommodation (AC/A) ratio.

For more detailed discussion of these and other problems at the reading distance, the reader is referred to the excellent review by Raskind.[206]

OCULAR TORTICOLLIS

Torticollis refers to habitual abnormal head position that may be due to congenital musculoskeletal anomalies, such as fibrous shortening of the sternocleidomastoid muscle, occipitocervical stenosis, or Klippel-Feil syndrome; or to acquired traumatic or inflammatory cervical myositis. *Ocular torticollis* indicates an unnatural head posture assumed to maintain binocularity (as with face-turn and head-tilt that compensates for superior oblique palsies), or to optimize visual acuity in congenital or acquired nystagmus by adopting a head-turn that places the eyes in a conjugate gaze direction (*i.e.*, the null point) that dampens the nystagmus (see Chapter 11). The nystagmus "blockage" syndrome is a type of congenital nystagmus that is reduced or absent with adduction of the fixating eye, so that a convergent position is assumed.[97] Nystagmus increases on attempts at abduction of either eye and, when an eye is occluded, the face turns in the direction of the fixating eye. Children may also adopt an anomalous head position in the presence of a hemianopia, with the head turn toward the blind hemifield (see Rubin and Wagner's[207] comprehensive review of ocular torticollis).

REFERENCES

1. Mayer DL, Beiser AS, Warner AF et al: Monocular acuity norms for the Teller acuity cards between ages one month and four years. Invest Ophthalmol Vis Sci 36:671, 1995
2. Mash C, Dobson V, Carpenter N: Interobserver agreement for measurement of grating acuity and interocular acuity differences with the Teller acuity card procedure. Vision Res 35:303, 1995
3. Quinn GE, Berlin JA, James M: The Teller acuity card procedure: three testers in a clinical setting. Ophthalmology 100:488, 1993
4. Kushner BJ, Lucchese NJ, Morton GV: Grating visual acuity with Teller cards compared with Snellen visual acuity in literate patients. Arch Ophthalmol 113:485, 1995
5. Kushner BJ: Editorial: Grating acuity tests should not be used for social service purposes in preliterate children. Arch Ophthalmol 112:1030, 1994
6. Holmes JM, Archer SM: Vernier acuity cards: a practical method of measuring vernier acuity in infants. J Pediatr Ophthalmol Strabismus 30:312, 1993
7. Hoyt CS: The clinical usefulness of the visual evoked response. J Pediatr Ophthalmol Strabismus 21:231, 1984
8. Roy MS, Barsoum-Homsy M, Orquin J, Benoit J: Maturation of binocular pattern visual evoked potentials in normal full-term and preterm infants from 1 to 6 months of age. Pediatr Res 17:140, 1995
9. Tychsen L: Development of vision. In Isenberg SJ (ed): The Eye in Infancy, pp 121–130. St. Louis, CV Mosby, 1994
10. Thorn F, Gwiazda J, Cruz AAV et al: The development of eye alignment, convergence, and sensory binocularity in young infants. Invest Ophthalmol Vis Sci 35:544, 1994
11. Aiello A, Wright KW, Borchert M: Independence of optokinetic nystagmus asymmetry and binocularity in infantile esotropia. Arch Ophthalmol 112:1580, 1994
12. Fielder AR, Fulton AB, Mayer DL: Visual development of infants with severe ocular disorders. Ophthalmology 98:1306, 1991
13. Bradford GM, Kutschke PJ, Scott WE: Results of amblyopia therapy in eyes with unilateral structural abnormalities. Ophthalmology 99:1616, 1992
14. Willshaw HE: Assessment of nystagmus. Arch Dis Child 69(a):102, 1993
15. Gelbart SS, Hoyt CS: Congenital nystagmus: a clinical perspective in infancy. Graefes Arch Clin Exp Ophthalmol 226:178, 1988
16. Cibis GW, Fitzgerald KM: Electroretinography in congenital idiopathic nystagmus. Pediatr Neurol 9:369, 1993
17. Lambert SR, Taylor D, Kriss A: The infant with nystagmus, normal appearing fundi, but an abnormal ERG. Surv Ophthalmol 34:173, 1989
18. Heher KL, Traboulsi EI, Maumenee IH: The natural history of Leber's congenital amaurosis. Ophthalmology 99:241, 1992
19. Bouzas EA, Caruso RC, Drews-Bankiewicz MA et al: Evoked potential analysis of visual pathways in human albinism. Ophthalmology 101:309, 1994
20. Kushner BJ: Infantile uniocular blindness with bilateral nystagmus: a syndrome. Arch Ophthalmol 113:1298, 1995
21. Brodsky MC, Glasier CM: Optic nerve hypoplasia: clinical significance of associated central nervous system abnormalities on magnetic resonance imaging. Arch Ophthalmol 111:66, 1993
22. Zeki SM, Hollman AS, Dutton GN: Neuroradiological features of patients with optic nerve hypoplasia. J Pediatr Ophthalmol Strabismus 29:107, 1992
23. Siatkowski RM, Sanchez JC, Andrade R, Alvarez A: The clinical, neuroradiographic, and endocrinologic profile of patients with bilateral optic nerve hypoplasia. Ophthalmology 104:493, 1997
24. Brodsky MC, Hoyt WF, Hoyt CF et al: Atypical retinochoroidal coloboma in patients with dysplastic optic discs and transsphenoidal encephalocele. Arch Ophthalmol 113:624, 1995
25. Eustis HS, Sanders MR, Zimmerman T: Morning glory syndrome

in children: association with endocrine and central nervous system anomalies. Arch Ophthalmol 112:204, 1994

26. Good WV, James EJ, DeSa L et al: Cortical visual impairment in children. Surv Ophthalmol 38:351, 1994

27. Wong VC: Cortical blindness in children: a study of etiology and prognosis. Pediatr Neurol 7:178, 1991

28. Fielder AR, Mayer DL: Delayed visual maturation. Semin Ophthalmol 6:182, 1991

29. Herzau V, Bleher I, Joos-Kratsch E: Infantile exotropia with homonymous hemianopia: a rare contraindication for strabismus surgery. Graefes Arch Clin Exp Ophthalmol 226:148, 1988

30. Göte H, Gregersen E, Rindziunski E: Exotropia and panoramic vision compensating for an occult congenital homonymous hemianopia: a case report. Binocular Vision Eye Muscle Surg Q 8(3):125, 1993

31. Farris BK, Pickard DJ: Bilateral postinfectious optic neuritis and intravenous steroid therapy in children. Ophthalmology 97:339, 1990

32. Kennedy C, Carroll FD: Optic neuritis in children. Arch Ophthalmol 63:747, 1960

33. Kennedy C, Carter S: Relation of optic neuritis to multiple sclerosis in children. Pediatrics 28:377, 1961

34. Taylor D, Cuendet F: Optic neuritis in childhood. In Hess RF, Plant FT (eds): Optic Neuritis, pp 73–85. Cambridge, Cambridge University Press, 1986

35. Johns DR et al: Leber's hereditary optic neuropathy. Arch Ophthalmol 111:495, 1993

36. Dubois LG, Feldon SE: Evidence for a metabolic trigger for Leber's hereditary optic neuropathy: a case report. J Clin Neuroophthalmol 12:15, 1992

37. Mackey DA, Buttery RG: Leber hereditary optic neuropathy in Australia. Austr NZ J Ophthalmol 20:177, 1992

38. Newman NJ, Lott MT, Wallace DC: The clinical characteristics of pedigrees of Leber's hereditary optic neuropathy with the 11778 mutation. Am J Ophthalmol 111:750, 1991

39. Dutton JJ: Gliomas of the anterior visual pathway. Surv Ophthalmol 38:427, 1994

40. Hoffman HJ, Humphreys RP, Drake JM et al: Optic pathway/hypothalamic gliomas: a dilemma in management. Pediatr Neurosurg 19(4):186, 1993

41. Liu GT, Lessell S: Spontaneous visual improvement in chiasmal gliomas. Am J Ophthalmol 114:193, 1992

42. Brzowski AE, Bazan C, Mumma JV et al: Spontaneous regression of optic glioma in a patient with neurofibromatosis. Neurology 42(3 Pt 1):679, 1992

43. Hoyt CS, Billson F, Ouvrier R et al: Ocular features of Aicardi's syndrome. Arch Ophthalmol 96:291, 1978

44. DelPero RA, Mets MB, Tripathi RC et al: Anomalies of retinal architecture in Aicardi syndrome. Arch Ophthalmol 104:1659, 1986

45. Hoyt WF, Nachtigaller H: Anomalies of ocular motor nerves: neuroanatomic correlates of paradoxical innervation in Duane's syndrome and related congenital ocular motor disorders. Am J Ophthalmol 60:443, 1965

46. Magath TB: A variation in distribution of the nervus abducens in man. Arch Ophthalmol 48:67, 1919

47. Phillips WH, Dirion JK, Graves GO: Congenital bilateral palsy of abducens. Arch Ophthalmol 8:355, 1932

48. Blodi FC: Electromyographic evidence for supranuclear gaze palsies. Trans Ophthalmol Soc UK 90:451, 1970

49. Huber A: Electrophysiology of the retraction syndromes. Br J Ophthalmol 58:293, 1974

50. Gross SA, Tien DR, Breinin GM: Aberrant innervational pattern in Duane's syndrome type II without globe retraction. Am J Ophthalmol 117:348, 1994

51. Matteucci P: I difetti congeniti di abduzione ("congenital abduction deficiency") con particolare riguardo alla patogenesi. Rass Ital Ottal 15:345, 1946

52. Hotchkiss MG, Miller NR, Clark AW, Green WR: Bilateral Duane's retraction syndrome: a clinical-pathologic case report. Arch Ophthalmol 98:870, 1980

53. Miller NR, Kiel SM, Green WR, Clark AW: Unilateral Duane's retraction syndrome (type 1) 100:1468, 1982

54. Hickey WF, Wagoner MD: Bilateral congenital absence of the abducens nerve. Virchows Arch Pathol Anat 402:91, 1983

55. Jay WM, Hoyt CS: Abnormal brainstem auditory-evoked potentials in Stilling-Turk-Duane retraction syndrome. Am J Ophthalmol 89:814, 1980

56. Taylor MJ, Polomeno RC: Further observations on the auditory brainstem response in Duane's syndrome. Can J Ophthalmol 18:238, 1983

57. Parkinson J, Tompkins C: Auditory response in Duane's retraction syndrome. Am J Orthopt 32:121, 1982

58. Gourdeau A, Miller N, Zee D, Morris J: Central ocular motor abnormalities in Duane's retraction syndrome. Arch Ophthalmol 99:1809, 1981

59. Metz HS: Duane's retraction syndrome. Arch Ophthalmol 100:843, 1982

60. Hedera P, Friedland RP: Duane's syndrome with giant aneurysm of the vertebral basilar arterial junction. J Clin Neuroophthalmol 13:271, 1993

61. Saad N, Lee J: Medial rectus electromyographic abnormalities in Duane syndrome. J Pediatr Ophthalmol Strabismus 30:88, 1993

62. Scott AB, Wong GY: Duane's syndrome: an electromyographic study. Arch Ophthalmol 87:140, 1972

63. Pressman SH, Scott WE: Surgical treatment of Duane's syndrome. Ophthalmology 93:29, 1986

64. Raab EL: Clinical features of Duane's syndrome. J Pediatr Ophthalmol Strabismus 33:64, 1986

65. Hoffman RJ: Monozygotic twins concordant for bilateral Duane's retraction syndrome. Am J Ophthalmol 99:563, 1985

66. Chew CKS, Foster P, Hurst JA et al: Duane's retraction syndrome associated with chromosome 4q27-31 segment deletion. Am J Ophthalmol 119:807, 1995

67. Cullen P, Rodgers CS, Callen DF et al: Association of familial Duane anomaly and urogenital abnormalities with a bisatellited marker derived from chromosome 22. Am J Med Genet 47:925, 1993

68. Tredici TD, von Noorden GK: Are anisometropia and amblyopia common in Duane's syndrome? J Pediatr Ophthalmol Strabismus 22:23, 1985

69. Rogers GL, Bremer DL: Surgical treatment of the upshoot and downshoot in Duane's retraction syndrome. Ophthalmology 91:1380, 1984

70. Pfaffenbach DD, Cross HE, Kearns TP: Congenital anomalies in Duane's retraction syndrome. Arch Ophthalmol 88:635, 1972

71. Regenbogen L, Stein R: Crocodile tears associated with homolateral Duane's syndrome. Ophthalmologica 156:353, 1968

72. Isenberg S, Blechman B: Marcus Gunn jaw-winking and Duane's retraction syndrome. J Pediatr Ophthalmol Strabismus 20:235, 1983

73. Miller MT, Folk ER: Strabismus. In Renie WA (ed): Goldberg's Genetic and Metabolic Eye Disease, p 269. Boston, Little, Brown & Co, 1986

74. Osher RH, Schatz NJ, Duane TD: Acquired orbital retraction syndrome. Arch Ophthalmol 98:1798, 1980

75. Miller GR, Glaser JS: The retraction syndrome and trauma. Arch Ophthalmol 76:662, 1966

76. Kivlin JD, Lundergan MK: Acquired retraction syndrome associated with orbital metastasis. J Pediatr Ophthalmol Strabismus 22:109, 1985

77. DeRespinis PA, Caputo AR, Wagner RS et al: Duane's retraction syndrome. Surv Ophthalmol 38:257, 1993

78. Rubenstein AE, Lovelace RE, Behrens MM, Weisburg LA: Möbius syndrome in association with peripheral neuropathy and Kallman syndrome. Arch Neurol 32:480, 1975

79. Wishnick MM, Nelson LB, Huppert L, Reich EW: Möbius syndrome and limb abnormalities with dominant inheritance. Ophthalmic Pediatr Genet 2:77, 1983

80. Elsahy N: Möbius syndrome associated with mother taking thalidomide during gestation. Plast Reconstr Surg 51:93, 1973

81. Traboulsi EI, Maumenee IH: Extraocular muscle aplasia in Moebius syndrome. J Pediatr Ophthalmol Strabismus 23:20, 1986

82. Pitner SE, Edwards JE, McCormick WF: Observations on the pathology of the Moebius syndrome. J Neurol Neurosurg Psychiatry 28:362, 1965

83. Towfighi J, Marks K, Palmer E, Vannucci R: Möbius syndrome: neuropathologic observations. Acta Neuropathol 48:11, 1979

84. Beerbower J, Chakeres DW, Larsen PD, Kapila A: Radiographic findings in Moebius and Moebius-like syndromes. AJNR 7:364, 1986

85. D'Cruz OF, Swisher CN, Jaradeh S et al: Möbius syndrome: evidence for a vascular etiology. J Child Neurol 8:260, 1993

86. MacDermot KD, Winter RM, Taylor D et al: Oculofacialbulbar palsy in mother and son: review of 26 reports of familial transmission within the 'Möbius spectrum of defects.' J Med Genet 28:18, 1991

87. Konkol RJ, D'Cruz O, Splaingard M: Central respiratory dysfunction in Möbius syndrome. J Child Neurol 6:278, 1991

88. Gilmore RL, Falace P, Kanga J et al: Sleep-disordered breathing in Möbius syndrome. J Child Neurol 6:73, 1991

89. Szajnberg NM: Möbius syndrome: alternatives in affective communication. Dev Med Child Neurol 36:459, 1994

90. Ziffer AJ, Rosenbaum AL, Demer JL et al: Congenital double elevator palsy: vertical saccadic velocity utilizing the scleral search coil technique. J Pediatr Ophthalmol Strabismus 29:142, 1992

91. Metz HS: Double elevator palsy. Arch Ophthalmol 97:910, 1979

92. Jampel RS, Fells P: Monocular elevation paresis caused by a central nervous system lesion. Arch Ophthalmol 80:45, 1968

93. Ford CS, Schwartze GM, Weaver RG, Troost BT: Monocular elevation paresis caused by an ipsilateral lesion. Neurology 34:1264, 1984

94. Muñoz M, Page LK: Acquired double elevator palsy in a child with a pineocytoma. Am J Ophthalmol 118:810, 1994

95. Lessell S: Supranuclear paralysis of monocular elevation. Neurology 25:1134, 1975

96. Kirkham TH, Kline LB: Monocular elevator paresis, Argyll Robertson pupils and sarcoidosis. Can J Ophthalmol 11:330, 1976

97. von Noorden GK: Burian and von Noorden's Binocular Vision and Ocular Motility: Theory and Management of Strabismus, pp 417–418, 480–481. St. Louis, CV Mosby, 1996

98. Jacobs L, Heffner RR, Newman RP: Selective paralysis of downward gaze caused by bilateral lesions of the mesencephalic periaqueductal gray matter. Neurology 35:516, 1985

99. Scassellati-Sforzolini G: Una sindroma molto rare: diffeto congenito monolaterale della elevazione con retrazione del globe. Riv Otoneurooftalmol 33:431, 1958

100. Khodadoust AA, von Noorden GK: Bilateral vertical retraction syndrome: a family study. Arch Ophthalmol 78:606, 1967

101. Pruksacholawit K, Ishikawa S: Atypical retraction syndrome: a case study. J Pediatr Ophthalmol 13:215, 1976

102. Thomas R, Mathai A, Gieser SC et al: Bilateral synergistic divergence. J Pediatr Ophthalmol Strabismus 30:122, 1993

103. Jimura T, Tagami Y, Isayama Y, Yamamoto M: A case of synergistic divergence associated with Horner's syndrome. Folia Ophthalmol Jpn 34:477, 1983

104. Wilcox LM, Gittenger JW, Breinin GM: Congenital adduction palsy and synergistic divergence. Am J Ophthalmol 91:1, 1981

105. Wartenberg R: Inverted Marcus Gunn phenomenon. Arch Neurol Psychiatry 60:584, 1948

106. Carmicheal EA, Critchley M: The relations between eye movements and other cranial muscles. Br J Ophthalmol 9:49, 1925

107. Sano K: Trigemino-oculomotor synkineses. Neurologia 1:29, 1959

108. Wartenberg R: Associated movements in the oculomotor and facial muscles. Arch Neurol Psychiatry 55:439, 1946

109. Beyer-Machule CK, Johnson CC, Pratt SG, Smith BR: The Marcus-Gunn phenomenon. Orbit 4:15, 1985

110. Doucet TW, Crawford JS: The quantification, natural course, and surgical results in 57 eyes with Marcus Gunn (jaw-winking) syndrome. Am J Ophthalmol 92:702, 1981

111. Mrabet A, Oueslati S, Gazzah H et al: Clinical and electrophysiological study of 2 familial cases of Marcus Gunn phenomenon [transl. French]. Rev Neurol 147:215, 1991

112. Dryden RM, Fleming JC, Quickert MH: Levator transposition and frontalis sling procedure in severe unilateral ptosis and the paradoxically innervated levator. Arch Ophthalmol 100:462, 1982

113. Dillman DB, Anderson RL: Levator myectomy in synkinetic ptosis. Arch Ophthalmol 102:422, 1984

114. Lubkin V: The inverse Marcus-Gunn phenomenon: an electromyographic contribution. Arch Neurol 35:249, 1978

115. McLead AR, Glaser JS: Deglutition-trochlear synkinesis. Arch Ophthalmol 92:171, 1974

116. Pang MP, Zweifach PH, Goodwin J: Inherited levator-medial rectus synkinesis. Arch Ophthalmol 104:1489, 1986

117. Brown HW: True and simulated superior oblique tendon sheath syndromes. Doc Ophthalmol 34:123, 1973

118. Katz NNK, Whitmore PV, Beauchamp GR: Brown's syndrome in twins. J Pediatr Ophthalmol Strabismus 18:32, 1981

119. Catford GV, Dean-Hart JC: Superior oblique tendon sheath syndrome: an electromyographic study. Br J Ophthalmol 55:155, 1971

120. Papst W, Stein JH: Zur Atiologie des Musculus-obliquus-superior Sehnenscheidensyndroms. Klin Monatsbl Augenheilkd 154:506, 1969

121. Sevel D: Brown's syndrome: a possible etiology explained embryologically. J Pediatr Ophthalmol Strabismus 18:26, 1981

122. Beck M, Hickling P: Treatment of bilateral superior oblique tendon sheath syndrome complicating rheumatoid arthritis. Br J Ophthalmol 64:358, 1980

123. Wang FM, Wertenbaker C, Behrens MM, Jacobs JC: Acquired Brown's syndrome in children with rheumatoid arthritis. Ophthalmology 91:23, 1984

124. Moore AT, Morin JD: Bilateral acquired inflammatory Brown's syndrome. J Pediatr Ophthalmol Strabismus 22:26, 1985

125. Clarke WN, Noel LP, Agapitos PJ: Traumatic Brown's syndrome. Am Orthoptic J 37:100, 1987

126. Blanchard CL, Young LA: Acquired inflammatory superior oblique tendon sheath (Brown's) syndrome. Arch Otolaryngol 110:120, 1984

127. Wesley RE, Pollard ZF, McCord CD: Superior oblique paresis after blepharoplasty. Plast Reconstr Surg 66:283, 1980

128. Hermann JS: Acquired Brown's syndrome of inflammatory origin. Arch Ophthalmol 96:1228, 1978

129. Booth-Mason S, Kyle GM, Rossor M, Bradbury P: Acquired Brown's syndrome: an unusual cause. Br J Ophthalmol 69:791, 1985

130. Hertle RW, Katowitz JA, Young TL et al: Congenital unilateral fibrosis, blepharoptosis, and enophthalmos syndrome. Ophthalmology 99:347, 1992

131. Gillies WD, Harris AJ, Brooks AMV et al: Congenital fibrosis of the vertically acting extraocular muscles. Ophthalmology 102:607, 1995

132. Harley RD, Rodriguez MM, Crawford JS: Congenital fibrosis of the extraocular muscles. Trans Am Ophthalmol Soc 76:197, 1978

133. Duke-Elder S, Wybar K: System of Ophthalmology, Vol 6, Ocular Motility and Strabismus, pp 736–740. St. Louis, CV Mosby, 1973

134. Dell'Osso LF, van der Steen J, Steinman RM et al: Foveation dynamics in congenital nystagmus: I. Fixation. Doc Ophthalmol 79:1, 1992

135. Dell'Osso LF, van der Steen J, Steinman RM et al: Foveation dynamics in congenital nystagmus: II. Smooth pursuit. Doc Ophthalmol 79:25, 1992

136. Dell'Osso LF, Weissman BM, Leigh RJ et al: Hereditary congenital nystagmus and gaze-holding failure: the role of the neural integrator. Neurology 43:1741, 1993

137. Abel LA, Williams IM, Levi L: Intermittent oscillopsia in a case of congenital nystagmus: dependence upon waveform. Invest Ophthalmol Vis Sci 32:3104, 1991

138. Gresty MA, Bronstein AM, Page NG et al: Congenital-type nystagmus emerging in later life. Neurology 41:653, 1991

139. Safran AB, Gambazzi Y: Congenital nystagmus: rebound phenomenon following removal of contact lenses. Br J Ophthalmol 76:497, 1992

140. Zubcov AA, Störk N, Weber A et al: Improvement of visual acuity after surgery for nystagmus. Ophthalmology 100:1488, 1993

141. Helveston EM, Ellis FD, Plager DA: Large recession of the horizontal recti for treatment of nystagmus. Ophthalmology 98:1302, 1991

142. Gresty MA, Metcalfe T, Timms C et al: Neurology of latent nystagmus. Brain 115(Pt 5):1303, 1992

143. Kommerell G, Zee DS: Latent nystagmus: release and suppression at will. Invest Ophthalmol Vis Sci 34:1785, 1993

144. Liu C, Gresty M, Lee J: Management of symptomatic latent nystagmus. Eye 7(Pt 4):550, 1993

145. Abadi RV, Pascal E: Periodic alternating nystagmus in humans with albinism. Invest Ophthalmol Vis Sci 35:4080, 1994

146. Smith JL, Flynn JT, Spiro HJ: Monocular vertical oscillations of amblyopia: the Bielschowsky phenomenon. J Clin Neuroophthalmol 2:85, 1982

147. Pritchard C, Flynn JT, Smith JL: Wave form characteristics of vertical oscillations in longstanding vision loss. J Pediatr Ophthalmol Strabismus 25:233, 1988

148. Prasad P, Nair S: Congenital ocular motor apraxia: sporadic and familial: support for natural resolution. J Neuroophthalmol 14:102, 1994

149. Churchyard A, Stell R, Mastaglia FL: Ataxia telangiectasia presenting as an extrapyramidal movement disorder and ocular motor apraxia without overt telangiectasia. Clin Exp Neurol 28:90, 1991

150. Steinlin M, Thun-Hohenstein L, Boltshauser E: Congenital oculomotor apraxia. Presentation—developmental problems—differential diagnosis [transl. German]. Klin Monatsbl Augenheilkd 200:623, 1992

151. Young TL, Weis JR, Summer G, Esbert JE: The association of strabismus, amblyopia, and refractive errors in spasmus nutans. Ophthalmology 104:112, 1997

152. Gottlob IF, Zubcov AA, Wizov SS et al: Head nodding is compensatory in spasmus nutans. Ophthalmology 99:1024, 1992

153. Gottlob I, Wizov SS, Reinecke RD: Spasmus nutans. Invest Ophthalmol Vis Sci 36:2768, 1995

154. Gottlob I, Wizov SS, Reinecke RD: Quantitative eye and head movement recordings of retinal disease mimicking spasmus nutans. Am J Ophthalmol 119:374, 1995

155. Lambert SR, Newman NJ: Retinal disease masquerading as spasmus nutans. Neurology 43:1607, 1993

156. Shawkat FS, Harris CM, Wilson J et al: Eye movements in children with opsoclonus-polymyoclonus. Neuropediatrics 24:218, 1993

157. Wang PY: Acute cerebellitis with ocular flutter and truncal ataxia: a case report. Chin Med J (Engl) 50(2):169, 1992

158. De Graaf JH, Tamminga RY, Kamps WA: Paraneoplastic manifestations in children. Eur J Pediatr 153:784, 1994

159. Koh PS, Raffensperger JR, Berry S et al: Long-term outcome in children with opsoclonus-myoclonus and ataxia and coincident neuroblastoma. J Pediatr 125(5 Pt 1):712, 1994

160. Fisher PG, Wechsler DS, Singer HS: Anti-Hu antibody in a neuroblastoma-associated paraneoplastic syndrome. Pediatr Neurol 10:309, 1994

161. Wilfong AA, Parke JT, McCrary JA III: Opsoclonusmyoclonus with Beckwith-Wiedemann syndrome and hepatoblastoma. Pediatr Neurol 8:77, 1992

162. Pranzatelli MR et al: Antibodies to ACTH in opsoclonus-myoclonus [review]. Neuropediatrics 24:131, 1993

163. Yee RD et al: Voluntary saccadic oscillations, resembling ocular flutter and opsoclonus. J Neuroophthalmol 14:95, 1994

164. Schultz RT, Cho NK, Staib LH et al: Brain morphology in normal and dyslexic children: the influence of sex and age. Ann Neurol 35:732, 1994

165. Irlen H: Improving reading problems due to symptoms of scotopic sensitivity syndrome using Irlen lenses and overlays. Education 109:413, 1989

166. Menacker SJ, Breton ME, Breton ML et al: Do tinted lenses improve the reading performance of dyslexic children? Arch Ophthalmol 111:213, 1993

167. Metsahonkala L, Sillanpaa M: Migraine in children: an evaluation of the IHS criteria. Cephalalgia 14:285, 1994

168. Katerji MA, Painter MJ: Infantile migraine presenting as colic. J Child Neurol 9:336, 1994

169. Norton G: Letter to the Editor: Migraine and somnambulism. Austr NZ J Med 23:715, 1993

170. Shevell MI, Silver K, Watters GV et al: Transient oculosympathetic paresis (group II Raeder paratrigeminal neuralgia) of childhood: migraine variant. Pediatr Neurol 9:289, 1993

171. Good PA, Taylor RH, Mortimer MJ: The use of tinted glasses in childhood migraine. Headache 31:533, 1991

172. Battistella PA, Ruffilli R, Cernetti R et al: A placebo-controlled crossover trial using trazodone in pediatric migraine. Headache 33:36, 1993

173. MacDonald JT: Treatment of juvenile migraine with subcutaneous sumatriptan. Headache 34:581, 1994

174. Ottman R, Lipton RB: Comorbidity of migraine and epilepsy. Neurology 44:2105, 1994

175. Lessell S: Pediatric pseudotumor cerebri (idiopathic intracranial hypertension) [review]. Surv Ophthalmol 37:155, 1992

176. Kodsi SR, Younge BR: Acquired oculomotor, trochlear, and abducent cranial nerve palsies in pediatric patients. Am J Ophthalmol 114:568, 1992

177. Hamed LM: Associated neurologic and ophthalmologic findings in congenital oculomotor nerve palsy. Ophthalmology 98:708, 1991

178. Ing EB, Sullivan TJ, Clarke MP et al: Oculomotor nerve palsies in children. J Pediatric Ophthalmol Strabismus 29:331, 1992

179. Wolin MJ, Saunders RA: Aneurysmal oculomotor nerve palsy in an 11-year-old-boy. J Clin Neuroophthalmol 12:178, 1992

180. Branley MG, Wright KW, Borchert MS: Third nerve palsy due to cerebral artery aneurysm in a child. Austr NZ J Ophthalmol 20:137, 1992

181. Hamed LM, Fang EN, Fanous MM et al: The prevalence of neurologic dysfunction in children with strabismus who have superior oblique overaction. Ophthalmology 100:1483, 1993

182. Hamed LM, Maria BL, Quisling RG et al: Alternating skew on lateral gaze. Ophthalmology 100:281, 1993

183. Seaber JH: The effect of supranuclear midbrain lesions on ocular motility. In Ravault AP, Lenk M (eds): Transactions of the Fifth International Orthoptic Congress, pp 105–118. Lyon, LIPS, 1984

184. Lepore FE: Disorders of ocular motility following head trauma. Arch Neurol 52:924, 1995

185. Pratt-Johnson JA, Tillson G: Acquired central disruption of fusional amplitude. Ophthalmology 86:2140, 1979

186. Stanworth A, Mein J: Loss of fusion after removal of cerebellar tumor. Br J Orthopt 28:97, 1971

187. MacLellan AV: A case of recovery from traumatic loss of fusion. Br J Orthopt 31:102, 1974

188. Kushner BJ: Unexpected cyclotropia simulating disruption of fusion. Arch Ophthalmol 110:1415, 1992

189. Miller MM, Guyton DL: Loss of fusion and the development of A or V patterns. J Pediatr Ophthalmol Strabismus 31:220, 1994

190. Morris RJ, Scott WE, Dickey CF: Fusion after surgical alignment of longstanding strabismus in adults. Ophthalmology 100:135, 1993

191. Kushner BJ, Morton GV: Postoperative binocularity in adults with longstanding strabismus. Ophthalmology 99:316, 1992

192. Daw NW: Mechanisms of plasticity in the visual cortex. Invest Ophthalmol Vis Sci 34:4168, 1994

193. Boyd TAS, Budd GE: The monofixation syndrome: heterophoria and asthenopia. Am J Orthopt 26:43, 1976

194. Parks MM: Monofixation syndrome. In Tasman W, Jaeger EA (eds): Duane' Clinical Ophthalmology, Vol 1, pp 1–14. Philadelphia, JB Lippincott, 1990

195. Burgess D, Roper-Hall G, Burde RM: Binocular diplopia associated with subretinal neovascular membranes. Arch Ophthalmol 98:311, 1980

196. Bixenman WW, Joffe L: Binocular diplopia associated with retinal wrinkling. J Pediatr Ophthalmol Strabismus 21:215, 1984

197. Goldman HD, Nelson LB: Acute acquired comitant esotropia. Ann Ophthalmol 17:777, 1985

198. Burian HM, Miller JE: Comitant convergent strabismus with acute onset. Am J Ophthalmol 45:55, 1958

199. Stark N, Walther C: Cyclische esotropie bei einem erwaschenen. Klin Monatsbl Augenheilkd 184:553, 1984

200. Troost BT, Abel L, Noreika J, Genovese FM: Acquired cyclic esotropia in an adult. Am J Ophthalmol 91:8, 1981

201. Friendly DS, Manson RA, Albert DG: Cyclic strabismus: a case study. Doc Ophthalmol 34:189, 1973

202. Roper-Hall MJ, Yapp JMS: Alternate day squint. In The First

International Congress of Orthoptics, pp 262–271. St. Louis, CV Mosby, 1968

203. Windsor CE, Berg EF: Circadian heterotropia. Am J Ophthalmol 67:656, 1969
204. Hugonnier R, Maynard P: Les desequilibres oculomoteur observes en cas de myopie forte. Ann Ocul 202:713, 1969

205. Lieppman ME: Accommodative and convergence insufficiency after decompression sickness. Arch Ophthalmol 99:453, 1981
206. Raskind RH: Problems at the reading distance. Am J Orthopt 26:53, 1976
207. Rubin SE, Wagner RS: Ocular torticollis. Surv Ophthalmol 30:366, 1986

CHAPTER 14

Orbital Disease and Neuro-ophthalmology

Part I: An Overview

Joel S. Glaser

History-Taking
Orbital Examination
Diagnostic Considerations
  Graves' Disease
  Inflammations

Vascular Lesions
Neoplasms
Trauma
Diagnostic Procedures
Surgery of the Orbit

The orbits vary much in position depending on whether the eyes look frontally or laterally; their capacity compared with the size of the globe also varies within wide limits. . . . Even among the Primates themselves the size of the orbit varies only very loosely with that of the globe, large Primates having a relatively small orbital capacity.

Sir Stewart Duke-Elder
The Eye in Evolution, 1958

That diseases of the orbit may be conjoined with neuro-ophthalmology should come as no surprise. These two domains of ophthalmologic interest are integrated by common symptoms, signs, and anatomic structures. The orbit shares bony partitions with the sinuses medially and inferiorly, with the anterior cranial fossa above, with the superior orbital fissure and cavernous sinus at the orbital apex, and with the sphenoid complex and middle cranial fossa posteriorly (Figs. 14–1 and 14–2). Moreover, there are congenital, inflammatory, neoplastic, vascular, and traumatic processes that bridge the orbito-cranial junction. Clinically, orbital lesions that cause double vision are regularly mistaken for intracranial problems. In evidence, one need look no further than the single most common cause of spontaneous diplopia in the adult, that is, the restrictive myopathy of Graves' disease, which is so frequently misdiagnosed as cranial nerve palsies or myasthenia. And while proptosis is so compelling an indicator of orbital masses, passive orbital congestion with exophthalmos is also a sign of

arteriovenous fistula, of intracranial obstruction of venous flow, or of tumor growth in the middle cranial fossa or paranasal sinuses.

This chapter elucidates the communal turf shared by diseases of the orbit and neuro-ophthalmologic disorders, with emphasis on the clinical means by which strictly neurologic dilemmas may be distinguished from pathologic processes predominantly of the orbit. The material here is intended to provide a pragmatic approach to diagnosis of orbital disease, with special accent on the physical examination; orbital lesions causing diplopia are discussed at length in Chapter 12. Neither the specifics of orbito-cranial anatomy (Figs. 14–1 and 14–2) nor an exhaustive commentary on all orbital diseases is included, but common surgical procedures are discussed in Chapter 14, Part II. The reader is referred to the several excellent anatomic atlases available, and especially to Rootman's[1] *Diseases of the Orbit.*

HISTORY-TAKING

As with other fields of clinical medicine, accuracy in diagnosis and appropriateness of management depend on an orderly protocol that begins with historical documentation (Table 14–1). Review of the personal medical history is an essential part of the assessment of orbital and neuro-ophthalmologic problems. For example, failure to uncover a past history of dysthyroidism is to ignore a substantial clue to the single most common cause of uni- or bilateral proptosis. Likewise, a rapidly progressive orbital congestive syndrome with ophthalmoplegia, occurring in a patient with diabetes, should

J. S. Glaser: Departments of Neurology and Ophthalmology, Bascom Palmer Eye Institute, University of Miami School of Medicine, Miami; and Neuro-ophthalmology, Cleveland Clinic Florida, Ft. Lauderdale, Florida

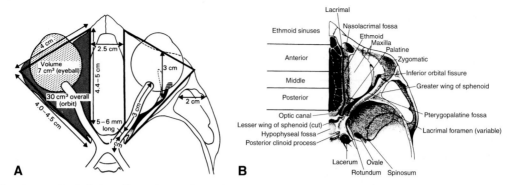

Fig. 14–1. A. Relative dimensions of orbital and adnexal structures. **B.** Bones of the orbital floor, from above. Note relationship of ethmoidal sinus complex medially and sphenoid wing posteriorly. (From ref. 1)

suggest the possibility of an opportunistic fungus such as mucormycosis. Clearly, any previous tumor surgery is suspect, although metastases constitute only 3% to 7% of biopsied orbital masses[2]; nasopharyngeal and sinus neoplasms accounted for 23% of secondary orbital masses in the British Columbia series.[3] A history of cranial or facial trauma likewise must be assessed, but is usually not obscure or forgotten.

In a similar vein, family medical history is important and occasionally of diagnostic value. It is recognized, for instance, that optic glioma is a relatively frequent manifestation of neurofibromatosis (see Chapter 5). Therefore, in a child with unexplained chronic proptosis, the occurrence of skin lesions (birthmarks, skin lumps, or tumors), seizures, or central nervous system (CNS) masses in blood relatives is critical information. Ideally, such family members should be examined or further details obtained. Dysthyroidism also has a distinct familial predilection.

The sudden onset of rapidly progressive proptosis in childhood (Fig. 14–3) should be considered an orbital emergency, the clinician's responsibility being to rule out a life-threatening tumor such as rhabdomyosarcoma or metastatic neuroblastoma. A similar picture may evolve with acute orbital congestion associated especially with ethmoidal or maxillary sinusitis, in children with or without fever.[4,5] In the adult, with the exception of metastatic tumors, most orbital neoplasms produce insidiously progressive exophthalmos. Inflammatory orbital "pseudotumor"[6] is the only common cause of relatively abrupt, usually painful, proptosis with diplopia in the otherwise well adult, and myositis occurs in children or adults.[7] In contrast, intermittent painful proptosis, at times accompanied by spontaneous subconjunctival hemorrhage or lid ecchymoses, is practically pathognomonic of venous varices or lymphangiomas.[8] An acute phase of Graves' disease may mimic other orbital congestive syndromes (see below), but usually this most common orbitopathy is chronic and not characterized by significant pain.

Over a wide age spectrum, with severe coughing or prolonged retching, or during protracted obstetrical labor, pressure in intra-orbital veins may be momentarily raised to the point of rupture with formation of a usually painful retrobulbar hematoma.[9,10] These Valsalva orbital hemorrhages usually resolve spontaneously.

In situations where the duration of proptosis is not clear, review of antecedent photographs (driver's license, family snapshots, etc.) may be extremely helpful. The clinician should be aware that proptosis may be suddenly discovered rather than actually occurring rapidly, so that the evidence provided by review of previous photographs is helpful in dating true onset. Such photographs may be scrutinized with the illumination and magnification provided by the slit lamp.

As a rule, insidiously progressive orbital masses that produce axial (straightforward) displacement of the globe tend not to produce diplopia until proptosis is relatively marked. Inflammatory pseudotumor is an exception, because of the propensity for infiltration of extraocular muscles (myositis),[7,11] and the restrictive myopathy of congestive Graves' disease regularly results in concomitant diplopia. Tumors located superiorly in the orbit commonly produce deficits in upward gaze, nasal masses produce adduction deficits, and temporal masses produce abduction deficits. Under ideal conditions these physical observations should be confirmed by enhanced computed tomography (CT) or magnetic resonance imaging (MRI); standardized ultrasonography is an ideal complementary procedure.

Defects in visual function are due to compression of the optic nerve by intra- or extra-conal masses but, as with neural structures elsewhere, if tumor growth is insidious, remarkably large masses are compatible with normal nerve function. Retrobulbar masses that indent

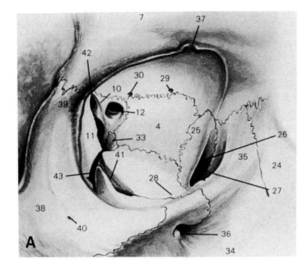

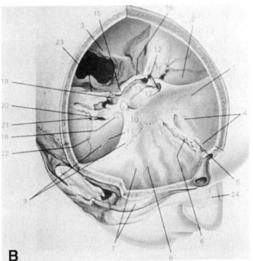

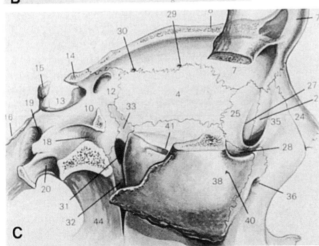

Bony structures

1 Anterior cranial fossa
2 Middle cranial fossa
3 Posterior cranial fossa
4 Ethmoid bone
5 Crista galli
6 Cribriform plate
7 Frontal bone
8 Orbital plate
9 Sphenoid bone
10 Lesser wing of sphenoid
11 Greater wing of sphenoid
12 Optic canal
13 Hypophyseal fossa
14 Anterior clinoid process
15 Posterior clinoid process
16 Dorsum sellae
17 Tuberculum sellae
18 Foramen rotundum
19 Foramen lacerum
20 Foramen ovale
21 Foramen spinosum
22 Groove for middle meningeal artery
23 Groove for superior petrosal sinus
24 Nasal bone
25 Lacrimal bone
26 Lacrimal fossa
27 Lacrimal crest
28 Fossa for inferior oblique muscle
29 Anterior ethmoid foramen
30 Posterior ethmoid foramen
31 Pterygopalatine foramen
32 Pterygopalatine fossa
33 Palatine bone
34 Maxillary bone
35 Frontal process of maxilla
36 Infraorbital foramen
37 Supraorbital notch
38 Zygomatic bone
39 Frontal process of zygomatic bone
40 Zygomaticofacial foramen
41 Infraorbital groove
42 Superior orbital fissure
43 Inferior orbital fissure
44 Lateral pterygoid lamina

Fig. 14–2. A. Front view of orbital bones constituting rims and posteromedial structures. **B.** Anterosuperior view of orbital roof (*8*) (*i.e.*, anterior cranial fossa) and middle cranial fossa (*9,11*) at posterior aspect of orbit. **C.** Bony details of medial orbital wall and posterior relationships at orbitocranial junction. (All numbers refer to accompanying table.) (From ref. 1)

**TABLE 14–1. History of Illness:
Orbit**

Medical history
    Dysthyroidism
    Diabetes mellitus
    Tumor surgery (breast, lung, etc.)
    Sinus disease
    Facial trauma
Family history
    Dysthyroidism
    Neurofibromatosis
Onset
    Insidious
    Sudden
    Traumatic
Symptoms
    Proptosis
    Diplopia
    Visual defect: fixed, transient
    Pain
Progression
    Rapid
    Slow
    Intermittent

the posterior pole of the globe may induce relative hyperopia, requiring additional plus lenses to improve acuity. Transient blurring of vision in extremes of gaze, especially abduction or noted during reading,[12] can be produced by any orbital mass, including dysthyroidism.

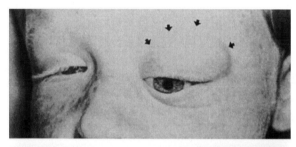
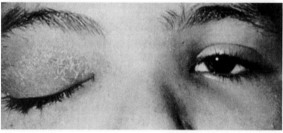

Fig. 14–3. Acute proptosis in childhood. **Top.** A 5-year-old boy with 6-day history of massive firm swelling in upper lid and downward displacement of globe by rhabdomyosarcoma occupying orbital roof. **Bottom.** A 7-year-old boy with 3-day course of painful red swelling and complete ptosis of right lid; orbital cellulitis secondary to ethmoiditis resolved quickly on antibiotic therapy.

This phenomenon may be related to compression of the optic nerve as it is dynamically stretched over a mass, compressed by contracting muscles, as the posterior wall of the globe becomes deformed, or as vascular flow is compromised (or combinations of these mechanical effects).

Proptosis with true orbital pain (as opposed to ocular irritation or foreign body sensation) is relatively rare, with the following exceptions: acute orbital inflammation, including myositis; metastases; elevated venous pressure due to arteriovenous fistulas or malformations; acute thrombosis of venous varices; and acute thrombosis of enlarged orbital veins associated with arteriovenous fistulas or vascular malformations. Of course, orbital and eye pain may be a symptom associated with the ophthalmoplegia of orbital apex and cavernous sinus syndromes (see Chapter 12), or referred from dural structures.

Atta et al[13] have elaborated a syndrome of venous stasis orbitopathy, composed of proptosis, ophthalmoplegia, and injected conjunctival vessels, of vascular (arteriovenous fistulas) and non-vascular etiologies. These authors note the usefulness of standardized echography, especially with measurement of extraocular muscle diameters, to distinguish fistulas from mass lesions.

ORBITAL EXAMINATION

The ophthalmologist is secure in his or her ability to directly visualize the anterior segment of the globe, and the fundus in most instances may be similarly brilliantly illuminated and observed. But the orbit is a bête noire (or better yet, a "black box") that does not allow the direct inspection that the transparent ocular media so easily permit, and if the ophthalmologist is uncomfortable in orbital diagnosis, how much more so the neurologist? Nonetheless, office evaluation of the orbit is not as limited as one might think. In addition to standard assessment of visual function and ocular motility, the physical examination of the orbit may be conducted as outlined in Table 14–2.

Since Graves' disease represents the most common orbital ailment, the lids must be carefully evaluated for spontaneous retraction (Fig. 14–4; see also Fig. 3–11) or for induced lag on slow ocular pursuit movements from upward to downward. Preliminary observations of the lids should be made during history-taking, before the patient's attention is called to the actual examination; some patients will stare during intense concentration or conscious effort to cooperate. True stare should be spontaneous, and lag reproducible. Lid position and movement defects must be assessed before sympathomimetic agents are instilled for pupil dilation; for example, phenylephrine (Neosynephrine) will induce moderate

TABLE 14–2. Orbit: Physical Examination

Lids
  Position: ptosis, retraction
  Movement: lag, levator function
  Swelling
  Mass
Conjunctiva
  Vessels
  Edema
  Infiltrate
Globe
  Position: proptosis, displacement
  Resistance to retropulsion
  Pulsation
Palpation of anterior orbital tissues
Auscultation
Valsalva maneuver
Forced (passive) ductions
Intraocular tension
Fundus

to marked lid retraction that masks pathologic lid position.

Anomalies of lid position and movement need not be bilateral. Ptosis is quite rare in Graves' disease, but is fairly common with inflammatory pseudotumor. Ptosis, in the absence of pain or other congestive orbital signs, should always bring to mind the possibility of myasthenia. Unilateral ptosis may account for contralateral lid retraction; thus, a patient with right partial ptosis may show relative retraction of the left upper lid, due to increased effort in an attempt to overcome the ptosis (Hering's law of equivalent innervation is applicable to the two levator palpebrae).[14] If the eye with ptosis is occluded, or the lid mechanically raised, the opposite retracted lid will assume a normal position. The causes of lid retraction are the following:

1. Graves' ophthalmopathy
2. Aberrant third nerve regeneration
3. Unilateral ptosis, with contralateral overaction of levator palpebrae (*e.g.*, myasthenia)
4. Collier's sign of dorsal midbrain (Parinaud) syndrome—bilateral

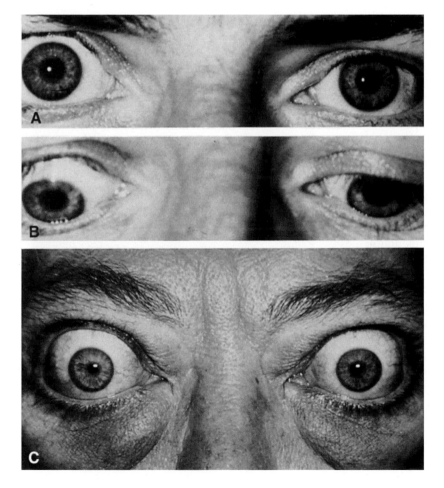

Fig. 14–4. A. Graves' disease with unilateral right lid retraction. **B.** Lid lag on downward gaze. **C.** Patient shows more profound bilateral "stare," proptosis, and edema of four lids.

5. Hyperkalemic periodic paralysis
6. Chronic systemic corticosteroid therapy

Lid swelling regularly results from the congestive edema of Graves' disease, but also typically occurs in pre-septal or orbital cellulitis, inflammatory pseudotumor, arteriovenous fistulas, and with acute viral conjunctivitis. For obscure reasons, chronic orbital neoplasms may cause intermittent lid edema. Most lid edema is accentuated by sleep, during which time the head is maintained in a relatively dependent position. Palpation of a discrete mass in the lids is exceedingly helpful, since potential biopsy is facilitated.

Veins may be visible within the thin lid tissues, either passively dilated by diffusely increased orbital pressure, or engorged by arterialization of orbital and adnexal vessels fed by arteriovenous communications. In the latter case, audible bruits and palpable thrills are evidence of turbulent, increased blood flow.

Abnormalities of the conjunctiva may serve as clues to orbital diagnosis. In general, edema (chemosis) is too nonspecific a finding to be very helpful, being common in Graves' disease, inflammatory pseudotumor, and arteriovenous fistulas. Any retrobulbar mass may produce chronic or intermittent chemosis, presumably by interfering with venous drainage in the orbit. In Graves' ophthalmopathy, the vessels overlying the insertions of especially the medial and lateral recti muscles are commonly enlarged, and indeed the muscle insertions themselves may be visibly hypertrophied (Fig. 14–5). These two conjunctival signs are exceedingly useful in identifying Graves' orbitopathy and should be sought in cases of unexplained proptosis and/or diplopia. Also, engorgement of orbital vessels may be reflected as hypervascularity of conjunctival and scleral vessels, which take on a more-or-less specific pattern in the presence of arteriovenous fistula (see Fig. 17–14).

Diffuse or focal hyperemia of scleral and episcleral vessels (especially in the superior lateral quadrant of the globe) is seen in anterior scleritis (episcleritis), or as an anterior component of posterior scleritis that accompanies the painful ophthalmoplegia syndrome of idiopathic orbital inflammation (Fig. 14–6).

The position of the globes relative to the orbital rims is subject to considerable individual and racial variations. Not the least problem is accuracy and reproducibility of measurements as obtained by a number of exophthalmometric techniques, of which the Hertel exophthalmometer is the most common, and probably the most accurate (Fig. 14–7). In a study of 681 normal adults ranging in age from 18 to 91 years, mean normal protrusion values were 15.4 mm in white women, 16.5 mm in white men, 17.8 mm in black women, and 18.5 mm in black men; upper limits of normal were 20.1, 21.7, 23.0, and 24.7 mm,

respectively.[15] No normal individual showed more than 2 mm of asymmetry.

To reiterate, there is no clinically precise technique for quantitating proptosis, as minor deviations in positioning of exophthalmometers at the lateral orbital rim result in gross variations in readings. Depending on technique and experience, substantial interobserver variation is demonstrable.[16]

Subtle degrees of proptosis are difficult to detect and more difficult still to measure. The following techniques are useful in determining the presence of relative unilateral proptosis: viewing the position of the globes and lids from above the brows (Fig. 14–8, top); insertion of fingertips between inferior orbital rim and globe; and simultaneous palpation of corneal apices (Fig. 14–8, bottom).

The clinician should be aware of several situations in which proptosis is more apparent than real, that is, a condition of pseudo-exophthalmos: unilateral lid retraction, wherein the homolateral eye appears larger; unilateral mild ptosis, wherein the contralateral eye appears larger; asymmetry of facial bones including orbital rims;

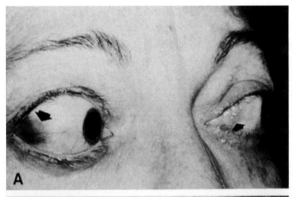
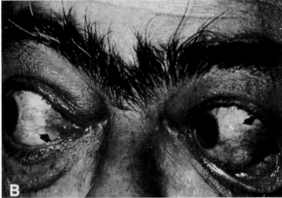

Fig. 14–5. Conjunctival signs of Graves' congestive orbitopathy. **A.** Characteristic fleshy hypertrophy of insertion of right lateral rectus (*large arrows*). Note localized chemosis of left caruncle (*small arrow*). **B.** Hypertrophy of insertion of medial rectus with hypervascularity of the vessels overlying the horizontal recti insertions (*arrows*).

and unilateral enophthalmos,[17] wherein the normal contralateral eye appears prominent (Fig. 14–9). The differential diagnosis of enophthalmos is included in Table 14–3.

In a small number of patients, differences in the axial lengths of the globes may account for relative unilateral proptosis. This situation is resolved by finding differences in the amount of myopia (*i.e.*, greater myopia in the apparently proptosed globe). Precise determination of axial globe lengths is afforded by ultrasonography.

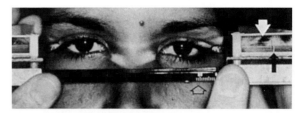

Fig. 14–7. Exophthalmometry with Hertel instrument. *White arrow* indicates cornea of left eye as viewed through right-angle prism. *Black arrow* indicates mires fixed at 18 mm. *Open arrow* indicates baseline gauge. Note position of footplates placed against lateral orbital rims.

There is little evidence to support the claim that a complete third nerve palsy results in sufficient relaxation of the muscle cone to produce detectable proptosis. As a rule, any significant degree of proptosis should not be attributed to extraocular muscle weakness. This dictum may be confirmed by performing exophthalmometry on patients with vascular-diabetic oculomotor palsies; one finds no meaningful difference between the two eyes at the time of most profound ophthalmoplegia, and no changes in exophthalmometry readings following complete recovery. Moreover, irreducible proptosis (increased resistance to retropulsion of

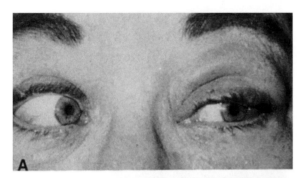
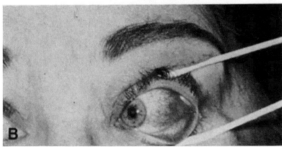
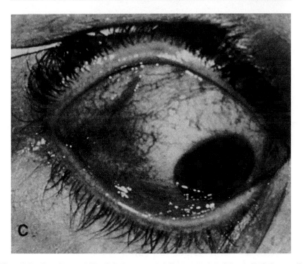

Fig. 14–6. A and **B.** A 60-year-old woman with painful swelling of left lids, abduction defect, and episcleral vascular suffusion. Results of ultrasonography were typical for idiopathic inflammation with thickened sclera. **C.** Second event involved right globe, as acute episcleritis. No underlying systemic disorder was found; both episodes were relieved dramatically with a course of oral corticosteroid therapy.

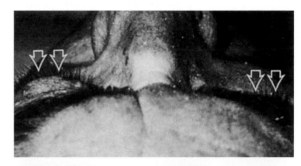
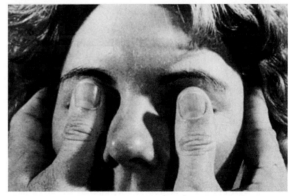

Fig. 14–8. Subtle degrees of proptosis detected by viewing the relative position of the lids and lashes as seen from over the brows **(top)**. By placing the thumbs against the orbital rims, relative position of corneas may be assessed **(bottom)**; also, with gentle pressure, relative resistance to retropulsation of the globes is determined.

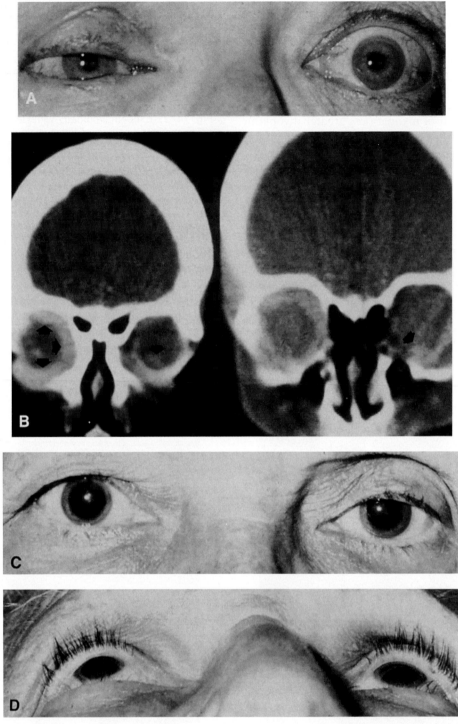

Fig. 14–9. Enophthalmos. **A.** A 56-year-old woman with right enophthalmos and fixation of the globe, and proptosis of the left eye. **B.** Bilateral orbital metastases of scirrhous breast carcinoma were disclosed by CT scan. **C.** Patient was referred for right proptosis but actually had left enophthalmos caused by simple senile atrophy of orbital fat pad, without history of facial trauma; note sunken superior lid sulcus on left **(C)**, and relative position of left globe and lids, as viewed from below **(D)**.

TABLE 14–3. Causes of Enophthalmos

Senile orbital fat atrophy
Traumatic fat atrophy
Traumatic orbital floor fracture
Sclerosing orbital metastases from stomach (linitis plastica) or breast (desmoplastic fibrosis)
Parry-Romberg (facial hemiatrophy; scleroderma) syndrome*
Facial osteomyelitis, fat necrosis
Maxillary sinus atelectasis (hypoplasia)†

* Data from ref. 18.
† Data from ref. 19.

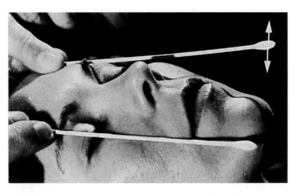

Fig. 14–10. To detect pulsation, cotton-tipped applicators are placed tangentially across closed lids. Pulsation is transmitted and amplified by length of stick (*arrows*).

the globe through closed lids) in the presence of motor deficits signifies Graves' disease, or a mass at the orbital apex or superior orbital fissure. If oculomotor nerve palsy could result in proptosis, there would be no resistance to globe retropulsion, there being no mass or congestion present.

Pulsation of the globe is encountered most commonly with acquired carotid-cavernous fistulas, and rarely in other conditions.[20] Causes of pulsation are listed in Table 14–4.

Biomicroscopical examination usually reveals even minimal pulsation, best seen during measurement of intraocular tension by Goldmann applanation tonometry. Cotton-swab sticks may be placed tangentially across the corneal apices, such that transmitted pulsations are amplified by the length of the swab (Fig. 14–10).

Exploration of the orbital rim by fingertip palpation (Fig. 14–11) may reveal masses lying in the tissues of the lids and also in the anterior portions of the orbit. Discovery of such masses is extremely helpful since biopsy via simple transseptal anterior orbitotomy is the most rapid route to tissue identification.

Auscultation of the globe and face is a useful maneuver to confirm the presence of vascular bruits, as encountered in acquired arteriovenous fistulas or congenital vascular malformations. Bruits may be more intense over zygoma or mastoid bones, where the diaphragm

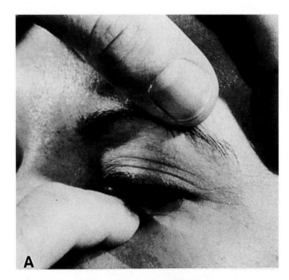

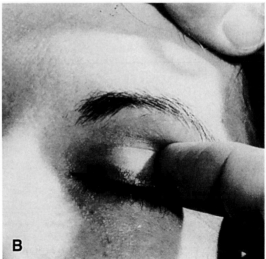

Fig. 14–11. A and **B.** Fingertip exploration 360°; palpation for anterior aspect of orbital mass.

TABLE 14–4. Causes of Globe Pulsation

Congenital sphenoidal dysplasia with partial orbitocranial encephalocele (in neurofibromatosis)
Transmission of pulsation of intracranial pressure via surgical or traumatic defects in the roof or posterior wall of the orbit
Arterial pulsation of orbital veins resulting from arteriovenous fistulas
Congenital arteriovenous malformations
Orbito-cranial venous varicocele complexes
Tricuspid regurgitation*

* Data from ref. 21.

of the stethoscope is more effective than the bell, with which the globe itself is better auscultated (Fig. 14–12). Symmetrical cranial or ocular bruits are commonly present in normal children and therefore must be evaluated with caution.

Forced expiration against resistance (Valsalva maneuver) raises venous pressure in the neck, face, and head, such that orbital masses with significant draining veins will increase in volume, evidenced by transient increase in proptosis (Fig. 14–13). This phenomenon is typically demonstrable in the presence of congenital venous varices or arteriovenous malformations, but may also be seen with acquired carotid-cavernous fistula or

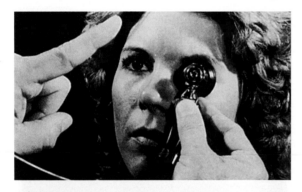
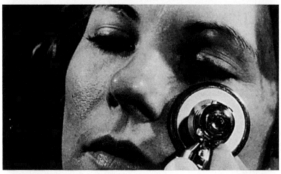
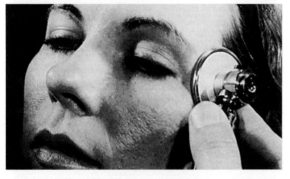

Fig. 14–12. Auscultation of globe and face. **Top.** Stethoscope bell used to auscultate globe and orbit; note that contralateral eye fixates finger to minimize lid movement. **Middle.** Stethoscope diaphragm was used to auscultate zygoma. **Bottom.** Stethoscope diaphragm used to auscultate temple. Vascular bruits may also be best heard at the mastoid.

with primary or secondary bony defects that permit transmission of intracranial pressure to orbital contents. Crying infants with such lesions may show this sign spontaneously or with head-hanging.

Where accompanying physical signs are absent or minimal, the single most useful technique in distinguishing neural ophthalmoplegia (cranial nerve palsies, myasthenia, chronic progressive external ophthalmoplegia) from local orbital disease (e.g., Graves' ophthalmopathy) is the forced (passive) duction test. In 1967, Stephens and Reinecke[22] reported a method for quantitation of the forced duction test, but no standardized accessible and practical instrument is currently available. There are various techniques to test for mechanical resistance to rotation of the globe; the test described here is that preferred by this author (see Fig. 3–6). Following topical conjunctival anesthesia with, for example, proparacaine (Ophthetic) or tetracaine (Pontocaine), cotton-tipped swabs are saturated with 10% aqueous cocaine and applied for about 1 minute to the area of the insertions of the four recti muscles of each eye. It is important to compare corresponding muscles in both eyes. For example, if the right eye lags in upward gaze, the insertion of the inferior rectus is grasped and, while the patient looks upward, an attempt is made to gently rotate the right globe upward. For comparison, the insertion of the left inferior rectus is then grasped, and the left globe rotated upward. With care, there is only slight discomfort, and the conjunctiva is minimally traumatized; minor subconjunctival hemorrhage is of no great consequence. Alternatively, the conjunctiva at the limbus may be grasped, or a cotton swab tip may be braced against the corneoscleral junction and used to "push the eye."

The forced duction test will be positive, that is, there will be resistance to mechanical rotation of the globe, in the following situations: Graves' restrictive myopathy, inflammatory pseudotumor (myositis), infiltrating carcinoma, incarceration of extraocular muscles and their surrounding soft tissue attachments that herniate into orbital floor, and medial wall fractures. Because of secondary fibrotic contractures of extraocular muscles, on rare occasions the forced duction test will be positive in the chronic fixed form of ocular myasthenia, in advanced chronic external ophthalmoplegia, or with extremely long-standing sixth or third nerve palsies.

In situations where the globe is mechanically restricted (again, Graves' disease is typical) intraocular tension may be spuriously elevated, or pressure may inordinately rise on attempted upward gaze.[23] There seems to be a correlation with higher ocular tensions and degree of proptosis; tension decreases in patients undergoing orbital decompression.[24] However, it must be recognized that intraocular pressure increases linearly with vertical excursions of the globe, changes of

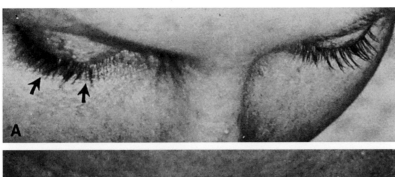

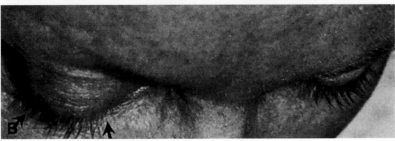

Fig. 14–13. A 46-year-old woman with recurrent right orbital pain. **A.** Minimal right proptosis detected by observing position of lids and lashes (*arrows*) from above the brow. **B.** Increasing right proptosis during Valsalva maneuver (*arrows*). Orbital venography demonstrated typical venous varix.

as much as 7 mmHg being recorded in normal subjects.[25] Indeed, this phenomenon in normal subjects brings into question the validity of this procedure as an adjunct in the diagnosis of Graves' orbitopathy.[26] Carotid cavernous or dural arterial fistulas also typically elevate intraocular tension by raising episcleral venous drainage pressure.

The ocular fundus may be altered by any retrobulbar mass in the following ways: indentations of the posterior wall of the globe produces chorioretinal striae (Fig. 14–14), while compression at the equator of the globe and

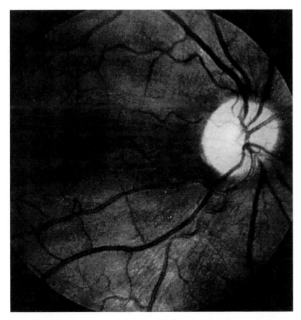

Fig. 14–14. Chorioretinal striae through fovea caused by retrobulbar mass, which in this case was an hemangioma.

beyond results in a more diffuse flattening, best appreciated by indirect ophthalmoscopy, and accentuated by rotation of the eye toward the quadrant(s) of the orbit occupied by the tumor; dilation and tortuosity of retinal veins (venous hemorrhages or occlusions suggest relatively high pressures, as encountered with arteriovenous fistulas); retinal arterial occlusions, especially in orbital phycomycoses such as mucormycosis; edema or frank elevation of the optic nerve head; optic atrophy in chronic compression; optociliary shunt vessels of the disk, especially with perioptic meningioma; retinal detachment or choroidal suffusion with inflammatory lesions or scleritis. De La Paz and Boniuk[27] have extensively reviewed the fundus manifestations of orbital disease.

Optic disc swelling (Table 14–5) does not necessarily suggest actual infiltration of the nerve or its meninges, this fundus finding being rather non-specific and observed potentially with any increase in retrobulbar mass. Indeed, in orbital context, disc edema is seen most commonly with Graves' orbitopathy. On rare occasions optic gliomas produce a picture of disc swelling with or without venous occlusion, and perioptic meningiomas may be characterized by a clinical triad of slowly progressive visual loss, pallor admixed with disk swelling, and papillary retino-ciliary venous shunts (See Chapter 5, Part II).

DIAGNOSTIC CONSIDERATIONS

After history-taking and thorough physical examination as outlined in the preceding sections, the clinician should be able to make at least a tentative but rational diagnosis, even before special diagnostic studies are un-

TABLE 14–5. Optic Disc Swelling with Orbital Lesions

Graves' orbitopathy
Perioptic meningioma*
Optic glioma
Carotid-cavernous fistula
Inflammatory pseudotumor
Any retrobulbar mass

* Proptosis may be minimal or absent.

dertaken. Excluding congenital dysostoses, malformations and cysts, and traumatic fractures and hematomas, which rarely cause diagnostic dilemmas, all orbital disease may in essence be classified into only four common types: (1) Graves' ophthalmopathy, (2) idiopathic inflammations, (3) vascular malformations and fistulas, and (4) true neoplasms. Large series of patients with orbital disorders show variable specific incidence rates, depending on referral patterns and age groups. Graves' orbitopathy may be underestimated since many clinicians do not regularly refer uncomplicated cases; the same is true for trauma and congenital anomalies (Table 14–6).

Graves' Disease

Graves' congestive orbitopathy is the single most common orbital disorder, with annual incidence rates ranging from 12 to 20 per 100,000 population, and with higher prevalence rates (42%) among Caucasian (European) groups than in Asians (8%). The age-specific incidence rates are greatest among middle-aged patients, and are approximately four times higher in women than in men. In patients with hyperthyroidism, ophthalmopathy is evident in 25% to 50%, but severe complications evolve in just 3% to 5%. Several studies have linked tobacco smoking to increased severity of Graves' orbitopathy,[28] possibly related to alterations in immunoregulatory cell function induced by smoking, and increased synthesis of glycosaminoglycans by orbital fibroblasts.

Thyroid eye disease is usually associated with hyperthyroidism, and less frequently with Hashimoto's thyroiditis, euthyroid states, thyroid carcinoma, or primary hyperthyroidism. About 80% of patients will develop signs of ophthalmopathy either during the year before or the year after a diagnosis of thyroid malfunction.[29] Tallstedt et al[30] demonstrated a two- to threefold increase in risk of developing orbitopathy when the thyroid disease was managed with radioactive iodine treat-

TABLE 14–6. Causes of Orbital Disease*

Disorder	Percentage	No. patients
Graves' disease	47%	
Inflammations	10%	
Infectious, sinus		52/144
Idiopathic, miscellaneous		92/144
Neoplasms	22%	314
Primary		
Optic glioma		15
Meningioma, perioptic		7
Meningioma, sphenoid		22
Mesenchymal/bone		35
Lacrimal		14
Lymphoproliferative		58
Nerve sheath		23
Contiguous (*e.g.,* sinus, eyelids, etc)		44
Metastatic		29
Vascular	7%	96
Neoplasms		56
Hemangioma		35
Lymphangioma		19
Arteriovenous shunts/malformations		18
Venous varices		15
Miscellaneous	10%	
Trauma		75
Dermoid/epidermoid		36
Mucocele		26

* Based on approximately 1400 cases.
Adapted from ref. 1.

ment as opposed to surgical or medical treatment; this effect may be related to the release of thyroid antigens and to subsequent enhancement of autoimmune response directed toward antigens shared by the thyroid and the orbit. Evolution of ophthalmopathy after radio-iodine therapy is often transient and may be ameliorated by the administration of prednisone.[28,31]

The principal signs are lid retraction and edema, proptosis, and diplopia. If congestive signs are slight, the ocular motor defects are regularly misdiagnosed, and unsuitable studies for intracranial disease follow. Eye movement defects with Graves' disease are discussed in detail in Chapter 12. Infrequently Graves' disease presents in an acute inflammatory form that mimics orbital cellulitis or idiopathic pseudotumor, including pain, lid swelling with ptosis, diplopia and infrequently visual loss.[32] Proptosis and restrictive myopathy also may occur in children with hyperthyroidism.[33]

Obscured by the more obvious external congestive signs and by symptoms of diplopia, the complication of compressive optic neuropathy may be overlooked. Although its incidence is said to be less than 5% among patients with typical thyroid disease, Graves' optic neuropathy is a treatable cause of potentially disabling visual loss (see also Chapter 5, Part II). Congestive symptoms always precede visual loss, which is usually gradual in onset and bilateral in most patients, but may occasionally be acute and asymmetrical. Presenting acuities are poorer than 20/60 in 50% of cases; central scotomas, at times combined with inferior field depression, are the predominant field defects. Congestive signs are usually of moderate intensity without severe proptosis or exposure keratopathy. Bilateral and symmetrical ductional restriction is the most commonly associated motility disturbance. Oral corticosteroids are often effective in restoring visual function, but steroid-unresponsive neuropathy may be improved promptly by supervoltage orbital irradiation or surgical decompression.[34,35] The medical management of Graves' disease is complex and demands a comprehensive approach, often requiring a variety of surgical (see below) and radiotherapeutic interventions.[36,37]

It is worth noting that Graves' ophthalmopathy frequently presents or worsens weeks to months after radioactive iodine ablative therapy, and that concomitant corticosteroid therapy may ameliorate this effect.[28,31,38] Char[39] has reviewed the immune mechanisms by which intrathyroidal clonally restricted B-cells secrete autoantibodies, with extraocular muscle and orbital tissues, including fibroblasts, acting as antigenic targets; fibroblasts in turn produce glycosaminoglycan that binds water, increasing orbital connective tissue volume. Prednisone, cyclosporine, and irradiation, in variable combinations, are all applicable forms of therapy. Indeed, in the Mayo Clinic experience[40] of therapies for Graves' ophthalmopathy, only 20% of patients required one or more surgical procedures; 7 of 120 patients (6%) developed optic neuropathy.

Inflammations

Orbital inflammatory disease may take several distinct forms. Acute orbital cellulitis is defined as infectious inflammation of soft tissues posterior to the orbital septum, characterized by distension and hyperemia of the lids and conjunctiva, pain, proptosis, and limitation of eye movements. Although sinus infections were formerly frequently associated, this is now a relatively rare condition, thanks to the availability of antibiotics. However, the condition is potentially life-threatening. Principal predisposing risk factors include ocular or adnexal surgical procedures (lid, strabismus, or retinal operations), facial or orbital trauma, especially with retained orbital foreign bodies, dacryocystitis or other periorbital infections, insect bite envenomization, diabetes, and immunosuppressive states. Especially in children and young adults, orbital cellulitis is still associated with ethmoidal and maxillary sinusitis. Those bacterial agents commonly responsible for sinusitis (predominantly *Streptococcus pneumoniae, Staphylococcus aureus,* and less frequently *Haemophilus influenzae*), not surprisingly are implicated in orbital cellulitis.[41] Rapidly progressive rhabdomyosarcoma may present a clinical picture of pseudocellulitis in children (Fig. 14–3).

CT scanning or MRI is mandatory, not only to disclose sinus disease, but also to determine the presence of meningitis, cavernous sinus thrombosis, or orbital abscess formation, which requires surgical drainage. Most associated abscesses occur in the medial orbit adjacent to the ethmoidal sinuses, with spread of infection via communicating veins (septic thrombophlebitis) or across the thin lamina papyracea. Chronic mucoceles may also be associated with cellulitis or abscess formation.

Rhino-orbital mucormycosis (genera *Mucor, Absidia,* or *Rhizopus*) is a catastrophic form of often fulminant, necrotizing orbital infection, most likely to occur in patients in ketoacidosis or immunosuppressed by chemotherapy, AIDS, or hemodialysis. Such infection is extremely rare in healthy individuals. A chronic form of rhino-cerebral mucormycosis is well described,[42] and is associated with carotid artery and cavernous sinus thrombosis. Rapid confirmation by nasopharyngeal mucosal aspiration and biopsy is essential. Wide debridement and amphotericin B infusion may be life-saving, and hyperbaric oxygen has been advocated.[43] Aspergillosis may also cause an indolent or acute orbital cellulitis (see also Chapter 12).

Allergic fungal sinusitis is a relatively uncommon form of chronic paranasal mycosis in immunocompetent individuals. This entity can involve the orbit without direct invasion or dire outcome, and is most frequently, but not exclusively, attributed to *Aspergillus*. Signs include nasal obstruction, focal pain, proptosis, diplopia, optic neuropathy, and facial deformity. Inflamed sinus mucosa shows hyperintense signal characteristics on both T1- and T2-weighted MRI, but isointense signal of sinus cavities, with involvement of multiple sinuses; peripheral eosinophilia and elevated total immunoglobulin E, as well as fungus-specific IgE and IgG, help establish the diagnosis.[44] In the differential spectrum are included invasive fungal sinusitis, orbital inflammatory pseudotumor, metastatic carcinoma, lymphoma, Wegener's granulomatosis, and systemic vasculitis.

Idiopathic orbital inflammation (orbital pseudotumor) is a frequent cause of acute, subacute, or chronic painful ophthalmoplegia, accompanied by variable orbital signs. This clinical term encompasses non-infectious processes that mimic cellulitis, Graves' disease, or neoplasm; thus, the term *orbital pseudotumor*. Inflammation may be diffuse, or localized to the posterior scleral coat (posterior scleritis), to single or multiple extraocular muscles (myositis; see Chapter 12), to the lacrimal gland (dacryoadenitis), or to perioptic meninges (perioptic neuritis), or present as a soft tissue mass. Signs and symptoms are determined by location and include severe to mild orbital ache, diplopia, lid swelling with ptosis, conjunctival chemosis, episcleral injection, proptosis, and ductional defects. Uveitis, uveal effusion, and optic neuropathy are rare, but account for visual loss.

Orbital pseudotumor and the Tolosa-Hunt syndrome are likely the same process, varying only in that the idiopathic inflammation involves predominantly the orbit in the former and predominantly the superior orbital fissure and/or the anterior cavernous sinus in the latter. Idiopathic inflammation is a diagnosis of exclusion, made only in a fairly circumscribed clinical context, and when other pathologic processes have been ruled out. In this regard, contrast-enhanced CT scan or MRI shows diffuse infiltration or focal lesions, usually with notable enhancement of the posterior wall of the globe (Fig. 14–15). With proper orbital imaging and ultrasonographic assessment as diagnostic procedures, tissue biopsy is rarely necessary, and the response to systemic corticosteroid administration is usually dramatic, if not diagnostic (see also Chapter 12).

Uncommonly, orbital inflammation takes the form of a non-caseating granuloma, suggesting sarcoidosis, but without other systemic implications. This seems principally a histologic variant, with some predilection for the lacrimal gland.[45] In contrast, Wegener's granulomatosis is locally destructive necrotizing vasculitis with respiratory and other systemic implications. The majority present as scleritis with or without orbital mass lesions, either uni- or bilateral, and commonly with nasal and sinus symptoms.[46] Also known as lethal midline granuloma, and causing destruction of midline facial tissues

including nasal septum, biopsy shows mixed inflammation with necrosis. Other orbital vasculitides include giant cell arteritis, zoster ophthalmicus, and lupus erythematosus.

Orbital lymphoid hyperplasia is a histopathologic quandry even when biopsy specimens show polyclonal T-cell lymphocyte proliferation (suggesting benign, reactive lymphoid hyperplasia), versus monoclonal proliferation of B cells typical of malignant lymphoma. Thus, lymphoid hyperplasia may possibly embrace simple pseudotumor inflammation, but in other instances is a harbinger of non-Hodgkins lymphoma.[47] Because of this potential outcome, some authors suggest complete systemic staging (hematologic survey), and strict clinical follow-up. Atypical features or monoclonality make more extensive immunotypic surface cell typing or DNA hybridization mandatory.[48] Therefore, biopsy specimens should not be placed in formalin! Both corticosteroids and radiation therapy are acutely effective, as is usually also the case with idiopathic inflammation. Therefore, clinical response to initial therapy cannot carry diagnostic inferences.

In the immunocompromised AIDS population, lymphoma is the most frequent orbital lesion, non-Hodgkin's lymphoma being well-documented,[49] as well as Burkitt small noncleaved; the importance of immunophenotypic (immunoglobulin light chain antigens) characteristics is stressed.[50] Also, orbital cellulitis from contiguous sites of fungal (*Aspergillus, Mucormycosis*)[51] and toxoplasmosis infection may be encountered.

The specifics of histologic and immunologic typing techniques for the classification of orbital lymphomatous and other hematopoietic tumors are reviewed by Jakobiec and Nelson.[52]

Vascular Lesions

Vascular lesions involving the orbit may be categorized as neoplastic (hemangiomas and lymphangiomas), congenital anomalies (simple venous varix, arteriovenous malformation), and acquired arteriovenous shunts such as the carotid-cavernous fistula. From the extensive Moorfields Eye Hospital Orbital Clinic experience, Wright[53] concludes that vascular abnormalities are the commonest space occupying lesions, of which primary congenital venous varix complexes constitute the largest category. Most series support the view that cavernous hemangioma is the most frequent primary orbital neoplasm. Otherwise, venous varices and lymphatic malformations (lymphangiomas) are of neuro-ophthalmologic interest because of orbital complications (enlargement during respiratory infections; spontaneous orbital hemorrhage) and their association with contiguous and noncontiguous facial and/or intracranial vascular anomalies[54] (see also Chapter 17).

In neuro-ophthalmologic context, carotid-cavernous

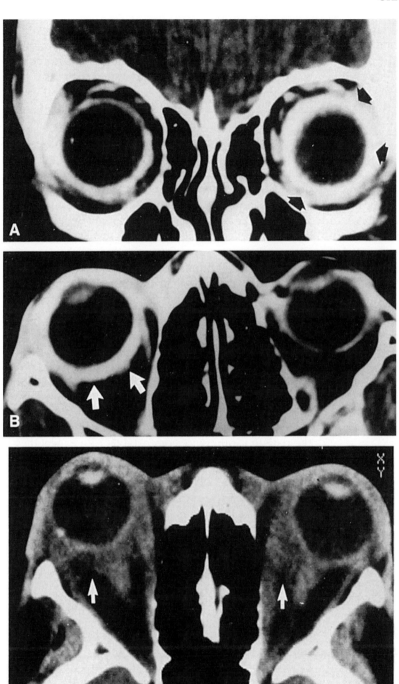

Fig. 14–15. Contrast-enhanced computed tomography (CT) scan in patient with painful ophthalmoplegia, lid swelling, and proptosis. In unilateral case, note enhancing envelope of thickened sclera (*arrows*) on coronal **(A)** and axial **(B)** sections of left globe. **C.** Bilateral orbital pseudotumor shows shaggy infiltration of orbital soft tissues (*arrows*) surrounding globes and optic nerves.

fistulas (CCFs) are of singular interest. CCFs are initiated by rupture of the wall of the carotid artery, or one of its branches, into the cavernous sinus. In the presence of a CCF, the cavernous sinus and its venous exits are exposed to arterial pressure that alters their hemodynamic state. The major orbital communication of the cavernous sinus is the superior ophthalmic vein, which may expand tremendously, engorging all orbital and conjunctival veins. These veins become arterialized, producing signs and symptoms of venous congestion. The classic, fully developed syndrome includes pulsating exophthalmos, ocular bruit that may be subjective and/ or objective, diplopia, headache, conjunctival chemosis, increased intraocular pressure, dilated conjunctival vessels, and visual decrease (see Fig. 17–13). To some degree bilateral orbital involvement is often present because of normally occurring venous communications between the cavernous sinuses. In some cases contralateral exophthalmos may exceed that present on the side of the fistula, because of ipsilateral orbital vein thrombosis.

Small meningeal arterial branches supplying the dural

walls of the cavernous sinus and its tributaries may rupture, creating a minor dural arteriovenous shunt. This type of fistula usually appears in middle-aged women as a distinctive syndrome and may account for most so-called spontaneous CCFs. The signs are usually mild and include dilated conjunctival veins, mild proptosis, and bruit. Transient sixth nerve palsy and unilateral headache frequently antedate orbital signs by many months. Chronic unilateral "red eye" is often misdiagnosed and treated as an inflammatory condition.[55] The diagnosis and management of arteriovenous fistulas is addressed in Chapter 17.

Arteriovenous fistulas are the prototypic cause of a venous stasis orbitopathy syndrome, combining engorgement and hypoxia of orbital soft tissues, and composed of clinical signs of proptosis, variable ophthalmoparesis, lid swelling, and conjunctival chemosis. Other mechanical obstruction obtains with venous blockage at the orbital apex, within the cavernous sinus and with middle cranial fossa masses.[13] In this setting, standardized A-scan echography has proven helpful in distinguishing fistulas from mass lesions, or from Graves' disease.

Orbital infarction with acute pain, visual loss, ophthalmoplegia, and anterior and posterior segment ischemia occurs with giant cell arteritis, mucormycosis, common carotid artery occlusion,[56] and carotid artery dissection.[57]

Neoplasms

The wide variety of primary and secondary neoplasms that affect the orbit and adnexal structures is too extensive a subject to be adequately covered in the present discussion; therefore, only a few generalizations will be attempted here.

As noted above, benign tumors such as cavernous hemangioma, neurilemoma (schwannoma), dermoid cysts, etc., constitute the commonest lesions, which are characterized by insidious growth with slowly progressive proptosis. Although termed benign, the mixed lacrimal gland tumor also progresses sluggishly, filling the lacrimal fossa, but authoritative consensus requires complete surgical extirpation of any lacrimal gland mass unless inflammatory signs are clinically predominant. While the advent of CT, MRI, and ultrasonography have added enormously to the previously vague radiologic assessment of orbital soft tissue disease, and certain tumors (e.g., hemangioma, dermoid) show rather typical images, nonetheless, surgical exploration with tissue confirmation is the most reasonable approach; this dictum is more emphatic in the presence of pain, visual loss, or a rapidly progressive course. In childhood, brisk evolution suggests rhabdomyosarcoma, acute leukemia, and histiocytosis especially where bone is eroded.[58] Other frequent orbital disorders in children include cysts, vascular lesions, optic gliomas and meningiomas, inflammatory masses, etc.; malignancies constitute

roughly 20%.[59] Again, inflammatory cellulitis with or without contiguous sinusitis must be investigated.

Orbital metastases are uncommon, constituting 2% to 7% of biopsied orbital lesions.[2] Most such cases have a previous diagnosis of primary malignancy, and orbital findings tend not to be necessarily suggestive of metastasis. The intraconal space, muscles, and adjacent bone, sinuses or brain may be involved. In adult women, of course, breast carcinoma metastases are most common, with at times remarkably long intervals between primary diagnosis and therapy, and subsequent orbital secondary lesions; the relationship may be cryptic. While proptosis is the rule, schirrhus breast carcinoma regularly produces a reactive fibrosis (desmoplasia) that causes soft tissue induration, severe eye movement limitation, and progressive enophthalmos.[17] Unless bone is involved, neither CT pattern nor ultrasound findings are suggestive. Fine-needle biopsy[60] is especially helpful when there is a strong suspicion, for example with known primary malignancy, that a focal orbital mass represents a metastasis and more extensive surgical manipulation is unwarranted.

Many orbital metastases will respond to palliative radiotherapy, but anterior segment complications, such as recurrent sloughing of corneal epithelium with ensuing chronic irritation, must be taken into account if the patient is otherwise comfortable. Life expectancy is limited, as determined principally by the primary malignancy type or other non-orbital metastases.

Trauma

Trauma accounts for orbital problems that take the following forms: fractures of orbital walls, commonly with floor fractures, but the medial wall may be the site of a "blowout" as well; hemorrhage into the orbital soft tissues, with extension usually into the lids and bulbar conjunctiva; occult hematoma; immediate or delayed signs of arteriovenous fistula. With the exception of the last-named complication, traumatic orbitopathy is usually not a diagnostic dilemma. However, diplopia may not necessarily be attributable to the common mechanism of entrapment of the inferior rectus or inferior oblique muscles in a floor fracture. Hematoma and edema, or direct injury to extraocular muscles or motor nerves, also produces double vision that, fortunately, may abate without surgical intervention. A negative forced duction test, that is, absence of mechanical restriction, suggests this second mechanism, and, in the absence of enophthalmos (due to major floor fracture), surgery may be deferred.[61]

Ophthalmologic signs and symptoms may divert attention from the possibility of complications of orbital roof fractures, and from potentially life-threatening intracranial injury. Furthermore, evidence of CNS involvement may be delayed and underestimated. Continuing headache, stiff neck, and other non-localizing features can indicate subdural hematoma, meningitis, or pyogenic abscess formation. CT scanning or MRI will reveal pneumocephalus, and most fracture sites are best visualized with CT bone-window settings. Neuro-surgical repair and broad-spectrum antibiotic therapy is indicated, as is scrupulous clinical and radiologic follow-up.[62] The general problems of diagnosis and management of orbital trauma, including fractures, are reviewed elsewhere.[63,64]

DIAGNOSTIC PROCEDURES: AN OVERVIEW

Detailed descriptions of diagnostic procedures are beyond the scope of this presentation. But a brief overview of available techniques (Table 14–7) and their rational application may provide pragmatic guidelines. The advent of elegant technical equipment in no way discharges the clinician's responsibility for astute history-taking and meticulous physical examination.

Any case of orbital disease, the cause of which is not obvious, arguably may profit from a preliminary plain skull x-ray series. With this initial radiologic procedure, the following features may be scrutinized: the general contour of the orbital bones; the condition of the paranasal sinuses, especially the ethmoid complexes, maxillary antra, and frontal sinuses; and the density and configuration of the sphenoid wings and superior orbital fissure.

Computed tomography (CT) is presently the single most productive modality for analyzing orbital bones, with which the following structures may be visualized: the bony confines of the orbit and surrounding sinus structures; the lacrimal bony canal; the globe and lens; the intraorbital portions of the optic nerve; and the extraocular muscles, especially the horizontal and superior recti (Fig. 14–16). Moreover, CT with contrast enhancement discloses the full configuration and location of masses with respect to other orbital structures, principally the relationships to muscle cone, optic nerve, and lacrimal gland. In several particular instances, the location, configuration, and degree of contrast enhancement of lesions may strongly suggest a distinctive tumor type (Fig. 14–17) or inflammation (*e.g.*, cavernous hemangioma, optic glioma, lacrimal gland tumor, dermoid cyst,

TABLE 14–7. Orbital Imaging Techniques

Plain skull series: antero-posterior, lateral, and Waters' views
Computed tomography, contrast-enhanced; bone-window (especially for fractures)
Ultrasonography
Magnetic resonance imaging; fat-suppression techniques
Arteriography
Venography
Radionuclide scan

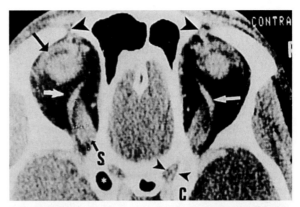

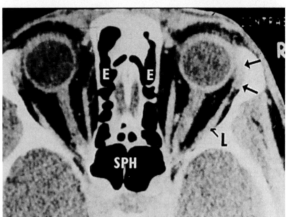

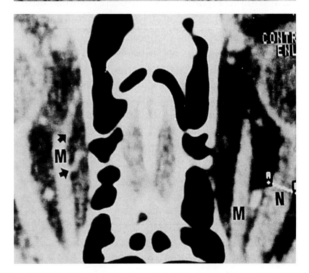

Fig. 14–16. Contrast-enhanced CT scan of normal orbits. **Top.** Superior orbit section shows superior ophthalmic veins (*white arrows*), superior rectus origin (*S*), left levator muscle complex (*black arrow*), position of trochlea and tendon of superior oblique muscles (*large arrowheads*), right optic canal (*small arrowheads*), and anterior clinoid (*C*). (**, pneumatized left anterior clinoid.*) **Middle.** Midorbital section shows ethmoidal sinus complex (*E*), sphenoidal sinus (*SPH*), lacrimal gland (*arrows*), and lateral rectus (*L*). **Bottom.** Enlargement shows left medial rectus (*M*), with anterior (*top arrow*) and posterior (*bottom arrow*) ethmoidal arteries; note cursor across optic nerve on right (*N*).

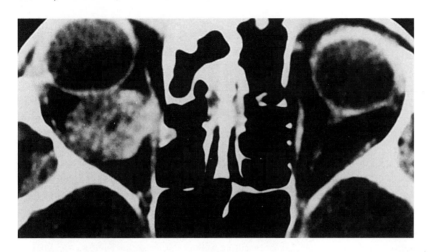

Fig. 14–17. CT scan shows typical configuration of intraconal hemangioma. Note slightly inhomogeneous content, rounded distinct borders, and clear apical space.

mucocele, perioptic meningioma, single or multiple muscle thickening),[65-67] but no firm histopathologic diagnosis may be inferred by CT characteristics alone.

Thin-section (1.5–3.0 mm) contiguous overlaps with bone-window settings provide a sensitive detector of orbital bone fractures, especially with regard to floor defects (blowout fracture),[60,68] and CT analysis of orbital volume and degree of soft tissue herniation may have prognostic value for risk of delayed enophthalmos.[69] Thin-section CT, thus, has replaced complex motion laminography in defining fractures, erosions, expansions, and hyperostosis of the bony walls of the orbit or skull base.

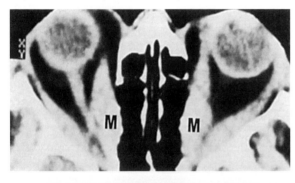

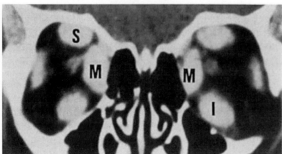

Fig. 14–18. CT scan in Graves' disease. **Top.** Axial section shows massively enlarged horizontal recti (*M, medial*) with packed apex. **Bottom.** Coronal section demonstrates enlarged medial (*M*), superior (*S*), and inferior (*I*) recti.

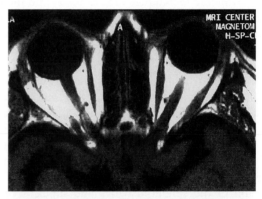

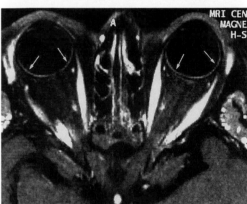

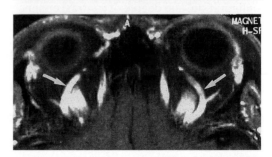

Fig. 14–19. MRI of orbits, axial sections. **Top.** T1-weighted: orbital fat is white (hyperintense), muscles are dark. **Middle.** Fat saturation with gadolinium through mid-orbit: orbital fat signal suppressed (*dark*), accentuates hyperintense muscles; note also choroid (*small arrows*). **Bottom.** Fat-saturation technique through superior aspect of orbit; note superior ophthalmic veins (*arrows*).

Graves' disease is the overwhelming single most common cause of single or multiple extraocular muscle thickening (Fig. 14–18; see also Figs. 12–28 and 12–30); inflammatory myositis is considerably less frequent, and muscle metastases are quite rare. Passive congestive myopathy also accompanies arteriovenous shunts and lesions of the superior orbital fissure and cavernous sinus, where orbital venous return is obstructed. The capacity of CT to detect minor to moderate changes in muscle diameter is perhaps limited,[70] and standardized A-scan ultrasonography seems more sensitive and practical.[71]

Now almost universally available, MRI is the preferable technique for imaging the soft tissue contents of the orbit, high-resolution 3-mm and thinner sections being available, as well as gadolinium contrast enhancement (Figs. 14–19, 14–20, and 14–21).

To facilitate maximal application of CT scanning or MRI procedures, the clinician must communicate to the technician or radiologist a specific request for multiple orbital sections and fat saturation protocols, and should indicate the principal clinical diagnostic considerations. As an anatomic guide for surgical exploration, neuroimaging provides critical spatial details, if not more precise diagnostic information. The ideal complementary comparison study to CT or MRI is standardized ultrasonography (echography), which not only defines gross

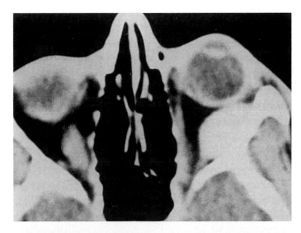

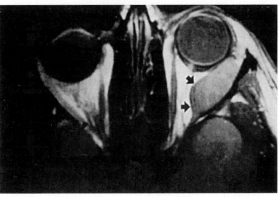

Fig. 14–21. Young patient had slowly evolving unilateral proptosis. **Top.** Enhanced CT scan shows laterally placed homogeneous mass. **Bottom.** MRI with contact coil shows mass well separated from optic nerve and splaying lateral rectus (*arrows*) on medial surface of lesion; tumor was a fibrous histiocytoma.

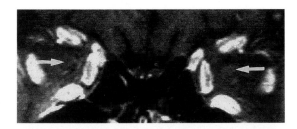

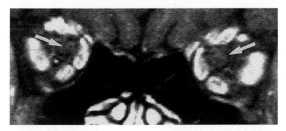

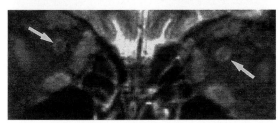

Fig. 14–20. MRI of orbits, coronal sections. Fat suppression. **Top.** Mid-orbit. **Middle.** Orbital apex. **Bottom.** T2-weighted. *Arrows* indicate optic nerve; note ring of CSF (*bottom*).

morphologic configuration, but also is most useful in classifying tumors by tissue-density groups. Whereas CT and MRI provide precise anatomic localization, ultrasonography roughly indicates tissue composition. Such categorization of typical inflammation or tumor patterns closely correlates with histologic diagnoses. Furthermore, standardized echography (combined A-scan, contact B-scan, and Doppler ultrasound) is an efficient and convenient diagnostic modality that sensitively detects changes in extra-ocular muscle size (see Fig. 12–30) and reflectivity (as noted above), accurately measures optic nerve size and sheath distension due to increased subarachnoid fluid, distinguishes abnormalities of vascular flow, and differentiates other orbital soft tissue changes.[67] Many tumors show quite characteristic, if not pathognomonic, reflectivity patterns. Enlargement of the superior orbital vein is detected by ultrasonography,[67,72] and by CT scan[73] and MRI,[74] the differential diagnosis of which includes carotid-cavernous fistula (see Fig. 17–16), Graves' orbitopathy, orbital inflammation, meningioma invading the cavernous sinus, vascular lesions of the orbit, and diffuse cerebral swelling associated with ruptured aneurysms or intracerebral hematomas.[75]

Arteriography has never been a particularly useful technique in orbital disease, with the exception of suspected arteriovenous fistula or malformation, and with the advent of MRI and standardized ultrasonography the indications for arterial contrast studies are few. Unlike the venous injections for enhanced CT scanning, where complications are limited to idiosyncratic reactions to iodinated contrast media, or benign gadolinium contrast for MRI studies, arterial injections or catheterizations run a small but significant risk of embolic sequelae. In the patient with suspected arteriovenous fistula prepared to undergo surgical correction, selective vessel catheterization is required, coupled with photographic subtraction of bone images (See Chapter 17).

The advent of CT, MRI, and ultrasonography has considerably simplified the radiodiagnostic assessment of orbital disease. Radionuclide scanning and positive contrast retrobulbar orbitography must now be considered obsolete, as are contrast studies of the venous system of the orbit and cavernous sinus.

By becoming familiar with those points of medical historical significance, by applying simple examination techniques and learning to recognize suggestive (if not pathognomonic) signs, and by the judicious use of diagnostic techniques (principally CT scan, ultrasonography, and now MRI), the clinician need not be overwhelmed by orbital disease. Nor should the distinction, even on strictly clinical grounds, between neural and orbital causes of ophthalmoplegia be an insurmountable problem.

Part II: Surgery of the Orbit and Optic Nerve

David T. Tse and Warren J. Chang

Anatomy: An Overview
Pre-Operative Management
Surgical Techniques: Orbitotomy
   Anterior
     Transseptal
     Transconjunctival
     Extraperiosteal
   Lateral
   Lateral Combined
   Superior-Craniotomy

Post-Operative Management
   Recovery Room
   Post-Operative Complications
Graves' Ophthalmopathy
   Clinical Features
   Orbital Decompression
   Lid Malposition
Idiopathic Intracranial Hypertension
Traumatic Optic Neuropathy

A number of excellent texts, atlases, and reviews of surgical procedures of the orbit are available, but an overview in the context of neuro-ophthalmology is pertinent to this text. The surgical procedures for neuro-ophthalmic and orbital diseases require a brief review of the relevant anatomy, especially applied to the evaluation and management of these conditions. The treatment of optic neuropathy associated with Graves' ophthalmopathy, pseudotumor cerebri, and traumatic optic neuropathy will be discussed with particular emphasis on the surgical techniques commonly used by the ophthalmologist.

ANATOMY: AN OVERVIEW

The bony orbit has contributions from seven bones: sphenoid, frontal, zygomatic, maxillary, lacrimal, palatine, and ethmoid (see Figs. 14–1 and 14–2). The orbits are closely related to the paranasal sinuses: the maxillary sinuses inferiorly, the ethmoid and sphenoid sinuses medially, and the frontal sinuses superiorly. The pear-shaped bony orbit is widest approximately 1 cm behind the orbital rim, then tapers toward the apex. The total volume is approximately 30 cm³. The medial walls of the orbits are parallel and are separated by the sphenoid and ethmoid sinuses. The lateral orbital walls form a 90° angle with one another, and a 45° angle with the medial walls.[1] The medial and superior walls extend posteriorly to the orbital opening of the optic nerve canal.

The orbital floor is composed of the maxillary, zygomatic, and palatine bones. The floor does not extend to the orbital apex, as it blends with the medial wall and extends posteriorly to the inferior orbital fissure at approximately the posterior wall of the maxillary sinus. Laterally the orbital floor is separated from the lateral wall by the inferior orbital fissure. The inferior orbital groove, containing the infraorbital neurovascular bundle, originates 2.5 to 3 cm posterior to the orbital rim and exits through the inferior orbital foramen of the anterior maxilla. The orbital floor medial to the infraorbital groove is thin and commonly involved in blowout fractures.

The medial wall of the orbit consists of the ethmoid, maxillary, lacrimal, and sphenoid bones. The ethmoid bone (lamina papyracea) is the principal component of the medial wall. The posterior aspect of the medial wall is formed by the sphenoid bone that contains the optic canal. Located at the anterior aspect of the medial wall is the fossa for the lacrimal sac, formed by the frontal process of the maxilla and the lacrimal bones. The frontoethmoidal suture and the anterior and posterior ethmoidal foramens are the superior limit of the medial orbital wall. This suture line marks the roof of the ethmoid sinus; bone removal superior to this suture during decompression surgery can expose the dura of the anterior cranial fossa. The anterior ethmoidal foramen is approximately 24 mm posterior to the anterior lacrimal crest, the posterior ethmoidal foramen is an additional 12 mm posterior, and the optic canal ring is an additional 6 mm posterior. The suture between the ethmoid and maxillary bone is the inferior border of the medial wall and marks the strut of bone that provides support for the inferomedial orbit. The thin lamina papyracea is a weak anatomic barrier to confine ethmoid sinus infections or neoplasms from encroaching into the orbit. The thin medial wall can also be the site of blowout fractures.

D. T. Tse and W. J. Chang: Bascom Palmer Eye Institute, University of Miami School of Medicine, Miami, Florida

The lateral wall of the orbit is triangular and consists of the zygomatic bone anteriorly and greater wing of the sphenoid posteriorly. The sphenoid bone separates the orbit from the middle cranial fossa. The lateral wall terminates posteriorly at the superior orbital fissure. The frontosphenoid suture forms the junction between the lateral and superior walls. The inferior aspect of the greater wing of the sphenoid and the posterior wall of the maxillary sinus forms the inferior orbital fissure. The pterygopalatine fossa lies just below the inferior orbital fissure.

The orbital roof is triangular in shape and is composed of the frontal bone and the lesser wing of the sphenoid. Posteriorly the intracranial roof tapers into the anterior clinoid process of the lesser sphenoid wing. Anteriorly, the superior orbital notch (foramen) is located at the medial one-third of the orbital rim and is approximately in vertical alignment with the inferior orbital foramen.

Within the lesser wing of the sphenoid the optic canal (see Fig. 4–5) extends from the middle cranial fossa to the superior, medial aspect of the orbital apex. The length of the bony canal varies from 5 to 11 mm and is angled superomedially toward the anterior clinoid. In contrast to the orbital portion of the optic nerve, which has some redundancy and is mobile, the intracanalicular portion is held firmly to the surrounding structures. The annulus of Zinn at the orbital apex forms a tight band around the nerve sheath, and the dural sheath is tightly adherent to the periosteum within the bony canal. As the nerve enters the middle cranial fossa, it is in apposition superiorly to a falciform dural fold of the planum.

The orbital apex contains the optic canal within the lesser wing of the sphenoid. The medial aspect of the canal is adjacent to the posterior ethmoid and sphenoid sinuses. Superior to the optic canal is the orbital roof with the anterior cranial fossa above. Just lateral to the optic foramen the superior orbital fissure is formed by a gap in the greater and lesser wings of the sphenoid. The superior orbital fissure transmits the lacrimal, frontal, trochlear, superior division of oculomotor, abducens, nasociliary, and inferior division of the oculomotor nerves. The inferior orbital fissure transmits the infraorbital nerve and artery.

The optic nerve can be separated into four portions: intraocular, orbital, canalicular, and intracranial. The optic nerve is surrounded by three meningeal sheaths identical to that of the central nervous system, the dura mater, the arachnoid, and the pia mater. The intraocular portion of the optic nerve, that is, anterior to, and including, the perforated scleral lamina cribrosa (see Fig. 4–4), is 1 mm in length. Just posterior to the lamina cribrosa, the nerve acquires a dural sheath that is slightly bulbous and less adherent to the optic nerve in comparison to the closer relationship of the nerve and dural sheath at the orbital apex. The intraorbital segment is 25 to 30 mm and the intracanalicular portion 9 to 10 mm; the

obliquely angled intracranial portion is about 15 to 17 mm. The vascular supply of the optic nerve is described in Chapter 4.

PRE-OPERATIVE MANAGEMENT

Sound knowledge of the anatomy, an understanding of the biologic behavior of the orbital diseases, and an ability to interpret orbital diagnostic imaging studies are prerequisites for successful orbital surgery. Pre-operatively, anatomic localization and a preliminary lesion diagnosis are the most important factors in selecting the appropriate surgical approach to the orbit. If the lesion appears to extend beyond the orbit, consultation with a neurosurgeon or an otolaryngologist is imperative.

Lesions that are palpable in the anterior orbit can usually be accessed through a transseptal orbitotomy approach. If imaging studies demonstrate the lesion to be in the posterior orbit, an extraperiosteal approach may be selected to safely gain entrance into the deep orbit. A transconjunctival medial orbitotomy approach may be most appropriate for an intraconal lesion situated within the medial central surgical space. A plan for total excision is formulated if a localized tumor is present. Diffuse infiltrative tumors are approached for diagnostic biopsy only.

Proper assessment of the biologic behavior as well as the location of the suspected lesion may modify the choice of surgical approach. Thus, a lacrimal gland lesion may be exposed via a transseptal anterior orbitotomy if biopsy of a suspected inflammatory or malignant process is anticipated. However, if a benign mixed tumor of the lacrimal gland is the likely diagnosis, lateral orbitotomy is necessary for *en-bloc* removal. Some disease processes that involve only the subperiosteal space, such as subperiosteal hematoma or abscess, floor fractures, and mucoceles, are best approached through a transperiosteal route that does not violate the periorbita. If a malignant or metastatic infiltrative tumor is suspected, extraperiosteal orbitotomy should be avoided and another route of access considered, which would maintain the periorbita as an intact barrier against tumor spread. The lateral approach provides the best access to the retrobulbar compartments inside and outside the muscle cone. It is especially useful for lesions in the lacrimal gland fossa, but may be inadequate for some lesions deeply situated at the orbital apex.

It is usually not necessary to prepare for blood transfusion for orbital surgery. However, this preoperative measure should be considered in patients with low hemoglobin or hematocrit, or in whom significant intraoperative bleeding is anticipated, such as in resection of arteriovenous malformation or in cannulating the superior ophthalmic vein for embolization of a cavernous-dural fistula. Patients taking anticoagulants, such as sodium warfarin (Coumadin), or inhibitors of platelet

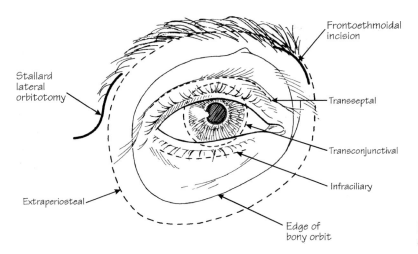

Fig. 14–22. Diagrammatic representation of anatomic incision locations for anterior orbitotomy.

aggregation, such as aspirin, should discontinue their medications at least 2 weeks prior to surgery, if possible. Several over-the-counter drugs contain aspirin, such as Alka-Seltzer, Sine-Off, and Midol, and they, too, should be discontinued. Fish oil, a product sold in health food stores for prevention of heart disease, is frequently not regarded as medication by patients, and their use of it may not be disclosed. Fish oil can interfere with platelet function and prolong bleeding time. Control of hypertension is important, and general medical evaluation is sought when necessary. The ingestion of alcoholic beverages may dilate periocular and periorbital vessels; thus patients are advised to abstain from alcohol intake a few days before surgery.

SURGICAL TECHNIQUES: ORBITOTOMY

Anterior

Transseptal

Anteriorly located tumors that are not subconjunctival but are visible within the substance of the eyelid or palpable within the anterior orbital space can be biopsied or removed completely through the transseptal approach, even with local anesthesia. The transseptal access may be performed in the upper eyelid or the lower eyelid (Fig. 14–22). This approach is most appropriate for well-demarcated lesions (*e.g.*, dermoid cyst or cavernous hemangioma) situated in the anterior orbit that tend to bulge the septum forward, drainage of an abscess, or for incisional biopsy of a diffuse, infiltrative lesion, such as lymphoma, pseudolymphoma, or metastasis. The transseptal anterior orbitotomy may be performed under local or general anesthesia.

In the upper eyelid, the transseptal orbitotomy incision is best camouflaged within the upper eyelid crease. A 4-0 black silk traction suture is passed through the tarsal plate in a lamellar fashion, avoiding the marginal vascular arcade. When secured to the surgical drape inferiorly, this traction suture puts all lid structures posterior to the orbicularis on stretch, while allowing the overlying skin and orbicularis to be mobilized. The skin is incised along the lid crease initially marked with a scalpel. Hemostasis is achieved with a bipolar cautery. The skin and orbicularis muscles are tented anteriorly and a vertical cut is made in the avascular postorbicular fascial plane. A Westcott scissors is used to open this plane medially and laterally along the length of the wound. Gentle pressure applied to the globe will prolapse the orbital fat forward, bulging the shiny orbital septum. The septum is incised across the entire width of the upper eyelid to fully expose the preaponeurotic fat pad. Gentle palpation and blunt dissection of the orbital fat, coupled with careful placement of retractors, will facilitate exposure of the orbital lesion. After biopsy, excision, or drainage, the wound is closed in layers. The orbital septum is not closed as a separate layer. The reformation of the crease is accomplished by suturing the pretarsal skin-muscle edge to the levator aponeurosis. Four to five sutures are usually adequate to form a good eyelid crease. The remainder of the incision is closed with a running suture.

In patients with unsuccessful transarterial embolization of cavernous-dural fistulas, a medial lid crease or a sub-brow incision can be used to locate the dilated anterior superior ophthalmic vein for transvenous embolization (Fig. 14–23; see also Fig. 17–21C). Sharp dissection is carried superiorly in the preseptal plane until the arcus marginalis is reached. The orbital septum is incised along the width of the skin incision. The trochlea and superior oblique tendon are identified and insulated with neurosurgical cottonoids. The orbital fat adjacent to the trochlea is moved laterally with a pair of malleable retractors. Orbital fat septa are bluntly dissected apart to prolapse the superior ophthalmic vein forward. Once identified, the vessel is insulated with ½-inch neurosurgical cottonoids to prevent herniating fat from obscuring the surgical field. Two 2-0 silk ligatures are placed

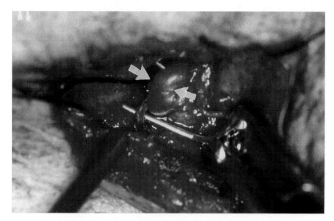

Fig. 14–23. Exposure of supraorbital vein (*arrows*) for endovascular interventional closure of cavernous sinus fistula.

around the vein for traction. A guidewire is introduced through a venipuncture between the two ligatures. An angiographic catheter is threaded over the guidewire and secured to the vessel with a silk suture. With successful closure of the shunt, the vessel is no longer arterialized. The silk ligatures are then loosened and the venipuncture site cauterized with a bipolar cautery.

Occasionally, hemangiomas, pseudolymphomas, or lymphomas will appear through the lower lid. The lower eyelid transseptal anterior orbitotomy is similar in principle to the upper eyelid approach, with an incision made within 1 to 2 mm below the lashes, identical to the standard transcutaneous blepharoplasty technique. A myocutaneous flap is fashioned using sharp and blunt dissection. Dissection within the postorbicular fascial plane is carried inferiorly until the inferior orbital rim is reached. The orbital septum is opened to prolapse forward the preaponeurotic fat pad. Surgical retractors are used to expose the lesion. After either excision or biopsy of the lesion, the subciliary incision is closed with a simple running suture. In patients with lower lid laxity, suspending the lid with either a Steri-strip or traction suture may help avert postoperative ectropion.

Transconjunctival

The transconjunctival approach provides direct access to subconjunctival lesions and for some anterior orbital lesions located outside the muscle cone. The more common subconjunctival masses include congenital dermoids, dermolipomas, epidermoids, pseudolymphomas, lymphoid tumors, prolapsed palpebral lobe of the lacrimal gland, and orbital fat. This anterior orbitotomy technique can be used to drain a localized abscess or to gain access to the intraconal space by disinserting the appropriate rectus muscle. Entrance to the intraconal space is most commonly performed medially and will be described in relation to papilledema in pseudotumor cerebri. Indications for the intraconal transconjunctival

orbitotomy with disinsertion of the medial rectus muscle include excision of localized cavernous hemangioma or neurilemoma, excision or biopsy of primary optic nerve tumors such as glioma or meningioma, and optic nerve sheath fenestration.

In general, an incision through conjunctiva and Tenon's capsule is made near the lesion and extended radially to expose the deep tissue. Rectus muscles in the quadrant of the tumor are isolated and tacked with 4-0 black silk sutures to facilitate traction. In some cases, disinsertion of the appropriate rectus muscle is necessary for better exposure. With the eye gently retracted in the direction opposite the lesion, careful blunt dissection with malleable retractors aided by neurosurgical cottonoids, is undertaken. A retinal cryoprobe can be applied to the lesion for traction and to facilitate extraction. The closure of the transconjunctival approach includes reattachment of the rectus muscle, if applicable, and suturing of the conjunctiva.

Another technique of exposing the inferior orbit is an inferior fornix approach utilizing a lateral canthotomy and cantholysis of the inferior limb of the lateral canthal tendon. Both the transconjunctival approach and the transcutaneous lower lid approach can give excellent exposure for the purpose of removing inferior orbital tumors, biopsy of tumors arising from the maxillary sinus, repair of blowout fractures of the orbital floor, and decompression of the bony orbit for thyroid-related orbitopathy (antral-ethmoidal decompression).

Extraperiosteal

Lesions located adjacent to the orbital roof, adjacent to the medial orbital wall, on the floor of the orbit, beneath the nasolacrimal sac, or within the frontal or ethmoid sinuses, including mucoceles of the frontal sinus, dermoids, and hemangiomas, are ideally suited for approach through extraperiosteal incisions. This incision is also useful for drainage of a subperiosteal hematoma or abscess.

For exposure of the superonasal and medial quadrants of the orbit, an outline is made in the brow beginning at the supraorbital notch and carried medially into the medial canthus, and further inferiorly into the alar region of the nose (Lynch incision). The area of the incision is infiltrated with 2% lidocaine with 1:100,000 dilution of epinephrine. Skin incision is made with a no. 15 Bard-Parker blade and carried through the subcutaneous tissue and orbicularis muscle layers. The periosteum is incised along the orbital rim, avoiding the supraorbital neurovascular bundle that exits the supraorbital foramen. The incised periosteum is reflected off the bone with a Freer periosteal elevator. After entering the extraperiosteal space, dissection is carried as far posteriorly as necessary to expose the lesion. Care must be taken to avoid unnecessary damage to the superior oblique muscle and trochlea. The trochlea may be elevated from its bony fossa with the attached periosteum reflected inward. Once the lesion is palpated, it is exposed by a longitudinal incision of periosteum. A biopsy is taken or the tumor is completely removed as described for the subconjunctival approach. If the mass is encapsulated, it should be extracted with blunt dissection. If the tumor is cystic and ruptures, the lining should be removed by careful dissection. After removal of the lesion, the periosteal edges are reapproximated with 5-0 polygalactin 910 (Vicryl) suture. The muscle layer is closed with 5-0 chromic suture. The skin is closed with 6-0 nylon suture in a vertical mattress fashion.

Mucoceles of the frontal or ethmoid sinuses are benign cystic lesions that may expand to displace the orbital bones and secondarily invade the orbit. If erosion of the posterior wall of the frontal sinus is present radiographically, neurosurgical consultation should be obtained. Most mucoceles are caused by obstruction of the sinus ducts and ostia through which fluid normally drains. Trauma or tumors that invade sinuses, or polyps obstructing the ostia, may lead to mucocele formation. Therefore, otolaryngologic consultation is advised. Surgical treatment of paranasal sinus mucoceles usually involves the evacuation of the mucoid contents with removal of the mucosal lining. Furthermore, since the formation of mucoceles is due to an obstructive sinus process, adequate drainage of the sinus into the intranasal cavity must be established. Surgical passage communicating the frontal sinus with the intranasal cavity can be made either through the ethmoids or the nasofrontal duct itself. Recurrence of frontal mucoceles is common if they are inadequately treated by intranasal drainage alone. For recurrent or bilateral mucoceles, effective surgery involves an osteoplastic mid-forehead flap approach, with removal of all sinus mucosa, followed by obliteration of the sinus cavity with abdominal fat transplantation. To avoid a conspicuous facial incision, a bicoronal forehead flap may be used to achieve exposure for superior, superior lateral, and superior nasal extraperiosteal orbitotomies.

Inferior extraperiosteal orbitotomy is similar to the superior approach, and is useful for masses on the orbital floor, blowout fracture, and decompression for Graves' ophthalmopathy. We describe the transconjunctival approach to the inferior extraperiosteal space, though some surgeons prefer a transcutaneous incision. Initially, a lateral canthotomy is performed, with an incision directed horizontally, extending 3 to 5 mm in length. The scissors blades are then rotated 90° inferiorly, and insinuated between skin and conjunctiva, cutting all the tissues of the lateral retinaculum in between. Several snips are required to cut through the lateral canthal tendon and the overlying orbicularis muscle until the lateral edge of the lid can be completely distracted from the orbital rim. The lid margin is then retracted, while the fused edge of conjunctiva and lid retractor muscle is severed from the inferior margin of tarsal plate. This incision is begun at the lateral canthotomy and carried medially to the inferior lacrimal punctum.

A silk suture is passed through the cut edge of conjunctiva and retractors, drawn superiorly, and clamped to the drapes. This maneuver facilitates the plane of dissection between conjunctiva and retractors posteriorly and orbicularis anteriorly, and also provides protection to the cornea. The plane of dissection is the same whether the percutaneous or transconjunctival approach is used. The only difference is that the plane is entered from the posterior surface if the transconjunctival approach is used. A scissors is used to dissect inferiorly between the orbicularis muscle and septum, down to the level of the orbital rim. During dissection, it is important to maintain traction on the lid margin to prevent folding of the skin and orbicularis. Otherwise, the plane of dissection may be obscured, which can result in full-thickness "button-holing" through the anterior lamella. Dissection performed within this plane also maintains an intact septum and prevents orbital fat from prolapsing into the surgical field. Dissection down to the inferior orbital rim is aided by frequent finger palpation to identify the position of the bony rim. After dissection to the rim, a Desmarres retractor can be used to retract the skin-muscle flap inferiorly. Soft tissue overlying the rim can be bluntly dissected with a Stevens scissors until the periosteum is exposed. While palpating the rim, the periosteum is incised with a scalpel blade. Incision is begun medially at the level of the punctum and carried across the rim, ending just below the lateral orbital tubercle. The incision is placed just below the rim on the anterior face of the maxilla, but care must be taken to avoid the infraorbital nerve. A periosteal elevator is used to reflect the posterior edge of the periorbita across the width of the rim, and the dissection continued posteriorly. Once the lesion is localized, an opening is made in the periorbita through which the tumor is biopsied or excised. The conjunctiva and lower eyelid retractors are reapproximated with a 6-0 plain suture. The lateral canthal tendon is sutured to the inner aspect of the lateral orbital rim with 4-0 Vicryl sutures. The lateral canthal skin incision is closed with interrupted 6-0 nylon sutures.

This same approach may be used for floor fracture (blowout) repair or decompression for Graves' ophthalmopathy.

Lateral

The lateral approach provides the best access to the retrobulbar compartments inside and outside the muscle cone. It is especially useful for lesions in the lacrimal fossa, but may be inadequate for lesions at the orbital apex. General endotracheal anesthesia is preferred when the retrobulbar area is explored. Induced intraoperative hypotension, though not usually required, may be considered to control hemostasis that facilitates tissue dissection.

A fiberoptic headlight and magnifying loupes are essential to provide illumination and magnification of fine orbital structures during lateral orbitotomy. The patient is placed in a slight reverse Trendelenburg position to reduce orbital venous pressure. A suture tarsorrhaphy of the lids is not advisable, as it will prevent forward displacement of the globe and preclude monitoring of pupillary reaction during orbital manipulation.

An S-shaped Stallard skin incision (Fig. 14–22) is preferred because it gives excellent exposure and eliminates the necessity to reconstruct the lateral canthal angle. The lateral canthal region and the temporalis muscle are infiltrated with lidocaine 2% with 1:100,000 dilution of epinephrine prior to draping and scrubbing of hands. This allows the vasoconstrictive effect of epinephrine to work before an incision is made. After the surgical site has been prepped, the S-shaped skin outline is inscribed with a marking pen. The marking begins beneath the lateral one-third of the eyebrow, extending inferolaterally along the superior and lateral bony orbital rim, past the level of the lateral commissure to terminate over the zygomatic arch (Fig. 14–22).

The initial incision is carried down to, but not through, the periosteum. Subcutaneous tissues and orbicularis oculi muscles are bluntly dissected with a Freer periosteal elevator to expose the periosteum and fascia of the temporalis muscle. Bleeding from orbicularis muscle is controlled by bipolar cautery. Traction sutures of 4-0 black silk are positioned in both sides of the skin-muscle flaps and secured to the surgical drapes with hemostats.

The periosteum is then incised with a no. 15 Bard-Parker parallel to and approximately 2 mm lateral to the orbital rim. The periosteal incision is carried superiorly above the zygomaticofrontal suture line and inferiorly past the superior aspect of the zygomatic arch. Periosteal relaxing incisions are made at the superior and inferior ends of the incision. The periosteum and temporalis muscles are reflected from the zygomatic process of the frontal bone and the frontal process of the zygomatic bone. This maneuver is accomplished by using either a Woodson or Freer periosteal elevator. Once the dissection is carried into the temporalis fossa, the separation of the periosteum and temporalis muscle is facilitated by forcing an opened 4 × 4 gauze into the dissection plane with a Freer elevator to just behind the sphenozygomatic suture line. By bluntly dissecting the temporalis muscle off its bony attachment with a gauze, shredding of the muscle by the sharp tip of the periosteal elevator can be avoided. Brisk bleeding may be encountered in the bed of the temporalis muscle or from avulsion of the zygomaticotemporal artery. This can be controlled either by pressure or with bipolar cautery. Oozing from the bony surface can be stopped with bone wax.

After the periosteum and temporalis muscle have been separated from the external aspect of the lateral orbital wall, the periorbita is gently reflected away from the inner aspect of the lateral wall with a Freer periosteal elevator. Within the orbit, the periorbita is loosely adherent and can be easily separated from the bone. Care should be taken to maintain the integrity of the periorbita. The zygomaticotemporal or the zygomaticofacial artery may be seen as it penetrates the lateral wall from within the orbit. This vessel should be cauterized before further posterior dissection. It is unnecessary to dissect beyond the sphenofrontal suture line since removal of the lateral wall often stops short of this landmark.

Once the full dimension of the lateral orbital wall has been delineated and hemostasis assured, the anticipated bony incisions are then determined. The superior bone incision is positioned about 5 mm above the zygomaticofrontal suture line, and the inferior bone cut is made above the upper margin of the zygomatic arch. If the inferior bone cut is made too low, there is a potential hazard of fracturing into the inferior orbital fissure during bone removal. Bone incisions are made with an oscillating saw, the vertical distance between the two cuts usually being 3 to 3.5 cm. To protect the periorbita and globe during the entire bone cutting process, a broad metal malleable retractor is positioned within the lateral wall of the orbit. Another malleable retractor is placed in the temporalis fossa to reflect and protect the temporalis muscle. The superior and inferior bone incisions should be parallel, and the posterior depth of incision usually does not exceed 1.5 cm. For the superior incision, the depth of the cut should terminate anterior to the sphenofrontal suture line. Before bone removal, holes are made with a pneumatic drill above and below the bone incision to allow fixation with sutures when the bone fragment is returned to its original position at the conclusion of the procedure.

The lateral orbital rim is then grasped with a large double-action bone rongeur and gently rocked laterally until posterior fracture is induced and the section of lateral wall disinserted. This bone fragment is then wrapped in saline-soaked gauze and preserved for later replacement. Further resection of the lateral wall in the depth of the temporalis fossa may be accomplished in a piecemeal fashion with a bone rongeur, until the thick cancellous bone of the spheroid is reached, marking the most posterior limit before entering the middle cranial fossa. Bleeding from the cancellous bone can be controlled with bone wax. Hemostasis must be assured before opening the periorbita.

The intact periorbita is now visualized and a T-shaped periorbital incision is made. The anteroposterior limb is made just above or below one side of the lateral rectus muscle and carried posteriorly as far as possible. The vertical incision is made beginning at the level of the lacrimal gland and extending inferiorly to below the lateral rectus. The incision can be started with a Bard-Parker blade, but is completed with a Westcott scissors to prevent injury to orbital tissues. The edges of the periorbital incisions are grasped with a forceps and gently reflected away from the orbital contents with a Freer elevator.

With the periorbita opened, the perimuscular fascial sheaths are bluntly dissected with periosteal elevators to locate the lateral rectus muscle. It is preferable to displace the lateral rectus medially, with the globe, rather than dissecting the surrounding fat or encircling the muscle with a suture or a vascular band. Overmanipulation of the lateral rectus muscle may result in transient postoperative motility dysfunction.

At this point, gentle finger palpation can usually locate the position of the orbital mass. For deeper exploration within the central surgical compartment (muscle cone), two malleable retractors are used to spread the orbital fat in a hand-over-hand fashion. Perhaps the most difficult feature of the dissection is the tendency of orbital fat to obscure normal anatomic landmarks. The fat is divided into lobules by fine connective-tissue septa; these lobules often billow over the edges of the retractors, screening the plane of dissection. Moistened ½-inch neurosurgical cottonoids, to which the orbital fat will adhere slightly, will prevent fat from billowing over the retractor edges, minimizing this problem. By gradually removing and reinserting the orbital retractor blades over the cottonoids, orbital fat can be kept away from the plane of dissection.

Once the lesion is located, a Freer periosteal elevator is used to bluntly dissect the orbital tissues away from the surface of the tumor. If the lesion is encapsulated, it may be engaged with a retinal cryoprobe while blunt dissection is continued around the capsule with the periosteal elevator. Dissection should be blunt and tangential to the plane of the tumor or capsule. Under no circumstances should there be blind cutting with a scissors. If the lesion is infiltrative and adherent to vital structures, frozen section examination of the tissue will determine whether intraconal dissection should continue. If tissue planes are not clearly defined, it may be wise to leave portions of the lesion rather than risk ocular dysfunction by overly aggressive extirpation.

After lesion removal, attention should be directed to meticulous hemostasis accomplished by pinpoint bipolar cautery with fine-tipped forceps. The use of unipolar Bovie cautery within the orbit is hazardous. Suction within the periorbita is to be avoided, as undue traction on orbital fat may cause bleeding from avulsed small blood vessels. Closure of an orbitotomy should not commence until complete hemostasis is assured. The use of microfibrillar collagen hemostat (Avitene) to stop bleeding within the orbit may cause tissue scarring. A regenerated oxidized cellulose hemostat (Surgicel) may be helpful in controlling slow ooze, but should be removed completely from within the orbit prior to closure after hemostasis. This material induces hemostasis, but it subsequently swells on contact with blood and may potentially exert considerable compressive force within the enclosed orbit, especially at the apex.

Following removal or biopsy of an intraorbital tumor, the periorbita is closed with interrupted 5-0 chromic catgut or 5-0 polygalactin 910 (Vicryl) sutures. The lateral orbital wall bone fragment is returned to its original position and anchored with a 4-0 Prolene suture through the preplaced drill holes. The suture knots are then rotated and buried into a drill hole on the external surface of the bony rim.

The periosteum and anterior temporalis fascia are reapproximated with 5-0 chromic sutures. Traction sutures are removed. Orbicularis muscle and subcutaneous tissues are also reapproximated with 5-0 chromic sutures in an interrupted fashion. The skin incision is closed with multiple interrupted vertical mattress sutures of 6-0 nylon.

Lateral Combined

An inferior-lateral approach combines a modified blepharoplasty incision with a lateral orbitotomy. This technique is useful for large lesions occupying both the muscle cone and the inferior lateral portion of the orbit. Also, a lateral orbitotomy with an inferior orbitotomy through a fornix incision may be combined (Reese-Burke). The lateral orbital wall is removed as described.

Medial-lateral orbitotomy is used for lesions occurring in the nasal apex of the orbit, or medial to the optic nerve in the deep orbit, which prove most difficult to remove. Examples include tumors such as gliomas or meningiomas at the nasal apex. Other common lesions located in the posterior nasal orbit are peripheral nerve tumors and hemangiomas. To obtain an adequate exposure, a combination of lateral orbitotomy and medial fornix approach allows the eye to be rotated laterally, exposing the medial retrobulbar space. After lateral orbitotomy, a lid speculum is placed in the fornices, and a nasal 180° limbal conjunctival peritomy is performed, followed by radial conjunctival relaxing incisions to expose the medial rectus muscle. The medial rectus is tacked with a double-armed 5-0 Vicryl suture and disinserted. With the medial rectus and conjunctival flap retracted medially and the globe laterally, retractors are inserted between the globe and the muscle to push billowing orbital fat away from the retrobulbar space. By carefully replacing and repositioning the retractors, the orbital lesion can usually be brought into view. Decompression of the optic nerve sheath or controlled excision or biopsy of a mass lesion is facilitated in this manner. Closure of transconjunctival medial orbitotomy and lateral orbitotomy incisions are as described previously.

Superior-Craniotomy

Superior-craniotomy combines orbitotomy with neurosurgical craniotomy and provides excellent exposure of cranio-orbital lesions located in the superior-posterior orbit and otherwise inaccessible masses at the orbital apex. Optic nerve tumors with and without intracranial extension, trauma (fractures, foreign bodies), and complex lesions simultaneously affecting the orbit, middle cranial fossa, temporalis, and pterygopalatine fossae are best served by this combined approach.

In most instances, a bicoronal skin incision is used and the scalp of the forehead, including the periosteum, is reflected anteriorly. The coronal scalp incision may be extended to just below the tragus for tumors extending into the pterygopalatine or inferotemporal fossa. At the superior orbital ridge, the periorbita, which is continuous with pericranium, is dissected off the surface of the orbital roof. The continuity of the periorbita and pericranium should be maintained. The supraorbital neurovascular bundle is carefully separated from the bony notch. Dissection must be done with particular care to prevent dehiscence of the periorbita and subsequent orbital fat herniation into the operative field. The orbital surgeon dissects the periorbita off the superior and lateral walls of the orbit. The dissection process extends toward the superior orbital fissure and lateral aspect of the inferior orbital fissure, or to the anterior limit of bone and soft tissue invaded by tumor. This allows the orbital surgeon to protect the periorbita during craniotomy by the neurosurgeon.

The extradural component of the procedure begins with placement of two burr holes, one placed in the midline at the level of the orbital ridge and the other just behind the arch of the zygomatic process.[76] The midline burr hole will often involve the frontal sinus. The two burr holes are then connected using a Gigli saw. This cut includes the superior orbital rim and part of the orbital roof. Using a craniotome, a bone flap is fashioned that incorporates the superior orbital rim and part of the orbital roof, ultimately permitting an excellent cosmetic closure. The remaining roof of the orbit and the lesser and greater wing of spheroid can be removed with rongeurs. While maintaining an intact dura, and with minimal retraction of the frontal lobe, a panoramic view of the superior orbit is achieved.

The optic canal may be opened with a burr in those cases requiring exploration or extirpation of tumor or optic nerve. Opening the periorbita provides a large field for intraorbital exploration. The orbital soft tissues are dissected using blunt malleable retractors and neurosurgical cottonoids. Following removal of the cranio-orbital tumor, a pericranial flap is then developed from the skin flap and is turned down to cover the opening in the frontal sinus that may have been created by the initial craniotomy. The cranial bone flap is then secured with sutures or microfixation osteosynthesis plates. The skin and galea are then closed in the usual manner.

POST-OPERATIVE MANAGEMENT

Recovery Room

After the patient awakens from anesthesia, visual acuity and pupillary reaction are assessed and the skin incisions inspected for evidence of bleeding. The head of the bed is elevated to a 45° position, and the patient is cautioned to report any deep orbital pain that might signal orbital hemorrhage. An ice pack is applied to the periorbital region, but an eye bandage is avoided since it obscures lid and conjunctival signs of retrobulbar bleeding. In the immediate postoperative period, an analgesic is given only for incisional pain. Any complaints of deep orbital pain should be investigated. A stool softener is used and the patient cautioned to avoid straining or Valsalva efforts.

Systemic corticosteroids are given if any inflammatory lesion has been biopsied, or if the optic nerve was manipulated during surgery. The dressing over the incision is removed in 24 hours. An antibiotic ointment is applied onto the incision t.i.d. for 1 week. Sutures are removed after 7 days and the wound reinforced with a Steri-strip.

Post-Operative Complications

One of the most dreaded complications of orbital surgery is post-operative hemorrhage with visual loss, most likely due to compression of the optic nerve or interruption of ocular perfusion and resultant ischemia of the eye. Older patients with hypertension are especially at risk. As orbital pressure approaches the systolic blood pressure, central retinal artery or posterior ciliary artery flow may be compromised, resulting in decreased retinal and choroidal perfusion. Concomitantly, elevated intraocular pressure (IOP) from direct transmission of high orbital tension, or from acute angle closure glaucoma, may contribute to retinal and optic nerve ischemia. Recovery of vision is unlikely if retinal ischemia persists for more than a few minutes. For these reasons, any compressive bandage compounds the situation, and masks physical monitoring of the pupil, vision, and lid ecchymoses.

In the worst case, therefore, maximum effort should be directed at detecting and restoring retinal and optic nerve perfusion within this vulnerable period. The main sources of bleeding are the temporalis muscle, bone incisions, and small vessels that traverse the orbital fat lobules. Treatment of an expanding orbital hematoma must be initiated without delay by surgical wound exploration. Blood clots are evacuated and the source of bleeding must be identified and cauterized. Intraocular pressure and retinal perfusion status should also be monitored and, in the presence of elevated IOP, medical therapy should commence. Topical timolol (Timoptic, 0.5%), intravenous acetazolamide (500 mg), and mannitol (1–2 g/kg of a 20% solution infused over 20 minutes) may be administered to decrease IOP and enhance retinal perfusion. Intravenous corticosteroids should also be given to reduce orbital swelling, decrease vascular permeability and to protect the optic nerve from ischemic damage.

GRAVES' OPHTHALMOPATHY

Clinical Features

The highly variable clinical course of thyroid ophthalmopathy ranges from no signs and symptoms to complete loss of vision and disfiguring exophthalmos. As discussed previously, ophthalmic evaluation includes standard assessment of visual function, with special attention to measurement of proptosis, eyelid morphology (edema), movement and position, corneal evaluation, and determination of motility. In situations of visual changes, optic nerve functions are included (see Chapter 5).

Signs and symptoms of Graves' ophthalmopathy arise from a discrepancy between the expanded volume of the retrobulbar tissues and the fixed volume of the bony orbit. Treatment strategy is directed at either shrinking the volume of the hypertrophied orbital tissues or expanding the volume of the orbit. The overall approach is one of conservatism in the early stages until the systemic disease is evaluated, treated, and stabilized over a period of 6 to 12 months. More immediate and aggressive therapy may be instituted in cases of compressive optic neuropathy or serious corneal exposure complications.

Management of the orbitopathy is mainly palliative to minimize ocular discomfort and prevent loss of vision and disfigurement. Nonsurgical measures used to reduce the expanded soft tissue volume include corticosteroids, cyclosporine, combinations of corticosteroids and cyclosporine,[77] or orbital radiation therapy. Extraconal and intraconal fat extirpation without bone removal is a surgical attempt to ease this volume disparity.

Mild to moderate corneal involvement can be treated with lubricants, moist chamber, and/or taping the eyelids at night. Severe corneal involvement may necessitate tarsorrhaphy or decompression surgery. During sleep, head elevation on more than one pillow or with other devices may reduce periorbital edema in the morning. Prisms in spectacles are effective in controlling double vision in primary gaze when the motility restriction is mild to moderate. Botox (botulinum toxin) injections have also been used to control strabismus in patients with restrictive strabismus. Corticosteroids are reserved for patients showing aggressive inflammatory signs (e.g., rapidly progressive proptosis, corneal exposure, and/or compressive optic neuropathy).[31] Strabismus, lid retraction, and modest proptosis usually do not improve much with steroid therapy. The potential risks and side effects of corticosteroids must be considered.

Radiation therapy is used to halt the progressive inflammatory component of the condition, rapidly progressive congestive orbitopathy, optic neuropathy, or where complications of corticosteroid therapy are intolerable, but is usually unproductive in chronic stable orbitopathy.[31–33] External beam radiation dosage of 1500 to 2000 cGy is given, 180 to 200 cGy per sessions. Corticosteroid therapy may be continued during irradiation, then gradually tapered. A response is usually seen over a 6-week period, with maximum improvement observed over the course of 4 months. In the case of compressive optic neuropathy, if the optic neuropathy is severe or rapidly progressive, orbital decompression should be considered. Soft tissue inflammatory signs and proptosis are usually reduced; however, strabismus is infrequently improved with radiotherapy.

Orbital radiation has been effective in about two-thirds of patients, although approximately 30% of these patients will require some surgical procedure at a later date. Orbital radiation is expensive to perform, and its potential complications include eyelid and facial erythema and dry eye; cataract, radiation retinopathy or optic neuropathy, and secondary malignancy are associated with doses greater than 5000 cGy, but are remote possibilities with low dosage used for Graves' or other inflammatory orbitopathies.

Surgical rehabilitation needs to be individualized and performed in stages. Corrective surgical measures should not be undertaken until the inflammatory process has abated and the condition has remained stable for at least 6 months. If more than one type of surgery is indicated, the order in which it should be undertaken is as follows: orbital decompression, strabismus surgery, eyelid retraction repair, and blepharoplasty.[78] This logical sequence is important because the first procedure could influence the indications and findings to be addressed by the following procedure. For example, orbital decompression may actually cause and worsen a pre-existing strabismus condition, and the subsequent muscle surgery would need to correct these abnormalities. If orbital decompression is not required prior to strabismus or eyelid surgery, strabismus surgery should be delayed until the orbits are no longer inflamed.

Orbital Decompression

Orbital decompression is indicated for the following conditions: apical compressive optic neuropathy that fails to reverse with high-dose corticosteroids and/or radiation therapy, severe corneal exposure refractory to medical treatment, disfiguring proptosis, recurrent spontaneous globe subluxation, and severe orbital inflammation inadequately treated by corticosteroids or radiation therapy.

Decompression has been described for all four walls of the orbit.[79–82] Orbital decompression for the treatment of compressive optic neuropathy must emphasize decompression of the orbital apex and optic nerve. The medial and superior walls are the only walls that extend posteriorly to the optic nerve canal; thus at least one of these walls should be decompressed in the treatment of compressive optic neuropathy. Laterally, decompression of the apex is limited by the temporal lobe of the brain. Inferior orbitotomy does not reach the orbital apex, as decompression is limited to the posterior wall of the maxillary sinus. The most common method of orbital expansion to relieve apical compression is a two-wall decompression into the ethmoidal sinus and the maxillary antrum. This is typically performed through a subciliary or transconjunctival approach. Removal of the lateral wall permits additional expansion into the temporalis fossa. Decompression of the orbital roof is associated with greater risks and is typically performed by neurosurgeons. Four-wall decompression is reserved for patients with extreme exophthalmos. An endoscopic transnasal approach has been described particularly appropriate for decompression of the posterior portion of the medial wall, perhaps best suited for relief of traumatic optic neuropathy.[83]

Evaluation of patients for orbital decompression should include CT scan to assess the paranasal sinuses and bony anatomy. Thyroid function and medical status should be stabilized, and anticoagulants or platelet aggregation inhibitors such as aspirin, Motrin, or ticlid should be discontinued 2 weeks prior to surgery.

Orbital decompression is performed under general anesthesia. The subciliary or transconjunctival approaches can be used to expose the bony orbit (the transconjunctival approach is described above). The subciliary incision is outlined with a marking pen and infiltrated with 2% lidocaine containing 1 : 100,000 epinephrine. A 4-0 silk traction suture is placed through the posterior lamella of the lower eyelid margin and anchored to the drape superiorly. The subciliary skin incision extends from the lateral canthus to just temporal to the punctum. Sharp dissection is then made inferiorly in the post-orbicularis tissue plane anterior to the orbital septum. The dissection is continued until the periosteum of the orbital rim is identified. The periosteum is incised 2 mm from the rim using a no. 15 blade. With a periosteal elevator, periosteum is elevated to expose the bones of the orbital floor. Care is taken to avoid opening the periorbita and exposing the orbital fat.

The orbital floor may be fractured medial to the infraorbital neurovascular bundle by using a hemostat or a periosteal elevator.[79] The bone resection of the orbital floor extends laterally to the inferior orbital fissure, posteriorly to the posterior wall of the maxillary sinus, and medially to the inferior-medial strut. A Takahashi rongeur is used for bone removal. Care should be taken to identify and preserve the infraorbital neurovascular bundle and the lacrimal sac fossa. Along the medial wall the anterior and posterior ethmoidal arteries are identified, cauterized, and incised. Cauterization of the perforating ethmoidal vessels early in the procedure will substantially reduce bleeding during ethmoid sinus exenteration. The bone resection of the medial wall extends superiorly to the frontoethmoidal suture line, and inferiorly to the inferior-medial strut. The ethmoid air cells and mucosa are removed using the Takahashi rongeur. Posteriorly, the bone removal extends to the posterior ethmoidal foramen, which is approximately 5 mm anterior to the optic foramen. The lateral wall may be decompressed independently or in addition to an inferomedial, medial wall, or floor decompression.[84] Through the lower lid incision, the lateral orbital wall can be removed with a burr. The periorbita is then opened in an anterior-posterior direction using a Wescott scissors. The surgical field is inspected for hemostasis prior to closing the incision. The periosteum is reapproximated with 5-0 polygalactin sutures and the subciliary incision closed with a running 7-0 nylon suture.

Potential complications of orbital decompression include infraorbital nerve hypesthesia, lid abnormalities, strabismus, hypoglobus, nasolacrimal duct obstruction, cerebrospinal fluid leaks, infection, bleeding, decreased vision, and loss of vision.[80–82,86,87] A review of 428 patients who underwent transantral decompressions at the Mayo Clinic[82] showed an improvement in vision in 65% and a decrease in 12%, new diplopia in 64%, entropion in 9%, cerebrospinal fluid (CSF) leak in 3.5%, and significant blood loss requiring transfusion in 2.5%; only 3% required additional decompressive surgery.

The natural history of compressive optic neuropathy is unclear; however, a number of eyes may spontaneously improve[34] (see also Chapter 5). In combined series of 26 eyes with untreated thyroid optic neuropathy, 19 (73%) spontaneously improved to 20/50 or better; however, 6 (23%) had significant visual loss with visual acuity of counting fingers or worse.[86] In a study by Hurwitz and Birt,[78] orbital decompression for optic neuropathy resulted in a significant improvement in visual acuity in 22 of 27 (81%) eyes; the five patients who did not improve had been treated with lateral orbital decompressions, and three of the five subsequently improved following subsequent medial wall decompressions. In this study significant improvement was defined as at least three lines from the pre-operative visual acuity. This study supports the efficacy of orbital decompression and the anatomic theory that lateral orbital decompression is not the most effective way to decompress the orbital apex.

Mourits and associates[79] described 25 patients who had inferomedial or inferomedial plus lateral wall decompressions for optic neuropathy; visual acuity and visual fields improved in 19 (76%); four of six patients who did not improve had diabetes mellitus. The authors noted that proptosis improved up to 6 months following decompression, with a mean reduction in proptosis of 2.0 mm (range 2–5 mm) for two-wall decompression and 4.3 mm (range 3–6 mm) for three-wall decompression. Warren et al[88] reviewed 305 cases of transantral inferomedial orbital decompression; 95% of patients had stable or improved visual acuity with a 4.0 mm mean reduction of proptosis (range 1–12 mm); strabismus surgery was subsequently performed in 69 of the patients for persistent diplopia following decompression. Carter et al[86] evaluated 13 patients with compressive optic neuropathy treated with transantral inferomedial wall decompressions; all patients with preoperative visual acuity of 20/40 or better retained vision within this range after surgery; 8 of 10 patients with preoperative visual acuity of 20/50 to 20/100 improved to 20/40 or better; four of seven patients with acuity of less than 20/200 improved to better than 20/40; visual field defects improved in all but one case. Acquired post-operative diplopia in primary gaze position follows inferomedial decompression in 5% to 25% with the transorbital approach, and 30% to 65% with the transantral approach.

Orbital decompression is an effective treatment for optic neuropathy and proptosis; however, there are other theories on how to effectively decompress the orbit. Harvey[89] examined the role of inferomedial decompressions, but with leaving periosteum intact in four eyes with compressive optic neuropathy; all had significant improvement in visual acuity. Olivari[87] advocated orbital decompression with removal of intraorbital fat only. He excised an average of 6 cm^3 of orbital fat in 10 patients with reduced visual acuity, with acuity increase in six patients and no change in the remaining four. Such series involve small numbers of patients, with somewhat limited documentation of ocular examinations, and therefore these surgical procedures are not widely accepted. Other immune-modifying treatments are being assessed, including the use of cyclosporine, plasmaphoresis, and immunoglobulin therapy.[76,90]

Orbital decompression establishes a more posterior globe position and alters the muscle cone position, inducing or worsening strabismus. The patient needs to understand that restoration of single vision in all fields of gaze may be extremely difficult, and the goal of stra-

bismus surgery is to achieve greatest range of fusion in both the primary and reading positions. Before contemplating muscle alignment surgery, it is imperative that the strabismus condition be stable for at least 6 months. Symptomatic diplopia may be treated with Fresnel prisms and patching, while ocular misalignment is still in evolution. Once ocular misalignment has reached a stable status, recession of the involved muscles can be performed using adjustable sutures. Superior oblique tenectomies or tenotomies may be necessary to correct torsional diplopia.

Lid Malposition

Eyelid retraction is one of the most common ophthalmic manifestations of Graves' ophthalmopathy. Eyelid malposition may occur with or without exophthalmos and is responsible for functional and cosmetic problems in many patients with thyroid-related eye disease. The etiology of eyelid retraction is not clear, but several factors seem to be contributory. In the upper lid, these factors include (1) Mueller's muscle overaction from sympathetic stimulation, (2) levator contraction from degeneration and thickening of the levator muscle or aponeurosis, (3) levator adhesions to the orbicularis muscle and orbital septum, and (4) overaction of the levator-superior rectus complex in response to a hypophoria produced by fibrosis and retraction of the inferior rectus.

In the lower eyelid, adrenergic stimulation of the Mueller's muscle may play some role, but fibrosis of the inferior rectus exerting a retraction action on the lower eyelid through its capsulopalpebral head appears to be more influential. Recession of a tight inferior rectus muscle to correct ocular misalignment will accentuate lower lid retraction. Surgical treatment of eyelid retraction is usually reserved for patients whose endocrine status and eyelid height have been stable for at least 6 months to 1 year, and in whom retraction causes significant exposure to keratopathy, lagophthalmos, chronic conjunctival injection, and cosmetic imperfection.

Muellerectomy along with recession of the fibrosed levator aponeurosis can be performed with or without the use of a spacer. In contrast to the upper eyelid, the lower eyelid often needs an interpositional graft, such as an ear cartilage or a hard palate, to achieve lid elevation. Normal lid function and closure is imperative to minimize exposure keratopathy.

In view of the remarkable variations in physical presentation and unpredictable clinical course, Graves' ophthalmopathy poses a genuine challenge in both diagnosis and management, for which the treating ophthalmologist must be prepared. Responsibility begins with accuracy of diagnosis, maximal support of emotions and

discomfort, [...]
lized, restora [...]

IDIOPATHI[...]
HYPERTEN[...]

The clinical [...] [...]symptoms [...]
raised intracranial pressure, including idiopathic intracranial hypertension (IIH), is discussed in detail in
Chapter 5, Part II. As noted, the natural history of
patients with IIH followed over a long period demonstrates that, in some older series, some 50% will have
some permanent visual deficit, with severe visual field
defects in 25%. It is essential that visual function be
carefully monitored in all patients with papilledema;
funduscopic appearance alone may be misleading.

Surgical decompression of the optic nerve should be
considered sooner rather than later, and certainly before
major field or acuity defects occur. To reiterate, because
early damage to the optic disc manifests as peripheral
visual field constriction, with normal visual acuity, progressive constriction of visual field is a consideration for
surgical intervention, even if central visual acuity is not
affected. Progression of visual loss despite maximum
medical therapy is sufficient reason for optic nerve
sheath decompression.

Neurosurgical craniectomy for subtemporal bone resection is now rarely performed, and various ventricular
shunt procedures are frought with risks of infection or
shunt blockage, with variable long-term results. Indeed,
the use of lumboperitoneal shunts has decreased, as
optic nerve sheath fenestration has proven to be more
effective, with fewer complications and with less morbidity.

Optic nerve sheath fenestration is a well-accepted
surgical technique employed to preserve vision in patients with papilledema that threatens vision. Indeed,
DeWecker[91] first described optic nerve decompression
in 1872.

Preoperative screening for metabolic or electrolyte
abnormalities must be performed in patients who have
been receiving long-term medical therapy, especially
carbonic anhydrase inhibitors or diuretics. Systemic hypertension may contribute to optic disc damage and
visual morbidity in these patients. Although systemic
hypertension should be treated, abrupt or drastic reduction of blood pressure must be avoided since it may
result in hypoperfusion to the optic disc in the presence
of marked disc edema.

Access to the optic nerve sheath can be achieved
either through the medial transconjunctival approach,
via a lateral orbitotomy, or by a combination of these
two methods. The optimal optic nerve exposure is
achieved by performing a lateral orbitotomy with bone
removal.[92] This approach is useful in patients with failed

[...]proach, or for patients with a previous scleral
[...] [...]at limits optic nerve exposure.

[...]dial approach involves disinsertion of the me-
[...]s muscle to access the intraconal space and
[...]nerve. A lid speculum is used to retract the
[...]d a protective shield is placed over the other
[...])° conjunctival peritomy is performed along
the medial limbus from the 12 o'clock to 6 o'clock positions. A tenotomy scissors is used to bluntly dissect
along the sclera in the superonasal and inferonasal quadrants. The medial rectus muscle is isolated with a muscle
hook and the intramuscular attachments are severed.
A double-armed 5-0 polygalactin suture is passed partial
thickness through the medial rectus muscle just behind
the insertion, with locking full-thickness suture bites at
the upper and lower muscle margins, as is standard
in muscle displacement strabismus surgery. The medial
rectus muscle is disinserted and retracted medially using
the aforementioned suture. While good exposure is key
for all orbital surgery, it is especially important for medial exploration of the intraconal space. It is critically
important to recognize important anatomic landmarks.
The vortex veins number between four and eight and
lie 5 to 8 mm posterior to the equator of the globe.
They are close to the vertical meridian and are most
commonly seen in the temporal quadrants. The short
posterior ciliary arteries branch from the ophthalmic
artery to encircle the optic nerve. The paired long posterior ciliary arteries also course on either side of the optic
nerve. Violation of any of these vascular structures can
lead to serious hemorrhaging, which could jeopardize
the surgical procedure or visual function of the eye.

The intraconal space is now accessible by following
the space between the sclera and the medial rectus. Two
malleable ribbon retractors (1 cm in width) are bent 90°
to form a right angle. The two retractors are used to
enter the medial orbit oriented and in alignment with
the medial rectus. Once the malleable retractors are in
the intraconal space just behind the globe they are rotated 90° so that the retractors are oriented superiorly
and inferiorly. The retractors are then separated to expose the intraconal space with the retraction away from
the optic nerve and medial rectus muscle (Fig. 14–24).
Neurosurgical cottonoids are used to assist in retracting
the orbital fat superiorly and inferiorly. The optic nerve
sheath may still be obscured by surrounding orbital fat,
which is separated just behind the globe using two periosteal elevators. The malleable retractors and cottonoids are repositioned to retract the separated fat.
The fat dissection is performed carefully until the optic
nerve sheath is exposed. Throughout the procedure all
retraction is directed superiorly and inferiorly to eliminate traction on the globe or optic nerve. The pupil is
monitored for dilation during the procedure, which
would indicate manipulation of the posterior ciliary
nerves. If this occurs, dissection is stopped and the mal-

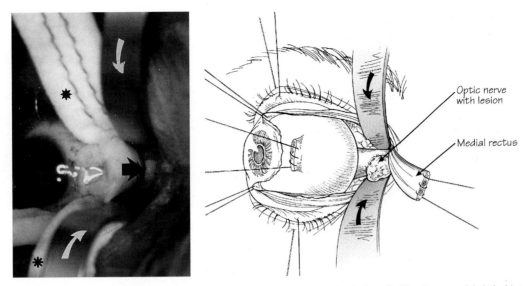

Fig. 14–24. Medial exposure of intraconal surgical space: surgical view (**left**), diagram (**right**). Note position of malleable metal retractors (*curved arrows*); neurosurgical cottonoids (*asterisks*); and optic nerve (*black arrow*) on surgical view.

leable retractors are repositioned to reduce traction against the ciliary nerve fibers.

Once the retrobulbar portion of the optic nerve is exposed, a binocular-operating microscope mounted on a Contraves (Contraves, Zurich) stand is moved into position. This stand provides a unique balancing system, allowing rapid, stable adjustments for different viewing angles during surgery. Under microscopic visualization, adipose tissue surrounding the bulbous portion of the nerve immediately behind the globe is gently retracted. The short ciliary nerve, the posterior ciliary arteries, and the fine vascular plexus made up of collateral branches of the ophthalmic artery on the epidural surface should be identified (Fig. 14–25). Extreme care

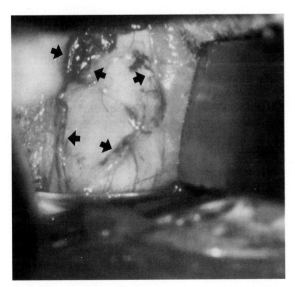

Fig. 14–25. Fine vascular plexus of collateral capillaries (*arrows*) of ophthalmic artery, on surface of epidura of optic nerve. Retractor blade (*right*).

must be exercised to preserve the fine vasculature surrounding and supplying the nerve; these vessels should be neither manipulated nor cauterized. Blood vessels and ciliary nerves are brushed behind the cottonoids to delineate an area on the optic nerve sheath for incision.

The dura of the distal bulbous portion of the optic nerve sheath is best grasped with a fine neurosurgical microforceps and incised with a bayonet microsurgical scissors (Fig. 14–26). As the dura is incised, arachnoid bulges slightly through the incision. The arachnoid and the edge of the dura are then regrasped together with the forceps, and the subarachnoid space is entered by snipping the arachnoid with the microscissors. Because CSF escapes once the arachnoid is incised, it is important to prevent the arachnoid from collapsing onto the pia. The arachnoid and dura should be excised without touching the pia. One blade of the microscissors is inserted into the subarachnoid space, and a rectangular window at least 3 × 5 mm is excised from the sheath (Fig. 14–27). If an epidural vessel is inadvertently cut, hemostasis can be obtained by gentle pressure on the cut edge of the vessel with a cotton-tip applicator; bipolar cauterization is often not necessary. The dural edge of the window is examined with a microforceps; two distinct cut edges should be seen: the arachnoid and the overlying dura. The arachnoid layer within the sheath window must be excised since an intact arachnoid is an effective barrier to CSF egress. The malleable retractors and cottonoids are then removed from the wound. Some surgeons prefer to use a blade and make several slits on the nerve sheath instead of a window, but there are no data that show any advantage. Once hemostasis has been assured, the medial rectus is re-attached at its insertion with the preplaced polygalactin muscle margin

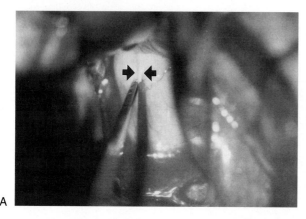
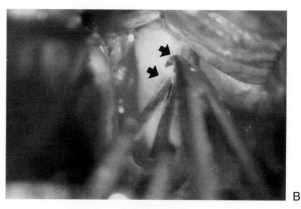

Fig. 14–26. Incision of optic nerve sheath. **A.** Dura of bulbous distal portion of optic nerve grasped and elevated (*small arrows*) with fine neurosurgical microforceps. **B.** Incision of tented dura with microsurgical scissors (*arrows*).

sutures. The conjunctiva is closed with interrupted 6-0 plain gut suture.

The lateral orbitotomy is patterned after that described by Stallard, which was described earlier. After en bloc removal of the bone of the lateral orbital wall, a T-shaped periorbital incision is made. Dissection within the central surgical space to gain access to the optic nerve is performed with malleable orbital retractors. As with the medial approach, the most difficult feature of lateral access is the tendency of orbital fat to obscure normal anatomic landmarks. The fat lobules often billow over the edges of the retractors, obscuring the plane of dissection. Using ½-inch (13-mm) neurosurgical cottonoids to insulate the billowing orbital fat lobules can eliminate this problem. By gradually removing and reinserting the orbital retractor blades over the cottonoids, the fat can be displaced from the plane of dissection. The optic nerve can be reached easily if posterior dissection follows the surface of the scleral wall. The nerve sheath fenestration is performed as described

above for the medial approach. After optic nerve fenestration is effected, the periorbita is reapproximated with interrupted 5-0 polygalactin sutures. The lateral orbital wall bone fragment is replaced and fixed with a nonabsorbable suture in the preplaced drill holes. The periosteum, muscle, subcutaneous tissues, and skin are closed in separate layers.

Kersten and Kulwin[93] described a lateral approach without bone removal. This approach begins with a lateral canthotomy, and sharp dissection is carried down to the periosteum at the lateral orbital rim. A 4-0 silk suture is passed beneath the lateral rectus muscle and used to adduct the eye. The periosteum at the lateral rim is incised from the frontozygomatic suture to the zygomatic arch. A periosteal elevator is used to elevate the periosteum and the periorbita approximately 2-mm posterior to the rim. A T-shaped incision is made in the periorbita and the flaps are retracted with 4-0 silk sutures. The lacrimal gland is then identified immediately within the periorbita and retracted superiorly with

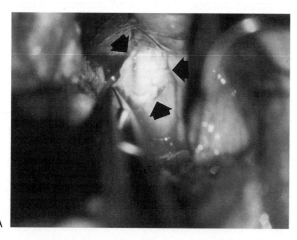
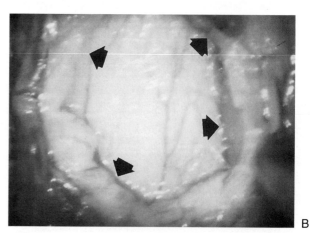

Fig. 14–27. Fenestration of optic nerve sheath. **A.** A window of dura is excised from optic nerve sheath (*arrows*). **B.** Enlarged view shows excision of arachnoid layer (*arrows*), baring optic nerve proper, with small nutrient vessels on surface.

a Sewell retractor. The lateral rectus muscle is then identified and retracted inferiorly. The plane of blunt dissection is between the lacrimal gland and the lateral rectus muscle. The retractors and cottonoids are repositioned as the dissection proceeds toward the nerve. Once the optic nerve is identified, the overlying ciliary nerves and blood vessels are cleared from the fenestration site; fenestration is performed in the same manner as described before. The lateral canthal angle is reapproximated with a double-armed 6-0 polygalactin suture and the skin is close with 7-0 nylon. The advantages of this technique are that bone does not need to be removed and the rectus muscle does not need to be disinserted.

The potential complications of optic nerve sheath fenestration include diplopia, pupillary dilation, angle closure glaucoma, conjunctival bleb, microhyphema, infection, decreased vision, and loss of vision. The most common complication of the medial approach is transient adduction deficit. A disadvantage of the lateral approach is the location of the ciliary ganglion on the lateral aspect of the optic nerve. Damage to the ganglion or to the ciliary nerves can result in pupillary and accommodation abnormalities. Another potential concern is the location of the papillomacular bundle nerve fibers along the lateral side of the optic nerve, although there is no evidence of different visual outcomes based on the surgical approach. The most severe complication of this procedure is permanent visual loss. This may be due to direct trauma to the optic nerve or central retinal artery occlusion. The incidence of permanent visual loss from optic nerve decompression has been reported as low as 2%. However, results of several clinical studies clearly have validated the efficacy of optic nerve sheath fenestration as an effective and safe surgical treatment to limit visual loss in idiopathic intracranial hypertension.[92-95]

Optic sheath fenestration may also have a role in the treatment of optic nerve sheath hemorrhage, acute retinal necrosis, and papilledema secondary to a nonresectable central nervous system mass. There is no substantial evidence to indicate that nerve sheath decompression is useful in the treatment of the progressive form of nonarteritic anterior ischemic optic neuropathy (see Chapter 5, Part II).

TRAUMATIC OPTIC NEUROPATHY

Traumatic optic neuropathy may occur by direct trauma in association with penetrating injury or by indirect closed-head orbitofacial trauma. An indirect injury to the optic nerve is usually associated with an anterofrontal impact with rapid deceleration of the head. Trauma can affect any portion of the optic nerve, from the intraocular segment to the intracranial.[96,97] The sinusoidal shaped intraorbital segment is redundant and cushioned by orbital fat. The surplus in its length allows the nerve to be displaced away from penetrating objects and makes it less liable to indirect injury. In contrast, the intracanalicular segment of the nerve is most vulnerable and subject to shearing forces, as it is tethered firmly to the bony optic canal entrance. Within the canal, the dural sheath of the nerve fuses with the periosteum of the lesser wing of the sphenoid. At the intracranial entrance of the optic foramen, the nerve is firmly adherent to the falciform dural fold superiorly. In the posterior indirect type of traumatic optic neuropathy, usually from a midfacial blow with rapid deceleration of the head, the brain and orbital contents continue to shift forward while the intracanalicular segment of the nerve remains immobile.[98] The shearing forces generated result in microscopic injuries to the optic nerve. Postulated mechanisms of injury include fracture of the canal with bone impingement of the optic nerve, edema or hemorrhage within the tight confines of the bony canal, contusion necrosis of the nerve fibers, and ischemia or infarction secondary to shearing of the nutrient pial vessels.[84,99-101]

In assessing a patient with possible traumatic optic neuropathy, the systemic search for life-threatening injuries must take priority. All patients should receive a thorough ophthalmic examination, emphasizing the assessment of optic nerve function. Traumatic optic neuropathy is a diagnosis of exclusion, so other ocular injuries or causes of decreased vision should be evaluated. The visual acuity in traumatic optic neuropathy patients can range from 20/20 to no light perception. A relative afferent pupillary defect with other signs of optic nerve dysfunction in association with an otherwise normal ocular examination is suggestive of traumatic optic neuropathy. It is important to note that a relative afferent pupillary defect does not rule out the possibility of bilateral traumatic optic neuropathy, and no relative afferent pupillary defect also does not rule out bilateral traumatic optic neuropathy.

In patients suspected of having traumatic optic neuropathy, orbital CT should be performed. The orbit, optic canal, and paranasal sinuses are assessed with axial and coronal projections, preferably with 1.5 mm or smaller sections. Fractures may be seen in up to 50% of indirect posterior traumatic optic neuropathies. The severity of the optic neuropathy is independent of the presence of an optic canal fracture.[97,98,102] In cases of suspected anterior optic nerve injury including avulsion of the optic nerve and optic nerve sheath hemorrhage, ultrasonography may be helpful in evaluating the globe and the anterior aspect of the orbit.

The management of traumatic optic neuropathy is controversial, with no clear consensus. Treatment options include observation, corticosteroids, and optic canal decompression. Spontaneous visual improvement has been reported in as high as 20% to 33% of patients with traumatic optic neuropathy.[99,103,104] High-dose corticosteroids have shown a beneficial effect in prospective studies involving spinal cord injuries. Therapy is usually instituted immediately following injury. In the National Acute Spinal Cord Injury Study, patients treated within 8 hours of injury had fewer permanent neurologic deficits than those whose treatment was initiated after 8 hours.[105] The corticosteroid therapy may be continued for up to 72 hours, although there is no clear evidence that treatment beyond 24 hours is beneficial. If clinical improvement is noted after 72 hours of intravenous corticosteroids, the patient is placed on oral prednisone and the prednisone is slowly tapered. If no improvement is noted after 72 hours, the corticosteroids may be discontinued and no prednisone taper is necessary. Patients are typically started on an H-2 blocking agent as gastric ulcer prophylaxis. It is important to note that it is unclear whether the conclusions of the spinal cord injury studies apply to traumatic optic neuropathy. The megadose corticosteroids treatment of traumatic optic neuropathy should only be considered empirical at this time. Once the diagnosis is made, the current suggested regimen is 30 mg/kg of methylprednisolone IV loading and 5.4 mg/kg/hour continuous IV infusion thereafter.[96,97,99]

Optic canal decompression has been shown in retrospective studies to be beneficial in cases of traumatic optic neuropathy.[106–111] This is a consideration in a patient whose vision deteriorates or fails to improve on megadose of corticosteroids within the first 48 hours, or in whom vision deteriorates on oral taper. This procedure is usually reserved for those cases in which a fracture of the optic canal is documented on imaging; however, some have advocated that the absence of a canal fracture on imaging is not a contraindication for decompression, as small fractures can be identified at the time of surgery.[97,98,106] Optic canal decompression may be more beneficial in patients younger than 40 years of age.[100] Extracranial access to the optic canal can be achieved through transorbital, transethmoidal, and transnasal approaches.[107–112] Optic canal decompression performed transcranially does not appear to be effective and is normally only performed if other intracranial procedures are necessary. An adequate canal decompression should fulfill the criteria of removing at least 50% of the circumference of the bony canal, bone removal along the entire length of the canal, and total longitudinal incision of the dural sheath including the annulus of Zinn.[96,112] This procedure should be performed by an experienced surgeon, as potential risks include carotid artery injury, cavernous sinus injury, hemorrhage, cerebrospinal fluid leak, diplopia, decreased vision, loss of vision, and death.

The literature regarding the management of traumatic optic neuropathy is limited to retrospective small series. Cook et al[113] performed a meta-analysis on all case series and case reports of traumatic optic neuropathy in the English-language literature. The authors iden-tified 244 cases of traumatic optic neuropathy of which 49 patients were treated only with observation. Visual acuity improved in 22% of patients who had no treatment. Patients were separated into three treatment groups: corticosteroids, 64 patients; extracranial decompression, 68 patients; and corticosteroids and decompression, 63 patients. Visual acuity improved 42% to 59% in the treatment groups; however, the data were insufficient to determine which treatment was most effective. The authors concluded that treatment with corticosteroids, extracranial decompression, or both was better than observation for traumatic optic neuropathy. The International Optic Nerve Trauma Study was supposed to prospectively examine the role of megadose corticosteroids in comparison to corticosteroids and extracranial canal decompression; however, the study was stopped due to limited enrollment.

REFERENCES

1. Rootman J: Diseases of the Orbit. Philadelphia, JB Lippincott, 1988
2. Char DH: Metastatic orbital tumors. Orbit 6:189, 1987
3. Katz SE, Rootman J, Goldberg RA: Secondary and metastatic tumors of the orbit. In Tasman W, Jaeger EA (eds): Duane's Clinical Ophthalmology, Vol 2, Chap 46. Philadelphia, JB Lippincott, 1996
4. Jarrett WH, Gutman FA: Ocular complications of infection in the paranasal sinuses. Arch Ophthalmol 81:683, 1969
5. Hornblass A, Herschorn BJ, Stern K et al: Orbital abscess. Survey Ophthalmol 29:169, 1984
6. Mombaerts I, Goldschmeding R, Schlingeman RO et al: What is orbital pseudotumor? Survey Ophthalmol 41:66, 1996
7. Siatkowski RM, Capo H, Byrne SF et al: Clinical and echographic findings in idiopathic orbital myositis. Am J Ophthalmol 118:343, 1994
8. Rootman J, Hay E, Graeb D et al: Orbital-adnexal lymphangiomas. A spectrum of hemodynamically isolated vascular hamartomas. Ophthalmology 93:1558, 1986
9. Katz B, Carmody R: Subperiosteal orbital hematoma induced by the Valsalva maneuver. Am J Ophthalmol 100:617, 1985.
10. Jacobson DM, Itani K, Digre KB et al: Maternal orbital hematoma associated with labor. Am J Ophthalmol 105:547, 1998
11. Mannor GE, Rose GE, Moseley IF et al: Outcome of orbital myositis. Clinical features associated with recurrence. Ophthalmology 104:409, 1997
12. Manor RS, Yassur Y, Hoyt WF: Reading-evoked visual dimming. Am J Ophthalmol 121:212, 1996
13. Atta HR, Dick AD, Hamed LM et al: Venous stasis orbitopathy: a clinical and echographic study. Br J Ophthalmol 80:129, 1996
14. Gay AJ, Salmon ML, Windsor CE: Hering's law, the levators, and their relationship in disease states. Arch Ophthalmol 77:157, 1967
15. Migliori ME, Gladstone GJ: Determination of the normal range of exophthalmometric values for black and white adults. Am J Ophthalmol 98:438, 1984
16. Musch DC, Frueh BR, Landis JR: The reliability of Hertel exophthalmometry. Observer variation between physician and lay readers. Ophthalmology 92:1177, 1985
17. Cline RA, Rootman J: Enophthalmos: a clinical review. Ophthalmology 91:229, 1984
18. Miller MT, Spencer MA: Progressive hemifacial atrophy. A natural history study. Trans Am Ophthalmol Soc 93:203, 1995
19. Soparkar CNS, Patrinely JR, Cuaycong MJ et al: The silent sinus syndrome: a cause of spontaneous enophthalmos. Ophthalmology 101:772, 1994
20. Bullock JD, Bartley GB: Dynamic proptosis. Am J Ophthalmol 102:104, 1986

21. Allen SJ, Naylor D: Pulsation of the eyeballs in tricuspid regurgitation. Can Med Assoc J 133:119, 1983
22. Stephens KF, Reinecke RD: Quantitative forced ductions. Trans Am Acad Ophthalmol Otolaryngol 71:324, 1967
23. Gamblin GT, Harper DG, Galentine P et al: Prevalence of increased intraocular pressure in Graves' disease. Evidence of frequent subclinical ophthalmopathy. N Engl J Med 308:420, 1983
24. Ohtsuka K: Intraocular pressure and proptosis in 95 patients with Graves' ophthalmopathy. Am J Ophthalmol 124:570, 1997
25. Reader AL: Normal variations of intraocular pressure on vertical gaze. Ophthalmology 89:1084, 1982
26. Spierer A, Eisenstein Z: The role of increased intraocular pressure on upgaze in the assessment of Graves' ophthalmopathy. Ophthalmology 98:1491, 1991
27. De La Paz M, Boniuk M: Fundus manifestations of orbital disease and treatment of orbital disease. Surv Ophthalmol 40:3, 1995
28. Keltner JL: Is Graves' ophthalmopathy a preventable disease. Arch Ophthalmol 116:1106, 1998
29. Burch HB, Wartofsky L: Graves' ophthalmopathy: current concepts regarding pathogenesis and management. Endocr Rev 14:747, 1993
30. Tallstedt L, Lundell G, Torring O et al: Occurrence of ophthalmopathy after treatment for Graves' hyperthyroidism. N Engl J Med 326:1733, 1992
31. Bartalena L, Marcocci C, Bogazzi F et al: Relation between therapy for hyperthyroidism and the course of Graves' ophthalmopathy. N Engl J Med 338:73, 1998
32. Sanders MD, Brown P: Acute presentation of thyroid ophthalmopathy. Trans Ophthalmol Soc UK 105:720, 1986
33. Liu GT, Heher KL, Katowitz JA et al: Prominent proptosis in childhood thyroid eye disease. Ophthalmology 103:779, 1996
34. Trobe JD, Glaser JS, Laflamme P: Dysthyroid optic neuropathy. Clinical profile and rationale for management. Arch Ophthalmol 96:1199, 1978
35. Kazim M, Trokel S, Moore S: Treatment of acute Graves' orbitopathy. Ophthalmol 98:1443, 1991
36. Harnett AN, Doughty D, Hirst A, Plowman PN: Radiotherapy in benign orbital disease. II: Ophthalmic Graves' disease and orbital histiocytosis X. Br J Ophthalmol 72:289, 1988
37. Kao SCS, Kendler DL, Nugent RA et al: Radiotherapy in the management of thyroid orbitopathy. Computed tomography and clinical outcomes. Arch Ophthalmol 111:819, 1993
38. Bartalena L, Marcocci C, Bogazzi F et al: Relation between therapy for hyperthyroidism and the course of Graves' ophthalmopathy. N Engl J Med 338:73, 1998
39. Char D: Thyroid eye disease. Br J Ophthalmol 80:922, 1996
40. Bartley GB, Fatourechi V, Kadrmas EF et al: The treatment of Graves' ophthalmopathy in an incidence cohort. Am J Ophthalmol 121:200, 1996
41. Donahue SP, Schwartz G: Preseptal and orbital cellulitis in childhood. Ophthalmology 105:1902, 1998
42. Harril WC, Stewart MG, Lee AG et al: Chronic mucormycosis. Laryngoscope 106:1292, 1996.
43. De La Paz MA, Patrinely JR, Marines HM et al: Adjunctive hyperbaric oxygen in the treatment of bilateral cerebro-rhino-orbital mucormycosis. Am J Ophthalmol 114:208, 1992
44. Klapper SR, Lee AG, Patrinely JR et al: Orbital involvement in allergic fungal sinusitis. Ophthalmology 104:2094, 1997
45. Mombaerts I, Schlingemann RO, Goldschmeding R et al: Idiopathic granulomatous orbital inflammation. Ophthalmology 103:2135, 1996
46. Perry SR, Rootman J, White VA: The clinical and pathologic constellation of Wegener granulomatosis of the orbit. Ophthalmology 104:683, 1997
47. Polito E, Leccisotti A: Prognosis of orbital lymphoid hyperplasia. Graefes Arch Clin Exp Ophthalmol 234:150, 1996
48. Jakobiec FA, Neri A, Knowles DM: Genotypic monoclonality in immunophenotypically polyclonal orbital lymphoid tumors: a model of tumor progression in the lymphoid system. Ophthalmology 94:980, 1987
49. Logani S, Logani SC, Ali BH et al: Bilateral intraconal non-Hodgkin's lymphoma in a patient with acquired immunodeficiency syndrome. Am J Ophthalmol 118:401, 1994
50. Reifler DM, Warzynski MJ, Blount WR et al: Orbital lymphoma associated with acquired immune deficiency syndrome (AIDS). Surv Ophthalmol 38:371, 1994
51. Peterson KL, Wang M, Canalis RF et al: Rhinocerebral mucormycosis: evolution of the disease and treatment options. Laryngoscope 107:855, 1997
52. Jakobiec FA, Nelson D: Lymphomatous, plasmacytic, and hematopoietic tumors of the orbit. In Tasman W, Jaeger EA (eds): Duane's Clinical Ophthalmology, Vol 2, Chap. 39. Philadelphia, JB Lippincott, 1993
53. Wright JE: Doyne lecture: current concepts in orbital disease. Eye 2:1, 1988
54. Katz SE, Rootman J, Vangveeravong S et al: Combined venous lymphatic malformations of the orbit (so-called lymphangiomas). Association with noncontiguous intracranial vascular anomalies. Ophthalmology 105:176, 1998
55. Phelps CD, Thompson HS, Ossoinig KC: The diagnosis and prognosis of atypical carotid-cavernous fistula (red-eyed shunt syndrome). Am J Ophthalmol 93:423, 1982
56. Borruat F-X, Bogousslavsky J, Uffer S et al: Orbital infarction syndrome. Ophthalmology 100:562, 1993
57. Galetta SL, Leahey A, Nichols CW et al: Orbital ischemia, ophthalmoparesis, and carotid dissection. J Clin Neuro-Ophthalmol 11:284, 1991
58. Erly WK, Carmody RF, Dryden RM: Orbital histiocytosis X. AJNR 16:1258, 1995
59. Kodsi SR, Shetlar DJ, Campbell RJ et al: A review of 340 orbital tumors in children during a 60-year period. Am J Ophthalmol 117:177, 1994
60. Kennerdell JS, Slamowitz T, Dekker A et al: Orbital fine needle aspiration biopsy. Am J Ophthalmol 99:547, 1985
61. Putterman AM: Management of blow-out fractures of the orbital floor: III. The conservative approach. Surv Ophthalmol 35:292, 1991
62. Flanagan JC, McLachlan DL, Shannon GM: Orbital roof fractures. Neurologic and neurosurgical considerations. Ophthalmology 87:325, 1980
63. Iwamoto MA, Iliff NT: Management of orbital trauma. In Tasman W, Jaeger EA, (eds): Duane's Clinical Ophthalmology, Vol 6, Chap. 135. Philadelphia, Lippincott, 1993
64. Meyer DR: Orbital fractures. In Tasman W, Jaeger EA, eds: Duane's Clinical Ophthalmology, Vol 2, Chap. 48. Philadelphia, Lippincott, 1996
65. Char DH, Norman D: The use of computed tomography and ultrasonography in the evaluation of orbital masses. Surv Ophthalmol 27:49, 1982
66. Moseley I: The contribution of X-ray computed tomography to the diagnosis and management of orbital disease. Orbit 5:149, 1985
67. Johnson MH, DeFilipp GJ, Zimmerman RA, Savino PJ: Scleral inflammatory disease. AJNR 8:861, 1987
68. Ball JB: Direct oblique sagittal CT of orbital wall fractures. AJNR 8:147, 1987
69. Gilbard SM, Mahmood FM, Lagouros PA et al: Orbital blowout fractures. The prognostic significance of computed tomography. Ophthalmology 92:1523, 1985
70. Holt JE, O'Connor PS, Douglas JP et al: Extraocular muscle size comparison using standardized A-scan echography and computerized tomography scan measurements. Ophthalmology 92:1351, 1985
71. Byrne SF, Glaser JS: Orbital tissue differentiation with standardized echography. Ophthalmology 90:1071, 1983
72. Jorgensen JS, Guthoff R: Differential diagnosis of the dilated superior ophthalmic vein by B-scan ultrasonography. Orbit 5:259, 1986
73. Peyster RG, Savino PJ, Hoover ED, Schatz NJ: Differential diagnosis of the enlarged superior ophthalmic vein. J Comput Assist Tomogr 8:103, 1984
74. Carr WA, Baker RS, Lee C et al: NMR imaging of the orbit. An initial evaluation and comparison with CT. Orbit 6:85, 1987
75. Khanna RK, Pham CJ, Malik GM et al: Bilateral superior ophthalmic vein enlargement associated with diffuse cerebral swelling. Report of 11 cases. J Neurosurg 86:893, 1997

76. Jane JA, Parks TS, Pobereskin LH et al: The supraorbital approach: technical note. Neurosurgery 11:537, 1982
77. Prummel MF, Mourits MP, Berghout A et al: Prednisone and cyclosporine in the treatment of severe Graves' ophthalmopathy. N Engl J Med 321:1353, 1989
78. Hurwitz JJ, Birt D: An individualized approach to orbital decompression in Graves' orbitopathy. Arch Ophthalmol 96:1199, 1978
79. Mourits M, Koornneef L, Wiersinga WM et al: Orbital decompression for Graves' ophthalmopathy by inferomedial, by inferomedial plus lateral, and by coronal approach. Ophthalmology 97:636, 1990
80. Lyons CJ, Rootman J: Orbital decompression for disfiguring exophthalmos in thyroid orbitopathy. Ophthalmology 101:223, 1994
81. Harting F, Koornneef L, Peeters HJ et al: Decompression surgery in Graves' orbitopathy—a review of 14 years' experience at the orbita centrum, Amsterdam. Dev Ophthalmol 20:185, 1989
82. Garrity JA, Fatourechi V, Bergstralh EJ et al: Results of transantral orbital decompression in 428 patients with severe Graves' ophthalmopathy. Am J Ophthalmol 116:533, 1993
83. Kennedy DW, Goodstein ML, Miller NR et al: Endoscopic transnasal orbital decompression. Arch Otolaryngol Head Neck Surg 116:275, 1990
84. Leone CR, Piest KL, Newman RJ: Medial and lateral wall decompression for thyroid ophthalmopathy. Am J Ophthalmol 108:160, 1989
85. Deleted in proof
86. Carter KD, Frueh BR, Hessburg TP et al: Long term efficacy of orbital decompression for compressive optic neuropathy of Graves' eye disease. Ophthalmology 98:1435, 1991
87. Olivari N: Transpalpebral decompression of endocrine ophthalmopathy by removal of intraorbital fat: experience with 147 operations over 5 years. Plast Reconstr Surg 187:627, 1991
88. Warren JD, Spector JG, Burde R: Long term follow up and recent observations on 305 cases of orbital decompression for dysthyroid orbitopathy. Laryngoscope 99:35, 1989
89. Harvey JT: Orbital decompression for Graves' disease leaving the periosteum intact. Ophthalmol Plast Reconstr Surg 5:199, 1989
90. Pitz GK, Muller-Forell W, Hommel G: Randomized trial of intravenous immunoglobulins versus prednisolone in Graves' ophthalmopathy. Clin Exp Immunol 106:197, 1996
91. DeWecker L: On incision of the optic nerve in cases of neuroretinitis. Rep Int Ophthalmol Congr 4:11, 1872
92. Tse DT, Nerad JA, Anderson RL et al: Optic nerve sheath fenestration in pseudotumor cerebri: a lateral orbitotomy approach. Arch Ophthalmol 106:1458, 1988
93. Kersten RC, Kulwin DR: Optic nerve sheath fenestration through a lateral canthotomy incision. Arch Ophthalmol 111:870, 1993
94. Corbett JJ, Nerad JA, Tse DT et al: Results of optic nerve sheath fenestration for pseudotumor cerebri: the lateral orbitotomy approach. Arch Ophthalmol 106:1391, 1988
95. Brourman ND, Spoor TC, Ramochi JM: Optic nerve sheath decompression provides long-term visual improvement for pseudotumor cerebri. Arch Ophthalmol 106:1378, 1988
96. Steinsapir KD, Goldberg RA: Traumatic optic neuropathy. Surv Ophthalmol 38:487, 1994
97. Bilyk JR, Joseph MP: Traumatic optic neuropathy. Semin Ophthalmol 9:200, 1994
98. Joseph MP: Traumatic optic neuropathy. Ophthalmol Clin North Am 8:693, 1995
99. Anderson RL, Panje WR, Gross CE: Optic nerve blindness following blunt trauma. Ophthalmology 89:445, 1982
100. Aitken PA, Sofferman RA: Traumatic optic neuropathy. Ophthalmol Clin North Am 4:479, 1991
101. Crompton MR: Visual lesions in closed head injury. Brain 93:785, 1970
102. Manfredi SJ, Raji MR, Sprinkle PM: Computerized tomographic scan findings in facial fractures associated with blindness. Plast Reconstr Surg 68:479, 1981
103. Miller NR. The management of traumatic optic neuropathy. Arch Ophthalmol 108:1086, 1990
104. Spoor TC, Hartel WC, Lensink DB et al: Treatment of traumatic optic neuropathy with corticosteroids. Am J Ophthalmol 110:665, 1990
105. Bracken MB, Shepard MJ, Collins WF et al: A randomized, controlled trial of methylprednisolone or naloxone in the treatment of acute spinal-cord injury results of the Second National Acute Spinal Cord Injury Study. N Engl J Med 322:1405, 1990
106. Call NB. Decompression of the optic nerve in the optic canal. Ophthalmic Plast Reconstr Surg 2:133, 1996
107. Takahashi M, Itoh M, Kaneko M, et al: Microscopic intranasal decompression of the optic nerve. Arch Otorhinolaryngol 246:113, 1989
108. Amrith S, Pham T, Chee C et al: Visual recovery following transethmoidal optic nerve decompression in traumatic optic neuropathy. Ophthalmic Surg 24:49, 1993
109. Knox BE, Gates GA, Berry SM. Optic nerve decompression via the lateral facial approach. Laryngoscope 100:458, 1990
110. Joseph MP, Lessell S, Rizzo J et al: Extracranial optic nerve decompression for traumatic optic neuropathy. Arch Ophthalmol 108:1091, 1990
111. Levin LA, Joseph MP, Rizzo JF et al: Optic canal decompression in indirect optic nerve trauma. Ophthalmology 101:566, 1994
112. Sofferman RA: Sphenoethmoidal approach to the optic nerve. Laryngoscope 91:184, 1981
113. Cook MW, Levin LA, Joseph MP et al: Traumatic optic neuropathy. Arch Otolaryngol Head Neck Surg 122:389, 1996

CHAPTER 15

The Pupils and Accommodation

Thomas L. Slamovits and Joel S. Glaser

Anatomical Considerations
  Light Reflex Pathway
  Ocular Sympathetic Pathways
  Near Reflex and Accommodation
The Patient with Abnormal Pupils
  Relative Afferent Pupillary Defect
  Argyll Robertson Pupils

Light-Near Dissociation Syndromes
Essential Anisocoria
Tonic Pupil Syndrome
Oculosympathetic Defects (Horner's Syndrome)
Pharmacologic Accidents: The Fixed Dilated Pupil
Episodic Dysfunction of the Pupil
Disorders of Accommodation

He sustained them in a desert land,
In an empty howling wasteland.
He encompassed them and raised them up,
Protecting them like the pupil* of His eye.
Deuteronomy 32:10

The pupil is a kinetic indicator of both ocular motor function and the special sensory apparatus, the retina, which it serves. The neural mechanisms that control pupil size and reactivity are highly complex, yet they may be sampled and evaluated by simple clinical procedures. Dr. Irene Lowenfeld's scholarly text *The Pupil* is recommended reading for encyclopedic information about the pupil.[1]

Pupillary function depends on the integrity of the structures along the course of the pupillomotor pathway (Fig. 15–1): retinal receptors; ganglion cell axons in the optic nerve, optic chiasm, and optic tract (but not the lateral geniculate body); brachium of the superior colliculus; pretectal area of the mesencephalon; the interconnecting neurons to pupilloconstrictor motor cells in the oculomotor nuclear complex; the efferent parasympathetic outflow accompanying the third cranial nerve; and the efferent sympathetic pathway from the hypothalamus to the pupillary dilator

T. L. Slamovits: Departments of Ophthalmology, Neurology, and Neurosurgery, Albert Einstein College of Medicine/Montefiore Medical Center, Bronx, New York

J. S. Glaser: Departments of Neurology and Ophthalmology, Bascom Palmer Eye Institute, University of Miami School of Medicine, Miami; and Neuro-ophthalmology, Cleveland Clinic Florida, Ft. Lauderdale, Florida

*Hebrew, ishon, little man.

muscle. In addition, the size of the pupils is influenced by the intensity of retinal illumination, the near-effort reflex, the state of retinal light adaptation, by supranuclear influences from the frontal and occipital cortex above the pretectal area, and from the reticular formation of the brain stem below.

At a given moment, any or all of the aforementioned factors may influence pupillary size and reactivity. It should be no wonder, then, that in the awake state, the pupil is rather constantly moving, a condition of physiologic unrest termed *hippus*. This incessant change in pupil size has no pathologic significance,[2] although it is described in diverse conditions ranging from encephalitis to schizophrenia and from cataracts to hemorrhoids. Age affects both pupillary size and reactivity.[3,4] The pupil of the neonate is miotic but increases in size during the first decade of life; from the second decade on, the pupil steadily becomes smaller (Fig. 15–2). Pupillary reactivity, at least to "long" (3-second) light flashes, also seems related to age; the range of amplitude of the light reflex declines with increasing age (Fig. 15–3).

The pupil may be considered to have three major optic functions: (1) to regulate the amount of light reaching the retina; (2) to diminish the chromatic and spherical aberrations produced by the peripheral imperfections of the optical system of the cornea and lens; and (3) to increase depth of field (analogous to the f-stop setting of a camera).

As pupillary size increases, so does chromatic and spherical aberration. As pupillary size decreases, light diffraction at the pupil edge becomes a more significant factor in reducing image quality; this generally outweighs any benefit of miosis-induced increase in focal depth. In their experiments of optical line-spread func-

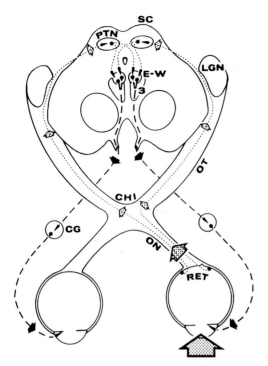

Fig. 15–1. Pupillary light reflex. Light in left eye (*dotted arrow*) stimulates retina (*RET*), whose afferent axons (*fine dashed lines*) ascend optic nerve (*ON*), decussate at chiasm (*CHI*), and terminate in pretectal nuclear complex (*PTN*). Lateral geniculate nucleus (*LGN*) is bypassed by these pupillomotor fibers. The PTN is connected by crossed and uncrossed intercalated neurons to both Edinger-Westphal parasympathetic motor nuclei (*E-W*), which comprise the dorsal aspect of the oculomotor nuclear complex (*3*). Preganglionic parasympathetic fibers (*heavy dashed lines*) leave ventral aspect of midbrain in the substance of the third cranial nerves. After synapsing in the ciliary ganglia (*CG*), the postganglionic fibers innervate the pupillary sphincter muscles. Note that uniocular light stimulus evokes bilateral and symmetric pupillary constriction. Brain stem diagram represents section through level rostral to superior colliculi (*SC*).

tion, Campbell and Gubisch[5] found the optimal pupil diameter to be 2.4 mm; scatter and focusing defects have an increasing effect with larger pupils.

ANATOMIC CONSIDERATIONS

Mechanically, the diameter of the pupil is determined by the antagonistic actions of the iris sphincter and dilator muscles, with the radially arranged dilator fibers playing the minor role. The dilator muscle inserts at the iris root and extends from there to an area about 2 mm from the pupillary margin. The sphincter muscle has circumferential fibers, is more superficial in the iris stroma, and occupies an area about 2 to 4 mm from the pupillary margin. The sphincter can be seen in light or atrophic irides. Rather than retracting toward one quadrant when severed or ruptured, the sphincter continues to function except in the altered segment. Therefore, with prudence, the pupillary reactions may be evaluated even in the presence of iris atrophy, traumatic rupture of the sphincter, and congenital or surgical coloboma.

Light Reflex Pathway

The pupillary light reflex pathway functionally may be considered a three-neuron arc (see Fig. 15–1): the afferent neurons from retinal ganglion cells to the pretectal area; an intercalated neuron from the pretectal complex to the parasympathetic motor pool (Edinger-Westphal nucleus) of the oculomotor nuclear complex; and the parasympathetic outflow with the oculomotor nerve to the ciliary ganglion, and from there to the pupillary sphincter.

Considerable evidence exists that the visual cells of the retina (*i.e.,* the rods and cones) also serve as light receptors, controlling pupillomotor activity. For exam-

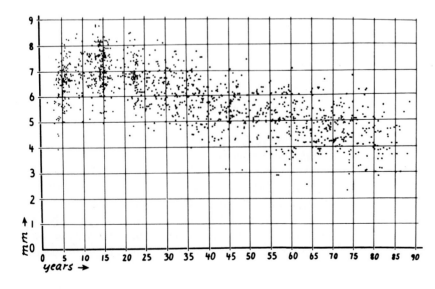

Fig. 15–2. Pupillary size in darkness of 1263 subjects chosen at random; average pupil size was used [(R + L)/2]. Abscissa shows horizontal diameters in millimeters, ordinate shows subjects' age in years. Note the wide scatter but obvious ages trend. See also Figure 15–3, top curve. (Reprinted with permission from Loewenfeld IE: Pupillary changes related to age. In Thompson HS, Daroff RB, Frisen L et al (eds): Topics in Neuro-ophthalmology, p 129. Baltimore: Williams & Wilkins, 1979)

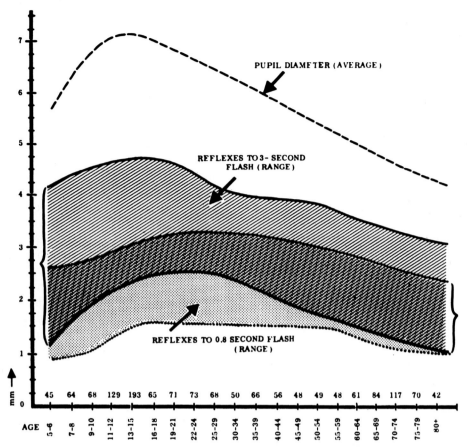

Fig. 15–3. Normal ranges of light reflex amplitude for long and for short flashes. Shaded area (*left bracket*) is normal range for 3-second flashes; stippled area is normal range for 0.8-second flashes. The numbers above the abscissa indicate the number of subjects per age group. Note early peak, followed by decline with age for reactions to long light flashes. In contrast, reflexes elicited by short flashes show relatively flat age curve. (Reprinted with permission from Loewenfeld IE: Pupillary changes related to age. In Thompson HS, Daroff RB, Frisen L et al (eds): Topics in Neuro-ophthalmology, p 137. Baltimore: Williams & Wilkins, 1979)

ple, pupillomotor light thresholds follow the same shifts in spectral sensitivity as visual thresholds, depending on the state of light adaptation of the retina (Purkinje shift). Pupillomotor sensitivity of the retina also parallels visual form sensitivity, which is highest at the fovea and lowest in the periphery. In our present state of knowledge, it seems that the same afferent axons in the optic nerve transmit pupillomotor information to the pretectal area and visual information to the lateral geniculate nuclei. It is suspected but unproved that this dual function is accomplished by axonal bifurcation in the optic tract in humans.[6] Therefore, we may consider two intimately related systems: retinogeniculate for visual perception and retinomesencephalic for pupillomotor control and foveation.

At the optic chiasm, slightly more than one half of the afferent axons in the optic nerve cross to the opposite optic tract, where they are mixed with noncrossing axons from the contralateral optic nerve. The ratio of crossed to uncrossed fibers is approximately 53:47.[7] From the chiasmal level posteriorly, afferent visual and pupillomotor information from either eye is divided into crossed fibers (from nasal retinal receptors of the contralateral eye) and uncrossed fibers (from temporal retinal receptors of the ipsilateral eye). In the posterior aspect of the optic tract (pregeniculate), the pupillomotor branches of the afferent axons gain the pretectal nuclear area by transversing the brachium of the superior colliculus into the rostral midbrain. Intercalated neurons interconnect from the preolivary nucleus of the posterior commissure and lentiform nucleus[8] to the Edinger-Westphal nuclei by crossing dorsal to the aqueduct in the posterior commissure and by coursing ventrally in the periaqueductal gray matter. This simplistic anatomic approach belies the true complexity of the neurophysiology and neuroanatomy of the pretectal nuclear complex. The reader is referred to articles by Smith and coworkers,[9] Carpenter and Pierson,[10] Benevento and associates,[11] and Burde.[12]

The organization of the oculomotor nuclear complex in the mesencephalon (midbrain) depicted by Warwick[13] in 1953 and Jampel and Mindel[14] in 1967 has been modified by Burde and Loewy[15] and Burde[12] with recognition of the anterior median nucleus rostrally and accessory cell columns caudally. The anteromedian nucleus is the source of special visceral efferent motor axons to the iris sphincter and ciliary musculature. This dorsal cell mass may be subdivided into a rostral portion associated with accommodation, a caudal portion—the stimulation of which produces pupil constriction, and a midportion associated with both accommodation and constriction. Direct input to the the iris sphincter and ciliary body also may be provided by the nucleus of Perlia.[8,15] The pretectal olivary nuclei receive direct retinal input and in turn provide direct input to the Edinger-Westphal nuclei. The exact location of the Edinger-Westphal nuclei is not known. Kourouyan and Horton[16] injected tritiated H-proline into macaque monkey eyes and found the primary pretectal retinal projections terminating in the olivary nuclei, ipsilaterally and contralaterally. The label for the Edinger-Westphal nucleus was found bilaterally in the midbrain, ventral to the cerebral aqueduct, in the central gray matter, in well-defined columns, corresponding to an area termed the lateral visceral column in the classic literature (Fig. 15–4). According to the degeneration studies by Warwick,[17] the ciliary ganglion contains more cells for innervation of the ciliary muscles than for innervation of the iris sphincter

(about 30:1). Presumably, that same ratio occurs in the Edinger-Westphal nucleus, although the presence of diffuse projections may argue against it.

From the parasympathetic nucleus, the pupillomotor and ciliary fibers join the outflow of the oculomotor nuclei and exit from the substance of the midbrain with the oculomotor nerves as multiple rootlets in the interpeduncular space. According to Kerr and Hollowell,[18] the pupillomotor fibers are located superficially in the nerve, lying just internal to the epineurium. It is believed that this superficial position makes the pupillomotor fibers especially vulnerable to compression. In a more rostral part of its projections and in more anterior segments (e.g., the cavernous sinus), however, pupillomotor fibers may be spared preferentially even in the presence of total oculomotor palsy. It is likely that involvement or "sparing" of the pupil sphincter reflects the nature and acuteness of the injury rather than merely the portion of the third nerve that is compromised.[19]

At about the level of the superior orbital fissure, the oculomotor nerve divides into superior and inferior divisions, with parasympathetic fibers traveling in the latter to the ciliary ganglion via the branch to the inferior oblique muscle. Although the ciliary ganglion contains

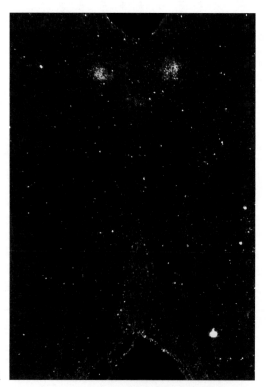
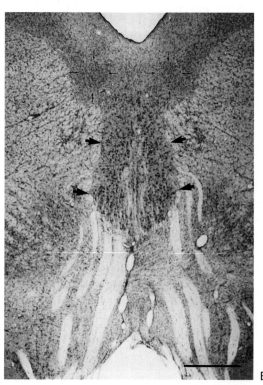

Fig. 15–4. A. Transneuronal autoradiographic label in the Edinger-Westphal nuclei, seen bilaterally adjacent to the midline, ventral to the cerebral aqueduct. **B.** The label seen in **(A)** corresponds on each side to the fairly distinct cell group, (*thin arrows*), the lateral visceral cell column of the Edinger-Westphal nucleus, shown in a Nissl-counterstained section. The somatic subnuclei of the oculomotor complex (*thick arrows*) contain larger nuclei. Fascicles from the oculomotor complex are seen streaming inferiorly toward the interpeduncular fossa. Scale bar = 1 mm. (Reprinted with permission from Kourouvan HD, Horton JC: Transneuronal retinal input to the primate Edinger-Westphal nucleus. J Comp Neurol 381:68, 1997)

afferent sensory fibers (nasociliary nerve) and sympathetic fibers to the vessels of the globe and dilator of the iris, only the parasympathetic fibers synapse here. The parasympathetic postganglionic fibers then pass to the globe via the short ciliary nerves.

The weight of anatomic evidence supports the view that the parasympathetic pupillomotor fibers synapse in the ciliary ganglion.[17,20] Some experimental studies in monkeys using horseradish peroxidase techniques suggest the presence of a nonsynapsing pathway between the midbrain and the eye,[21,22] but subsequent work by the same authors[23] ascribe their initial findings to transsynaptic passage of horseradish peroxidase. Parasympathetic denervation hypersensitivity does not occur solely with postsynaptic lesions. Preciliary ganglionic hypersensitivity to low-concentration methacholine and pilocarpine has been reported, with complete[24–26] and (inferior) divisional oculomotor palsies.[27] Warwick's proposed synapsing pathways remain accepted generally.[20]

The protectal pupilloregulator mechanism is subject to a variety of supranuclear influences, which may be summarized as follows: (1) excitatory, retinomesencephalic (light stimulus) and occipitomesencephalic (near reflex) and (2) inhibitory, corticomesencephalic and hypothalamomesencephalic pathways and the ascending reticulomesencephalic system. During sleep and obtunded states, these supranuclear inhibitory influences are diminished, with resultant miotic but reactive pupils. Arousal results because of the return of supranuclear inhibition, and sympathectomy does not eliminate this dilatation.

Ocular Sympathetic Pathways

Sympathetic outflow to the iris dilator muscles begins in the posterolateral area of the hypothalamus and descends uncrossed through the tegmentum of the midbrain and pons (Fig. 15–5). At the level of the medulla, the sympathetics lie laterally, where they may be af-

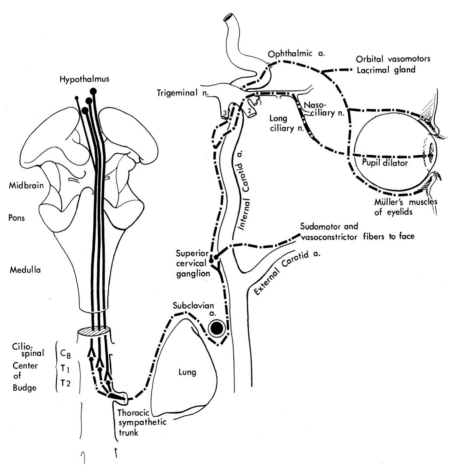

Fig. 15–5. Ocular sympathetic pathways. Hypothalamic sympathetic fibers comprise a polysynaptic (?) system as they descend to the ciliospinal center. This intra-axial tract is functionally considered the "first-order neuron." The second-order neuron takes a circuitous course through the posterosuperior aspect of the chest and ascends in the neck in relationship to the carotid system. Third-order neurons originate in the superior cervical ganglion and are distributed to the face with branches of the external carotid artery and to the orbit via the ophthalmic artery and ophthalmic division (*1*) of the trigeminal nerve.

fected in lateral medullary plate infarction (*i.e.,* Wallenberg's syndrome). The descending fibers, considered first-order preganglionic neurons, terminate in the intermediolateral cell column at the C8 to T2 cord level (the ciliospinal center of Budge). Second-order preganglionic fibers exit the cord primarily with the first ventral thoracic root (T1), but some pupillomotor sympathetics egress with C8 or T2. Via the white rami communicantes, the fibers enter the paravertebral sympathetic chain, which is closely related to the pleura of the lung apex. At this location, the sympathetics may be affected by neoplasms, (*i.e.,* the Pancoast's syndrome; see discussion of Horner's syndrome).

The fibers detour with the ansa subclavia around the subclavian arteries, ascend without synapsing through the inferior and middle cervical ganglia, and terminate in the superior cervical ganglion at the base of the skull. Third-order postganglionic oculosympathetic fibers ascend the internal carotid to enter the skull, whereas fibers for sweat and piloerection of the face follow the external carotid and its branches.

The intracranial sympathetics to the eye follow a circuitous course: (1) fibers to the tympanic plexus of the middle ear and petrous bone; (2) fibers temporarily joining the path of the intracavernous abducens nerve before anastomosing with the first division of the trigeminal nerve; (3) anastomoses with the ophthalmic-trigeminal nerve (the primary pupillomotor pathway via the nasociliary nerve); and (4) fibers to the ophthalmic artery and ocular motor nerves at the level of the cavernous sinus. Postganglionic sympathetics include (1) orbital vasomotor fibers, (2) pupillary dilators, (3) smooth muscles of the upper and lower lids (Müller), (4) the lacrimal gland, and (5) trophic fibers to uveal melanophores. Vasomotor sympathetics to the globe pass without synapse through the ciliary ganglion and short posterior ciliary nerves.

Near Reflex and Accommodation

With accommodative effort, caused either by a blurred retinal image or conscious visual fixation on a near object of regard, a "near synkinesis" is evoked, including (1) increased accommodation of the lens, (2) convergence of the visual axes of the eyes, and (3) pupillary constriction. The neural mechanisms of this motor triad are not understood as well as the pathways for pupillary light reactions or the saccadic and pursuit ocular motor systems. Awareness of decreased object distance probably evokes accommodative effort originating in frontal centers; blurred retinal images are sensed in the occipital cortex and corrected via occipitotectal tracts. Jampel[28] obtained increased bilateral accommodation, convergence, and usually miosis by unilateral stimulation of the peristriate cortex (area 19) in primates. A group of midbrain cells subserving conver-

gence has been identified in the monkey.[29] The anteromedian nucleus in the midbrain rostrally and the Edinger-Westphal nucleus caudally have been mapped stereotactically,[14] with the rostral portion concerned with accommodation, the caudal portion with pupillary constriction, and the middle segment with accommodation and constriction.

The final pathway for pupil constriction, whether evoked by light or accommodative effort, consists of the oculomotor nerve, ciliary ganglion, and short posterior ciliary nerves. The ratio of ciliary ganglion cells innervating ciliary muscle to cells innervating the iris sphincter is about 30:1.

Pupillary constriction evoked by the near reflex is not evaluated as easily as the light reaction. Accommodative vergence is under voluntary control, and the success of this maneuver is very much dependent on the patient's cooperation and capacity to converge. In the elderly, convergence is diminished and the near reflex is especially difficult to test. An accommodative target is helpful, including the use of the patient's own fingertips. Vision itself is not a requisite for the near response, which can be tested in the blind by proprioceptive "fixation" of the patient's fingertips. Indeed, accommodation and convergence may be held in abeyance by substituting plus lenses and base-out prisms, without eliminating pupillary constriction.

If pupillary reactions are brisk to light stimulus, the near reactions need not be examined. However, the student must learn this examination technique and become acquainted with the limits of normality. The light and near efforts are additive, that is, even with the eye brightly illuminated, further pupillary constriction is observed when gaze is shifted from distance to near. Therefore, when testing the light reflex, gaze (accommodation) should be controlled steadily by fixation on a distant target. If the pupil fails to react to light, the eye may be illuminated fully while the near reflex is examined.

THE PATIENT WITH ABNORMAL PUPILS

In office practice, patients present with relatively few isolated "pupil" problems, including the tonic pupil syndrome, pharmacologic accidents, sympathetic paresis (Horner's syndrome), pupillary light-near dissociation, Argyll Robertson pupils, and essential anisocoria (Table 15–1). It is extremely unlikely that a patient with a posterior communicating aneurysm or other basal tumor has only an abnormal pupil and no ocular motor or sensory disturbances. The reader is referred to the index to these volumes to locate a more detailed discussion of pupillary findings with posterior communicating artery aneurysms. Direct trauma to the anterior ocular segment, local disease of the iris (*e.g.,* cyst, melanoma, rubeosis, sphincter rupture, iritis), and angle-closure

TABLE 15-1. Characteristics of Pupils Encountered in Neuro-ophthalmology

	General characteristics	Responses to light and near stimuli	Room condition in which anisocoria is greater	Response to mydriatics	Response to miotics	Response to pharmacologic agents
Essential anisocoria	Round, regular	Both brisk	No change	Dilates	Constricts	Normal and rarely needed
Horner's syndrome	Small, round, unilateral	Both brisk	Darkness	Dilates	Constricts	Cocaine 4%, poor dilation Paredrine 1%, no dilation if third-order neuron damage
Tonic pupil syndrome (Holmes-Adie syndrome)	Usually larger* in bright light; sector pupil palsy, vermiform movement Unilateral or, less often, bilateral	Absent to light, tonic to near; tonic redilation	Light	Dilates	Constricts	Pilocarpine 0.1% or 0.125% constricts; Mecholyl 2.5% constricts
Argyll Robertson pupils	Small, irregular, bilateral	Poor to light, better to near	No change	Poor	Constricts	
Midbrain pupils	Mid-dilated; may be oval; bilateral	Poor to light, better to near (or fixed to both)	No change	Dilates	Constricts	
Pharmacologically dilated pupils	Very large,† round, unilateral	Fixed‡	Light		No‡	Pilocarpine 1% will not constrict
Oculomotor palsy (nonvascular)	Mid-dilated (6 mm–7 mm), unilateral (rarely bilateral)	Fixed	Light	Dilates	Constricts	

* Tonic pupil may appear smaller after prolonged near-effort or in dim illumination; affected pupil is initially large but with passing time gradually becomes smaller.

† Atropinized pupils have diameters of 8–9 mm. No tonic, midbrain, or oculomotor palsy pupil ever is this large.

‡ Pupils may be weakly reactive, depending on interim after instillation.

glaucoma are slit-lamp diagnoses that need not be discussed here, other than to point out that such local iris lesions have been misinterpreted as neurologic deficits.

Relative Afferent Pupillary Defect

When there is a significant unilateral or asymmetric visual deficit caused by retinal or optic nerve disease, the pupils show a subnormal response to light stimulation of the eye with the greater field or (generally) acuity loss. The pupils have a more extensive constriction response with light stimulation of the normal or less involved eye. It is this combination of subnormal direct pupillary light response and a normal indirect (consensual) response when the opposite eye is illuminated that constitutes the relative afferent pupillary defect (RAPD) (Fig. 15–6). The RAPD can be demonstrated clinically by the alternate cover test, also termed Gunn's pupillary test, as described by Kestenbaum,[30] or by the swinging flashlight test of Levatin.[31]

The swinging flashlight test is best performed in a dimly lit room, using a bright light, such as a muscle light or penlight. During the test, the patient must look at a distant fixation target to avoid accommodative miosis.

The test light is shone directly into the visual axis to illuminate first one pupil and then the other. The alternating or swinging light should pause 3 to 5 seconds in each eye, and this maneuver should be repeated several times. As a rule, the pupils are round and practically equal in diameter (see section on Essential Anisocoria) and briskly and symmetrically reactive to light stimuli. After an initial, prompt pupil constriction, a slight "release" dilation generally occurs. For example, in the presence of a right afferent defect (see Fig. 15–6), the following is observed with the swinging flashlight test: the pupillary diameters are equal and slightly larger bilaterally when the right eye is stimulated and bilaterally smaller when the normal left eye is illuminated. If only the illuminated pupil is observed—the other pupil

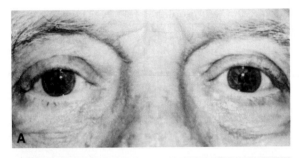

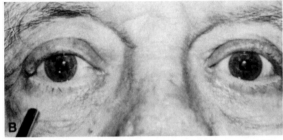

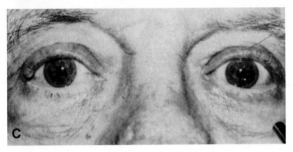

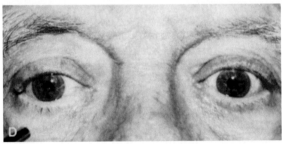

Fig. 15–6. Swinging flashlight test for afferent pupil defect. The patient is a 72-year-old man with right visual loss due to ischemic optic neuropathy. **A.** Pupils are equal in dim light. **B.** Illumination of right eye results in modest bilateral constriction. **C.** When the light swings to the left, there is more extensive constriction in both pupils. **D.** When the light swings back to the right, both pupils dilate.

being hidden in darkness—the following is seen: the normal left pupil constricts promptly on illumination; as the light is moved rapidly to the right, the right pupil actually is seen to dilate or "escape"; as the light moves again to the left, the left pupil again constricts briskly.

Afferent pupillary defects may be quantitated conveniently by the use of neutral-density filters placed before the normal eye to "balance" or neutralize a positive (asymmetric) swinging light test.[32] Whether a dim, bright, or brilliant light is best suited for pupil light-reaction testing is somewhat controversial,[33] but an indirect ophthalmoscope light set at 6 volts may be used as

a handy "standardized" light source. Thompson and Jiang[34] stress the importance of avoiding asymmetric retinal bleach, by maintaining a rhythmic "equal time" alternation of the light from one eye to the other and by not swinging the light too many times between the eyes. Thompson and others[32,35] provide detailed guidelines for proper performance of the pupillary examination and assessment of the RAPD. Computerized infrared pupillometry may allow the most reliable standardization of the swinging flashlight test.[36]

An afferent pupillary defect may be assessed even if one of the pupils is unreactive because of mydriatics, miotics, oculomotor palsy, trauma (Fig. 15–7), or synechia formation. In such cases, when performing the swinging flashlight test, the direct and consensual responses of the single reactive pupil must be compared. The reactive pupil's direct light response reflects the afferent function of the ipsilateral eye; its consensual response reflects the afferent function of the contralateral eye.

Even severe unilateral visual loss due to retinal or optic nerve diseases associated with an afferent pupillary defect is not of itself a cause of anisocoria, despite past statements to the contrary. If a patient with an RAPD also shows anisocoria, the pupillary inequality must be treated as a separate finding. The RAPD most typically provides objective evidence of optic nerve disease that is either unilateral or asymmetric, with more profound visual involvement on the side of the RAPD. In such cases, the RAPD is not specific and may reflect optic neuropathy due to demyelination, ischemia, compression, or asymmetric glaucoma.

Because slightly more fibers cross than remain uncrossed at the level of the chiasm, RAPDs also may be seen with optic tract lesions, where greater visual field loss occurs in one eye. An obvious example would be an optic tract lesion with a complete homonymous hemianopia. In such a case, a relative afferent pupillary defect would be expected in the eye with the temporal visual field loss (*i.e.,* the eye contralateral to the side of the optic tract lesion).[37] Theoretically, the same kind of RAPD could be present without any associated visual field defect if there is a contralateral lesion affecting the pupillomotor fibers between the optic tract and pretectal region. The eye with the RAPD should have normal visual acuity, color vision, and visual field, and no other (occult) cause for the pupillary defect (*i.e.,* no amblyopia, glaucoma, past optic neuritis). Ellis[38] has reported an afferent pupillary defect contralateral to a pineal region tumor, suggesting that this was due to involvement of afferent pupillary fibers between the optic tract and pretectal nucleus. Johnson and Bell[39] also have documented an RAPD in a pretectal lesion due to a pineal gland mixed-cell tumor.

RAPD also can be seen with diseases of the retina and macula. An extensive retinal detachment, such as two detached quadrants, should cause an obvious RAPD, as do arterial occlusions. With unilateral or

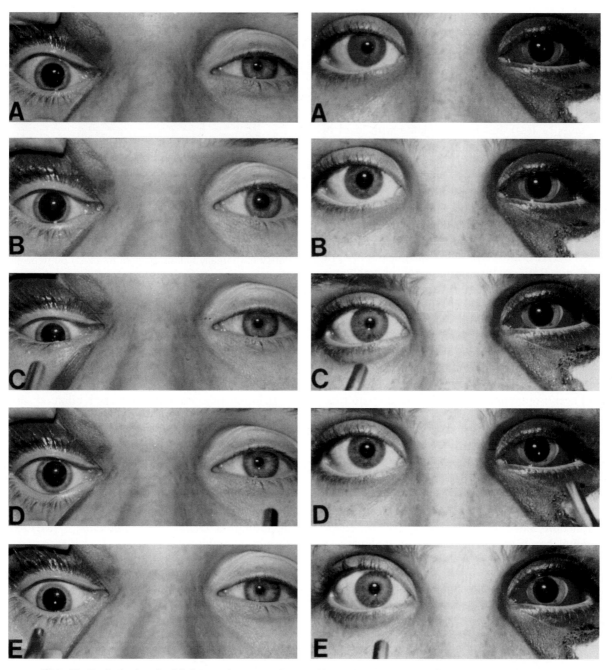

Fig. 15–7. Swinging flashlight test in two patients with mydriasis on side of orbital trauma. Pupils in bright **(A)** and dim **(B)** room lighting reveal normal responses on the uninjured side and minimal if any response on the affected side. As the flashlight is swung from right **(C)** to left **(D)** and again to right **(E)**, one can observe the normally reactive pupil. The patient on the left has no afferent pupillary defect, whereas the patient on the right has a left relative afferent pupillary defect.

markedly asymmetric retinitis pigmentosa, one should see an RAPD; however, usually the disease process is quite symmetric and thus an RAPD typically is not present.[40] RAPD in general is proportional to the extent of visual field loss, and the size of the visual field defect is more closely correlated with the extent of the RAPD than is visual acuity loss.[41,42] As a rule, strictly macular disease leads to a much less profound afferent pupillary defect than the bulk of diseases affecting the optic

nerve.[43] Patients with central choroidopathy, for example, show either a small or no RAPD[44] and the RAPD is much more likely to persist with resolved optic neuritis than resolved central serous choroidopathy.[45] Patients also have been reported to have an RAPD[46] with central retinal vein occlusion, the RAPD being more obvious (generally greater than 1 log unit) in the ischemic than in the nonischemic (all less than 1 log unit, most less than 0.3 log units) form of the disease. Thus, the RAPD may be helpful in distinguishing between ischemic and nonischemic central retinal vein occlusions. Interesting but rarely encountered in the usual clinical setting are RAPDs induced by contralateral monocular occlusion or resulting from dense contralateral cataracts.[47-49] An RAPD may be observed in strabismic or refractive amblyopia,[50,51] but the RAPD with amblyopia is small (most 0.3 log units or less) and not correlated with level of acuity.[50] Occasionally, a small (neutral density filter of 0.3 log unit or less) RAPD is detected and may be assumed to be benign if there are no etiologic clues from the history or clinical examination.[52] Follow-up with lack of progressive visual changes on subsequent examinations should provide further corroboration that the small isolated RAPD is indeed "benign."

Thus, the RAPD most typically is an indicator of optic nerve disease. Retinopathy, maculopathy, or amblyopia also can lead to RAPD. Even with very poor acuity, however, the latter diseases usually cause much less obvious RAPD than that found with optic neuropathy, even with minimal acuity or field depression. If a very obvious RAPD is seen in cases of amblyopia, advanced cataracts, retinopathy, or maculopathy, additional tests are recommended to rule out the possibility of a superimposed occult optic neuropathy that would better explain the pupillary findings.

Argyll Robertson Pupils

In 1869, Argyll Robertson described abnormal pupils characterized by miosis, unresponsiveness to light stimulus, and contraction on near-effort in eyes with intact visual function. Since that time, the Argyll Robertson (A-R) pupil has been recognized as the hallmark of late central nervous system syphilis. In 1969, an article commemorating Douglas Argyll Robertson appeared in the *Survey of Ophthalmology* and included an exhaustive scholarly review of the A-R pupil by Dr. Irene Loewenfeld.[53]

Although an absolute defect of light reaction was described initially, it is clear that the critical point in the light-near dissociation is simply a more extensive reaction to near than to light, although some degree of light reaction may be observed (Fig. 15–8). In fact, A-R pupils with impaired rather than absent light reaction are by far more common. Although it is tempting to consider that the incomplete A-R pupil with impaired light reaction represents an incipient form of the light-fixed pupil, there is no documentation of such progression.

An eye with reduced sensitivity to light, that is, an afferent pupil defect due to major retinal disease or optic nerve conduction defects, does show a better response to near-effort than to light stimulus. Therefore, the definition of light-near dissociation must be qualified to include the criterion of no significant visual deficit. In addition, the A-R syndrome must include miosis to exclude nonsyphilitic causes of light-near dissociation

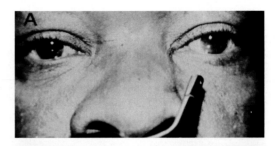
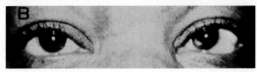

Fig. 15–8. The Argyll Robertson pupil. **A.** The pupils are small and irregular with no reaction to light. **B.** Pupils promptly constrict (partially hidden by light reflexes) on near-effort.

(*e.g.,* tonic pupils, amaurotic pupils, midbrain pupils). When viewed in darkness, the miotic feature is more striking because of the failure of the pupil to dilate. Thus, the A-R pupil neither constricts well to light stimulus nor, as a rule, dilates well in darkness. The characteristics of this syndrome are listed in Table 15–2.

In most cases, the A-R syndrome is bilateral, although not invariably so, and the pupils also tend to be irregular in shape. If the criteria listed in Table 15–2 are met, the diagnosis of neurosyphilis may be made. Serologic tests, including serum Venereal Disease Research Laboratory (VDRL) or rapid plasma reagin (RPR) tests, and the fluorescent treponemal antibody absorption (FTA-Abs) test or equivalent tests (*e.g.,* microhemagglutination-*Treponema pallidum* [MHA-TTP]) should be obtained.

Numerous causes of A-R–like pupils have been proposed, but if the criteria that have been elaborated are applied, especially miosis, the only remaining common denominator is some degree of light-near dissociation. Syphilis also is capable of producing large pupils that are fixed to both light and near-effort (Fig. 15–9).[54] These abnormalities typically occur in taboparesis. Fletcher and Sharpe[55] recommend that patients with bilaterally tonic pupils have serologic tests for syphilis. Of their five luetic patients with bilaterally tonic pupils, two had tabes dorsalis and another two had other manifestations of neurosyphilis.

TABLE 15–2. Characteristics of Argyll Robertson Syndrome

Visual function grossly intact
Decreased pupillary light reaction
Intact near response
Miosis
Pupils irregular
Bilateral, asymmetric
Poor dilation
Iris atrophy variable

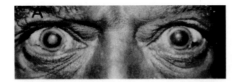
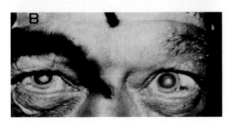
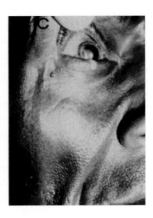

Fig. 15–9. Taboparetic pupils. **A.** Pupils show bilateral mydriasis (5 mm and 7 mm) that is fixed to near-effort **(B)** and the bright focal beam of the slit-lamp **(C)**.

When evaluating the pupillary reflex, testing errors can be introduced by using an insufficiently bright light source or an inadequate accommodative target, or by failing to ensure that the patient is exerting a maximal accommodative effort. A wristwatch face provides a pragmatic stimulus for near-effort.

Light-Near Dissociation Syndromes

With the exception of errors in testing techniques or poor patient cooperation, there is no pathologic situation in which pupillary light reflex is normal while the near response is defective. Therefore, if the pupils respond briskly to light, the near response need not be examined. Lack of direct and near responses, in the absence of ocular motility disturbance, should raise the question of bilateral pharmacologic pupillary dilation or local ocular disease, such as sphincter trauma or synechiae. Rarely such findings represent congenital mydriasis.[56] Paradoxical pupillary responses (pupillary constriction induced by darkness) have been reported in association with concomitant stationary night blindness and congenital achromatopsia and subsequently with other retinopathies and with optic neuropathies.[57] Dissociation of the light-near response, when certain other criteria are met (see Table 15–2), is diagnostic of neurosyphilis, as discussed in the preceding section. Other distinctive clinical syndromes include pupillary light-near dissociation. The tonic pupil is characterized by light-near dissociation but is distinguished from the A-R pupil by other characteristic features (see section on Tonic Pupil Syndrome). With rostral midbrain lesions in the area of the pretectal nuclear complex, interruption of retinotectal fibers with preservation of supranuclear accommodative pathways produces light-near dissociation associated with moderate mydriasis due to damage to the pretectal pupilloconstrictor nuclei (Fig. 15–10). These "midbrain" pupils usually are seen as part of the periaqueductal syndrome (Parinaud's syndrome),[58] which also includes supranuclear paralysis of upward gaze, lid retraction (Collier's sign), defective convergence with convergence-nystagmus on attempted

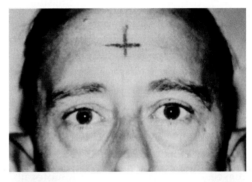
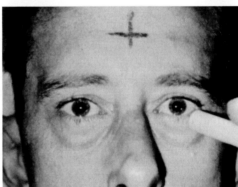
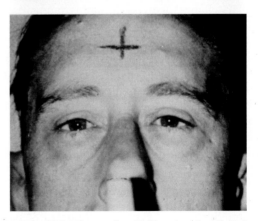

Fig. 15–10. Midbrain pupils. Unlike the Argyll Robertson pupils, midbrain pupils are mid-dilated. Constriction on near-effort is preserved until late stage, but the light reflex is defective early. Patient has pinealoma for which he is receiving radiation therapy.

upward gaze, retraction-nystagmus (also elicited on attempted rapid upgaze or as optokinetic targets are moved downward), and both accommodative paresis and accommodative "spasm" (failure of relaxation of accommodation following near-effort).

Any eye with a severe visual deficit due to retinal or optic nerve disease, with significant field loss, has a diminished pupillary response to light (RAPD) but an intact near-reflex. For example, an eye blind from glaucoma demonstrates a light-near dissociation. Patients with profound bilateral visual loss caused by anterior visual pathway disease have bilaterally poor pupillary light responses (RAPDs) but intact accommodative responses. Therefore, patients with bilateral end-stage glaucoma, total retinal detachments, or blindness resulting from bilateral optic nerve/chiasmal injuries should not be construed as having dorsal midbrain disease on the basis of their light-near dissociation. On occasion, patients with longstanding juvenile diabetes demonstrate moderate symmetric mydriasis with light-near dissociation that clearly is disproportionate to any concurrent retinopathy. Loewenfeld[53] suggests that such patients also may have typical A-R pupils, including miosis.

When aberrant regeneration follows oculomotor nerve palsies, fibers originally associated especially with the medial rectus (although other oculomotor fibers occasionally are responsible) may anomalously innervate the pupillary sphincter as well. In such cases, the light-paretic pupil constricts when the medial rectus acts, either in convergence or with conjugate lateral gaze. Therefore, a light-"near" (actually, gaze-evoked) pupillary dissociation is observed. Unlike the true A-R pupil, the aberrant-regeneration pupil is large rather than miotic and is accompanied by other signs of third-nerve palsy, some paretic and some with "misdirection" features.[59] Infrared videographic transillumination readily demonstrates denervated and aberrantly reinnervated sphincter segments.[60]

Pupillary changes seen on slit-lamp examination may provide the early evidence of aberrant oculomotor regeneration; segmental pupillary sphincter contractions may be seen with attempted eye movements in the field of action of oculomotor innervated muscles.[61] In more obvious cases, the pupillary constriction may be grossly visualized with attempted efforts by any of the muscles normally innervated by the oculomotor nerve.[59] Ohno and Mukuno[62] report anomalous pupillary innervation in 6 of 10 patients with aberrant oculomotor regeneration; pupillary constriction was seen most commonly with downgaze or adduction and less frequently with upgaze. In two patients, pupillary dilation was noted on abduction. Spiegel and Kardon[63] evaluated 24 patients with aberrant oculomotor regeneration. Clinically, involvement of the eyelid and pupil was evident much more commonly than that of ocular motility. Pupil signs

of aberrant behavior, such as eye movement-induced anisocoria, were most noticeable in dim illumination.

Essential Anisocoria

All pupils are *not* created equal. In fact, benign pupillary inequality exists in practically all individuals, but not necessarily all of the time. Using photographic techniques, Lam and associates[64] determined pupil size in 128 healthy individuals, measuring greatest pupil diameter twice each day for 5 consecutive days: 41% showed anisocoria of 0.4 mm or greater at one time or another: 80% showed anisocoria of 0.2 mm or greater at some time; that is, a majority of the subjects had anisocoria of some degree at one time or another (Fig. 15–11). Anisocoria is as common in men as in women, in the morning as in the afternoon, in the young as in the aged (although Loewenfeld[65] suggests that anisocoria is more common in the elderly), and in dark as in light irides. In a study of healthy neonates, anisocoria of 0.5 mm or more was found in about 20% of infants, but none had anisocoria greater than 1 mm.[66] The physician can detect regularly a pupil difference of as little as 0.2 mm in diameter, given that clinical judgment of inequality is based more on impressions of pupil area than on measured diameter. Because the percentage difference in area is greater for smaller than for larger pupils, for any given diameter difference, anisocoria is detected more easily in smaller pupil pairs. The prevalence of anisocoria decreases in bright conditions when measured as a difference in pupil diameter, but not when is assessed as a ratio of pupil areas.[67]

Essential or "central" anisocoria should be identified easily because the pupillary light and near reactions are normal and eye movement is full. The relative difference between pupil diameters is constant under various levels of illumination, unlike the Horner's pupil, where anisocoria is enhanced in dim lighting. Incidental ptosis due

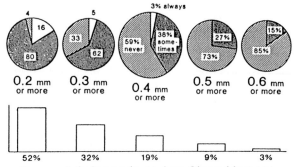

Fig. 15–11. Prevalence of simple anisocoria. (Data of Lam BL et al.[64] From Thompson HS: The pupil. In Lessell S, van Dalen JTW [eds]: Current Neuro-ophthalmology, p 214. Chicago: Year Book Medical Publishers, 1989)

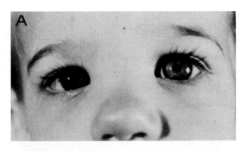

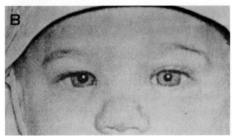

Fig. 15–12. A. Anisocoria noted at age 14 months in otherwise healthy infant. **B.** Photograph at age 6 months confirms chronicity and benign nature of finding. There was no iris heterochromia.

to traumatic or senile levator aponeurosis dehiscence and weakening, when ipsilateral to the smaller pupil of essential anisocoria, may be confused with a true Horner's syndrome.[68] When the distinction between true and pseudo-Horner's syndrome is difficult by simple inspection alone, pharmacologic testing usually solves the dilemma. With essential anisocoria, pupillary responses to pharmacologic agents, including topical cocaine, are normal bilaterally.

The evaluation of anisocoria is facilitated by the presence of the following associated signs (see Table 15–1): mild upper ptosis as well as lower lid elevation on the side of a relatively miotic pupil (Horner's syndrome); a dilated pupil fixed to light but with very slow constriction on prolonged near fixation (tonic pupil); and small irregular pupils that react better to near than to light (A-R pupil).

Some individuals with longstanding anisocoria may suddenly discover the condition while shaving or applying make-up or may have it called to their attention over the breakfast table. In such situations, inspection of previous photographs is an invaluable aid in determining the nature and duration of pupil anomalies. A hand magnifying glass, a trial frame lens, an indirect ophthalmoscope lens, or even the high magnification of the slit-lamp beam[69] may prove useful for examining pupil details in snapshot or portrait-quality photographs (Fig. 15–12).

Tonic Pupil Syndrome

High on the list of causes of isolated internal ophthalmoplegia is the tonic pupil (Adie's syndrome). Although symptoms of unilateral defective accommodation may prompt an office visit, the difference in pupil size usually is the more dramatic signal. Characteristically, the involved pupil is larger than its fellow, but if viewed in darkness, it actually may be the smaller one because the normal pupil is free to dilate widely: because both dilatation and constriction are defective in the involved eye, the diameter of the normal pupil may be smaller (in bright illumination) or larger (in dim illumination) than the tonic pupil. With the passage of time, the anisocoria becomes less marked (Table 15–3) as the initially large tonic pupil gradually becomes less dilated and eventually even miotic over the years[60,70] (Fig. 15–13).

As a rule, the tonic pupil is grossly defective in its reaction to light stimulus but may show some minimal degree of contraction. On slit-lamp examination, however, irregular spontaneous low-amplitude movements may be observed. Segmental sector contractions may be seen in the portions of the sphincter that either still are not denervated or are reinnervated. Also, areas of sector palsy of the iris sphincter are seen. With prolonged accommodative effort, the pupil slowly constricts, usually not extensively. When near-effort is relaxed, the dilation movement also is gradual, requiring minutes or hours for redilation. Therefore, with accommodative effort and before redilation is complete, the tonic pupil can be relatively miotic with respect to its normal opposite. These pupillary kinetics constitute "the tonic pupil," and pharmacologic testing (see Fig. 15–13) is additive rather than diagnostic.

Supersensitivity to the parasympathomimetic drug methacholine (Mecholyl) 2.5%, with pupillary constriction, is a good but not foolproof test. Thompson[71] suggests the use of 0.125% pilocarpine as a substitute for methacholine. Actually, because of its stronger miotic action, pilocarpine 0.125% is in some ways the preferable drug; supersensitivity is demonstrable in a greater proportion of patients with tonic pupils. It produces a more visible degree of anisocoria; a negative test is more valid. Some authors have used weaker solutions of pilocarpine, such as 0.0625% or 0.05%.[72] Weak-concentration arecoline, a pilocarpine-like drug, also has been used; its advantage, if any, may be that it brings about maximal miosis more quickly.[73] Pupillary parasympathetic hypersensitivity to

TABLE 15–3. Characteristics of Tonic Pupil Syndrome

Relative mydriasis in bright illumination
Poor to absent light reaction
Slow contraction to prolonged near-effort
Slow redilation after near-effort
Iris sphincter sector palsy
Segmental vermiform movements of iris border
Defective accommodation
Pupil constricts with Mecholyl 2.5%, pilocarpine 0.125%
Associated with diminished deep tendon reflexes

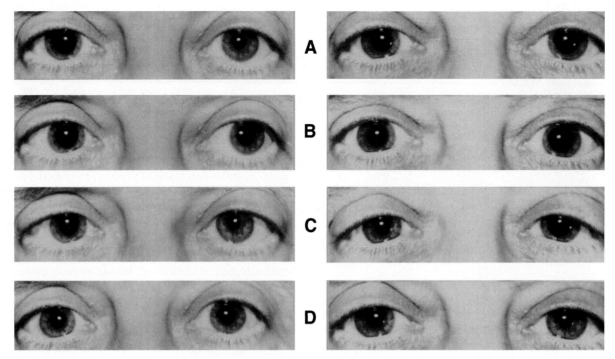

Fig. 15–13. A 52-year-old woman with right tonic pupil (*left*): 1 year later involvement of the left pupil developed as well (*right*). Pupils are shown in bright **(A)** and dim **(B)** room lighting after near-convergence attempt **(C)**, and in dim room lighting after instillation of 0.125% pilocarpine in both eyes **(D)**. Note that the right pupil is smaller 1 year later **(A)** (*right*) than when it was "fresh" **(A)** (*left*). With time, the right pupil also has become more responsive to near-accommodation effort **(C)** (*left* and *right*). Parasympatho-mimetic hypersensitivity is seen in the right pupil **(D)** (*left*) and 1 year later bilaterally **(D)** (*right*).

2.5% methacholine or low-concentration pilocarpine can occur not only with postciliary ganglionic but also with preciliary ganglionic lesions.[24–27,62]

Accommodation, like pupillary constriction–redilation, also is tonic and changes slowly from far to near gaze and from near to far gaze. Vision is blurred momentarily until the ciliary muscle "catches up," either while attempting to accommodate or after prolonged near-effort. If accommodation is measured, it will be found to be deficient.

Pupillotonia usually is one sided, but bilateral cases do occur in which the eyes are involved either simultaneously or separately (see Fig. 15–13). Unilateral Adie's syndrome becomes bilateral at the rate of about 4% per year.[74] Although all ages and both sexes are involved, there is an unexplained predilection for women in the third to fifth decades. In most instances the cause is unknown, although nonspecific viral illnesses have been incriminated. Orbital trauma, including surgery, is the most direct cause of pupillotonia. In the few pathologically studied cases, ganglion cells of the orbital ciliary ganglion are absent or grossly diminished.[75]

The tonic pupil's light-near dissociation (*i.e.,* slow constriction on near-effort and very poor reaction to light stimulation) is explained on the basis of misdirected regeneration and collateral sprouting of nerve fibers after injury to the ciliary ganglion and its postganglionic fibers.[76] Recall that some 97% of fibers from the ciliary ganglion innervate the ciliary muscle; the remaining 3% innervate the pupillary sphincter.[17] Because the great excess of neurons are destined to innervate the ciliary body, regenerated fibers and collateral sprouts also are much more likely to subserve accommodative function. This results in pupillary sphincter reinnervation almost entirely by fibers initially intended for accommodation. Kardon and colleagues,[60] using infrared transillumination, provide videographic demonstration of pupillary behavior in patients with Adie's tonic pupil (Fig. 15–14). They also show that with time-extensive reinnervation of the initially denervated pupillary sphincter can develop, leading to constant contraction and therefore a miotic ("little old Adie's") pupil. Impairment of the final postganglionic nerve supply to the iris sphincter accounts for denervation supersensitivity, with pupillary constriction produced by weak parasympathomimetic agents (methacholine 2.5%, pilocarpine 0.125%). An alternate explanation for the light-near dissociation in the tonic pupil syndrome has been offered:[77,78] the permanently denervated pupillary sphincter constricts with accommodation as acetylcholine leaks into the aqueous from cholinergic nerve fibers of the ciliary body. Loewenfeld and Thompson[79] convincingly rebutted this latter hypothesis by arguing that acetylcholine diffusion would not explain the iris reinnervation and segmental pupillary sphincter contractions that Anderson[80] reported after performing ciliary ganglionectomies in cats.

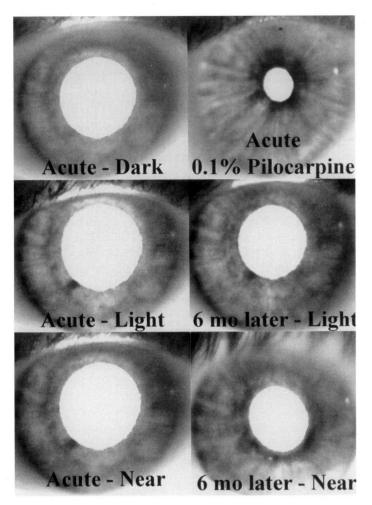

Fig. 15–14. Six infrared transillumination views of the same iris in a patient with acute Adie's pupil affecting all but one of the segments. The middle and lower photographs on the right are from the same eye 6 months later. The photographs on the left side show that there is only one small segment (the dark area at the pupil border at the 7:00 position) that still contracts appropriately to light and near. This example was chosen because all the rest of the iris sphincter-reacting segment can be discerned in the dark (captured during the latency period of the pupil light reflex), in light, and at near. In the acute-dark photograph (*top left*), the area at the 7:00 meridian cannot be seen but becomes dark in response to light (*middle left*, acute-light) and in response to low concentration pilocarpine (*top right*). All the denervated segments show darkening to the 0.1% pilocarpine except for the one segment that normally is innervated, and therefore presumably not supersensitive, which appears colored at the 7:30 meridian (*top right*, acute 0.1% pilocarpine). This same patient was examined 6 months later (*right side, middle,* and *bottom*) and shows a light-near dissociation with a darkening on near response. The pupil is slightly smaller in light that in the acute state because of some sustained firing of accommodative fibers that have started to reinnervate the sphincter areas. (Reprinted with permission from Kardon RH, Corbett JJ, Thompson HS: Segmental denervation and re-innervation of the iris sphincter as shown by infrared videographic transillumination. Ophthalmology 105:313, 1998)

Tonic pupil is a benign condition that, in the absence of other signs and symptoms, heralds no neurologic or systemic disease state. The association with diminished deep tendon reflexes is the well-known Holmes-Adie syndrome. Spinal cord dorsal column atrophy was documented in such a case.[81] Bilateral pupillotonia has been associated with other autonomic nervous system dysfunction, including orthostatic hypotension, progressive segmental hypohidrosis[82,83] *forme fruste* familial dysautonomia,[84] and the typical Riley-Day syndrome.[85] Autonomic neuropathy and chronic relapsing polyneuropathy due to paraneoplastic disease also have been reported to cause tonic pupils,[86,88] as has acute ophthalmoplegic polyneuritis (Fisher syndrome).[89] Bilateral pupillotonia, including denervation hypersensitivity to low-concentration pilocarpine, may be caused by syphilis; if so, other manifestations of neurosyphilis, such as tabes dorsalis, typically should be present as well.[54,55] More specifically, orbital ciliary ganglion ischemia is the proposed mechanism for a reported case of tonic pupils with giant cell arteritis.[90] Orbital surgery, such as optic nerve fenestration, especially when done by the temporal approach, can lead to ciliary ganglion injury and a secondary tonic pupil.

The dysfunction of both the pupillary sphincter and ciliary muscle can cause symptoms in patients with tonic pupils. Symptoms related to pupillary mydriasis almost never need treatment, although some patients seem to like the cosmetic effect brought about by topically applied low-concentration pilocarpine. The ciliary symptoms may at times be more troublesome and may manifest as unilateral accommodative paresis, induced astigmatism, and sometimes, ciliary spasms. Pharmacologic treatment of ciliary symptoms often is not effective, but on occasion, low-concentration anticholinesterase (physostigmine), low concentration cholinergic (pilocarpine), or anticholinergic (tropicamide, atropine) drops may help.[78,91]

The tonic pupil has been evaluated in detail by Loewenfeld and Thompson,[76] who also include a discussion of pathologic mechanisms and pupillographic analysis.

A dilated pupil rarely can develop as a sequela of uneventful intraocular surgery, whether keratoplasty or cataract surgery: the history of its onset after intraocular surgery makes it easy to recognize, and pilocarpine 1% fails to constrict the affected, atonic pupil.[92]

The use of parasympathomimetic agents—but not of

parasympatholytic agents—has an established role in pharmacologic pupillary assessment. Scinto and colleagues[93] reported that patients with Alzheimer's disease could be identified, perhaps even before the onset of symptoms of obvious dementia, on the basis of their pupillary hypersensitivity to dilute tropicamide, a cholinergic antagonist. In a well-designed study in which patients with potential corneal abnormalities or dry eye conditions were excluded, Loupe and associates[94] found that the dilute tropicamide test did not allow distinction between patients with Alzheimer's disease and control subjects.

Oculosympathetic Defects (Horner's Syndrome)

The complicated course of the oculosympathetic pathways has been outlined previously. In essence, the ocularsympathetic chain may be interrupted partially or totally in any location, from the hypothalamus down through the brain stem to the cervical cord, in the apex of the chest, in relationship to the carotid sheaths, or in the cavernous sinus or orbit. Causative lesions may be the result of cerebrovascular disease (Wallenberg's lateral medullary plate infarction syndrome), cervical trauma (Fig. 15–15), chest tumors, intracavernous lesions, or even a form of vascular headaches.

Heterochromia with Horner's syndrome (the lighter iris in the same eye) usually is considered a sign that the sympathoparesis is congenital or acquired in infancy. However, progressive heterochromia has been reported following acquired Horner's syndrome in adults.[95,96]

Horner's syndrome consists of mild to moderate ptosis of the upper lid due to paresis of Müller's muscle. The lid fold (see Fig. 15–15) also usually is lost and is a subtle confirmatory sign. The lower lid may be somewhat elevated because of paresis of smooth muscle attached to the inferior tarsal plate. This can be evaluated by noting the relationship of the lower lid margin to the corneoscleral junction (inferior limbus). With ptosis, the pupil is variably miotic, depending on the location, completeness, and chronicity of the defect. Anisocoria due to Horner's syndrome is more marked in dim illumination (evoking dilation) than in bright light. Painful stimuli or sudden loud noises increase the anisocoria. The miosis need not be marked, and usually the pupillary diameter is reduced by 0.5 mm to 1 mm.

Enophthalmos is more apparent than real[97,98]: the interpalpebral fissure is narrowed by ptosis of the upper lid and elevation of the lower lid. Thus, the eye may be described as looking "smaller" or seeming to be enophthalmic.

With the complete syndrome, the ipsilateral face is anhidrotic, warm, and hyperemic because of denervation of sweat and vasoconstrictor fibers that are distributed to the face through branches of the external carotid

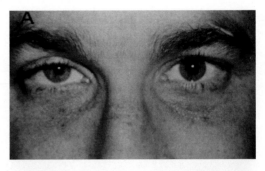
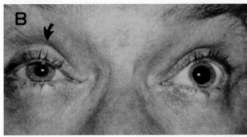
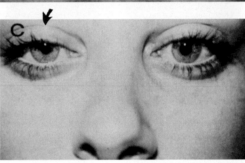

Fig. 15–15. Oculosympathetic paresis. **A.** Congenital right Horner's syndrome. Note partial ptosis, miosis, and lighter iris. **B.** Positive cocaine test in 45-year-old patient with right side headaches and oculosympathetic paresis (Raeder's syndrome). Note that cocaine 4% dilates normal left pupil only. **C.** High cervical ("Hengman's") fracture with quadriplegia and right Horner's syndrome. Note spontaneous sweating of left side of face only. In **(B)** and **(C)**, lid fold (*arrow*) is diminished.

artery. These defects are for the most part transient, being rapidly overcome by denervation hypersensitivity to circulating adrenergic substances. Ocular hypotony and defective accommodation have been described with sympathetic denervation, but these are at best transient and inconstant signs and are of little help in diagnosis. The pupillary reaction to light or near stimulus is normal, but slowed redilation can be documented photographically or pupillographically. The clinical manifestations of this syndrome are summarized as follows:

1. Miosis;
2. Partial ptosis;
3. Apparent enophthalmos;
4. Diminished sweat, drier skin;
5. Transient: dilated conjunctival and face vessels; facial flush; ocular hypotony; increased accommodation; and

6. Heterochromia: characteristic if congenital; rarely acquired by adults.

Although the pattern of facial sweating may be helpful in localizing Horner's lesions,[99] it is by pharmacologic means that the site of involvement most often is ascertained. Numerous pharmacologic tests have been used for the diagnosis or confirmation of oculosympathetic paresis. Cocaine 4% is the most widely used agent, although dilute solutions of epinephrine (0.001%) and hydroxyamphetamine 1% (Paredrine) also are useful.[100] Thompson believes that the use of dilute epinephrine is a poor test with inconclusive results, but that the use of phenylephrine 1% dramatically demonstrates supersensitivity in postganglionic Horner's syndrome. Ramsay[72] reports catecholaminergic hypersensitivity to 1% phenylephrine in 71% of tested patients with Horner's syndrome. Cocaine blocks the reuptake of norepinephrine released at the myoneural junction and therefore induces mydriasis when instilled in patients with intact oculosympathetic pathways. In Horner's syndrome, cocaine instillation results in poor or no dilation, regardless of the site of the lesion. The cocaine test therefore corroborates the diagnosis of Horner's syndrome, but does not allow distinction between a central (brain stem or cervical cord), preganglionic (chest or neck), or postganglionic (above superior cervical ganglion) cause of sympathetic denervation. A cocaine test that induces 1 mm or more of anisocoria is strongly supportive (>95% probability) of the diagnosis of Horner's syndrome.[101,102] Hydroxyamphetamine (Paredrine) causes release of norepinephrine stored in the presynaptic terminals of pupils with intact third-order (postganglionic) neurons and therefore causes pupillary dilation normally and with first-order (central) and second-order (preganglionic)—but not third-order (postganglionic)—oculosympathetic lesions. Therefore, the Paredrine test is useful in identifying patients whose Horner's syndrome is postganglionic.[103] A Paredrine test that induces 1 mm or more of anisocoria identifies postganglionic Horner's syndrome with high probability (90% or more).[104] Although a false-negative response to Paredrine can occur in congenital[105] and acute Horner's syndrome (of less than 2 weeks' duration),[106] the test generally is very useful and reliable clinically. Paredrine is no longer available commercially,[107] but hydroxyamphetamine hydrobromide 1% can be "special-ordered" from a number of pharmacies. Pholedrine has been used by some as a substitute for for pharmacologic testing of Horner's lesions.[108,109] There is no clinically useful pharmacologic test for distinction between central (first-order) and preganglionic (second-order) oculosympathetic lesions.

In all pharmacologic tests for sympathetic denervation, drops should be instilled in both eyes so that the reaction of the normal pupil serves as a control. Tonometry, testing of corneal sensitivity, or any procedures that may mechanically or chemically disturb corneal epithelium should not be performed before these drops are instilled. If cocaine is used, the hydroxyamphetamine reaction should not be tested before 48 hours have elapsed. Differences in observed pharmacologic reaction between the two pupils are more common than absolute dilation failure: the eye with partial sympathetic denervation may dilate less extensively than the normal pupil, rather than demonstrating no dilatation at all.

The topical diagnosis of Horner's syndrome is very much dependent on accompanying signs and symptoms. It is most unlikely that a patient with a brain stem lesion will present with an isolated Horner's syndrome. Sympathoparesis may accompany the lateral medullary syndrome of Wallenberg's syndrome (posterior inferior cerebellar artery syndrome), which includes dysphagia (laryngeal and pharyngeal paralysis), analgesia in ipsilateral face and contralateral trunk and extremities (spinal tract and nucleus of trigeminal nerve, and ascending lateral spinothalamic tracts), ipsilateral cerebellar ataxia, and rotary nystagmus; skew deviation may occur, with vertical diplopia. A central Horner's syndrome has been reported in association with cerebral and hypothalamic infarction caused by internal carotid artery occlusion.[110] The interruption of the hypothalamospinal tract leads to ipsilateral hemianhidrosis, ptosis, and miosis, and there is associated contralateral hemiplegia, sometimes homonymous hemianopsia or aphasia. This constellation of findings has been termed telodiencephalic ischemic syndrome by Schiffter.[111,112] Central Horner's syndrome also can be caused by cervical cord lesions, including trauma (see Fig. 15–15), syringomyelia, tumors, and rarely, demyelinating disease.

In the chest apex and superior mediastinum, destructive lesions may interfere with sympathetic fibers as they pass in close proximity to the apical pleura and great vessels. The Pancoast superior sulcus syndrome usually is caused by bronchogenic carcinoma, of which oculosympathetic paresis may be the first sign; also, such lesions typically cause pain in the shoulder and arm. Patients with an acquired, nontraumatic, preganglionic oculosympathetic paresis and arm or shoulder pain require appropriate radiologic studies of the pulmonary apex, chest, and cervical spine. Acquired preganglionic Horner's syndrome in combination with brachial plexopathy can be due not only to primary lung tumor, but also to breast cancer, lymphoma, sarcoma, or metastasis of other tumors. According to Kori and coworkers,[113] in patients with cancer and brachial plexopathy, Horner's syndrome appears more commonly with metastatic disease (52%) than with radiation injury (14%).

In the neck, as the sympathetic fibers ascend in relationship with the carotid sheath, oculosympathetic paresis may be caused by enlarged lymph nodes, tumors, abscess, trauma,[114,115] and even acute carotid thrombosis.[116] Ipsilateral neck, facial, or orbital pain[117] and, less frequently, amaurosis fugax, disagreeable taste (dysgeusia)[118] or facial numbness and dysesthesia[119] strongly suggest the possibility of spontaneous internal carotid artery dissection. Bougousslavsky and colleagues[120] report the presence of Horner's syndrome in 20% of their patients with spontaneous carotid dissection. Hydroxyamphetamine 1% provides rapid corroboration of a postganglionic (third-order neuron) level lesion, and cerebral angiography or—less invasively and perhaps preferably—cervical magnetic resonance imaging is diagnostic[121,122] (Fig. 15–16).

At the level of the brachial plexus, the sympathetic fibers may be damaged by birth trauma, and Horner's syndrome may accompany Klumpke's paralysis of the ipsilateral arm. Perinatal neck trauma is the proposed mechanism of a congenital postganglionic oculosympathetic lesion with associated carotid artery fibromuscular dysplasia.[123] It is possible that many congenital Horner's syndromes originate with trauma sustained during labor or delivery (see Fig. 15–15).

When Horner's syndrome is caused by lesions of the base of the skull or cavernous sinus, the accompanying cranial neuropathies frequently make localization possible. The coexistence of a postganglionic Horner's syndrome and ipsilateral abducens palsy should suggest a cavernous sinus lesion (Fig. 15–17). Parkinson[124] has provided an illustration of the theoretical location for such a lesion, where the intracavernous oculosympathetics temporarily run with the abducens nerve before joining the first division of the trigeminal division. Parkinson's syndrome—a Horner's syndrome and abducens nerve palsy in the absence of other cranial neuropathies—clinically is uncommon but has been documented with trauma, intracavernous carotid aneurysms, and metastasis.[125,126]

In an adult outpatient ophthalmology setting, isolated postganglionic oculosympathetic defects most frequently are the result of third-order neuron lesions, including status postendarterectomy, other neck surgery

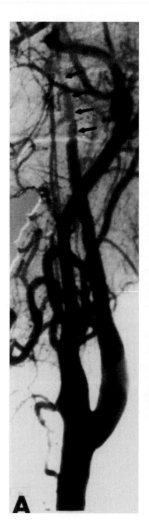
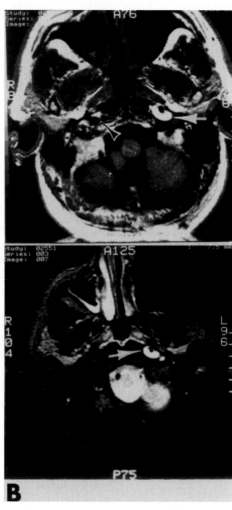

Fig. 15–16. Arteriogram and magnetic resonance imaging (MRI) scan of two patients with left spontaneous carotid artery dissections. **A.** Arteriogram (lateral view, left common carotid injection) shows a tapered narrowing (*black arrows*) of the left internal carotid artery with slow flow. The abnormal artery segment extends from the C_2 level to the base of the skull. (The patient, a 52-year-old woman, initially noted left amaurosis fugax and left upper lid ptosis as well as left eye injection. On examination, she also had facial and tongue weakness). **B. (Top)** T1-weighted MRI scan TR = 600, TE = 20). A bright signal, denoting blood (*white arrow*) surrounds a dark signal indicative of flow in the left internal carotid artery. The normal right internal carotid artery also is shown as a flow void (*arrowhead*). The bright signal anterior to the right carotid artery denotes fat, which on the T2-weighted images will be much less echo-intense. **(Bottom)** T2-weighted MRI scan (TR = 2500, TE = 75) shows persistence of the bright signal generated by blood (*white arrow*) surrounding the left internal carotid artery. The fat density anterior to the right carotid artery, which was bright and the T1-weighted image has practically disappeared on the T2-weighted scan. (The patient, a 53-year-old man, noted on acute onset, left-sided headache followed by speech and swallowing difficulties. Examination also revealed multiple left cranial neuropathies.) Arteriogram and MRI scan courtesy of Richard Latchaw, MD.

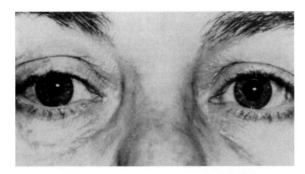
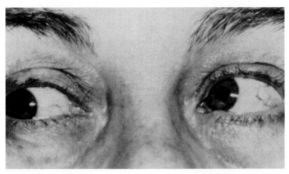
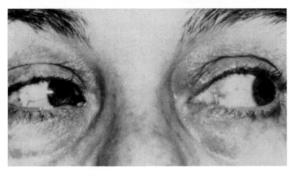

Fig. 15–17. Right Horner's syndrome and partial sixth nerve palsy due to cavernous sinus lesion. In addition, this patient had involvement of the right trigeminal divisions and therefore did not have a "pure" Parkinson's syndrome. (Reprinted with permission from Slamovits TL, Cahill KV, Sibony PA et al: Orbital fine-needle aspiration biopsy in patients with cavernous sinus syndrome. J Neurosurg 59:1037, 1983)

tion, possibly by means of the small caliber arterial branches arising from the carotid, of the vascular supply to the sympathetic plexus. Postganglionic oculosympathetic lesions do not include anhidrosis, but only ptosis and miosis. Unilateral recurrent cranial or facial pain in the trigeminal distribution, in combination with a third-order Horner's syndrome, constitutes a common enough variant of vascular-mediated headaches, the Raeder's syndrome. When not accompanied by parasellar cranial nerve deficits, this headache syndrome is likely to follow a benign course, with resolution within a few months.[128]

Whether first-, second-, or third-order sympathetic lesions are encountered most frequently is a function of whether outpatient ophthalmologic or inpatient neurologic data are assayed. Several authors have reported on their series.[103,129–132] Giles and Henderson's retrospective review[129] of 216 patients from the University of Michigan Hospital suggests that most frequently the Horner's syndrome is due to tumors (in about one third of all patients and in more than half of patients with a known cause for their Horner's syndrome); of all tumors, about three fourths were malignant and most were due to lesions in the neck, involving either the preganglionic or extracranial postganglionic sympathetic chain; about 10% of the cases were localized to the first-order neuron. In contradistinction, Keane's neurologic series[131] of 100 hospitalized patients found that most (approximately two thirds) of Horner's syndromes were first-order neuron lesions, mostly stroke related; about one fourth of the cases were preganglionic and an eighth were postganglionic; of all cases with known cause, approximately one fourth were due to tumors, about two thirds of which were preganglionic and one third postganglionic.

Grimson and Thompson's 120 cases[130] were rarely due to a central lesion; of all cases with known etiology, close to one half were preganglionic. More than one third were postganglionic, and only a minority were of central origin. In this series, about half of all preganglionic lesions were due to neoplasia, whereas postganglionic lesions mostly were caused by vascular headache or head trauma.

The subject population of Maloney and associates[132] consists of both inpatients and outpatients. Forty percent of the 450 patients studied had no known cause for the oculosympathetic defect. Of 270 patients with known cause of Horner's syndrome, Maloney found a minority to be central (13%) and about an equal number to be preganglionic (43%) and postganglionic (44%). Whereas 13% of the 450 patients had tumors, only 3% had occult malignancies. This suggests that it is rare for Horner's syndrome to be the presenting sign of an occult malignancy.

In the pediatric population, the implications may be more ominous because Horner's syndrome can be an

or trauma, or in the context of vascular headaches of the "cluster" type. Where the cause is inconclusive, undetected carotid disease is presumed. In cadaver studies, superior cervical ganglion compression has been demonstrated, caused by a tortuous atherosclerotic internal carotid artery that at times produced actual indentation of the ganglion (Fig. 15–18); perhaps this mechanism accounts for a benign postganglionic Horner's syndrome in elderly patients. Another autopsy study[127] disclosed that some internal carotid arteries give off small-caliber branches in their extracranial segments within 3 cm from the base of the skull. Typically, these branches were associated intimately with the sympathetic carotid plexus, and the authors suggested that isolated Horner's syndrome may result from interrup-

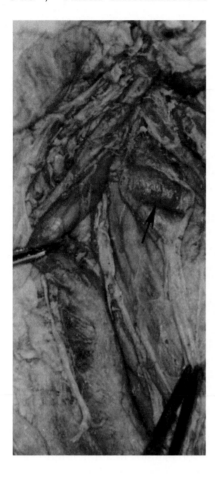
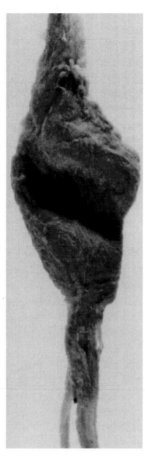

Fig. 15–18. Cadaver neck dissection (left), with the cervical carotid artery retracted away from the superior cervical ganglion. Note the groove (*arrow*) created by the carotid artery. Enlarged anterior-posterior view of the superior cervical ganglion (right) with obvious carotid indentation mark. (Courtesy of Dr. Yochanan Goldhammer; Goldhammer Y, Nathan H, Luchansky E: Compression of the Superior Cervical Sympathetic Ganglion by the Internal Carotid Artery Demonstrated by Anatomic Studies: A Possible Etiology of the Horner's Syndrome in the Elderly. Presented at the Fourth International Neuroophthalmology Society Meeting, Hamilton, Bermuda, June 1982)

important ocular sign of neuroblastoma[133] and often is associated with a severe underlying disease, such as tumor metastasis, leukemia, lymphoma, or aneurysm.[134] Unless an obvious and plausible precipitant, such as chest surgery, is present to explain a neonatal or acquired pediatric Horner's syndrome, appropriate testing, including imaging and 24-hour urinary catecholamine measurement, should be ordered to look for possible neuroblastoma.[135]

Thus, in the evaluation of patients with the Horner's syndrome, the most important clues to diagnosis are the clinical history and the accompanying neurologic signs and symptoms. When combined with cranial nerve palsies or other localizing signs and symptoms, sympathoparesis often is caused by tumor, trauma, or vascular disease. If any doubt exists about whether the patient has a false or true Horner's syndrome,[48] the cocaine test should be performed. If the clinical assessment shows a Horner's syndrome to be an isolated finding, 1% hydroxyamphetamine (Paredrine) is instilled in both eyes to pharmacologically distinguish a postganglionic lesion from a preganglionic or central one. In neonates and in the pediatric population, an isolated Horner's syndrome not considered congenital requires further assessment to search for neuroblastoma or other underlying malig-

nancy. In adults, truly isolated postganglionic lesions often remain unexplained: these are presumed to be of vascular origin and are compatible with a benign course. Isolated preganglionic Horner's lesions in adults require further investigation, with special attention to the pulmonary apex and chest. Appropriate consultations and radiologic studies (lordotic x-ray views of the chest, mediastinal computed tomography, cervical spine images) should be obtained. Several authors have provided guidelines for selective imaging of patients with oculosympathetic lesions.[136,137]

Pharmacologic Accidents: The Fixed Dilated Pupil

A mydriatic pupil, unresponsive to light or near reflex, occurring as an isolated sign unaccompanied by ptosis or any oculomotor dysfunction, is almost always caused by inadvertent or factitious application of a pharmacologic agent. Medical personnel, including nurses, physicians, and pharmacists, are especially liable to accidental instillation of a mydriatic agent (Fig. 15–19), which more often than not also leads to cycloplegia, photophobia, and even headache. These signs and symptoms should not be construed as an ominous warning of intracerebral disease.

Thompson[138] has reviewed the problem of the fixed dilated pupil and points out the practicality of identifying pharmacologic mydriasis by the use of weak solutions of miotics. If pilocarpine 1% is instilled in an eye with a dilated pupil because of parasympathetic denervation (*e.g.,* oculomotor palsy, tonic pupil), prompt miosis occurs. However, pilocarpine miosis is diminished or absent in patients with pharmacologic mydriasis (see Fig. 15–19). Both eyes should be subjected to pilocarpine instillation, with the normal eye serving as a control.

Accidental instillation of the fluid of many plants that contain belladonna and atropine-like alkaloids, such as jimson weed, may cause mydriasis. Since the introduction of retroauricular scopolamine patches for motion sickness, reports have appeared of associated unilateral mydriasis.[139–141] This probably occurs as a result of finger contamination with scopolamine, followed by inadvertent eye contact. Perfumes and cosmetics also may contain agents capable of dilating the pupil. On occasion, both young and elderly patients intentionally apply a mydriatic agent to the eye and subsequently deny such a maneuver.

Intraocular iron foreign bodies can lead to fixed dilated pupils, even before the development of heterochromia or visual loss. In a report of two such cases, the patients, both young boys, failed to report their past ocular injuries.[142] A dilated, atonic pupil rarely can develop after uncomplicated penetrating keratoplasty or cataract extraction.[92]

Episodic Dysfunction of the Pupil

Episodic unilateral mydriasis, lasting minutes to weeks and usually accompanied by blurred vision and headache, has been reported and reviewed by Hallett and Cogan.[143] This periodic phenomenon remains controversial and most of the time is not entirely free of suspicion of pharmacologic misadventure. However, there remain "pure" cases that lead credence to this dramatic if unexplained pupillary phenomenon (*i.e.,* the "springing pupil"). A clinical pattern may be defined as follows: (1) brief, episodic unilateral mydriasis occurring in young, otherwise healthy, females; (2) peculiar sensations in and about the affected eye, often progressing to headache (but not typical migraine); and (3) usually defective accommodation, but without any other signs of lid or extraocular muscle dysfunction.

Transient pupillary distortion with segmental iris dilator spasm has been reported by Thompson[144] and termed *tadpole pupil.* The condition probably represents a subset of the larger group of patients who carry the less precise diagnosis *springing pupil.* The clinical pattern and prognosis of patients with tadpole pupil appear to be similar to those described previously.

Periodic unilateral pupil dilation has been reported in association with migraine.[144–148] Suggested causes for the periodic mydriasis include transient sympathetic hyperactivity[144] or transient parasympatholytic activity,[146,147] or both,[149] perhaps as a variant of ophthalmologic migraine. Oculosympathetic spasm has been observed several months after spinal cord injury,[150] and, according to the authors, the pupillary dilation, brought on by elevation and stretch of the ipsilateral arm or leg, possibly represents a localized form of autonomic hyperreflexia.

Because a fixed dilated pupil in an unconscious patient usually is interpreted as a sign of temporal lobe herniation or aneurysmal compression, it should be noted that transient unilateral mydriasis on occasion may accompany convulsive disorders in children[151,152] or adults.[153]

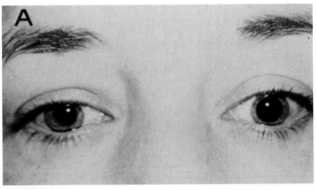
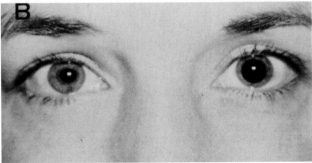

Fig. 15–19. Accidental atropinization. **A.** An 18-year-old student nurse presented with headache, blurred vision, and widely dilated, fixed left pupil. **B.** Pilocarpine 1% instilled in both eyes constricts right but not left pupil, corroborating pharmacologic origin of mydriasis.

DISORDERS OF ACCOMMODATION

As discussed previously, the neural pathways controlling the near reflex and accommodation are not defined precisely. As a rule, in those disorders that interrupt the parasympathetic supply to the pupil sphincter, accommodation also is defective because of denervation of the ciliary musculature. In certain situations, however, the convergence–accommodation mechanism is faulty while pupillary reflexes are spared or minimally involved.

The accommodative power of the eye is difficult to assess because of the subjective nature of the end point and the great dependency on cooperation of the patient. A unilateral accommodative deficiency is easier to define because the uninvolved eye serves as a normal "control." Accommodation usually is measured in terms of near point (the shortest distance from the naked eye at which an accommodative target can no longer be focused and appears blurred), or the maximum power of minus lenses that the eye can overcome to see clearly with best-corrected distance acuity may be used. In the presbyopic eye, accommodation is difficult to assess, but unilateral defects are rare.

Obviously, the most common defect of accommodation is related to aging because of the progressive deficiency of the lens in changing its refractive power. Unilateral or asymmetric lens opacities or brunescence may present as an "accommodative" symptom, but slit-lamp examination quickly resolves this diagnostic problem.

Occasionally, rapid changes in the refractive power of the eyes takes place during poorly controlled diabetes mellitus, with resulting increase in the refractive index of the lenses. In this case, the patient becomes more myopic and reports blurring of distant vision; however, presbyopic patients may suddenly be able to read without the aid of bifocals. This situation should immediately suggest a state of hyperglycemia.

Defective accommodation almost always accompanies pupillotonic syndromes and also peripheral oculomotor nerve palsies, in which instance blurred vision is the least dramatic aspect and may go unnoticed by both the patient and the physician. Local ocular disease, traumatic, inflammatory, or otherwise, need not be discussed. Patients using anticholinergic medications may complain of bilateral defective accommodation, and the use of preoperative atropine in surgical patients often produces transient accommodative insufficiency.

Many individuals complain of rather vague problems of "focusing" the eyes, and as a rule, nothing is found. Fortunately, these patients usually are well equipped with other aches, pains, and ill-defined asthenopic symptoms. In some instances, however, symptoms of accommodative and convergence insufficiency appear to be valid residue of cerebral concussion or cervicocranial hyperextension injury ("whiplash"). These symptoms may extend from weeks to years in duration and are at times miraculously relieved by litigation settlements. Here the physician is at the mercy of variations in patient cooperation and strictly subjective end points. It may be impossible to separate the patient with true post-traumatic accommodative–convergence insufficiency from the dissembler unless objective signs are present or a positive response to therapy excludes the latter possibility.

Paralysis of accommodation classically occurs in children with diphtheria, a disorder encountered rarely in the United States. Postdiphtheritic paralysis is attributed to a demyelinating toxin with a special predilection for cranial nerves.

Contamination of food with *Clostridium botulinum* is responsible for a serious form of food poisoning (*i.e.,* botulism). Typically, botulism is caused by ingestion of toxin that has been produced in contaminated foods. In infants and rarely in adults, botulism also can be caused by *in vivo* toxin production after colonization of the gastrointestinal tract by *C. botulinum* organisms.[154] The elaborated exotoxin interferes with cholinergic transmission, resulting in the clinical picture of an alert patient with dilated nonreactive pupils, accommodative paralysis, dry mouth, and respiratory distress. Tyler[155] has pointed out that in only one third of patients does an acute gastrointestinal episode occur (nausea, vomiting, and diarrhea). Dizziness, headache, blurred vision, diplopia, and swallowing difficulties should alert the physician to the possibility of botulism.[156]

The pupillary and ciliary musculature may be paretic in the ophthalmoplegic form of acute idiopathic polyneuritis. Clinical involvement of the internal ocular muscles in myasthenia probably does not occur, although this is a controversial subject. The presence of internal ophthalmoplegia as a rule makes a diagnosis of ocular myasthenia untenable (unless the patient has another cause of the internal ophthalmoplegia).

Rostral-dorsal midbrain lesions may result in a state of spastic-paretic accommodation, usually accompanied by moderately dilated, light-near dissociated pupils, upgaze palsy, and retraction nystagmus (the periaqueductal syndrome). When shifting gaze from distance to near, accommodation is paretic; on attempted upward gaze, accommodative spasms occur such that distant vision is blurred because of momentary myopia (see previous discussion of periaqueductal syndrome).

Spasm of the near reflex may be associated with organic disease.[157-159] However, even then there may be an element of functional disturbance superimposed on the organic process. In most instances, spasms of accommodation are of functional origin. Some degree of convergence excess is common, such that an esotropic deviation may mimic a unilateral or bilateral abduction deficiency (Fig. 15–20). Pupils that become constricted on lateral gaze attempts should be the clue to such hysterical "spasm of the near reflex." Atropinization, nonspecific "eye exercises," time, and litigation settlements all may have salutary effects.

Transient myopia may occur as a toxic reaction to sulfa-derived drugs (including sulfonamides and acetazolamide), tetracycline, prochlorperazine (Compazine), promethazine (Phenergan), autonomic blocking agents used to treat hypertension,[160] and isosorbide dinitrate (Isordil), an organic nitrate used to treat angina.[161]

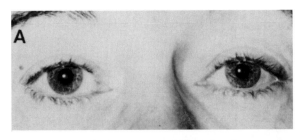

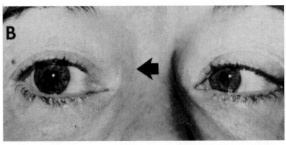

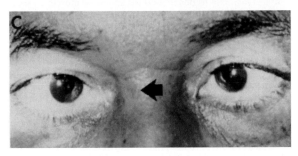

Fig. 15–20. Spasm of near reflex of volitional origin. **A.** Gaze forward in a young woman after an automobile accident. Note 4-mm pupils. **B.** Gaze right attempt shows abduction defect on right but constricted pupils. **C.** Another patient shows bilateral abduction "palsies" when asked to follow near target to either side. Note extreme pupillary miosis. While reading an acuity chart at 6 m, eyes were straight and full abduction was present with face turn to either side.

REFERENCES

1. Loewenfeld IE: The Pupil. 1st ed. Ames and Detroit: Iowa State and Wayne State University Press, 1993
2. Thompson HS, Franceschetti AT, Thompson PM: Hippus, semantic and historic considerations of the word. Am J Ophthalmol 71:1116, 1971
3. Loewenfeld IE: Pupillary changes related to age. In Thompson HS (ed): Topics in Neuro-ophthalmology, pp 124–150. Baltimore: Williams & Wilkins, 1979
4. Bourne PR, Smith SA, Smith SE: Dynamics of the light reflex and the influence of age on the human pupil measured by television pupillometry. J Physiol 293:1P, 1979
5. Campbell FW, Gubisch RW: Optical quality of the human eye. J Physiol 186:558, 1966
6. Bowling DB, Michael CR: Projection patterns of simple physiologically characterized optic tract fibers in the cat. Nature 286:899, 1980
7. Kupfer C, Chumbley L, Downer J: Quantitative histology of optic nerve, optic tract and lateral geniculate nucleus of man. J Anat 101:393, 1967
8. Breen L, Burde RM, Loewy AD: Brainstem connections to the Edinger–Westphal nucleus of the cat, a retrograde tracer study. Br Res 261:303, 1983
9. Smith JD, Masek GA, Ichinose LY et al: Single neuron activity in the pupillary system. Brain Res 24:219, 1970
10. Carpenter MB, Pierson RJ: Protectal region and the pupillary light reflex. J Comp Neurol 149:271, 1973
11. Benevento LA, Rezak M, Santos-Anderson RM: An autoradiographic study of the projections of the pretectum in the Rhesus monkey (*Macaca mulatta*): Evidence for sensorimotor links to the thalamus and oculomotor nuclei. Brain Res 127:197, 1977
12. Burde RM: The visceral nuclei of the oculomotor complex. Trans Am Ophthalmol Soc 81:532, 1983
13. Warwick R: Representation of the extra-ocular muscles in the oculomotor complex. J Comp Neurol 98:449, 1953
14. Jampel RS, Mindel J: The nucleus for accommodation in the midbrain of the macaque. Invest Ophthalmol 6:40, 1967
15. Burde RM, Loewy AD: Central origin of the oculomotor parasympathetic neurons in the monkey. Br Res 198:434, 1980
16. Kourouyan HD, Horton JC: Transneuronal retinal input to the primate Edinger–Westphal nucleus. J Comp Neurol 381:68, 1997
17. Warwick R: The ocular parasympathetic nerve supply and its mesencephalic sources. J Anat 88:71, 1954
18. Kerr FWL, Hollowell OW: Location of pupillomotor and accommodation fibers in the oculomotor nerve: Experimental observations on paralytic mydriasis. J Neurol Neurosurg Psychiatry 27:473, 1964
19. Nadeau SE, Trobe JD: Pupil sparing in oculomotor palsy: A brief review. Ann Neurol 13:143, 1983
20. Ruskell GL: Accommodation and the nerve pathway to the ciliary muscle: a review. Ophthalmic Physiol Opt 10:239, 1990
21. Jaeger RJ, Benevento LA: Innervation of eye internal structures. Invest Ophthalmol Vis Sci 19:575, 1980
22. Parelman JJ, Fay MT, Burde RM: Confirmatory evidence for a direct parasympathetic pathway to internal eye structures. Trans Am Ophthalmol Soc 84:371, 1985
23. Burde RM: Direct parasympathetic pathways to the eye: Revisited. Brain Res 463:158, 1988
24. Ponsford JR, Bannister R, Paul EA: Methacholine pupillary responses in third nerve palsy and Adie's syndrome. Brain 105:583, 1982
25. Slamovits TL, Miller RN, Burde RM: Intracranial oculomotor nerve paresis with anisocoria and pupillary parasympathetic hypersensitivity. Am J Ophthalmol 104:401, 1987
26. Jacobson DM: Pupillary responses to dilute pilocarpine in preganglionic 3rd nerve disorders. Neurology 40:804, 1990
27. Franklin AI, Cruz-Flores S, Chung S et al: Cholinergic supersensitivity associated with inferior division oculomotor nerve palsies. Abstract presented at the 23rd Annual North American Neuroophthalmology Society Meeting, Keystone, CO, February 1997.
28. Jampel RS: Representation of the near-response on the cerebral cortex of the Macaque. Am J Ophthalmol 48:573, 1959
29. Mays LE: Neurophysiological correlates of vergence eye movements. In Schor CM, Ciuffreda KJ (eds): Vergence eye movements: Basic and clinical aspects, pp 649–670. Woburn, MA: Butterworth Publishers Inc, 1983
30. Kestenbaum A: Clinical Methods of Neuro-ophthalmologic Examination, p 344–357. New York: Grune & Stratton, 1961
31. Levatin P: Pupillary escape in disease of the retina or optic nerve. Arch Ophthalmol 62:768, 1959
32. Finsberg E, Thompson HS: Quantitation of the afferent pupillary defect. In Smith JL (ed): Neuro-ophthalmology Focus 1980, pp 25–29. New York, Masson, 1979
33. Browning DJ, Tiedeman JS: The test light affects quantitation of the afferent pupillary defect. Ophthalmology 94:53, 1987
34. Thompson HS, Jiang MQ: Letter to the editor. Ophthalmology 94:1360, 1987
35. Thompson JS, Corbett JJ, Cox TA: How to measure the relative afferent pupillary defect. Surv Ophthalmol 26:39, 1981
36. Kawasaki A, Moore P, Kardon RH: Variability of the relative afferent pupillary defect. Am J Ophth 120:622, 1995
37. Newman SA, Miller NR: Optic tract syndrome: Neuro-ophthalmologic considerations. Arch Ophthalmol 101:1241, 1983
38. Ellis CJK: Afferent pupillary defect in pineal region tumour. J Neurol Neurosurg Psychiatry 47:739, 1984
39. Johnson RE, Bell RA: Relative afferent pupillary defect in a

lesion of the pretectal afferent pupillary pathway. Can J Ophthalmol 22:282, 1987

40. Jiang MQ. Thompson HS: Pupillary defects in retinitis pigmentosa. Am J Ophthalmol 99:607, 1985
41. Thompson HS, Montague P, Cox TA et al: The relationship between visual acuity, pupillary defect and visual loss. Am J Ophthalmol 93:681, 1982
42. Johnson LN, Hill RA, Bartholomew MJ: Correlation of afferent pupillary defect with visual field loss on automated perimetry. Ophthalmology 95:1649, 1988
43. Thompson HS, Watsky RC, Weinstein JM: Pupillary dysfunction and macular disease. Trans Am Ophthalmol Soc 78:311, 1980
44. Folk JC, Thompson HS, Han DP et al: Visual function abnormalities and central serous retinopathy. Arch Ophthalmol 102:1299, 1984
45. Han DP, Thompson HS, Folk JC: Differentiation between recently resolved optic neuritis and central serous retinopathy. Arch Ophthalmol 103:394, 1985
46. Servais EG, Thompson HS, Hayreh SS: Relative afferent pupillary defect in central retinal vein occlusion. Ophthalmology 93:301, 1986
47. Lam BL, Thompson HS: Relative afferent pupillary defect induced by patching. Am J Ophthalmol 107:305, 1989
48. DuBois LG, Sadun AA: Occlusion-induced contralateral afferent pupillary defect. Am J Ophthalmol 107:306, 1989
49. Lam BL, Thompson HS: A unilateral cataract produces a relative afferent pupillary defect in the contralateral eye. Ophthalmology 97:334, 1990
50. Portnoy JZ, Thompson HS, Lennarson L, Corbett JJ: Pupillary defects in amblyopia. Am J Ophthalmol 96:609, 1983
51. Greenwald MJ, Folk ER: Afferent pupillary defects in amblyopia. J Pediatr Ophthalmol Strabismus 20:63, 1983
52. Kawasaki A, Moore P, Kardon RH: Long-term fluctuation of relative afferent pupillary defect in subjects with normal visual function. Am J Ophthalmol 22:875, 1996
53. Loewenfeld IE: The Argyll Robertson pupil, 1869–1969: A critical survey of the literature. Surv Ophthalmol 14:199, 1969
54. Sundaram MBM: Pupillary abnormalities in congenital neurosyphilis. Can J Neurol Sci 12:134, 1985
55. Fletcher WA, Sharpe JA: Tonic pupils in neurosyphilis. Neurology 36:188, 1986
56. Caccamise WC, Townes PL: Congenital mydriasis. Am J Ophthalmol 81:515, 1976
57. Seybold ME, Yoss RE, Hollenhorst RW et al: Pupillary abnormalities associated with tumors of the pineal region. Neurology 21:232, 1971
58. Frank JW, Kushner RJ, France TD: Paradoxic pupillary phenomena—a review of patients with pupillary constriction to darkness. Arch Ophthalmol 106:1564, 1988
59. Olsen T, Jakobsen J: Abnormal pupillary function in third nerve regeneration (the pseudo Argyll Robertson pupil): A case report. Acta Ophthalmol 62:163, 1984
60. Kardon RH, Corbett JJ, Thompson HS: Segmental denervation and re-innervation of the iris sphincter as shown by infrared videographic transillumination. Ophthalmology 105:313, 1998
61. Cox TA: Czarnecki's sign as the initial finding in acquired oculomotor synkinesis. Am J Ophthalmol 102:543, 1986
62. Ohno S, Mukumo K: Studies on synkinetic pupillary phenomena resulting from aberrant regeneration of the third nerve. Jpn J Clin Ophthalmol 27:229, 1973
63. Spiegel P, Kardon RH: Features of eye, eyelid and pupil movement critical to the recognition of aberrant regeneration of the oculomotor nerve revealed by infrared and color videography. Abstract presented at the 23rd Annual North American Neuro-ophthalmology Society Meeting, Keystone, CO, 1997
64. Lam BL, Thompson HS, Corbett JJ: The prevalence of simple anisocoria. Am J Ophthalmol 104:69, 1987
65. Loewenfeld IE: "Simple central" anisocoria: A common condition seldom recognized. Trans Am Acad Ophthalmol/Otolaryngol 83:832, 1977
66. Roarty JD, Keltner JL: Normal pupil size and anisocoria in newborn infants. Arch Ophthalmol 108:94, 1996
67. Lam BL, Thompson HS, Walls RC: Effect of light on the prevalence of simple anisocoria. Ophthalmology 103:790, 1996
68. Thompson BM, Corbett JJ, Kline LB et al: Pseudo-Horner's syndrome. Arch Neurol 39:108, 1982
69. Safran AB, Roth A: Using a slit lamp for the neuroophthalmologic evaluation of old photographs. Am J Ophthalmol 95:558, 1983
70. Thompson HS, Bell RA, Bourgon P: The natural history of Adie's syndrome. In Thompson HS, Daroff RB, Frisen L et al (eds): Topics in Neuro-ophthalmology, pp 96–99. Baltimore: Williams & Wilkins, 1979
71. Pilley SFJ, Thompson HS: Cholinergic supersensitivity in Adie's syndrome: Pilocarpine vs. Mecholyl. Am J Ophthalmol 80:955, 1975
72. Ramsay DA: Dilute solutions of phenylephrine and pilocarpine in the diagnosis of disordered autonomic innervation of the iris. J Neurol Sci 73:125, 1986
73. Babikian PV, Thompson HS: Arecoline miosis. Am J Ophthalmol 98:514, 1984
74. Thompson HS: Adie's syndrome: Some new observations. Trans Am Ophthalmol Soc 75:587, 1977
75. Harriman DGF, Garland H: The pathology of Adie's syndrome. Brain 91:401, 1968
76. Loewenfeld IE, Thompson HS: The tonic pupil: A reevaluation. Am J Ophthalmol 63:46, 1967
77. Wirtschafter JD, Volk CR, Sawchuk RJ: Transaqueous diffusion of acetylcholine to denervated iris sphincter muscle: A mechanism for the tonic pupil syndrome (Adie syndrome). Ann Neurol 4:1, 1978
78. Wirtschafter JD, Horman WK: Low concentration eserine therapy for the tonic pupil (Adie) syndrome. Ophthalmology 87:1037, 1980
79. Loewenfeld IE, Thompson HS: Mechanism of tonic pupil. Ann Neurol 10:275, 1981
80. Anderson HK: The paralysis of involuntary muscle: Part III, on the action of pilocarpine, physostigmine and atropine upon the paralysed iris. J Physiol (Lond) 33:414, 1905
81. Selhorst JB, Madge G, Ghatak M: The neuropathology of the Holmes-Adie syndrome. Ann Neurol 16:138, 1984
82. Lucy DD, Van Allen MW, Thompson HS: Holmes-Adie syndrome with segmental hypohidrosis. Neurology 17:763, 1967
83. Spector RH, Bachman DL: Bilateral Adie's tonic pupil with anhidrosis and hyperthermia. Arch Neurol 41:342, 1984
84. Esterly NB, Cantolino SJ, Alter BP et al: Pupillotonia, hyporeflexia, and segmental hypohidrosis: Autonomic dysfunction in a child. J Pediatr 73:852, 1968
85. Goldberg MF, Payne JW, Brunt PW: Ophthalmologic studies of familial dysautonomia: The Riley-Day syndrome. Arch Ophthalmol 80:732, 1968
86. Maitland GC, Scherokman BJ, Schiffman J et al: Paraneoplastic tonic pupils. J Clin Neuro-ophthalmol 5:99, 1985
87. Van Lieshout JJ, Wieling W, Van Montfrans GA et al: Acute dysautonomia associated with Hodgkin's disease. J Neurol Neurosurg Psychiatry 49:830, 1986
88. Bell TAG: Adie's tonic pupil in a patient with carcinomatous neuromyopathy. Arch Ophthalmol 104:331, 1986
89. Keane JR: Tonic pupils with acute ophthalmoplegic polyneuritis. Ann Neurol 2:393, 1977
90. Currie J, Lessell S: Tonic pupil with giant cell arteritis. Br J Ophthalmol 68:135, 1984
91. Thompson HS: Discussion of Wirtschafter JD, Herman WK: Low concentration eserine therapy for the tonic pupil. Ophthalmology 87:1043, 1980
92. Lam S, Beck RW, Hall D et al: Atonic pupil after cataract surgery. Ophthalmology 96:589, 1989
93. Scinto LFM, Daffner KR, Dressler D et al: A potential noninvasive neurobiological test for Alzheimer's disease. Science 266:1051, 1994
94. Loupe DN, Newman NJ, Green RC et al: Pupillary responses to tropicamide in patients with Alzheimer disease. Ophthalmology 103:495, 1996
95. Makley MA, Abbott K: Neurogenic heterochromia: A report of an interesting case. Am J Ophthalmol 59:927, 1965
96. Diesenhouse MC, Palay DA, Newman NJ et al: Acquired heterochromia with Horner's syndrome in two adults. Ophthalmology 99:1815, 1992

97. Lapore FE: Enophthalmos and Horner's syndrome. Arch Neurol 40:460, 1983

98. Van der Wiel HL, Van Gijn J: Letter to the editor: No enophthalmos in Horner's syndrome. J Neurol Neurosurg Psychiatry 50:498, 1987

99. Morris JGL, Lee J, Lim CL: Facial sweating in Horner's syndrome. Brain 107:751, 1984

100. Thompson HS, Mensher JM: Adrenergic mydriasis of Horner's syndrome: Hydroxyamphetamine test for diagnosis of postganglionic defects. Am J Ophthalmol 72:472, 1971

101. Kardon RH, Dennison CE, Brown CK et al: Critical evaluation of the cocaine test in the diagnosis of Horner's Syndrome. Arch Ophthalmol 108:384, 1990

102. Wilhelm H, Ochsner H, Kopycziok E et al: Horner's Syndrome: a retrospective analysis of 90 cases and recommendation for clinical handling. J Ophthalmol 1:76, 1992

103. Grimson BS, Thompson HS: Drug testing in Horner's syndrome. In Glaser JS, Smith JL (eds): Neuro-ophthalmology Symposium Vol VIII, pp 265–270, St. Louis: CV Mosby, 1975

104. Cremer SA, Thompson HS, Digre KB et al: Hydroxy amphetamine mydriasis in Horner's Syndrome. Am J Ophthalmol 110:71, 1990

105. Weinstein JM, Zweifel TJ, Thompson HS: Congenital Horner's syndrome. Arch Ophthalmol 98:1074, 1980

106. Donahue SP, Lavin PJ, Digre K: False-negative hydroxyamphetamine (Paredrine) test in acute Horner's syndrome. Am J Ophthalmol 122:900, 1996

107. Burde RM, Thompson HS: Hydroxyamphetamine: A good drug lost? Am J Ophthalmol 111:100, 1991

108. Wilhelm H, Schaffer E: Pholedrine for determining the site of Horner's syndrome. Klin Monatsbl Augenheilk 204:169, 1994

109. Bates AT, Chamberlain SY, Champion M et al: Pholedrine: A substitute for hydroxyamphetamine as a diagnostic eyedrop test in Horner's syndrome. J Neurol Neurosurg Psychiatry 58:215, 1995

110. Stone WM, de Toledo J, Romanul FCA: Horner's syndrome due to hypothalamic infarction: Clinical radiologic and pathologic correlation. Arch Neurol 43:199, 1986

111. Schiffter R: Letter to the editor: Telodiencephalic ischemic syndrome. Arch Neurol 44:1218, 1987

112. Schiffter R, Reinhart K: The telodiencephalic ischemic syndrome. J Neurol 222:265, 1980

113. Kori SH, Foley KM, Posner JB: Brachial plexus lesions in patients with cancer: 100 cases. Neurology 31:45, 1981

114. Yang PT, Seeger JF, Carmody RF et al: Horner's syndrome secondary to traumatic pseudoaneurysms. AJNR Am J Neuroradiol 7:913, 1986

115. Teich SA, Halprin SL, Tay S: Horner's syndrome secondary to Swan-Ganz catheterization. Am J Med 78:168, 1985

116. O'Doherty DS, Green JB: Diagnostic value of Horner's syndrome in thrombosis of the carotid artery. Neurology 111:842, 1958

117. Mokri B, Sundt TM Jr, Houser OW: Spontaneous internal carotid dissection, hemicrania, and Horner's syndrome. Arch Neurol 36:877, 1979

118. Kline LB, Vitek JJ, Raymon BC: Painful Horner's syndrome due to spontaneous carotid artery dissection. Ophthalmology 94:226, 1987

119. Francis KR, Williams DP, Troost BT: Facial numbness and dyesthesia: New features of carotid artery dissection. Arch Neurol 44:345, 1987

120. Bougousslavsky J, Deepland PA, Regli F: Spontaneous carotid dissection with acute stroke. Arch Neurol 44:137, 1987

121. Goldberg HI, Grossman RI, Gomori JM et al: Cervical internal carotid artery dissecting hemorrhage: Diagnosis using MR. Radiology 158:157, 1986

122. Assaf M, Sweeney PJ, Kosmorsky G et al: Horner's syndrome secondary to angiogram negative, subadventital carotid artery dissection. Can J Neurol Sci 20:62, 1993

123. Reader AL III, Massey EW: Fibromuscular dysplasia of the carotid artery: A cause of congenital Horner's syndrome? Ann Ophthalmol 12:326, 1980

124. Parkinson D: Bernard, Mitchell, Horner's syndrome and others? Surg Neurol 11:221, 1979

125. Abad JM, Alvarez F, Munoz J et al: Un sindrome neurologico no reconocido: Paralisis del sexto par y sindrome de Bernard Horner's debido a lesiones traumaticas intracavernosas. Rev Clin Esp 165:135, 1982

126. Gutman I, Levartovski S, Goldhammer Y et al: Sixth nerve palsy and unilateral Horner's syndrome. Ophthalmology 93:913, 1986

127. Havelius ULF, Hindfelt B: Minor vessels leaving the extracranial internal carotid artery: Possible clinical implications. Neuro-ophthalmology 5:51, 1985

128. Grimson BS, Thompson HS: Raeder's syndrome: A clinical review. Surg Ophthalmol 24:199, 1980

129. Giles CL, Henderson JW: Horner's syndrome: An analysis of 216 cases. Am J Ophthalmol 46:289, 1958

130. Grimson BS, Thompson HS: Horner's syndrome: Overall view of 120 cases. In Thompson HS, Daroff RB, Frisen L et al (eds): Topics in Neuro-Ophthalmology, pp 151–156. Baltimore: Williams & Wilkins, 1979

131. Keane JR. Oculosympathetic paresis: Analysis of 100 hospitalized patients. Arch Neurol 36:13, 1979

132. Maloney WF, Younge BR, Moyer NJ: Evaluation of the causes and accuracy of pharmacologic localization in Horner's syndrome. Am J Ophthalmol 90:394, 1980

133. Musarella MA, Chan HS, deBoer G et al: Ocular involvement—Neuroblastoma: Prognostic implications. Ophthalmology 91:936, 1984

134. Sauer T, Levinsohn M: Horner's syndrome in childhood. Neurology 26:216, 1976

135. Woodruff G, Buncic JR, Morin JD: Horner's syndrome. J Pediatr Ophthalmol Strabismus 25:40, 1988

136. Digre KB, Smoker WRK, Johnston P et al: Selective MR imaging approach for evaluation of patients with Horner's syndrome. AJNR Am J Neuroradiol 13:223, 1992

137. Lee AG, Hayman LA, Tang RA et al: An imaging guide for Horner's syndrome. Int J Neuroradiol 2:196, 1996

138. Thompson HS, Newsome DA, Loewenfeld IE: The fixed dilated pupil: Sudden iridoplegia or mydriatic drops? A simple diagnostic test. Arch Ophthalmol 86:21, 1971

139. Lepore FE: Letter to the editor: More on cycloplegia from transdermal scopolamine. N Engl J Med 307:284, 1982

140. Verdier D, Kennerdell J: Letter to the editor: Fixed dilated pupil resulting from transdermal acopolamine. Am J Ophthalmol 93:803, 1982

141. Johnson SF, Moore RJ: Transderm pupil and confusion in a 10 year old. Ann Neurol 13:583, 1983

142. Monteiro ML, Ulrich RF, Imes RK et al: Iron mydriasis. Am J Ophthalmol 97:794, 1984

143. Hallett M, Cogan DG: Episodic unilateral mydriasis in otherwise normal patients. Arch Ophthalmol 84:130, 1970

144. Thompson HS, Zackon DH, Czarnecki JSC: Tadpole-shaped pupils caused by segmental spasm of the iris dilator muscle. Am J Ophthalmol 96:467, 1983

145. Edelson RN, Levy DE: Transient benign unilateral pupillary dilation in young adults. Arch Neurol 31:12, 1974

146. Woods D, O'Connor PS, Fleming R: Episodic unilateral mydriasis and migraine. Am J Ophthalmol 98:229, 1984

147. Purvin VA: Adie's tonic pupil secondary to migraine. J Neuroophthalmol 15:43, 1995

148. Miller NR: Intermittent pupillary dilation in a young woman: Comments by Keltner JL, Gittinger JW Jr, Burde RM. Surv Ophthalmol 31:65, 1986

149. Jacobson DM: Benign episodic unilateral mydriasis-clinical characteristics. Ophthalmology 102:1623, 1995

150. Kline LB, McCluer SM, Bonikowski FP: Oculosympathetic spasm with cervical spinal cord injury. Arch Neurol 41:61, 1984

151. Pant SS, Benton JW, Dodge PR: Unilateral pupillary dilatation during and immediately following seizures. Neurology 16:337, 1966

152. Gadoth N, Margalith D, Bechar M: Unilateral pupillary dilatation during focal seizures. J Neurol 225:227, 1981

153. Zee DS, Griffin J, Price DL: Unilateral pupillary dilatation during adversive seizures. Arch Neurol 30:403, 1974

154. Chia JK, Clark JB, Ryan GA et al: Botulism in an adult associated

with food-borne intestinal infection with Clostridium botulinum. N Engl J Med 315:239, 1986

155. Tyler HR: Botulism. Arch Neurol 9:652, 1963

156. Cherington M: Botulism: Ten-year experience. Arch Neurol 30:432, 1974

157. Dagi LR, Chrousos GA, Cogan DC: Spasm of the near reflex associated with organic disease. Am J Ophthalmol 103:582, 1987

158. Tijssen CC, Goor C, Van Woerkom TCAM: Spasm of the near reflex: Functional or organic disorder? Neuroophthalmology 3:59, 1983

159. Safran AB, Roth A, Gauthier G: Le syndrome des spasmes de convergence "plus." Klin Monatsbl Augenheilkd 108:471, 1982

160. Maddalena MA: Transient myopia associated with acute glaucoma and retinal edema. Arch Ophthalmol 80:186, 1968

161. Dangel ME, Weber PA, Leier CB: Transient myopia following isosorbide dinitrate. Ann Ophthalmol 15:1156, 1983

CHAPTER 16

Migraine and Other Headaches

B. Todd Troost

Description of the Migraine Attack
    Prodrome
    Aura
    Headache Phase
    Termination and Postdrome
Pathophysiology
Migraine without Aura (Common)
Migraine with Aura (Classic)
Migraine with Prolonged Aura and Migrainous Infarctions
    Cerebral Migraine
    Ophthalmoplegic Migraine
    Retinal Migraine
    Basilar Artery Migraine
    Other Varieties
Cluster Headache
Migraine in Childhood

Other Headaches
    Facial Pain
    Temporal Arteritis
    Intracranial Mass Lesions
    Muscle Contraction
    Post-Traumatic Headache
    Aneurysm and Arteriovenous Malformation
    Ocular Headache
    Carotid Dissection
Differential Diagnosis
Therapy
    Symptomatic Treatment
        Sumatriptan
    Prophylactic Treatment
        Calcium Channel Blockers
        β-Blockers
        Tricyclic Antidepressants
        Serotonin Antagonists

When you're lying awake
With a dismal headache
And repose is taboo'd by anxiety,
I conceive you may use
Any language you choose
To indulge in without impropriety.
          "Iolanthe"—W. S. Gilbert

Headache in a variety of forms is one of the most common complaints addressed by the clinician. A new classification of headache has been proposed by the International Headache Society (IHS) and is summarized in Table 16–1.[1]

This chapter addresses the neuro-ophthalmologic aspects of migraine and provides a brief review of other common headaches, such as facial and ocular pains. Migraine is a periodic and paroxysmal protean disorder that affects more than 17% of women and 6% of men in the United States.[2,3] Neuro-ophthalmologic symptoms and signs are common in migraine and should be recognized by the clinician. The term *hemicrania* evolved from a variety of older descriptions and was one of the first names for this disorder; this was later changed by

the French in the 13th century to the word "migraine." More than 300 years ago, Thomas Willis wrote the first modern description of migraine and its possible causes. Historical figures believed to have had migraine include Julius Caesar, Emmanuel Kant, Alexander Pope, and Sigmund Freud. Throughout the 18th and 19th centuries, descriptions of the clinical phenomena and suggestions for therapy continued to appear in the writings of many prominent men in the medical professions. Sacks[4] pays homage to Edward Liveing's masterful treatise *On Megrim, Sick Headache, and Some Allied Disorders* (1873) as an unequaled description of the disorder. Further detailed clinical descriptions are found in the writings of Gowers.[5]

In contemporary medicine, Dalessio, Raskin, Sacks, Silberstein, Lipton, Stewart, Saper, and Welch are among those who could be singled out for their contributions to the study of migraine. One central theme seems to decry the simplistic view that migraine is defined by a unilateral (hemicranial) headache. As Sacks[4] wrote, "It is necessary to state that headache is never the sole symptom of a migraine, nor indeed is it the necessary feature of migraine attacks." Another quotation emphasizes this belief: "Migraine is diagnosed by the entire history, not by physical findings or by the presence of headache alone."[6] It is unfortunate that many have lim-

B. T. Troost: Department of Neurology, Wake Forest University School of Medicine; and Department of Neurology, North Carolina Baptist Hospital, Winston-Salem, North Carolina

TABLE 16–1. New International Headache Society Classification of Headache

1. Migraine	**8. Headache associated with substances or their withdrawal**
1.1 Migraine without aura	8.1 Headache induced by acute substance use or exposure
1.2 Migraine with aura	8.2 Headache induced by chronic substance use or exposure
1.3 Ophthalmoplegic migraine	8.3 Headache from substance withdrawal (acute use)
1.4 Retinal migraine	8.4 Headache from substance withdrawal (chronic use)
1.5 Childhood periodic syndromes that may be precursors to or associated with migraine	8.5 Headache associated with substances but with uncertain mechanism
1.6 Complications of migraine	
1.7 Migrainous disorder not fulfilling above criteria	**9. Headache associated with noncephalic infection**
	9.1 Viral infection
2. Tension-type headache	9.2 Bacterial infection
2.1 Episodic tension-type headache	9.3 Headache related to other infection
2.2 Chronic tension-type headache	
2.3 Tension-type headache not fulfilling above criteria	**10. Headache associated with metabolic disorders**
	10.1 Hypoxia
3. Cluster headache and chronic paroxysmal hemicrania	10.2 Hypercapnia
3.1 Cluster headache	10.3 Mixed hypoxia and hypercapnia
3.2 Chronic paroxysmal hemicrania	10.4 Hypoglycemia
3.3 Cluster headache–like disorder not fulfilling above criteria	10.5 Dialysis
	10.6 Headache related to other metabolic abnormality
4. Miscellaneous headaches not associated with structural lesions	**11. Headache or facial pain associated with disorder of cranium, neck, eyes, ears, nose, sinuses, teeth, mouth, or other facial or cranial structures**
4.1 Idiopathic stabbing headache	11.1 Cranial bone
4.2 External compression headache	11.2 Neck
4.3 Cold stimulus headache	11.3 Eyes
4.4 Benign cough headache	11.4 Ears
4.5 Benign exertional headache	11.5 Nose and sinuses
4.6 Headache associated with sexual activity	11.6 Teeth, jaws, and related structures
	11.7 Temporomandibular joint disease
5. Headache associated with head trauma	
5.1 Acute posttraumatic headache	**12. Cranial neuralgias, nerve trunk pain, and deafferentation pain**
5.2 Chronic posttraumatic headache.	12.1 Persistent (in contrast to tic-like) pain of cranial nerve origin
	12.2 Trigeminal neuralgia
6. Headache associated with vascular disorders	12.3 Glossopharyngeal neuralgia
6.1 Acute ischemic cerebrovascular disorder	12.4 Nervus intermedius neuralgia
6.2 Intracranial hematoma	12.5 Superior laryngeal neuralgia
6.3 Subarachnoid hemorrhage	12.6 Occipital neuralgia
6.4 Unruptured vascular malformation	12.7 Central causes of head and facial pain other than tic douloureux
6.5 Arteritis	12.8 Facial pain not fulfilling criteria in groups 11 or 12
6.6 Carotid or vertebral artery pain	
6.7 Venous thrombosis	**13. Headache not classifiable**
6.8 Arterial hypertension	
6.9 Headache associated with other vascular disorder	
7. Headache associated with nonvascular intracranial disorders	
7.1 High CSF pressure	
7.2 Low CSF pressure	
7.3 Intracranial infection	
7.4 Intracranial sarcoidosis and other noninfectious inflammatory diseases	
7.5 Headache related to intrathecal injections	
7.6 Intracranial neoplasm	
7.7 Headache associated with other intracranial disorders	

CSF, cerebrospinal fluid
(Olesen J: Headache Classification Committee of the International Headache Society: Classification and diagnostic criteria for headache disorders, cranial neuralgia, and facial pain. Cephalalgia 8[suppl 7]:1, 1988)

ited their concept of migraine to a stereotyped syndrome of visual disturbance followed by unilateral throbbing headache, which is diagnosed by the response to ergot preparations. Migraine gives rise to a number of well-recognized syndromes, as well as a variety of "equiva-lents" less commonly considered migraine. The symptom-complexes or syndromes of migraine include migraine without aura, migraine with aura, ophthalmoplegic migraine, retinal migraine, and others (see Table 16–1). The clinical features of migraine will be discussed according to the formal criteria published by the IHS in 1988.[7]

Other conditions and syndromes discussed include cluster headache, trigeminal neuralgia, atypical facial pain, temporal arteritis, and the headaches produced by intracranial mass lesions, muscle contraction, trauma, vascular anomalies, and ocular lesions.

DESCRIPTION OF THE MIGRAINE ATTACK

Blau[8] divided the migraine attack into five phases: the prodrome, occurring hours or days before the headache; the aura, which comes immediately before the headache; the headache itself; the headache termination; and the postdrome. As pointed out by Silberstein and Lipton,[9] "although most people experience more than one phase, no one particular phase is required for the diagnosis of migraine." The following is a description of these five phases of migraine.

Prodrome

Premonitory phenomena occur in approximately 60% of migraineurs, often hours to days before the onset of headache. These phenomena include psychological, neurologic, constitutional, and autonomic features. Psychological symptoms include depression, euphoria, irritability, restlessness, mental slowness, hyperactivity, fatigue, and drowsiness. Neurologic phenomena include photophobia, phonophobia, and hyperosmia. The generalized or constitutional symptoms include a stiff neck, a cold feeling, sluggishness, increased thirst, increased urination, anorexia, diarrhea, constipation, fluid retention, and food cravings. Some patients just report a poorly characterized feeling that they know a migraine attack is coming.

Aura

An aura refers to the appearance of focal neurologic symptoms that precede or even accompany an attack of migraine. Approximately 20% of migraine sufferers experience auras. Most aura symptoms develop over a course of 5 to 20 minutes and usually last less than 60 minutes. The aura can be characterized by visual, sensory, or motor phenomena, and may also involve language or brainstem disturbances. When a headache follows, it most often occurs within 60 minutes of the end of the aura. The appearance of isolated auras without headache is known as *migraine dissociée*. The most common aura is visual, previously termed classic migraine. It usually has a distribution in a single hemifield.

Sensory disturbances involve one side of the body and are characterized by descriptions of numbness or tingling on the face and in the hand. (For further neuro-logic symptomatology, see section titled Migraine with Prolonged Aura and Migrainous Infarction.)

Headache Phase

The typical migraine headache is unilateral and throbbing. It may be bilateral and constant at first and later become throbbing. As pointed out by Lipton and colleagues,[10] pain is characterized as throbbing in 85% of migraineurs. It should be noted, however, that throbbing is also described in other types of headaches.[11] The pain of migraine is almost always accompanied by other features, such as anorexia. Up to 90% of migraineurs experience nausea, and about one third have vomiting.[10]

Many patients experience photophobia, phonophobia, and osmophobia and seek seclusion in a dark, quiet room. Additional generalized symptoms include blurry vision, nasal stuffiness, anorexia, hunger, tenesmus, diarrhea, abdominal cramps, polyuria (followed by decreased urinary output after the attack), facial pallor (or, less commonly, redness), sensations of heat or cold, and sweating.[9] Localized edema of the scalp, face, or periorbital regions may occur with tenderness. There may also be tenderness of the scalp, a special prominence of a vein or artery in the temple, or a stiffness or tenderness of the neck. Impaired concentration is common; memory impairment occurs less frequently. Depression, fatigue, anxiety, nervousness, and irritability are common. A sensation of lightheadedness may be experienced. The IHS selects particular associated features as cardinal manifestations for diagnosis.

Termination and Postdrome

In the termination phase, the pain wanes. The patient, thereafter, may feel listless, tired, or "washed out" and not be themselves for 24 to 48 hours. Rarely, patients feel unusually refreshed or euphoric after an attack, but it is more common for patients to experience depression and malaise.[9]

PATHOPHYSIOLOGY

Although there is some understanding of the mechanism of migraine, its precise underlying causes are unknown. Extensive reviews and volumes have been published on the pathophysiology of headache, particularly migraine.[12–15]

It was primarily through the work of Wolff and coworkers that vascular phenomena were recognized as a mechanism responsible for the headache of migraine.[15] Research to date suggests that the initiation of a migraine attack is a primary neuronal phenomenon with subsequent hemodynamic consequences.[16–18] Wolff divided the migraine attack into four phases: preheadache,

headache, late headache, and postheadache. The *pre-headache phase* is characterized by the constriction of certain blood vessels that supply the brain. Then, the beginning of the *headache phase* is characterized by vascular dilatation, particularly involving branches of the external carotid, such as the temporal, occipital, and middle meningeal arteries. Local tenderness of the scalp ensues, and the scalp vessels may become rigid. The nature of the headache then changes from a pulsatile type to a more constant dull ache (*late headache*). Alleviation of the early headache phase with vasoconstrictors (*e.g.*, ergotamine) is cited as evidence that this pain is related to vasodilatation.

In their most simplistic form, these concepts can be reduced to the idea that the cerebral symptomatology, including the auras of classic migraine, is due to cerebral ischemia secondary to intracranial vessel spasm, and the ensuing headache phase is initiated by vasodilatation. However, vasodilatation may occur without pain, and additional factors are involved in the production of the headache. Local tissue changes take place (*e.g.*, vessel edema, scalp swelling, conjunctival chemosis) that may continue after vasodilatation has ceased. A wide variety of substances have causative roles in the production of large and small vessel dilatation as well as local tissue changes. Among the substances most frequently considered are the kinins (neurokinin and bradykinin), acetylcholine, histamine, serotonin, and reserpine. Sicuteri[19] hypothesized that the following sequence occurs: the initial event is a local release of catecholamines (with vasoconstriction and increased urinary excretion of vanillylmandelic acid); during subsequent reactive hyperemia, serotonin is released (documented by plasma serotonin decrease[20] and increased urinary 5-hydroxyindoleacetic acid[21]), presumably from platelets or mast cells, which sensitizes cranial pain receptors perhaps also affected by the kinins.

Additional evidence suggests that there are nervous system connections between the trigeminal ganglia and cerebral blood vessels, termed the *trigeminovascular system*.[22] Trigeminovascular neurons and their peripheral unmyelinated nerve fibers contain the neurotransmitter peptide substance P. Stimulation of this system by a variety of mechanisms would cause the release of substance P, which is postulated to increase vascular permeability and dilate cerebral blood vessels. The role of this system in the generation of human vascular headache may account for the effects of hormones or other circulating substances that change the receptive field properties of trigeminal ganglion cells. Persons prone to chemically induced headaches from ingestion of tyramine, alcohol, phenylethyamine, monosodium glutamate, nitroglycerin, wine, or chocolate also experience spontaneous headaches.[23] Extensive studies of the reactivity of blood vessels in migraine[24] and cerebral blood flow[17,18,25,26] suggest that abnormal vasomotor responses

may be present in migraine patients between, as well as during, migraine attacks.

There are several lines of indirect evidence that suggest a relationship between serotonin and migraine, making the understanding of the pharmacology of serotonin very important for understanding the pharmacology of the new serotonin agonist in migraine therapy.[9] The serotonin or 5-HT receptors consist of at least three distinct types of molecular structures: guanine nucleotide G protein–coupled receptors, ligand-gated ion channels, and transporters. At least five 5-HT$_1$ receptor subtypes are present in humans. Headaches bearing resemblance to migraine can be triggered by serotonergic drugs, such as reserpine (a 5-HT releaser and depleter) and m-chlorophenylpiperazine (a serotonin agonist).[27,28]

Other metabolic and endocrine factors also influence migraine attacks. According to Friedman and Merritt,[29] 80% of female migraineurs either stop having attacks or have improved symptoms during pregnancy. Callahan,[30] however, found an increase in the severity of migraine during pregnancy. The use of oral contraceptives appears to increase the incidence and severity of migraine.[31,32] Whitty and colleagues[33] suggested that migraine might be precipitated by withdrawal of progesterone, whereas Somerville[34] found from a study of three women with regular menstrual migraine that their attacks were related to estradiol withdrawal, rather than to falling levels of progesterone. Tyramine has also been invoked as a precipitating factor, especially in the so-called allergic migraine.[35] Only approximately 5% of migraine subjects notice having headaches precipitated by food; however, some patients are unusually sensitive to chocolate or alcohol, particularly red wine. Recent therapeutic trials of dietary therapy designed to avoid hypoglycemia suggest that glucose and/or insulin metabolism may play a role in the generation of vascular headache.

The role of trauma in the production or exacerbation of a preexisting migrainous tendency is still incompletely defined. Many persons experience vascular headaches of the common migraine type after even minor head trauma.[36] A previously well-controlled migraineur can experience a recrudescence of prior symptomatology after a head trauma. Such exacerbations are usually short lived, and a return to preinjury status usually occurs within weeks to a few months. Some patients, however, experience post-traumatic migraine headaches for years after a head injury. Other triggering events preceding migraine attacks include bright light, especially sunlight reflected from water, exercise or exertion, and high altitude. Vascular headache of the migraine type may also follow orgasm.[37] The role of stress is less clear. Migraine headache appears to be more likely to occur after a period of psychological stress than during a stressful event.

The pathophysiology of the migraine aura itself has

also been studied extensively. Wolff showed that the use of amyl nitrate, a potent vasodilator, could abort the migraine scotoma (Fig. 16–1), supporting the vasoconstrictor hypothesis. Milner[38] suggested that the scotomas of migraine may be related to the neurophysiologic phenomenon termed *Leão's spreading depression*. The spreading depression progresses across the cortex at approximately 3 mm/minute, similar to the slow evolu-

tion of the visual phenomena detailed by Lashley,[39] and is estimated to spread over the occipital cortex at a rate of 3 mm/minute. Unfortunately, the concept of spreading depression cannot explain much of the symptomatology in migraine. The rate of spread of the visual phenomena is not always consistent with a uniform spread of 3 mm/minute over the occipital cortex. Many patients experience just a "glare," and some have a continuously

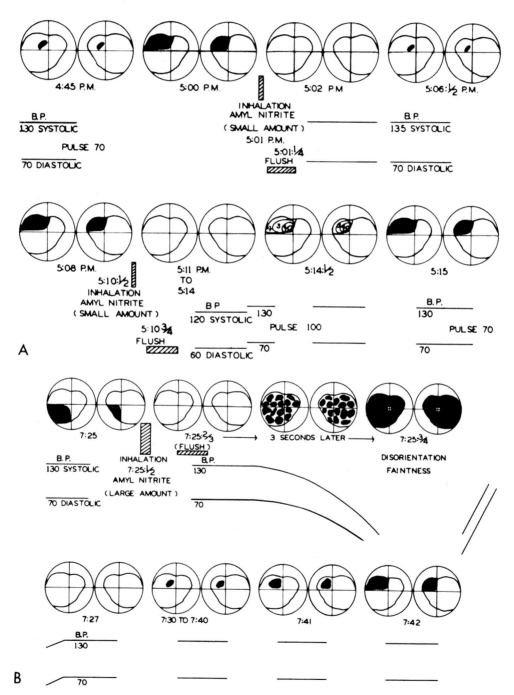

Fig. 16–1. A. Effect of inhalation of small amount of amyl nitrite on preheadache scotomas in migraine subject. The amount was insufficient to cause a drop in blood pressure or "light-headedness." **B.** With inhalation of a large amount of amyl nitrite, a drop in pressure occurred with amblyopia and faintness. (Wolff HG: Headache and Other Head Pain, 2nd ed. New York, Oxford University Press, 1963)

migrating visual form. The visual experiences in "retinal migraine" (see later discussion), which are strictly monocular, cannot be readily explained by the occipital cortex changes. No clearly analogous "spreading depression" is apparent in the retina, which is quite different from the cerebral cortex in terms of functional anatomy, biochemistry, and information processing. Wilkinson and Blau[40] observed that Leão's spreading depression has not been encountered in man or monkey by a variety of neurosurgeons and experts in cerebral blood flow. Raskin[14] discussed spreading depression further, indicating that there are many problems with the hypothesis linking spreading depression to migraine, but nonetheless has focused interest on neuronal rather than vascular, pathogenetic possibilities. In short, factors more complex than spreading depression must be invoked to explain most of what is observed in migraine.

MIGRAINE WITHOUT AURA (COMMON)

The IHS classification has improved the diagnosis of headaches. It has also facilitated clinical research on migraine. To establish a diagnosis of migraine without aura, five attacks are needed (Table 16–2). Each attack must last 4 to 72 hours and have two of the following four pain characteristics: (1) unilateral location, (2) pulsating quality, (3) moderate to severe intensity, and (4) aggravation by routine physical activity. In addition, the at-

TABLE 16–2. Migraine without Aura

1.1 Migraine without aura
Previously used terms: common migraine, hemicrania simplex

Diagnostic criteria
A. At least five attacks fulfill B through D
B. Headache lasts 4 to 72 h (untreated or unsuccessfully treated)
C. Headache has at least two of the following characteristics:
 1. Unilateral location
 2. Pulsating quality
 3. Moderate or severe intensity (inhibiting or prohibiting daily activities)
 4. Aggravation by walking stairs or performing a similar routine physical activity
D. At least one of the following occurs during headache:
 1. Nausea and/or vomiting
 2. Photophobia and phonophobia
E. At least one of the following is true:
 1. History, physical, and neurologic examinations do not suggest one of the disorders listed in groups 5 through 11.
 2. History and/or physical and/or neurologic examinations do suggest such disorder, but it is ruled out by appropriate investigations.
 3. Such disorder is present, but migraine attacks do not occur for the first time in close temporal relation to the disorder.

tacks must be associated with at least one of the following: (1) nausea, (2) vomiting, or (3) photophobia and phonophobia. With these criteria, no single characteristic is mandatory for a diagnosis of migraine. A patient who has severe pain aggravated by routine activity, photophobia, and phonophobia meets these criteria, as does the more typical patient with unilateral throbbing pain and nausea.

Migraine usually lasts several hours or the entire day. When the migraine persists for longer than 3 days, the term *status migrainosus* is used. The frequency of attacks varies widely from a few per lifetime to several per week.[9] The average migraineur has one to three headaches per month.[3] A precise location ascribed to migraine, such as unilateral or temporal, is misleading, for as Wolff[24] wrote:

> The sites of migraine are notably temporal, supraorbital, frontal, retrobulbar, parietal, postauricular, and occipital . . . They may as well occur in the malar region, in the upper and lower teeth, at the base of the nose, in the median wall of the orbit, in the neck, and in the region of the common carotid arteries and down as far as the tip of the shoulder.

The prodromes of common migraine are vague, preceding the attack by hours or days, and include psychic disturbances (such as depression or hypomania), gastrointestinal manifestations, and changes in fluid balance. Usually the onset of the common migraine headache is unilateral, but the pain often becomes holocephalic. In an individual patient the headache is commonly more prominent on a single side, with occasional or rare alternation. Some patients always experience a unilateral headache, whereas in approximately one third the headache is diffuse from onset. The character of the headache is traditionally described as throbbing, but this may be a feature only at onset, with the discomfort soon changing to a steady ache. Patients can often relieve unilateral headache by compressing the carotid or temporal artery, only to experience resurgence of the pain after releasing pressure.

Nausea in some degree almost always accompanies common migraine. Vomiting can occur at the height of an attack, sometimes with relief of the headache, but more often only signals an intensifying phase of the episode, which continues for many minutes or hours. Usually the migraine sufferer becomes pallid and seeks seclusion, darkness, quiet, and a cold towel or ice bag for the head. Frequently at the time of nausea with vomiting, a diuretic phase with polyuria ensues, the consequence of fluid retention that occurred in the hours or days preceding the acute headache.

Ocular signs and symptoms may occur in common migraine, such as conjunctival injection, periorbital swelling, excessive tearing, foreign body sensation, and photophobia; however, these phenomena are more prominent in cluster headache.

TABLE 16–3. Migraine with Aura

1.2 Migraine with aura

Previously used terms: classic migraine; classical migraine; ophthalmic, hemiparesthetic, hemiplegic, or aphasic migraine

Diagnostic criteria

A. At least two attacks fulfill B
B. At least three of the following four characteristics are present:
   1. One or more fully reversible aura symptoms indicate focal cerebral cortical and/or brainstem dysfunction.
   2. At least one aura symptom develops gradually over more than 4 min, or two or more symptoms occur in succession.
   3. No aura symptom lasts more than 60 min; if more than one aura symptom is present, accepted duration is proportionally increased.
   4. Headache follows aura with a free interval of less than 60 min (it may also begin before or simultaneously with the aura).
C. At least one of the following is present:
   1. History, physical, and neurologic examinations do not suggest one of the disorders listed in groups 5 through 11.
   2. History and/or physical and/or neurologic examinations do suggest such a disorder, but it is ruled out by appropriate investigations.
   3. Such a disorder is present, but migraine attacks do not occur for the first time in close temporal relation to the disorder.

1.2.1 Migraine with typical aura

Diagnostic criteria

A. Fulfills criteria for 1.2, including all four criteria listed under B
B. One or more aura symptoms of the following types are present:
   1. Homonymous visual disturbance
   2. Unilateral paresthesias and/or numbness
   3. Unilateral weakness
   4. Aphasia or unclassifiable speech difficulty

MIGRAINE WITH AURA (CLASSIC)

Diagnosis of migraine with aura, the new term for classic migraine, requires at least two attacks with any three of the following four features (Table 16–3): (1) one or more fully reversible aura symptoms; (2) aura developing over a course of more than 4 minutes; (3) aura lasting less than 60 minutes; and (4) headache following aura within 60 minutes. Migraine with aura has a more well-defined clinical constellation compared with migraine without aura. The episodes are characterized by definite prodrome or aura, which is usually a visual sensation; however, sometimes motor or other sensory phenomena precede the headache. The headaches of classic migraine tend to be more compact and intense, rarely lasting more than 12 hours (usually 2 to 3 hours).

Many general characteristics are shared by common and classic migraine. Both varieties affect men and women and can occur at any age, often seemingly triggered by a significant event, such as puberty, school graduation, or marriage. A family history is usually present both in classic and common migraine, and there may be an earlier history of colic as a baby or car sickness as a small child. The full history of a complete migraineur would include migraine with aura in the teens, migraine without aura with nausea and vomiting in the second and third decades, followed by simple periodic headache or isolated migrainous auras in later life.

Migraine with aura is subclassified as follows: migraine with typical aura (homonymous visual disturbance, unilateral numbness or weakness, or aphasia); migraine with prolonged aura (or lasting longer than 60 minutes); familial hemiplegic migraine; basilar migraine; migraine without headache; and migraine with acute-onset aura.

The primary feature of migraine with aura is the visual aura. Extensive reviews of this phenomenon are found throughout the literature.[4,5,24,41–43] Although many variations occur, the following description by Richards[44] summarizes the most common type of visual phenomenon (Figs. 16–2 and 16–3):

> The visual disturbance usually precedes the headache . . . [it] begins near the center of the visual field as a small gray area with indefinite boundaries. If this area first appears during reading, as it often does, then the migraine is first noticed when words are lost in a region

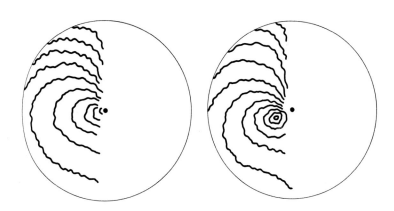

Fig. 16–2. Successive arcs expand across half of visual field, as shown in two diagrams based on Airy. The spectra may take 20 to 25 minutes to expand from a fuzzy gray area near the fixation point (*dot*) to the outer limit of the visual field. (Richards W: The fortification illusions of migraines. Sci Am 224:88, 1971)

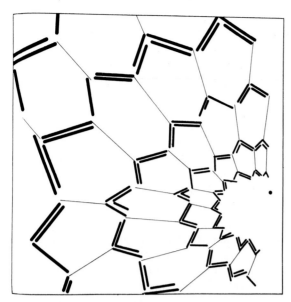

Fig. 16–3. Emerging honeycomb pattern from plotting data derived from visual phenomena in migraine subjects. Honeycomb and tendency for inner angle between lines to approximate 60° suggest a hexagonal organization of occipital cortical cells. (Richards W: The fortification illusions of migraine. Sci Am 224:88, 1971)

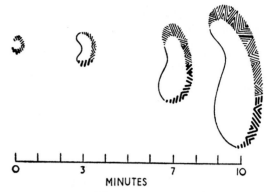

MINUTES

Fig. 16–4. Successive maps of a scintillating scotoma to show characteristic distribution of the fortification figures. (Modified from Lashley KS: Patterns of cerebral integration indicated by scotomas of migraine. Arch Neurol Psychiatry 46:333, 1941. Copyright © 1941, American Medical Association)

of "shaded darkness." During the next few minutes the gray area slowly expands into a horseshoe with bright zigzag lines appearing at the expanding outer edge. These lines are small at first and grow as the blind area expands and moves outward toward the periphery of the visual field.

One important aspect of the visual disturbance just described is that it expands slowly, over a period of 10 to 20 minutes. The initial region of visual abnormality is most often near fixation and then, as described by Lashley,[39] "with increase in size the disturbed area moves or 'drifts' across the visual field so that its central margin withdraws from the macular region as its peripheral margin invades the temporal . . . the area may be totally blind (negative scotoma), amblyopic or outlined by scintillations."

The scintillations surrounding the negative scotoma make "fortification" figures or spectrums, so called because of the appearance of a "map of the bastions of a fortified town."[39] The scintillations are brilliant, with the intensity of a bright fluorescent bulb flickering at a rate of 5 to 10 cycles/second (Figs. 16–4 and 16–5).

Gowers,[45] commenting on the descriptions by the British astronomer Sir George Airy and his physician son Dr. Hubert Airy (both migraineurs), was particularly impressed with the intensity of the visual sensation. Many migraine sufferers can recall their own vivid visual experiences well enough to describe them precisely or even, on occasion, to paint them (Figs. 16–6 and 16–7). Not all migraine visual disturbances begin near the fixa-

tion point: some patients consistently experience scotomas starting eccentrically in the visual field, and these sensations can appear alternately or simultaneously in both hemifields (Fig. 16–8). Other less dramatic visual auras also occur: just the sensation of peripheral brightness or awareness of a rhythmicity or pulsating character in the intensity of the ambient light. The duration of these visual symptoms is measured in minutes rather than the brief few seconds of flashing, bright moving spots or transient flickering phenomena characteristic of occipital epileptic discharges.[6,45] Additional visual disturbances categorized by Klee and Willanger[42] consist of metamorphopsia, diplopia, polyopia, and apparent movement of stationary objects. Variations in the scotomas of migraine, including their occurrence in patients with acquired blindness, are well described.[41,46]

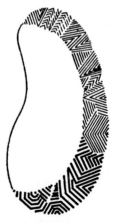

Fig. 16–5. Variations in fortification figures. Coarser and more complicated figures are generally in lower part of field. (Lashley KS: Patterns of cerebral integration indicated by scotomas of migraine. Arch Neurol Psychiatry 46:333, 1941; copyright © 1941, American Medical Association)

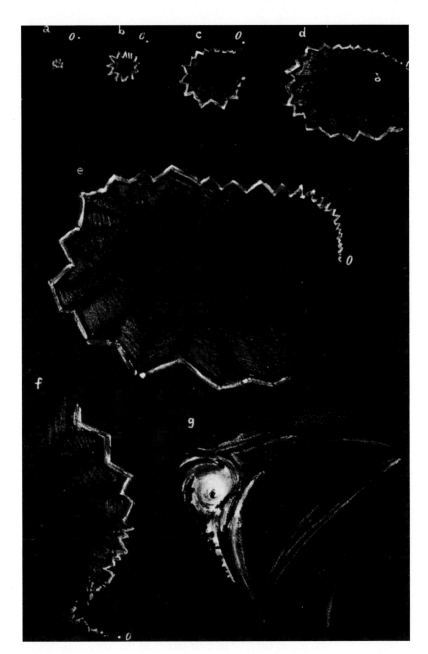

Fig. 16–6. Left-sided fortification spectrum of migraine. Illustration by Dr. Hubert Airy of his own scotomas. A bright stellate object (*a*) appeared suddenly below and to the left side of fixation (*o*). It rapidly enlarged, first as a circular zigzag, but on the inner side the zigzag was faint (*b*); as arc increased in size, it was broken centrally (*c*). In *d*, original circular outline had become oval. Rectangular lines that made up the fortification spectrum became longer as the process extended peripherally. When spectrum had extended through greater portion of the field (*e*), upper portion also began to expand (*f*). At this time the lower part of spectrum disappeared. The phenomenon ended in a whirling focus of light (*g*) 20 minutes after it began. At this time a headache appeared on the right side. (Gowers WR: Visual sensations in migraine. In Subjective Sensations of Sight and Sound: Abiotrophy and Other Lectures. London, Churchill, 1907)

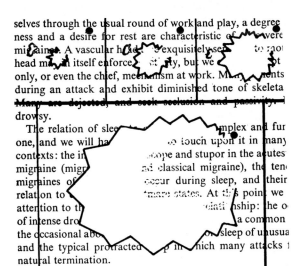

selves through the usual round of work and play, a degree
ness and a desire for rest are characteristic of ... were
migraines. A vascular h... exquisitely se... to ...
head m... in itself enforce... ...ly, but we ... ...t
only, or even the chief, me...ism at work. M... ...ents
during an attack and exhibit diminished tone of skeleta
~~Many are dejected, and seek seclusion and passivity~~
drowsy.

The relation of slee... ...mplex and fur
one, and we will ha... ... touch upon it in many
contexts: the i... ...ope and stupor in the acutes
migraine (migr... ...classical migraine), the ten...
migraines of ... ...ccur during sleep, and their
relation to ... ...more states. At this point we
attention to t... ...ship: the o
of intense dro... ...a common
the occasional ab... ...sleep of unusua
and the typical pro... ...p in which many attacks
natural termination.

Nowhere in the literature can we find more vivid and
descriptions of migrainous stupor than in Liveing's monogr

Fig. 16–7. Inhibitory character within angled oval of an expanding fortification spectrum. Outside the limiting line, vision is preserved; within it, vision is lost. This occurs at first over the whole area; afterwards, when the sphere is broken and has become oval, loss is most intense close to the limiting line and becomes less toward the middle. (Gowers WR: Visual sensations in migraine. In Subjective Sensations of Sight and Sound: Abiotrophy and Other Lectures. London, Churchill, 1907)

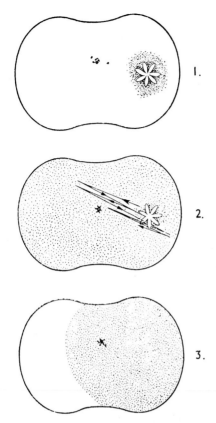

Fig. 16–8. Radial movement of a visual stellate object that itself remained unchanged throughout the episode. Stellate form appeared near edge of right half of field just below the horizontal and consisted of approximately six pointed leaf-like projections alternately red and blue. It appeared on a small area of darkness, moved slowly toward the left and upward, passing above the fixation point to beyond the middle line. Then it returned to its starting place, retraced this path once or twice and passed to the right edge of the field, suddenly disappearing at the spot where it began. (Gowers WR: Visual sensations in migraine. In Subjective Sensations of Sight and Sound: Abiotrophy and Other Lectures. London, Churchill, 1907)

The auras of migraine, although most commonly only visual, have many other associated manifestations, such as hemihypesthesias, perioral anesthesia, vertigo, and transient aphasia. The auras or prodromes of classic migraine may be precipitated by intense stimuli: bright lights, loud noises, head trauma, or the intake of certain foods in susceptible individuals.

In the usual sequence of migraine with aura, the sensory prodrome precedes the onset of the headache (in accord with the traditional concept of vasoconstriction followed by vasodilatation). In rare instances, the visual disturbance may have a simultaneous onset with headache or, once having disappeared, may recur following the onset of headache. Such unusual patterns, or strict unilaterality for all attacks, should increase suspicion of a mass lesion or vascular malformation. As opposed to definite periodicity with symptom-free intervals and

predictable circumstances, as in migraine without aura, migraine with aura may occur "out of the blue" and in multiple attacks over a few days.

Migraine with aura attacks tend to diminish in the third and fourth decades. Although most migraine patients experience a stereotypic clinical pattern, there is a well-recognized group who have an admixture of both classic and common migraine attacks.[47] Some patients with classic migraine may lose the headache component eventually and experience only isolated auras thereafter. This monosymptomatic pattern stresses the importance of taking an accurate history of patients presenting with isolated visual phenomena (migraine dissociée). Haas[48] emphasized the occurrence of *migraine aura status*. The differential diagnosis should include consideration of vertebrobasilar transient ischemic attacks. Symptomatology that favors migraine has been reviewed by Fisher,[49] and includes luminous visual images, build-up of images, progression from one aura to another, and benign outcome.

MIGRAINE WITH PROLONGED AURA AND MIGRAINOUS INFARCTIONS

In the new classification of migraine, subtype 1.6 indicates complications of migraine. This includes all of the permanent defects discussed in this section.

Focal symptoms and signs of the aura may persist beyond a headache phase. In the previous classification, this was termed "complicated migraine." It is now defined by the IHS classification with two labels with increased specificity. If the aura lasts for longer than 1 hour but less than 1 week, the term *migraine with prolonged aura* is applied. If the signs persist for more than 1 week or a neuroimaging procedure demonstrates a stroke, a *migrainous infarction* has occurred. As pointed out previously, in mid or later life the aura may not be followed by headache and has been termed *migraine accompagnée* or *migraine dissociée*. Migraine with aura (classic) in early reports was sometimes referred to as "ophthalmic migraine" (to be differentiated from ophthalmoplegic migraine, a subtype of migraine with aura).

Cerebral Migraine

A variety of cerebral symptoms may occur in migraine with aura, including motor, visual, and other sensory defects. As pointed out previously, if the aura lasts for more than 1 hour, but less than 1 week, the term migraine with prolonged aura is applied. If, however, the signs persist for more than 1 week or a neuroimaging procedure shows a stroke, the term *migrainous infarction* is used. Welch[16] classified migraine-related stroke into four subtypes (Table 16–4), briefly described as follows:

TABLE 16–4. Classification of Migraine-Related Stroke

Category	Feature
I	Coexisting stroke and migraine
II	Stroke with clinical features of migraine
	A. Symptomatic migraine
	B. Migraine mimic
III	Migraine-induced stroke
	A. Without risk factors
	B. With risk factors
IV	Uncertain

I. *Coexisting stroke and migraine:* A clearly defined clinical stroke syndrome must occur remotely in time from a typical migraine attack. Stoke in the young is rare; in contrast, migraine is common. As pointed out by Welch, the two conditions should coexist, but migraine should not be a contributing risk factor for stroke.

II. *Stroke with clinical features of migraine:* A structural lesion that is unrelated to migraine pathogenesis presents with clinical features of a migraine attack.

   A. *Subtype A (symptomatic migraine):* In these patients, established structural central nervous system (CNS) lesions or cerebral vessels cause episodic symptoms typical of migraine with neurologic aura, although infrequently. Cerebral arteriovenous malformation (AVM) exemplifies this concept and may masquerade as migraine with aura.[6,50]

   B. *Subtype B (migraine mimic):* In this category, stroke caused by acute and progressive structural disease is accompanied by headache and a constellation of progressive neurologic signs and symptoms. These situations are difficult to distinguish from those of migraine, hence the term *migraine mimic*. The diagnosis can be most difficult in patients who continue to have migraine late in life, when the incident of cerebrovascular disease increases.[16]

III. *Migraine-induced stroke:* For this diagnosis, the following criteria must be met:

   A. Neurologic deficit must be identical to the migraine symptoms of previous attacks.

   B. The stroke must occur during the course of a typical migraine attack.

   C. All other causes of stroke must be excluded, although stroke risk factors may be present.

IV. *Uncertain classification:* Welch has indicated that many migraine-related strokes cannot be categorized with certainty. For example, the IHS definition of migraine-induced stroke does not prevent the diagnosis in patients with migraine without aura. Migraine-induced stroke associated with treatment of the attack is appropriately classified

in this category. In addition, there are occasional cases of migraine-like symptoms and persistent neurologic deficit associated with cerebrospinal fluid protein and pleocytosis.[51,52] Other rare syndromes and types of migraine-related stroke include migraine associated with mitochondrial encephalopathies[53] and "migraine coma."[54] Intracerebral hemorrhage has been reported[55]; according to Welch, most of these cases are subtype B (migraine mimic). Whether antiphospholipid antibodies play a role is still to be determined.[56]

Permanent homonymous visual field defects are well documented in migraine patients.[43,57–59] The defects almost always occur in patients who have previously had migrainous attacks with transient scintillating scotomas. Computed tomography (CT) and magnetic resonance imaging (MRI) of the cranium have documented a number of cerebral infarctions, usually in the occipital and parietal regions. Rothrock and associates[60] evaluated 22 patients with migraine-associated stroke: 91% were women, and 23% had a prior history of presumed migrainous stroke. They concluded that extracranial and intracranial vasospasm played a major role in some cases that were documented angiographically. One controlled study of migraine with aura reported that 91% of patients who had stroke during an attack had no arterial lesions. This is in contrast to 9% of classic migraine patients who had a stroke remote from a migraine attack, and 18% of patients who had a stroke without a history of migraine.[61] In a rigorous case-controlled study, no overall association between migraine and ischemic stroke was found, but among women younger than 45 years, migraine and stroke were significantly associated; the risk was increased four fold, and it became even greater in women who smoked.[62]

According to Hollenhorst,[63] approximately 4% of patients who have a typical sequence of visual aura followed by hemicranial headache experience transient hemianopsia lasting up to 15 minutes. Much rarer are patients with permanent hemianopia. Bilateral upper quadrantic defects have been reported.[64,65]

Other sensory disturbances, such as paresthesias, particularly involve hands, fingers, and lips.[64–66] Various aspects of cerebral migraine with aura are illustrated by the following case history:

A 26-year-old woman was seen with a complaint of difficulty with vision. She had a history of migraine since age 12, characterized by an aura of "black spots" slowly spreading over the field of vision for 20 minutes, occasionally accompanied by numbness in the right hand and arm. Thereafter, throbbing headache would occur that was left-sided 90% of the time. Her father had a history of classic migraine as a young man. Ten days before first being seen, she had a typical attack of migraine, but with persistent difficulty in vision following the episode. Examination was entirely normal except for a congruous right

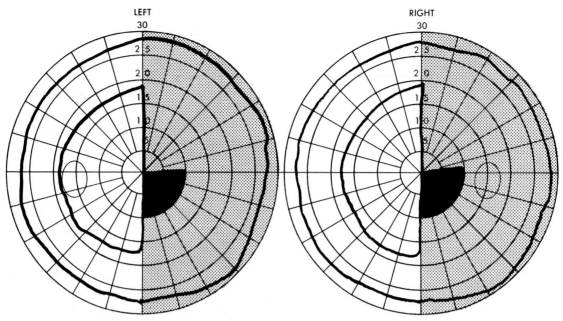

Fig. 16–9. Visual field defect in complicated migraine. Defect cleared completely. Visual acuity 20/20 OU. Relative homonymous hemianopia (2, 5/1000 w; scotoma out to 30/1000 w).

homonymous visual field defect (Fig. 16–9). Ten days later, she again developed her visual aura, but with a moderate right hemiparesis as well, during her headache. Brain scan and cerebral arteriography were normal. During the next week all neurologic abnormality, including her visual field defect, cleared completely.

Frequently a disturbance of language occurs with migraine, as pointed out by Sir George Airy in 1865, who described his own inability to speak during an attack.

A typical history related to me by my brother is as follows:

> While reading, I become aware that I am unable to understand what I have just read. After rereading a paragraph two or three times, I begin to realize that I cannot understand the sense of words. The letters can be identified but the words are unintelligible . . . At this point, a numb feeling occurs in my right hand and I finally realize that I am at the start of another migraine attack.

A wide variety of language difficulties, sensory defects, and motor abnormalities have been described (most often transient, but in rare instances permanent) from presumed cerebral infarction. Caplan and co-workers[67] reported on 12 patients with transient global amnesia and prior migraine; in 3 patients, the classic migrainous phenomenon accompanied the amnestic attack.

Electroencephalographic (EEG) findings are variable.[65,68,69] There is general lack of agreement as to the incidence and significance of abnormalities in the EEGs of patients with migraine. Some authors report a normal EEG,[70] but various abnormal patterns have been recorded.[68,69] In a detailed review of 560 migraine patients, Hockaday and Whitty[71] found an EEG abnormality rate

of 61%. The highest frequency of abnormality occurred in patients with transient lateralized motor or sensory auras.

Friedman[72] was the first to report the results of angiography during an attack of migraine; there were no abnormalities. Although the majority of patients in reported cases have normal arteriograms, others have demonstrated some abnormality during an attack (see Cluster Headache section). Some, however, believe angiography places patients with migraine[43,73] at increased risk, and the procedure has not yet provided useful information on the pathophysiology of complicated migraine.[74–76]

Hemiplegic migraine occurs both sporadically and as a familial syndrome. This entity is defined as a "vascular headache," featuring sensory and motor phenomena that persist during and (for a brief time) after the headache.[77] A narrower view would be to use the term "hemiplegic migraine" when there is only motor involvement (*i.e.*, weakness, paralysis).

The first mention of transient hemiparesis during an attack of migraine was made by Liveing,[4] and multiple reviews and case reports have appeared since.[78,79] Heyck[80] reviewed the neurologic complications of 980 of 3890 patients with migraine. The majority of these patients complained of unilateral tingling or numbness that invariably involved the hand and sometimes spread to the arm, face, and tongue, and in rare cases to the leg. The symptoms seldom lasted more than 30 minutes and could occur before or at the peak of the headache. Twelve of these patients had unilateral motor disturbances ranging from minimal loss of function to complete paralysis. There have been few permanent sequelae attributed to hemiplegic migraine; progressive dementia and permanent hemiplegia have been reported.[65,74,80]

Reports of hemiplegic migraine in the literature seem to indicate that most cases are familial. Heyck,[74] however, pointed out the tendency to report familial cases: if unselected patients with the syndrome are reviewed, most do not occur in families with hemiplegic migraine, but rather in "families with ordinary migraine as often as common or classic migraine." Familial hemiplegic migraine is well documented,[78,81,82] at times in kindred with associated neuro-ophthalmologic findings, such as retinal degeneration and nystagmus.[83] In an interesting report, Dooling and Sweeney[84] described a blind woman whose attacks were precipitated by breastfeeding her infant. This led to the speculation that oxytocin (chemically similar to ergotamine) could exercise a complex effect on cerebral vessels predisposed to vasospasm.

Ophthalmoplegic Migraine

In this rare variety of complicated migraine, the headaches are associated with ocular motor nerve palsies.[85,86] Although the ophthalmoplegia is usually transient, it can become permanent, especially after repeated attacks. Major controversy has surrounded the diagnostic and nosologic position of ophthalmoplegic migraine since its initial recognition in the mid 1880s. A detailed review of the early history of the disorder is admirably presented by Bruyn.[66] Until the 1930s and 1940s, when angiography was introduced and practiced, it was impossible in many cases to rule out aneurysms and other lesions in the vicinity of the cavernous sinus. Multiple etiologies were cited as underlying causes of "ophthalmoplegic migraine," including aneurysm, basilar arachnoiditis, and tumors. Indeed, many physicians believed that no separate clinical syndrome of ophthalmoplegic migraine existed, but that all patients had specific organic lesions.

As pointed out by Walsh and Hoyt,[43] "at the root of the problem has been a lack of strict criteria for the clinical diagnosis of ophthalmoplegic migraine and insufficient knowledge of the pathophysiologic events that occur during a migraine attack." Walsh and O'Doherty[87] presented specific criteria for the diagnosis of the syndrome:

1. A history of typical migraine headache: a severe throbbing headache, usually unilateral, but occasionally bilateral or alternating. It is typically of the crescendo type, and may last several hours or days.
2. Ophthalmoplegia including one or more nerves and possibly alternating sides with attacks. Extraocular muscle paralysis may occur with the first attack of headache or, rarely, precede it. However, the paralysis usually appears subsequent to an established migraine pattern.
3. Other causes must be excluded by arteriography, surgical exploration, or autopsy.

Alpers and Yaskin[75] presented the case of a patient with this clinical syndrome in whom no organic lesion was found at autopsy. Additional cases that fulfill all the clinical criteria for ophthalmoplegic migraine have been recorded.[88-90]

In a review of 5000 migraine patients, Friedman and associates[91] found 8 patients with ophthalmoplegic migraine, thus attesting to its rarity. All eight patients (five male, three female) had periodic migraine headaches and unilateral ophthalmoplegia. Three patients had persistent ophthalmoplegia after years, and one had a definite family history of migraine. Six patients had arteriograms during the attacks; all results were normal. The details of this review are listed below:

Number of attacks: four patients with 20+ attacks; two patients with 5 to 10 attacks; two patients with less than 5 attacks; and 1 patient with a single attack
Age at onset: 2, 2, 3, 3, 5, 8, 17, and 30 years
Clinical findings: Oculomotor paresis in all patients; pupillary involvement in seven
Pain: Always on same side as ophthalmoplegia
Paresis: Occurred 3 to 5 days after onset of headache in six patients
Recovery: 1 to 4 weeks
Arteriogram: Normal during attack in six of six patients
Therapy: Limited success

In most patients with well-defined cases, the onset of ophthalmoplegia occurs before age 10.

Woody and Blaw[92] reported two cases of ophthalmoplegic migraine occurring in infants 5 and 7 months old. The infants had recurrent attacks with almost complete clearing between episodes. During subsequent attacks both children were treated with prednisone, which seemed to shorten the duration of the episodes.

In ophthalmoplegic migraine, the third nerve is most frequently involved. Walsh and Hoyt[43] stated that abducens palsy occurs one tenth as frequently as third nerve palsy, with even rarer affliction of the fourth nerve. In most cases there is a negative family history. Thus, a typical clinical syndrome emerges: (1) a child or young adult with periodic headache has ophthalmoplegia involving all functions of the third nerve, beginning at the height of an attack of cephalgia, which is primarily unilateral and in the orbital region; (2) the paresis lasts for days to weeks after the cessation of headache; and (3) recovery is gradual and tends to be less complete after repeated attacks. The following case report is considered exemplary:

A 3-year-old boy presented with a complete left oculomotor palsy. The day before, he had complained of head-

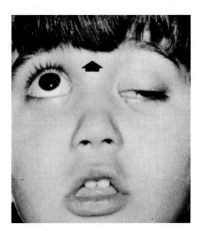

Fig. 16–10. Third nerve paresis in 3-year-old boy with ophthalmoplegic migraine. Pupil was sluggishly reactive to light. Note failure of elevation, abducted position of left eye, and ptosis.

ache, was lethargic, and went to bed early. The following morning he awakened with complete ptosis of the left upper lid, but his headache was gone. On examination, the left pupil was 6 mm and slightly reactive to light; all muscles supplied by the left third nerve were profoundly affected (Fig. 16–10). The neurologic examination and plain skull x-rays were entirely normal. The child recovered completely in 3 weeks. A similar episode occurred 20 months later, also with rapid spontaneous resolution, and a third episode occurred 1 year after that. The child is now well and has only occasional headaches.

In the differential diagnosis, consideration should be given to aneurysm, tumor, diabetes, and sphenoid sinus mucocele. The age at onset, negative glucose tolerance test, and radiologic studies will usually rule out the listed possibilities. Other clinical entities confused with ophthalmoplegic migraine have included myasthenia gravis and Tolosa-Hunt syndrome. The former condition is ruled out if the pupil is involved (and actually should not be considered in the presence of pain) and with response to edrophonium chloride (Tensilon); the latter possibility should be considered if pain persists. On rare occasions, there is only limited involvement of the third nerve.

Reports of transient, otherwise unexplained unilateral pupillary mydriasis have been tentatively attributed to migraine in young patients.[93–95] One should be careful to exclude intermittent angle-closure glaucoma with mydriasis, as pointed out by Sarkies and colleagues.[96] They reported on a 31-year-old man with an 18-month history of episodic periorbital pain who, during an attack, noted blurred vision and a dilated pupil. He was found to have a sector palsy in the upper nasal quadrant of the left iris, an intraocular pressure of 16 mmHg between attacks, and on gonioscopy a narrow angle with a plateau-type iris. During an attack, his intraocular pressure increased to 26 mmHg. After a provocative dark-room test, a typical headache developed; the patient was found to have an intraocular pressure of 45 mmHg and

a closed angle on gonioscopy. This report is important because it points out a condition that must be eliminated before considering episodic mydriasis with ocular pain to be a part of ophthalmoplegic migraine.

Rarely, ophthalmoplegic migraine may occur without headache. Durkan and associates[97] described two children with isolated, recurrent, painless oculomotor palsy in whom neurodiagnostic investigations were all normal.

In the differential diagnosis, suspicion would be raised by (1) the absence of a migraine history; (2) severe, persistent headache with total ophthalmoplegia; (3) onset after age 20; and (4) symptoms and signs of subarachnoid hemorrhage. Angiography is not warranted in a young patient who strictly fulfills the clinical criteria. Because this is a diagnosis of exclusion, noninvasive imaging tests such as MRI or magnetic resonance angiography (MRA) should be performed in all cases to exclude the possibility of aneurysm.[86] The finding of an entirely normal MRI in a child with a third cranial nerve palsy after a 4-day history of headache, who is otherwise well, should complete the workup. This is because aneurysmal third nerve palsies are extremely rare in children younger than 14 years of age.[98] In third nerve palsy involving pupillomotor function, however, serious consideration should be given to angiography. The usual cause will be a posterior communicating artery aneurysm, which is best excluded by conventional angiography; however, newer techniques (*e.g.*, MRA, spiral contrast-enhanced CT) may soon provide sufficient resolution to exclude aneurysm as a cause.[86]

The pathophysiology of ophthalmoplegic migraine remains obscure. Theories include swelling of the posterior cerebral artery, pituitary swelling, vascular anomaly with compression of the third nerve, and unilateral brain swelling. None of these theories has been documented, and cerebral angiography is unrevealing. Walsh and O'Doherty[87] suggested that a swollen intracavernous carotid artery would compress adjacent cranial nerves within the cavernous sinus. Such swelling would also narrow the vessel, which they attempted to document angiographically. Subsequent negative arteriograms during attacks, however, do not support this theory.[91] In Nigeria, ophthalmoplegic migraine has been associated with an abnormal hemoglobin.[99]

Ideally, prophylactic therapy would prevent the occurrence of repeated episodes and prevent the development of permanent eye muscle palsies, but reports suggest that therapy has met with only limited success.[91] A trial with calcium channel blockers (*e.g.*, verapamil) or β-blockers (*e.g.*, propranolol [Inderal], methysergide maleate [Sansert]) may be warranted if the attacks are frequent.

Retinal Migraine

The IHS code for retinal migraine is 1.4. According to the Headache Classification Committee, retinal migraine consists of repeated attacks of monocular scotoma or blindness that lasts less than 1 hour and is associated with headache. Other ocular or structural vascular disorders must be ruled out. Additional terms include ocular migraine, anterior visual pathway migraine, and ophthalmic migraine. This condition may be broadly defined as a transient or permanent monocular visual disturbance accompanying a migraine attack or occurring in a person with a strong history of migrainous episodes. One term applicable to all such attacks would be "ocular migraine"; however, to include optic nerve dysfunction as well, a more general term such as "anterior visual pathway migraine" may be preferable. This last phrase would include reported defects such as ischemic papillitis, retinal hemorrhage, vitreous hemorrhage, central serous retinopathy, pigmentary changes of the retina, and optic nerve atrophy.

Retinal migraine occurs more frequently than ophthalmoplegic migraine. We estimate that the frequency of strictly monocular visual phenomena occurring in conjunction with migraine is 1 in 200 migraine sufferers. Frequently, however, homonymous visual field phenomena in migraineurs is incorrectly attributed to a single eye. For example, a patient with transient right homonymous hemianopia might think that the right eye is affected, because normally the right temporal hemifield is 30° to 40° larger than the left nasal hemifield.[100]

The exact genetic predisposition to this subtype of migraine headache is unknown. The familial occurrence is similar to that expected in all patients with migraine preceded by visual aura (i.e., familial history is positive in an estimated 25% of cases). Retinal migraine is expected to be more common in women than men, which is true of migraine headaches in general, but this also has not be documented.

There are two forms of anterior visual pathway migraine: (1) transient monocular blindness; and (2) permanent unilateral visual loss, a much less common occurrence. The transient form has a relatively stereotypic presentation, consistent with retinal or optic nerve hypoperfusion from spasm of the central retinal or ophthalmic artery. For example, 10 of 24 patients reported by Tomsak and Jergens[101] described concentric contraction of vision, and only 5 of their patients had an altitudinal or quadratic visual change consistent with spasm of the retinal artery branch. Kline and Kelley[102] studied a patient with a history of cluster headache and documented a reduction in central retinal artery blood flow during an attack of ocular migraine by intravenous fluorescein angiography. They noted no change in choroidal perfusion, also suggesting selective spasm of the central retinal artery. Others have noted retinal artery constriction during episodes of migrainous transient monocular blindness[103,104] or normal arterial caliber.[105] It is of interest to note that in the case reported by Wolter and Burchfield,[105] a review of the fundus photographs depicts venous vasoconstriction as well as retinal opacification during an episode (Fig. 16–11). Recently, Burger and co-workers[106] reported amaurosis fugax episodes due to documented vascular constriction in the retina. These cases did not involve retinal migraine, but demonstrated the ability of retinal vascular constriction to produce monocular episodes of amaurosis in the absence of embolic phenomena.

Permanent unilateral visual loss from anterior visual path migraine is well documented, but uncommon. In addition to arterial or venous retinal vascular occlusions,[72,104,107,108] central serous retinopathy, vitreous hemorrhage, retinal hemorrhage, and ischemic optic neuropathy have been noted.[109,110] Newman and colleagues[111] reported bilateral central retinal artery occlusions, disk drusen, and migraine, and other descriptions of anterior visual path migraine and vascular retinopathy have been

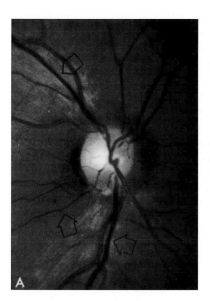
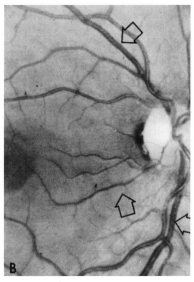

Fig. 16–11. Retinal migraine. **A.** During amaurotic episode. Note dusky appearance of fundus, increased retinal opacity (edema?), and dark, narrowed veins (*arrows*). Disc is hyperemic. **B.** Fundus after episode. Note normal caliber of veins (*arrows*). (Courtesy of Dr. J Reimer Wolter)

reported.[112,113] A recent unconfirmed report suggested that up to one third of migraineurs are found to have visual field defects of the retinal or optic nerve type when tested with automated perimetry.[114]

Clinical Features of Retinal Migraine

The IHS diagnostic criteria for retinal migraine are as follows:

A. At least two attacks fulfilling criteria B and C
B. Fully reversible monocular scotoma or blindness lasting less than 60 minutes and confirmed by examination during attack or (after proper instruction) by patient's drawing of monocular field defect during an attack
C. Headache following visual symptoms with a free interval of less than 60 minutes, but sometimes preceding them
D. Normal ophthalmologic examination outside of attack; embolism ruled out by appropriate investigations

A typical history is that of a young adult with a pattern of common or classic migraine, who has recurrent episodes of monocular visual loss or monocular scintillating scotomas. The visual loss is often one-sided, stereotypic in nature, and tends to affect the entire monocular visual field,[101] although any of the visual patterns described in migraine with aura may occur on a monocular basis in "retinal" migraine. Carroll[115] suggested that such transient episodes never have a preceding fortification spectra, that the *absence of accompanying headache was invariable, and that the visual disturbance never lasted more than 10 minutes. Permanent visual loss is the exception rather than the rule. Transient anterior visual pathway migraine is not associated with other neurologic symptoms, but may be precipitated by postural change or exercise. Approximately one third of patients have a prior history of migraine.*[101]

Ocular migraine as a cause of transient monocular blindness should be a diagnosis of exclusion. This was highlighted by a recent case in which a young medical student had episodes of amaurosis fugax, occasionally accompanied by headache, and was considered to have retinal migraine. He turned out to have a large pituitary tumor![116]

Walsh and Hoyt[43] stated that "the eye itself can be involved in the angiospastic circulatory disturbance of a migraine attack" and that subsequent visual disturbance is due to retinal hypoxia. The retinal arterioles have been reported by some authors[43,103] to be constricted during such an episode, or to be normal despite an ischemic retina.[105]

McDonald and Sanders[117] presented a case of ischemic papillopathy in migraine, in which a migraine patient had sudden monocular visual loss after experiencing multiple bouts of transient amaurosis of the same eye. A typical nerve fiber bundle defect was present on visual field testing, and fluorescein angiography showed areas of delayed choroidal filling in the peripapillary region.

Typical case histories of "retinal migraine" are presented below:

CASE HISTORY 1. The patient was a 22-year-old college student who complained of decreased vision in the left eye. He had a 7-year history of classic migraine headaches, which had been much less frequent in the previous 3 years. Three years before the examination, he awakened to discover decreased vision in the temporal quadrant of the left eye. One year later, he again noticed an abrupt onset of a negative scotoma in the inferior nasal periphery of the same eye. Neuro-ophthalmologic examination was normal except for a slight afferent pupillary defect in the left eye and the visual fields (Fig. 16–12A). Fundus photography revealed an absence of the nerve fiber bundle layer in the superior portion of the left optic disc corresponding to the inferior visual field defect demonstrated on perimetry (Fig. 16–12B).

CASE HISTORY 2. A 24-year-old right-handed carpenter complained of "blackouts" in the right eye occurring over the previous 3 months. The patient stated that he had nine episodes of diminished vision in the right eye unassociated with other neuro-ophthalmologic signs. These episodes began as a "blur" starting in the right temporal field and were characterized by distinct "lines and angles," or like "a fish net." There was a subjective appreciation of increased brightness during the phenomenon, but no particular color. As the effect intensified, the entire field of the right eye became gray such that the patient "could not see anything," and the vision subsequently diminished to bare perception of light. This sensation lasted 10 to 15 minutes and then slowly cleared in reverse fashion. There was no previous history of migraine, transient neurologic phenomena, or family history of migraine. His neurologic and neuro-ophthalmologic examinations were entirely normal. The patient appeared to have experienced a retinal migraine.

The pathogenesis of such episodes is not well defined. It would appear in most instances that the visual disturbances are due to constriction in either the central retinal artery or the ophthalmic artery, with resultant ischemia of the optic nerve or retina. One proponent of the argument that vasoconstriction occurs in vessels proximal to the retina itself is Laties,[118] who demonstrated the absence of adrenergic innervation to the intraocular branches of the central retinal artery. Additional clinical descriptions of anterior visual pathway migraine and vascular retinopathy associated with this condition are presented by Corbett[112] and Coppeto and associates.[119]

In general, the prognosis for retinal migraine is similar to that of migraine headache with typical aura. Recurrent attacks are expected with a variable interval. As the true incidence of retinal migraine is unknown, it is uncertain whether there is a higher incidence of permanent neuroretinal injury. The visual field data presented previously suggest that there is a higher incidence of end-arteriolar distribution infarction and a higher incidence of permanent visual field defects in retinal mi-

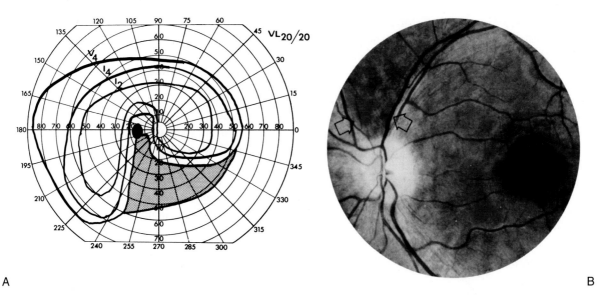

Fig. 16–12. Patient with permanent retinal nerve fiber bundle defect attributed to migraine. **A.** Visual field. **B.** Visible attenuation of retinal nerve fiber layer (*between arrows*) corresponding to field defect. Compare with visible nerve fibers entering inferior aspect of disc.

graine than in clinically manifest cerebral infarctions in migraine with aura.[114] In migraineurs with visual aura who are studied by MRI, however, there may be a higher incidence of cerebral infarctions than expected. In effect, these infarctions would be silent strokes revealed by neuroimaging that were clinically unsuspected. An infarction in the retina, however, is usually apparent to the patient.

A recent study of transient ischemic attacks in young patients, who comprise a large proportion of migraineurs, suggested a benign prognosis for stroke and myocardial infarction as long as other cardiovascular risk factors are not present.[120] Another study of retinal strokes in persons younger than 30 years of age found that 8 of 27 had migraine. Only two patients, however, had migraine as the *only* association; the others had other systemic and/or ocular risk factor as well.[121]

We believe that all patients with retinal migraine should be placed on prophylactic antimigrainous therapy, such as calcium channel blockers or β-blockers. There is a report of the salutary effects of isoproterenol inhalation on anterior visual pathway migraine and other migrainous visual phenomena,[122] but we have not had personal experience with this treatment. Newman and co-workers[111] reported bilateral central retinal artery occlusions, disk drusen, and migraine.

Basilar Artery Migraine

Basilar artery migraine is not a separate category in the new IHS classification, but it is described separately because of its clinical manifestations.

Bickerstaff[123] introduced the concept of basilar artery migraine, including the following symptomatology: bi-

lateral disturbance of vision, ataxia, dysarthria, vertigo, tinnitus, and facial or limb paresthesias, followed by a severe, throbbing headache, usually in the occipital region. Although a definite diagnosis of migraine was impossible to prove, the mode of onset, the associated headache, the relatively brief duration of the attack, the family history of migraine, the occurrence of other attacks more typically migrainous, and the absence of any neurologic abnormality between episodes made the diagnosis of migraine most likely. Of 34 described patients, 26 were adolescent girls. The symptoms lasted 2 to 45 minutes and then disappeared rapidly; however, if there had been complete loss of vision, this symptom disappeared more gradually, with a period of "graying" of vision. The attacks occurred infrequently, but tended to be associated with menses in the young girls. The episodes subside over ensuing years and are replaced by more common varieties of migraine.

The visual symptoms described included vivid flashes of light throughout the entire visual field, intense enough to obscure vision completely, and sudden bilateral visual loss occurring over seconds and persisting up to 15 minutes, with a gradual return of vision to normal. None of these patients' symptoms of brainstem ischemia were accompanied by the characteristic fortification spectra of classic migraine.

Later, Bickerstaff[124] described a group of patients in whom consciousness was impaired during attacks of migraine, and he suggested that the mechanism was transient ischemia of the reticular activating system of the brainstem secondary to vasomotor disturbance in the distribution of the basilar artery. Loss of consciousness in migraine was reviewed by Lees and Watkins,[125] with particular reference to the association between migraine and epilepsy. Basser,[126] in an analysis of 1800 migraine patients, demonstrated an increased incidence of epilepsy when compared with a control group. Bickerstaff[127] suggested that two mechanisms could lead to loss of consciousness in migraine: (1) brainstem ischemia of the reticular activating system; and (2) ischemia producing seizure in a potentially epileptic brain, the latter being much less common.

Basilar artery migraine is regarded as a rare but definite clinical variant of the migraine spectrum, with signs and symptoms similar to those seen in transient ischemic attacks of the posterior circulation, as observed in elderly patients with cerebrovascular disease. This syndrome occurs primarily in young women and usually has a benign prognosis; however, one reported fatality with migraine was probably due to an attack of basilar artery migraine.[128]

Basilar artery migraine was reviewed by Swanson and Vick.[129] Ten of the 12 patients reported were female. The age of onset ranged from 8 to 46 years. All but one patient had onset before age 25. Symptoms included typical classic migraine visual auras, diplopia, ptosis, ataxia, and brief (1- to 10-minute) episodes of unconsciousness. One illustrative case is abstracted as follows:

> The patient had cyclic vomiting and car-sickness as a young girl. At age 20 she had episodes of bilateral loss of vision associated with vertigo, but no headaches or other migrainous symptoms. At age 21, and twice at age 23, she became unconscious without warning. Two attacks occurred in a brightly lighted environment while she was standing at the foot of an upward-moving elevator. The third attack occurred at home while she was reading quietly. In each attack she suddenly lost vision and quickly became unconscious, slumping to the floor. Upon awakening she had a severe, generalized, throbbing headache; nausea; and vomiting. Truncal ataxia was severe and lasted 15 minutes. Her father had common migraine and her mother had classic migraine. At age 24, photic stimulation during an EEG induced a fourth attack similar to the others.

Therapy for these patients included ergonovine maleate, propranolol, phenytoin, and primidone. It is of interest that anticonvulsants were effective in half of the patients.

Other Varieties

Less common varieties of migraine are the so-called migraine equivalents and unusual varieties of complicated migraine. *Migraine equivalent* is a term used to denote conditions or symptomatology believed to be migrainous in origin, but without the typical history of either classic or common migraine headache. While the idea of migraine equivalents has not always been well received, according to Sacks[4] the concentrated experience of working with migraine patients must convince the physician, whatever his previous beliefs, that many patients do suffer repeated, discrete, paroxysmal attacks of abdominal pain, chest pain, fever, and other symptoms, which will fill every clinical criteria of migraine save the presence of headache.

The most well-recognized type of migraine equivalent is abdominal migraine, in which cyclic vomiting, periodic attacks of nausea, or abdominal pain occur (usually in children or adolescents). These patients experience more typical attacks of migraine in later life. If the past history of migraine patients is investigated, a history of cyclic vomiting is far more commonly found than in a control headache population.[130] Very rarely true abdominal migraine occurs in adult life. In this situation there may be sudden severe abdominal pain with vomiting and even abdominal rigidity. The usual brevity of the attack or previous similar benign episodes or strong history of migraine help confirm the diagnosis.[131] Other migraine equivalents include periodic diarrhea, fever, mood changes, and possibly attacks of chest pain known as *precordial migraine*. Acute confusional states have been attributed to migraine in juveniles.[132]

Migraine attacks may clearly occur without headache. Whitty[133] detailed the case histories of 16 patients who experienced auras of different varieties, with and without headache, in whom strong family histories of migraine, other migraine attacks, or otherwise asymptomatic follow-up allowed the diagnosis of migraine. Other atypical symptoms of complicated migraine have been separated into subgroups such as facioplegic migraine, cerebellar migraine, dysphrenic migraine, and migraine with involuntary movements.[66] Such unusual cases must be reviewed individually and carefully evaluated before it can be concluded that such episodes truly are migrainous.

CLUSTER HEADACHE

Cluster headache is classified as headache type 3.1 in the IHS classification (see Table 16–1). The diagnostic criteria for cluster headache are outlined in Table 16–5.

The term *cluster headache* denotes a characteristic type of cephalgia defined as severe unilateral head or facial pain lasting minutes to hours; it is often associated with ipsilateral lacrimation, nasal congestion, and facial flushing. The headaches tend to occur in separate bouts or clusters in one or more attacks daily for periods of weeks to months.[134–139] Often during an attack, and sometimes persisting beyond it, there is ipsilateral miosis and ptosis (*i.e.*, oculosympathetic paresis [Horner's syndrome]).

In 1840 Romberg described "ciliary neuralgia" as recurrent pain in the eye with injection and pupillary constriction.[140] Harris described the same syndrome in 1926 as "periodic migrainous neuralgia"[141] and later, in 1928, as ciliary (migrainous) neuralgia.[142] Multiple redescriptions and rediscoveries of the syndrome have resulted

TABLE 16–5. Cluster Headache

3.1.1 Cluster headache

Diagnostic criteria
A. At least five attacks fulfill B through D
B. Severe unilateral orbital, supraorbital, and/or temporal pain lasts 15 to 180 min untreated
C. Headache is associated with at least one of the following signs, which have to be present on the side of the pain:
  1. Conjunctival injection
  2. Lacrimation
  3. Nasal congestion
  4. Rhinorrhea
  5. Forehead and facial sweating
  6. Miosis
  7. Ptosis
  8. Eyelid edema
D. Frequency of attacks ranges from one every other day to eight per day
E. At least one of the following is true:
  1. History, physical, and neurologic examinations do not suggest one of the disorders listed in groups 5 through 11.
  2. History and/or physical and/or neurologic examinations do suggest such a disorder, but it is ruled out by appropriate investigations.
  3. Such a disorder is present, but cluster headache does not occur for the first time in close temporal relation to the disorder.

3.1.2 Episodic cluster headache

Description: occurs in periods lasting 7 d to 1 y, separated by pain-free periods lasting 14 d or more

Diagnostic criteria
A. All the letter headings of 3.1
B. At least two periods of headaches (cluster periods) last (in untreated patients) from 7 d to 1 y, separated by remissions of at least 14 d

3.1.3 Chronic cluster headache

Description: Attacks occur for more than 1 y without remission or with remissions lasting less than 14 D

Diagnostic criteria
A. All the letter headings of 3.1
B. Absence of remission phases lasts for 1 y or more, with remissions lasting less than 14 d

TABLE 16–6. Cluster Headache and Variants

Synonyms
Periodic migrainous neuralgia
Ciliary neuralgia
Harris' neuralgia
Symonds' "particular variety of headache"
Cluster headaches
Autonomic faciocephalgia
Erythromelalgia of the head
Histaminic cephalgia
Horton's cephalgia or syndrome
Petrosal neuralgia
Raeder's neuralgia (type 2)

Syndromes bearing possible relationship
Erythroprosopalgia
Some cases of vidian neuralgia
Some cases of Sluder's neuralgia
Some cases diagnosed as "supraorbital neuralgia"

Syndromes bearing no relationship
Reader's neuralgia
Most cases of vidian neuralgia
Most cases of Sluder's neuralgia
Trigeminal neuralgia
Atypical facial pain
Tension headaches

(Modified from Bickerstaff EB: Cluster headaches. In Vinken PJ, Bruyn GW [eds]: Handbook of Clinical Neurology, Vol 5, Headache and Cranial Neuralgias. New York, American Elsevier, 1968)

---

in a host of synonymous terms as well as confusion with other entities not related to this particular headache syndrome (Table 16–6).

The pain in cluster headache is very severe, being described as "boring," "sharp," "unbearable," and "the worst pain I have ever felt." The headache usually appears in or around one eye or on the cheek and then can spread to the temple, frontal region, occiput, or the ipsilateral neck. It rapidly builds to a peak within a few minutes, with an intensity greater than most other headache varieties. It usually lasts for 30 minutes to a few hours. Rather than lying down in seclusion, as preferred by most migraine sufferers, the cluster headache victim often paces about, holds onto his face, or

applies very hot or cold water to the affected region, even to the point of self-injury. The attacks usually occur once in a 24-hour period, often at a specific time, and frequently in the early morning hours awakening the patient from sleep. Men are affected much more commonly than women, by a ratio of approximately 5:1. Usually the episodes begin in the second or third decade and, according to Bickerstaff,[135] frequently are ipsilateral to previous head trauma. The headache tends to remain on the same side in a given cluster but rarely may alternate in subsequent clusters. Typical migraine headache is frequently found in family members. Although most patients have cluster headaches occurring over weeks or months (often in the same season of the year), other patients have sporadic attacks or irregular episodes for indeterminate periods of time.

Typical migraine headaches may occur in persons with cluster headaches, sometimes waning as the cluster commences. In the cluster attacks just described, it is extremely rare that any organic pathology is ever demonstrated; however, variants of the syndrome require more detailed analysis. When the pain becomes persistent or bilateral, or when additional neurologic abnormalities are present (such as fifth nerve or optic nerve involvement), other conditions must be ruled out.

Regarding the mechanism of cluster headache, few specifics are known. Ekbom and Greitz,[143] however, demonstrated a localized narrowing of the extradural portion of the internal carotid artery distal to its exit from the carotid canal in a patient during an attack of cluster headache. They speculated that, in addition to the headache, the partial Horner's syndrome might be due to repeated dilatation and edema of the internal carotid artery, resulting in damage to the sympathetic nerves surrounding the vessel.

Bickerstaff[135] reviewed the variety of terms used to describe cluster headache and their relationship to other types of facial and cranial neuralgias. Vail[144] described *vidian neuralgia* as recurrent, aching pain affecting the nose, eye, face, neck, and shoulder on one side, but he also included recurrent episodes that would clearly conform to the cluster headache syndrome. The facial pain described originally by Sluder included clinical variants, but primarily referred to a constant pain affecting eye, upper jaw, hard palate, and teeth on one side, usually in menopausal women.[145]

In 1924, Raeder described five patients with Horner's syndrome, but without facial anhydrosis (oculosympathetic paresis), who had pain or numbness in the distribution of the ophthalmic branch of the trigeminal nerve, which he termed "paratrigeminal neuralgia."[146] Some of his patients, however, had other cranial nerve signs, and additional findings suggested specific intracranial lesions.

Boniuk and Schlezinger[147] divided Raeder's syndrome into two groups: (1) hemicrania, ipsilateral oculosympathetic paresis, and parasellar cranial nerve (III, IV, V, and VI) involvement, the additional cranial nerve signs suggesting disease in the middle cranial fossa and indicating appropriate diagnostic studies; and (2) hemicrania and Horner's syndrome, the most common cause of which is a cluster headache variant,[148–150] and further diagnostic studies including arteriography are unwarranted. In Raeder type 2 neuralgia, however, aneurysm[151,152] and fibromuscular dysplasia of the carotid artery[153] have been reported. In patients with such demonstrable lesions, unilateral facial pain was persistent, rather than the episodic excruciating variety described in the classic cluster headache syndrome.

Therapy recommended for cluster headache has been quite variable and has often been tailored to the suspected condition. Harris[142] injected the gasserian ganglion, Horton[154] tried to desensitize his patients to histamine, and others have recommended sphenopalatine ganglionectomy.[155] Histamine is indeed elevated in serum during a cluster attack, with minimal change in serotonin (in contrast to depressed levels of serotonin in typical migrainous episodes).[156] Ergotamine preparations have been widely used, parenterally in the acute attack and orally as a prophylactic agent.[156] The prophylactic use of methysergide maleate (Sansert) has been employed successfully,[157] and currently propranolol (20 to 40 mg two to four times daily) may serve as an effective preventive.[158] Calcium channel blockers may also be effective in cluster headache, particularly nimodipine.[159] Therapy for cluster headaches, as well as their relationship to other forms of vascular headache, was reviewed by Lance.[160]

MIGRAINE IN CHILDHOOD

All forms of migraine, with the exception of cluster headache, occur in childhood. Childhood migraine would also include the childhood periodic syndromes that may be precursors to or associated with migraine (1.5 in the IHS classification). Some of the periodic syndromes were discussed earlier (see Other Varieties section). The incidence of migraine in childhood has been estimated at between 2% and 5.7%.[161,162] It is probable that most migrainous episodes actually begin early in childhood,[163,164] but the diagnosis is not often made until the child is old enough to describe the symptoms. Holguin and Fenichel[165] reviewed the characteristics of migraine in a group of 55 children. They stated that the clinical picture of migraine in school-age children is only slightly different from that in adults, and abdominal symptoms are often more prominent.

The visual symptoms experienced by children may be striking. Hachinski and colleagues[166] reviewed the symptomatology of 100 children with migraine. Of the 100 patients, 77 had transient visual impairment or binocular scotomas. Total obscuration of vision was more common that hemianopia. Altitudinal or quadrantic defects were unusual but did occur. Sixteen children experienced distortions of vision, including micropsia, macropsia, inversion of vision, alterations in perception of motion, and even elaborate hallucinations. Seven children had uniocular visual impairment.

A particularly unusual type of migraine, with recurrent attacks of impairment of time sense, body image, and visual analysis of the environment, has been termed the *Alice in Wonderland syndrome*. Golden[167] reported on two children with this syndrome, both of whom retained a clear state of consciousness during recurrent episodes. The following is an excerpt from the description of an 11-year-old girl:

> As I started to go into Mommy's room I grabbed my door—it felt about one foot thick in my hand. As I went through the hall, it felt as if I was going too fast. (Like you want to stop but energy is keening up inside of you. You feel like you're going to burst and your eyes are going to pop out—like you're going to explode.) Things were going too fast. I felt like my hands were made of tiny twigs with a little mushy flesh on the outside. I felt like I was holding things in my hands.

In children, migraine may be triggered by head trauma, and some of the post-traumatic syndromes may also be related to migraine.[168] It has been suggested that transient blindness following head injury in childhood[169] may occur primarily in children with a history of migraine.[170] Acute confusional states in juveniles may also represent migraine.[132]

The treatment of childhood migraine is similar to that of adult migraine (see Therapy section) and is theoretically directed toward preventing vascular dilatation.[171] The prognosis in childhood migraine is thought to be good,[172] but a complete follow-up study has not been reported.[165]

OTHER HEADACHES

A host of other conditions are associated with headache (see Table 16–1), including specific syndromes such as trigeminal neuralgia, systemic diseases such as temporal arteritis, and entities such as muscle contraction, intracranial neoplasms, and vascular anomalies. Some of these conditions are described briefly in the following sections, but they are covered in more detail in standard textbooks[14,15,173,174] and reviews of the headache literature.[175,176]

Facial Pain

Trigeminal neuralgia, or tic douloureux, is a facial pain characterized by repetitive attacks of lightening-like jabs of lancinating pain in the maxillary and mandibular divisions of the trigeminal nerve. The ophthalmic division may be involved, but it is rarely the sole location. The onset is usually in the sixth or seventh decade, and women are affected at a slightly higher rate than men (3:2). The usual cause is vascular cross-compression of the sensory root entry zone of the fifth nerve as it enters the pons, but multiple sclerosis and cerebellopontine angle tumors may also produce the syndrome. In rare cases, both sides of the face are involved, with pains occurring asynchronously on opposite sides. Bilaterality in a person younger than 50 years of age suggests multiple sclerosis.

The paroxysmal attacks last only seconds, reaching maximal intensity immediately; often a deep, aching pain persists between the paroxysms. The pain is often described as "electric" and is frequently triggered by talking, chewing, touching the lips, or by cold exposure. Most of these patients have a normal neurologic examination, but some, even those with classic tic, have a small area of numbness medially on the upper lip. Any neurologic deficit or the presence of the condition in a patient younger than 50 years of age necessitates that MRI be ordered to rule out tumor or multiple sclerosis.

Medical therapy is successful in the majority of patients and includes carbamazepine, baclofen, phenytoin, clonazepam, and valproic acid alone or in combination.[14,177] Surgical therapy includes vascular decompression[178–180] and a variety of percutaneous procedures aimed at destruction of the pain fibers of the trigeminal nerve.[14,180,181]

Atypical facial pain is a less well-defined complex involving pain in the face. The pain tends to be deep, aching, more diffuse, and sometimes superficial, but longer in duration than attacks of trigeminal neuralgia. Facial sensation is sometimes altered. The pain is not necessarily localized to the sensory distribution of the trigeminal nerve and is often poorly characterized by the patient. The pain responds poorly to medical or surgical therapy and is usually accompanied by various degrees of psychological impairment. Such patients should be thoroughly evaluated to rule out organic causes, such as nasopharyngeal neoplasm and dental abnormality. In the absence of defined pathology, however, these patients may be treated symptomatically with nonaddictive analgesics, antidepressants, and psychotherapy.

Temporal Arteritis

Temporal arteritis, or giant cell arteritis, is a systemic disorder of unknown cause characterized by an inflammatory obliterative arteritis particularly, but not exclusively, involving branches of the external carotid and ophthalmic arteries. It is well known as a cause of anterior ischemic optic neuropathy and less well recognized as a cause of ophthalmoplegia. The most common initial symptom is headache, often accompanied by diffuse aches and pains (polymyalgia rheumatica).[182] Other common symptoms include jaw claudication, fever, anemia, and weight loss. In the study of Vilaseca and co-workers,[183] the simultaneous presence of recent-onset headache, jaw claudication, and abnormalities of the temporal arteries on physical examination had a specificity of 94.8% compared with the histologic diagnosis and 100% with respect to the final diagnosis (see also Chapter 5, Part II).

Solomon and Cappa[184] pointed out that the headache of temporal arteritis may clearly involve more than the temporal area and include pain in the temporal, frontal, vertex, and occipital regions. The headache is characterized by gradual onset, progressing to a diffuse, often severe, aching. The headache may be intermittent, but usually becomes a prominent, if not daily, feature of patients with the disorder. The headache usually is constant and perceived as superficial in the scalp. There may be exquisite tenderness of the scalp and blood vessels, particularly in the temporal region. The headache is usually worse at night and may be especially aggravated by exposure to cold.[14]

Sixty-five percent of patients are women, and the average age at onset is 70 years (range, 50 to 85). It is a common disorder and must be actively sought in any headache patient presenting after the age of 50, particularly in those with systemic symptoms.[185] Allen and Studenski[182] emphasized additional symptoms, such as extremity and tongue claudication, ear pain, stroke, and angina, as well as systemic panarteritis involving the peripheral nervous system and abdominal or pelvic viscera.

Other ocular complaints associated with temporal arteritis include tonic pupils due to ischemia of the ciliary ganglia,[186] and bilateral uveitic glaucoma, which may be an immunologic manifestation.[113] Although most attention has been drawn to vascular complications in the distribution of the external carotid and ophthalmic arteries, rarely patients present with vertebral basilar symptomatology.[187] The following are among the protean manifestations of temporal arteritis: bilateral carotid artery occlusion,[188] renal disease,[189] aortic arch arteritis,[190] temporal mandibular joint pain,[191] painful facial swelling,[192] jaw claudication,[193] and sudden death due to arteritis in the coronary arteries, dissection of the aorta, and major cerebrovascular accident.[194]

Some consider an elevated erythrocyte sedimentation rate (ESR) indispensable in diagnosing temporal arteritis. Without an elevated ESR, even in patients with a classic history and clinical findings, the diagnosis might be abandoned without proceeding to a temporal artery biopsy.

Nonetheless, it is now estimated that up to 9% of patients with temporal arteritis may have normal ESRs.[195,196] Wong and Korn[195] identified 37 reported cases of biopsy-proven temporal arteritis who had a normal Westergren ESR (less than 40 mm/hour in patients older than 50 years of age).

Up to one third of temporal artery biopsies may be falsely negative, especially when one fails to examine a long segment of vessel by serial sections. As recently stated by Plum, "because of the danger to vision, most authorities would start steroid treatment when they suspect the diagnosis clinically. Any response other than prompt and striking improvement in clinical well-being and symptoms, however, speaks against the diagnosis."[197] Raskin and others[14,182] believe that steroid therapy should start immediately, before confirmation by laboratory and pathologic determinations. They have suggested that in very ill patients, intravenous methylprednisolone may be a better choice than oral steroids.

Intracranial Mass Lesions

The headache associated with an intracranial mass is nonspecific and often not localizing. It is estimated that almost two thirds of patients with brain tumors complain of headache, and that half consider headache to be the primary complaint.[14] The headache of an intracranial mass lesion is believed to be due to traction on pain-sensitive structures within the cranium, including the meninges and dural venous sinuses. The typical headache has a dull, nonthrobbing quality, is of moderate intensity, is worsened by physical activity (especially change in posture), and is intermittent. The headache is often associated with nausea and vomiting, as is a typical migraine headache. Ten percent of adults and two thirds of children with brain tumors are awakened from sleep by headaches. Brain tumor headache may be more prominent upon arising. *Supratentorial headaches* tend to have some localization to the side of the tumor; *posterior fossa tumor headaches* tend to be bilateral, especially posterior. Any focal finding on neurologic examination or presence of papilledema in a patient with new-onset headache requires neuroimaging and follow-up.

Cough headache describes the sudden, transient occurrence of a diffuse, often severe, headache precipitated by a Valsalva maneuver (*e.g.*, coughing, sneezing, bending, lifting). It is usually benign, but approximately 10% of such patients have intracranial abnormalities, usually in the posterior fossa. The Arnold-Chiari malformation, in particular, may present with cough headache, and therefore all patients with this condition must have MRIs performed.

Increased intracranial pressure alone, in the absence of a mass lesion, may be responsible for headache, as in the syndrome of benign increased intracranial pressure, or *pseudotumor cerebri*. These headaches tend to be diffuse, daily, and mildly to moderately severe, and they are usually relieved after the increased intracranial pressure is reduced—either by drugs, such as acetazolamide, or by lumbar puncture. Raskin[14] was impressed by the frequency of "migrainous" symptoms in persons with pseudotumor cerebri, and indicated that many have persistent headaches even after resolution of papilledema and increased intracranial pressure. It is my experience that headache improvement is a good guide to efficacy of therapy in most patients. Given the overall frequency of migraine in young women, it is not surprising that many with pseudotumor cerebri may have migraine as a concomitant condition.

Muscle Contraction

Tension-type headache is classified as headache type 2 in the IHS classification and is further subclassified as follows: 2.1, episodic tension-type headache; 2.2, chronic tension-type headache; and 2.3, tension-type headache not fulfilling the above criteria.

Muscle contraction or tension headache has been characterized as head pain without migrainous features. Typically, these headaches are described as bilateral, commonly in an occipital or posterior neck location; variable in intensity; dull, with pressure and tightness in muscles; and associated with emotional conflict.[14,198] They tend to occur on a daily basis, but may be intermittent or periodic. On careful analysis, there are many overlapping features common to migraine. Features once believed to be specific for tension headache, such as neck muscle contraction and precipitation by stress and anxiety, are now known to occur just as often in migraine.[199] Indeed, many patients with daily constant headache, without throbbing and having a "band-like" tightness, may respond to antimigrainous therapy. At one point an ad hoc committee on the classification of headache recommended separate categories for "headaches of delusional, conversion, or hyperchondriacal states" and "muscle-contraction headaches." Others, however, prefer to combine these into the category "psychogenic headaches," which include the following subtypes: depression (overt or masked), delusional (psychotic), somatoform disorder, chronic post-traumatic, chronic atypical facial pain, and muscle contraction pain (when due to a psychogenic factor, rather than unusual postures or strains).[198] In the present classification, there is no separate category for headaches of psychogenic origin, and they would be classified as 13 (headache not classifiable).

Clearly there are patients with major psychological problems who have psychogenic headaches as a feature of their disorder, but in a majority without features that permit a diagnosis of probable or definite migraine, the distinction is often difficult. Muscle contraction or tension headaches do overlap significantly with migraine, as indicated earlier, and may respond to similar therapy. Tricyclic antidepressants may be helpful for both muscle contraction and migraine headaches.

Post-Traumatic Headache

In the IHS classification, section 5 is devoted to headache associated with head trauma. This section is further subdivided into 5.1, acute post-traumatic headache; and 5.2, chronic post-traumatic headache. Post-traumatic headaches are a regular feature of the post-traumatic or postconcussion syndrome, which follows significant head injury. The syndrome is not necessarily associated with definable central nervous system injury and can occur whether or not unconsciousness occurred at the time of trauma.[14] The syndrome is characterized by headache, vertigo, impairment of memory and concentration, and variable degrees of emotional impairment. Headache lasting more than 2 months occurs in up to 60% of patients hospitalized after head injury.[200] The degree of apparent disability may seem to outweigh the amount of objective evidence of central nervous system or musculoskeletal injury. Some believe that persistent symptoms relate to the patient's desire to seek compensation, but most believe that this occurs in only a small percentage. There is evidence that an organic mechanism is operative in a large proportion of these patients.[14,201]

The headache in postconcussional states usually occurs within a day of the injury, but may be delayed for weeks. It is characterized by a dull, aching, generalized discomfort with localized exacerbation in bifrontal, bioccipital, or bitemporal locations that may last for hours.

The headache tends to be on a daily basis, but may be periodic and throbbing, quite characteristic of migraine. The usual course is gradual improvement in all symptoms when there is no severe organic impairment, but the headache may persist for many months.

Both common and classic migraine may be significantly exacerbated after a closed head injury; uncommonly, typical migraine attacks may follow injury in a previously headache-free person. The incidence of post-traumatic migraine is higher in persons with a strong family history of migraine headache.

Aneurysm and Arteriovenous Malformation

Headaches associated with vascular disorders are IHS category 6 (see Table 16–1). A sudden, severe, "blinding," excruciating headache with stiff neck, vomiting, and altered mental status is the classic presentation of a ruptured berry aneurysm. Subarachnoid blood is usually found on lumbar puncture, if performed, and the majority of CT scans reveal evidence of blood. Focal neurologic deficits may occur after rupture of berry aneurysms, such as the third nerve palsy that often follows rupture of a posterior communicating artery aneurysm or hemiparesis following middle cerebral artery aneurysm rupture. The syndrome of "occipital apoplexy" (sudden headache, stiff neck, and a homonymous field defect) is almost pathognomonic for a ruptured occipital lobe AVM.[6] Any patient with sudden-onset severe headache, with or without stiff neck or focal neurologic signs, must be evaluated for the possibility of a ruptured or unruptured vascular anomaly, such as aneurysm or AVM. The other neuro-ophthalmologic signs and symptoms of aneurysms, AVMs, and related vascular anomalies are detailed in Chapter 17.

Unruptured aneurysms and AVMs may also produce headache. A headache pattern that is completely stereotypic throughout life is strongly suggestive of an AVM, rather than migraine with aura.[50] Sentinel headaches are reported to occur in approximately 50% of patients days to weeks preceding subarachnoid hemorrhage from a berry aneurysm.[47] About half of such headaches are reported to be abrupt in onset and severe and have been believed to be due to an initial leak from a partial rupture. Such patients should probably be evaluated with arteriography, even if the cerebrospinal fluid does not disclose blood, as Day and Raskin have documented that thunderclap headache episodes may occur as symptoms of an unruptured aneurysm.[202]

Ocular Headache

Several ocular lesions are important and treatable as causes of headache, including conjunctivitis, corneal lesions, anterior uveitis, angle closure glaucoma, optic neuritis, metastatic orbital tumors, orbital pseudotumors, and Tolosa-Hunt syndrome. Paratrigeminal syndrome, ocular motor nerve paralysis, small vessel disease, carotid cavernous fistulas, and nasopharyngeal carcinomas may all have eye pain as a presenting symptom. Patients with dissection of the internal carotid artery can also present with eye pain (see later discussion). Photophobia is often seen with subarachnoid hemorrhage, meningitis, retrobulbar neuritis, and migraine and probably has its basis in central cortical and brainstem reflexes.[203]

Carlow[202] noted that the eye and periorbital regions are common points of headache, but that the eye is rarely responsible if ophthalmic signs are not obvious. He also suggested that refractive disorders and muscle imbalance are overemphasized as the cause of headache and that correction of these problems seldom provides resolution, the exception being convergence insufficiency. *Ocular neurosis* is the usual cause of eye-strain headache that begins abruptly with use of the eyes, which appear normal on ophthalmologic examination.

Carotid Dissection

Another type of unusual facial pain that initially may be thought to be temporal arteritis is caused by spontaneous dissection of the carotid and/or vertebral arteries.[204] The vascular dissection may occur spontaneously, especially in those with unsuspected fibromuscular dysplasia. Carotid and/or vertebral artery dissection may follow head and neck injury caused by "whiplash," blows to the neck, and neck manipulation. The clues to making the diagnosis include pain over the angle of the jaw and hemicranium, oculosympathetic paresis, dysgeusia, and altered facial sensation, as in the following case:

> A 46-year old mildly hypertensive woman experienced "lightening pains" that radiated to her face from the left side of her neck. The following day, the pain had become dull and was localized behind her left eye. She noted slight drooping of her left eyelid; a strange, persistent metallic taste; and discomfort over the left side of her forehead. Her unilateral neck and face pain then increased in intensity, and the entire left side of her face became "numb and disagreeable." Examination showed a left oculosympathetic paresis and a marked decrease in sensation to light touch and pinprick over all three divisions of the left trigeminal nerve. Testing facial sensation evoked an unpleasant sensation. The remainder of her examination was normal, as were CT and MRI scans. Cerebral angiography demonstrated a dissection of the left internal carotid artery extending intracranially to the cavernous sinus and a 2-cm dissection of the left vertebral artery.[205]

Carotid dissection can mimic Raeder's paratrigeminal syndrome (see earlier discussion), but requires angiography for diagnosis.

DIFFERENTIAL DIAGNOSIS

In the differential diagnosis of the migraine headache syndromes, one should first consider the classification of headaches presented in Table 16–1, as well as comments on the new headache classification.[198]

Headaches in general should be considered a serious medical problem only when they become continuous or recur frequently, as almost everyone suffers from occasional headaches. In discussing the approach to diagnosing a severe headache, Dalessio[1] made the following statement: "Although headache remains one of the most common medical complaints, even its most severe and chronic manifestations are rarely caused by organic disease. In a given year, nearly three quarters of Americans have headaches, but of these, only 5% seek medical help."[1] When the complaint concerns a persistent or recurrent headache, the history becomes of primary importance in establishing the proper diagnosis. Additional descriptions of the characteristics of nonmigrainous headaches are found in standard references on headache.[14,15,174] The question arises as to which conditions are confused with migraine, and when one should reasonably proceed to a more detailed investigation or referral to a specialist.

In assessing the specific history of the headache, important facts to determine are onset, duration, periodicity, timing, localization, intensity, character, precipitating factors, accompanying symptoms and signs, and response to therapy. Often the exact description alone of the nature, duration, and timing of the headache permits the correct diagnosis. This is particularly true with migraine headache characterized by periodicity and associated symptoms.

When a new headache occurs, particularly in an adult who has never been prone to headache and in whom atypical features are present, such as persistent focal pain, then disorders other than migraine should be carefully ruled out. When obvious disease of cranial or extracranial structures accompanies the headache, little diagnostic confusion results. However, when cephalgia persists without readily apparent reason, further evaluation is needed.

General physical and neurologic examinations in patients with migraine, aside from the complicated varieties, are normal. Conditions that may be confused with each of the migraine syndromes described previously will be briefly reviewed.

Migraine without aura (common migraine), as emphasized earlier, should not be diagnosed simply based on the presence of headache. Tension or muscle-contraction headache alone or in combination with a vascular component is most often confused with common migraine. The periodicity, associated symptoms (*e.g.*, nausea, photophobia, fluid retention), and family history all weigh in favor of migraine. Persistent pain, absent family history, muscle tenderness, and bizarre descriptions, such as "a knife being driven through the skull," raise the possibility of muscle contraction or psychogenic headache. Any neurologic abnormality on examination (*e.g.*, mild hemiparesis, consistent sensory defect, reflex asymmetry) again suggests the possibility of intracranial disease and traction headache. Headache from intracranial sources is most often produced by inflammation, traction and displacement, or distension of pain-sensitive structures, usually dura and blood vessels. Exact correlation of the headache site with intracranial mass lesions is often misleading; however, in general, lesions of the posterior fossa produce an occipital headache, and hemispheric tumors produce a more anterior, frontal headache. In the absence of increased intracranial pressure, the headache tends to be localized to the side of the lesion.

Cranial arteritis, a disorder of the elderly, often produces headache, frequently without overt signs. The headache can be severe and accompanied by tenderness of the extracranial arteries. In the older patient, the investigation of a new headache should always include an ESR as a screening test for cranial arteritis.

Migraine with aura (classic migraine), in its complete form with slowly progressive visual aura, is virtually never caused by an organic process. A question is frequently raised as to the possibility of AVM. Although headaches may indeed be present with AVM, such vascular lesions more commonly present as subarachnoid hemorrhage or seizure. In a review of occipital lobe AVMs, Troost and Newton[6] determined that the characteristic visual phenomena represent occipital epilepsy, and the nonalternating, unilateral character of the headache, as well as the history of a seizure, always distinguishes these vascular malformations from migraine. Rarely, an AVM may produce clinical symptomatology, which in a single episode is indistinguishable from an episode of classic migraine.[50] The invariant nature of the attack, lack of response to therapy, and presence of abnormality on examination (*e.g.*, cranial bruit) should lead to additional diagnostic studies in these unusual patients. A normal physical examination, family history, and response to therapy should eliminate the need to perform neuroradiologic studies in the vast majority of patients with migraine.

Common, classic, and complicated migraine may be precipitated by trauma. If the typical clinical pattern of one of the migraine syndromes follows head trauma, other additional causes (*e.g.*, subdural hematoma) need not be sought. Complicated migraine can present some of the most difficult diagnostic problems, particularly in the absence of prior episodes or family history. The acute onset of neurologic dysfunction and headache in this setting must always be regarded initially as caused by another process (*e.g.*, cerebrovascular disease, rapidly growing tumor) and must be fully investigated.

Again, prior history of uncomplicated common or classic migraine may lessen the suspicion of another process in a given patient.

Ophthalmoplegic migraine should be diagnosed only in the typical clinical setting described in the previous section: a young patient with a history of recurrent ophthalmoplegic episodes or known migraine. Sudden oculomotor nerve palsy associated with previous chronic headache, or with a new, acute, severe headache, should be considered caused by aneurysm until it is proved otherwise. With aneurysm, the history is not one of recurrent episodes of ophthalmoplegia with full recovery. Occasionally other congenital vascular anomalies, meningeal inflammation, or neoplastic disease may produce painful ophthalmoplegia. Diabetic oculomotor palsy usually occurs in older diabetics, spares the pupil, and is rarely recurrent. Sphenoid sinus mucocele may present as a recurrent headache and third nerve palsy[206]; radiologic studies should clarify the diagnostic dilemma.

Cranial nerve abnormality other than oculosympathetic paresis in a patient with "cluster headache" should alert the physician to an intracranial mass lesion (Raeder's paratrigeminal neuralgia, type 1). Persistent, localized pain most often makes this cluster atypical and points to a different etiology.

In general, a knowledge of the different headache varieties other than migraine and a careful history and examination will lead to the appropriate diagnosis.

THERAPY

Appropriate and effective treatment for migraine first assumes an accurate diagnosis. In general, the treatment of migraine may be divided into two general pharmacologic approaches: (1) treatment of the acute attack (abortive, symptomatic); or (2) preventative (prophylactic) therapy aimed at preventing the recurrence of headache. Patients often may need both treatments if their headaches are frequent and severe. As pointed out by Silberstein and Lipton,[9] symptomatic treatment is appropriate for most acute attacks and should be used a maximum of 2 to 3 days/week. If attacks occur more frequently, treatment strategy should emphasize decreasing attack frequency with prophylactic medications. A full discussion of migraine therapy can be found in a review by Baumel.[207]

Medications used in acute headache treatment include analgesics, antimedicanzietyalytics, nonsteroidal anti-inflammatory drugs (NSAIDs), ergots, steroids, major tranquilizers, narcotics, and more recently, the selective 5-HT$_1$ (serotonin) agonists. The primary serotonin agonist is sumatriptan, which was originally introduced in the United States in subcutaneous form but recently became available in oral dosage.[208–211] Preventive therapy includes a broad range of medications, most notably calcium channel blockers, β-blockers, antidepressants, serotonin antagonists, and anticonvulsants.

Headaches similar to migraine can be triggered by serotonergic drugs, such as reserpine and m-chloralphenalpiprazine (serotonergic agonist).[27,28] Two agents are effective in the acute treatment of migraine: sumatriptan,[212–214] a serotonin analogue; and dihydroergotamine (DHE),[215,216] an ergot derivative. These agents block the development of neurogenically induced inflammation in rat dura mater. This, in turn, blocks the release of neuropeptides, including substance P and calcitonin gene–related peptide, preventing neurogenic inflammation.[9] The NSAIDs may also block neurogenic inflammation; the mechanism of this action, however, is less certain.

Symptomatic Treatment

There are a wide variety of acute treatments available for migraine (Table 16–7). A further listing of abortive and symptomatic therapies for migraine is adapted from the review by Baumel[207] (Tables 16–8 and 16–9). As pointed out by Silberstein and Lipton,[9] the choice of acute treatment depends on the severity and frequency of headaches, the pattern of associated symptoms, comorbid illnesses, and the patient's treatment response profile. The simplest treatment is achieved with analgesics (prescription or nonprescription). Many patients find headache relief with compounds such as aspirin or acetaminophen, taken either alone or in combination with caffeine. butalbital, a short-acting barbiturate, is often added to the combination of simple analgesics and caffeine. The combination of acetaminophen, isometheptene (a sympathomimetic), and dichloralphenazone (a chloral hydrate derivative) is also safe and effective in headache treatment.[217,218] When simple analgesics fail, consideration may be given to combining them with more potentially habit-forming medications (e.g., codeine). The nausea is often effectively treated with prochlorperazine.

More potent narcotic analgesics, such as propoxyphene, meperidine, morphine, hydromorphone, and oxycodone, are available alone and in combination. Because of medication overuse and rebound, however, these agents should be used sparingly and only for patients who experience infrequent headaches.[14] Further discussion about the use of opioids and transnasal opioids are discussed by Silberstein and Lipton.[9]

Ergotamine and DHE can be used to treat moderate to severe migraine.[219] Ergot preparations were once the mainstay of acute therapy. It was once said that "if a headache does not respond to ergotamine tartrate, it is not true migraine."[220] This agent, derived from *Claviceps purpurea,* a fungus that grows in rye and other grains, is the major compound effective as a specific agent in an acute migraine attack. Ergotamine is one of the naturally occurring alkaloids in crude ergot; all the ergot alkaloids are derivatives of lysergic acid.[221] One of the major pharmacologic properties of ergotamine is its ability to produce peripheral vasoconstriction; in higher

TABLE 16–7. Drugs Used for Acute Migraine Therapy

Trade name (Manufacturer)	Composition	Route and dosage
Cafergot tablets and suppositories (Sandoz)	1 mg ergotamine tartrate 100 mg caffeine	Orally: 2 tablets at onset; 1 additional tablet every 30 min if needed to maximum 6/attack, 10/wk
	2 mg ergotamine tartrate 100 mg caffeine	Rectally: 1 suppository at onset, second in 1 h if needed; maximum 2/attack, 4/wk
Gynergen tablets (Sandoz)	1 mg ergotamine tartrate	2 tablets orally at onset, 1/30 min to maximum 6/attack, 10/wk
Gynergen injection (Sandoz)	0.5 mg/mL ergotamine tartrate	0.5 mL SC or IM at onset; repeat at 40 min; maximum 2 mL/wk
D.H.E. 45 injection	1 mg/mL dihydroergotamine	1 mL IM at onset; repeat every hour to total of 3 mL if needed; may be given IV 0.5 mg or 1 mg every 8 h
Ergotrate maleate tablets (Lilly)	0.2 mg ergonovine maleate	1 tablet at onset; 1 every hour to 6/attack
Wigraine tablets and suppositories (Organon)	1 mg ergotamine tartrate 100 mg caffeine 0.1 mg belladonna 130 mg phenacetin	1 tablet at onset; 1 every hour to 6/attack 1–2 tablets or suppositories at onset with 1–2 after 15 min to maximum of 6/attack or 12/wk
Stadol NS (Bristol-Myers Squibb)	1 mg butorphanol tartrate spray	1 mg at onset; 1 mg in 60–90 min
Imitrex (Glaxo)	6 mg sumatriptan	1 SC injection at onset; may repeat in 1 hour
	25 or 50 mg sumatriptan	Oral tablets; 1 at onset, repeat in 2 hours if necessary; maximum dose 300 mg/d

IM, intramuscularly; *SC,* subcutaneously.

TABLE 16–8. Abortive Therapy for Migraine

Drug	Route of administration	Dosage
Serotonin-receptor agonists		
Dihydroergotamine	IM, SC, IV	0.5–1 mL
Ergotamine derivatives		
Ergotamine and caffeine*	PO	2 tablets; repeat in 1 h if necessary; limit, 4 per attack
Ergotamine*	Sublingual	1 tablet (let dissolve); may repeat in 30 min; limit, 2 per attack
Ergotamine and caffeine*	Suppository	½–1 suppository; repeat in 1 h if necessary; limit, 2 doses
Sympathomimetic agents		
Isometheptene, acetaminophen, dichloral-phenazone	PO	2 capsules, may repeat in 1 h; limit, 3 times per wk
Corticosteroids		
Dexamethasone	PO†	2–6 mg; may repeat in 3 h if necessary
	IM†	4 mg
All NSAIDs		
Mixed barbiturate analgesics (see Table 8)		

* Wait 3 days between dosing with ergotamine in patients with frequent migraine or daily headache.
† For protracted migraine.
IM, intramuscular; NSAIDs, nonsteroidal anti-inflammatory drugs; PO, by mouth; SC, subcutaneous.

TABLE 16–9. Symptomatic Therapy for Migraine

Drug	Route of administration	Dosage
NSAIDs		
Naproxen	PO	550–750 mg with repeat in 1–2 h; limit, 3 times per wk
Meclofenamate	PO	100–200 mg with repeat in 1–2 h; limit, 3 times per wk
Flurbiprofen	PO	50–100 mg with repeat in 1–2 h; limit, 3 times per wk
Ibuprofen	PO	200–300 mg with repeat in 1–2 h; limit, 3 times per wk
Mixed barbiturate analgesics		
Butalbital, aspirin or acetaminophen, and caffeine; butalbital and acetaminophen	PO	1–2 tablets q 4–6 h; limit, 4 tablets per day up to twice per wk
Narcotics (codeine-containing compounds, oxyco-done, propoxyphene, meperidine)	PO	Sparingly and infrequently, if at all, in patients with chronic headaches
Antiemetics*		
Promethazine	PO, IM	50–125 mg/d
Prochlorperazine	PO	1–25 mg/d
	Suppository	2.5–25 mg/d
	IM/IV	5–10 mg/d
Trimethobenzamide	PO	250 mg/d
	Suppository	200 mg/d
Metoclopramide	PO	5–10 mg/d
	IM	10 mg/d
	IV	5–10 mg (diluted)
Dimenhydrinate	PO	50 mg

* Given 10–20 minutes before ingestion of oral abortive migraine medication.
IM, intramuscular; *PO*, by mouth.

doses, it can damage the capillary endothelium. Inasmuch as ergotamine is neither a sedative nor an analgesic and other forms of pain are not relieved by the drug, its action is believed to be directly related to the pathophysiology of migraine. In the classic experiments of Graham and Wolff,[222] the intensity of pain was directly related to the amplitude of the temporal artery pulsation, and both decline in response to intravenous ergotamine tartrate (Fig. 16–13).

DHE is available in 1 mg/mL ampules, which can be administered intramuscularly, subcutaneously, or intravenously.[14] A nasal spray with 40% bioavailability is awaiting approval by the US Food and Drug Administration. Dosage for individual attacks should be limited to 1 mg intramuscularly or intravenously, with a maximum of 3 mg/day. Monthly limits, according to Silberstein and Lipton,[9] are 18 ampules or 12 events.

The oral combination of 1 mg ergotamine tartrate with 100 mg caffeine (Cafergot) remains widely used. The oral absorption of ergotamine is erratic. Although often effective, it shares the disadvantage of most of the oral ergotamine preparations in that it can produce nausea and vomiting itself. However, patients who cannot tolerate ergotamine because of nausea can be pretreated with metoclopramide,[223] prochlorperazine, promethazine,[224] or a mixture of a barbiturate and a belladonna alkaloid. For patients with intractable migraine, intravenous DHE has been recommended.[225]

It should be noted that pregnant women should not use ergot preparations because of their potent oxytocic effects. Fortunately, pregnancy usually causes a diminution in the symptoms of migraine. Ergot preparations in high doses can cause peripheral capillary endothelial damage, peripheral paresthesias, pain, and even gangrene. These preparations are generally not recommended for patients in septic states or who have coronary artery disease, obliterative peripheral vascular disease, or cardiac conditions.

Is it advisable to use vasoconstricting agents during a complicated migraine prodrome, such as mild hemiparesis or dysphasia? If the cerebral event is indeed vasoconstriction, will ergot preparations potentiate the possibility of permanent cerebral infarction? Theoretically, the preparations act only peripherally and not on the intracranial vasculature. However, since little is really known about the actual effects of ergot alkaloids on the central nervous system,[221] it may be wise to be cautious with their use if prominent central nervous system symptoms precede the headache attack.

Sumatriptan

Sumatriptan is a relatively new acute treatment for migraine. It is a selective 5-HT$_1$ receptor agonist. Cady and associates[226] found that sumatriptan (6 mg subcutaneously) was more effective than placebo in reducing

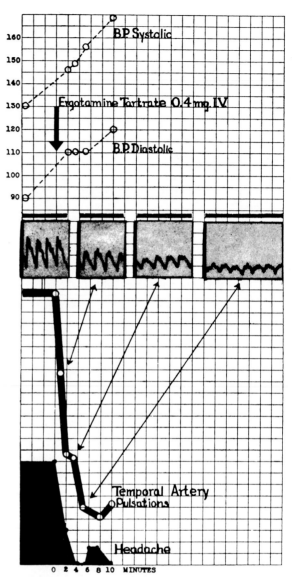

Fig. 16–13. Relation of amplitude of pulsations of temporal artery to intensity of headache after administration of ergotamine tartrate. The sharp decrease in the amplitude of pulsation following injection of ergotamine closely paralleled the rapid decrease in intensity of headache. Representative sections of photographic record are inserted. The average amplitude of pulsations for any given minute before and after administration of ergotamine was ascertained by measuring individual pulsations from the photographic record. The points on the heavy black line (lower half) represent these averages, expressed as percentages. Initial or "control" amplitude was taken as 100%. (Dalessio DJ: Wolff's Headache and Other Head Pain, 3rd ed. New York, Oxford University Press, 1972)

pain from being moderate or severe to being mild or absent (70% vs 22%), and in completely relieving pain (49% vs 9%) after 1 hour. Sumatriptan is now one of the most widely used acute abortive agents.[207] The efficacy of oral sumatriptan in a 100-mg dosage is comparable with that of the subcutaneous injection, but the onset of treatment effects is longer.[208,227] The initial starting dose of oral sumatriptan is 25 mg taken with fluids. The maximum recommended single dose is 100 mg. If a satisfactory response is not obtained in 2 hours, a second dose of up to 100 mg may be given. If headache returns, additional doses may be taken at intervals of at least 2 hours up to a maximum daily dosage of 300 mg.[208-211] Specific contraindications to the use of sumatriptan include ischemic heart disease, Prinzmetal's angina, and vertebrobasilar migraine. Side effects include pain at the injection site, tingling, flushing, burning, and warm or hot sensations. Dizziness, heaviness, neck pain, and dysphoria can occur. These side effects generally abate within 45 minutes. An intranasal form is being investigated.

Prophylactic Treatment

Preventive therapy should be based on general principles including the following[9]:

1. When two or more attacks occur per month and produce disability lasting more than 3 days
2. When symptomatic medications are contraindicated or ineffective
3. When abortive medication is required more than twice a week or when special circumstances exist (*e.g.*, a rare headache attack that produces profound disruption)

The major medication groups include calcium channel antagonists, β-adrenergic blockers, antidepressants, serotonin antagonists, and anticonvulsants (Table 16–10). For cluster headache, if these drugs fail, methysergide or lithium may be used. Methysergide is an extremely effective agent for cluster. It is related chemically to ergotamine tartrate and closely to lysergic acid, but it is relatively free of vasoconstrictor effects and is believed to be an antagonist of serotonin. Acutely, it may in rare cases cause a confusional state requiring its withdrawal. The major concern as to its chronic use is the development of retroperitoneal fibrosis.[228,229] This complication develops after long-term (usually more than 1 year) continuous methysergide therapy, often at doses of 8 to 16 mg/day. It is currently believed that such complications can be avoided by gradually discontinuing the drug (to avoid rebound) over a 2- to 3-week period and stopping it for 3 to 4 weeks every 6 months.

Calcium Channel Blockers

Specific calcium channel blockers were originally intended for use in cardiovascular disease, but show great promise as prophylactic agents in the treatment of migraine. Diltiazem,[230] verapamil,[231] nifedipine,[232] nimodipine,[160,233,234] and flunarizine[235] have all been reported to be effective in migraineurs. The mechanism of action of this class of drug in headache is unknown, but may

TABLE 16–10. Preventive Therapy for Migraine

Drug	Daily oral dosage range
β-Blockers	
Propranolol*	40–240 mg
Nadolol*	20–80 mg
Atenolol†	50–150 mg
Timolol*	20–60 mg
Metoprolol†	50–300 mg
Calcium channel blockers	
Verapamil	120–480 mg
Diltiazem	90–180 mg
Nifedipine	30–120 mg
Serotonin antagonists/agonists	
Cyproheptadine	4–8 mg
Methysergide	4–6 mg
Methylergonovine maleate	0.2 mg tid or qid
Tricyclic antidepressants	
Amitriptyline	10–200 mg
Nortriptyline	10–150 mg
Doxepin	10–200 mg
Imipramine	10–200 mg
MAO inhibitors	
Phenelzine	30–90 mg
Serotonin-reuptake inhibitors	
Fluoxetine	10–30 mg
Trazodone	50–300 mg
Anticonvulsants	
Phenytoin	300–800 mg
Carbamazepine	200–800 mg
Divalproex sodium	250–1500 mg
NSAIDs	
Naproxen	550–1100 mg (*e.g.,* 275 mg tid)
Meclofenamate sodium	100–400 mg (*e.g.,* 50 mg tid)
Flubiprofen	50–200 mg
Ibuprofen	300–1200 mg
α-Adrenergic blockers	
Clonidine	0.1 mg bid or tid

* Nonselective.
† Selective.
MAO, monoamine oxidase; *NSAIDs,* nonsteroidal anti-inflammatory drugs.

relate to its antivasoconstrictor activity[236] or to nonvascular processes such as inhibition of platelet aggregation, serotonin release,[231] or serotonin and histamine receptor blockade. Calcium channel blockers do not necessarily share common molecular structures and may act at different sites on the calcium channel. For instance, nimodipine, nifedipine and nitrendipine are dihydropyridines; flunarizine is a piperazine derivative; and verapamil is structurally related to papaverine. It is now known that many other drugs have calcium channel blocking activity, including some that are useful for migraine (*e.g.*, amitriptyline, cyproheptadine).[236]

Data suggest that there may be a delay of up to 8 weeks before any response to these agents is seen.[160,230,233]

Verapamil may be an exception, with improvement occurring within 1 or 2 weeks of initiation. Currently, verapamil is my first choice for most patients with migraine headaches. Therapy is initiated according to the following regimen: 80 mg/day for 2 days, then 80 mg twice daily for 2 days, and then 80 mg three times daily for 2 days, followed by a switch to the 240-mg sustained-release form. Sometimes patients report an initial increase in headache, but headache improvement often requires weeks of treatment. The dose of verapamil may then be increased to 240 mg sustained release in the morning and 120 mg sustained release in the evening, and later to 240 mg sustained release twice daily. The primary side effect of verapamil is constipation, which may be avoided with the use of stool softeners. Other side effects vary depending on the individual drug, but include dizziness, headache (particularly with nifedipine), depression, vasomotor changes, tremor, orthostatic hypotension, and bradycardia. Calcium channel blockers are especially useful in patients who have comorbid hypertension or in whom β-blockers are contraindicated, such as those with asthma or Raynaud's disease. These agents, particularly verapamil, may have a particular advantage in patients with prolonged aura or basilar artery migraine. There is a lack of comparative data on the efficacy of various calcium channel blockers.

β-Blockers

β-Blockers, particularly propranolol, have been the most widely used prophylactic agents in migraine. They have proved 60% to 80% effective in producing a greater than 50% reduction in attack frequencies. Many controlled studies[237] have shown that propranolol, metoprolol, timolol, nadolol, and atenolol reduce the frequency of attacks in patients who have migraine with or without aura.[158,219] All β-blockers do have side effects, such as drowsiness, fatigue, lethargy, sleep disorders, nightmares, depression, and in rare cases, esophageal spasm. Less common side effects include orthostatic hypotension, significant bradycardia, impotence, and aggravation of intrinsic muscle disease. Such drugs have specific contraindications, including asthma, heart block, and congestive heart failure. Long-acting forms of propranolol may be helpful in some patients, but are significantly more expensive and less flexible in dosage. Studies of other β-blocking agents have been carried out, but none have been superior to propranolol. There are clearly some patients who are responsive to one drug in this class and not to others, so if a patient does not respond to propranolol it is reasonable to proceed with nadolol (80 to 240 mg), atenolol (50 to 100 mg), or timolol (20 to 60 mg). Determination of plasma propranolol concentrations have demonstrated that different responses to the same oral dose do not depend on different plasma levels of the drug.[238] Therefore, clinical response

to such agents would seem to be linked to individual sensitivity. Several articles and texts discuss the overall approach to the treatment of vascular headaches.[14,15,207,238]

Tricyclic Antidepressants

Ziegler and colleagues[239] compared propranolol to amitriptyline and found them to be equally effective, but that has not been my experience. Many regard amitriptyline to be the drug of choice in mixed headache, particularly when there is a muscle contraction and depression factor. Time and experience will indicate whether tricyclic antidepressants are really as effective as the β-blocking drugs in pure vascular headaches. The study by Diamond and associates[240] included the following statement: "The ideal prophylactic agents for the therapy of migraines should be early active, possess long-term efficacy with few side effects and a convenient dosing schedule, and truly prevent attacks from occurring rather than merely decreasing their severity." The fact is that no such ideal agent has been found.

The tricyclic antidepressants most commonly used for migraine and tension-type headache prophylaxis include amitriptyline, nortriptyline, doxepin, and protriptyline.[219] Side effects of tricyclic antidepressants are common and involve antimuscarinic effects such as dry mouth and sedation. These drugs also increase appetite and therefore cause weight gain. One should also be aware of potential cardiac toxicity and orthostatic hypotension. Tricyclics have also been used cautiously in combination with monoamine oxidase (MAO) inhibitors or β-blockers. Selective serotonin reuptake inhibitors, such as fluoxetine and sertraline, are the newest types of antidepressants that may be effective in some headache patients.

Serotonin Antagonists

Methysergide is a semisynthetic ergot 5-HT$_2$ receptor antagonist that displays affinity for the 5-HT$_1$ receptor.[9] Methysergide is an effective migraine prophylactic in 60% or more of migraineurs and may be especially effective in cluster headache. Its side effects include transient muscle aching, claudication, abdominal distress, nausea, weight gain, and hallucination. The major complication is the rare (1 in 5000) development of retroperitoneal, pulmonary, or endocardial fibrosis.[241,242] It is believed that this major complication may be prevented by having a medication-free interval of 4 weeks after each 6-month period of continuous treatment. The dosage should not exceed three 2-mg pills daily (i.e., 6 mg/day total).

Discussion on the use of other agents, such as cyproheptadine and pizotifen, as well as anticonvulsant medications, can be found elsewhere.[9,207]

Another approach to migraine therapy is vigorous

bilateral compression and massage of the frontal branch of the superficial temporal artery, started at the first sign of visual aura. The technique was successful in blocking 81% of attacks in 15 patients.[243] The authors speculated that the blood vessels of the extracranial circulation, as well as those of the circle of Willis, have perivascular nerve fibers of trigeminal origin. It may well be that these nerve fibers, rather than the dilation of blood vessels with release of vasoactive substances, mediate the pain syndrome of migraine. Digital massage might stimulate the nerve endings and somehow stop the ensuing pain phase of the headache.

As pointed out by Silberstein and Lipton,[9] the goals of treatment are to relieve or prevent pain and the associated symptoms of migraine and to optimize the patient's ability to function normally. The patient should learn to identify and avoid headache triggers. The wide variety of drug therapies available (more than 400) attest to the fact that no particular therapy or combination of drugs is completely effective. The management of the patient with migraine is a complex problem requiring evaluation and elimination of possible precipitating factors, including psychogenic ones, as well as vigorous management of the acute attack and attempts at prevention of recurrent episodes. The care of the migraine patient continues to represent, in many instances, a major therapeutic challenge.

REFERENCES

1. Dalessio DJ: Diagnosing the severe headache. Neurology 44(suppl 3):6, 1994
2. Lipton RB, Stewart WF: Migraine in the United States: epidemiology and health care utilization. Neurology 43(suppl 3):6, 1993
3. Stewart WF, Lipton RB, Celentano DD et al: Prevalence of migraine headache in the United States. JAMA 267:64, 1992
4. Sacks OW: Migraine, the Evolution of a Common Disorder. Los Angeles, University California Press, 1970
5. Gowers WR: Subjective visual sensations. Trans Ophthalmol Soc UK 15:1, 1895
6. Troost BT, Newton TH: Occipital lobe arteriovenous malformations: clinical and radiologic features in 26 cases with comments on the differentiation from migraine. Arch Ophthalmol 93:250, 1975
7. Headache Classification Committee of the International Headache Society: Classification and diagnostic criteria for headache disorders, cranial neuralgia, and facial pain. Cephalalgia 8(suppl 7):1, 1988
8. Blau JN: Migraine prodromes separated from the aura: complete migraine. Br Med J 281:658, 1980
9. Silberstein SD, Lipton RB: Overview of diagnosis and treatment of migraine. Neurology 44(suppl 7):6, 1994
10. Lipton RB, Stewart W, Celentano DD et al: Undiagnosed migraine: a comparison of symptom-based and self-reported physician diagnosis. Arch Intern Med 156:1, 1992
11. Stewart WF, Schecter A, Lipton RB: Migraine heterogeneity: disability, pain intensity, attack frequency, and duration. Neurology 44(suppl 4):24, 1994
12. Amery WK, Van Neueten JM, Wauquier A: The Pharmacological Basis of Migraine Therapy. London, Pitman, 1984
13. Rose CF: Progress in Migraine Research Vol 2. London, Pitman, 1984
14. Raskin NH: Headache, p 1. New York, Churchill Livingstone, 1988
15. Dalessio DJ: Wolff's Headache and Other Head Pain, p 1. New York, Oxford University Press, 1993
16. Welch KMA: Relationship of stroke and migraine. Neurology 44(suppl 7):33, 1994
17. Olesen J, Larsen B, Lautitzen M: Focal hyperemia followed by spreading oligemia and impaired activation of rCBF in classic migraine. Ann Neurol 9:344, 1981
18. Skyhoj-Olesen TS, Friberg L, Lassen NA: Ischemia may be the primary cause of the neurologic deficits in classic migraine. Arch Neurol 44:156, 1987
19. Sicuteri F: Vasoneuroactive substances in migraine. Headache 6:109, 1966
20. Lance JW, Anthony M, Gonski A: Serotonin, the carotid body, and cranial vessels in migraine. Arch Neurol 16:553, 1967
21. Curran AC, Hinterberger H, Lance JW: Total plasma serotonin, 5-hydroxyindoleacetic acid and p-hydroxy-m-methoxymandelic acid excretion in normal and migrainous subjects. Brain 88:997, 1966
22. Moskowitz MA: The neurobiology of vascular head pain. Ann Neurol 16:157, 1984
23. Raskin NH: Chemical headaches. Annu Rev Med 32:63, 1981
24. Dalessio DJ: Wolff's Headache and Other Head Pain, p 1. New York, Oxford University Press, 1993
25. O'Brien M: Cerebral blood changes in migraine. Headache 10:139, 1971
26. Simard D, Pauson OB: Cerebral vasomotor paralysis during migraine attack. Arch Neurol 29:207, 1973
27. Brewerton TD, Murphy DL, Mueller EA et al: Induction of migraine-like headaches by the serotonin agonist m-chlorophenylpiperazine. Clin Pharmacol Ther 43:605, 1988
28. Gordon ML, Lipton RB, Brown SL et al: Headache and cortical responses to m-chlorophenylpiperazine are highly correlated. Cephalalgia 13:400, 1993
29. Friedman AP, Merritt HH: Headache: Diagnosis and Treatment. Philadelphia, FA Davis, 1959
30. Callahan N: The migraine syndrome in pregnancy. Neurology 18:197, 1968
31. Shafey S, Scheinberg P: Neurological syndromes in patients receiving synthetic steroids. Neurology 16:205, 1966
32. Phillips BM: Oral contraceptive drugs and migraine. Br Med J 2:99, 1968
33. Whitty CWM, Hockaday KM, Whitty MM: The effect of oral contraceptives on migraine. Lancet 1:856, 1966
34. Somerville BW: Estrogen-withdrawal migraine: I. Duration or exposure required and attempted prophylaxis by premenstrual estrogen administration. Neurology 25:235, 1975
35. Hanington E, Horn M, Wilkinson M: Further observations on the effects of tyramine. In Cochrane AL (ed): Background to Migraine, Third Migraine Symposium, pp 113–119. London, Heinemann, 1969
36. Haas DC, Pindela GS, Lourie H: Juvenile head trauma syndromes and their relationship to migraine. Arch Neurol 32:727, 1975
37. Paulson GW, Klawans HL: Benign orgasmic cephalgia. Headache 13:1, 1974
38. Milner PM: Note on a possible correspondence between the scotomas of migraine and spreading depression of Leão. Electroencephalogr Clin Neurophysiol 10:705, 1958
39. Lashley KS: Patterns of cerebral integration indicated by scotomas of migraine. Arch Neurol Psych 46:333, 1941
40. Wilkinson M, Blau JN: Are classical and common migraine different entities? Headache 25:211, 1985
41. Alverez WC: The migrainous scotoma is studied in 618 persons. Am J Ophthalmol 49:389, 1960
42. Klee A, Willanger R: Disturbance of visual perception in migraine. Acta Neurol Scand 42:400, 1966
43. Walsh FB, Hoyt WF: Clinical Neuro-Ophthalmology. Baltimore, Williams & Wilkins, 1969
44. Richards W: The fortification illusions of migraines. Sci Am 224:88, 1971
45. Gowers WR: Visual sensations in migraine. In Gowers WR (ed): Subjective Sensations of Sight and Sound, Abiotrophy and Other Lectures, pp 18–41. London, Churchill, 1907

46. Peatfield C, Rose F: Migrainous visual symptoms in a woman without eyes. Arch Neurol 38:466, 1981
47. Day JW, Raskin NH: Thunderclap headache: symptoms of un-ruptured aneurysm. Lancet 2:1247, 1986
48. Haas DC: Prolonged migraine aura status. Ann Neurol 11:197, 1982
49. Fisher CM: Late-life migraine accompaniments as a cause of unexplained transient ischemic attacks. Can J Neurol Sci 7:9, 1980
50. Troost BT, Mark LE, Maroon JC: Resolution of classic migraine following removal of an occipital lobe arteriovenous malformation. Ann Neurol 5:199, 1979
51. Bartleson JD: Transient and persistent neurological manifestations of migraine. Stroke 15:383, 1984
52. Berg MJ, Williams LS: The transient syndrome of headache with neurologic deficits and CSF lymphocytosis. Neurology 45:1648, 1995
53. Dvorkin GS, Andermann F, Carpenter S et al: Classical migraine, intractable epilepsy, and multiple strokes: A syndrome related to mitochondrial encephalomyopathy. In Andermann F, Lugaresi E (eds): Migraine and Epilepsy, pp 203–232. Stoneham, MA, Butterworth, 1987
54. Fitzsimons R, Wolfenden WH: Migraine coma: menigitic migraine with cerebral edema associated with a new form of autosomal dominant cerebellar ataxia. Brain 108:555, 1985
55. Caplan L: Intracerebral hemorrhage revisited. Neurology 38:624, 1988
56. Levine SR, Joseph R, D'Andrea G et al: Migraine and the lupus anticoagulant. Cephalalgia 7:93, 1987
57. Ormond AW: Two cases of permanent hemianopsia following severe attacks of migraine. Ophthalmol Rev 32:192, 1913
58. Butler TH: Scotoma in migrainous subjects. Br J Ophthalmol 17:83, 1933
59. Butler TH: Uncommon symptoms of migraine. Trans Ophthalmol Soc UK 61:205, 1941
60. Rothrock JF, Walicke P, Swenson MR et al: Migrainous stroke. Arch Neurol 45:63, 1988
61. Bougousslavsky J, Regli F, Van Melle G et al: Migraine stroke. Neurology 38:223, 1988
62. Tzourio C, Iglesias S, Hubert J et al: Migraine and risk of ischemic stroke: a case-controlled study. Br Med J 307:289, 1993
63. Hollenhorst RB: Ocular manifestations of migraine: report of 4 cases of hemianopsia. Proc Staff Meeting Mayo Clinic 28:686, 1958
64. Rich WM: Permanent quadrantanopia after migraine. Br Med J 116:592, 1948
65. Connor RCR: Complicated migraine: a study of permanent neurological and visual defects by migraine. Lancet 2:1072, 1962
66. Bruyn GW: Complicated migraine. In Vinken PJ, Bruyn GW (eds): Handbook of Clinical Neurology, pp 59–95. New York, American Elsevier, 1968
67. Caplan L, Chedru F, Lhermitte F et al: Transient global amnesia and migraine. Neurology 31:1167, 1981
68. Selby G, Lance JW: Observations on 500 cases of migraine and allied vascular headache. J Neurol Neurosurg Psych 23:23, 1960
69. Smyth VOG, Winter AL: The EEG and migraine. Electroencephalogr Clin Neurophysiol 16:194, 1964
70. Boudin G, Pepin B, Barbizet J et al: Migraine and EEG disturbances. Electroencephalogr Clin Neurophysiol 14:141, 1962
71. Hockaday JM, Whitty CWM: Factors determining the electroencephalogram in migraine: a study of 560 patients according to clinical type of migraine. Brain 92:769, 1969
72. Friedman MW: Occlusion of central retinal vein in migraine. Arch Ophthalmol 45:678, 1951
73. Heyck H: Pathogenesis of migraine. In Friedman AP (ed): Research and Clinical Studies in Headache, pp 1–28. New York, Karger, 1969
74. Heyck H: Varieties of hemiplegic migraine. Headache 14:135, 1973
75. Alpers BJ, Yaskin HE: Pathogenesis of ophthalmoplegic migraine. Arch Ophthalmol 45:555, 1951
76. Patterson RH, Goodell H, Dunning HS: Complications of carotid arteriography. Arch Neurol 10:513, 1964
77. Friedman AP, Finley KH, Graham JR et al: Classification of headache. Neurology 12:173, 1962
78. Whitty CWM: Familial hemiplegic migraine. J Neurol Neurosurg Psychiatry 16:172, 1953
79. Blau JN, Whitty CWM: Familial hemiplegic migraine. Lancet 2:1115, 1955
80. Heyck H: Die neurologischen Begleiterscheinungen der Migraine und das Problem des "angiospastischen Herninsults." Nervenarzt 33:193, 1962
81. Rosenbaum HE: Familial hemiplegic migraine. Neurology 10:164, 1960
82. Ohta M, Araki S, Kuroiwa Y: Familial occurrence of migraine with hemiplegic syndrome and cerebellar manifestations. Neurology 17:813, 1967
83. Young GF, Leon-Barth CA, Green J: Familial hemiplegic migraine, retinal degeneration, deafness, and nystagmus. Arch Neurol 23:201, 1970
84. Dooling EC, Sweeney VP: Migrainous hemiplegia during breast feeding. Am J Obstet Gynecol 118:568, 1974
85. Troost BT, Tomsak RL: Ophthalmoplegic migraine and retinal migraine. In Olesen J, Tfelt-Hansen P, Welch KMA (eds): The Headaches, pp 421–426. New York, Raven, 1993
86. Tomsak RL, Masaryk TJ, Bates JH: Magnetic resonance angiography (MRA) of isolated aneurysmal third nerve palsy. J Clin Neuro Ophthalmol 11:16, 1991
87. Walsh JP, O'Doherty DS: A possible explanation of the mechanism of ophthalmoplegic migraine. Neurology 10:1079, 1960
88. Verbrugghen A: Pathogenesis of ophthalmoplegic migraine. Neurology 5:311, 1955
89. Lincoff H, Cogan D: Unilateral headache and oculomotor paralysis not caused by aneurysm. Arch Ophthalmol 57:181, 1957
90. Donahue HC: Migraine and its ocular manifestations. Arch Ophthalmol 43:96, 1950
91. Friedman AP, Harter DH, Merritt HH: Ophthalmoplegic migraine. Arch Neurol 7:320, 1962
92. Woody RC, Blaw ME: Ophthalmoplegic migraine in infancy. Clin Pediatr 25:82, 1986
93. Hallet M, Cogan DG: Episodic unilateral mydriasis in otherwise normal patients. Arch Ophthalmol 84:130, 1970
94. Edelson RN, Levy DE: Transient benign unilateral pupillary dilatation in young adults. Arch Neurol 31:12, 1974
95. Woods D, O'Connor PS, Fleming R: Episodic unilateral mydriasis and migraine. Am J Ophthalmol 98:229, 1984
96. Sarkies NJC, Sanders MD, Gautier-Smith PC: Letter to the Editor: Episodic unilateral mydriasis and migraine. Am J Ophthalmol 99:217, 1985
97. Durkan GP, Troost BT, Slamovits TL et al: Recurrent painless oculomotor palsy in children: a variant of ophthalmoplegic migraine. Headache 21:58, 1981
98. Gabianelli EB, Klingele TG, Burde RM: Acute oculomotor nerve palsy in childhood: is arteriography necessary? J Clin Neuro Ophthalmol 9:33, 1989
99. Osuntoken O, Osuntoken BO: Ophthalmoplegic migraine and hemoglobinopathy in Nigerians. Am J Ophthalmol 74:451, 1972
100. Anderson DR: Perimetry: With and without automation. St Louis, CV Mosby, 1987
101. Tomsak RL, Jergens PB: Benign recurrent transient monocular blindness: a possible variant of acephalgia migraine. Headache 27:66, 1987
102. Kline LB, Kelley CL: Ocular migraine in a patient with cluster headache. Headache 20:253, 1980
103. Gronvall A: On changes in the fundus oculi and persisting injuries to the eye in migraine. Acta Ophthalmol 16:602, 1938
104. Cassen JH, Tomsak RL, DeLuise VP: Mixed arteriovenous occlusive disease of the fundus. J Clin Neuro Ophthalmol 5:164, 1985
105. Wolter JR, Burchfield WJ: Ocular migraine in a young man resulting in unilateral transient blindness and retinal edema. J Pediatr Ophthalmol 8:173, 1971
106. Burger SK, Saul RF, Selhorst JB, Thurston SE: Transient monocular blindness caused by vasospasm. N Engl J Med 325:870, 1991
107. Graveson GS: Retinal arterial occlusion in migraine. Br Med J 2:838, 1949

108. Krapin D: Occlusion of the central retinal artery in migraine. N Engl J Med 270:359, 1964
109. Miller NR: Walsh and Hoyt's Neuro-Ophthalmology, 4 ed, p 220. Baltimore, Williams & Wilkins, 1982
110. Hupp SL, Kline LB, Corbett JJ: Visual disturbance of migraine. Surv Ophthalmol 33:221, 1989
111. Newman NJ, Lessell S, Brandt M: Bilateral central retinal artery occlusions, disk drusen, and migraine. Am J Ophthalmol 107:236, 1989
112. Corbett JJ: Neuro-ophthalmic complications of migraine and cluster headaches. In Smith CH, Beck RW (eds): Neurologic Clinics. Symposium on Neuro-Ophthalmology, pp 973–995. Philadelphia, WB Saunders, 1983
113. Coppeto JR, Monteiro MLR, Sciarra R: Giant cell arteritis with bilateral uveitic glaucoma. Ann Ophthalmol 17:299, 1985
114. Lewis RA, Vijayan N, Watson C et al: Visual field loss in migraine. Ophthalmology 96:321, 1989
115. Carroll D: Retinal migraine. Headache 10:9, 1970
116. Dirr LY, Janton FJ, Troost BT: Non-benign amaurosis fugax in a medical student. Neurology 40:349, 1990
117. McDonald WI, Sanders MD: Migraine complicated by ischemic papillopathy. Lancet 2:521, 1971
118. Laties AM: Central retinal artery innervation: absence of adrenergic innervation to the intraocular branches. Arch Ophthalmol 77:405, 1967
119. Coppeto JR, Lessell S, Sciarra R et al: Vascular retinopathy in migraine. Neurology 36:267, 1986
120. Larsen BH, Sorensen PS, Marquardsen J: Transient ischaemic attacks in young patients, a thromboembolic or migrainous manifestation? A ten year follow up of 46 patients. J Neurol Neurosurg Psychiatry 53:1029, 1990
121. Brown GC, Margargal LE, Shields JA et al: Retinal arterial obstruction in children and young adults. Ophthalmology 88:18, 1981
122. Kupersmith MJ, Hass WK, Chase NE: Isoproterenol treatment of visual symptoms in migraine. Stroke 10:299, 1979
123. Bickerstaff ER: Basilar artery migraine. Lancet 1:15, 1961
124. Bickerstaff ER: Impairment of consciousness in migraine. Lancet 2:1057, 1961
125. Lees F, Watkins SM: Loss of consciousness in migraine. Lancet 2:647, 1963
126. Basser LS: The relation of migraine and epilepsy. Brain 92:285, 1969
127. Bickerstaff ER: The basilar artery and the migraine-epilepsy syndrome. Proc R Soc Med 55:167, 1962
128. Guest IA, Woolf AL: Fatal infarction of the brain in migraine. Br Med J 1:225, 1964
129. Swanson JW, Vick NA: Basilar artery migraine, 12 patients, with an attack recorded electroencephalographically. Neurology 28:782, 1978
130. Lance JW: The Mechanisms and Management of Headache. London, Butterworth, 1969
131. Whitty CWM: Migraine variants. Br Med J 1:38, 1971
132. Gascon G, Barlow C: Juvenile migraine, presenting as an acute confusional state. Pediatrics 45:628, 1970
133. Whitty CWM: Migraine without headache. Lancet 2:283, 1967
134. Kunkle EC, Pfeiffer JB, Wilhoit WM et al: Recurrent brief headache in "cluster" pattern. Trans Am Neurol Assoc 77:240, 1967
135. Bickerstaff EB: Cluster headaches. In Vinken PJ, Bruyn GW (eds): Handbook of Clinical Neurology, pp 111–118. New York, American Elsevier, 1968
136. Eggleston DJ: Periodic migrainous neuralgia. Oral Surg 29:524, 1970
137. Nelson RF: Cluster migraine: an unrecognized common entity. Can Med Assoc J 103:1026, 1970
138. Lance JW, Anthony M: Migrainous neuralgia or cluster headache. J Neurol Sci 13:401, 1971
139. Ekbom K: A clinical comparison of cluster headache and migraine. Acta Neurol Scand 46:1, 1970
140. Romberg MH: A Manual of the Nervous Disease of Man, p 56. unknown publisher, 1853
141. Harris W: Neuritis and Neuralgia, pp 145–146. Oxford, Oxford University Press, 1926
142. Harris W: Ciliary (migrainous) neuralgia and its treatment. Br Med J 1:457, 1938
143. Ekbom K, Greitz T: Carotid angiography in cluster headache. Acta Radiol 10:177, 1970
144. Vail HH: Vidian neuralgia, with special reference to eye and orbital pain in suppuration of petrous apex. Ann Otolaryngol 41:837, 1932
145. Aubry M, Pialoux P: Sluder's syndrome. In Vinken PJ, Bruyn GW (eds): Handbook of Clinical Neurology, pp 326–332. New York, American Elsevier, 1968
146. Raeder JG: "Paratrigeminal" paralysis of oculopupillary sympathetic. Brain 47:149, 1924
147. Boniuk M, Schlezinger NS: Raeder's paratrigeminal syndrome. Am J Ophthalmol 54:1074, 1962
148. Ford FR, Walsh FB: Raeder's paratrigeminal syndrome: a benign disorder, possibly a complication of migraine. Bull Johns Hopkins Hosp 103:296, 1958
149. Smith JL: Raeder's paratrigeminal syndrome. Am J Ophthalmol 46:194, 1958
150. Kunkle EC, Anderson WB: Significance of minor eye signs in headaches of migraine type. Arch Ophthalmol 65:504, 1961
151. Davis RH, Daroff RB, Hoyt WF: Hemicrania, oculosympathetic paresis, and subcranial carotic aneurysm: Raeder's paratrigeminal syndrome (group 2). J Neurosurg 29:94, 1968
152. Law WR, Nelson ER: Internal carotid aneurysm as a cause of Raeder's paratrigeminal syndrome. Neurology 18:43, 1968
153. Cohen DN, Zakov ZN, Salanga VD et al: Raeder's paratrigeminal syndrome: a new etiology. Am J Ophthalmol 79:1044, 1975
154. Horton BT: Histaminic cephalgia: differential diagnosis and treatment. Proc Mayo Clin 31:325, 1956
155. Meyer JS, Binns PM, Ericsson AD et al: Sphenopalatine ganglionectomy for cluster headache. Arch Otolaryngol 92:475, 1970
156. Anthony M, Lance JW: Histamine and serotonin in cluster headache. Arch Neurol 25:225, 1971
157. Graham JR: Methysergide for prevention of headache. N Engl J Med 270:67, 1964
158. Weber RB, Reinmuth OM: The treatment of migraine with propranolol. Neurology 22:366, 1972
159. Gelmers HJ: Nimodipine, a new calcium antagonist, in the prophylactic treatment of migraine. Headache 23:106, 1983
160. Lance JW: Headache. Ann Neurol 10:1, 1981
161. Vahlquist B: Migraine in children. Int Arch Allergy Appl Immunol 7:348, 1955
162. Bille B: A study of the incidence and short term prognosis, and a clinical, psychological and encephalographic comparison between children with migraine and matched controls. Acta Pediatr Scand 51:1, 1962
163. Michael MI, Williams JM: Migraine in children. J Pediatr 41:18, 1952
164. Krupp GR, Friedman AP: Recurrent headache in children: a study of 100 clinical cases. NY State J Med 53:43, 1933
165. Holguin J, Fenichel G: Migraine. J Pediatr 70:290, 1967
166. Hachinski VC, Porchawka J, Steele JC: Visual symptoms in the migraine syndrome. Neurology 23:570, 1973
167. Golden GS: The "Alice in Wonderland syndrome" in juvenile migraine. Pediatrics 63:517, 1979
168. Haas DC, Souner RD: Migraine attacks triggered by mild head trauma and their relation to certain post-traumatic disorders of childhood. J Neurol Neurosurg Psychiatry 32:548, 1969
169. Griffith JF, Dodge PR: Transient blindness following head injury in children. N Engl J Med 278:638, 1968
170. Greenblatt SH: Post-traumatic transient cerebral blindness: association with migraine and seizure diathesis. JAMA 225:1073, 1973
171. Forsyth WI, Gillies D, Sills MA: Propanolol ("Inderal") in the treatment of childhood migraine. Develop Med Child Neurol 26:737, 1984
172. Hinrichs WL, Keith HM: Migraine in childhood: a follow-up report. Mayo Clin Proc 40:593, 1965
173. Diamond S, Dalessio DJ: The Practicing Physician's Approach to Headache, p 1. Baltimore, Williams & Wilkins, 1986
174. Anonymous: The Headaches, p 1. New York, Raven Press, 1993
175. Troost BT, McCormick GM: Migraine and facial pain. In Lessell S, Van Dalen JTW (eds): Current Neuro-Ophthalmology, pp 269–287. Chicago, Year Book, 1989

176. Troost BT: Migraine and facial pain. In Lessell S, Van Dalen JTW (eds): Current Neuro-Ophthalmology, pp 269–287. New York, Year Book, 1988

177. Swerdlow M: Anticonvulsant drugs and chronic pain. Clin Neuropharmacol 7:51, 1984

178. Janetta PJ: Microsurgical approach to the trigeminal nerve for tic douloureux. Progr Neurol Surg 7:188, 1976

179. Janetta PJ: Microsurgical management of trigeminal neuralgia. Arch Neurol 42:800, 1985

180. Zorman G, Wilson CB: Outcome following microsurgical vascular decompression or partial sensory rhizotomy in 125 cases of trigeminal neuralgia. Neurology 34:1362, 1984

181. Sweet WH: The treatment of trigeminal neuralgia. N Engl J Med 316:692, 1987

182. Allen NB, Studenski SA: Polymyalgia rheumatica and temporal arteritis. Med Clin North Am 79:369, 1986

183. Vilaseca J, Gonzalez A, Cid MC et al: Clinical usefulness of temporal artery biopsy. Ann Rheum Dis 46:282, 1987

184. Soloman S, Cappa KG: The headache of temporal arteritis. J Am Geriatr Soc 35:163, 1987

185. Wall M, Corbett JJ: Arteritis. In: Olesen J, Tfelt-Hanson P, Welch KMA (eds): The Headaches, pp 653–663. New York, Raven Press, 1993

186. Currie J, Lessell S: Tonic pupil giant cell arteritis. Br J Ophthalmol 68:135, 1984

187. Monteiro MLR, Coppeto JR, Greco P: Giant cell arteritis of the posterior cerebral circulation presenting with ataxia and ophthalmoplegia. Arch Ophthalmol 102:407, 1984

188. Howard GF, Ho SU, Kim KS et al: Bilateral carotid artery occlusion resulting from giant cell arteritis. Ann Neurol 15:204, 1984

189. Truong L, Kopelman RG, Williams GS et al: Temporal arteritis and renal disease. Am J Med 78:171, 1985

190. Perruquet JL, Davis DE, Harrington TM: Aortic arch arteritis in the elderly: an important manifestation of giant cell arteritis. Arch Intern Med 146:289, 1986

191. Selsky IJ, Nirankari VS: Temporomandibular joint pain as a manifestation of temporal arteritis. South Med J 78:1249, 1985

192. Accetta DD, Kelley JF, Tubbs RR: An elderly black woman with a painful "swollen" face. Ann Allergy 55:819, 1985

193. Goodman BW, Shepard FA: Jaw claudication: Its value as a diagnostic clue. Postgrad Med 73:177, 1983

194. Save-Soderbergh J, Malmvall BE, Andersson R et al: Giant cell arteritis as a cause of death: report of nine cases. JAMA 255:493, 1986

195. Wong RL, Korn JH: Temporal arteritis and normal sedimentation rates. Am J Med 80:959, 1986

196. Villalta J, Estrach T: Letter to the Editor: Temporal arteritis with normal erythrocyte sedimentation. Ann Intern Med 103:808, 1985

197. Plum F: Temporal arteritis with normal sedimentation rate. Neurology Alert 4:46, 1986

198. Daroff RB: New headache classification. Neurology 38:1138, 1988

199. Ziegler DK: Tension-muscle contraction headaches: A review. In Pfaffenrath V, Lundberg PO, Sjaastad O (eds): Updating Headache, pp 315–320. Berlin, Springer-Verlag, 1985

200. Jakobsen J, Baadsgaard SE, Thompsen S et al: Prediction of post-concussional sequelae by reaction time test. Acta Neurol Scand 75:341, 1987

201. Leblanc R: The minor leak preceding subarachnoid hemorrhage. J Neurosurg 66:35, 1987

202. Carlow TJ: Headache and the eye. In Dalessio DJ (ed): Wolff's Headache and Other Head Pain, pp 304–320. New York, Oxford University Press, 1987

203. Mokri B, Sundt TM, Houser OW et al: Spontaneous dissection of the cervical internal carotid artery. Ann Neurol 19:126, 1986

204. Vinken PJ, Bruyn GW: Handbook of Clinical Neurology. New York, American Elsevier, 1968

205. Francis KR, Williams DP, Troost BT: Facial numbness and dysesthesia. Arch Neurol 44:345, 1987

206. Pincus JH, Daroff RB: Sphenoid sinus mucocele: a curable cause of the ophthalmoplegic migraine syndrome. JAMA 187:459, 1964

207. Baumel B: Migraine: a pharmacologic review with newer options and delivery modalities. Neurology 44(suppl 3):13, 1994

208. Edmeads J: Advances in migraine therapy: focus on oral sumatriptan. Neurology 45(suppl 7):3, 1995

209. Cutler N, Mushet GR, Davis R et al: Oral sumatriptan for the acute treatment of migraine: evaluation of three dosage strengths. Neurology 45(suppl 7):5, 1995

210. Sargent J, Kirchner JR, Davis R, Kirkhart B: Oral sumatriptan is effective and well tolerated for the acute treatment of migraine: results of a multicenter study. Neurology 45(suppl 7):10, 1995

211. Rederich G, Rapoport A, Cutler N et al: Oral sumatriptan for the long-term treatment of migraine: clinical findings. Neurology 45(suppl 7):15, 1995

212. Humphrey PPA, Feniuk W, Perren MJ: Anti-migraine drugs in development: advances in serotonin receptor pharmacology. Headache 30(suppl 1):12, 1990

213. Peroutka SJ: Developments in 5-hydroxytryptamine receptor pharmacology in migraine. Neurol Clin 8:829, 1990

214. Peroutka SJ: The pharmacology of current antimigraine drugs. Headache 30(suppl 1):12, 1990

215. Callaham M, Raskin N: A controlled study of dihydroergotamine in the treatment of acute migraine headache. Headache 26:168, 1986

216. Silberstein SD: Review: serotonin 5-HT and migraine. Headache 34:408, 1994

217. Ryan RE: A study of Midrin in the symptomatic relief of migraine headache. Headache 14:33, 1974

218. Tfelt-Hansen P, Lipton RB: Miscellaneous drugs. In Olesen J, Tfelt-Hansen P, Welch KMA (eds): The Headaches, pp 353–358. New York, Raven Press, 1993

219. Silberstein SD, Saper J: Migraine: Diagnosis and treatment. In Dalessio D, Silberstein SD (eds): Wolff's Headache and Other Head Pain, pp 96–170. New York, Oxford University Press, 1993

220. Wilkinson M: Migraine: treatment of acute attack. Br Med J 2:754, 1971

221. Goodman LS, Gilman A: The Pharmacological Basis of Therapeutics, p 1. New York, Pergamon Press, 1990

222. Raskin NH, Raskin KE: Repetitive intravenous dihydroergotamine for the treatment of intractable migraine. Neurology 34(suppl 1):245, 1984

223. Sanders SW, Haering N, Mosberg H et al: Pharmacokinetics of ergotamine in healthy volunteers following oral and rectal dosing. Eur J Clin Pharmacol 30:331, 1986

224. Volans GN: Research review: migraine and drug absorption. Clin Pharmacokinet 3:313, 1978

225. Sicuteri F, Franchi G, Del Bianco PL: An antaminic drug, BC-105, in the prophylaxis of migraine. Int Arch Allergy Appl Immunol 31:78, 1967

226. Cady RK, Wendt JK, Kirchner JR et al: Treatment of acute migraine with subcutaneous sumatriptan. JAMA 265:2831, 1991

227. The Oral Sumatriptan International Multiple-Dose Study Group: Evaluation of a multiple-dose regimen of oral sumatriptan for the acute treatment of migraine. Eur Neurol 31:306, 1991

228. Slugg PH, Kunkel RS: Complications of methysergide therapy: retroperitoneal fibrosis, mitral regurgitation, edema, and hemolytic anemia. JAMA 213:297, 1970

229. Cortelli P, Sacquegna T, Albani F et al: Propranolol plasma levels and relief of migraine: relationship between plasma propranolol and 4-hydroxypropranolol concentrations and clinical effects. Arch Neurol 42:46, 1985

230. Solomon GD, Steel JD, Spaccavento LJ: Verapamil prophylaxis of migraine: a double-blind, placebo-controlled study. JAMA 250:2500, 1983

231. Kahan A, Weber S, Amor B et al: Nifedipine in the treatment of migraine in patients with Raynaud's phenomenon. N Engl J Med 308:1102, 1983

232. Meyer JS, Hardenberg J: Clinical effectiveness of calcium entry blockers in prophylactic treatment of migraine and cluster headaches. Headache 23:266, 1983

233. Havanka-Kanniainen H, Hokkanen E, Myllyla VV: Efficacy of minodipine in the prophylaxis of migraine. Cephalalgia 5:38, 1985

234. Louis P: A double-blind placebo-controlled prophylactic study of flunarizine (Sibelium) in migraine. Headache 21:235, 1981

235. Amery WK, Caers LI, Aerts TJL: Flunarizine, a calcium entry blocker in migraine prophylaxis. Headache 25:249, 1985

236. Ryan RE Sr, Ryan RE Jr, Sudilovsky A: Nadolol: its use in the prophylactic treatment of migraine. Headache 23:26, 1983

237. Andersson K, Vinge E: Adrenoceptor blockers and calcium antagonists in the prophylaxis and treatment of migraine. Drugs 39:355, 1990

238. Daroff RB, Whitney CM: Treatment of vascular headaches. Headache 26:470, 1986

239. Ziegler DK, Hurwitz A, Hassanein RS et al: Migraine prophy-laxis: a comparison of propranolol and amitriptyline. Arch Neurol 44:486, 1987

240. Diamond S, Solomon GD, Freitag FG et al: Long-acting propranolol in the prophylaxis of migraine. Headache 27:70, 1987

241. Elkind AH, Friedman AP, Bachman A et al: Silent retroperitoneal fibrosis associated with methysergide therapy. JAMA 206:1041, 1968

242. Graham J: Cardiac and pulmonary fibrosis during methysergide therapy for headache. Am J Med Sci 254:1, 1967

243. Lipton SA: Prevention of classic migraine headache by digital massage of the superficial temporal arteries during visual aura. Ann Neurol 19:515, 1986

CHAPTER 17

Aneurysms, Arteriovenous Communications, and Related Vascular Malformations

B. Todd Troost, Joel S. Glaser, and P. Pearse Morris

Aneurysms
  Saccular Aneurysms
    Intracavernous Carotid
    Carotid-Ophthalmic Artery
    Carotid-Supraclinoid
    Ophthalmic Artery
    Posterior Communicating Artery
    Middle Cerebral Artery
    Anterior Communicating Artery
    Vertebrobasilar System
    Posterior Cerebral Artery
  Childhood Aneurysms
  Traumatic Aneurysms
  Fusiform Aneurysms
    Carotid System
    Vertebrobasilar System
Arteriovenous Malformations
  Supratentorial
  Infratentorial
Cavernous Malformations

Carotid-Cavernous Sinus Fistulas
Endovascular Interventional Procedures
  Dural Arteriovenous Malformations and Carotid-Cavernous Fistulas
  Aneurysms of the Carotid Siphon
  Embolization of Tumors of the Cavernous Sinus
Oculocephalic Vascular Anomalies
  Retinocerebellar Angiomatosis (von Hipple-Lindau Disease)
  Encephalotrigeminal Angiomatosis (Sturge-Weber Syndrome)
  Racemose Hemangiomas of Retina, Thalamus, and Midbrain
  Cavernous Angiomas of Retina and Brain
Orbital Vascular Anomalies
  Venous Varices, Lymphangiomas, and Related Lesions
  Vascular Defects Related to Trauma

I've had migraine but this was an explosion in my head! The pain was unbearable and I went down, first to my knees, then face-forward. Above me there were two refrigerators . . . and then I died.

> Patient RMK survived rupture of a posterior communicating artery aneurysm.

Aneurysms and arteriovenous communications of the cranial blood vessels, both congenital and acquired, commonly produce signs and symptoms in the ocular motor and visual sensory systems. They are of particular importance in neuro-ophthalmologic diagnosis and should be considered as etiologic possibilities in clinical profiles characterized by chronic mass effect, as well as in the more dramatic acute hemorrhagic episodes.

Vascular defects present from birth may suddenly become manifest in adult life as, for example, an oculomotor palsy resulting from an aneurysm at the origin of the posterior communicating artery or as a homonymous visual field defect from occipital lobe arteriovenous malformation (AVM). Acquired vascular lesions may become evident immediately following trauma or after some interval, as in the case of carotid-cavernous sinus fistulas.

B. T. Troost: Department of Neurology, Wake Forest University School of Medicine; and Department of Neurology, North Carolina Baptist Hospital, Winston-Salem, North Carolina

J. S. Glaser: Departments of Neurology and Ophthalmology, Bascom Palmer Eye Institute, University of Miami School of Medicine, Miami; and Neuro-ophthalmology, Cleveland Clinic Florida, Ft. Lauderdale, Florida

P. P. Morris: Department of Ophthalmology, Wake Forest University School of Medicine, Winston-Salem, North Carolina

ANEURYSMS

Intracranial saccular aneurysms are acquired lesions that occur principally at arterial bifurcations of the circle of Willis at the base of the brain, this location accounting for perhaps some 80% to 90% of all aneurysms. Most present as sudden, non-traumatic subarachnoid hemorrhage, with high morbidity and mortality rates. Unruptured asymptomatic aneurysms are discovered in 5% of autopsied adults, and about 10% present with neurologic deficits related to mass effects, such as visual loss. The age- and sex-adjusted annual incidence rate is 9.0/100,000, more frequent in women, and incidence of rupture increases with age, peaking in the 2 decades between 55 and 75 years. Risk of hemorrhage in unruptured aneurysms is 1% to 2% annually.[1] The annual incidence of subarachnoid hemorrhage from aneurysm is approximately 1/100,000, and multiple intracranial aneurysms are found in 20% to 30% of patients.[2]

In addition to the common saccular ("berry") aneurysm, the other morphologic type is *fusiform,* which most frequently, but not exclusively, involves the posterior vertebrobasilar system. Fusiform aneurysms are characterized by tortuous dilatation and elongation (dolichoectasia) of an artery and are usually associated with atherosclerosis, hence the synonymous term "atherosclerotic aneurysm."

The intracranial arteries have thin media and poorly developed or absent internal elastic lamina; they are particularly prone to develop small outpouchings at arterial branch junctions where developmental defects in the media exist. Histologic study of the saccular aneurysm often demonstrates a defect in the elastic and muscular coat, beginning at the point of origin (neck) from the parent artery. This finding has supported the concept of a developmental origin and has created the term "congenital aneurysm" to designate saccular aneurysms, although these lesions are not present at birth. Factors such as hypertension, degenerative changes in the arterial wall, and heritable connective tissue disorders as in the Ehlers-Danlos syndrome and neurofibromatosis-1, all play roles in the subsequent development of aneurysms. There is firm evidence of aneurysm disease in first- or second-degree relatives, and there is a distinct association with polycystic kidney disease and aortic coarctation.[2]

As noted, multiple saccular aneurysms of the carotid or vertebrobasilar system occur 20% to 30% of the time, frequently with identical or "mirror" sites found in the left-sided and right-sided circulations. Most aneurysms arise from the carotid system on the anterior communicating, middle cerebral, and internal carotid arteries, or they arise in the region of the origins of the posterior communicating arteries (Fig. 17–1A). Only some 5% of saccular aneurysms arise on the vertebrobasilar system (Fig. 17–1B).

Usually, clinical symptoms are due to rupture of an aneurysm, resulting in extravasation of blood under arterial pressure into the subarachnoid or intraventricular spaces or into the brain parenchyma, with intracerebral hematoma formation. Subarachnoid and intraventricular blood causes depression of consciousness; intracerebral hematoma and vascular spasm produce focal

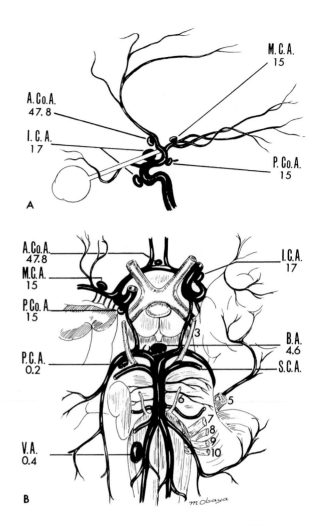

Fig. 17–1. Common aneurysm sites in lateral **(A)** and basal **(B)** views. Numbers indicate percentage of aneurysms in each location. *A.Co.A.,* anterior communicating artery; *M.C.A.,* middle cerebral artery; *I.C.A.,* internal carotid artery; *P.Co.A.,* posterior communicating artery; *P.C.A.,* posterior cerebral artery; *V.A.,* vertebral artery; *B.A.,* basilar artery. (Data from Krayenbuhl O: Kassifikation and Klinische Symptomatologie der zerebralen Aneurysmen. Ophthalmologica 167:122, 1973)

neurologic signs and even cerebral herniation with compression of the third nerve. The subsequent sudden increase in the intracranial pressure may result in sixth nerve palsies, in subretinal, intraretinal, or preretinal hemorrhage, and in conjunctival and, rarely, orbital hemorrhage.

About 100 years ago, Terson recorded the occurrence of vitreous hemorrhage after spontaneous subarachnoid bleeding. Such ocular hemorrhage is believed to result from transmission of intracranial pressure through the subarachnoid communication between the optic nerve sheath and the intracranial cavity, with subsequent nerve sheath dilation and rupture of dural and bridging vessels (Fig. 17–2). Intraocular hemorrhage is possibly the result of retinal venous hypertension brought on by obstruction of both the central retinal vein and the

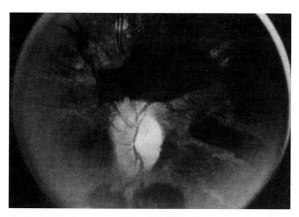

Fig. 17–2. Terson's syndrome. Multiple preretinal hemorrhages accompanying subarachnoid bleeding.

retinochoroidal anastomoses. Kuhn et al[3] reviewed Terson's syndrome, including the role of pars plana vitrectomy; these authors noted the high incidence of preceding coma and the efficacy of surgical intervention in visual recovery.

Aneurysms, either saccular or fusiform, also cause neurologic deficits by progressive enlargement rather than by rupture, for example, visual loss caused by compression of the optic nerve from fusiform distortion of the supraclinoid carotid or ophthalmic artery, or saccular enlargement of the intracavernous carotid artery that produces chronic ocular motor palsies. Symptoms in patients with aneurysmal compression of the anterior visual pathway may include visual loss that can be acute, gradual, or fluctuating.

Saccular Aneurysms

Intracavernous Carotid

Intracavernous carotid aneurysms constitute only 2% to 3% of all intracranial aneurysms and are unique because of their location. These aneurysms arise from the internal carotid artery as it traverses the cavernous sinus[4] (Fig. 17–3) and therefore produce a specific constellation of ocular and neurologic signs and symptoms. Rupture of such aneurysms, which are almost always saccular, may possibly result in carotid-cavernous sinus fistula, but subarachnoid hemorrhage is rare.[5] However, slowly progressive enlargement is the rule, usually occurring within the cavernous sinus, with compression of the third, fourth, and sixth cranial nerves and later involving the first and second divisions of the fifth nerve (see Chapter 12).[6]

Progressive enlargement of the aneurysm forms a mass in the floor of the middle cranial fossa, compromising motor as well as sensory functions of the trigeminal nerve. Anterior expansion of the aneurysm erodes the anterior clinoid, optic foramen, and superior orbital fissure, eventually producing unilateral visual loss and exophthalmos. Posterior expansion, which occurs later,

can erode the petrous portion of the temporal bone, causing ipsilateral facial palsy and, rarely, deafness. The sphenoidal sinus and the nasopharynx may infrequently be involved by inferior expansion, and medial extension erodes into the sella and may simulate a pituitary tumor[7] or cause bilateral ophthalmoplegia.[8] Bilateral saccular intracavernous aneurysms occur uncommonly.[9]

The onset of signs and symptoms is usually insidious, at times accompanied by pain about the eye and frontal area on the involved side. The pattern of serial involvement of the cranial nerves within the cavernous sinus is usually as follows: sixth, third, fifth, and fourth. Occasionally, palsies evolve simultaneously, and the ipsilateral optic nerve may eventually be encroached on by superior expansion of the aneurysm. The pupil is often not dilated maximally, as in the usual acute third nerve palsy; it may be relatively small (rarely immobile) because of simultaneous involvement of the oculosympathetic fibers.[6] Barr and associates[4] believed that such aneurysms usually arise as a weakness in the lateral wall of the carotid artery within the cavernous sinus and that the aneurysm tends to expand laterally between the third and fourth nerves superiorly and the sixth nerve inferiorly, finally compressing the nerves on the medial wall of the aneurysmal sac rather than laterally. Late involvement of the fifth nerve is emphasized by the findings that, in the three studied cases, this nerve was not splayed over the lateral aspect of the aneurysm, but it lay mainly inferior, lateral, and posterior in the region where late expansion of the aneurysm occurs. Although periocular pain has been often emphasized as a prominent symptom, it may not occur until ophthalmoplegia has been present for years.

Intracavernous aneurysms are suspected by the clinical presentation of a chronic cavernous sinus syndrome and are diagnosed by enhanced computed tomography (CT), magnetic resonance imaging (MRI), and arteriography (see Fig. 17–3). Because of the location and configuration within the cavernous sinus, direct surgical approaches to cavernous carotid aneurysms are hazardous. In recent years, intravascular occlusion of the internal carotid by detachable balloon has evolved as a safe and successful procedure, often with relief of pain and improvement in ophthalmoplegia.[10]

Carotid-Ophthalmic Artery

The carotid-ophthalmic aneurysm arises from the superior or medial surface of the carotid artery above the cavernous sinus and below the origin of the posterior communicating artery. Such aneurysms have an intimate relation to the anterior clinoid and optic nerve, which tends to cover their point of origin. They are rare in reported series: Pool and Potts[11] cited only 2 examples in 157 cases, and there was a 5.4% incidence in 2672 patients with single aneurysms in the Cooperative Study of Intracranial Aneurysms and Subarachnoid Hemor-

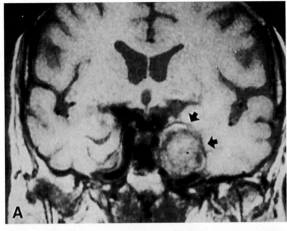

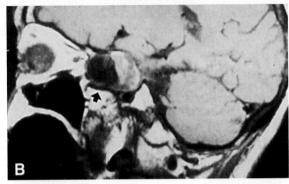

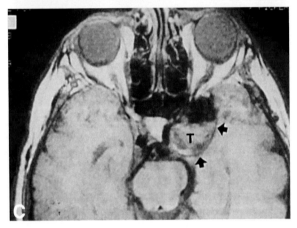

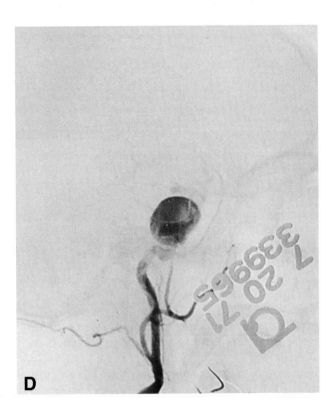

Fig. 17–3. Magnetic resonance images of intracavernous aneurysm in a 72-year-old woman with left retrobulbar pain and sixth nerve palsy. **A.** Coronal section (TR, 800 milliseconds; TE, 30 milliseconds). **B.** Parasagittal section (TR, 1000 milliseconds; TE, 20 milliseconds). **C.** Axial section (TR, 800 milliseconds; TE, 30 milliseconds). Note partial occlusion by thrombus (*T*). **D.** In a similar patient, carotid arteriogram (subtracted, lateral view) demonstrates a large intracavernous aneurysm.

rhage.[12] Ferguson and Drake[13] reported 32 such aneurysms; Guidetti and LaTorre[14] reported 16 cases. A high incidence of concurrent cerebral aneurysms has been reported: 67% in 1 series[14] and 37.5% in another.[15]

There is a striking correlation between aneurysmal projection and visual impairment. With superior-medial projection, optic nerve compression with monocular visual loss is often present. Eight of 16 patients reported by Guidetti and LaTorre[14] had prominent visual symptomatology with reduced vision and optic atrophy. Larger aneurysms may involve both optic nerve and chiasm. However, Ferguson and Drake[13] reported 32 patients with preoperative visual deficits. Whereas

involvement of the anterior visual pathway is the most frequent neuro-ophthalmologic presentation, paralysis of the third cranial nerve was reported in a single case. Although deemed a rare event,[13] visual loss occurs in approximately one-third of patients with carotid-ophthalmic aneurysms.[15]

Carotid-Supraclinoid

One of the more insidious and potentially treatable causes of progressive visual loss is unruptured aneurysm of the *supraclinoid* portion of the internal carotid artery. Here, the term "supraclinoid" seems more a function of

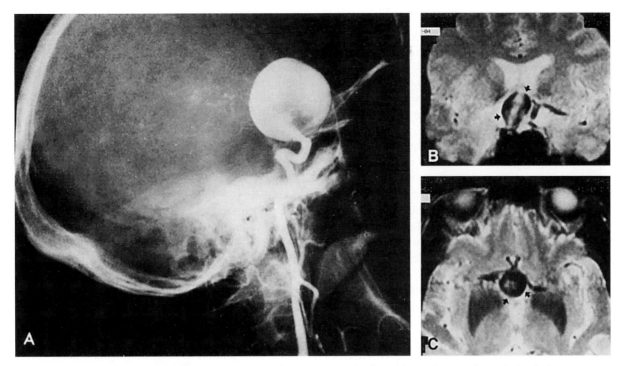

Fig. 17–4. Giant suprasellar (supraclinoidal) aneurysms. **A.** Carotid arteriogram (lateral view) shows a huge aneurysm of the internal carotid artery in a 59-year-old woman with progressing visual loss. Coronal **(B)** and axial **(C)** magnetic resonance imaging sections of a similar case. Note partial thrombus formation (TR, 2100 milliseconds; TE, 80 milliseconds).

size than of specific site or origin, and distinction between "ophthalmic" and supraclinoidal types is unclear. Of 3123 giant (larger than 25 mm) intracranial aneurysms in one series,[16] 93 involved the internal carotid above the cavernous sinus, thus qualifying as supraclinoid. Sixty-five were carotid-ophthalmic, 16 were at the bifurcation of the middle cerebral artery, and 12 were carotid-posterior communicating-anterior choroidal in location. Bilateral carotid-ophthalmic aneurysms were found in 19 cases, with a female predominance and average age of 48 years. The visual system was compressed in all but 6 cases, and 14 aneurysms presented as subarachnoid bleeding. Most of these giant aneurysms occur in women in the fifth and sixth decades of life, and their effects are primarily the result of compression of the optic nerves and chiasm.[16] For the most part, involvement of the visual system represents the only neurologic complication. Such aneurysms may rarely rupture, but most commonly they present as insidious visual loss, or they are uncovered during angiography for other sister aneurysms.[17] The pattern of visual field loss with supraclinoid aneurysm and its temporal profile tend to differ from that occurring with primary intrasellar or parasellar tumors. Vision is usually affected in a single eye, commonly with nasal field depression, and at times progressing to blindness before the second eye is involved.[18] These aneurysms arise below the optic nerve, which is stretched and flattened before subsequent involvement of the chiasm and the opposite nerve.

Most such aneurysms expand upward and forward, becoming located primarily anteriorly (Fig. 17–4). The optic nerves rise upward from the optic canal and may be inclined at a 45° angle such that the chiasm is more superiorly, as well as posteriorly, placed. It may be expected that uniocular ipsilateral visual loss would occur and progress before the contralateral field is involved, owing to chiasmal compression and before opposite nerve damage ensues. Although rapid visual loss has been reported, a longer duration (even years) is the rule. Rarely, the aneurysm may be more posteriorly placed or the chiasm more anteriorly fixed, resulting in initial involvement of the optic tract.[19]

Large aneurysms also arise from or involve the origins of the middle or anterior cerebral arteries, and they may precisely mimic a slowly growing suprasellar neoplasm. Similarly, large aneurysms of the supraclinoid carotid can simulate a pituitary tumor,[7] including prolactinemia.[20] *That aneurysms may mimic other masses underscores the need for MRI or arteriography in the evaluation of some sellar or parasellar syndromes.*

Ophthalmic Artery

Intracranial ophthalmic artery aneurysms are rare and in many series are not distinguished from supraclinoid aneurysms,[16,18] already discussed. The symptoms are quite similar, consisting of monocular progressive visual loss due to vascular compression from beneath the optic nerve. The pattern of visual loss begins as a unilateral scotoma usually involving fixation and then depression of the nasal and upper field, progressing to blindness. Further expansion involves the lateral aspect of the chiasm, causing temporal field loss in the opposite eye. Rarely, such aneurysms extend to involve the more distal aspects of the ophthalmic artery, producing enlargement of the optic foramen and even erosion into the orbit.[18,21] Jain[22] reported an unusual presentation of a true saccular aneurysm of the ophthalmic artery with projection into the optic foramen in a patient with monocular papilledema. Again, the intimate relationship of the ophthalmic artery origin from the internal carotid, and the size of the aneurysm, may blur distinctions among "ophthalmic," carotid-ophthalmic, and supraclinoid types.

Intraorbital ophthalmic artery "aneurysm" was the clinical diagnosis given to the first cases of carotid-cavernous fistula described by Travers[23] in 1809. All such previous cases reported before modern angiography must be suspect, with the majority probably being misdiagnosed carotid-cavernous fistulas or arteriovenous communications involving the orbital circulation. However, cases proved arteriographically do exist. Rubinstein and associates[24] reported the case of a 36-year-old man who experienced monocular burning and lacrimation with progressive loss of vision fluctuating over weeks; angiography demonstrated a 7-mm aneurysm arising intraorbitally, 12 mm distal to the origin of the ophthalmic artery. Rarely, direct penetrating trauma may produce aneurysmal dilation of the intraorbital ophthalmic artery.[25]

Posterior Communicating Artery

Aneurysms that primarily arise from the carotid system at the origin of the posterior communication artery are of special interest to neurologists, neurosurgeons, and ophthalmologists because they tend to involve the oculomotor nerve. The classic presentation is sudden onset of severe unilateral frontal headache, ptosis, limitation of adduction, depression and elevation of the eye, and dilated and fixed pupil. The cerebrospinal fluid is grossly bloody, and arteriography is diagnostic (Fig. 17–5). Pain in and around the eye in the trigeminal-ophthalmic distribution is a conspicuous symptom, but sensory defects are absent. Clinical and pathologic evidence indicates that impairment of function by a contiguous aneurysm usually occurs in conjunction with hemorrhage into the oculomotor nerve that, along with sudden distortion, can produce referred pain.[26]

Oculomotor palsy due to posterior communicating artery aneurysm typically shows maximal involvement of all third nerve functions. Although an individual extraocular muscle may be partially paretic, it is quite

uncommon for any single extraocular muscle to be entirely spared (lateral rectus and superior oblique excepted). Relative pupillary sparing and pupillary involvement is of considerable importance in differential diagnosis. The common situation is total pupillary paralysis with ruptured or unruptured posterior communicating aneurysms that involve the third nerve, but important exceptions exist. Of course, in the clinical setting of sudden onset of a painful third nerve palsy, with severe headache and nuchal rigidity, angiography is indicated whether or not the pupil is involved.

In approximately one half of patients with ruptured posterior communicating artery aneurysms, third nerve palsy develops either immediately or within a day. Before actual rupture the aneurysms by compression can cause ipsilateral frontal headache and third nerve palsy. Approximately 70% of symptomatic, but unruptured, aneurysms show a third nerve palsy, and by far the most common location is at the origin of the posterior communication artery.[12] The incidence of oculomotor palsy with posterior communicating artery aneurysms varies from 34% to 56%.[27]

Following third nerve palsy, especially when caused by aneurysm or trauma, if recovery does not begin within a few weeks, the phenomenon of "misdirection" usually occurs (see Chapter 12). Hepler and Cantu[28] assessed the ultimate ocular status in 25 patients with third nerve palsies secondary to aneurysms and found that all patients had some residual abnormality of third nerve function, but it was usually of trivial importance to the patient. Only 5 of 25 patients in this series complained of significant difficulty with diplopia, and 1 patient had a persistent complete third nerve palsy. In another study of patients treated by a direct surgical approach to the posterior communicating artery aneurysm within 10 days of symptomatic onset, a better prognosis existed for recovery of third nerve function than in those operated on after a longer interval.[27,29]

Middle Cerebral Artery

Aneurysms in the distribution of the middle cerebral artery are common and have a relatively good prognosis even following rupture. These lesions arise at the bifurcation or trifurcation of the middle cerebral artery within the sylvian fissure and usually do not give rise to neuro-ophthalmologic symptoms until they hemorrhage. Thereafter, blood may dissect into brain parenchyma, producing intracerebral hematomas with resultant contralateral paralysis, sensory loss, and homonymous visual field defect. Rarely, an isolated visual field defect may be the only focal neurologic sign of a bleeding aneurysm located distally on a posterior branch of the middle cerebral artery, with the hematoma having dissected into the visual radiations. Ipsilateral hemicranial, hemifacial, or

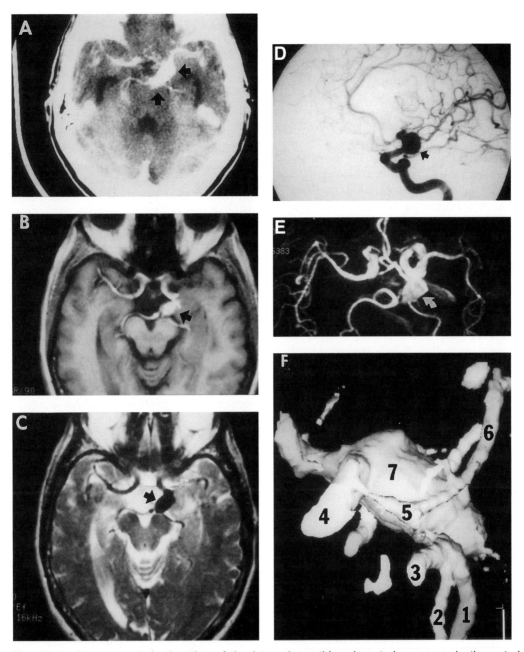

Fig. 17–5. Aneurysm at the junction of the internal carotid and posterior communicating arteries. **A.** Contrast-enhanced axial computed tomography (CT) shows a large aneurysm (*arrows*). Magnetic resonance imaging (MRI) studies effectively demonstrate the aneurysm. **B.** T$_1$-weighted MRI with gadolinium. **C.** T$_2$-weighted (*arrow* indicates black flow void). **D.** Selective internal carotid angiogram. **E.** MR angiogram (*curved arrow*) shows the same aneurysm. **F.** Helical image-intensified CT technique provides quasi–three-dimensional mold of arteries: *1.* right posterior cerebral; *2.* posterior superior cerebellar; *3.* basilar; *4.* internal carotid; *5.* posterior communicating; *6.* left posterior cerebral; *7.* supraclinoid aneurysm, same as depicted in **A** through **E**. (Courtesy of Dr. Raphael Aponte)

periorbital pain may herald minor leakage preceding frank subarachnoid hemorrhage.[30]

Anterior Communicating Artery

The anterior communicating artery is the most common single location of intracranial aneurysm, but these aneurysms rarely produce focal neurologic signs before rupture despite being situated just above the optic nerves. Chan et al[31] reported six cases collected over 37 years that caused monocular blindness by rupture of downward pointing aneurysmal sacs; with rupture, bleeding occurs into the optic nerve with symptoms of severe headache and monocular blindness.

Vertebrobasilar System

From 5% to 15% of all intracranial aneurysms are located in the posterior fossa, but these are often not clinically suspected until rupture. Most such aneurysms are at or about the bifurcation of the basilar artery. This location approaches the brain stem exit of the oculomotor nerves, but it is rare that third nerve palsy occurs before aneurysm rupture. Only those aneurysms found just distal to the basilar bifurcation on the proximal posterior cerebral arteries are likely to compromise the oculomotor nerve. When such aneurysms enlarge, they can exert pressure beneath the third ventricle and chiasm, thereby simulating the signs of a parasellar tumor, or the aneurysm may invaginate the third ventricle and thus may mimic a colloid cyst.[32] Saccular vertebrobasilar aneurysms usually present with subarachnoid hemorrhage, without concurrent or premonitory focal neurologic signs and symptoms. Among the 28 patients reported by Hööke et al,[33] only 8 patients had pre-rupture symptoms (headache), and 4 had pre-rupture signs. However, prodromal signs that falsely suggest either vertebrobasilar insufficiency or a posterior fossa mass lesion have been amply documented. We have seen 2 patients who presented with mild subarachnoid hemorrhage from a basilar artery aneurysm but who developed Parinaud's syndrome as the predominant symptomatology, presumably resulting from dorsal midbrain ischemia secondary to vessel spasm. McKinna[34] reviewed eye signs in a series of 611 posterior fossa aneurysms and found diplopia, major field defects, retinal or vitreous hemorrhage, or papilledema present in 50%. The double vision (present in 35%) was due to cranial nerve palsy, skew deviation, defective upward gaze, and bilateral external ophthalmoplegia.

In a series of 50 patients with basilar artery aneurysm, Nijensohn and associates[35] found 27 patients with saccular aneurysms and 23 with fusiform basilar dilations. In the former group, symptoms such as episodic diplopia, transient hemiplegia, and paresthesia mimicked the signs and symptoms of vertebrobasilar vascular disease. Various brain stem signs, such as progressive quadriparesis, nystagmus, and multiple cranial nerve involvement, occur with such aneurysms even before rupture. Isolated oculomotor paralysis has been reported with both saccular and fusiform aneurysms of the basilar system.[36] Posterior fossa aneurysms can thus mimic mass lesions, with progressive cranial nerve palsies and hydrocephalus.[37]

Saccular basilar aneurysms tend to present at a younger age (less than 60 years) and are most common in middle-aged women, whereas fusiform ectasia is associated with arteriosclerosis in hypertensive men in the sixth and seventh decades. In one study,[35] the majority of patients with saccular aneurysms died of rupture, as opposed to those with fusiform basilar artery aneurysms in whom death tended to occur from myocardial infarction. Treatment of such aneurysms presents a formidable technical problem well described elsewhere.[38]

Posterior Cerebral Artery

Aneurysms of the posterior cerebral artery are rare lesions. Their incidence in the Cooperative Study of Intracranial Aneurysms and Subarachnoid Hemorrhage was 0.8%.[12] Although such aneurysms arise in vessels supplying the major portions of the visual radiations and cortex, Pool and Potts[11] remarked that they knew of no instance in which visual symptoms occurred before rupture of the aneurysms. Drake and Amacher[39] reported their experience in eight patients, only one of whom had a temporary homonymous field defect after hemorrhage. Rarely, such aneurysms arise from the first portion of the posterior cerebral artery near the junction of the posterior communicating artery; more commonly, they occur at the first major branching of the posterior cerebral artery as it courses around the midbrain. In the former location, ruptured aneurysms are associated with third nerve palsy and contralateral hemiparesis. These signs may be anticipated because the proximal segment of the posterior cerebral artery is closely related to the cerebral peduncle and third nerve at its emergence between the posterior cerebral artery and superior cerebellar artery.

Childhood Aneurysms

Intracranial aneurysms uncommonly become symptomatic in children, in whom hemorrhage is less frequent and mass effect is more likely. Most intracranial arterial aneurysms seen in children are saccular, and heritable connective tissue disorders may be associated, including autosomal dominant polycystic kidney disease, Ehlers-Danlos syndrome type IV, neurofibromatosis-1, and Marfan's syndrome.[2] Amacher and Drake[40] noted that pediatric aneurysms may reach giant size, may be fusiform in configuration, especially in the vertebrobasilar system, and can be causally related to bacterial endocarditis or other infections. Such "mycotic" aneurysms are the result of arterial damage from a septic embolus.[41] Neurofibromatosis-1 is associated with proliferation of Schwann's cells within arteries, with secondary degenerative changes; in this disorder, there is a predilection for arterial occlusions or aneurysms of the cervical carotid and anterior communicating arteries.[42] Fusiform aneurysms of the basilar or carotid arteries, although a common sequel of atheromatous degeneration of the intracranial arteries in adult patients, are rare in children and may be associated with neurofibromatosis-1[43] or have another pathologic basis.

Patel and Richardson[44] found 58 patients younger

than 19 years of age (1.9%) among 3000 cases of ruptured intracranial aneurysms. Of 2951 patients with cerebral aneurysm in the Cooperative Study of Intracranial Aneurysms and Subarachnoid Hemorrhage summarized by Locksley, only 41 patients showed evidence of aneurysmal rupture by the age of 19 years.[12] Because of their rarity in pediatric patients, aneurysms are infrequently suspected in children with signs of intracranial hemorrhage or mass lesions. Yet, early diagnosis and treatment of aneurysms in children, as in adults, can be lifesaving.

Although there is no doubt that intracranial aneurysm is the most frequent source of subarachnoid hemorrhage in adults, it is a long-established maxim that AVM more commonly leads to subarachnoid hemorrhage in children than does aneurysm. Yet, when large series of patients up to 20 years of age with subarachnoid hemorrhage are considered, aneurysm is a more common cause than AVM. In the 124 young patients with subarachnoid hemorrhage reported by Sedzimir and Robinson,[45] for example, 50 patients had aneurysms and 33 had AVMs. These authors also summarized 321 patients through 20 years of age, including their own patients and those from 3 other series, and found 36% with aneurysm and 27% with AVM. Thus, if patients up to age 20 years are included, intracranial aneurysms cause subarachnoid bleeding more frequently than do vascular malformations. AVMs predominate if only preadolescent patients with subarachnoid hemorrhage are considered, because symptomatic aneurysms are rare in younger groups. There appears to be a biphasic presentation of intracranial aneurysms of the first 2 decades, with the lesions most often becoming symptomatic after age 10 or before age 2.[46] Aneurysms in children rarely become symptomatic between 2 and 10 years of age.

Intracranial aneurysms in children are more common than has previously been recognized, owing to a greater awareness and to safety of arteriography. There are clinical tendencies in children with intracranial aneurysms that differ from those in adults: (1) multiple aneurysms are less common in children; (2) associated congenital anomalies, especially coarctation of the aorta and polycystic kidneys, are more commonly seen in children with symptomatic aneurysms; (3) the mortality from initial hemorrhage in children admitted to hospital is less than in adults; and (4) children tend to recover more quickly and completely from neurologic defects. The usual presentation is intracranial hemorrhage, but ophthalmoplegia, diabetes insipidus, and other signs mimicking tumor have rarely been reported with aneurysms.[41]

Traumatic Aneurysms

Secondary ("false") aneurysms usually occur following blunt head injury, with or without basilar skull fracture, and also after penetrating injuries to the face or cranium. Traumatic aneurysms of the intracavernous segment of the internal carotid artery come to attention because of recurrent, often massive, epistaxis, with variable involvement of the ocular motor nerves.[47] Postsurgical aneurysms are documented following sinus surgery, transsphenodial pituitary resection, and yttrium-90 implantation.[48] Despite the large number of transsphenoidal procedures, this complication appears unusual. Paullus and co-workers[49] reported an extraordinary case of progressive bilateral ophthalmoplegia due to false aneurysm complicated by a carotid-cavernous fistula component. It is to be recalled that, according to microdissections of Rhoton and associates,[50] the carotid arteries may approach the midline within the sella to as small a distance as 4 mm, and adherence to a strictly midline approach seems advisable.

Aneurysms of the extracranial carotid system are distinctly uncommon and may follow trauma or may be associated with atherosclerosis or fibromuscular dysplasia.[51] Neuro-ophthalmologic signs are rare, including headache or ipsilateral oculosympathetic palsy. Penetrating orbital trauma with false aneurysm of the ophthalmic artery has been noted.[25]

Fusiform Aneurysms

Fusiform aneurysms are actually tortuous dilatations and elongations (dolichoectasia) of pre-existing arteries, usually associated with advanced, but not necessarily caused by, atheromatous degeneration, which accounts for the term "atherosclerotic ectasia." The neurologic complications of such dilatations, which can involve either the carotid or vertebrobasilar systems, are most often secondary to direct pressure effects, rather than to rupture and subarachnoid hemorrhage.

Carotid System

Fusiform carotid aneurysms involve the intracavernous or internal carotid artery. A dilated and tortuous carotid may flatten the optic nerve against the falciform dural fold above the opening of the optic canal. Such compression rarely may be responsible for instances of slowly progressive visual loss with eventual optic atrophy, some instances of which may be mistakenly diagnosed as "soft" or "normal tension" glaucoma.

Hilton and Hoyt[52] reported a case of bitemporal hemianopia associated with fusiform dilation of the internal carotid and anterior cerebral arteries. The latter actually prolapsed between the optic nerves. The slowly progressive bitemporal hemianopia and optic atrophy, with normal sella, was not believed to be due to compression by the dilated vessels but was considered more likely due to impaired circulation caused by traction on, and obstructions of, the small vessels supplying the anterior aspect of the chiasm. Colapinto et al[53] also described optic nerve compression by fusiform ectasia of internal carotid artery demonstrated by MRI and cerebral angiography (see Chapter 5, Part II).

As noted above, fusiform aneurysms have been described even in young children and have been associated with connective tissue diseases and neurofibromatosis.[2,40,42,43,54] Thus, congenital causes must be suspect in youth, as well as in the situation of spontaneous arterial dissections.

Vertebrobasilar System

Tortuous or redundant basilar arteries are not uncommon in the older age group. Occasionally, gross dilation or ectasia develops so that the basilar artery acts as a mass in the posterior fossa. This phenomenon produces signs of low-pressure hydrocephalus, cranial nerve palsies, and long tract and sensory signs and may even simulate a cerebellopontine angle tumor or tumor at the foramen magnum.[55] It is possible to diagnose such lesions with CT[56] or MRI,[57] but angiography is definitive (Fig. 17–6). The association of insidious multiple cranial nerve palsies and long tract signs referable to a brain stem level, in an elderly patient with evidence of atherosclerosis, should make fusiform basilar artery dilation a diagnostic consideration.

As opposed to saccular basilar aneurysms, fusiform aneurysms tend to occur in the older age group (older than 60 years) and are found predominately in men.[2,35] They are commonly associated with hypertension and atherosclerotic cardiovascular disease, and a notable association with abdominal aortic aneurysms also exists.

ARTERIOVENOUS MALFORMATIONS

AVMs are developmental anomalous communications between the arterial and venous systems without intervening capillary beds, with an incidence of 0.04% to 0.52% in large autopsy series.[58] AVMs have been described by such terms as *tumor circoidius, aneurysm racemosum, circoid aneurysm, angiomatous malformation, and racemose angioma.* The generic term AVM is used here to describe all such developmental vascular anomalies, although it is possible pathologically to differentiate AVMs into capillary telangiectases, cavernous angiomas, pure venous malformations, and AVMs.[59] The most common, the true AVM, is a tortuous mass of both arteries and veins, abnormally developed in caliber and length. Blood is shunted directly from the arterial to the venous circulation without an intervening capillary bed.

Although many AVMs remain silent, the signs and symptoms of AVMs may be classified broadly into two groups: (1) those produced primarily by the abnormal blood vessels, depending primarily on the location of the AVM; and (2) the effects that occur as complications of subarachnoid and intracerebral hemorrhage. The

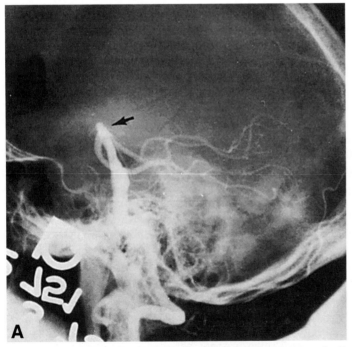
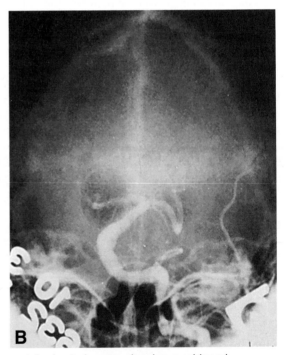

Fig. 17–6. Fusiform basilar dilation. **A.** Lateral projection vertebral arteriogram showing a widened basilar artery (*arrow*) projecting beyond level of dorsum sellae. **B.** Anteroposterior projection showing a widened and tortuous basilar artery.

general clinical features of congenital AVMs have been extensively documented.[60-62] The most common manifestations are convulsions, headaches, progressive hemispheric neurologic deficit, and mental change. These clinical phenomena are due to hemorrhage, but some effects of large AVMs may be due to shunting of blood away from otherwise normal brain. Subarachnoid hemorrhage is the common mode of presentation, with a classic history of sudden headache and depression of consciousness accompanied by stiff neck, but without localizing signs. Untreated AVMs have an annual hemorrhage rate of 2% to 4%, with combined annual morbidity and mortality of about 3%.[58]

Seizures are the next most frequent presenting feature and are nonfocal in approximately 40% of patients, but almost 90% of patients with AVMs that bleed have no history of a previous seizure. The initial symptoms of AVM usually present between the second and third decades of life, but they also occur in children[63]; hemorrhage, when it occurs, is most often evident between the ages of 10 and 40 years. Although debatable, it would appear that pregnancy has a deleterious effect on AVMs, with an increased likelihood of hemorrhage, such that cesarean section and sterilization have been advised by some investigators,[64] but stereotactic radiosurgery is currently an evolving alternative.[58]

According to Ondra et al,[62] of 160 patients with AVM, the average age at presentation was 33 years, most with hemorrhage. Forty percent of patients experienced hemorrhagic events during follow-up, with a 4% per year risk, and mean interval to hemorrhage of 7.7 years. Hemorrhage and death rates were equal regardless of initial AVM presentation. Pollock et al[58] found a mean age of 35 ± 15.2 years with an annual re-bleeding rate of 7.45%. Factors affecting outcome include age and gender, pregnancy, size and location, and mode of presentation; the risk of recurrent hemorrhage increases with age.

Supratentorial

From 85% to 90% of AVMs are in the supratentorial compartment and are supplied primarily by the carotid circulation (Figs. 17–7 and 17–8). The remainder are supplied by the vertebrobasilar system. The approximate frequency of location is as follows: frontal, 22%; temporal, 18%; parietal, 27%; occipital, 5%; and deep intraventricular or paraventricular, 18%. The intracerebral site of the malformation does not necessarily indicate that there will be signs referable to that area simply from the mass effect of the malformation. Clinical features primarily result from subarachnoid hemorrhage or intraparenchymal hemorrhage with hematoma formation.

In general, when hemorrhage occurs involving a portion of the visual radiations, a homonymous visual field

defect is to be expected. Selective involvement of the anterior visual pathways may occur either with extensive venous angiomas at the base of the brain or as part of the Wyburn-Mason syndrome (see below), with direct involvement of the optic nerve, chiasm, or tract. Other variants such as congenital cavernous hemangiomas may involve the anterior visual pathways,[65] as may intraparenchymal cryptic AVMs,[66] and may present as symptomatic visual loss also resulting from hemorrhage and hematoma. Amaurosis fugax may even be the presenting symptom of supratentorial AVMs when blood is shunted to the meningeal circulation from the ophthalmic artery.[67] When supratentorial AVMs drain into dural venous sinuses or the vein of Galen, distant ocular effects evolve, such as proptosis[68] or ophthalmoplegia,[69] owing to arterialization of cavernous sinus complex.

Of particular interest are those AVMs that involve the occipital lobe (Fig. 17–9). The clinical differentiation of migraine from a cerebral AVM was previously regarded as difficult, because the clinical features of occipital lobe AVMs include visual phenomena or headaches. However, in most cases, the clinical distinction is possible. In 26 cases with occipital AVM, 2 distinct syndromes were defined in 18 patients: "occipital epilepsy," and "occipital apoplexy."[70] Focal seizures with occipital malformations consist of elementary visual sensations similar to the phenomena evoked by direct cortical stimulations. When seizure activity occurs in the striate cortex (area 17), the patient usually reports sensations of moving lights in the right or left homonymous fields. The sensations are poorly formed, episodic, usually brief, sometimes colored, and unassociated with the angular, scintillating figures so characteristic of migrainous cortical phenomena. Epileptic discharges from areas 18 and 19 cause photopsias that are unlikely to remain stationary and to flicker rapidly. The epileptic photopsias usually last only seconds; occasionally they last for a few minutes before the onset of a generalized seizure. In other instances, only the brief visual episodes occur without spreading to produce a generalized seizure. Momentary dimming or blindness in one or both homonymous fields may be experienced with seizure activity in the occipital areas.

Occipital apoplexy results from hemorrhage and hematoma formation within the occipital lobe and is characterized by sudden severe headache and homonymous visual field loss. Homonymous hemianopia is the most important sign produced by vascular malformations of the occipital lobe. Compression and necrosis of visual pathways by an intracerebral hematoma are the principal mechanisms. Usually, the hematoma is large and tends to split or dissect longitudinally through the white matter of the occipital lobe. The effects of compression may be reversed by prompt, surgical evacuation of the hematoma.[70] With hemorrhage into one occipital

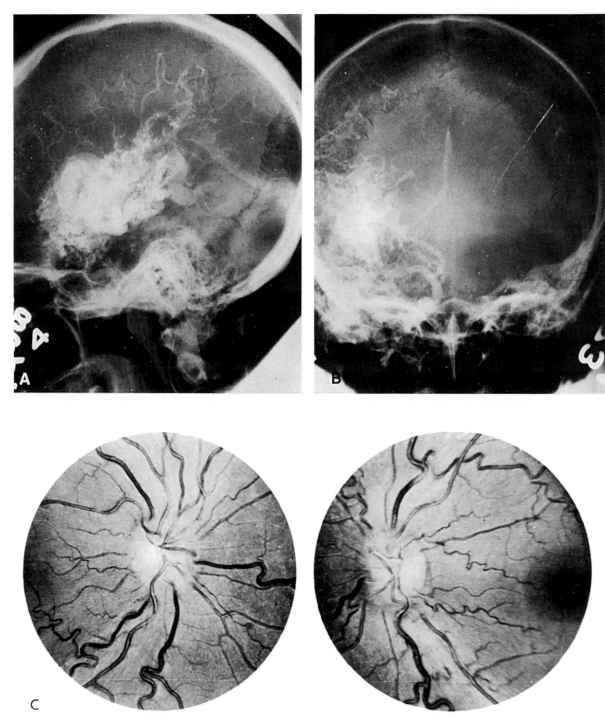

Fig. 17–7. Supratentorial arteriovenous malformation in a 28-year-old woman with a history of focal motor seizures for many years and a recent subarachnoid hemorrhage. **A.** Lateral projection carotid arteriogram demonstrating a huge deep hemispheral arteriovenous malformation. **B.** Frontal projection. **C.** Fundus photograph showing anomalous tortuous vasculature in each eye. No retinal arteriovenous shunt was detectable.

lobe, hemianopia in the visual field of the contralateral "normal" occipital lobe may develop, producing *total* blindness that can last for several days. The rapidly expanding hematoma may shift the damaged hemisphere anteriorly, or across the midline, with downward herniation of the uncus through the tentorial incisura. This shift compresses the posterior cerebral arteries and accounts for bilateral occipital lobe dysfunction. Arrest of function in the undamaged occipital lobe may be due to an interhemispheral inhibitory phenomenon termed

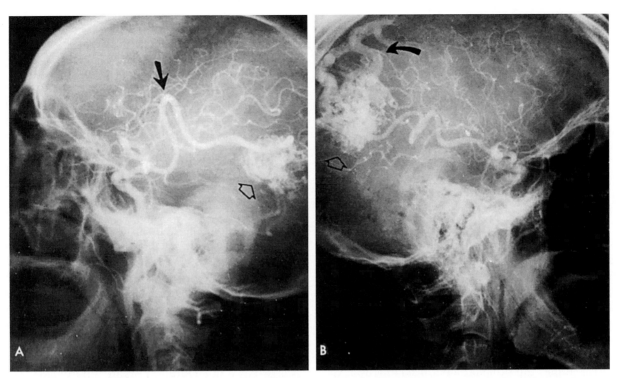

Fig. 17–8. Multiple supratentorial arteriovenous malformations (AVMs). **A.** Lateral projection of left carotid arteriogram shows dilated afferent artery (*solid arrow*) feeding the right hemispheric parietal AVM (*open arrow*). **B.** Right carotid injection fills a second, more posteriorly located, parieto-occipital AVM (*open arrow*), which drains immediately to markedly dilated cortical veins (*curved arrow*).

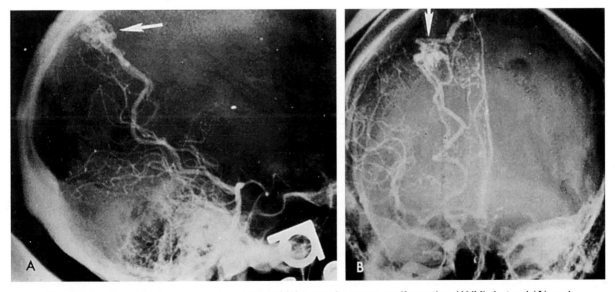

Fig. 17–9. Carotid arteriogram of an occipital lobe arteriovenous malformation (AVM). Lateral (**A**) and frontal (**B**) projections demonstrating a small occipital AVM (*arrow*). The patient was a 23-year-old woman who presented with severe apoplectic unilateral headache, total left homonymous hemianopia, and mild nuchal rigidity. Despite xanthochromic cerebrospinal fluid, she was initially diagnosed elsewhere as having migraine. An AVM was successfully resected, and a small occipital lobe hematoma was removed.

diaschisis. Visual field defects with occipital AVMs are regularly due to hemorrhage and hematoma formation. Congenital AVMs can occupy the entire occipital pole (the macular projection area) for decades without producing visual field defects.

Although migraine aura is often cited as a symptom of AVM, it is extremely rare that classic migraine is mimicked by occipital AVM. None of the patients in the above series[70] described the 15- to 20-minute episodes that characterize the visual aura of classic migraine. The headaches of AVM differ from migraine in that they are constantly localized to the same side of the head, and intermittent visual phenomena, if present, can persist throughout the headache or even after, whereas in migraine the visual phenomena usually precede the headache. Bruyn[71] has reviewed the clinical features of 57 reported and 7 personal cases of AVM, concluding that the "migraine" of AVM is late onset, nonfamilial, and brief. *Rarely,* the complete clinical symptomatology of classic migraine can be mimicked by an occipital lobe AVM (see Chapter 16).[72] In addition to hemianopia, other visual disturbances can occur after hemorrhage into the occipital lobe, including dyslexia without agraphia (see Chapter 7).

Infratentorial

AVMs within the posterior fossa may be classified by location or by type of blood supply, but the cerebellar hemispheres are more common sites than the brain stem. Verbiest[73] classified these lesions anatomically as follows: (1) intraparenchymous, including cerebellar, pontine, and mixed forms; (2) subarachnoid, including the cerebellopontine angle and those in the region of the vein of Galen; and (3) those within the walls of the posterior fossa, which are principally intradural.

The clinical features of the intraparenchymous malformations are extremely varied, and, occasionally, these AVMs are discovered only at post-mortem examinations, with the patient being entirely asymptomatic during life. Otherwise, such malformations may determine an acute or chronic neurologic syndrome or a course of chronic evolution interrupted by a sudden apoplectic event. Acute manifestations result from subarachnoid, cerebellar, or brain stem hemorrhage. In the nine patients reviewed by Logue and Monckton,[74] two patients with cerebellar AVM experienced apoplectic-onset subarachnoid hemorrhage, combined with bilateral sixth nerve paresis and ataxia. However, other patients in the series had a fluctuating course extending as long as 15 years, with involvement of cranial nerves II through XII, pyramidal tract signs, Parinaud's syndrome, and ataxia. Ocular signs and symptoms otherwise have included palsies of cranial nerves III, IV, and

VI, horizontal gaze palsy, and nystagmus,[75] as well as ocular skew deviation.[76]

Lessell and associates[77] suggested that brain stem AVMs may be suspected in the following clinical settings: (1) subarachnoid hemorrhage with focal brain stem signs; (2) subarachnoid hemorrhage without focal signs; (3) tic douloureux or hemifacial spasm in a young adult; (4) hydrocephalus with or without signs of increased intracranial pressure; (5) recurrent occipital or hemicranial headache; (6) progressive posterior fossa signs; and (7) remitting multifocal brain stem signs. Pedersen and Troost[78] presented a single patient who had all such features over a lifetime, including nystagmus, skew deviation, and optic atrophy.

Arteriovenous anomalies involving the dural venous sinuses constitute a special situation. Central nervous system signs and symptoms are related to passive venous hypertension or congestion as a result of increased pressure in the superior sagittal sinus or to venous sinus thromboses. Seizures, transient ischemic attacks, motor weakness, and brain stem or cerebellar symptoms accrue with cortical vein thrombosis, and subarachnoid hemorrhage may occur. Dural AVMs are reported to comprise 6% to 15% of intracranial AVMs and may be congenital or acquired.[79] Houser and colleagues[80] have angiographically demonstrated sigmoid and transverse sinus occlusions that preceded the development of "spontaneous" AVMs, and Chaudhary and co-workers[81] documented AVMs following head trauma. Therefore, the origin of an AVM may include the combined influence of congenital anomalies, trauma, and coagulopathic states. Most patients become symptomatic in the fifth and sixth decades, and the condition has no gender preference.

Clinical findings are determined by the volume, direction, and route of venous drainage. Of neuro-ophthalmologic interest are the presence of papilledema,[82] cranial nerve palsies, pulse-synchronous bruit, and (rarely) tinnitus[83]; proptosis may be bilateral.[84]

The detection of intracranial AVMs is facilitated by CT scanning and MRI (Fig. 17–10),[85] but optimal management requires selective angiography that assesses the size and configuration of the mass, the number and location of feeding arteries, the flow characteristics and degree of steal from brain parenchyma, and the pattern of venous drainage.

The natural history of unruptured intracranial AVMs is somewhat controversial,[62,64] the issue being conservative management or interventional therapy using refined microsurgical or embolization techniques. Brown and associates[86] reviewed the experience of the Mayo Clinic, Rochester, Minnesota, from 1974 through 1985, with a minimal follow-up of at least 4 years after diagnosis (mean follow-up time, 8.2 years). Of 168 patients, 18.5% had an intracranial hemorrhage, with an overall risk of hemorrhage of 2.25% per year (vs. 4%[62]), and observed

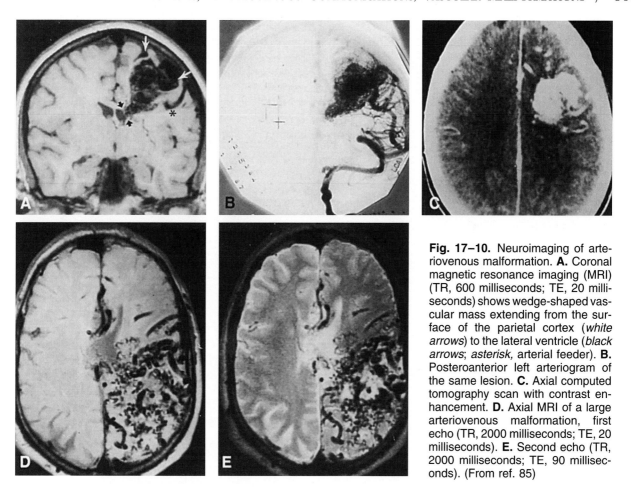

Fig. 17–10. Neuroimaging of arteriovenous malformation. **A.** Coronal magnetic resonance imaging (MRI) (TR, 600 milliseconds; TE, 20 milliseconds) shows wedge-shaped vascular mass extending from the surface of the parietal cortex (*white arrows*) to the lateral ventricle (*black arrows*; *asterisk,* arterial feeder). **B.** Posteroanterior left arteriogram of the same lesion. **C.** Axial computed tomography scan with contrast enhancement. **D.** Axial MRI of a large arteriovenous malformation, first echo (TR, 2000 milliseconds; TE, 20 milliseconds). **E.** Second echo (TR, 2000 milliseconds; TE, 90 milliseconds). (From ref. 85)

annual rates of hemorrhage increased over time. The mortality rate from hemorrhage was 29%. Of 22 patients with nonfatal intracranial hemorrhages, 14 did not undergo treatment, and none of these had recurrent hemorrhage during the mean follow-up of 58 months. No radiologic or clinical features seem consistently helpful in predicting rupture. According to Pollock et al,[58] analysis of clinical and radiologic features revealed 6 significant risk factors for hemorrhage: (1) history of prior bleeding; (2) deep location; (3) deep venous drainage; (4) increasing patient age; (5) diffuse morphology (versus compact nidus); and (6) single draining vein. Based on these findings, these authors concluded that annual bleeding for the low-risk group was 1.0%, and it was 9.0% for the highest risk group.

The therapy for AVMs has been reviewed elsewhere,[60] and it most often includes a direct surgical approach to the malformation. However, various intravascular techniques employ embolization[87,88] with materials such as Silastic and isobutyl-2-cyanoacrylate (Fig. 17–11). Complications of intravascular embolotherapy include pulmonary emboli and the histotoxicity of

bucrylate. Radiation therapy includes conventional irradiation and stereotactic heavy-ion Bragg peak radiosurgery.[89] Pollock et al[58] believe that stereotactic radiosurgery is 80% effective for AVMs less than 3 cm in average diameter, within a latency period of 2 to 3 years, but the patient is at risk during the interval until obliteration of the lesion.

CAVERNOUS MALFORMATIONS

Cavernous malformations (cavernous angiomas, hemangiomas) are congenital vascular anomalies of brain parenchyma, many times found incidentally on neuroimaging for unrelated symptoms. Histopathologically, these anomalies are characterized by dilated thin-walled vascular channels lined by simple endothelium and fibrous adventitia, but without major arterial feeders or draining venous channels; typically, no brain parenchyma is found within the lesion.[90] Annual bleeding rates are lower than for AVM, being roughly 1%, but such incidents are rarely life-threatening. These lesions may be familial. In a series of 122 patients,[91] mean age

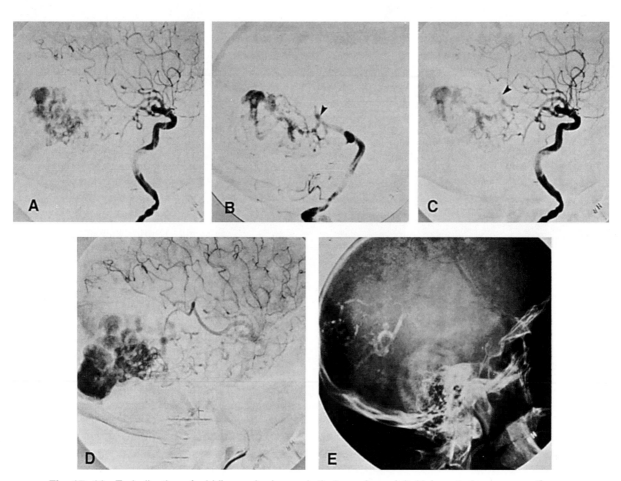

Fig. 17–11. Embolization of middle cerebral vessels that supply occipital lobe arteriovenous malformation (AVM). The patient had a subarachnoid and intraparenchymal hemorrhage that produced a left homonymous field defect. **A.** Right carotid arteriogram demonstrates contribution via posterior communicating artery to a right occipital lobe AVM. **B.** Vertebral injection. The *arrow* points to the enlarged right posterior cerebral artery that is a major feeder of the AVM. **C.** Right carotid arteriogram during glue embolization procedure. The *arrow* points to a catheter as it traverses the segment seen in (**B**). The catheter was advanced via the internal carotid artery but is positioned far posteriorly. **D.** Upper branches to the AVM now are occluded, with residual low-flow vascularization via the middle cerebral artery. **E.** Skull film showing radiopaque glue within the AVM and blood vessels previously supplying it. The patient had a persistent visual field defect but greatly reduced headache and no persistence of subjective bruit. (Courtesy of Dr. Joseph Horton)

was 37 years (range, 4 to 82 years), 35% of the angiomas were located in the brain stem, 17% in basal ganglia or thalamus, and were hemispheric in 48%; 50% of patients had not had a symptomatic hemorrhage. Stereotactic radiosurgery is beneficial, especially for lesions that have bled.[91]

Cerebral developmental venous anomalies (DVAs) are relatively rare lesions associated with head, cervicofacial, or orbital venous malformations, but they are improperly called *cerebral venous angiomas* or *cavernoma*.[92] Blue cutaneous "staining," increased by dependent position or Valsalva maneuver, is caused by ectatic dermal venous channels, without thrill or bruit.

Intraoral mucosal malformations are common. Located in paraventricular or subcortical sites, cerebral DVAs are usually incidental findings without preceding hemorrhage or neurologic deficits and are discovered at the time of angiography for facial venous malformations. MRI and MR angiography are considered reliable noninvasive techniques to elucidate the superficial venous malformations as well as the occult cerebral DVAs.[92]

CAROTID-CAVERNOUS SINUS FISTULAS

Arteriovenous communications in the region of the cavernous sinus include the classic, and often dramatic, internal carotid-cavernous fistula and the more elusive syndrome of spontaneous shunts in the dural-meningeal circulation. These dynamic shunts are dilemmas not only in clinical diagnosis but also in the management of ocular complications and in the application of diagnostic and therapeutic techniques.

The S-shaped intracavernous segments of the internal carotid arteries lie within a bilateral plexus of freely communicating venous channels that comprise the paired, extradural parasellar cavernous sinuses. An extensive arterial anastomosis interconnects the two intracavernous carotid arteries, which are also in communication with the meningeal arterial system arising from the external carotid arteries (ascending pharyngeal and internal maxillary arteries), internal carotid arteries, and vertebral arteries. The three major intracavernous branches of the internal carotid artery are the meningohypophyseal trunk, the inferior cavernous sinus artery, and the superior hypophyseal arteries (Fig. 17–12).

Venous flow from the face (frontal and angular veins) enters the superior ophthalmic vein at the superior-medial orbital rim, thence to the cavernous sinus via the superior orbital fissure. The cavernous complex drains posteriorly via superior and inferior petrosal dural sinuses, and the basal clival plexus, to the internal jugular system.

Arteriovenous shunts involving the cavernous sinuses are rarely congenital. Some 25% of arteriovenous fistulas occur spontaneously, especially in middle age to elderly women, and atherosclerosis may be considered the substrate for such dural arterial leaks. Cerebral trauma accounts for some 75% of carotid-cavernous fistulas, usually in the younger age group, producing the classic clinical picture of pulsating exophthalmos. Other traumatic causes include penetrating orbito-cranial wounds, including knife injuries. Iatrogenic fistulas are reported following transsphenoidal pituitary surgery,[49] after injury to the internal carotid during endarterectomy,[93] after ethmoidal sinus surgery,[94] or after percutaneous gasserian and retro-gasserian procedures.[95] Connective tissue disorders such as Ehlers-Danlos syndrome have been associated with spontaneous carotid-cavernous fistula,[96] and fistulas are documented during otherwise uncomplicated pregnancy.[97]

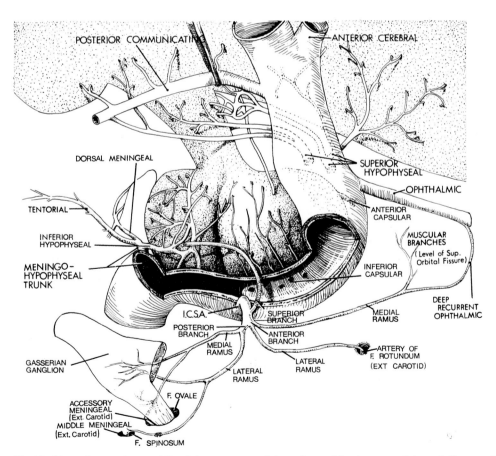

Fig. 17–12. Vascular anatomy of the intracavernous internal carotid artery supplying pituitary, sellar, and parasellar structures.

The classification of carotid-cavernous fistulas is problematic, but these lesions may be sorted according to several criteria: pathogenetically, into spontaneous or traumatic; angiographically, into direct (cavernous carotid) or dural (external carotid); and hemodynamically, into high-flow and low-flow, although no objective criteria exist for this distinction, except severity of clinical findings. Barrow and co-workers[98] suggest that all carotid-cavernous fistulas may be categorized into one of four angiographic types: type A, direct shunts between the internal carotid artery and the cavernous sinus, including most traumatic carotid-cavernous fistulas that are characterized by high venous pressure and flow; type B, dural shunts between meningeal branches of the internal carotid artery and cavernous sinus; type C, dural shunts between meningeal branches of the external carotid artery and cavernous sinus; and type D, dural shunts between meningeal branches of both internal and external carotid arteries and cavernous sinus.

Carotid-cavernous fistulas are initiated by traumatic or spontaneous rents in the walls of the intracavernous internal carotid artery or its branches, with short-circuiting of arterial blood into the venous complex of the cavernous sinuses. The two cavernous sinuses are connected across the sphenoid, including the sellar floor and clivus, so that any signs and symptoms may be bilateral. The major anterior outflow structures of the cavernous sinus are the orbital veins, which become engorged, with secondary congestion of orbital soft tissues (Figs. 17–13 and 17–14). With raised venous pressure and lowered arterial perfusion, stagnant hypoxic changes also contribute to soft tissue swelling, some degree of ophthalmoplegia, and anterior segment ischemia.

In the fully evolved state, this syndrome includes lid swelling and orbital pain, varying degrees of pulsating exophthalmos, subjective or objective ocular or cephalic bruit, diplopia, engorged and chemotic conjunctiva, and raised intraocular tension. The fundus may show dilated veins without spontaneous pulsations, disc edema, retinal hemorrhages, venous stasis retinopathy or vein occlusions, and, rarely, choroidal effusions.[99–101] The ophthalmoplegia with carotid-cavernous fistulas is believed to be due to enlarged muscles or to damage of cranial nerves within the cavernous or petrosal sinus. Enlarged extraocular muscles are demonstrable by ultrasonography in this form of "venous stasis orbitopathy"; ultrasonography also uncovers reversal of flow in the superior ophthalmic vein.[102] Sudden pain with increased swelling, followed by improvement, suggests thrombosis of the superior ophthalmic vein, an event that may be documented by orbital MRI[103] or by standardized orbital

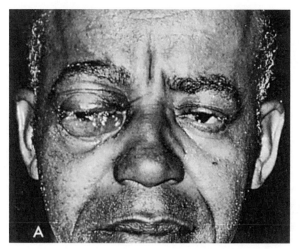
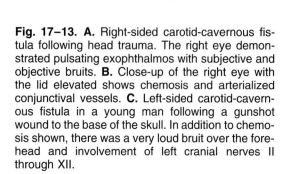
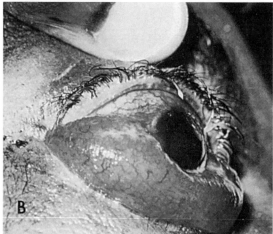
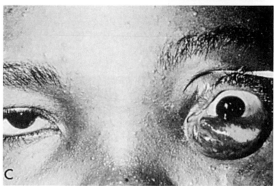

Fig. 17–13. A. Right-sided carotid-cavernous fistula following head trauma. The right eye demonstrated pulsating exophthalmos with subjective and objective bruits. **B.** Close-up of the right eye with the lid elevated shows chemosis and arterialized conjunctival vessels. **C.** Left-sided carotid-cavernous fistula in a young man following a gunshot wound to the base of the skull. In addition to chemosis shown, there was a very loud bruit over the forehead and involvement of left cranial nerves II through XII.

echography. In addition, proptosis that improves on one side, only to increase on the opposite side, produces a picture of signs and symptoms more marked contralateral to the fistula.[104]

Anterior segment hypoxia may include protein flare and cells in aqueous, corneal edema, glaucoma, iris rubeosis, rapidly progressive cataract, and venous stasis retinopathy, that is, a hypoxic eyeball syndrome. Lesser degrees of congestion with mild conjunctival "arterialization" (Fig. 17–15), ocular hypertension, and small abduction defect all hint at the slower-flow, lower-pressure situation that accrues usually spontaneously with dural circulation fistulas.[99,101] Bruit is less likely.

Although the clinical constellation described above implies the great likelihood of carotid-cavernous fistula, definitive diagnosis depends on complete angiographic evaluation with selective opacification of bilateral internal and external carotid arteries and vertebral circulation. Prominence of the superior ophthalmic vein is frequently detected on CT scan and MRI, and less frequently extraocular muscle enlargement and lateral bulging of the cavernous sinus are seen by MRI.[105] Standardized orbital echography regularly confirms enlargement of the superior ophthalmic vein and increased flow (Fig. 17–16),[102,106] in both direct and indirect fistulas.

Therapy for carotid-cavernous fistula is directed toward relieving ocular symptoms, especially when visual loss is threatened, with the goal being thrombosis of the fistula with normalization of orbital hemodynamics. Various arterial ligatures, "trapping" procedures, controlled embolizations, and even direct intracranial attacks have been advocated, but the current trend indicates the great advance represented by intravascular closure using detachable balloon microcatheterization techniques (Fig. 17–17)[101] or embolization with isobutyl-2-cyanoacrylate or polyvinyl alcohol particles.[107] Com-

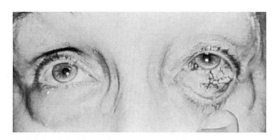

Fig. 17–15. Dilated tortuous conjunctival vessels in a 63-year-old woman with a presumed dural carotid-cavernous fistula. She presented with a 2-week history of "red eye," mild retro-orbital headache, and double vision. On examination, a left sixth nerve paresis, 3 mm of proptosis, a faint orbital bruit, and slightly elevated intraocular pressure were found. All signs and symptoms resolved spontaneously in 6 weeks, while angiography was being contemplated.

plications of these techniques include transient or fixed hemispheral dysfunction, cranial nerve palsies, field loss, and pseudoaneurysm formation.[101,107]

Spontaneous thrombosis of some fistulas does occur, especially with the slow-flow dural variety. In a series of 20 patients, 12 fistulas closed spontaneously within 3 months and 3 closed at between 6 to 18 months,[108] whereas in other reviews, closure rates range from 10% to 60%.[101] Therefore, a period of observation may afford the least harmful management. Precise indications for intervention are unclear, but surely they include visual deterioration due to glaucoma, iris rubeosis or ischemic retinopathy, transient ischemic attacks, intolerable subjective bruit, or head or eye pain not otherwise amenable to conservative therapy. Halbach and co-workers[109] suggested that increased intracranial pressure, rapidly progressive proptosis, visual loss, and varix-like distortion of the cavernous sinus itself all constitute indications for urgent intervention. We have seen a case of a young

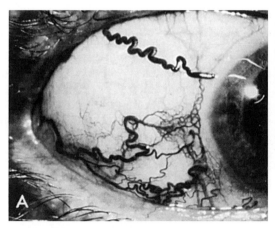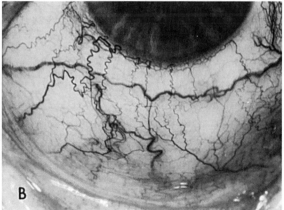

Fig. 17–14. Conjunctival vessels in two patients with carotid-cavernous fistulas. **A.** Large dilated veins in a patient with a major post-traumatic fistula. **B.** "Corkscrew" vessel tortuosity in a 55-year-old woman with a dural carotid-cavernous fistula.

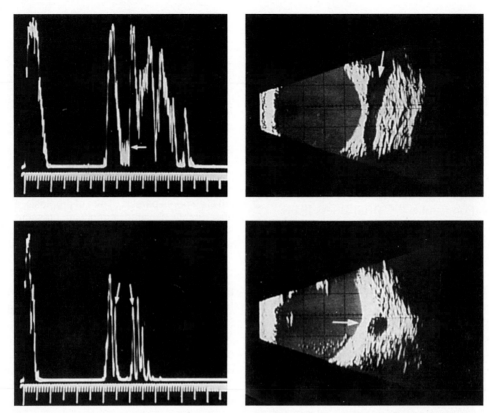

Fig. 17–16. Orbital ultrasonography. Transocular A-Scans **(left)** and B-scans **(right)** in a carotid-cavernous fistula with dilated arterialized superior ophthalmic vein. **Top left.** Blurred spikes (*arrow*) within the dilated vessel indicate fast blood flow. **Bottom left.** Distinct spikes (*arrows*) from vessel walls, at low system sensitivity. **Top right.** Dilated superior ophthalmic vein (*arrow*), at low sensitivity setting. **Bottom right.** Cross-section of enlarged superior ophthalmic vein. (From Byrne SF, Glaser JS: Orbital tissue differentiation with standardized echography. Ophthalmology 90:1071, 1983)

man with traumatic fistula and cavernous sinus enlargement to the point of intracranial compression of the ipsilateral optic nerve, with reversal of blindness after balloon occlusion, and Mirabel et al[110] reported a giant suprasellar varix of the superior petrosal sinus associated with a dural arteriovenous fistula, with chiasmal compression. It bears repetition that few carotid-cavernous fistulas are life-threatening, and cautious individual case assessment seems reasonable.

ENDOVASCULAR INTERVENTIONAL PROCEDURES

The risks of direct surgical vascular repairs within the cavernous sinus are formidable, owing to the complexity of basal skull anatomy, the multitude of cranial nerves traversing that area, and the complexity of the anterior arterial system. Furthermore, in the setting of a dural AVM (dAVM) or carotid cavernous fistula (CCF), the venous structures in the region of the cavernous sinus become distended and tense, making surgical exploration in these conditions difficult and hazardous. Similar, and other, mechanical difficulties can be encountered in surgical exposure or resection of tumors of the caver-

nous sinus or of aneurysms of the carotid siphon. Fortunately, in the past decade, there has been rapid growth in the development of catheter technology that permits endovascular approaches for blood flow abnormalities of the cavernous sinus and related structures.

Dural Arteriovenous Malformations and Carotid-Cavernous Fistulas

The pathogenic effects of a dAVM are mediated primarily through the elevation in venous pressure that accrues in this condition.[101,109,111] This venous pressure may be transmitted anteriorly into the orbit causing signs and symptoms associated with chronic orbital congestion and hypoxia. Because of the rich intercavernous basisphenoidal venous anastomoses, venous hypertension usually develops bilaterally, and both orbits may be affected.

The decision to treat is problematic. Retinal hypoxia ("venous stasis retinopathy"), with declining vision, field loss, elevation of intraocular pressure, significant proptosis, and worsening chemosis, raises concern for the long-term preservation of vision and for the need for treatment. Frequently, milder symptoms and signs

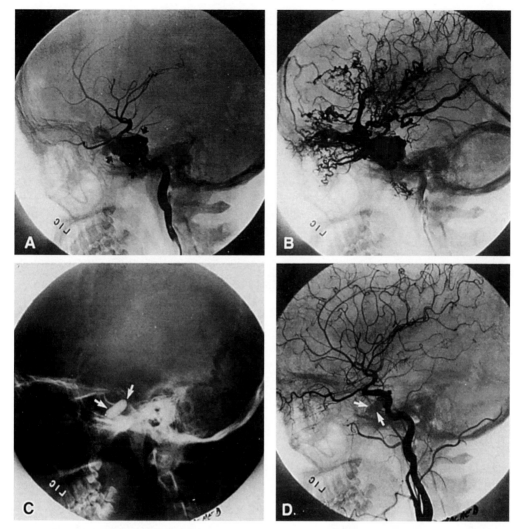

Fig. 17–17. A 32-year-old woman was accidentally shot in the right eye with a low-velocity missile. The initial recovery was excellent, except for loss of the right eye. Five days after the injury, left proptosis and bruit developed. Two weeks after the injury, she developed paralysis of the left sixth and fourth nerves, and visual acuity dropped to 20/400 (6/120) in her remaining (left) eye. An interventional neuroradiologic procedure was performed with complete return of function in the left eye. **A.** Left carotid arteriogram with immediate opacification of entire cavernous sinus (*arrows*). **B.** One-half second after **(A)** there was extensive filling of dural venous channels and orbital veins. **C.** Detachable flow-guided balloon (*arrows*) placed in the fistula under fluoroscopic control and opacified with contrast medium. **D.** Follow-up left carotid arteriogram after balloon (*arrows*) placement. The fistula was completely closed with preservation of carotid flow. (Courtesy of Dr. Charles Kerber)

may be managed conservatively, while the patient practices ipsilateral carotid compression with the contralateral hand for 5 minutes per hour every day.[112] Reports in the literature cite a response rate to this regimen, or of spontaneous dAVM thrombosis, as high as 20% to 30%. However, our experience with this technique has been less favorable, and there is some question that damage may be done to pre-existing atherosclerotic neck vessels.

In some persons, the cavernous sinuses have existing or potential connections to the deep venous system of the brain. Indeed, this may be the preferential route of venous drainage from all or part of the cavernous basal

sinus complex. Therefore, the clinical appearance of orbital venous hypertension associated with a cavernous dAVM may be relatively minimal, but arterialized flow is instead transmitted chiefly via venous dural channels draining the medial aspects of the temporal lobes and the basal vein of Rosenthal. The latter drains an extensive deep parenchymal territory, including part of the posterior fossa. This effluent pattern explains how some cavernous dAVMs or CCFs present with relatively minor outward physical signs, but with serious complications from cortical venous hypertension (Fig. 17–18), elevated intracranial pressure (a form of secondary "pseudotumor cerebri syndrome"; see Chapter 5, Part

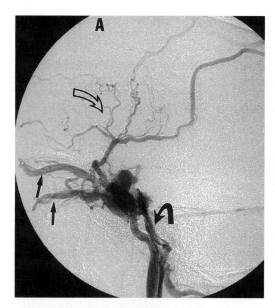

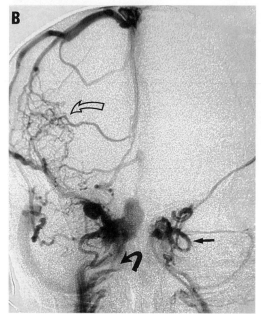

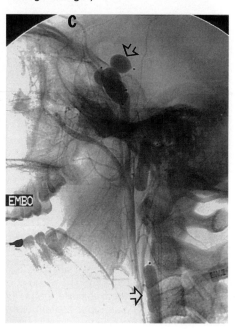

Fig. 17–18. A 25-year-old man developed severe right-sided proptosis and a loud bruit at the time of a vehicular accident. Lateral projection of the right internal carotid artery in the **(A)** early arterial phase and **(B)** late arterial phase in anteroposterior projection demonstrate immediate opacification of the superior and inferior ophthalmic veins (*straight arrows*), the inferior petrosal sinuses (*curved arrows*) and of the deep parenchymal veins of the right hemisphere (*open curved arrows*). The fistula was related to a large carotid laceration involving the cavernous and supraclinoid segments of the right internal carotid artery. The artery could not be preserved at the time of treatment. **C.** Latex balloons (*open-ended arrowheads*) were placed in the fistula and within the carotid artery at the time of treatment. (Courtesy of Frank Huang-Hellinger)

II), temporal lobe seizures, brain parenchymal hemorrhage due to venous infarction or venous rupture (Fig. 17–19), or edema of the posterior fossa structures.[111]

The anatomic substrate for the vascular chain of complications can be defined best by timely conventional selective angiography alone, even in patients presenting with seemingly mild signs. The decision to intervene and the mode of treatment can only be based on the precise angiographic details.

Endovascular treatment of fistulous lesions in the cavernous sinus can be pursued via transarterial or transvenous routes.[113–116] In the case of direct CCFs, the laceration of the carotid artery is usually most easily

sealed with a transarterial detachable balloon (see Fig. 17–17).[117] If possible, this technique is performed by detaching the balloon on the venous side of the fistula to close it, while preserving flow in the carotid artery. Occasionally, such precise balloon positioning may not be possible, or the laceration of the carotid artery may be complex. Therefore, assuming that adequate collateral intracranial circulation has been demonstrated, a trapping procedure using detachable balloons may be necessary, that is, closing the carotid artery above, below, and at the site of the fistula. Detachable balloons are manufactured from silicone or latex, and their placement can be difficult, sometimes requiring a shift in

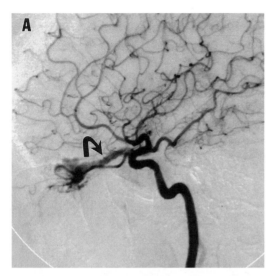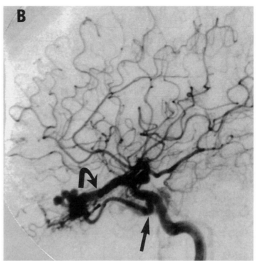

Fig. 17–19. A 30-year-old woman presented with headaches. Lateral views of left **(A)** and right **(B)** internal carotid arteriograms demonstrate developmental venous malformation of the cribriform plate supplied by both ophthalmic arteries. Note subarachnoid veins of the anterior cranial fossa (*curved arrows*). In addition, the right ophthalmic artery **(B)** has a cavernous origin (*arrow*), a vestige of the dorsal ophthalmic artery that usually atrophies in fetal development.

mid-procedure to alternative techniques. Spontaneous deflation over a period of weeks occurs in both types of balloons when the inflating material is conventional radiographic contrast. By this time, however, the fistula site will, one hopes, have thrombosed and become endothelialized. Delayed recanalization of the fistula site after balloon closure is not a common problem, although these sites have a 20% to 30% rate of pouch or pseudoaneurysm formation on delayed follow-up.[115] However, clinical sequelae of these pouches or pseudoaneurysm sites seem to be uncommon.

The major alternative to balloon closure of a CCF is coil placement.[118,119] This can be accomplished transarterially, similar to the technique for balloon placement across a fistula. Alternatively, transvenous catheterization with closure of the fistula using coils, similar to transvenous embolization of a dAVM, is also well established as a viable technique. This has particular application in patients in whom the fistula hole is too small to allow passage of a balloon or in whom the hole has a configuration that prevents stable positioning of a balloon.

The more effective therapy consists in transvenous packing of the cavernous sinus using fibered thrombogenic 0.018-inch coils placed via a coaxial microcatheter system. By tightly packing the venous side of a dAVM with a thrombogenic mesh of platinum coils, flow through the dAVM ceases, and the arterial feeders regress. Access to the cavernous sinus can be gained in more than 80% of such patients via the inferior petrosal sinus. A 5- to 7-French introducer catheter is advanced

from a femoral vein to the jugular bulb. Within the introducer catheter, a co-axial microcatheter is then directed into the inferior petrosal sinus and cavernous sinus (Fig. 17–20). Various coil types and sizes, most made of platinum, are available and may be deployed in this location. These are advanced in the introducer microcatheter with an 0.018-inch pusher wire until they extrude from the tip of the microcatheter. Some fibered coils are also available in the Guglielmi Detachable Coil range. These coils are soldered to a stainless steel wire pusher. When the coil is in a satisfactory location, the coil is detached by passing an electrolytic 9-V current that dissolves the solder. This coil type carries the advantage of allowing more precise placement and greater control, distinctly advantageous in a high-flow fistula.

Occasionally, transvenous access to the cavernous sinus is thwarted by variations in otherwise normal native anatomy. For example, some compartments of the cavernous sinus involved with the shunt may be completely separated from the inferior petrosal sinus, with exclusive drainage to the superior ophthalmic vein. In such patients, transvenous access can be gained by retrograde catheterization of the superior ophthalmic vein (Fig. 17–21), either directly or by puncture of the facial vein.[120] When the venous drainage from the cavernous sinus is directed exclusively to the veins of the temporal lobes or to the basal vein of Rosenthal, surgical exposure of the cavernous sinus and intraoperative venous packing with coils may be necessary.

Transarterial embolization therapy of dAVMs of the

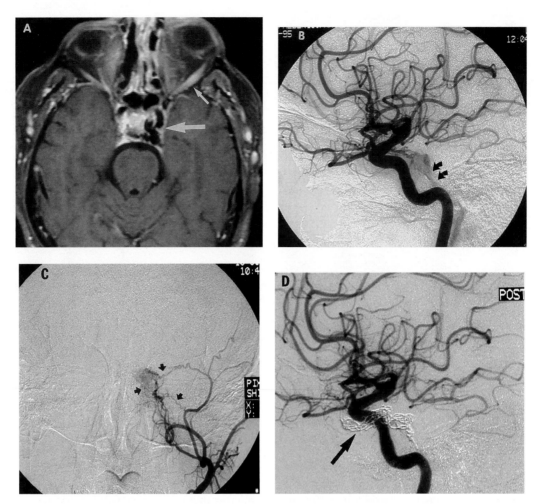

Fig. 17–20. A 54-year-old man presented with worsening proptosis and chemosis of his left eye following endoscopic sinus surgery. **A.** Contrast-enhanced T_1-weighted axial magnetic resonance imaging demonstrates an asymmetric dilation of veins (*large arrow*) in the left cavernous sinus; note enlarged lateral rectus muscle (*small arrow*). Lateral view of selective left internal carotid arteriogram **(B)** and frontal view of selective left external carotid arteriogram **(C)** demonstrate opacification of the cavernous sinus through numerous small vessel shunts; note opacification of the inferior petrosal sinus (*small arrows* in **B**), indicating a potential route for transvenous approach. The cavernous sinus was packed with fibered coils using transvenous access via the inferior petrosal sinus. **D.** Lateral view of post-embolization angiogram of the left internal carotid artery shows complete closure of the malformation. The mesh of packed coils is seen on the subtracted image (*arrow*).

cavernous sinus is less satisfactory in efficacy and safety profile than is transvenous embolization. Dural AVMs in this region typically draw arterial supply from a myriad of distal branches of the external carotid artery, ophthalmic artery, and internal carotid artery. Quite apart from the difficulty of closing all these small vessels with particulate polyvinyl alcohol or coils, the hazards of inadvertent embolization of the ophthalmic artery or internal carotid artery are considerable. Aggressive embolization in this territory with more noxious agents such as alcohol or cyanoacrylate also carries a high risk of ischemic injury to the cranial nerves of the cavernous sinus. More recently, radiosurgery ("gamma knife") was

proposed by Guo et al[121] as an alternative treatment for dAVFs of the cavernous sinus, with obliteration of fistulas in 12 of 15 patients reported in this series.

Aneurysms of the Carotid Siphon

Aneurysms in the region of the carotid siphon fall into two major categories. Intradural aneurysms, including those related to the carotid-ophthalmic junction, occur above the carotid dural ring. Extradural aneurysms occur below the dural ring and are synonymous with "cavernous" aneurysms. From a neurosurgical point of view, intradural aneurysms are more dangerous in that their

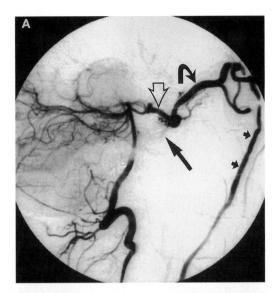

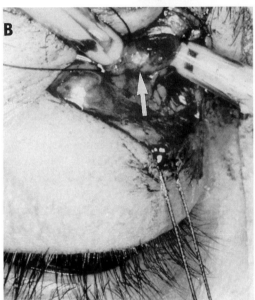

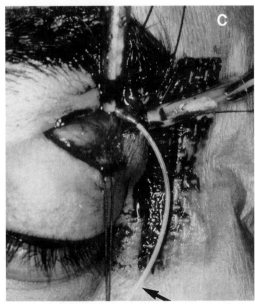

Fig. 17–21. A 35-year-old man with a right carotid cavernous fistula (CCF) following head trauma. Therapeutic alternatives in this case were limited by the presence of an occlusive dissection of the ipsilateral right internal carotid artery and absence of venous access to the fistula via the inferior petrosal sinus. The lesion was embolized initially via the ipsilateral posterior communicating artery (*arrow* in **A** indicates coils from the first procedure). However, the fistula recanalized, and the patient presented with recurrent symptoms. **A.** Lateral projection of the left vertebral artery at the start of the second procedure demonstrates opacification of the supraclinoid right internal carotid artery (*open arrow*), with fistulous flow to the superior ophthalmic vein (*curved arrow*), draining inferiorly via the facial veins (*small arrows*). The second procedure was performed with surgical exposure of the superior ophthalmic vein under general anesthesia in the angiography suite. **B.** The tense distended vein (*white arrow*) has been dissected and secured with two vascular ties. **C.** A small venotomy was performed between the vascular ties through which a Tracker 18 microcatheter (*small arrow*) was inserted. This was then guided over a wire into the cavernous sinus in the region of the fistula, where a further packing of coils resulted in complete occlusion of the CCF. (Courtesy of Dr. Peter Rubin)

rupture is associated with sudden onset of subarachnoid hemorrhage and its attendant morbidity and mortality. Rupture of cavernous aneurysms rarely causes subarachnoid or subdural hemorrhage and is even most unlikely to result in the sudden presentation of a spon-

taneous CCF. Most small cavernous aneurysms are discovered incidentally during angiography performed for other reasons, and they do not require therapy.

Large cavernous aneurysms often present to the ophthalmologist, when expansion of the aneurysm causes

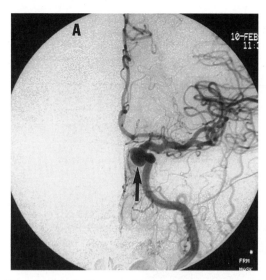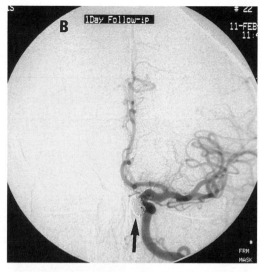

Fig. 17–22. A 63-year-old woman presented with a 3-month history of severe left-sided retro-orbital headaches. **A.** Frontal view of the left carotid angiogram shows a 7-mm rounded aneurysm of the left cavernous segment projecting medially (*arrow*). **B.** Following virtually complete obliteration of the aneurysm with Guglielmi detachable coils (*arrow*), the symptoms improved significantly.

severe dural headache, or when mass-effect causes compression of the intracavernous cranial nerves with diplopia (see Chapter 12). Typically, patients present with retro-orbital pain and an ipsilateral VI palsy, later progressing to involve cranial nerve III. In these patients, treatment may be warranted, especially for pain. Intervention may also be recommended in certain asymptomatic patients when the location of the aneurysm is on the medial aspect of the carotid genu. In this site, the "carotid cave," the precise location of the dural ring can be difficult to discern, and some uncertainty may exist about whether an aneurysm of this site is intradural or extradural. Some "transitional" aneurysms in this position straddle both compartments, and, therefore, there is a risk of subarachnoid hemorrhage.

Because of the difficulties in surgical exploration of the cavernous sinus, as with dAVFs, endovascular therapy for aneurysm in the region of the cavernous sinus has evolved rapidly.[122,123] Furthermore, intradural aneurysms related to the carotid-ophthalmic junction, or along the proximal supraclinoid carotid artery, may present a difficult surgical exposure. The anatomy of the anterior clinoid process, the falciform dural fold extending medially from the anterior clinoid process to the tuberculum sellae, and the middle and posterior clinoid ligaments can be variable. These variations further confound surgical exposure and closure of aneurysms in this location. Consequently, growing numbers of such patients are being referred for endovascular therapy.

Endovascular therapy of aneurysms of the carotid siphon depends on two questions: Can the aneurysm be obliterated while preserving anterograde flow in the carotid artery? If the aneurysm cannot be obliterated safely, then does the clinical profile of the patient warrant a consideration of carotid artery closure, and is there adequate intracranial collateral flow to tolerate such a maneuver? Reconstructive endovascular therapy of aneurysms in the carotid siphon consists of transarterial packing of the aneurysm with platinum Guglielmi Detachable Coils (Fig. 17–22). These coils are manufactured in a range of helix-diameters and lengths, in 0.010- and 0.018-inch diameters. When satisfactorily placed, the coils are detached from the stainless steel pusher with a 9-V battery current. The procedure is performed with the patient under general anesthesia and with full heparinization.

The object of the procedure is to achieve a tight packing of the aneurysm lumen to stop inflow of blood, while preserving flow in the parent (carotid) artery. The configuration of the neck of the aneurysm is therefore of some concern in that a small-shouldered neck is more likely to retain the coil loops within the aneurysm. Aneurysms with wide, gaping necks are less favorably disposed to this technique. However, a newer technique has now been described whereby two catheters are placed in the carotid artery at once.[123] One microcatheter is placed in the aneurysm while a balloon-catheter is placed along the mouth of the aneurysm. The balloon is inflated gently for a short period at the time of each coil placement, resulting in satisfactory preservation of the carotid lumen during aneurysm packing.

For giant aneurysms (larger than 2.5 cm) of the carotid siphon, or those with other complicating anatomic features, coil obliteration of the aneurysm with preservation of the carotid artery may not be possible.[124] A temporary balloon test occlusion of the carotid artery can be conducted to test the feasibility of arterial sacrifice as definitive therapy. Ideally, it is preferable to place balloons or occluding coils above and below the aneurysm site, so-called aneurysm "trapping." However, this may not always be possible, and proximal occlusion of the artery may be necessary. This maneuver probably has a slightly higher risk of embolization into the intracranial circulation from the long-remaining artery stump and is therefore a second choice in this type of procedure. Intra-arterial detachable balloons are the easiest and least expensive means of executing arterial sacrifice. It can also be accomplished by packing the lumen of the artery with thrombogenic coils. However, this is a lengthy procedure, and the number of coils necessary contributes significantly to the comparative expense.

Embolization of Tumors of the Cavernous Sinus

Preoperative embolization of meningiomas and other tumors in the region of the cavernous sinus is a commonly performed procedure, depending on the preferences of the operating neurosurgeon. Extremely vascular meningiomas, or vascular metastases to the skull base from renal cell or thyroid carcinoma, can be problematic because of blood loss at the time of surgery. Preoperative devascularization of such lesions with particulate embolization can contribute significantly to the ease and efficacy of surgery. Such embolization therapy is somewhat hazardous and requires considerable training and experience in order to be performed safely. The numerous common or rare variants of anastomoses between the ophthalmic artery, internal carotid artery, and the external carotid artery add to risks, which may can include stroke, blindness, and cranial nerve palsy.

OCULOCEPHALIC VASCULAR ANOMALIES

Associated congenital vascular anomalies of the eye and brain, although infrequently encountered, are an area of special interest to ophthalmologists, neurologists, and neurosurgeons. The incidence of co-existence of such malformations cannot be stated with accuracy: many patients with retinal lesions are neurologically asymptomatic and are not subjected to MRI, angiography, or other neuroimaging procedures, and in patients with an intracranial AVM, careful scrutiny

of the fundus is often bypassed. A long list of eponymic oculocephalic congenital vascular syndromes has developed, perhaps sharing more features in common than characteristics that truly separate the various forms into any useful system of classification. The widespread availability of CT scanning and MRI has allowed more precise correlations and accurate diagnosis.[125,126]

Retinocerebellar Angiomatosis (Von Hippel-Lindau Disease)

After von Hippel's description of *angiomatosis retinae,* Lindau synthesized the clinical entity, which includes angiomas of the retina, brain, spinal cord, and viscera. Although the retinal lesion may be the clue that identifies the disease (and causes loss of vision), it is the cerebellar hemangioblastoma (cystic or solid) or renal carcinoma that potentially dooms the patient.[127] The disorder is inherited, in the majority of instances, in an autosomal dominant pattern with variable and incomplete penetrance, the gene mapped on the short arm of Cr3. The penetrance of this disease is age and tumor dependent, most patients presenting in the second and third decades. When angiomatous lesions become symptomatic, a careful family history is mandatory, and examination of first- and second-degree relatives is ideal. Symptoms are usually related to the retinal or cerebellar lesions, but spinal cord hemangioblastomas occur, and other *visceral* hamartomas should be sought; these include the following: pancreatic, lung epididymal, and renal cysts; renal cell carcinoma; pheochromocytoma; and multiple visceral angiomas.[127] Indeed, the lifetime risk for renal clear cell carcinoma amounts to 70% and is the most frequent cause of death. Pheochromocytomas affect 7% to 20% of reported patients and can be bilateral and malignant.

The retinal lesions (von Hippel's tumor) may take the form of a fully developed elevated angioma in the mid-periphery (Fig. 17–23), an incipient small nodule,[128] or minuscule anomalies on the disc.[129] Hemangioblastoma of the optic nerve is reported, associated with cerebellar and visceral cysts.[130] Most central nervous system lesions are found in the cerebellum, spinal cord, and brain stem; there is special predilection for the craniocervical junction and *conus medullaris.* Supratentorial lesions are rare, but chiasmal hemangioblastomas are documented.[131] The larger retinal lesions are characterized by single enlarged and tortuous retinal arterial afferents and similarly dilated venous efferents. Yellowish retinal and subretinal exudate is seen, somewhat mimicking the exudative retinopathy of Coats' retinal telangiectasia. Macular exudate or retinal detachment

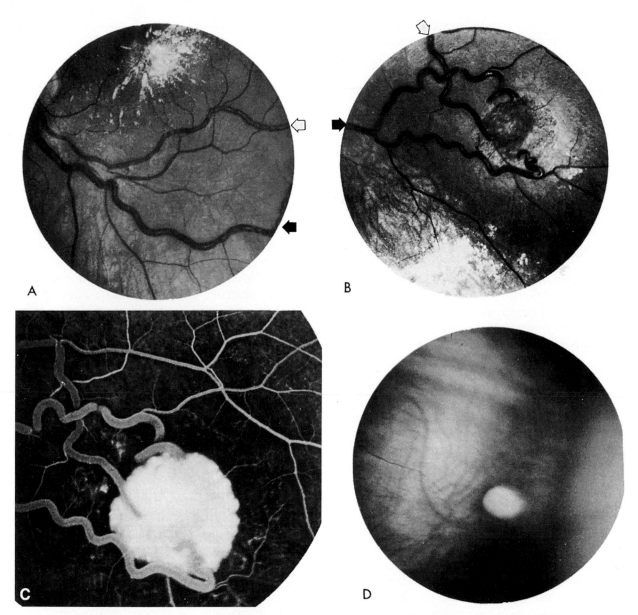

Fig. 17–23. Angiomatosis retinae (von Hippel's tumor). **A.** A 23-year-old man presented with diminished vision from exudative retinopathy involving the left macula. **B.** Typical retinal angioma was noted in inferotemporal midperiphery. *Open arrows* indicate feeding retinal arteriole; *closed arrows* indicate draining vein. **C.** Fluorescein angiogram demonstrates arteriovenous shunt through angioma. **D.** Small berry-like angioma in far retinal periphery. (**A** through **C**, Courtesy of Dr. J. D. M. Gass)

accounts for visual symptoms and may progress to proliferative retinopathy and secondary glaucoma. Multiple angiomas may occur in the same or contralateral eye. Indirect ophthalmoscopy and fluorescein angiography are exceedingly helpful in discovering small or incipient lesions.

It is impossible to predict which patients with retinal angiomas harbor co-existing cerebellar lesions or other systemic harmartomas. In extensive and excellent reviews,[127,132] the average age at onset of symptoms, whether ocular or neurologic, occurs in the early thirties, but surely younger than 50 years of age. The cerebellar lesions present as chronic posterior fossa masses, with signs and symptoms of chronic headaches, vertigo, vomiting, and ataxia. In addition, 10% to 20% of cerebellar hemangioblastomas are associated with polycythemia. If polycythemia does not diminish following resection of the cerebellar lesion, it is likely that the mural nodule (Lindau's tumor) was overlooked or that the patient harbors a renal cell carcinoma or pheochromocytoma.[132]

Neurodiagnostic studies in the presence of a cerebellar mass may be expected to show dilation of the ventricular system and signs of posterior fossa mass. These lesions, especially when small, are amenable to surgery, and therefore the prognosis is good. Hydrocephalus may

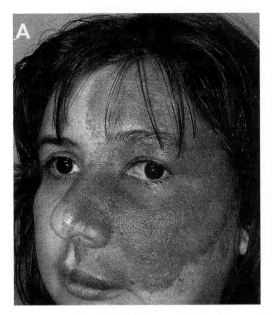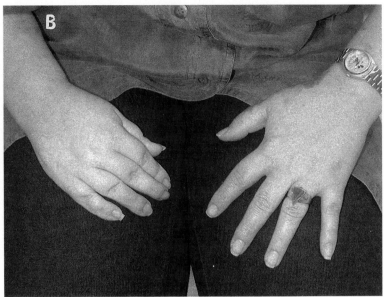

Fig. 17–24. Sturge-Weber disease. A 34-year-old woman with life-long seizures and with right homonymous hemianopia. **A.** Verrucous facial nevus flammeus; note that cutaneous angioma in this case precisely outlines right ophthalmic and maxillary divisions of the trigeminal nerve. **B.** Relative somatic hypoplasia on the right (small right hand) owing to a left cerebral vascular lesion.

dilate the third ventricle and produce chiasmal compression with bitemporal field defect.[133]

Once a retinal angioma is diagnosed, all efforts should be directed to uncover the possibility of a cerebellar lesion and occult renal cell carcinoma. The Cambridge screening protocol,[127,134] outlined by Maher, recommends the following: annual physical examination and urinalysis; annual indirect ophthalmoscopy, with fluorescein angiography; MRI of brain every 3 years to age 50 years, and every 5 years thereafter; annual renal ultrasound, with CT every 3 years; annual 24-hour urine collection for vanillylmandelic acids.

Encephalotrigeminal Angiomatosis (Sturge-Weber Syndrome)

Among the most striking of the neurocutaneous vascular syndromes are those that include facial hemangiomas. In its complete form, Sturge-Weber syndrome is characterized by the following: (1) "port-wine angioma" (*nevus flammeus*) of the face, commonly involving the distribution of the ophthalmic division of cranial nerve V (Fig. 17–24), but not limited to it; (2) seizure disorder beginning early life; (3) gyriform cortical calcifications associated with leptomeningeal angiomatosis; (4) homolateral buphthalmos or glaucoma, especially when the nevus extends to the lid; and (5) intellectual retardation. In addition, hemiplegia or hemianopia may be seen contralateral to the cerebral lesion. Familial occurrence is unsubstantiated. In a series of 51 patients seen at the Hospital for Sick Children, Toronto,[135] 71% had glau-

coma, 69% had conjunctival or episcleral hemangiomas, and 55% had choroidal hemangiomas, almost half of which were bilateral.

Choroidal hemangiomas may diffusely involve the entire uvea, or the hemangioma may be more localized (Fig. 17–25). For example, a minimally elevated, nonpigmented, poorly circumscribed subretinal lesion is seen. These tumors are easily overlooked, even with indirect ophthalmoscopy. The appearance resembles metastatic choroidal carcinoma. Visual symptoms are caused by cystoid degeneration of the fovea and exudative retinal detachment. The rare occurrence of a cilio-optic vein may provide a clue to diagnosis.[136] MRI can disclose diffuse choroidal hemangiomas.

The facial nevus is congenital and does not change with age, except for a tendency to become verrucous (see Fig. 17–24). The supraorbital area is monotonously involved, but the angioma does not lie strictly within the boundaries of the trigeminal distribution. The differential diagnosis and therapy for facial hemangiomas and port- wine stains have been extensively discussed.[137] Leptomeningeal venous angioma of the homolateral cerebral hemisphere constitutes the lesion that accounts for convulsions, contralateral hemiparesis, and somatic hemiatrophy. Calcification of the cerebral cortex accounts for radiologic findings of tortuous double lines ("railroad tracks"). At present, gadolinium-enhanced MRI provides sensitive documentation of leptomeningeal enhancement (see Fig. 17–24), the principal radiologic sign of Sturge-Weber syndrome, and enhancing choroidal angiomas also are demonstrable (Fig. 17–26); bilateral choroidal lesions infer bilat-

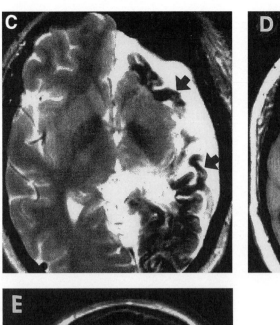
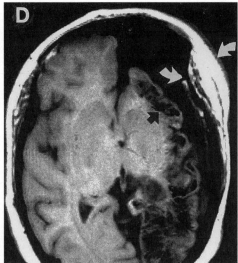
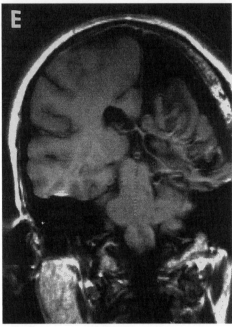

Fig. 17–24. (*continued*). **C.** T$_2$-weighted magnetic resonance imaging (MRI) shows hemicerebral atrophy, thickening of meninges due to venous angioma, and calcification (*black areas, arrows*) that occurs in outer layers of cortex and in meningeal arteries. **D.** T$_1$-weighted MRI. Note calcified gyri (*black areas*) and compensatory thickening of overlying cranium (*arrows*). **E.** MRI, coronal section.

eral cerebral hemisphere abnormalities.[138] The most frequent site of cerebral angiomatosis is the occipital or occipitoparietal region of one hemisphere. For more extensive description, the reader is referred to the chapter by Alexander in *Handbook of Clinical Neurology*[139] and to Font and Ferry[140] for a discussion of ocular histopathology.

Racemose Hemangiomas of Retina, Thalamus, and Midbrain

In the continuum of oculocephalic vascular anomalies, racemose hemangiomas of the retina, thalamus, and midbrain, also known as Bonnet-de Chaume-Blanc syndrome or Wyburn-Mason syndrome, are quite rare. This syndrome is included in the group of "neurophakomatoses" with fundus vascular anomalies and associated intracranial AVM. Theron and associates[141] recorded only 25 cases from the literature that met the criteria of angiographic or pathologic verification. Other additional cases have since been described,[142–144] including involvement of the optic nerve and chiasm. In 1937, Bonnet and associates[145] recognized the coexistence of retinal and cerebral AVMs and, in 1943, Wyburn-Mason,[146] recorded arteriovenous aneurysms of the midbrain and retina, facial nevi, and mental changes.

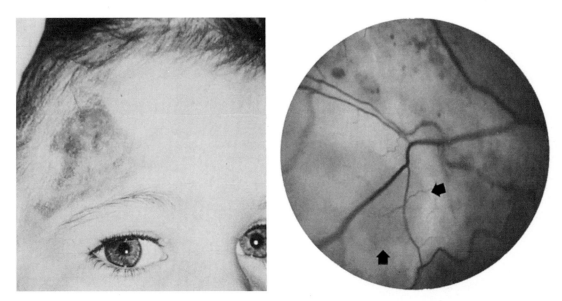

Fig. 17–25. Sturge-Weber disease in a 5-year-old girl with congenital angioma above the right brow and loss of vision in the right eye. An orange-red choroidal hemangioma (*arrows*) could be partially visualized beneath the detached retina. Note that the cutaneous angioma in this instance does not involve the lids.

The classic ocular lesion is a unilateral arteriovenous retinal shunt, usually with greatly dilated tortuous vessels (Fig. 17–27). Arteriovenous shunting results in similar coloration of arteries and veins, but fluorescein angiography is helpful in elucidating complicated flow patterns. The lesions are congenital and nonprogressive, with symptoms of lowered vision appearing in the second and third decades of life. Rarely is vision completely spared, and the eye may be totally blind. The retrobulbar structures, including the optic nerve and chiasm, are involved by vascular malformation in a large percentage of cases, and the nerve may be almost entirely replaced by dilated vascular channels.[141] Instances are described with neovascular glaucoma that followed retinal ischemia or hemorrhage from the retinal vascular malformation.[144] Some retinal AVMs have been treated successfully with xenon laser photocoagulation (Fig. 17–28).

The clinical characteristics of the syndrome are elaborated in Table 17–1. Involvement of the nervous system

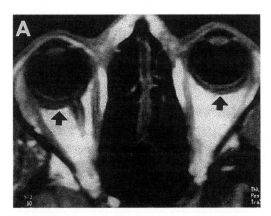
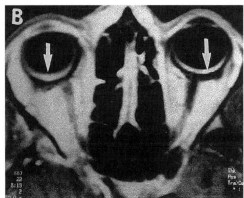

Fig. 17–26. Sturge-Weber. Axial magnetic resonance imaging sections. **A.** T_1-weighted axial image shows thickening of posterior aspect of both globes (*arrows*). **B.** T_1-weighted image with contrast shows bilateral diffuse choroidal hemangiomas (*arrows*). (From ref. 138)

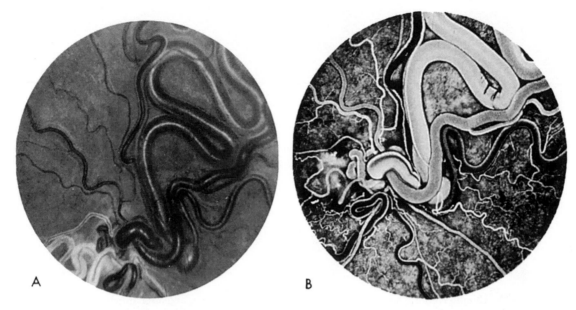

Fig. 17–27. Racemose angioma of the retina. **A.** Knot of retinal tissues at the inferior aspect of the photograph represents the area of the optic disc. Visual acuity is finger-counting. **B.** Fluorescein angiogram demonstrates complex flow patterns, including rapid arteriovenous shunting. The patient had an arteriovenous malformation of the right maxilla. (Case reported as von Hippel's disease by LaDow CS, McFall TA: Central hemangioma of the maxilla, with von Hippel's disease: report of case. J Oral Surg 22:252, 1964. Copyright by American Dental Association. Reprinted by permission. Photographs courtesy of Mr. John Justice)

takes the form of deep AVMs, which have special predilection for the visual pathways, including the optic nerve, chiasm, hypothalamus, basal ganglia, and mesencephalon. Midbrain and other posterior fossa signs may be encountered, including cranial nerve palsies, Parinaud's syndrome, internuclear ophthalmoplegia, and nystagmus. Obstructive hydrocephalus may result from periaqueductal lesions. The symptomatology of posterior fossa AVM has been previously discussed. Deep hemispheral and basicranial lesions are not usually amenable to direct surgical intervention, and ligation of extracranial afferent vessels is not effective.

Cavernous Angiomas of Retina and Brain

Certain disorders link congenital vascular anomalies of the eye and brain, including familial cavernous angiomas of the retina and central nervous system, more com-

TABLE 17–1. Clinical Characteristics of Bonnet-De Chaume-Blanc (Wyburn-Mason) Syndrome*

Ocular
  Unilateral retinal arteriovenous malformations: 25
  Acuity: normal, 5; blind, 8
  Fields: homonymous hemianopia, 8
  Dilated conjunctival vessels: 3
Orbital (including optic nerve or perioptic tissue)
  Arteriovenous malformations.
  Proptosis: 13 (1 with pulsation)
  Enlarged optic canal: 9
Neurologic
  Mental disturbances: 7
  Hemiparesis, hemiplegia: 13

Cerebral/subarachnoid hemorrhage: 4
Subjective bruit: 4
Cerebellar dysfunction: 2
Seizures: 1
Miscellaneous
  Cutaneous vascular nevus: 6 (3 "port-wine")
  Facial asymmetry: 3
  Head angiomas: cheek/nose, 6; mandible, 3; palate, 2;
    maxilla, 1; buccal mucosa, 1
  Recurrent epistaxis: 5
  Gingival/tonsillar bleeding: 3

*Specific clinical information not recorded in all 25 cases.
Adapted from ref. 141.

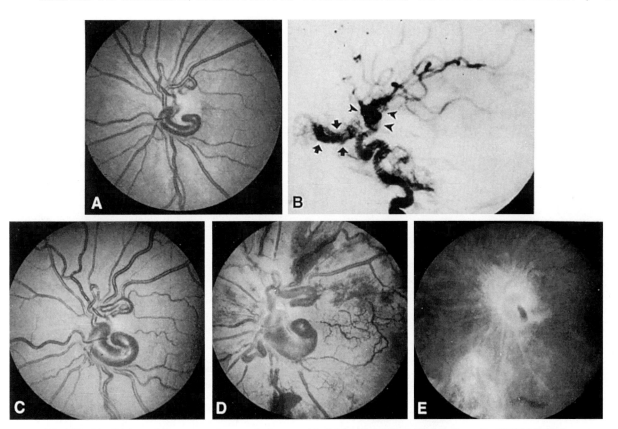

Fig. 17–28. Wyburn-Mason syndrome. A 4-year-old child with left "amblyopia," acuity 20/200 (6/60). **A.** Dilated venous anomaly, left disc. **B.** Subtracted left internal carotid angiogram shows both an arteriovenous malformation along course of ophthalmic artery (*arrows*) and a suprasellar vascular anomaly (*arrowheads*). **C.** Progressive enlargement of venous complex. **D.** Within 20 months, vision reduced to finger-counting, the fundus appearance was that of hemorrhagic ischemic retinopathy, and neovascular angle-closure glaucoma developed with applantation tension of 54 mmHg. Panretinal xenon laser photocoagulation was performed. **E.** Repeat fluorescein angiography shows clearing of retinopathy and diminished perfusion of anomalous vessels. Applanation tension was reduced to 10 mmHg. (From Effron L, Zakov ZN, Tomsak RL: Neovascular glaucoma as a complication of the Wyburn-Mason syndrome. J Clin Neuro Ophthalmol 5:95, 1985)

monly in the supratentorial space than posterior fossa. As a rule, this syndrome is transmitted as an autosomal dominant trait and is characterized by seizures, headache, and intracranial hemorrhages.[147,148] Gass[149] believes the retinal lesion to be a vascular hamartoma (*i.e.,* a cavernous hemangioma) but not angiomatosis retinae, retinal telangiectasia, or racemose angioma. The lesion appears as a "cluster of saccular aneurysms filled with venous blood" at the nerve head or mid-retina (Fig. 17–29). Such cases are variably associated with small cutaneous angiomas, and bilateral retinal involvement has been documented as well as familial occurrence.[150,151] Neither retinal nor cerebral lesion need be symptomatic. Rigamonti and associates[148] demonstrated the superiority of MRI over CT in discovering the cerebral cavernous angiomas, characterized by small-caliber feeding vessels with slow circulation and thrombosis.

In general, it should be recognized that there is a wide and confounding spectrum of both hereditary and nonfamilial neurocutaneous angiomatoses, including various AVMs or hemangiomas of the skin and ocular fundus, associated with AVMs and venous anomalies of the brain. Leblanc et al[152] suggested a useful classification of vascular neurocutaneous syndromes (Table 17–2). Fortunately, MRI and MR venous angiography have evolved as practical and precise techniques in elucidating occult cerebral lesions and at least serve as preliminary studies that direct decisions for more elaborate selective arteriography.

ORBITAL VASCULAR ANOMALIES

A detailed discussion of hemangiomas, hemangiopericytomas, and other vascular tumors occurring in the

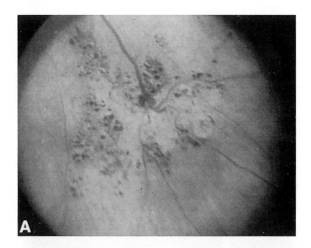

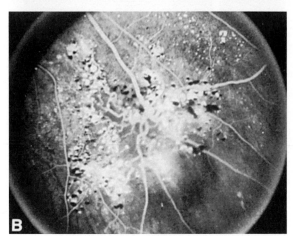

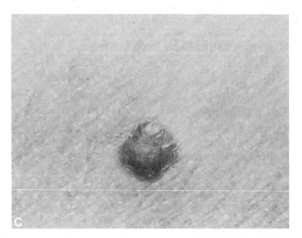

Fig. 17–29. Cavernous hemangioma of the retina. Fundus appearance **(A)** and fluorescein angiogram **(B)** of segmental angiomatous malformation of retina. Note saccular dilation of capillary shunts with pooling of dye. **C.** Cutaneous angioma in same patient. (Courtesy of Dr. J. D. M. Gass)

TABLE 17–2. Vascular Neurocutaneous Syndromes

Phakomatoses
  Hereditary hemorrhagic telangioectasia (Rendu-Osler-Weber)
  Encephalotrigeminal angiomatosis (Sturge-Weber)
  von Hippel-Lindau disease
  Neurofibromatosis
  Ataxia-telangiectasia (Louis-Bar)
  Hereditary neurocutaneous angiomatosis
Neurocutaneous Vascular Hamartomas
  Cerebroretinal arteriovenous malformations (Wyburn-Mason)
  Multiple systemic hemangiomatosis
  Blue rubber bleb nevus syndrome
  Cutaneomeningospinal angiomatosis (Cobb syndrome)

From ref. 152.

orbit related to trauma. Cutaneous hemangiomas of head and neck with associated vascular brain anomalies are discussed previously.

Venous Varices, Lymphangiomas, and Related Lesions

According to Wright,[153] venous anomalous malformations are by far the most common variety of vascular lesion of the orbit, and the clinical behavior and prevalence in infancy and childhood imply a hamartomatous condition. In the Moorfields series,[153] presentation occurred in patients younger than 16 years in 60% of cases, and two-thirds of the lesions enlarged slowly, painfully, and with hemorrhage, often showing bruising in the lids. There may be clinical clues such as bluish swelling especially at the superomedial aspect of the orbit, some proptosis and, as noted, distinct tendency to spontaneous hemorrhage; most enlarge with the Valsalva maneuver (see Fig. 14–13) and calcified phleboliths may be present, demonstrable by CT.

Other radiologic findings include enlargement of orbit and venous lakes or vascular marking of the frontal bone. Diagnosis may be affirmed by orbital venography, which typically delineates single or multiple complex varices (Fig. 17–30), and ultrasonography shows a linear echolucency that is compressible and enlarges with the Valsalva maneuver. In addition, enlargement with the Valsalva maneuver may be documented with CT, especially with short scan time "spiral" technique.[154]

Conjunctival vessels may be dilated, and anomalies of the retinal vascular tree are occasionally observed (see Fig. 17–30). Pulsation is not invariable, but its presence may mimic acquired arteriovenous shunts, such as seen with carotid-cavernous fistulas. Objective bruit or thrill is uncommon, unlike in fistula, and the proptosed globe may be retropulsed into the orbit by applying steady pressure on the eye through closed lids. Most

orbit is beyond the intent of this chapter. Specific lesions of neuro-ophthalmic interest, especially those clinically confused with acquired arteriovenous fistulas, are considered and include venous varices and lymphangiomas, complicated venous varices, and vascular lesions of the

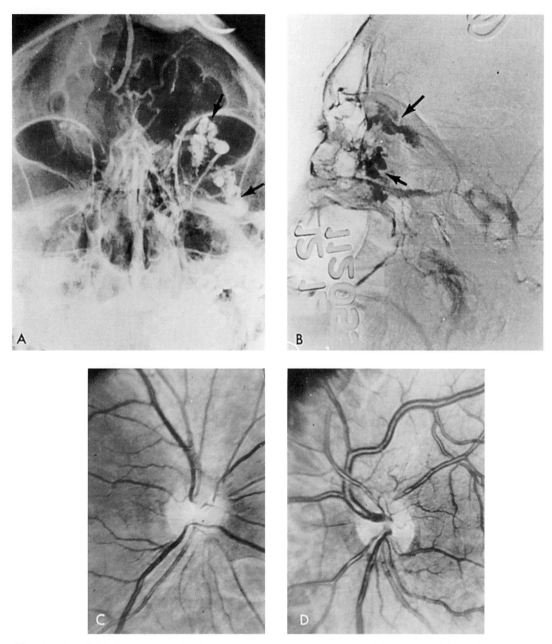

Fig. 17–30. Orbital venous varix. A 27-year-old man was evaluated for two episodes of severe left orbital pain; the last episode was accompanied by spontaneous hemorrhage in the lower lid. Motility and vision were normal, but 3 mm of proptosis was present. Orbital venography was performed. The unsubtracted frontal projection **(A)** shows two lobulated venous varices (*arrows*), which are also demonstrated by the lateral subtracted view **(B)**. **C.** Right fundus is normal. **D.** Left fundus shows anomalous dilated and tortuous veins.

patients enjoy normal vision, but venous varices may be associated with recurrent episodes of orbital pain, motility disturbances, and optic neuropathy (Fig. 17–31).

Conservative therapy frequently suffices, and surgery is complicated by arborization of vessels in orbital soft tissues, tendency to bleeding, and extension into the posterior aspect of the orbit. Surgery is usually indicated for cosmesis or complications of multiple hemorrhages.

Meddlesome operative intervention or injection of "sclerosing" agents may produce greater deficits and discomfort than those signs and symptoms that occur spontaneously. Radiation therapy is of no known value.

There is considerable controversy concerning origin and nomenclature. Wright[153] suggested that such anomalies with venous connections are *varices,* and those without are *lymphangiomas.* On the basis of hemodynamic

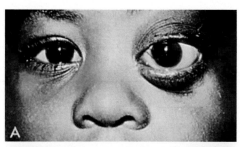

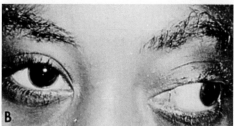

Fig. 17–31. Orbital venous varix. **A.** A 2-year-old child with left intermittent exophthalmos associated with extensive venous varix. The attempt to excise orbital varices was accompanied by massive blood loss. **B.** Ten years later, the eye is blind and exotropic. Venous anomalies of the kidneys were also discovered.

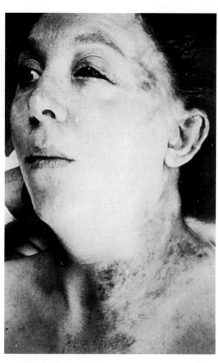

Fig. 17–32. Orbital venous varix with subcutaneous venous anomalies of temple, ear, neck, and superior chest wall. (Courtesy of Dr. Dan Boghen)

distinctions, Rootman[155] argued that varices and lymphangiomas are distinct, the latter characterized by avascular pooling without arterial or venous connections, and nondistensibility. The histologic distinction between lymphatic channels and small veins is often difficult, and endothelial-lined spaces with lymphocytic aggregates may be seen in tissue specimens from patients with orbital varices. Concensus opinion[156] dictates that orbital vascular malformations be classified according to hemodynamic characteristics: no flow, venous flow, and arterial flow lesions. These distinctions are germane to management.

Rootman and Graeb[157] provided an excellent discussion on the clinical spectrum of orbito-adnexal lymphangiomas, categorized principally by location in the orbit: superficial (lids and conjunctiva); deep (associated with orbital hemorrhage); and combined. In this series, connections with systemic venous circulation were found, suggesting relative hemodynamic isolation, and clinical and histologic distinction from venous varix was reported.

No clear line of demarcation exists where the simple orbital venous varix ends and more complicated venous vascular malformations begin. For example, involvement of the hard palate is occasionally noted to accompany an otherwise uncomplicated orbital varix or lymphangioma.[157] However, other soft tissue structures of the face and neck may be involved as well (Fig. 17–32). Orbito-frontal varices have been reported in association with limb osteohypertrophy, cutaneous hemangiectases, and extremity varicosities, a complex

known as the Klippel-Trenaunay-Weber syndrome.[158] Combined venous lymphatic malformations of the orbit (so-called lymphangiomas) may rarely be associated with non-contiguous intracranial venous developmental anomalies.[159]

Cutaneovisceral hemangiomatosis (blue rubber bleb nevus syndrome; Bean's syndrome) is a rare congenital disorder with hallmark skin lesions (blue blebs) and gastrointestinal bleeding. Ocular involvement includes lid blebs, iris and retinal angiomas,[160] and orbital hemangiomas that may present with lid ecchymoses or intermittent proptosis.[161]

Vascular Defects Related to Trauma

The involvement of orbital veins with arteriovenous fistulas at the level of the cavernous sinus has been discussed previously. On rare occasions, shunts of the ophthalmic artery may follow blunt or penetrating injury to the orbit itself. Orbital and ocular signs following such lesions are similar to those of carotid-cavernous fistulas. Internal carotid arteriography shows enlargement of the ophthalmic artery and immediate opacification of either the superior or the inferior ophthalmic vein (Fig. 17–33).

Post-traumatic arteriovenous shunts involving the intraorbital portion of the ophthalmic artery,[25] or its branches, traditionally have been confused with primary arterial aneurysms of the orbit. The latter lesion is ex-

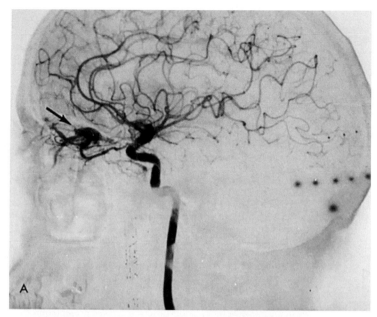

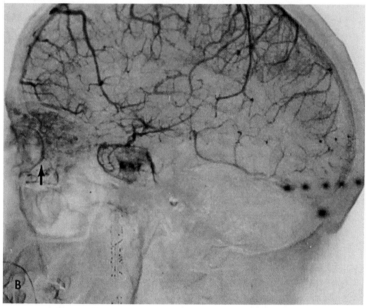

Fig. 17–33. Orbital arteriovenous fistula. A 58-year-old man noted redness of the left eye, blurred vision, and diplopia 3 years following head trauma, which had resulted in brief unconsciousness and amnesia for 2 hours. The left eye was initially red but recovered fully, and the patient was asymptomatic in the interval. Examination showed proptosis, slight limitation of motion of globe, and bruit over orbit. **A.** Left carotid arteriogram demonstrates vascular mass in the roof of the left orbit (*arrow*) with marked arteriovenous shunting from the ophthalmic artery. **B.** Venous phase shows choroidal crescent of the globe (*arrow*), slightly flattened and displaced anteriorly. Surgical excision at the University of California, San Francisco, was successful, with disappearance of all signs and symptoms. (Courtesy of Dr. Gene Coin)

ceeding rare. However, the case presented by Rubinstein and colleagues[24] fulfills the angiographic criteria for acceptance.

REFERENCES

1. Menghini VV, Brown ND, Sicks MS et al: Incidence and prevalence of intracranial aneurysms and hemorrhage in Olmsted County, Minneapolis, 1965 to 1995. Neurology 51:405, 1997
2. Schievink WI: Intracranial aneurysms. N Engl J Med 336:28, 1997
3. Kuhn F, Morris R, Witherspoon CD et al: Terson syndrome: results of vitrectomy and the significance of vitreous hemorrhage in patients with subarachnoid hemorrhage. Ophthalmology 105:472, 1998
4. Barr HWK, Blackwood W, Meadows SP: Intracavernous carotid aneurysms: a clinical pathological report. Brain 94:607, 1971
5. Lee AG, Mawad ME, Baskin DS: Fatal subarachnoid hemorrhage from the rupture of a totally intracavernous carotid artery aneurysm: case report. Neurosurgery 38:596, 1996
6. Trobe JD, Glaser JS, Post MJD: Meningioma and aneurysms of the cavernous sinus: neuro-ophthalmologic features. Arch Ophthalmol 96:457, 1978
7. Arseni C, Ghitescu N, Cristescu A et al: Intrasellar aneurysms simulating hypophyseal tumors. Eur Neurol 3:321, 1970
8. Hancock DO: A case of complete bilateral ophthalmoplegia due to an intrasellar aneurysm. J Neurol Neurosurg Psychiatry 26:81, 1963
9. Wilson CB, Meyers FK: Bilateral saccular aneurysms of the internal carotid artery in the cavernous sinus. J Neurol Neurosurg Psychiatry 26:174, 1963
10. Kupersmith MJ, Berenstein A, Choi IS et al: Percutaneous transvascular treatment of giant carotid aneurysms: neuro-ophthalmologic findings. Neurology 34:328, 1984
11. Pool JL, Potts DG: Aneurysms and Arteriovenous Anomalies

of the Brain: Diagnosis and Treatment. New York: Harper & Row, 1965

12. Locksley HB: Report on the Cooperative Study of Intracranial Aneurysms and Subarachnoid Hemorrhage. Section V. Part I. Natural history of subarachnoid hemorrhage, intrancranial aneurysms and arteriovenous malformations. J Neurosurg 25:219, 1966

13. Ferguson GG, Drake CG: Carotid-ophthalmic aneurysms: visual abnormalities in 32 patients and the results of treatment. Surg Neurol 16:1, 1981

14. Guidetti B, LaTorre E: Carotid-ophthalmic aneurysms: a series of 16 cases treated by direct approach. Acta Neurochir 22:289, 1970

15. Ferguson GG, Drake CG: Carotid-ophthalmic aneurysms: the surgical management of those cases presenting with compression of the optic nerves and chiasm alone. Clin Neurosurg 27:263, 1980

16. Vinuela F, Fox A, Chang JK: Clinico-radiological spectrum of giant superclinoid internal carotid artery aneurysms: observations in 93 cases. Neuroradiology 26:93, 1984

17. Kumon Y, Sakaki S, Kohno K et al: Asymptomatic, unruptured carotid-ophthalmic aneurysms: angiographical differentiation of each type, operative results and indications. Surg Neurol 48:465, 1997

18. Day AL: Aneurysms of the ophthalmic segment: a clinical and anatomic analysis. J Neurosurg 72:677, 1990

19. Savino PJ, Paris M, Schatz NJ et al: Optic tract syndrome: a review of 21 patients. Arch Ophthalmol 96:656, 1978

20. Mindel JS, Sachdev VP, Kline LB et al: Bilateral intracavernous aneurysms mimicking a prolactin-secreting pituitary tumor. Surg Neurol 19:163, 1983

21. Goldin RR, Silver ML: Ophthalmic artery aneurysm. Radiology 68:727, 1957

22. Jain KK: Saccular aneurysm of the ophthlamic artery. Am J Ophthlamol 69:997, 1970

23. Travers B: A case of aneurysm by anastomosis cured by ligation of the common carotid artery. Med Chir Travail 2:1, 1809

24. Rubinstein MK, Eilson G, Levin DC: Intraorbital aneurysms of the ophthalmic artery: report of a unique case and review of the literature. Arch Ophthalmol 80:42, 1968

25. Rahmat H, Abbassioun K, Amirjamshidi A: Pulsating unilateral exophthalmos due to traumatic aneurysm of the intraorbital ophthalmic artery. J Neurosurg 60:630, 1984

26. Hyland HH, Barnett HJM: The pathogenesis of cranial nerve palsies associated with intracranial aneurysms. Proc R Soc Med 47:141, 1954

27. Soni SR: Aneurysms of the posterior communicating artery and oculomotor paresis. J Neurol Neurosurg Psychiatry 37:475, 1974

28. Hepler RS, Cantu RC: Aneurysms and third nerve palsies. Arch Ophthalmol 77:604, 1967

29. Grayson MC, Soni SR, Spooner VA: Analysis of the recovery of third nerve function after direct surgical intervention for posterior communicating aneurysms. J Ophthalmol 58:118, 1974

30. Leblanc R: The minor leak preceding subarachnoid hemorrhage. J Neurosurg 66:35, 1987

31. Chan JW, Hoyt WF, Ellis WG et al: Pathogenesis of acute monocular blindness from leaking anterior communicating artery aneurysms: report of six cases. Neurology 48:680, 1997

32. Bull J: Massive aneurysms at the base of the brain. Brain 92:535, 1969

33. Hööke O, Norlen G, Guzman J: Saccular aneurysms of the vertebral-basilar arterial system: a report of 28 cases. Acta Neurol Scand 39:271, 1963

34. McKinna AJ: Eye signs in 611 cases of posterior fossa aneurysms: their diagnosis and prognostic value. Can J Ophthalmol 18:3, 1983

35. Nijensohn DE, Saiz RJ, Regan TJ: Clinical significance of basilar artery aneurysms. Neurology 24:301, 1974

36. Trobe JD, Glaser JS, Quencer RC: Isolated oculomotor paralysis: the product of saccular and fusiform aneurysms of the basilar artery. Arch Ophthalmol 96:1236, 1978

37. Arseni C, Ghitescu N, Cristescu A et al: The pseudotumoral form of aneurysms of the posterior cranial fossa. Neurochirurgia 12:123, 1969

38. Drake CG, Peerless SJ, Hernesniemi JA: Surgery of Veterobasilar Aneurysms. Vienna, Springer-Verlag, 1996

39. Drake CG, Amacher AL: Aneurysms of the posterior cerebral artery. J Neurosurg 30:468, 1969

40. Amacher AL, Drake CG: Cerebral artery aneurysms in infancy, childhood and adolescence. Childs Brain 1:72, 1975

41. Bell WE, Butler C: Cerebral mycotic aneurysms in children. Neurology 18:81, 1968

42. Sobata E, Ohkuma H, Suzuki S: Cerebrovascular disorders associated with von Recklinghausen's neurofibromatosis: a case report. Neurosurgery 22:544, 1988

43. Benatar MG: Intracranial fusiform aneurysms in von Recklinghasen's neurofibromatosis. J Neurol Neurosurg Psychiatry 57:1279, 1994

44. Patel AN, Richardson AE: Ruptured intracranial aneurysms in the first two decades of life: a study of 58 patients. J Neurosurg 35:571, 1971

45. Sedzimir CB, Robinson J: Intrancranial hemorrhage in children and adolescents. J Neurosurg 38:269, 1973

46. Orozco M, Trigueros F, Quintana F et al: Intracranial aneurysms in early childhood. Surg Neurol 9:247, 1978

47. Mahmoud NA: Traumatic aneurysms of the internal carotid artery and epistaxis: review of literature and report of a case. J Laryngol Otol 93:629, 1979

48. Awad I, Sawhny B, Little JR: Traumatic postsurgical aneurysm of the intracavernous carotid artery: a delayed presentation. Surg Neurol 18:54, 1982

49. Paullus WS, Norwood CW, Morgan HW: False aneurysms of the cavernous carotid artery and progressive external ophthalmoplegia after transsphenoidal hypophysectomy. J Neurosurg 51:707, 1979

50. Rhoton AL, Hardy DG, Chambers SM: Microsurgical anatomy and dissection of the sphenoid bone, cavernous sinus and sellar region. Surg Neurol 12:63, 1979

51. Mokri B, Piepgras DG, Sundt TM et al: Extracranial internal carotid artery aneurysms. Mayo Clin Proc 57:310, 1982

52. Hilton GF, Hoyt WF: An arteriosclerotic chiasmal syndrome: bitemporal hemianopia associated with fusiform dilatation of the anterior cerebral arteries. JAMA 196:1018, 1966

53. Colapinto EV, Cabeen MA, Johnson LN: Optic nerve compression by a dolichoectatic internal carotid artery: case report. Neurosurgery 39:604, 1996

54. Johnston SC, Halbach VV, Smith WS et al: Rapid development of giant fusiform cerebral aneurysms in angiographically normal vessels. Neurology 50:1163, 1998

55. Sacks JG, Lindenberg R: Dolicho-ectatic intracranial arteries. Johns Hopkins Med J 125:95, 1969

56. Corkill G, Sarwar M, Virapongse C: Evolution of dolichoectasia of the vertebro-basilar system as evidenced by serial computed tomography. Surg Neurol 18:262, 1982

57. Naseem N, Leehey P, Russell E et al: MR of basilar artery dolichoectasia. AJNR Am J Neuroradiol 9:391, 1988

58. Pollock BE, Gorman DA, Schomberg PJ, Kline RW: The Mayo Clinic gamma knife experience: indications and initial results. Mayo Clinic Proc 74:5, 1999

59. McCormick WF, Hardman JM, Boulter TR: Vascular malformations ("angiomas") of the brain with special reference to those occurring in the posterior fossa. J Neurosurg 28:241, 1968

60. Wilson CB, Stein BM: Intracranial Arteriovenous Malformations. Baltimore, Williams & Wilkins, 1984

61. Perret G, Nishioka H: Report on the cooperative study of intracranial aneurysm and subarachnoid hemorrhage. VI. Arteriovenous malformations: an analysis of 545 cases of craniocerebral arteriovenous malformations and fistulae reported to the cooperative study. J Neurosurg 25:467, 1966

62. Ondra SL, Truupp H, George ED et al: The natural history of symptomatic arteriovenous malformations of the brain: a 24 year follow-up assessment. J Neurosurg 73:387, 1990

63. Celli P, Ferrante L, Palma L et al: Cerebral arteriovenous malformations in children. Surg Neurol 22:43, 1984

64. Horton JC, Chambers WA, Lyons SL et al: Pregnancy and the risk of hemorrhage from cerebral malformations. Neurosurgery 27:867, 1990

65. Manz HJ, Klein LH, Fermaglich J et al: Cavernous hemangioma

of the optic chiasm, optic nerves and right optic tract. Virchows Arch A 383:225, 1979

66. Roski RA, Gardner JH, Spetzler RF: Intrachiasmatic arteriovenous malformation: case report. J Neurosurg 54:540, 1981
67. Bogousslavsky J, Vinuela F, Barnett HJM et al: Amaurosis fugax as the presenting manifestations of dural arteriovenous malformation. Stroke 16:891, 1985
68. Eckman P, Fountain E: Unilateral proptosis: associated with arteriovenous malformation involving the galenic system. Arch Neurol 31:350, 1974
69. Brunquell PJ, Rosenberger PB: Recurrent cavernous sinus syndrome complicating supratentorial arteriovenous malformation: report of a case. Stroke 13:865, 1982
70. Troost BT, Newton TH: Occipital lobe arteriovenous malformations: clinical and radiologic features in 26 cases with comments on the differentiation from migraine. Arch Ophthalmol 93:250, 1975
71. Bruyn GW: Intracranial arteriovenous malformation and migraine. Cephalgia 4:191, 1984
72. Troost BT, Mark LE, Maroon JC: Resolution of classic migraine following removal of an occipital lobe arteriovenous malformation. Ann Neurol 5:199, 1979
73. Verbiest H: Arteriovenous aneurysms of the posterior fossa. Prog Brain Res 30:383, 1968
74. Logue V, Monckton G: Posterior fossa angiomas: a clinical presentation of nine cases. Brain 77:252, 1954
75. Newton TH, Weidner W, Greitz T: Dural arteriovenous malformation in the posterior fossa. Radiology 90:27, 1968
76. Delman M: Posterior fossa arteriovenous malformation: with reference to ocular symptoms. Am J Ophthalmol 56:409, 1963
77. Lessell S, Ferris EJ, Feldman RG et al: Brainstem arteriovenous malformations. Arch Ophthalmol 86:255, 1971
78. Pedersen RA, Troost BT: Neuro-ophthalmic manifestations of posterior fossa AVM. Neuroophthalmology 1:185, 1981
79. Graeb DA, Dolman CL: Radiologic and pathological aspects of dural arteriovenous fistulas. J Neurosurg 64:962, 1986
80. Houser OW, Campbell JK, Campbell RJ et al: Arteriovenous malformation affecting the transverse dural venous sinus: an acquired lesion. Mayo Clin Proc 54:651, 1979
81. Chaudhary MY, Sachdev VP, Cho SH et al: Dural arteriovenous malformation of the major venous sinuses: an acquired lesion. Am J Neuroradiol 3:13, 1982
82. Gans M, Kline L, Glaser JS et al: Pailledema and cranial bruits: signs of dural arteriovenous malformation. In Smith JL, Katz RS (eds): Neuro-ophthalmology Enters the Nineties, p 55. Hialeah, FL, Dutton Press, 1988
83. Sila CA, Furlan AJ, Little JR: Pulsatile tinnitus. Stroke 18:252, 1986
84. Buchanan TAS, Harper DG, Hoyt WF: Bilateral proptosis, dilatation of conjunctival veins, and papilledema: a neuro-ophthalmological syndrome caused by arteriovenous malformation of the torcular Herophili. Br J Ophthalmol 66:186, 1982
85. Smith HJ, Strother CM, Kikuchi Y et al: MR imaging in the management of supratentorial intracranial AVMs. AJNR Am J Neuroradiol 9:225, 1988
86. Brown RD, Wiebers DO, Forbes G et al: The natural history of unruptured intracranial arteriovenous malformations. J Neurosurg 68:352, 1988
87. Purdy PD, Sampson D, Batjer HH et al: Preoperative embolization of cerebral arteriovenous malformations with polyvinyl alcohol particles: experience in 51 adults. AJNR Am J Neuroradiol 11:501, 1990
88. Dion JE, Mathis JM: Cranial arteriovenous malformations: the role of embolization and stereotactic surgery. Neurosurg Clin North Am 5:459, 1994
89. DeSalles AAF: Radiosurgery for arteriovenous malformations of the brain. J Stroke Cerebrovasc Dis 4:277, 1997
90. Kondziolka D, Lunsford LD, Kestle JRW: The natural history of cerebral cavernous malformations. J Neurosurg 83:820, 1995
91. Kondziolka D, Lunsford LD, Flickinger JC et al: Reduction of hemorrhagic risk after sterotactic radiosurgery for cavernous malformations. J Neurosurg 83:828, 1995
92. Boukobza M, Enjolras O, Guichard J-P et al: Cerebral developmental venous anomalies associated with head and neck venous malformations. AJNR Am J Neuroradiol 17:987, 1996
93. Kushner FH: Carotid-cavernous fistula as a complication of carotid endarterectomy. Ann Ophthalmol 13:979, 1981
94. Pedersen RA, Troost BT, Schramm VL: Carotid-cavernous sinus fistula after ethmoid-sphenoid surgery: clinical course and management. Arch Otolaryngol 13:979, 1981
95. Sekhar LN, Heros RC, Kerber CW: Cartoid-cavernous fistula following percutaneous retrogasserian procedures: report of two cases. J Neurosurg 51:700, 1979
96. Farley MK, Clark RD, Fallor MK: Spontaneous carotid-cavernous fistula and the Ehler-Danlos syndromes. Ophthalmology 90:1337, 1983
97. Toya S, Shiobara R, Izumi J: Spontaneous carotid-cavernous fistula during pregnancy or in the postpartum stage: report of two cases. J Neurosurg 54:252, 1981
98. Barrow DL, Spector RH, Braun I et al: Classification and treatment of spontaneous cartoid-cavernous sinus fistulas. J Neurosurg 62:248, 1985
99. Phelps CD, Thompson HS, Ossoinig KC: The diagnosis and prognosis of atypical carotid-cavernous fistula (red-eyed shunt syndrome). Am J Ophthalmol 93:423, 1982
100. Kupersmith MJ, Berenstein A, Flamm E et al: Neuro-ophthalmic abnormalities and intravascular therapy of traumatic carotid cavernous fistulas. Ophthalmology 93:906, 1986
101. Keltner JL, Satterfield D, Dubin AB et al: Dural and carotid cavernous sinus fistulas: diagnosis, management and complications. Ophthalmology 94:1585, 1987
102. Atta HR, Dick AD, Hamed LM et al: Venous stasis orbitopathy: a clinical and echographic study. Br J Ophthalmol 80:129, 1996
103. Sergott RC, Grossman RI, Savino PJ et al: The syndrome of pardoxical worsening of dural-cavernous sinus arteriovenous malformations. Ophthalmology 94:205, 1987
104. Bynke HG, Efsina HO: Carotid-cavernous fistula with contralateral exophthalmos. Acta Ophthalmol 48:971, 1970
105. Elster AD, Chen MYM, Richardson DN et al: Dilated intercavernous sinuses: an MR sign of carotid-cavernous and carotid-dural fistulas. AJNR Am J Neuroradiol 12:641, 1991
106. Spector RK: Echographic diagnosis of dural carotid-cavernous sinus fistulas. Am J Ophthalmol 111:77, 1991
107. Kupersmith MJ, Berenstein A, Choi IS: Management of nontraumatic vascular shunts involving the cavernous sinus. Ophthalmology 95:121, 1988
108. Guthoff R, Jorgensen J: Long-term follow-up in patients with spontaneous A-V fistulas affecting the orbit. Orbit 6:229, 1987
109. Halbach VV, Hieshima GB, Higashida RT et al: Carotid cavernous fistulae: indications for urgent treatment. AJNR Am J Neuroradiol 8:627, 1987
110. Mirabel S, Lindblom B, Halbach VV et al: Giant suprasellar varix: an unusual cause of chiasmal compression. J Clin Neuroophthalmol 11:268, 1991
111. Lasjaunias P, Chiu M, Ter Brugge K: Neurological manifestations of intracranial dural arteriovenous malformations. J Neurosurg 64:724, 1986
112. Magidson MA, Weinberg PE: Spontaneous closure of dural arteriovenous malformation. Surg Neurol 6:107, 1976
113. Halbach VV, Higashida RT, Hieshima GB: Transvenous embolization of direct carotid cavernous fistulas. AJNR Am J Neuroradiol 9:741, 1988
114. Guglielmi G, Vinuela F, Duckwiler G et al: High-flow, small-hole arteriovenous fistulas: treatment with electrodetachable coils. AJNR Am J Neuroradiol 16:325, 1995
115. Lewis AI, Tomsick TA, Tew JM: Management of 100 consecutive direct carotid cavernous fistulas: results of treatment with detachable balloons. Neurosurgery 36:239, 1995
116. Desal H, Leaute F, Auffray-Calvier E et al: Direct carotid-cavernous fistula. Clinical, radiologic and therapeutic studies: a propos of 49 cases. J Neuroradiol 24:141, 1997
117. Phadke RV, Jumar S, Sawlani V et al: Traumatic carotid cavernous fistula: anatomical variations and their treatment by detachable balloons. Australas Radiol 42:1, 1998
118. Irie K, Fujiwara T, Kuyama H et al: Transvenous embolization of traumatic carotid cavernous fistula with mechanical detachable coils: minimally invasive. Neurosurgery 39:28, 1996

119. Siniluoto T, Seppanen S, Kuurne T et al: Transarterial embolization of a direct cartoid cavernous fistula with Guglielmi detachable coils. AJNR Am J Neuroradiol 18:519, 1997

120. Goldberg RA, Goldey SH, Duckwiler G et al: Management of cavernous sinus-dural fistulas: indications and techniques for primary embolization via the superior ophthalmic vein. Arch Ophthalmol 114:707, 1996

121. Guo WY, Pan DHC, Wu HM, et al: Radiosurgery as a treatment alternative for dural arteriovenous fistulas of the cavernous sinus. AJNR Am J Neuroradiol 19:1081, 1998

122. Cognard C, Pierot L, Boulin A et al: Intracranial aneurysms: endovascular treatment with mechanical detachable spirals in 60 aneurysms. Radiology 202:783, 1997

123. Moret J, Cognard C, Weill A et al: Reconstruction technic in the treatment of wide-neck intracranial aneurysms. Long-term angiographic and clinical results: a propos of 56 cases. J Neuroradiol 24:30, 1997

124. Graves VB, Perl J, Strother CM et al: Endovascular occlusion of the carotid or vertebral artery with temporary proximal flow arrest and microcoils: clinical results. AJNR Am J Neuroradiol 18:1201, 1997

125. Gardeur D, Palmieri A, Mashaly R: Cranial computed tomography in the phakomatoses. Neuroradiology 25:293, 1983

126. List A, Frisk b, Westberg NG: Computed tomography in von Hippel-Lindau disease. Acta Radiol 24:97, 1983

127. Maher ER, Kaelin WG: von Hippel-Lindau disease. Medicine 76:381, 1997

128. Welch RB: Von Hippel-Lindau disease: the recognition and treatment of early angiomatosis retinae and the use of cryosurgery as an adjunct to therapy. Trans Am Ophthalmol Soc 68:367, 1970

129. Imes RK, Monteiro MLR, Hoyt WF: Incipient hemangioblastoma of the optic disk. Am J Ophthalmol 98:116, 1984

130. Rubio A, Meyers SP, Powers JM et al: Hemangioblastoma of the optic nerve. Hum Pathol 25:1249, 1994

131. Balcer LJ, Galetta SL, Curtis M et al: Von Hippel-Lindau disease manifesting as a chiasmal syndrome. Surv Ophthalmol 39:302, 1995

132. Melmon KL, Rosen SW: Lindau's disease: review of the literature and study of a large kindred. Am J Med 36:595, 1964

133. Kupersmith MJ, Berenstein A: Visual disturbances in von Hippel-Lindau disease. Ann Ophthalmol 13:295, 1981

134. Maher ER, Yates JR, Harries R et al: Clinical features and natural history of von Hippel-Lindau disease. Q J Med 77:1151, 1990

135. Sullivan TJ, Clarke MP, Morin JD: The ocular manifestations of the Sturge-Weber syndrome. J Pediatr Ophthalmol Strabismus 29:349, 1992

136. Zaret CR, Choromokos EA, Meisler DM: Clio-optic vein associated with phakomatosis. Ophthalmology 87:330, 1980

137. Wisnicki JL: Hemangiomas and vascular malformations. Ann Plast Surg 12:41, 1984

138. Griffiths PD, Boodram MB, Blaser S et al: Abnormal ocular enhancement in Sturge-Weber syndrome: correlation of ocular MR and CT findings with clinical and intracranial findings. AJNR Am J Neuroradiol 17:749, 1996

139. Alexander GL: Sturge-Weber syndrome. In Vinken PJ, Bruyn GW (eds): Handbook of Clinical Neurology, p 223. New York: Elsevier, 1972

140. Font RL, Ferry AP: The phakomatoses. Int Ophthalmol Clin 12:1, 1972

141. Theron J, Newton TH, Hoyt WF: Unilateral retinocephalic vascular malformations. Neuroradiology 7:185, 1974

142. Hopen G, Smith JL, Hoff JT et al: The Wyburn-Mason syndrome. J Clin Neuroophthalmol 3:53, 1983

143. Danis R, Appen RE: Optic atrophy and the Wyburn-Mason syndrome. J Clin Neuroophthalmol 4:91, 1984

144. Bloom PA, Laidlaw A, Easty DL: Spontaneous development of retinal ischemia and rubeosis in eyes with retinal racemose angioma. Br J Ophthalmol 77:124, 1993

145. Bonnet P, de Chaume J, Blanc E: L'aneurysme cirsoide de la rétine (aneurysme racemeux), ses rélations avec l'aneurysme cirsoide de la face et avec l'aneurysme cirsoide du cerveau. J Med Lyon 18:165, 1937

146. Wyburn-Mason R: Arteriovenous aneurysm of midbrain and retina, facial naevi and mental changes. Brain 66:163, 1943

147. Dobyns WB, Michels VV, Groover RV et al: Familial cavernous malformations of the central nervous system and retina. Ann Neurol 21:578, 1987

148. Rigamonti D, Hadley MN, Drayer BP et al: Cerebral cavernous malformations: incidence and familial occurrence. N Engl J Med 319:343, 1988

149. Gass JDM: Cavernous hemangioma of the retina: a neuro-oculo-cutaneous syndrome. Am J Ophthalmol 71:799, 1971

150. Goldberg RE, Pheasant TR, Shields JA: Cavernous hemangioma of the retina: a four-generation pedigree with neurocutaneous manifestations and an example of bilateral retinal involvement. Arch Ophthalmol 97:2321, 1979

151. Bell D, Yang HK, O Brien CA: A case of bilateral cavernous hemangioma associated with intracerebral hemangioma. Arch Ophthalmol 115:818, 1997

152. Leblanc R, Melanson D, Wilkinson RD: Hereditary neurocutaneous angiomatosis: report of four cases. J Neurosurg 85:1135, 1996

153. Wright JE, Sullivan TJ, Garner A et al: Orbital venous anomalies. Ophthalmology 104:905, 1997

154. Rubin PAD, Remulla H: Orbital venous anomalies demonstrated by spiral computed tomography. Ophthalmology 104:1463, 1997

155. Rootman J: Orbital venous anomalies. Ophthalmology 105:387, 1998

156. Harris GJ: Orbital vascular malformations: a consensus statement on terminology and its clinical implications. Am J Ophthalmol 127:453, 1999

157. Rootman J, Graeb DA: Vascular lesions. In Rootman J (ed): Diseases of the Orbit, p 525. Philadelphia, JB Lippincott, 1988

158. Rathbun JE, Hoyt WF, Beard C: Surgical management of orbitofrontal varix in Klippel-Trenaunay-Weber syndrome. Am J Ophthalmol 70:109, 1970

159. Katz SE, Rootman J, Vangveeravong S et al: Combined venous lymphatic malformations of the orbit (so-called lymphangiomas): association with non-contiguous intracranial vascular anomalies. Ophthalmology 105;176, 1998

160. Crompton JL, Taylor D: Ocular lesions in the blue rubber naevus syndrome. Br J Ophthalmol 65:133, 1981

161. McCannel CA, Hoenig J, Umlas J et al: Orbital lesions in the blue rubber bleb nevus syndrome. Ophthalmology 103:933, 1996

CHAPTER 18

The Dizzy Patient: Disturbances of the Vestibular System

Ronald J. Tusa

Vestibular System: An Overview
    Normal Function: The Vestibular Reflexes
Pathophysiology
    Peripheral Structures
        Semicircular Canals
        Otoliths
Clinical Assessment
    History
        Tempo
        Symptoms
            Vertigo
            Disequilibrium
            Light-headedness
            Floating, Swimming, Rocking, and Spinning
                Inside of Head
            Oscillopsia
        Circumstance
        Medications
    Office Examination
        Eye Movements
            Vestibulo-ocular Reflex
            Smooth Pursuit and Vestibulo-ocular
                Reflex Cancellation
            Nystagmus
        Stance and Gait

Special Apparatuses
    Electronystagmography
        Rotary Chair
        Caloric Test
    Posturography
    Audiometry
    Brainstem Auditory-Evoked Response
    Neuroimaging
        Computed Tomography
        Magnetic Resonance Imaging
Abnormalities and Their Management
    Acoustic Neuroma
    Acute Vestibular Neuritis and Labyrinthitis
    Benign Paroxysmal Positional Vertigo
    Dizziness in Children
    Disequilibrium
    Head Trauma
    Meniere's Disease
    Migraine
    Motion Sickness
    Orthostatic Hypotension
    Panic Attacks and Hyperventilation
    Perilymphatic Fistula
    Seizures
    Transient Ischemic Attacks

There can be few physicians so dedicated to their art that they do not experience a slight decline in spirits on learning that their patient's complaint is of dizziness (giddiness). This frequently means that after exhaustive inquiry it will not be entirely clear what it is that the patient feels wrong or even less so why he feels it.

W.B. Matthews in *Practical Neurology*

VESTIBULAR SYSTEM: AN OVERVIEW

The vestibular system serves to stabilize eye position and movements during changes in head rotation and is

R. J. Tusa: Department of Neurology, Bascom Palmer Eye Institute; and Dizziness and Eye Movement Center, Department of Neuro-ophthalmology, Anne Bates Leach Hospital, Miami, Florida

an essential mechanism for clear vision. In fact, patients with bilateral vestibular defects must interrupt walking in order to see, and while reading a book they must even brace the head against the wall to prevent the smallest head movements transmitted from each heart beat. A classic article written by a physician describes the problems he experienced from ototoxicity.[1] This chapter describes the pathophysiology of vestibular function, elaborates the clinically relevant symptoms, and reviews treatment and management options.

Normal Function: The Vestibular Reflexes

Vestibular reflexes are triggered by head movements. Imagine a bird watcher standing in a rocking boat travel-

629

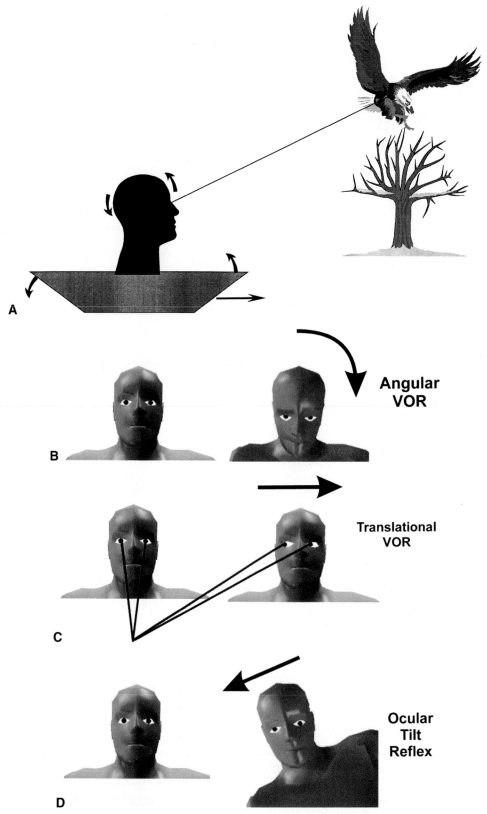

Fig. 18–1. Illustration of vestibulo-ocular reflex (*VOR*) and ocular tilt reflex (*OTR*). **A.** Bird-watcher standing in a rocking boat traveling downstream. **B.** As the boat pitches up and down, the angular VOR moves the eyes in the opposite direction, synchronous with the angular motion of the head. **C.** As the boat moves down the river toward the bird, the linear VOR moves the eyes horizontally in the opposite direction, synchronous with the linear motion of the boat. **D.** As the boat tilts to the left and right, the OTR tilts the eyes and head in the opposite direction to maintain an earth-horizontal plane. The figure shows what happens with tilt to the right. The right eye is elevated in the orbit and the left eye is depressed (skew deviation); both eyes undergo torsion to the left within the orbit (counter-roll deviation) and the head is tilted to the left on the body.

TABLE 18–1. Vestibular Reflexes

Vestibular reflex	Sensory organ	Motor output
Angular VOR	Semicircular canals (SCCs) Horizontal Posterior Anterior	Eyes move opposite to angular movement (rotation) of the head. Shaking the head up and down (yes) is termed *pitch* and is sensed by the anterior and posterior SCCs. Shaking the head horizontally (no) is termed *yaw* and is sensed by the horizontal SCCs.
Linear VOR	Otoliths Saccule Utricle	Eyes move opposite to linear movement of the head. Linear movement up and down (riding in an elevator) is sensed by the saccule. Linear movement horizontally (riding in a train on a straight track) is sensed by the utricle.
Ocular tilt reflex	Otolith Utricle	Eyes and head move opposite to tilt of the head. Tilt left causes elevation of the left eye, depression of the right eye, torsion of both eyes to the right, and rightward tilt of the head.

VOR, vestibulo-ocular reflex.

ing downstream (Fig. 18–1A). To identify a bird roosting on a tree, the image of the bird must be kept stable on the retina by three separate vestibular reflexes (see Fig. 18–1B). As the boat pitches up and down the eyes must move in the opposite direction and synchronously with the angular motion of the head to keep the eyes stable in space. This is accomplished by the angular vestibulo-ocular reflex (VOR), which is sensed by the semicircular canals in the inner ear (see Fig. 18–1B). As the boat moves down the river toward the bird, the eyes must move horizontally in the opposite direction synchronously with the linear motion of the boat. This is accomplished by the linear VOR, which is sensed by the otoliths in the inner ear (see Fig. 18–1C). Figure 18–1D shows the most complicated reflex as the boat tilts left and right. To keep the head and eyes level during tilt to the right, the right eye is elevated in the orbit and the left eye is depressed (skew deviation). Both eyes undergo torsion to the left within the orbit (counter-roll deviation) and the head is tilted to the left on the body (head tilt). This is accomplished by the ocular tilt reflex, which is sensed by the otoliths. Without these vestibular reflexes, visual acuity would be degraded and diplopia would occur. Table 18–1 lists the three vestibular reflexes, the sensory organs involved, and the motor output for each reflex.

PATHOPHYSIOLOGY

Peripheral Structures

The vestibular sensory organs lie within the membranous labyrinth of the inner ear, protected in the petrous portion of the temporal bone. The membranous labyrinth consists of three semicircular canals (SCCs)—the *anterior, posterior, and horizontal*—that lie 90 degrees (orthogonal) to each other, and two otoliths, the *utricle* (horizontally aligned) and the *saccule* (vertically aligned) (Fig. 18–2). The labyrinth is innervated by the vestibular nerve, which is part of the VIIIth nerve. The vestibular nerve contains two fascicles, the superior and inferior divisions. The cell bodies of each axon of the

VIIIth nerve lie in Scarpa's ganglion, located in the internal auditory canal. The superior division innervates the utricle and the anterior and horizontal SCCs. The inferior division innervates the saccule and posterior SCCs. Within each semicircular canal is an area of hair cells that protrude their processes into a gelatinous matrix called the cupula. Angular head acceleration imposes inertial forces on the endolymph fluid within the canal, which causes relative fluid flow through the canal in the direction opposite to that of head acceleration. This flow deflects the cupula and bends the hair cells (Fig. 18–3). During head acceleration, these hair cells bend in proportion to head acceleration and change the neuronal firing rate in the VIIIth nerve. Because each Scarpa's ganglion is spontaneously "firing" at 100 spike/sec, head motion (acceleration or deceleration) modulates this firing rate. The firing rate is increased for ipsilateral angular head movements and decreased for contralateral angular head movements. The otoliths also contain a local region of hair cells. The hair cells protrude their processes into a gelatinous matrix called the macula, which is covered by a surface of calcium carbonate crystals, the otoconia. The otolith organs respond to linear acceleration and sustained head tilt relative to gravity. Linear acceleration (including tilt of the head) causes these crystals to move, which bends the hair cells and modulates the firing rate in the VIIIth

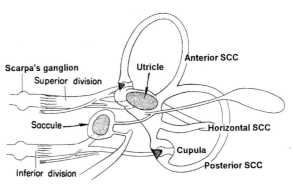

Fig. 18–2. Labyrinth. See text for details.

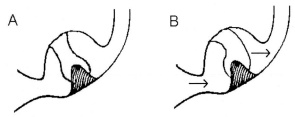

Fig. 18–3. A. Enlarged view of cupula of the horizontal semicircular canal when the head is still. **B.** The arrows indicate direction of endolymph flow during head rotation to the left.

nerve. The firing rate is increased for ipsilateral linear head movement or tilt, and is decreased for contralateral linear head movement and tilt.

Semicircular Canals

Each SCC innervates two eye muscles by means of a three-neuron arc. The central connections of the horizontal and anterior SCCs on one side are shown in Figure 18–4. The projections of these two SCCs are shown together because usually they are both involved in vestibular neuritis, the most common cause of severe vertigo. The pathophysiology of vestibular neuritis is diagrammed in Figure 18–5. This disorder disrupts the

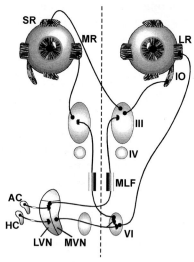

Fig. 18–4. Central connections of the horizontal and anterior semicircular canals mediating angular vestibulo-ocular reflex. Primary afferents of the horizontal semicircular canal (*HC*) project to the medial vestibular nucleus (*MVN*). Neurons in the medial vestibular nucleus project across the midline to terminate in the VIth nerve nucleus. Two types of neurons are in the VIth nerve nucleus, abducens neurons that project to the lateral rectus (*LR*) muscle, and interneurons that cross the midline and travel up the medial longitudinal fasciculus (*MLF*) to innervate the medial rectus subnuclei of the IIIrd nerve nucleus. Primary afferents of the anterior semicircular canal (*AC*) project to the lateral vestibular nucleus (*LVN*) and MVN, which in turn project across the midline and travel up the MLF to terminate in the superior rectus and inferior oblique subnuclei of the IIIrd nerve nucleus.

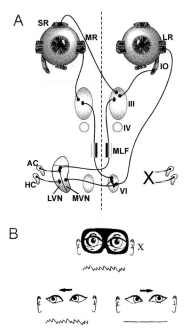

Fig. 18–5. Acute unilateral loss of semicircular canal function causing vestibular nystagmus. **A.** Disruption of the left superior division of the VIIIth nerve from vestibular neuritis. Loss of spontaneous neural activity from the left side causes slow phases to the left from relative excitation of the right horizontal semicircular canal (*HC*). **B.** Features of nystagmus. By convention, right eye position is up and left eye position is down. As the eyes move across the orbit, a quick phase resets the eyes back to the right. Quick phases are generated by burst cells, which are not part of the vestibular system. Nystagmus is labeled according to the direction of the quick phases. Consequently, this would be called a right-beating nystagmus. The lesion also disrupts spontaneous neural activity from the left anterior semicircular canal (*AC*), which results in right torsional nystagmus (the superior pole of each eye beats right). The intensity of nystagmus increases when the patient looks in the direction of the quick phases (**B**, *bottom*). If fixation is blocked by Frenzel glasses, nystagmus also increases and is seen clearly even in primary gaze (**B**, *top*).

superior division of the vestibular nerve.[2] Because the Scarpa's ganglion on each side normally is firing at 100 spikes/sec, any loss of activity on one side results in relative *excessive excitation* from the intact side. This large bias in neural activity causes nystagmus. The direction of nystagmus is determined according to the quick phase, but the vestibular deficit is actually driving the slow phase of the nystagmus. Vestibular neuritis results in a mixed horizontal and torsional nystagmus. This pattern of nystagmus is caused by the innervation pattern of the superior division of the VIIIth nerve on the intact side (recall that the superior division innervates the horizontal and anterior semicircular canals; see Fig. 18–2). Relative excitation of the horizontal SCC causes horizontal nystagmus with the slow phase toward the side of the lesion. Figure 18–5 depicts a left-sided lesion, which would cause a right-beating nystagmus. Relative excitation of the anterior SCC causes torsional nystagmus (counterclockwise nystagmus for a left-sided lesion). Because of the confusion over whether to label torsional nystagmus from the perspective of the observer or the patient, the current trend is to assess torsional nystagmus according to the direction of the quick phases toward which the superior poles of both eyes are beating. Thus, a left-sided lesion results in right beating and right torsional nystagmus (see Fig. 18–5B). There are two other key features of vestibular nystagmus. The intensity of nystagmus is increased when fixation is blocked (Fig. 18–5B depicts increased nystagmus when the subject looks through Frenzel or 20-diopter lenses), and the intensity of nystagmus also increases when the patient looks in the direction of the quick phases.

Otoliths

Each otolith innervates four eye muscles by means of a three-neuron arc. The central connections of the utricle on one side are shown in Figure 18–6.[3] The pro-

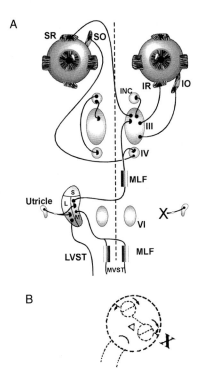

Fig. 18–7. Unilateral loss of the utricle, causing pathologic ocular tilt reflex. **A.** Disruption of the left utricular division of the VIIIth nerve from vestibular neuritis. **B.** The pathologic ocular tilt reflex from this lesion. Relative excitation of the right medial vestibular nucleus (*M*) causes elevation and intorsion of the right eye (mediated by the right superior rectus and right superior oblique muscles), and causes depression and extorsion of the left eye (mediated by the left inferior rectus and left inferior oblique muscles). Excitation of the neck muscles innervated by the intact vestibulospinal tract causes a left head tilt.

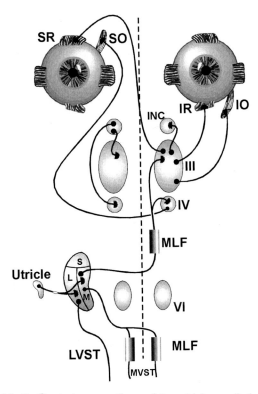

Fig. 18–6. Central connections of the utricle mediating the ocular tilt reflex. This figure illustrates the projections from the right utricle. Primary afferents of the utricle project to the lateral (*L*) and medial (*M*) vestibular nuclei. Neurons in the lateral vestibular nucleus cross the midline and travel up the medial longitudinal fasiculus (*MLF*) to project to the IVth and IIIrd nerve nuclei, which innervate eye muscles involved with vertical and torsional eye movements. The IIIrd nerve nucleus also innervates the interstitial nucleus of Cajal (*INC*). The INC in turn projects back to the IIIrd and IVth nerve nuclei. Neurons in the L and M vestibular nucleus also project to the spinal cord through the lateral and medial vestibular spinal tracts (*LVST* and *MVST*).

jection to the vertical muscles causes vertical eye deviation and torsion during head tilt. The projections in the lateral and medial vestibulospinal tracts mediate the head tilt during the ocular tilt reflex. Acute loss of function of the utricle on one side from the VIIIth nerve section or vestibular neuritis causes a pathologic ocular tilt response because of the unopposed excitation of the intact utricle. Figure 18–7 depicts the results of a left-sided lesion.[4] Excitation of the right superior rectus and oblique muscles causes elevation and intorsion of that eye. Excitation of the left inferior rectus and oblique muscles causes depression and extorsion of that eye. Excitation of the neck muscles innervated by the intact vestibulospinal tracts causes a left head tilt.

CLINICAL ASSESSMENT

History

Determining a patient's history is by far the most important part of a clinical evaluation. Unfortunately, taking a good history can be tedious because complaints by patients with dizziness are often vague and frequently confounded with anxiety-provoked symptoms. For these reasons a preliminary questionnaire is helpful. Three key items of the history are most helpful in determining the cause of dizziness.

Tempo

It must be determined whether the patient is suffering from an acute attack of dizziness (3 days or less), chronic dizziness (more than 3 days), or episodes of dizziness. An acute attack frequently is caused by vestibular neuritis, labyrinthitis, Meniere's disease, or brainstem infarct. Chronic dizziness often is caused by an uncompensated unilateral vestibular defect, bilateral vestibular hypofunction (ototoxicity, sequential vestibular neuritis), or disequilibrium from a variety of different causes, or psychological problems. If the patient suffers from episodic symptoms, the average duration of the dizziness spells should be determined. Spells that last for seconds are usually caused by benign paroxysmal positional vertigo (BPPV) or orthostatic hypotension; spells that last for minutes are usually caused by transient ischemic attacks (TIAs) or migraine; and spells that last for hours are usually from migraine or Meniere's disease.

Symptoms

What the patient means by "dizziness" should be expanded on. Dizziness is an imprecise term used to describe a variety of symptoms including vertigo, disequilibrium, light-headedness, floating, and rocking, each of which has a different pathophysiologic mechanism and significance (Table 18–2).

Vertigo

Vertigo is the illusion of movement (rotation, linear movement, or tilt) and is caused by a sudden imbalance of tonic neural activity in the vestibular nucleus. It may be caused by either normal head movements or disease in the labyrinth, VIIIth nerve, vestibular nucleus, vestibular cerebellum (nodulus and flocculus), or central otolith pathways (from the medial longitudinal fasciculus

to the interstitial nucleus of Cajal). The causes of vertigo may be simply divided into those lesions that cause a mechanical problem to the inner ear (e.g., BPPV), and those that cause loss of function (ablation) of the inner ear or central pathways (e.g., vestibular neuritis).

Disequilibrium

This is an imbalance or unsteadiness while standing or walking. It is caused by a variety of factors including diminished or double vision, loss of vestibular function, defects in proprioception from peripheral neuropathy or spinal cord lesions, defects in motor function from central nervous or peripheral nervous system abnormalities, joint pain or instability from arthritis or weakness, and psychological factors.

Light-headedness

Also called presyncope, light-headedness usually is related to a momentary decrease in blood flow to the brain.

Floating, Swimming, Rocking, and Spinning Inside of Head

These frequently are symptoms of psychological disorders, which include anxiety (panic attacks, agoraphobia, obsessive-compulsive disorder), somatiform disorders (including conversion), and depression.

Oscillopsia

This is the subjective illusion of visual motion. Patients with acquired nystagmus report apparent motion of the visual scene caused by movement of the retina (retinal slip). Patients occasionally interpret oscillopsia as dizziness, although it differs from true vertigo in that it only occurs with the eyes open. Patients with congenital nystagmus usually do not report oscillopsia because of compensatory neural mechanisms, including the foveation period, during which the eye is relatively stable, and the feedback of involuntary eye movement to the

TABLE 18–2. Symptoms

Term	Symptoms	Mechanism
Vertigo	Rotation, linear movement, or tilt	Sudden imbalance of tonic neural activity to vestibular nucleus
Dysequilibrium	Imbalance or unsteadiness while standing or walking	Loss of vestibulospinal, proprioception, visual, and motor function; joint pain or instability; and psychological factors
Light-headedness	Presyncope	Decreased blood flow to the brain
Psychologically induced	Floating, swimming, rocking, and spinning inside of head	Anxiety, depression, and somatiform disorders
Oscillopsia	Illusion of visual motion	Spontaneous: acquired nystagmus Head-induced: severe, bilateral loss of the vestibulo-ocular reflex

central nervous system (efference copy). Another form of oscillopsia occurs in patients with severe, bilateral loss of the VOR, which is frequently caused by ototoxicity from aminoglycosides. This form of oscillopsia occurs only during head movements and is caused by the lack of stabilizing features of the VOR; it is sometimes referred to as head-induced oscillopsia to differentiate it from oscillopsia caused by spontaneous nystagmus.

Circumstance

The circumstances under which dizziness occurs should be well defined. When dizziness occurs without provocation (spontaneously) and is vestibular in origin, it frequently is exacerbated by head movements. Dizziness may be provoked only by certain movements, such as standing up after reclining for at least 10 minutes (suggesting orthostatic hypotension), or may occur when the head is moved into certain vertical or oblique head positions (lying down or sitting up), suggesting BPPV.

Medications

Several medications may cause subjective symptoms of dizziness, especially in patients older than 65 years of age.[5,6] Table 18–3 lists common medications and their primary effects. Certain drugs cause disequilibrium and light-headedness. These include anticonvulsants, anti depressants, antihypertensives, antiinflammatory agents, hypnotics, muscle relaxants, tranquilizers, and (when used chronically) vestibular suppressants. Sensitization to meclizine and scopolamine may occur after a few days of continuous use, and withdrawal symptoms occur when the medication is discontinued; this may be misinterpreted as a recurrence of the disorder itself, so physicians should be cautious about restarting these medications. It is suggested that meclizine, scopolamine, and other vestibular suppressants be used for only a few days during acute vestibular hypofunction caused by vestibular neuritis or labyrinthitis. These drugs should then be discontinued because they interfere with central compensation within the denervated vestibular nucleus. Patients with brainstem medullary lesions may have nausea lasting for weeks and may require medication for a longer time. Certain drugs may cause vestibular ototoxicity and spare hearing, yet lead to disequilibrium. These include certain aminoglycosides (streptomycin, gentamicin, tobramycin), furosemide, and ethacrynic acid.

Office Examination

Eye Movements

Vestibulo-ocular Reflex

There are three bedside tests of the VOR (Table 18–4). The *vestibular dynamic visual acuity* test com-

pares static acuity with the head still to dynamic acuity with the head moving. First, distance visual acuity is measured using a Snellen chart. The patient is then asked to read the smallest possible line on the chart while the examiner manually oscillates the patient's head horizontally at 2 Hz, with the face moving about 1 to 2 inches in each direction; this is greater than the frequency at which smooth eye movements pursuit can track a target. If the VOR is normal, the patient's eyes move smoothly in the opposite direction of the head such that ocular fixation is always maintained. The patient should be able to read the same line that was readable when his or her head was still, or the adjacent line with larger letters. If the patient can read only letters more than three lines above his or her initial static visual acuity, the patient most likely has a vestibular defect. Second, VOR is examined using *head thrust*. Have the patient fixate on a target and observe the eyes after passive horizontal and vertical head thrusts. After a head thrust, an observed refixation saccade indicates decreased VOR.[7] Third, determine whether *head-shaking nystagmus* is present. Have the patient close his or her eyes, pitch the head down 30 degrees, and then oscillate the head 20 times horizontally. Elicitation of nystagmus during this procedure indicates a vestibular imbalance.[8] This sign may persist indefinitely after a peripheral or central unilateral vestibular lesion.

In very young children and babies, VOR can be assessed by picking up the child and rotating him or her in outstretched arms while observing the eyes for nystagmus. During this test, visual fixation should be blocked by having the patient wear Frenzel glasses (20- to 30-diopter lenses) to prevent the optokinetic response.

Smooth Pursuit and Vestibulo-ocular Reflex Cancellation

The patient is asked to track a slowly moving target, both horizontally and vertically, with the head still (smooth pursuit) and with the head moving synchronously with the target (VOR cancellation). Lesions in the parieto-occipital cortex, pons, and cerebellum cause deficits in smooth pursuit (catch-up saccades are observed) and VOR cancellation (inappropriate VOR) for targets moving toward the side of the lesion.

Nystagmus

Selective lesions in the peripheral and central vestibular pathways result in spontaneous nystagmus because of the unopposed higher spontaneous neural activity in the intact vestibular pathways (Table 18–5). For example, vestibular neuritis on one side results in peripheral vestibular nystagmus because of the unopposed activity of the lateral and posterior SCCs on the intact side. These two SCCs project to the medial vestibular nu-

TABLE 18–3. Drug-Induced Dizziness

	Drugs that can cause dizziness	Drugs that interfere with vestibular compensation	Ototoxic (vestibular) drugs
Antiarrythmics			
Amiodarone			X (synergistic)
Quinine			X (synergistic)
Anticonvulsants			
Barbiturates	X		
Carbamazepine	X		
Phenytoin	X		
Ethosuximide	X		
Antidepressants			
Amitriptyline	X		
Imipramine	X		
Antihypertensive agents			
Diuretics			
Hydrochlorthiazide	X		
Furosemide			X (synergistic)
Ethacrynic acid			X (synergistic)
α_1-Blockers			
Prozosine	X		
Terosine	X		
β-Blockers			
Atenolol	X		
Propranalol	X		
Calcium antagonists			
Nifedipine	X		
Verapamil	X		
Antiinflammatory drugs			
Ibuprofen			
Indomethacin	X		
Acetylsalicylic acid			X (reversible)
Antibiotics			
Streptomycin			X
Gentamicin			X
Tobramycin			X
Chemotherapeutics			
Cisplatin			X
Hypnotics			
Flurazepam	X		
Triazolam	X		
Muscle relaxants			
Cyclobenzaprine	X		
Orphenidrine	X		
Methocarbamol	X		
Tranquilizers			
Chlordiazepoxide	X		
Meprobamate	X		
Vestibular suppressants			
Meclizine	X	X	
Scopalamine	X	X	
Chlordiazepoxide	X	X	
Diazepam	X	X	

TABLE 18–4. Bedside Tests of the Vestibulo-Ocular Reflexes

Test	Procedure	Result
Vestibular dynamic visual acuity	Static, distant visual acuity is determined with the head still. Dynamic visual acuity is then determined while the patient's head is oscillated manually at 2 Hz.	A dynamic visual acuity of 3 or more lines above static visual acuity indicates a vestibular defect.
Head thrust	The patient fixates a distant visual target, and eye position is observed immediately after a small thrust of the head to the left and right.	A refixation saccade after the head thrust indicates decreased vestibulo-ocular reflex.
Head-shaking nystagmus	Patient's head is pitched down 30° and the head is oscillated horizontally 20 times.	Elicitation of jerk nystagmus after this procedure indicates a vestibular imbalance.

cleus. Dorsolateral medullary lesions (Wallenberg syndrome) result in torsional nystagmus caused by involvement of the anterior and posterior SCC pathways centrally on one side.[9] The presence of spontaneous nystagmus should be assessed with and without fixation because peripheral causes of nystagmus usually can be suppressed with fixation, whereas central causes cannot be suppressed. An easy way to test this is during the ophthalmoscopic examination, with the other eye fixating on a target.[10] During this procedure, the fixating eye can be covered with the hand. Torsional nystagmus is the only form of central vestibular nystagmus that is associated with vertigo. This may be because the lesions that cause other types of nystagmus are located between the vestibular nuclei and oculomotor nuclei. In contrast, lesions that cause vertigo lie within the vestibulothalamocortical system.

Certain maneuvers that may evoke nystagmus also should be performed. Results of the Hallpike-Dix test are positive in patients with BPPV. During this test the patient is seated on a flat table with the head rotated 45 degrees to one side. The patient is then quickly moved backward into a supine position with the head still deviated and hanging over the side of the table. Nystagmus from BPPV should begin within 30 seconds and lasts

less than 30 seconds. If nystagmus persists while the patient is in this position, and is not present while he or she is sitting, it is likely caused by a central disorder (central positional vertigo), although there are exceptions.[17] Nystagmus or a drift of the eyes also should be assessed after positive and negative pressure directed to the external auditory canal (Hennebert sign), valsalva, or loud noise (Tullio's phenomenon).[18,19] A positive response is found in patients with perilymphatic fistula or hypermobile stapes, and occasionally in patients with posttraumatic endolymphatic hydrops.

Stance and Gait

The Romberg, "sharpened" Romberg (heel-to-toe tandem stance), Fukuda stepping test, normal gait, and tandem gait should be examined. In the Romberg tests, the patient is asked to stand with feet slightly apart, first with eyes open, and then with eyes closed. The patient is asked to fold his or her arms across the chest for 30 seconds with eyes open and then 30 seconds with eyes closed. A *positive* Romberg is one in which the patient is stable with eyes open but looses balance with eyes closed. A positive Romberg may be found in patients with acute vestibular defects or proprioceptive defects

TABLE 18–5. Spontaneous Vestibular Nystagmus due to Peripheral and Central Lesions

Nystagmus	Pathology	Possible mechanism
Peripheral vestibular nystagmus	Labyrinth, vestibular nerve or root entry zone lesion	Decreased tonic neural activity to the MVN from horizontal and anterior SCC pathways on one side
Torsional nystagmus	Dorsolateral medulla lesion[9]	Decreased tonic neural activity to the INC from central anterior and posterior SCC pathways on one side
Downbeat nystagmus	Cerebellular flocculus lesion or floor of fourth ventricle lesion[11]	Decreased tonic neural activity to the INC from central posterior SCC pathways on both sides
Upbeat nystagmus	Brachium conjunctivum lesion Dorsal upper medulla lesion[12,13]	Decreased tonic neural activity to INC from central anterior SCC pathways on both sides
Seesaw nystagmus	Unilateral lesion of INC[14]	Unilateral inactivation of INC on one side
Periodic alternating nystagmus	Cerebellar nodulus lesions[15]	Unstable (high gain) neural activity in the MVN
Latent nystagmus	Loss of cortical binocular visual input to the NOT usually from congenital esotropia[16]	Decreased tonic neural activity to MVN from the NOT on one side when one eye is covered (NOT provides all of the visual input into the MVN)

MVN, medial vestibular nucleus; *SCCs*, semicircular canals; *INC*, interstitial nucleus of Cajal; *NOT*, nucleus optic tract.

from a peripheral neuropathy. A *positive* sharpened Romberg also is found in these circumstances, as well as in patients with chronic vestibular defects, and in some normal individuals over the age of 65 years. For the Fukuda stepping test, the patient steps in place for 50 steps with arms extended and eyes closed.[20] Progressive turning of more than 30 degrees toward one side is abnormal. A *positive* Fukuda stepping test frequently is found in patients with a unilateral vestibular defect, but it also is found in patients with a leg-length discrepancy or other structural abnormalities of the legs.

The Romberg test also is useful in identifying a functional component (nonorganic), which is suggested when patients rock backward on their heels yet remarkably do not fall. Other features of stance and gait help identify a functional component, including knee-buckling without fall, small-amplitude steps, uneconomical posture and movement, exaggerated sway during the Romberg test without fall, excessive slowness in gait, and fluctuations in levels of impairment.[21,22]

Special Apparatuses

Electronystagmography

Electronystagmography consists of eye movement recordings during visual tracking and during vestibular testing (rotary chair or caloric stimulation). It is objective and quantitative and ideally should be performed on all patients who exhibit a vestibular defect during the clinical examination.

Rotary Chair

This is the most sensitive test for assessing vestibular function and can be performed in children of any age, although calibrations usually are obtainable only in infants 6 months or older (by using a "happy face" or similar stimulus). Children less than 4 years of age can sit in a parent's lap during the test. Eye movements are measured by electro-oculography. After calibration, peak slow phase eye velocity is measured during either sinusoidal chair rotations or constant-velocity step rotations in the dark to assess VOR gain (eye velocity/chair velocity). VOR gain normally is near 1.0 at birth and decreases to about 0.7 in adults. Values less than 0.4 are abnormal and indicate vestibular hypofunction.

Caloric Test

Compared with rotary chair, the caloric test is a less sensitive but more specific test of peripheral vestibular function. This is the best method for determining whether a vestibular defect is peripheral or central, and also for indicating the side of the defect. This test usually is not well tolerated in children less than 8 years of age. Before the caloric test is performed, the internal auditory canal is examined with an otoscope, and any wax or debris blocking the canal is removed. If there is a tympanic membrane perforation, different temperatures of air instead of water should be used as the stimulus. The caloric test uses a nonphysiologic stimulus (water) to induce endolymphatic flow in the semicircular canals by creating a temperature gradient within each canal. Each ear canal is irrigated for 40 seconds, with a constant flow rate of water at two temperatures (30° and 44°C). Eye movements are recorded for 2 minutes after each irrigation. At the end of this period, the ear is emptied of any remaining water and sufficient time is allowed for the nystagmus to stop before proceeding with the next irrigation (usually 5 minutes).

Posturography

Postural sway is quantified with dynamic posturography that measures sway in conditions in which visual and somatosensory cues are absent or altered. Automatic postural responses also can be measured in response to perturbations of the support platform. Deficits in a variety of different neural systems can be identified, including the cerebral cortex, anterior cerebellum, and spinal cord. The test is not specific for vestibular disorders, although patients with uncompensated or severe vestibular deficits typically have difficulty maintaining their balance when both visual and somatosensory cues are altered. This test is also useful in demonstrating objective signs of a functional component.[23,24]

Audiometry

Audiometry should include both pure-tone and speech audiometry, and test acoustic reflexes and middle ear function. Audiometry should be performed on all individuals who complain of hearing loss. Acoustic neuromas usually present with unilateral hearing loss or tinnitus. Nonpulsatile and constant tinnitus without documented hearing loss is extremely rare. A nonorganic loss of hearing can be determined by the inconsistency of the audiogram (more than a 10-dB change in threshold on successive trials), which occurs in up to 10% of head-injured patients.[25]

Brainstem Auditory-Evoked Response

The brainstem auditory-evoked response (BAER) is recorded with scalp electrodes and represents the averaged surface-recorded activity of the auditory neural generators of the peripheral and central auditory pathways in the pons and midbrain. It can be used to determine auditory threshold when standard audiography cannot be performed. It also is an excellent screening test for abnormalities involving VIIIth nerve and central auditory brainstem pathways. The BAER has been reported to be abnormal in patients with postconcussive syndrome even when all other studies are normal.[26]

Neuroimaging

Computed Tomography

High-resolution computed tomography (CT) of the temporal bone is highly sensitive for evaluating petrous bone and ossicular chain abnormalities, including petrous bone fractures, cholesteatoma, and congenital defects.[27] The cause of conductive hearing loss and peripheral sensorineural hearing loss usually can be identified by the type of temporal bone fracture indicated by CT.[28] The location of cerebrospinal fluid leaks also is best determined with a high-resolution CT scan of the temporal bone after intrathecal injection of water-soluble contrast material.

Magnetic Resonance Imaging

Magnetic resonance imaging (MRI) with gadolinium-enhanced sections through the VIIIth nerve clearly defines the internal auditory canal, cerebellopontine angle, and brainstem.[29] Enhancement on MRI has been reported in patients with inflammation of the labyrinth,[30] but the significance of these findings is not yet clear.

ABNORMALITIES AND THEIR MANAGEMENT

Acoustic Neuroma

Acoustic neuroma is a benign tumor of the myelin sheaths of the vestibular nerve (VIII) and usually is characterized by unilateral hearing loss or tinnitus. Rarely does it cause vertigo or disequilibrium. Audiography shows features consistent with a retrocochlear process, which consists of poor speech discrimination relative to the degree of tone loss and recruitment in which increments in tone intensity cause a higher than expected increase in perceived tone loudness. The diagnostic procedure of choice for acoustic neuroma is gadolinium-enhanced MRI sections of the posterior fossa that include the VIIIth nerve and other cerebellopontine angle structures (Fig. 18–8).

Surgery is the treatment of choice, either by middle cranial fossa approaches (for tumors confined to the internal auditory canal, with usable hearing), by suboccipital craniotomy (for large tumors or those adherent to the brainstem, with usable hearing), or by a translabyrinthine approach (for small tumors, with no usable hearing).[31] With questionable or small intracanalicular tumors, especially in elderly patients or in those in poor medical condition, watchful waiting is prudent, with neuroimaging repeated at 6- to 12-month intervals. Focal radiosurgery may be ideal for recurrent tumors and for patients in poor medical condition who cannot tolerate posterior fossa surgery.[31] Tumor control is achieved in 95% of patients, but approximately 25% to 30% develop 5th and 7th cranial nerve loss and hearing loss caused by involvement of the vascular supply.[31,32]

Acute Vestibular Neuritis and Labyrinthitis

Acute vestibular neuritis and labyrinthitis are associated with intense vertigo, nausea, and disequilibrium that persist for days. It is caused by a viral infection of the superior portion of the vestibular nerve (neuritis) or of the endolymph of the labyrinth (labyrinthitis). A viral etiology has been postulated, and recent data suggest a reactivation of dormant herpes infection in Scarpa's ganglia.[33,34] Diagnosis of these entities is based primarily on clinical presentations. If associated with significant hearing loss (frequently with tinnitus), the

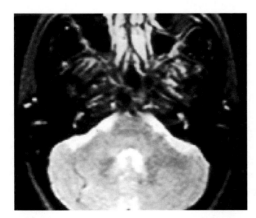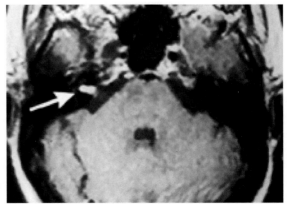

Fig. 18–8. Small acoustic neuroma revealed in an enhanced MRI of the head. **Left.** Axial T2 MRI through the cerebellar pontine angle. **Right.** Same section in a gadolinium-enhanced T1 MRI. The intracanalicular portion of the VIIIth nerve on the right side is enhanced (*arrow*) consistent with an acoustic neuroma.

disorder is labeled labyrinthitis; otherwise it is labeled vestibular neuritis. Viral serologic studies are superfluous and their results do not alter treatment. Differential diagnoses include infarcts of the labyrinth and a first attack of Meniere's disease. Audiography should be obtained when patients complain of hearing loss. After several days, caloric testing may document the extent of vestibular defects. In appropriate circumstances, serum fluorescent treponemal antibody absorption testing and erythrocyte sedimentation rate are used are performed to rule out otic syphilis and giant cell arteritis.

Admission to a hospital may be required for extreme dehydration from vomiting or when a central disorder is suspected. During the first few days, vestibular suppressants should be used, such as intramuscular promethazine (Phenergan; 25 to 50 mg) in the office and promethazine suppositories at home. Ondansetron (Zofran) may also be appropriate for patients with severe vertigo and nausea, but currently it is approved only for chemotherapy-induced nausea.[35] Keeping patients on vestibular suppressants too long is a common error because these drugs delay vestibular adaptation. Consequently, these medications should be discontinued and vestibular exercises started as soon as possible. The patient should be reassessed after a few days to make certain that symptoms are resolving. After an acute insult, the imbalance of spontaneous neural activity in the vestibular nucleus usually corrects itself within several days, possibly through commissural pathways between the vestibular nuclei. What remains is a low gain in the VOR from which patients perceive vertigo or unsteadiness *during head movements*. This defect can be treated with vestibular rehabilitation (see Disequilibrium).

Benign Paroxysmal Positional Vertigo

Benign paroxysmal positional vertigo is characterized by vertigo that lasts less than 1 minute. It usually occurs in the morning upon arising or even when turning over in bed. Symptoms also may be caused by reclining or extending the head backward. After a severe attack, patients frequently complain of disequilibrium that lasts for several hours. BPPV usually is idiopathic but also may occur after head trauma, labyrinthitis, or ischemia in the distribution of the anterior inferior cerebellar artery. The pathophysiologic mechanism of BPPV is related to portions of otoconia from the utricle that are displaced and free floating (canalithiasis) in the posterior SCC. Occasionally it is caused by otoconia attached to the cupula of this canal (cupulolithiasis). Both these conditions cause inappropriate neural afferent discharge from the posterior SCC after the head stops moving backward. The diagnosis is secured by eliciting a torsional-upbeat nystagmus associated with vertigo during the Hallpike-Dix test when the affected ear is inferior. In this test, the patient is seated on an examina-tion table with the head rotated 45 degrees to one side; he or she is then quickly moved backward into a lying position with the head still deviated and hanging over the side of the table (Fig. 18–9). BPPV also may occur from debris in the anterior or horizontal SCC, but the nystagmus induced by the Hallpike-Dix test is downbeat and horizontal, respectively. The nystagmus found in BPPV usually has a latency of 3 to 20 seconds, fatigues within 1 minute, and decreases with repeat testing.

BPPV is best treated by a maneuver called the canalith repositioning maneuver,[36] which moves the otoconia out of the posterior SCC and back into the utricle, where it is reabsorbed into the calcium matrix. Total remission or significant improvement from BPPV occurs in 90% of patients using theis maneuver,[37] and complications are rare.[38] During the canalith repositioning maneuver, the patient is seated with the head rotated toward the side that elicited nystagmus during the Hallpike-Dix maneuver. The patient is then moved backward into a lying position with the head hanging over the side of the table and kept is there until the vertigo and nystagmus stop. The head is then rotated toward the unaffected side, and the patient is rolled over onto this side until the face is pointed down. The patient is kept in this position for 1 minute. With the head deviated toward the unaffected side, the patient then slowly sits up. To make certain that the debris does not move back toward the cupula, the patient is fitted with a soft collar and told not to bend over or look up or down for 1 or 2 days. In addition, the patient is told to sleep sitting up during this period. For the subsequent 5 days the patient is allowed to lie down, but only on the unaffected side. After 7 days the patient is reevaluated. If the initial treatment does not work, then the patient is retreated. In patients that cannot tolerate sleeping upright for 1 or 2 days, a different maneuver is used.[39] In this maneuver, the patient sits on a table sideways, rotates the head 45 degrees horizontally, and then rapidly lies on his or her side in the opposite direction and waits until the vertigo has resolved or for 10 seconds if the vertigo does not resolve. The patient then rapidly sits up and waits for the same amount of time. He or she next performs the movement in the opposite direction. This can be repeated 5 to 10 times, 1 or 2 times each day. Unlike the single treatments described earlier, this latter treatment usually takes 1 to 2 weeks before symptoms resolve. The maneuver works either by habituation or by dislodging debris from the cupula of the posterior SCC. Vestibular suppressant drugs do not have a role in the treatment of BPPV unless excessive vertigo and nausea prevent the patient from doing the maneuvers.

Dizziness in Children

Dizziness in children is uncommon but alarming to parents. The most common cause is periodic dizziness

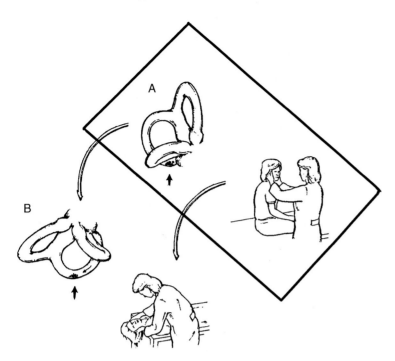

Fig. 18–9. Hallpike-Dix maneuver for benign paroxysmal positional vertigo. This figure shows the maneuver of the head and body during the test, along with the labyrinth (enlarged). **A.** The patient sits on the examination table with the head turned 45 degrees horizontally. **B.** The head and trunk are quickly brought straight back en bloc so that the head is hanging over the edge of the examination table by 20 degrees. The patient is assessed for nystagmus and is asked whether he or she has vertigo. Although not shown in the figure, the patient is then brought up slowly to a sitting position, with the head still turned 45 degrees, and nystagmus is sought again. This test is then repeated with the head turned 45 degrees in the other direction. This figure also shows movement of free-floating otoconia in the right posterior semicircular canal (*large black arrows*) during the Hallpike-Dix test. In this example, the patient has nystagmus and vertigo when the test is performed on the right side but not when the test is performed on the left side.

(ataxia) of childhood, which is a migraine aura.[40] Meniere's disease and BPPV usually do not present in childhood. The clinical evaluation of the dizzy child is the same as that of the adult.[41] A neurologic examination is performed to rule out a CNS defect, and reassurance and follow-up visits usually are sufficient.

Disequilibrium

Disequilibrium is an imbalance or unsteadiness while standing or walking. It may be caused by a number of problems, including loss of normal vestibular function, peripheral neuropathies, motor weakness, poor vision, disabling arthritis, or fear of falling. Normal balance is maintained through a complex integration of sensory input (vestibular, somatosensory, and visual) and appropriate automatic postural responses involving the frontal lobe, basal ganglia, cerebellum, spinal cord, and peripheral nerves. Patients with vestibular and proprioceptive loss in the feet complain that their balance is worse in the dark.[42] The clinical examination can be helpful in the diagnosis of bilateral or static unilateral vestibular defects. Frequently demonstrable are refixation saccadic eye movements following head thrust, caused by a decrease in the VOR (Table 4). Unilateral defects frequently produce nystagmus after horizontal head shaking, and bilateral lesions usually result in more than a four-line decrease in visual acuity during 2-Hz head oscillation and subjective oscillopsia. The diagnosis may be assured by demonstrating a decreased VOR during rotary chair testing, and the peripheral nature of the defect is identified by a decreased caloric response.

The treatment of unilateral vestibular defects is based on animal studies.[43,44] The chronic problem after a unilateral vestibular lesion is a dynamic deficit that can be repaired only by vestibular adaptation. Vestibular adaptation results when a mismatch occurs between head motion sensed by the vestibular system and head motion sensed by the visual system. To facilitate vestibular adaptation, the patient is encouraged to move the head while viewing a still target. Eventually these exercises should be done with the target moving in the opposite direction of the head. In addition, postural control is improved by having the patient stand with feet together, then in tandem, and then with the head moving. Similarly, the patient is encouraged to walk normally, then in tandem, and finally with the head moving back and forth. Controlled studies have shown that early intervention (on the second or third day after onset) with exercises speeds recovery, especially from imbalance and perception of disequilibrium.[45] Near complete recovery may be anticipated within 6 weeks. Supervised therapy and home exercises usually are sufficient treatment. Although vestibular neurectomy has been advocated for treatment of patients with posttraumatic unsteadiness and associated hearing impairment,[46] there is no conclusive evidence that neurectomy facilitates vestibular compensation. There is no physiologic basis for this surgical treatment except for intractable spells of vertigo caused by posttraumatic endolymphatic hydrops.

The treatment of bilateral vestibular defects includes avoidance of all ototoxins that may cause further permanent peripheral vestibular damage. These include gentamicin, streptomycin, tobramycin, ethacrynic acid, furosemide, quinine, and cisplatin. Drugs that may transiently impair balance (sedatives, anxiolytics, antiepileptics, and antidepressants) also should be avoided. Vestibular rehabilitation may be helpful for these patients. For bilateral defects, the same vestibular exercises described for unilateral vestibular defects can be used to improve any remaining vestibular function. Most recovery occurs with exercises that facilitate the substitution of other ocular motor systems (*e.g.*, the cervico-ocular reflex) and somatosensory and visual cues to recover postural stability.[47] Plateau in recovery should occur within 3 to 6 months. Several controlled studies[48–52] have demonstrated that supervised exercises are significantly more effective in improving balance and perceived dizziness in patients with unilateral and bilateral vestibular deficits than giving patients instruction sheets of exercises to perform on their own at home.

The treatment of disequilibrium that is not caused by vestibular defects depends on its specific etiology. Treatable causes of neurologic illnesses include Parkinson's disease, early normal pressure hydrocephalus, inflammatory peripheral neuropathies, compressive myelopathies, and certain types of myopathies. Chronic use of antivestibular drugs (meclizine [Antivert] and benzodiazepines) also may cause chronic dizziness, and these should be tapered. Exercises to improve static balance and dynamic postural stability often are very helpful in patients with disequilibrium.[49] Additional physical therapy to strengthen muscle and increase range of motion is helpful in patients with weakness, arthritis, and joint limitations. Patients who have a fear of falling often improve with supervised exercise; dynamic posturography is helpful in determining appropriate physical therapy. Patients with a psychological disorder may complain of chronic disequilibrium. A combination of counseling and physical therapy can decrease the problem in some patients.

Head Trauma

Head trauma frequently is associated with dizziness from a variety of causes.[53] BPPV is the most common cause, either from a direct blow to the head or from the shear forces from a flexion-extension injury to the neck ("whiplash"). Other causes of dizziness from head trauma include perilymphatic fistula from barotrauma (scuba diving or pressure force to the ear), interruption of the labyrinth or vestibular nerve from petrous bone fracture, and axon swelling and interruption within the brainstem. A CT scan of the petrous bone should disclose bone fractures. Caloric stimulation can confirm loss of vestibular function, and MRI may reveal central posterior fossa injury. BPPV and vestibular loss caused by petrous bone fractures respond well to therapy described earlier (for BPPV and acute vestibular neuritis and labyrinthitis).

Meniere's Disease

Meniere's disease causes spells of roaring sounds (tinnitus), ear fullness, and hearing loss often associated with vertigo that last for hours to days. With repeated attacks, a sustained low-frequency sensorineural hearing loss and constant tinnitus usually develops. The cause is believed to be decreased reabsorption of endolymph in the endolymphatic sac (see Fig. 18–2), which can occur after ear trauma or viral infection or which can be idiopathic. The diagnosis depends on documentation of fluctuating hearing loss by audiography.

The frequency of attacks of Meniere's disease can be significantly reduced by restricting the diet to 2000 mg or less of sodium per day[54,55]; some patients require the additional use of a diuretic. Acetazolamide may be the optimal diuretic because this drug may decrease osmotic pressure within the endolymph, but chlorthalidone and other diuretics also have been quite effective.[56,57] Less proven prophylactic therapy includes elimination of alcohol and caffeinated products (including chocolate). During acute attacks the patient is treated as with any other attack of acute vertigo, except extensive laboratory investigation and vestibular exercises usually are not necessary because the patient recovers quickly. Medical therapy may not control the disease. Endolymphatic shunts may be used, but are not always effective or may fail after a few years. Labyrinthectomy is appropriate in patients without evidence of contralateral disease in whom there is a severe preexisting hearing loss on the side of the defective labyrinth. Vestibular neurectomy is used for patients in whom hearing is preserved.[58]

Migraine

Migraine is a common but poorly recognized cause of dizziness. Dizziness caused by migraine usually lasts 4 to 60 minutes and may or may not be associated with a headache. The International Headache Society criteria for the diagnosis of migraine applies. Because migraine is a diagnosis of exclusion, a positive response to treatment is essential.

Spells of vertigo caused by migraine respond to the same types of treatment as those used for headaches.[59] After the diagnosis is established and the patient is reassured, he or she should be given a list of risk factors and foods that may precipitate an aura. Hypoglycemia should be avoided by eating every 6 to 8 hours, the use of nicotine and exogenous estrogen should be discontinued, and a regular sleep schedule should be maintained. If strict avoidance of these risk factors does not significantly reduce the frequency of dizziness episodes, based on a diary, then daily medication is used.[60] Beta-blockers (atenolol or propranolol) are among the most effective prophylactic drugs for migraine.

Motion Sickness

Motion sickness consists of episodic dizziness, tiredness, pallor, diaphoresis, salivation, nausea, and occasionally vomiting induced by passive locomotion (*e.g.*, riding in a car) or motion in the visual surrounding while standing still (*e.g.*, the motion of trains, traffic, flowing water). Motion sickness is believed to be a sensory mismatch between vision and vestibular cues.[61] Patients with migraine disorder are particularly prone to motion sickness, especially during childhood. Twenty-six to 60% of patients with migraine have a history of severe motion sickness compared with 8% to 24% of individuals without migraine.[62,63] The reason for this correlation is not clear. Diagnosis is based on careful history taking, and symptoms often are reproduced with the use of moving full-field visual targets such as optokinetic devices.

Treatment consists of reassurance, reduction of circumstances that cause sensory mismatch, and medication, if necessary. Intramuscular promethazine immediately relieves space motion sickness in 90% of individuals, compared with a resolution of symptoms in 72 to 96 hours in untreated individuals.[64] Cinnarizine, a calcium-channel blocker, is the drug most commonly used in Europe to treat dizziness. In a double-blind crossover study with scopolamine, scopolamine was shown to be more effective in protecting against seasickness, but Cinnarizine was better tolerated.[65]

Orthostatic Hypotension

Orthostatic hypotension produces symptoms that range from light-headedness when standing up to chronic fatigue, mental slowing, dizziness, nausea, and impending syncope. Common causes include medications (diuretics, antihypertensive medications, tricyclic antidepressants), prolonged bed rest, and neurogenic disorders (autonomic neuropathy from diabetes, multisystem atrophy, Parkinson's disease). Diagnosis is confirmed by recording a drop in systolic pressure of 20 mm Hg or more associated with reproduction of symptoms.

Potentially offending drugs should be discontinued if possible, and increased salt and fluid intake (5 g each day and five glasses of water) should be encouraged. Fludrocortisone (0.1 to 0.6 mg/day) may be required. If this fails 10 mg midodrine is given three times a day. In a double-blind, placebo-controlled study, midodrine significantly increased standing systolic blood pressure (by 22 mm Hg; p < .001) and decreased orthostatic dizziness, fatigue, and weakness (p < .05).[66] When these medications are used, the head of the patient's bed should be elevated to reduce supine hypertension.

Panic Attacks and Hyperventilation

Panic attack is an anxiety disorder that causes intense fear or discomfort that reaches a crescendo within 10 minutes and is frequently associated with dizziness, nausea, shortness of breath, and sweating. These symptoms may occur unexpectedly or may be situationally provoked. This disorder may be initiated by an organic cause of vertigo such as BPPV, especially in patients with a family history for panic attacks. Hyperventilation associated with chronic anxiety also may cause vague complaints of dizziness. This is associated with shortness of breath or chest tightness and paresthesia.

Imipramine is very effective in controlling panic attacks, but in a placebo-controlled study alprazolam was just as effective and better tolerated during a 6-month maintenance program.[67] Paroxetine (Paxil) may be an ideal medication because it is not habit-forming and because many patients with panic disorder have concomitant depression. Behavioral modification also has been shown to be effective in a recent clinical outcome study in which 96.1% of patients remained in remission at 2 years and 67.4% were in remission for at least 7 years.[68]

Perilymphatic Fistula

Perilymphatic fistula is a hole between the inner and middle ears caused by barotrauma (scuba diving), a tumor in the middle ear (cholesteatoma), head trauma, or displacement of a prosthetic middle ear bone into the inner ear. Any pressure changes to the inner or middle ear causes a flow of fluid between these two compartments and distorts the utricle or semicircular canal. Distortion of these end-organs frequently causes transient vertigo, nystagmus, or skew deviation. Nystagmus or drift of the eyes should be assessed after positive and negative pressure directed to the external auditory canal (Hennebert's sign), Valsalva maneuver, or loud noises (Tullio's phenomenon).[18,19] Diagnosis requires middle ear exploration. The oval and round windows are examined for the leak, which may be increased with the Valsalva maneuver. Surgical repair with autogenous tissue, followed by bed rest, usually is effective.

Seizures

Seizures commonly cause vague dizziness described as confusion, disorientation, or light-headedness, but they rarely cause vertigo.[69-71] Seizures also can cause head or eye deviation, and occasionally nystagmus, but there usually is associated mild confusion.[72] Electroencephalography is performed only when there is a strong suspicion of seizures, and ideally is recorded during the actual spell of dizziness. Therapy depends on the type of seizure.

Transient Ischemic Attacks

Caused by vertebrobasilar insufficiency, TIAs provoke episodes of dizziness that are abrupt and usually last only a few minutes. TIAs frequently are associated with other symptoms of vertebrobasilar insufficiency, most commonly visual disturbance, drop attacks, unsteadiness, and weakness.[73] A small percentage of patients with vertebrobasilar insufficiency may present with isolated spells of vertigo, presumably caused by ischemia in the distribution of the anterior vestibular artery. This small artery perfuses the anterior and lateral SCCs and the utricular macula, and spares the cochlea. These patients usually have known cerebrovascular disease or risk factors for this disease. Magnetic resonance arteriography can be performed to assess posterior circulation vessels and transcranial doppler may detect decreased flow in the basilar artery. Treatment includes reduction of risk factors for cerebrovascular disease and antiplatelet therapy. Warfarin (Coumadin) is used when there is significant vertebrobasilar artery stenosis.[74]

REFERENCES

1. JC: Living without a balancing mechanism. N Engl J Med 246:458, 1952
2. Fetter M, Dichgans J: Vestibular neuritis spares the inferior division of the vestibular nerve. Brain 119:755, 1996
3. Uchino Y et al: Utriculoocular reflex arc of the cat. J Neurophysiol 76:1896, 1996
4. Halmagyi GM, Gresty MA, Gibson WPR: Ocular tilt reaction with peripheral vestibular lesions. Ann Neurol 6:80, 1979
5. Ballantyne J, Ajodhia J: Iatrogenic dizziness. In Dix MR, Hood JD (eds): Vertigo, p 217. New York: John Wiley and Sons, 1984
6. Wennmo K, Wennmo C: Drug-related dizziness. Acta Otolaryngol [Suppl] 455:11, 1988
7. Halmagyi GM, Curthoys IS: A clinical sign of canal paresis. Arch Neurol 45:737, 1988
8. Hain TC, Fetter M, Zee DS: Head-shaking nystagmus in patients with unilateral peripheral vestibular lesions. Am J Otolaryngol 8:36, 1987
9. Morrow M, Sharpe JA: Torsional nystagmus in the lateral medullary syndrome. Ann Neurol 24:390, 1988
10. Zee DS: Ophthalmoscopy in examination of patients with vestibular disorders. Ann Neurol 3:373, 1978
11. Baloh RW, Spooner JW: Downbeat nystagmus: A type of central vestibular nystagmus. Neurology 31:304, 1980
12. Nakada T, Remler MP: Primary position upbeat nystagmus: Another central vestibular nystagmus? J Clin Neuro Ophthalmol 1:185, 1981
13. Ranalli PJ, Sharpe JA: Upbeat nystagmus and the ventral tegmental pathway of upward vestibulo-ocular reflex. Neurology 38:1329, 1988
14. Halmagyi GM et al: Jerk-waveform see-saw nystagmus due to unilateral meso-diencephalic lesion. Brain 117:789, 1994
15. Leigh RJ, Robinson DA, Zee DS: A hypothetical explanation for periodic alternating nystagmus: Instability in the optokinetic-vestibular system. Ann NY Acad Sci 374:619, 1981
16. Tusa RJ, Becker JL, Mustari MJ et al: Brief periods of impoverished visual experience during infancy impairs the development of specific gaze-holding systems in monkeys. In Fuchs A, Brandt T, Büttner U et al (eds): Contemporary Ocular Motor and Vestibular Research: A Tribute to Dave A. Robinson, p 345. Stuttgart: George Thieme Verlag, 1994
17. Baloh RW, Yue Q, Jacobson K et al: Persistent direction-changing positional nystagmus: Another variant of benign positional vertigo. Neurology 45:1297, 1995
18. Daspit CP, Churchill D, Linthicum FH: Diagnosis of perilymph fistula using ENG and impedance. Laryngoscope 90:217, 1980
19. Pyykko I, Ishizaki H, Aalto H et al: Relevance of the Tullio phenomenon in assessing perilymphatic leak in vertiginous patients. Am J Otol 13:339, 1992
20. Fukuda T: The stepping test: Two phases of the labyrinthine reflex. Acta Otolaryngol 50:95, 1959
21. Keane JR: Hysterical gait disorders: 60 cases. Neurology 39:586, 1989
22. Lempert T, Brandt T, Dieterich M et al: How to identify psychogenic disorders of stance and gait. J Neurol 238:140, 1991
23. Cevette MJ et al: A physiologic performance on dynamic posturography. Otolaryngol Head Neck Surg 112:676, 1995
24. Allum JHJ, Huwiler M, Honegger F: Identifying cases of nonorganic vertigo using dynamic posturography. Gait Posture 4:52, 1996
25. Berman JM, Fredrickson JM: Vertigo after head injury: A five year follow-up. J Otolaryngol 7:237, 1978
26. Noseworthy JH, Miller J, Murray TJ et al: Auditory brainstem responses in post-concussive syndrome. Arch Neurol 38:275, 1981
27. Hasso AN, Ledington JA: Traumatic injuries of the temporal bone. Otolaryngol Clin North Am 21:295, 1988
28. Momose KJ, Davis KR, Rhea JT: Hearing loss in skull fractures. Am J Neuroradiol 4:781, 1983
29. Swartz JD, Harnsberger HR: The temporal bone: Magnetic resonance imaging. Top Magn Reson Imag 2:1, 1990
30. Mark AS, Seltzer S, Nelson-Drake J et al: Labyrinthine enhancement on gadolinium-enhanced magnetic resonance imaging in sudden deafness and vertigo: Correlation with audiologic and electronystagmographic studies. Ann Otol Rhinol Laryngol 101:459, 1992
31. Kartush JM, Brackmann DE: Acoustic neuroma update. Otolaryngol Clin North Am 29:377, 1996
32. Flickinger JC et al: Radiosurgery of acoustic neurinomas. Cancer 67:345, 1990
33. Furuta Y et al: Latent herpes simplex virus type 1 in human vestibular ganglia. Acta Otolaryngol [Suppl] 503:85, 1993
34. Davis LE, Johnsson, LG: Viral infections of the inner ear: Clinical, virologic and pathologic studies in humans and animals. Am J Otolaryngol 4:347, 1983
35. Rice GPA, Ebers GC: Ondansetron for intractable vertigo complicating acute brainstem disorders. Lancet 345:1182, 1995
36. Epley JM: The canalith repositioning procedure: For treatment of benign paroxysmal positional vertigo. Otolaryngol Head Neck Surg 107:399, 1992
37. Herdman SJ, Tusa RJ, Zee DS et al: Single treatment approaches to benign paroxysmal positional vertigo. Arch Otolaryngol Head Neck Surg 119:450, 1993
38. Herdman SJ, Tusa RJ: Complications of the canalith repositioning procedure. Arch Otolaryngol 122:281, 1996
39. Brandt T, Daroff RB: Physical therapy for benign paroxysmal positional vertigo. Arch Otolaryngol 106:484, 1980
40. Basser LS: Benign paroxysmal vertigo of childhood. Brain 87:141, 1964
41. Tusa RJ, Saada AA, Niparko JK: Dizziness in childhood. J Child Neurol 9:261, 1994
42. Baloh RW, Honrubia V: Clinical Neurophysiology of the Vestibular System, p 101. Philadelphia: FA Davis, 1990
43. Igarashi M et al: Further study of physical exercise and locomotor balance compensation after unilateral labyrinthectomy in squirrel monkeys. Acta Otolaryngol 92:101, 1981
44. Fetter M, Zee DS: Recovery from unilateral labyrinthectomy in rhesus monkeys. J Neurophysiol 59:370, 1988
45. Herdman SJ, Clendaniel RA, Mattox DE et al: Vestibular adaptation exercises and recovery: Acute stage after acoustic neuroma resection. Otolaryngol Head Neck Surg 113:77, 1995
46. Sanna M, Ylikosky J: Vestibular neurectomy for dizziness after head trauma: A review of 28 patients. ORL J 45:216, 1983
47. Herdman SJ, Borello-France D, Whitney S: Treatment of vestibular hypofunction. In Herdman SJ (ed): Vestibular Rehabilitation. Philadelphia: FA Davis, 1994
48. Horak FB, Jones-Rycewicz C, Black FO et al: Effects of vestibular rehabilitation on dizziness and imbalance. Otolaryngol Head Neck Surg 106:175, 1992
49. Krebs DE, Gill-Body KM, Riley PO et al: Double-blind, placebo-controlled trial of rehabilitation for bilateral vestibular hypofunction: Preliminary report. Otolaryngol Head Neck Surg 109:735, 1993
50. Szturm T, Ireland DJ, Lessing-Turner M: Comparison of different

exercise programs in the rehabilitation of patients with chronic peripheral vestibular dysfunction. J Vest Res 4:461, 1994

51. Shepard NT, Telian SA: Programmatic vestibular rehabilitation. Otolaryngol Head Neck Surg 112:173, 1995

52. Cass SP, Borello-France D, Furman JM: Functional outcome of vestibular rehabilitation in patients with abnormal sensory-organization testing. Am J Otol 17:581, 1996

53. Tusa RJ, Brown SB: Neuro-otological trauma and dizziness. In Rizzo M, Tranzel D (eds): Head Injury and Post-Concussive Syndrome, p 177. New York: Churchill Livingstone, 1996

54. Boles R, Rice DH, Hybels R et al: Conservative management of Meniere's disease: Furstenberg regimen revisited. Ann Otol Rhinol Laryngol 84:513, 1975

55. Proctor C, Proctor TB, Proctor B: Etiology and treatment of fluid retention (hydrops) in Meniere's syndrome. Ear Nose Throat J 71:631, 1992

56. Klockhoff I, Lindblom U, Stahle J: Diuretic treatment of Meniere disease: Long-term results with chlorthalidone. Arch Otolaryngol 100:262, 1974

57. Shinkawa H, Kimura RS: Effect of diuretics on endolymphatic hydrops. Acta Otolaryngol 101:43, 1986

58. Molony TB: Decision making in vestibular neurectomy. Am J Otol 17:421, 1996

59. Tusa RJ: Diagnosis and management of neuro-otological disorders due to migraine. In Herdman SJ (ed): Vestibular Rehabilitation. Philadelphia: FA Davis, 1994

60. Peroutka SJ: The pharmacology of current anti-migraine drugs. Headache [Suppl] 30:5, 1990

61. Brandt T, Daroff RB: The multisensory physiological and pathological vertigo syndromes. Ann Neurol 7:195, 1980

62. Kuritzky A, Ziegler DK, Hassanein R: Vertigo, motion sickness and migraine. Headache 21:227, 1981

63. Kayan A, Hood JD: Neuro-otological manifestations of migraine. Brain 107:1123, 1984

64. Davis JR, Jennings RT, Beck BG et al: Treatment efficacy of intramuscular promethazine for space motion sickness. Aviat Space Environ Med 64:230, 1993

65. Pingree BJ, Pethybridge RJ: A comparison of the efficacy of cinnarizine with scopolamine in the treatment of seasickness. Aviat Space Environ Med 65:597, 1994

66. Jankovic J et al: Neurogenic orthostatic hypotension: A double-blind, placebo-controlled study with midodrine. Am J Med 95:38, 1993

67. Schweizer E, Rickels K, Weiss S et al: Maintenance drug treatment of panic disorder: I. Results of a prospective, placebo-controlled comparison of alprazolam and imipramine. Arch Gen Psychiatry 50:51, 1993

68. Fava GA, Zieezny M, Savron G et al: Long-term effects of behavioural treatment for panic disorder with agoraphobia. Br J Psychiatry 166:87, 1995

69. Nielsen JM: Tornado epilepsy simulating Ménière's syndrome. Neurology 9:794, 1959

70. Furman JMR, Crumrine PK, Reinmuth OM: Epileptic nystagmus. Ann Neurol 27:686, 1990

71. Kaplan PW, Tusa RJ: Neurophysiologic and clinical correlation of epileptic nystagmus. Neurology 43:2508, 1993

72. Tusa RJ, Kaplan PW, Hain TC: Ipsiversive eye deviation and epileptic nystagmus. Neurology 40:662, 1990

73. Grad A, Baloh RW: Vertigo of vascular origin. Arch Neurol 46:281, 1989

74. Gomez CR et al: Isolated vertigo as a manifestation of vertebrobasilar ischemia. Neurology 47:94, 1996

75. Schuknecht HF: Pathology of the Ear. Cambridge, UK: Harvard University Press, 1974

76. Brandt T: Vertigo: Its Multisensory Syndromes. London: Springer-Verlag, 1991

Subject Index

Page numbers in *italic* indicate figures.
Page numbers followed by "t" indicate tables.

A

Abdominal migraine, 570
Abducens nerve, anatomy, 406, 409
Abducens nucleus, horizontal gaze control
    and, 346
Abducens palsy, 409–413, 409t
    isolated, 411–413
Abduction deficits, causes of, 409t
    diagnostic studies for, 412t
Abiotrophies, retina, 97–99
Accommodation, 532
    disorders of, 548–549
Accommodative effort syndrome,
    pediatric, 483
Acetazolamide, transient myopia from,
    549
    treatment of intracranial hypertension,
    144
Acetylsalicylic acid, carotid atheromatous
    disease, dizziness, 636
Achiasma, nystagmus, 390–391
Achromacy, 15
Achromatopsia, cerebral, 262, 276. *See
    also* Rod, monochromatism
    pediatric, 464
Acoustic neuroma
    dizziness and, 639
    facial nerve, 311–312
    nystagmus, 390
Acoustically elicited eye movement, 53
Acquired immunodeficiency syndrome,
    152
    neuritis and, 152
    ocular flutter and, 394
    retinal disease and, 111
    Parinaud syndrome, 454
Acquired ocular motor apraxia, 271
Acromegaly, optic chiasm, 209–210
ACTH. *See* Adrenocorticotropic
    hormone

Acuity
    in alexia, 268
    definition, 10
    testing, 17
Acute zonal occult outer retinopathy, 96
Acyclovir, for herpes zoster, 70
Addison's disease
    with papilledema, intracranial pressure,
    143
    pseudotumor cerebri and, 145
Adenohypophysitis, lymphocytic, 232
    optic chiasm, 232
Adenoma, pituitary, 205–211
Adie's syndrome, (Tonic pupil syndrome)
    internal ophthalmoplegia and, 539
Adrenocorticotropic hormone, opsoclonus
    and, 394
Adrenoleukodystrophy, neonatal, 464
Afferent pupillary defect, relative, 21,
    533–536
Afferent visual symptoms, 2–4, 136
Afterimages, eye movement, 340–341
Agnosia, visual, 264–266
    apperceptive, 264
    associative, 264
Agraphia
    alexia without, 17
    literal alexia, 269
Aicardi's syndrome, 123
    optic disc, 123
    pediatric, 467
AIDS. *See* Acquired immunodeficiency
    syndrome
Akinetopsia, cerebral, 272–274
Albinism, nystagmus, 390–391
Alcohol
    elimination of, for Meniere's disease,
    642
    nystagmus induced by, 390
Alcohol amblyopia, 183–185
Alexander's law, 370, 381
    downbeat nystagmus, 386
Alexia
    acquired, 267–270

with agraphia, 269
Broca's aphasia, 269
Gerstmann's syndrome, 269
hemifield slide and, 269
literal, 269
pure, 267–268
secondary, 269
without agraphia, 17
Alice in Wonderland syndrome, in
    childhood migraine, 572
Alpha-blockers, dizziness, 636
Alternate cover test, diplopia, 56
Alzheimer's disease
    cerebral akinetopsia and, 272
    cerebrovisual loss and, 241
    motion sensitivity and, 47
    occipital cortex, 89
    pupil and, 542
    reading ability and, 270
Amaurosis
    congenital, Leber's, 97
    Leber's congenital, pediatric, 464
Amaurosis fugax, retinal arterial
    occlusion, 102, 103
    transient obscurations, diagnoses, 104t
Amblyopia, strabismic, 480
Amenorrhea, 206
Aminoglycosides, myasthenia-like
    symptoms with, 442
Amiodarone, dizziness from, 636
    optic neuropathy, 185
Amitriptyline, dizziness from, 636
    migraine therapy, 581
Aneurysm, 179–181, 589–598
    carotid siphon, 612–615
    in childhood, 596–597
    fusiform aneurysm, 597–598
        carotid system, 598
        vertebrobasilar system, 598
    headache and, 575
    saccular, 591–596
        anterior communicating artery, 596
        carotid-ophthalmic artery, 591–593
        carotid-supraclinoid, 593–594

Aneurysm (contd.)
  intracavernous carotid, 591
  middle cerebral artery, 595–596
  ophthalmic artery, 594
  posterior cerebral artery, 596
  posterior communicating artery,
    594–595
  vertebrobasilar system, 596
Anisocuviz, essential 538–539, 533t
Anterior ischemic optic neuropathy, 137,
  155–166
Antiarrythmics, dizziness from, 636
  optic neuropathy, 185
Antibiotics
  dizziness, 636
  myasthenia-like symptoms with, 442
  optic neuropathies, 185
Anticonvulsants
  dizziness from, 636
  hallucinations with, 278
  nystagmus induced by, 390
Antidepressants
  dizziness from, 636
  tricyclic, migraine, 582
Antihypertensive agents, dizziness, 636
Antiinflammatory drugs, dizziness, 636
Antiphospholipid antibody syndrome, 108
Anton's syndrome, 260
Aperiodic alternating nystagmus, 385
Aphasia
  Broca's, 269
  Wernicke's, 243
Apoplexy, pituitary, optic chiasm,
  210–211
Apperceptive agnosia, 264
Apraxia
  acquired ocular motor, 271
  congenital ocular motor, 477–478
  lid opening, 63, 322
  ocular motor, 361–362
Aqueductal stenosis, with papilledema,
  143
Arachnoid cyst, optic chiasm, 225–227
Argyll Robertson pupil, 536, 536–537
  characteristics of, 536t
Arnold-Chiari malformation
  divergence paralysis and, 413
  downbeat nystagmus and, 386
  nystagmus and, 384
Arterial dissection, carotid, 544, 544
Arterial occlusion, retina, 102–109
  Barlow's syndrome, 107
  carotid atheromatous disease, 102–107,
    104t
  chronic ocular hypoxia, 105
  factor V Leiden, 108

fibromuscular dysplasia, 107
  pulseless disease, 107
  transient obscuration of vision, 104t
  venous stasis retinopathy, 105
Arteriovenous fistula carotid-cavernous,
    605, 608
  orbit and, 504
Arteriovenous malformation, 598–605
Arteritis, cranial (giant-cell, temporal),
    162–166
  diplopia, 428t, 429
  headache, 573–574
  ischemic optic neuropathy, 160, 162,
    164
Associative agnosia, 264
Atenolol, dizziness, 636
Atheromatous disease of carotid, 102–107
Attentional dyslexia, 269
Audiometry, dizziness, 638
Aura
  migraine with, 555, 559t, 559–562
  migraine without, 558t, 558–559
  prolonged, migraine with, 562–570
Autoimmune vasculitis
  optic neuropathies, 151, 170
  retinal vasculitis and, 110
Automated static threshold perimetry,
    37–38
  visual field testing, 37–40
Automated visual field, blue-on-yellow
    stimulus, 42
Automated visual field interpretation,
    40–42
AZOOR. See Acute zonal occult outer
    retinopathy

B
B-complex vitamins
  dietary deficiency and optic neuropathy,
    183
Baclofen for periodic alternating
    nystagmus, 386
  withdrawal, visual hallucinations with,
    277
Bálint's syndrome, 270–272
  Gerstmann's syndrome and, 271
  optic ataxia, 270
  spatial disorder of attention, 270
Ballistic, defined, 402
Bandwidth, defined, 402
Barbiturates
  dizziness from, 636
  intoxication, with coma, 71, 73
  nystagmus induced by, 390
  ophthalmoplegia and, 454
Bardet-Biedl syndrome, 467

Barlow's syndrome, retinal artery
    occlusion and, 107
Bartonella, see Catscratch disease
Basal ganglia infarction, bilateral, 319
Basal ganglionic control, 355–363
Basilar artery, aneurysm, 596
  migraine, 569–570
Bassen-Kornzweig syndrome, 449
  in child, 467
Batten-Mayou syndrome, 101
Battle's sign, with temporal bone fracture,
    312
Bee sting, and optic neuropathy, 15
Behçet's disease
  retinal vasculitis and, 110, 111t
Behr's syndrome, 127
  optic atrophy and, 127, 128
Bell's palsy, 58–59, 306–307, 315–317
Benedikt syndrome, fascicular lesions,
    417–418
Benign paroxysmal positional nystagmus,
    640
Benton Facial Recognition Test, 265
Beta-blockers
  dizziness, 636
  migraine, 582
Bielschowsky-Jansky disorder, 101
Bjerrum's scotoma, 206
Blepharospasm, 319
  botulinum, use of, 319–320
  Huntington's chorea, 318
  Meige's syndrome, 318
  Parkinson's disease, 318
Blindness
  cerebral, 245
    pediatric, 259
      causes of, 260t
    transient, 259
      causes of, 259t
    post-traumatic, 259
  cortical, 245
  infant, 464–467
  monocular, transient, 96, 103, 104t, 105
  night
    congenital stationary, 464
Blindsight, residual vision, 260
Blindspot syndromes, 99–100
Blink reflex, facial nerve, 304–305
Blurred vision, symptoms, 16
Bobbing, ocular, 396
Bonnet-de Chaume-Blanc syndrome, 619
Borreliosis. See Lyme disease
Botulinum
  blepharospasm and, 319–320
  myasthenia-like symptoms with, 442
Botulism, facial nerve, 314–315

Brainstem
  auditory-evoked response, dizziness,
      638–639
  control, vergence eye movements,
      352–353
    disorders, 353
      divergence paresis, paralysis, 353
      motor commands, 352–353
      paramedian pontine reticular
          formation (PPRF), 346, 347,
          348, 354
      spasm of near reflex, 353
Broca's aphasia, 269
Bromocriptine, and prolactinoma, 206
Brown tendon sheath syndrome, 475–476
  after orbital trauma, 416
  collagen vascular disease and, 416
  hypogammaglobulinemia and, 416
  juvenile rheumatoid arthritis and, 416
  systemic lupus erythematosus and, 416
Brucellosis, with papilledema, 143
Bulbar polyneuritis, *424*
  facial palsy, 306
  ophthalmoplegia, 423–425
Bupropion, visual hallucinations with,
      277
Burns, thermal, and optic neuropathy, 188

C
Cafergot. *See* Migraine, therapy
Caffein, elimination of, for Meniere's
      disease, 642
Calcium antagonists, dizziness, 636
Calcium channel blockers, migraine,
      581–582
Caloric nystagmus, 388
Caloric test, dizziness, 638
Capgrass syndrome, palinopsia and, 276
Carbamazepine, dizziness from, 636
  treatment of facial pain, 573
  hemifacial spasm, 320
  ocular neuromyotonia, 452
  migraine, 581t
Carcinoma associated retinopathy, 112
  optic neuropathy and, 175
Cardiac glycosides
  ocular symptoms of, 112
  retina, 112
Carotid artery atheromatous disease,
      102–107, 104t
  dissection headache, 576
  endarterectomy, 106
Carotid-cavernous sinus fistula, 605–608
Carpal tunnel syndrome, acromegaly and,
      209
Cat-scratch disease, optic neuropathy, 153

Cavernous angioma of retina and brain,
      620–622
Cavernous malformation, 605
Cavernous sinus
  anatomy, *408, 431, 432*
  aneurysms, 430–433. *See also*
      Aneurysm, carotid siphon
  lesions, 420, 428t
  ophthalmoplegia, 427
  parasellar syndromes, 430
  Tolosa-Hunt, 429
Central scotoma
  Uhthoff's phenomenon, 3
  visual acuity testing, 18
Central scotoma syndromes, 185–187
Cerebellar migraine, 570
Cerebellar vermis hypoplasia. *See* Joubert
      syndrome
Cerebellopontine angle, facial nerve,
      anatomy, 301
Cerebellum
  eye movement and, 353–355
  lesions
    effects of, 354
    ocular motor disorders caused by,
        353t
  vascular syndromes of, 354–355
Cerebral achromatopsia, 262, 276
  akinetopsia, 272–274
  Alzheimer's disease and, 272, 273
  blindness, 245
  causes, 240–241
  cortical blindness, usage of term, 245
  pediatric, 259
    causes of, 260t
  transient, 259
    causes of, 259t
    post-traumatic, 259
  dyschromatopsia, 262
  macropsia, 281
  metamorphopsia, 282
  micropsia, 281
  migraine, 562–565
  polyopia, 276
Cerebral visual loss, 239–241. *See also*
      Cerebral blindness
  Alzheimer's disease, 241
  cerebrovascular disease, 240–241
Ceroid lipofuscinoses, 101, 464
Cervical nystagmus, 387
Chapman Speed of Reading Test, *265*
Charcot-Marie-Tooth disease, 135, 136
Charles Bonnet syndrome, 277–278
Chemotherapeutics, dizziness and, 636
  optic neuropathy, 185
Cherry-red spot, *100,* 101t

gangliosidoses, 100
  myoclonus syndrome, 102
Chiasm. *See* Optic chiasm
Chickenpox
  facial nerve, 311
  optic neuritis and, 151
Child. *See also* Pediatrics
  blindness, 464–467
  aneurysm, 596–597
  dizziness, 641
  examination of eye movement, 53
  examination of visual acuity, 462–467,
      461, 463t
  examination of visual field, 27–29, *30*
  migraine in, 572–573
    Alice in Wonderland syndrome, 572
  oculomotor palsies of, 426
  proptosis in, *492*
Childhood, acquired visual loss in, 467
Chlordiazepoxide, dizziness and, 636
Chorio-retinal inflammations, 99–100
Choroidal infarction, intraoperative globe
      compression and, 168
Choroidal ischemia, cranial arteritis and,
      163
Circular nystagmus, 387
Cisplatin
  dizziness and, 636
  optic neuropathy, 185
Claudication, jaw, cranial arteritis and, 165
Closed-loop system, defined, 402
Cluster headache, 570–572, 571t
Cocaine, test for Horner syndrome, 533t,
      543
  visual hallucinations with, 277
Cogan's lid twitch, myasthenia with, 439
Colitis, ulcerative, retina, 110
Collagen vascular disease. *See also*
      Vasculitis
Brown's syndrome and, 416
  optic neuritis and, 15
  retinal artery occlusion, 108
Collicular-burst neurons, superior
      colliculus, 358
Colloid cyst, optic chiasm, 225
Colobomas, optic disc, 121–123
Color comparison, visual field testing,
      31–32
Color vision, 14–15, 20–21
  achromacy, 15
  anomaloscope, 14
  cerebral defects, 262, 267
  deutan defect, 15
  dyschromatopsias, 14
  Farnsworth-Munsell 100-hue test, 21
  Hardy-Rand-Rittler, color plates, 20

Color vision (*contd.*)
  optic nerve disease and, 137
  protan defect, 15
  symptoms, 16
  trichromacy, 14
  tritan defect, 15
  dominant optic atrophy and, 130, *131*
Coma, 70–73
  barbiturate intoxication, 71, 73
  examination, 70
  Hutchinson's pupil, 70
  ocular signs in, 70–72, 72t, *71*
Comitance, spread of, 57
  diplopia and, 57
Compazine, transient myopia from, 549
Complicated migraine. *See* Migraine
Cone retinal
  anatomy, 8–9
  and color vision, 14
  degeneration, progressive, 99
  dystrophies, 97–99
Confrontation visual field testing, 27–28
Congenital gaze palsy, 361
Conjugate gaze, 52
  spasticity, 58–59
Constricted visual field, with retained
      acuity, 97t
Continuous, defined, 402
Contraceptives, pseudotumor cerebri and,
      145
Contrast, defined, 12
Contrast sensitivity, 12–13, *13, 19*, 19–20,
      261
  optic neuritis, 20
  Pelli-Robinson chart, 19
  Regan, Neima acuity charts, 19
  sine wave grating, 13, 19
  Vistech wall chart, 20
Control system, defined, 402
Convergence, 52–53
Convergence-accommodative micropsia,
      281
Convergence/convergence-evoked
      nystagmus, 385
Convergence insufficiencies, 353
  pediatric, 482–483
Convergence nystagmus, 385
Convergence spasm, 353
  abduction defects, 409
  pupils and, 548, *549*
Corneal reflexes, 67–68, 341
Corneal sensation, 64, 67, 67t
Corneo-mandibular reflex, 6
Corrective eye movements, 336–337
Cortex, occipital, anatomy, 85–86 *86, 87,*
      90

  vascular supply, 91–92, *91.*
    See also Cerebral visual loss; Visual
        cortex
Cortical blindness, usage of term, 245
Cortical function, higher, 239–290
Corticosteroids
  lid retraction and, 61, *62*
  in treatment of
    cranial arteritis, 166
    optic neuritis, 150, 169
    optic neuropathy, traumatic, 188
    orbital inflammations, 428, 501
    pseudotumor cerebri, 144
    sarcoidosis, 154, 225, 455
    Tolosa-Hunt syndrome, 429
    trigeminal neuralgia, herpes, 70
Cough headache, 574
Cover test, for diplopia 55, *56*
Cranial arteritis, 162–166
  diplopia in, 429
  headache in, 573
Cranial nerves, anatomy, *408, 431, 432.*
    See also specific nerves, i.e., facial
Craniopharyngioma, 215–218, *217,*
      215,
  age distribution, 215
Craniostenosis, with papilledema, 143
C-reactive protein, arteritis and, 165
Crescents, optic disc, 123, *122*
  field defects, *125*
Creutzfeldt-Jakob disease
  cerebrovisual loss and, 241
  myoclonus, 395
  rebound nystagmus and, 387
Crocodile tears. *See* Gustatory tearing
Cryptococcosis, central nervous system
      infection with, 152, *157* 436
Cyclic oculomotor palsy, 426–427
Cyclobenzaprine, dizziness and, 636
Cyclopean eye, defined, 402
Cyst
  arachnoid, 225–227
  colloid, 225
  epithelial, 225–227
  Rathke's, cleft, 226
  Rathke's pouch, 225
Cytomegalovirus, retina, 110, 111
  optic nerve, 152

D

Damped, damping, defined, 402
Danazol, pseudotumor cerebri and, 143
Dandy-Walker cyst, 123
de Morsier's syndrome. *See* Septo-optic
      dysplasia
Delayed maturation of vision, 467

Demyelinative disease, optic nerve, 150.
    See also Multiple sclerosis
  chiasm, 222–225
Dermatomyositis
  retinal vasculitis and, 110
Devic's disease, 223
  optic nerve, 151
  optic chiasm, 223
D. H. E. *See* Migraine, therapy
Diabetes mellitus and ischemic optic
      neuropathy, 15
  and optic atrophy, 128
  and optic nerve hypoplasia, 119
  papillopathy, 166–167
Diabetic oculomotor palsy, 420–421
Diaschisis, cerebral, 602
Diamox. *See* Acetazolamide
Diazepam, dizziness and, 636
Differentiation, defined, 402
Diphtheria, facial nerve, 311
Diplopia, 55–58
  after ocular surgery, 454–455
  alternate cover test, 56
  esotropia, 56
  examination, 55–58
  forced duction test, 57
  Hering's law, 56
  Maddox rod, 56
  monocular, 55
  polyopia, 55
  cerebral, 276
  spread of comitance, 57
Dipping (bobbing), ocular, 396
Disc, optic
  anatomy, 77
  dysplasia, congenital, 118–127
    aberrant myelination, 119, *122*
    Aicardi's syndrome, 123
    colobomas, 121–123, *122*
      Dandy-Walker cyst and, 123
    disc elevations, 124–127
    dysversions, 123, *122*
    hyaline bodies (drosen), 124
      field defects with, *126*
    nerve hypoplasia, 119–121
      septo-optic dysplasia, 121
      true aplasia, 121
    pseudoneuritis, 124
    pseudopapilledema, 124
    retro-bulbar arachnoid cysts, 123
  masses, 172
  swollen
    diagnosis, 138–139
    etiology, 138t
Discontinuous, defined, 402
Discrete, defined, 402

Disequilibrium, 634, 641–642. *See also* Dizziness
Displacement, defined, 402
Dissociated nystagmus, 384
Diuretics
  dizziness from, 636
  for Meniere's disease, 642
Divergence paralysis, 353
  Arnold-Chiari malformation and, 413
Dizziness (vertigo)
  acetylsalicylic acid, 636
  acoustic neuroma, 639
  alpha-blockers, 636
  amiodarone, 636
  amitriptyline, 636
  antiarrythmics, 636
  antibiotics, 636
  anticonvulsants, 636
  antidepressants, 636
  antihypertensive agents, 636
  antiinflammatory drugs, 636
  atenolol, 636
  audiometry, 638
  barbiturates, 636
  beta-blockers, 636
  brainstem auditory-evoked response, 638–639
  calcium antagonists, 636
  caloric test, 638
  carbamazepine, 636
  chemotherapeutics, 636
  in children, 641
  chlordiazepoxide, 636
  cisplatin, 636
  clinical assessment, 633–639
  Coumadin, 644
  cyclobenzaprine, 636
  diazepam, 636
  disequilibrium, 641–642
  diuretics, 636
  drug-induced, 636t
  electronystagmography, 638
  ethacrynic acid, 636
  ethosuximide, 636
  flurazepam, 636
  Fukuda stepping test, 638
  furosemide, 636
  gait, 637–638
  gentamicin, 636
  Hallpike-Dix maneuver, *641*
  head trauma, 642
  hydrochlorothiazide, 636
  hyperventilation and, 643
  hypnotics, 636
  ibuprofen, 636
  imipramine, 636

  indomethacin, 636
  labyrinthitis, 639–640
  management, 639–644
  meclizine, 636
  with medications, 635
  Menière's disease, 642–643
  meprobamate, 636
  methocarbamol, 636
  migraine, 643
  motion sickness, 643
  muscle relaxants, 636
  neuroimaging, 639
    computed tomography, 639
    magnetic resonance imaging, 639
  nifedipine, 636
  nystagmus, 635–637
  office examination, 635–638
  orphenidrine, 636
  orthostatic hypotension, 643
  otolinks, 633
    vestibular system, 633
  overview, 629–631
  panic attacks, 643
  paroxysmal positional vertigo, benign, 640
  pathophysiology, 631–633
  patient history, 633–634
    tempo, 634
      attack frequency, 634
      more than 3 days, 634
  perilymphatic fistula, 643–644
  peripheral structures, 631–632
  phenytoin, 636
  posturography, 638
  propranolol, 636
  prozosine, 636
  quinine, 636
  reflexes, 631t
    normal, 629–631
  Romberg test, 637, 638
  rotary chair, 638
  scopolamine, 636
  seizures, 644
  semicircular canals, 632–633
  smooth pursuit vestibulo-ocular reflex cancellation, 635
  stance, 637–638
  streptomycin, 636
  symptoms, 634t, 634–635
    disequilibrium, 634
    floating, 634
    light-headedness, 634
    oscillopsia, 634–635
    rocking, 634
    spinning, 634
    swimming, 634

  vertigo, 634
  terosine, 636
  tobramycin, 636
  tranquillizers, 636
  transient ischemic attacks, 644
  triazolam, 636
  verapamil, 636
  vestibular neuritis, 639–640
  vestibular suppressants, 636
  vestibulo-ocular reflex, 635
  Warfarin, 644
Doll's head phenomenon, in infant, 53
Dolichoectasia, and optic neuropathy, 17, *18*
Dorsal midbrain syndrome (Parinaud), 60, 53, 351, 452–454, *453*
Double elevator palsy, in child, 473
Double saccadic pulses, 394
Downbeat nystagmus, 386–387
  Alexander's law, 386
  Arnold-Chiari malformation, 386
  spinocerebellar degeneration, 386
Downgaze palsy, 351
Drugs
  accidents with, pupil, 546–547
  dizziness from, 636t
  for migraine, 578t
  nystagmus from, 390
  optic nerve and, 185
Drusem of disc. *See* Hyaline bodies
Dry eye syndrome, 68
  with facial palsy, 323
Duane syndrome, pediatric, 468–471, 474
Dural arteriovenous malformation and carotid-cavernous fistula, 609–612
Dyschromatopsia, 14
  cerebral, 262
Dysdiadocokinesia, 272
Dysgerminomas, optic chiasm, 222
Dyslexia
  attentional, 269
  central, 269–270
  deep, 270
  hemianopic, 269
  neglect, 269
  pediatric, 478
  phonologic, 270
  surface, 270
Dysmetria, 394
Dysmetropsia, 281–282
  macropsia, 281
    cerebral, 281
    retinal, 281
  metamorphopsia, 282
    cerebral, 282
    retinal, 282

Dysmetropsia (*contd.*)
micropsia, 281
cerebral, 281
convergence-accommodative, 281
retinal, 281
Dysthyroidism. *See also* Graves' disease, 442–446, 500, 517
lid retraction, 60, *61, 494, 495*
optic neuropathy, 178, *181*
surgery for, 518–520
myasthenia with, 437

E

Eale's disease, 110
Ear infections, facial nerve and, 310–311
Eaton-Lambert syndrome, 442
Echography. *See* Ultrasonography
Edrophonium chloride (Tensilon) test. *See* Myasthenia
Ehler-Danlos syndrome, 107
Electro-oculography, 342
Electromagnetic search coil, 342
Electromyography, ocular, 343
Electronystagmography, dizziness, 638
Electrophysiology tests, 42–47
dark adaptation, 46–47
Electroretinography, 15, 42–45
focal electroretinography, 43–44
standard electroretinography, 43
Elevator deficiencies, pediatric, 472–474
Elliptic nystagmus, 387
Embolization, retinal artery, 102–105, *103*
Embolization, endovascular procedures, 609–615
Embolization of tumors of cavernous sinus, 615
Empty sella syndrome, 233–234, *232, 233*
cyclic, pediatric, 482
Encephaloceles, basal, and disc colobomas, 123
Encephalomyelitis, acute disseminated (ADEM), and optic neoritis, 151
Encephalotrigeminal angiomatosis (Sturge-Weber), 112, 617–619, *617, 618, 619*
Endarterectomy, carotid, 106
End-point nystagmus, 383
Enophthalmus, 495, 496t, *497*
Entero-vioform, optic neuropathy, 185
Enterovirus, polyneuropathy, 436
Entoptic phenomena, 2
EOG. *See* Electro-oculograph
Epithelial cysts, and chiasm, 225–227
ERG. *See* Electroretinography
Ergostat, etc. *See* Migraine, therapy
Erythema migrans, Lyme disease and, 152

Erythrocyte sedimentation rate (ESR), 165, 163t
Esotropia, 56. *See also* Abduction deficits
ESR. *See* Erythrocyte sedimentation rate
Esthesioneuroblastoma, paranasal sinus disease and, 178
Ethacrynic acid
disequilibrium from, 635
dizziness and, 636
Ethambutol hydrochloride (Myambutol), optic neuropathy and, 185, 181t, *186*
Ethosuximide, dizziness from, 636
Examination, visual sensory system, 7–49
Exophthalmos (Proptosis), 494–496
Exophthalmometry, *495*
Exotropia, 56
pediatric, 479
Exponential, defined, 402
Extrageniculate visual systems, 88–89
Extrapyramidal system, facial nerve, anatomy, 299–301
Eye movement, 327–343
acoustically elicited, 53
anatomy and, 340
bilateral, bilateral, yoked, independent control, 340
unilateral, bilateral, yoked control, 340
brain stem control, 346
lesions, 346
characteristics, 340t
classifications, 329t
corrective movements, 336–337
diplopia, tests, 55–58
examination, clinical, 51–59
fast, 329–333
fixation, 334
functional classes of, 346t
horizontal gaze, 346
infranuclear disorders, 405–460
abducens palsy, 409
isolated, 411–413
abduction deficits, causes of, 409t
isolated, diagnostic studies for, 412t
Brown's syndrome, 416
cavernous sinus lesions, 420, 420t.
See also Cavernous sinus
childhood, oculomotor palsies of, 426
cranial nerve palsies, with human immunodeficiency virus infection, 436t
cyclic oculomotor palsy, 426–427
diabetic oculomotor palsy, 420–421

diplopia, after ocular surgery, 454–455
dorsal midbrain syndrome, 452–454
dysthyroidism, 442–446
etiology, 409–411
fascicular lesions, 417–418
Graves' disease, 442–446, *443, 444*
hemorrhage, in ocular muscles, 455
herpes zoster, 423
infectious polyneuropathy
acute, 423–425
bulbar polyneuritis, *424*
Fisher's syndrome, 424
Guillain-Barré syndrome, 424
interpeduncular lesions, 418–420
Parasellar syndrome, 420
ischemic oculomotor palsy, 420–421
Kearns-Sayre-Daroff syndrome, 446, 446t
lymphoma, non-Hodgkin's, 455
mitochondrial disease, 449t
myasthenia, 437–442, 63, *60, 438, 440*
edrophonium (Tensilon) test, 63
myasthenia-like syndromes, 442
myositis, orbital, 455
myotonic dystrophy, 451–452
ocular signs of, 452t
neuroanatomy, 405–409
neuromuscular junction, disorders of, 437t, 437–455
non-Hodgkin's lymphoma, 455
nuclear lesions, 416–417
ocular motor palsies, painful ophthalmoplegias, combined, 427
ocular neuromyotonia, 452
oculomotor palsy, 416
causes of, 417t
of childhood, 426
cyclic, 426–427
oculomotor synkinesis, 422–423
ophthalmoplegia, external, progressive, 446–450
conditions simulating, 450–451
ophthalmoplegic migraine, 425–426
orbital lesions, 420, 427–429
orbital myositis, 455
pain, ophthalmoplegia syndromes, 428t
parasellar syndromes, 430–436
polyneuritis, bulbar, *424*
polyneuropathy, infectious, acute, 423–425
progressive external ophthalmoplegia, 446, *447*

sixth nerve palsies, causes of, 409t
superior oblique paresis, causes of, 415t
thyroid gland, autonomous, 445
thyroid-related myopathy, 442–446
thyrotropin-releasing hormone, 445–446
Tolosa-Hunt syndrome, 429–430
trochlear palsies, 413–416
internal monitor, 336
micromovements, 339–340
near triad, 338–339
optokinetic reflex, 335–336
parasellar syndromes, 420
physiologic organization, 327–329
plasticity, 332–333
pursuit, 333
recording techniques, 340–343
  afterimages, 340–341
  contact lens, 342
  corneal reflection, 341
  electro-oculography, 342
  electromagnetic search coil, 342
  mechanical transducers, 341
  ocular electromyography, 343
  photoelectric oculography, 342
  photography, 341
  video, 342–343
slow, 333–336
subsystem synergism, 337
supranuclear disorders, 345–368
  brain stem, saccade circuits, cortical projections, 357–358
  caudate nucleus, saccade, 358
  cerebellar influences, 353–355
  cerebellum
    lesions, 354, 353t
    vascular syndromes of, 354–355
  cerebral control, eye movements, 355–363
  collicular-burst neurons, 358
  colliculus, superior, 358–359
  frontal eye fields, saccade generation, 357
  frontoparietal lesions, acute, bilateral, ocular motor apraxia, 361–362
  gaze
    functional disturbances of, 363
    holding, 360
  hemispheric lesions, unilateral, disturbances of gaze with, 360–361
  horizontal gaze, brain stem control, 346–349, 347
    internuclear ophthalmoplegia, 346, 347, 348t, 406, 408

internuclear ophthalmoplegia, causes of, 348t
MLF, 346, 405, 406, 407
medulla, lesions, horizontal gaze and, 346–349
motor commands, conjugate horizontal movements, 346
pons, lesions, horizontal gaze and, 346–349
saccades, slow, causes of, 347t
Huntington disease, 363
oculomotor apraxia, congenital, 361
paramedian pontine reticular formation (PPRF) 346, 347, 348, 354
parietal eye fields, saccade generation, 356
Parkinson disease, 362–363
prefrontal cortex, dorsolateral, saccade generation, 357
pursuit system, 359–360
riMLF, 349, 349, 350, 354
saccade
  generation, cortical areas, 355–357
  role, 355
saccadic palsy, congenital, 361
saccadic system, 355–357
substantia nigra pars reticulata, 358
supplemental eye fields, saccade generation, 357
torsional movements, brain stem connections, 349–352
vergence eye movements, brain stem control, 352–353
  disorders, 353
  divergence paresis, paralysis, 353
  motor commands, 352–353
  spasm of near reflex, see also convergence spasm, 353
vertical movements, brain stem connections, 349–352
  dorsal midbrain syndrome, 351
  midbrain lesions, 350
  skew deviation, 351
  supranuclear palsy, progressive, 351–352
  sustained vertical deviations, 350–351
vestibulo-ocular system, 360
Wallenberg syndrome, 354
vestibulo-ocular reflex, 334–335
visual-vestibulo-ocular response, 336
visually elicited, for visual field testing, 29
Eyelid, 59–63
apraxia of lid opening, 63

Cogan's lid twitch, 439
compensatory unilateral lid retraction, 59
edrophonium chloride (Tensilon), test, for myasthenia 63, 60, 438, 440
Graves' disease, 59, 60
Horner's syndrome, 62
lagophthalmos, 63
Müller's muscle, 59
Marcus-Gunn phenomenon, 61
myokymia, benign, 4, 320
myopathic ptosis, 63
neuroanatomy, 59–60
nystagmus, 63, 388
  astrocytoma, 388
  lateral medullary syndrome, 388
  Pick's sign, 63
opening, 322
Parinaud's syndrome, 60
physiology, 59–60
ptosis, 61–63
retraction, 59–61, 493

F

Face perception, anterograde prosopagnosia, 267
Facial embryopathies, 317, 316, 318t, 318
Facial hemiatrophy (Parry-Romberg), 315
Facial myokymia, 321–322
Facial nerve, blood supply, 302–304
  Guillain-Barré syndrome and, 321
Facial nerve, 293–326
  anatomy, 295–304, 296–297t
    blood supply, 302–304
    cerebellopontine angle, 301
    cortex, 295–299
    extracranial segment, 302
    extrapyramidal system, 299–301
    pons, 301
    supranuclear pathway, 295–299
    temporal bone, 301–302
  assessment, 304–306
  atrophy (hemiatrophy), 315
  blepharospasm, 321, 319
  botulism, 314–315
  childhood palsies, 317
  embryology, 293–295, 294t
    anomalies, 295
    extramedullary segment, 294
    intramedullary segment, 294
    intratemporal segment, 294–295
  embryopathies, 317, 317t
  facial myokymia, 321–322
  facial synkinesis, 320–321
  function, 304–306
    blink reflex, 304–305

Facial nerve, function (*contd.*)
  idiopathic facial palsy, 306–307
  motor evaluation, 304
  physiologic facial synkinesis,
    305–306
  taste, 304
  tear function, 304
Guillain-Barré syndrome, 308, 315
gustatory sweating, 321
gustatory tearing, 321
hemifacial spasm, 319–320, *320*
Huntington's chorea, 319
hyperkinetic facial disorders, 317–322
idiopathic palsy, 315
immune-mediated neuropathies,
  307–308
infectious disorders, 307–308
  chickenpox, 311
  diphtheria, 311
  ear infections, 310–311
  encephalitis, brain stem, 311
  enterovirus, 311
  herpes zoster cephalicus, 307–308,
    308
  infectious mononucleosis, 309
  influenza, 311
  leprosy, 311
  Lyme disease, 309–310
  mucormycosis, 311
  mumps, 311
  polio, 311
  polyradiculopathy, 308–311
  syphilis, 311
  tetanus, 311
  tuberculosis, 311
leukemia, 315
lid opening, 322
  apraxia of, 322
Lyme disease, 315
Meige's syndrome, 319
Melkerson-Rosenthal syndrome, 316,
  316
meningeal carcinomatosis, 315
Mobius' syndrome, 315, *318*
myasthenia gravis, 314, 315
myotonic dystrophy, 315
paresis, bilateral, 315–317
Parkinson's disease, 319
polio and, 315
porphyria, 315
porphyrias, acute, 314
postencephalitic parkinsonism, 319
progressive hemifacial atrophy, 315
sarcoidosis, 314, 315
skull fracture and, 315
Todd's paralysis, 319

trauma, 311
tumor, 311–314
  acoustic neuroma, 311–312
  facial neuroma, 312–313
  metastatic lesions, 313–314
Facial neuroma, 312–313
Facial pain, 573
  atypical, 69–70
Facial palsy. *See also* Facial nerve
  idiopathic, 306–307
  management of, 323–324
Facial synkinesis, 305–306, 320–321
  Bell's phenomenon, 304–306
  jaw-winking phenomenon,
    distinguishing, 321
Factitious fields
  hysteria, 36
  malingering, 36
  visual field testing, 36
Factor V Leiden, 108
False aneurysm, following blunt head
  injury, 597
Familial fibrosis syndrome, pediatric,
  476
Farnsworth-Munsell 100-hue test, 21
Fast eye movement, 329–333
Feedback
  defined, 402
  negative, defined, 402
  positive, defined, 402
Fibromuscular dysplasia, retinal artery
  occlusions and, 107
Fibrosis syndrome, pediatric, 476
Finger counting, visual field testing, 29
Finger mimicking, visual field testing,
  29
Fisher syndrome, 424
  facial palsy, 308
  infectious polyneuropathy, 424–425
  ophthalmoplegia, 427
Fistula, arterio-venous. *See also* Carotid-
  cavernous sinus fistula
  perilymphatic, dizziness and, 643–644
Fixation, visual, 51–52, 334
  losses, visual field testing, 40
Fixational eye movements, 52
Flurazepam, dizziness and, 636
Flutter, ocular, 394
  dysmetria, 394
  pediatric, 478
Folate deficiency, optic neuropathy and,
  183
Forced duction test, 57
Form recognition, 261
Foster Kennedy syndrome, 140
Four Diopter Base-out test, 23

Foveate (foveation, refoveation), defined,
  402
Foveation reflex, 29
Foville's syndrome, 301
Fragile X syndrome, myotonic dystrophy
  and, 451
Frequency, defined, 402
Frey syndrome (Gustatory sweating), 321,
  422
Friedreich's ataxia, 97
  neurodegeneration and, 135
Fukuda stepping test, dizziness, 638
Furosemide
  dizziness and, 636
  treatment of pseudotumor cerebri,
    144
Fusiform aneurysm, 597–598
  carotid system, 598
  vertebrobasilar system, 598
Fusional mechanism failure, 480–482
  acquired central defects, 480–481
  congenital anomalies, 481
  convergence insufficiency, 481
  microtropia, 481

G
Gain, defined, 402
Gait, dizziness and, 637–638
Galactorrhea, 206
  treatment of CMV, 111
Gancyclovir, visual hallucinations with,
  277
Ganglion cells, retinal, 8
Gaze palsy, congenital, 361
Generator, defined, 402
Geniculate nucleus, lateral
  anatomy, 83–85
  lesions, 242–243
Geniculocalcarine radiations. *See* Optic
  radiation
Gentamicin
  disequilibrium from, 635
  dizziness and, 636
Germ cell tumor, optic chiasm, 222
Germinoma, optic chiasm, 222
Gerstmann's syndrome
  agraphia with, 269
  Balint's syndrome and, 271
Geshwin's syndrome, occipital cortex, 88
Ghost image, 16
Giant-cell arteritis. *See* Cranial arteritis
Giant cell myocarditis, 455
Glaucoma
  angle-closure, pain, 3
  motion sensitivity and, 47
  optic nerve, 169

Glioblastoma
multiforme, malignant, optic chiasm, 227
of visual pathway, malignant, 221
Glioma
anterior visual pathway, pediatric, 467
optic chiasm, 218–222
optic nerve, 172
visual pathway, malignant, 221
Glioma, in child, 467
Glissade. See Eye movement
Globe pulsation, causes, 496t
Glue-sniffing, nystagmus induced by, 390
Glycosides, cardiac, retina, 112
Goldenhar's syndrome, 123
in child, 471
Goldmann kinetic perimetry, visual field testing, 36–37
Gonadotropic hormone deficiency, craniopharyngioma and, 215–216
Goodpasture's syndrome
retinal vasculitis and, 110
Gradenigo syndrome, 308, 410
Granulomas, of ocular muscles, therapy, 45
lethal midline. See Wegener syndrome
Graphs
contrast sensitivity, 19
in visual field testing, 40
Graves' disease, 178–179, 442–446, 443, 444, 494, 517–520, 510
vs. abducens palsy, 411
clinical features, 517–518
diagnosis, 500–501, 506
eyelid, 59, 60
lid malposition, 519–520
orbital decompression, 518–519
orbital resistance in, 427
ptosis with, 493
vs. trochlear palsy, 413
verticle deviation and, 416
Gray-scale symbols, in visual field testing, 40
Growth hormone
acromegaly and, 209
visceromegaly and, 209
Guillain-Barré syndrome, 308–311, 424
facial myokymia and, 321
facial nerve paresis and, 316
infectious polyneuropathy, 423, 424
optic neuritis and, 151
papilledema, 143
verticle deviation and, 416
Gustatory sweating, 321, 422
Gustatory tearing, 321
parasympathetic fibers and, 303

H

Hallerman-Streiff syndrome, 62
Hallpike-Dix maneuver, dizziness, 641
Hallucinations, 3
migrainous, 279–280
peduncular, 280–281
release, 277–278, 278
visual, 276–281
Hallucinogens, palinopsia and, 276
Hamartoma, 112–114
Klippel-Trenaunay-Weber syndrome, 112
neurofibromatosis, 114
phakomatoses, 113
retina, congenital, 112–114
neurofibromatosis, 114
tuberous sclerosis, 113–114
Sturge-Weber disease, 112
tuberous sclerosis, 113–114
von Hippel-Lindau disease, 112
Hand comparison, visual field testing, 29–31
Hardy-Rand-Rittler, color plates, 20
Hashimoto's thyroiditis, and Tolosa-Hunt syndrome, 430
Head-rest syndrome, optic neuropathy and, 168
Head trauma, dizziness and, 642
Headache
aneurysm, 575
arteriovenous malformation, 575
carotid dissection, 576
classification of, 554t
cluster, 570–572, 571t
cough headache, 574
cranial arteritis, 573–574
facial pain, 573
intracranial mass lesions, 574
migraine without, 570
muscle contraction, 574–575
ocular headache, 575–576
pediatric, 479
migraine, 479
post-traumatic headache, 575
posterior fossa tumor headache, 574
supratentorial headache, 574
tension, 574
trigeminal neuralgia, 573
Headache phase, of migraine, 555, 556
Heimann-Bielschowsky phenomenon, 477
Hemiachromatopsia, 262
Hemialexias, 268–269
Hemianopic dyslexia, 269
Hemianopia, 17. See also Cerebral visual loss

Hemianopia(s)
anatomic considerations, 25
lateral geniculate and, 243
migraine aura, 559, 564
optic chiasm. See Optic chaism
optic radiations and, 243, 251, 252, 253
optic tracts and, 241, 247
striate cortex and, 244, 254, 257, 258
symptoms, 17, 17
visual field tests, 29–36, 31, 33, 35, 37
Hemicrania, usage of term, 553
Hemidyschromatopsia, 262
Hemifacial atrophy, progressive, 315
Hemifacial spasm, 319–320
Hemifield slide, with chiasmal syndrome, 269, 482
Hemophilia, with papilledema, 143
Heredodegenerations, retina, 97–99. See also Optic nerve
Hering's law, 56, 439
Herpes, facial palsy and, 307
Herpes zoster, 5, 69, 423
acyclovir, 70
cephalicus, 295
facial nerve, 307–308, 308
optic neuritis and, 151, 158
Hertel exophthalmometer, use of, 495
Hertz. See Frequency, defined
Hex A defiency, 100
High gain instability, nystagmus, 370
Hippus, pupil, 527
HIV. See Human immunodeficiency virus
Homonymous hemianopia. See Hemianopia
Hooper Visual Organization Test, 266
Horizontal gaze
brain stem control, 346–349
Horizontal jerk nystagmus, 381–383
gaze-evoked nystagmus, 382–383
vestibular, 381–382
Horner's syndrome (oculosympathetic defects), 62, 70, 107, 301, 420, 542–546, 533t, 542
interpeduncular lesions, 419
pharmacologic tests, 543
sixth nerve palsy and, 410, 544, 545
sympathetic pathways, 531, 531
Human immunodeficiency virus, 152
cranial nerve palsy, 436t
facial palsy and, 307
optic neuritis and, 152
retina, 111
Humphrey Visual Field Analyser, 37–38
Huntington disease, 363
blepharospasm and, 318
choxea, 318

Hutchinson's pupil, 70
Hyaline bodies Drusenul of disc, optic
    disc, 124, *126, 127*
Hydrocephalus, 60
    optic chiasm, 232
Hydrochlorothiazide, dizziness and, 636
Hyperacuity
    measurement of, 12
    Vernier alignment, 12
Hyperglycemia, palinopsia and, 276
Hyperhidrosis, acromegaly and, 209
Hyperkinetic facial disorders, 317–322
Hyperprolactinemia
    causes of, 206
    empty sella syndrome and, 234
Hypertension
    intracranial, idiopathic, 520–523
    pain and, 5
Hyperventilation, dizziness and, 643
Hypervitaminosis A, with papilledema,
    143
Hypnotics, dizziness and, 636
Hypogammaglobulinemia, Brown's
    syndrome and, 416
Hypogenitalism, and Bardet-Biedl
    syndrome, 467
Hypogonadism, and bulbar palsy, 471
Hypoplasia, optic nerve, 119–121, *120*
    septo-optic dysplasia, 121, *121*
    true aplasia, 121
Hypotension, orthostatic, dizziness and,
    643
Hypothalamic glioma
    optic chiasm, 218–222
    precocious sexual development and, 219
Hypoxia, ocular, chronic, 105
Hysteria, factitious field, 36
Hz. (Hertz). *See* Frequency, defined

I

Ibuprofen, dizziness and, 636
Idiopathic facial palsy, 306–307
Idiopathic intracranial hypertension. *See*
    Papilledema, pseudotumor cerebri
Illumination. *See also* Light
    reduced, electrophysiology test, 47
Imipramine
    dizziness from, 636
    for panic attack, 643
Immune-mediated optic neuritides, 151
Immunodeficiency
    acquired immunodeficiency syndrome,
        152
    human immunodeficiency virus, 152
    optic neuropathy, 152t
Indomethacin, dizziness and, 636

Infant. *See also* Pediatrics
    blind, 464–467
    examination of, 53
    nystagmus, 372–381
        acquired, 380–381
            secondary to visual loss, 380–381
            spasmus nutans, 381
        characteristics of, 373t
        congenital, 372–379
        lateral/manifest latent, 379–380
        nystagmus blockage syndrome, 380
        therapies for, 375t
Infective optic neuropathies, 151–154
Inflammatory optic neuropathies, 145
Influenza, facial nerve, 311
    vaccination and optic neuropathy, 151
Infranuclear disorders, eye movement,
    405–460
    abducens palsy, 409
        isolated, 411–413
    abduction deficits, causes of, 409t
    abduction palsy, isolated, diagnostic
        studies for, 412t
    Brown's syndrome, 416
    childhood, oculomotor palsies of, 426
        cranial nerve palsies, with human
            immunodeficiency virus
Infection, 436t
    cyclic oculomotor palsy, 426–427
    diabetic oculomotor palsy, 420–421
    diplopia, after ocular surgery, 454–455
    dorsal midbrain syndrome, 452–454
    dysthyroidism, 442–446
    etiology, 409–411
    fascicular lesions, 417–418
        orbital lesions, 420
    giant cell myocarditis, 455
    granulomas, corticosteroid therapy, 455
    Graves' disease, 442–446, *443, 444*
    hemorrhage, 455
    herpes zoster, 423
    infectious polyneuropathy
        acute, 423–425
        bulbar polyneuritis, *424*
        Fisher's syndrome, 424
        Guillain-Barré syndrome, 424
    interpeduncular lesions, 418–420
        cavernous sinus lesions, 420
        Horner syndrome, 420
        Parasellar syndrome, 420
    ischemic oculomotor palsy, 420–421
    Kearns-Sayre-Daroff syndrome, 446t
    lymphoma, non-Hodgkin's, 455
    mitochondrial disease, 449t
    myasthenia, 437–442
    myasthenia-like syndromes, 442

myocarditis, giant cell, 455
myotonic dystrophy, 451–452
    ocular signs of, 452t
neuroanatomy, 405–409
neuromuscular junction, disorders of,
    437t, 437–455
non-Hodgkin's lymphoma, 455
nuclear lesions, 416–417
ocular neuromyotonia, 452
oculomotor palsy, 416, 426
    causes of, 417t
    cyclic, 426–427
    painful ophthalmoplegias, combined,
        427
oculomotor synkinesis, 422–423
ophthalmoplegia, external, progressive,
    446–450
    conditions simulating, 450–451
ophthalmoplegic migraine, 425–426
orbital lesions, 427–429
orbital myositis, 455
pain, ophthalmoplegia syndromes, 428t
parasellar syndromes, 430–436
polyneuritis, bulbar, 424, *424*
polyneuropathy, infectious, acute,
    423–425
sixth nerve palsies, causes of, 409t
superior oblique paresis, causes of,
    415t
thyroid-related myopathy, 442–446
thyrotropin-releasing hormone, 445–446
Tolosa-Hunt syndrome, 429–430
trochlear palsies, 413–416
Innervation, motor anomalies, congenital,
    468–475
    synkinesis, defined, 474
Input, defined, 402
Integrator (integral, integrate), defined,
    402
Integrator leak, nystagmus, 371
Interferon therapy, ocular symptoms of,
    112
Interhemispheric connections, anatomy,
    86–88
Internuclear opthalmoplegia, 346, 348t,
    406, *408*
Interpeduncular lesions, 418–420
Intracavernous aneurysms. *See* Cavernous
    sinus, aneurysms
Intracranial hypertension, idiopathic,
    520–523
Intracranial mass lesions, and headache,
    574
Intracranial pressure, papilledema with,
    139
Intrusions, saccadic, 391–396

Iodochlorhydroxyquin, optic neuropathy and, 185
Iodoquinol, optic neuropathy and, 185
Ischemic optic neuropathy, 35, 155–169, 163t, *164*
  anterior, 137
  common, 159, *160*
  cranial arteritis and, 16
Ishihara, pseudo-isochromatic plates, 20
Island of vision model, by Traquair, 24, 26–27
Isonaizid, optic neuropathy and, 185
Isordil, transient myopia from, 549

J

Jamaican optic neuropathy, 185
Jaw claudication, cranial arteritis and, 165
Jaw-winking phenomenon, facial synkinesis, distinguishing, 321
Jeune syndrome
  pediatric, 464
  retina, 464
Joubert syndrome
  pediatric, 464
  retina, 464
Juvenile rheumatoid arthritis, Brown's syndrome and, 416

K

Kallman syndrome, and bulbar palsy, 471
Kearns-Sayre-Daroff syndrome (progressive external phthalmoplegia), 466, 446t
  in child, 467
Kepone, pseudotumor and, 14
Keratitis sicca, 68
  facial palsy and, 323
Keratoconus, monocular diplopia, 4
Kernicterus, ophthalmoplegia and, 454
Klippel-Feil syndrome
  ocular torticollis, 483
  Wildervanck cervico-oculoacoustic, symptoms in, 471
Klippel-Trenaunay-Weber syndrome, hamartoma and, 112
Krabbe's disease, 101

L

Labyrinthectomy, for Meniere's disease, 643
Labyrinthitis, dizziness and, 639–640
Lagophthalmos, 63
Latency, defined, 402
Latent nystagmus. *See* Nystagmus
Lateral geniculate nucleus
  anatomy, 83–85

magnocellular layer, 84
parvocellular layer, 84
retino-cortical visual pathway, 9
visual defects, 243
Lateral medullary syndrome
  eyelid nystagmus, 388
  nystagmus, 390
Leão's spreading depression, in migraine, 557
Leber's congenital amaurosis, 97, 464
Leber's hereditary optic neuropathy, 97, 133–135, 467, 128t, *134, 135, 136*
Leigh's disease, 99
Leprosy, facial nerve, 311
Lethal midline granuloma. *See* Wegener's disease
Leukemia
  disc swelling and, 176
  facial nerve, 315
    paresis and, 316
  optic nerve, 176
Leukodystrophy, metachromatic, 101
LHON. *See* Leber's disease
Lid. *See* Eyelid
Light adaptation, electrophysiology test, 46–47
Light-headedness, 634
Light-near dissociation syndromes, pupil, 537
Light reflex pathway, pupil, 528–531
Light stress test, 22, *22*
Linear (nonlinear), defined, 403
Lipofuscinosis, neuronal ceroid, 101, 464
Lisch's iris nodules, neurofibromatosis and, 114
Literal alexia, 269
Lithium
  nystagmus induced by, 390
  pseudotumor cerebri and, 143
logMAR optotype acuity test, 15
  chart, 11
LSD, visual hallucinations with, 277
Lupus erythematosus
  optic neuropathy and, 169
  retinal vasculitis and, 110
Lyme disease, 152
  central nervous system infection with, 437
  facial nerve, 309–310, 315
    paresis, 316
  facial palsy, 307
    Bell's palsy, distinguishing, 310
  optic neuritis and, 152
Lymphangiomas, orbital, 502, 622, 624
Lymphocytic adenohypophysitis, 232
  pregnancy and, 232

Lymphoma, 175
  non-Hodgkin's, 455
Lysergic acid. *See* LSD

M

Macropsia, 16, 281
  cerebral, 281
  retinal, 281
Macro-saccadic oscillations, 393
Macula
  anatomy, 8, 76, *34*
  central field defects and, 25
  cherry-red spot, 100, 102, 101t
  cone-rod dystrophies, 97–99, *96, 99*
  lateral geniculate projection, 83, *84*
  striate cortex projection, 85, *87*
  tests of function, 17
Macula-splitting homonymous hemianopia, 244
Macular changes, storage diseases with, 101t
Macular function, tests of, 17–21
Macular sparing, homonymous hemianopia, 17, 244
Maddox rod, test for diplopia, 56, *57*
Magnetic resonance imaging. *See specific chapters*
Magnocellular layer, lateral geniculate nucleus, 84
Magnocellularis, subnucleus, 66
Malignant glioblastoma multiforme, 227
Malingering, factitious field, 36
Malnutrition, optic neuropathy, 183, *184*
Marcus Gunn jaw-winking synkineses, 61, *63*, 474–475
Marcus Gunn pupil. *See* Pupil, afferent pupillary defect, relative
Marfan's syndrome, 107
Marijuana, visual hallucinations with, 277
Maroteaux-Lamy syndrome, 102
Maturation of vision, delayed, 467
Mechanical transducers, eye movement recording, 341
Mecholyl, pupil test, 539, 533t
Meclizine, dizziness and, 636
Median longitudinal fasciculus (MLF), 346, 405, *406, 407*
Medications. *See* Drugs
Medulla, lesions, horizontal gaze and, 346–349
Meige's syndrome, 298, 319
  blepharospasm and, 318
Melkerson-Rosenthal syndrome, facial nerve, 316, *316*
Menière's disease, dizziness and, 642–643

Menière's disease
  alcohol, elimination of, 642
  caffein, elimination of, 642
  diuretics for, 642
  labyrinthectomy, 643
  sodium restriction, 642
Meningeal carcinomatosis, 436
  facial nerve, 315
  ophthalmoplegia, 436
  optic nerve, 137
Meningioma
  ophthalmoplegia and, 433, 434
  optic chiasm, 211–215, 214
  perioptic, 174, 175
Meningitis
  cerebral blindness, 259, 260t
  with HIV infections, 436, 436t
  infectious, optic chiasm, 224
  Lyme disease and, 152
  ophthalmoplegia, 419
  optic neuropathy, 154, 155
  pachymeningitis, 155, 159
  polyneuropathies, 436
  with tuberculosis, 225
  upbeat nystagmus and, 387
Meprobamate, dizziness and, 636
Mestinon, treatment of myasthenia, 441
Metabolic storage disorders, 100–102,
    101t
  Batten-Mayou syndrome, 101
  Bielschowsky-Jansky disorder, 101
  ceroid lipofuscinoses, 101
  cherry-red spot myoclonus syndrome,
    102
  Hex A defiency, 100
  Maroteaux-Lamy syndrome, 102
  metachromatic leukodystrophy, 101
  mucopolysaccharidoses, 101
  Tay-Sachs disease, 100, 100
  Vogt Spielmeyer syndrome, 101
Metachromatic leukodystrophy, 101
Metamorphopsia, 16, 19, 282
  cerebral, 282
  retinal, 282
Metastatic disease
  cavernous sinus, 429, 435
  facial nerve, 313–314
  meninges, 436
  ophthalmoplegia and pain, 428t
  optic nerve, 175
  orbit, 504, 500t
Methanol intoxication, optic neuropathy
    and, 185
Methocarbamol, dizziness and, 636
Micromovements, eye, 339–340
Micropsia, 16, 281

cerebral, 281
convergence-accommodative, 281
retinal, 281
Microtropia, 481
Middle-ear infection, in Gradenigo
    syndrome, 410
Migraine, 5, 17, 553–587
  abdominal, 570
  accompagnée, 562
  acephalgic, 570
  attack description, 555
  aura, 555, 559t, 559–562
    visual, 279, 557, 559, 560, 561, 562
  basilar artery, 569–570
  beta-blockers, 582
  calcium channel blockers, 581–582
  cerebellar, 570
  cerebellar migraine, 570
  cerebral, 562–565
  complicated, with infarction, 562–570,
    563t
  differential diagnosis, 576–577
  dissociée, 555
  dizziness and, 643
  dysphrenic, 570
  dysphrenic migraine, 570
  equivalent, 570
  facioplegic, 570
  hallucinations, 279–280
  headache phase, 555, 556
  infarction, 562–570
  with involuntary movements, 570
  Leão's spreading depression, 557
  motion sickness and, 425
  nonsteroidal anti-inflammatory drugs,
    577
  ophthalmoplegic, 425, 425, 565–566
  optic neuropathy, 168, 109
  pathophysiology, 555–558
  pediatric, 479, 572–573
    Alice in Wonderland syndrome, 572
  postdrome, 555
  pre-headache phase, 556
  precordial, 570
  preventive therapy, 581t
  prodrome, 555
  with prolonged aura, 562–570
  prophylactic treatment, 581–583
  retina, 108–109, 566–569, 109
    clinical features, 568–569
  scintillating scotoma, 279
  serotonin antagonists, 582–583
  sumatriptan, 580–581
  termination, 555
  therapy, 577–583, 578t, 579t
  tricyclic antidepressants, 582

trigeminovascular system and headache,
    556
  vidian neuralgia and, 572
  without aura, 558t, 558–559
Migraine, dysphrenic, 570
Migraine facioplegic, 570
Millard-Gubler syndrome, 301
Miller Fisher syndrome. See Fisher
    syndrome
Mitochondrial disease with Friedreich
    ataxia, 99, 449t
  and ophthalmoplegia, 446
  and optic neuropathy, 133
  with retinal degenerations, 99
Mitral valve prolapse syndrome, 107
MLF. See Median longitudinal fasciculus
Müller's muscle, 59
Möbius syndrome
  in child, 469, 471–472, 472, 409t
  facial nerve, paresis, 294, 316, 317, 318
Monocular diplopia, 4, 55
  "ghost image," 16
Monocular metamorphopsia, 19
Monofixation syndrome, 481. See also
    Microtropia
Mononucleosis
  facial nerve, 309
  optic neuritis and, 151
Motility, normal, ocular, 51–59
  disordered, symptoms, 4–5
  range, 51–53
Motion perception, tests of, 273
Motion sensitivity, electrophysiology test,
    47
Motion sickness
  dizziness and, 643
  migraine and, 425
Motor anomalies, congenital, 468–476
  restrictive syndromes, 475–476
    Brown tendon sheath syndrome,
      475–476
    familial fibrosis syndrome, 476
Moya-moya collateralization, and disc
    culoboma, with dolochoectasia,
    123
MRI. See specific chapters
Mucoceles, sphenoidal, and optic
    neuropathy, 177, 178
Mucopolysaccharidoses, 100–101, 101t
Mucormycosis
  facial palsy, 311
  ophthalmoplegia, 428
  orbit, 501, 502
Multiple sclerosis. See also Demyelinative
    disease
  chiasm, 222

nystagmus and, 384
optic neuritis, 150
with phlebitis, retinal vasculitis and, 110
MRI, *149, 224*
Mumps
facial nerve, 311
optic neuritis and, 151
Muscle contraction headache, 574–575
Muscle-paretic nystagmus, 387–388
Muscle relaxants, dizziness and, 636
Myasthenia, 63, 437–442, *60, 438, 440,*
abduction defect, 411
edrophonium (Tensilon) test, 63
facial weakness, 314–316
superior oblique palsy and, 413
Myasthenia-like syndromes, 442
antibiotics, 442
antineoplastic agents, 442
Eaton-Lambert syndrome, 442
other pharmaceuticals, 442
toxins, 442
Myasthenic nystagmus, 387–388
Mydriasis, swinging flashlight test, *535*
Myelination, optic disc dysplasia, 119
Myocarditis, giant cell, 455
Myoclonus, 395
anoxic encephalopthay and, 395
Creutzfeldt-Jacob disease, 395
startle, 395
usage of term, 395
Myokymia, 396
facial, 321–322
superior, oblique, 395–396
Myopathic ptosis, eyelid, 63
Myopathy, ocular, thyroid-related,
442–446
Myopia, with esotropia, 482
Myositis, orbital, 428, 455
Myotonic dystrophy, 451–452, *452*
facial nerve, 315
paresis, 316
ocular signs of, 452t

N

Nalidixic acid and pseudotumor cerebri,
143
Nasopharyngeal tumors ophthalmoplegia
and, 435
Near reflex, pupil, 532
Near triad, eye movement, 338–339
Neglect dyslexia, 269
Neima acuity charts, 19
Neomycin, myasthenia-like syndrome, 442
Neoplasms
optic chiasm, 204–222
acromegaly, 209–210

choriocarcinoma, 222
craniopharyngioma, 215–218
dysgerminomas, 222
embryonal carcinoma, 222
germ cell tumor, 222
germinoma, 222
glioma, 218–222
meningioma, 211–215
mixed tumor, 222
pituitary apoplexy, 210–211
pituitary tumor, 205–209
adenoma, 205–209
Russell's diencephalic syndrome, 219
suprasellar aneurysm, 222
yolk sac tumor, 222
ophthalmoplegia and. *See* Cavernous
sinus
optic nerve
meningioma, perioptic, 174, *175*
optic glioma, 172, *173*
secondary, 175–176
orbit, diagnosis, 504, 500t
Nerves, cranial. *See specific nerves*
Neural density filter, pupillary light
response, 21
Neuralgia, 69–70
herpes zoster, 69
postherpetic, 5
Ramsey Hunt syndrome, 70
trigeminal, 5
headache, 573
Neurasthenia, 441
Neuro-degenerative syndromes, and optic
neuropathies, 135–136
Neurodevelopmental milestones, in child,
462t
Neurofibromatosis (von Recklinghausen's
disease), 114, 218
chiasmal glioma and, 218–222, 218t,
220
diencephalic syndrome (Russell), 219
hypothalamic syndromes, 218
globe pulsation, 496t
optic glioma and, 172, *173*
precocious sexual development, 219
Neuromuscular junction disorders. *See*
Myasthenia; Myasthenia-like
syndromes
Neuromyelitis, optica (Devic's disease),
223
optic chiasm, 223
optic nerve, 151
Neuromyotonia, 452
Neuronal ceroid lipofuscinosis, 101, 464
Neuroretinitis, 147, *148*
Neutral zone, defined, 403

Nifedipine, dizziness and, 636
migraine therapy, 581
Night-blindness
congenital stationary, 464
Non-Hodgkin's lymphoma, 455
Nonsteroidal anti-inflammatory drugs, for
migraine, 577
North American Symptomatic Carotid
Endarterectomy Trial, 106
NSAIDs. *See* Nonsteroidal anti-
inflammatory drugs
Null, defined, 403
Nutritional optic neuropathies, 181, 183,
184
Nystagmus, 369–391, 371t
achiasma, 390–391
acoustic neuroma, 390
albinism, 390–391
aperiodic alternating, 385
Arnold-Chiari malformation, 384
ataxic, 384
cerebellum, 391
cervical nystagmus, 387
circular, elliptic, and oblique nystagmus,
387
clockwise, 384
congenital, 464
convergence/convergence-evoked, 385
dissociated, 384
with dizziness, 635–637
downbeat nystagmus, 386–387
reading
assessment of, 270
attention and, 269
eye movements and, 269
visual loss and, 269
visual agnosia, 264–267
face perception, disorders of, 267
prosopagnosia, 266–267
Nystagmus ataxic, 384
Nystagmus fatigue, 383
Nystagmus induced, 388–390

O

Octopus Visual Field Analyser, 37–38
Octreotide, with acromegaly, 209
Ocular bobbing, 396
Ocular flutter, 394
Ocular headache, 575–576
Ocular ischemia, 105–106
Ocular motility. *See also* Eye movement
character, eye movement, 51–53
fixational movements, 52
Ocular muscles, disorders
Myasthenia. *See* myasthenia
physiology, 55, *56*

Ocular muscles, disorders (*contd.*)
  thyroid-related myopathy, 442–446, *443, 445*
Ocular pain, 68, 69t
Ocular tilt reaction, 348, *352*
Ocular torticollis, sternocleidomastoid
  muscle, fibrous shortening of, 483
Oculocephalic vascular anomalies,
  615–622
Oculomotor apraxia, 361–362, *362*
Oculomotor nerve
  anatomy, 405, *407, 408*
  neuroma, 420, *420*
Oculomotor palsy, 416–421
  aneurysm and, 418, *418*
  causes of, 417t
  of childhood, 426
  cyclic, 426–427
  diabetic, 420–421
  fascicular, 417
  interpeduncular, 418
  ischemic, 420–421
  nuclear, 416, *417*
  painful ophthalmoplegias, combined,
    427
Oculomotor synkinesis, 422–423
Oculopalatal myoclonus, 295
Oculosympathetic defects, 542–546. *See
  also* Horner syndrome
Olivopontocerebellar degeneration, 97
One-and-a-half syndrome, 348
Open loop, defined, 403
Ophthalmoplegia, external, progressive,
    446–450
  conditions simulating, 450–451
Ophthalmoplegic migraine, 425–426,
    565–566
Opsoclonus, 394–395
  adrenocorticotropic hormone, 394
  pediatric, 478
Optic atrophy
  chiasmal syndrome, 213
  with Foster Kennedy syndrome, 140
  glaucoma
    vs. non-glaucoma, 169
    normal tension, 179, *182*
  heredodegenerative, 127–136, 128t
    dominant, 129, *130, 131, 132*
    Leber, 133, *134, 135*
    recessive, 127
      complicated, 127
      simple, 127
      Wolfram syndrome, with diabetes,
        128, *129*
  with ischemic optic neuropathy, 161,
    160

pseudo-Foster Kennedy syndrome,
    161
  Jamaican optic neuropathy, 185
  with metabolic storage disorders, 100
  with neurodegenerative syndromes, 135,
    137
  with lateral geniculate lesions, 243
  with optic tract lesions, bow-tie, 242
  papilledema, and, 140, 142, *141*
  perioptic meningioma, 174, *175*
  "secondary," 142
Optic chiasm
  anatomy, 80–83, 90, *82, 84, 90*
  aneurysm and, 222
  arachnoid cyst, 225–227, *226*
  arachnoiditis, 223
  arteriography, 204
  clinical manifestations, 200–203
  colloid cyst, 225
  congenital chiasmal dysplasia, 82, 204
  cyst of Rathke's pouch, 225
  demylinative disease, 222–225, *224*
  Devic's syndrome, 223
  diencephalic syndrome, Russell's, 219
  empty sella syndrome, 233–234, *232,
    233*
  endocrine defects and, 205
  epithelial cyst, 225–227
  glioblastoma
    multiforme, malignant, 227
    of visual pathway, 221
  glioma of visual pathway, malignant,
    221
  hydrocephalus, 232, *231*
  hypothalamic glioma, 218–222
  inflammation, 222–225
  lymphocytic adenohypophysitis, 232
  lymphoma, 227, *227*
  malignant glioma of visual pathway,
    221
  meningitis, infectious, 224
  metastastic disease, 227
  neoplasms, 204–222
    with acromegaly, 209–210
    choriocarcinoma, 222
    craniopharyngioma, 215–218, *215,
      216, 217*
    dysgerminomas, 222, *223*
    embryonal carcinoma, 222
    germ cell tumor, 222
    germinoma, 222
    glioma, 218–222, 218t, *220*
    meningioma, 211–215, *214*
    mixed tumor, 222
    pituitary apoplexy, 210–211, *211, 213*
    pituitary tumors, 205–209, *207, 212*

adenomas, 205–209
    prolactinomas, 206, *207*
    bromocriptine, 206
    Russell's diencephalic syndrome, 219
    yolk sac tumor, 222
  neuroimaging procedures, 203–204,
    210, *211, 213*
  neuritis, 223
  neuromyelitis optica, 223
  optic, anatomy, 80–83
  paraneoplastic autoimmune
    demyelination, 225
  pituitary metastases, 227
  pregnancy, 232–233
  radiation therapy, complications,
    229–232, *229, 230*
  Rathke's cleft cyst, 226
  Russell's diencephalic syndrome, 219
  sarcoidosis, 224, *225*
  sphenoidal mucocele, 227–228, *228*
  trauma, 228–229, *229*
  tuberculosis, 225
  vasculitis, 169, *170*
  visual field defects, 200–203, 205, *201,
    202, 203*
  visual loss, 3
Optic disc. *See also* Ischemic optic
    neuropathy; Optic atrophy; Swollen
    disc
  anatomy, 77, 91, *78, 80*
  hypoplasia, 119, *120, 121*
    and septo-optic dysplasia, 121, *121*
  dysplasias, congenital, 118–127
    colobomas, 121, *122*
      and encephalocele, 123
    crescents, 123, *122, 125*
    hyaline bodies, 124
    pits, 121–123
    pseudopapilledema, 124
  hyaline bodies, drusen, 124
  myelinated fibers, *122*
  papilla, usage of term, 77
  papillitis, 147, *148*
  papillopathy, diabetic, 166, *167*
Optic nerve. *See also specific entities*
  anatomy, 77–80, 91, *77, 78, 80, 81, 119*
  enlargement, 176, 177t
  neuroimaging techniques, 137
  retino-cortical visual pathway, 9
  topical diagnosis, 118, 197
  trauma and, 187–188, 523–524
  vascular supply, 157
Optic neuritis, 25, 35, 75, 148t, 145–155,
    149, 153
  causes, 148t
  contiguous inflammations, 154

and demyelinative disease, 150
and HIV, 151, 152t
immune mediated, 151
infective, 151
papillitis, 147
pediatric, 467
progressive, 154
symptoms, 147
venous sheathing, 150
visual fields, 146, *146*
Optic (Geniculo-calcarine) radiations, 76, 85, 243–244
Optic tracts. *See also* Hemianopia
anatomy, 70, 241–242, 83, *83, 84*
Optical abberation, 10
Optokinetic nystagmus, 53–55, *54,* 389–390
Optokinetic reflex, 335–336
Optotypes, on acuity chart, 17
Oral contraceptives
pseudotumor cerebri and, 145
Orbit, 489–508
anatomy, 509–510, *81, 490, 491, 505, 506, 507*
diagnosis, 500–505, *500t*
Grave's disease, 500–501
inflammation, 428, 501–502, *495*
neoplasm, 504
trauma, 504–505
vascular lesions, 502–504
diagnostic procedures, 505–508
enophthalmos, 497, *497*
causes, 496t
examination, 493–500, 493t, *498*
exophthalmometry, *495*
fundus changes, 499, *499,* 500t
globe pulsation, causes, 496t
Grave's disease, *494,* 517–520
clinical features, 442–446, *443, 444, 445,* 493, 506, 517–518
lid malposition, 60, *61, 494,* 519–520
orbital decompression, 518–519
history taking, 489–493, 492t
lesions, 427–429, 500t
mucormycosis. *See* Mucormycosis
myositis, 455
orbitotomy, 511–516
anterior, 511–514
lateral, 514–516
superior craniotomy, 516
pseudotumor. *See* Orbit, diagnosis, inflammation
postoperative management, 516–517
complications, 517
recovery room, 516
pre-operative management, 510–511

proptosis, 492–493, 496, *492*
surgery, 509–526
nerve sheath decompression, for pseudotumor cerebri, 520–523
traumatic optic neuropathy, 523
trauma, 504
vascular anomalies, 622–625
lesions, 502–504
Orbito-cranial injuries, optic neuropathy, 187–188, 523–524
Orbitopathies, optic nerve and, 178–179
Orbitotomy. *See* Orbit, orbitotomy
Organophosphate poisoning, upbeat nystagmus and, 387
Orphenidrine, dizziness, 636
Orthostatic hypotension, dizziness and, 643
Oscillations, saccadic, 391–396
Oscillopsia, 634–635
Osteopetrosis
pediatric, 464
retina, 464
Otitis media, facial paralysis and, 308
Gradenigo syndrome, 308
papilledema and, 145
Otoliths
dizziness and, 633
vestibular system, 633
Output, defined, 403

P

Pachymeningitis. *See* Meningitis
Paget's disease, with papilledema, 143
Pain, 5–6, 64–70, 69t
angle-closure glaucoma, 3
cranial arteritis, 3, 573
dry eye syndrome, 68
facial, atypical, 68–70
headache syndromes, 553–583
herpes zoster, 5
ophthalmoplegia syndromes, 427, 427t, 428t
postherpetic neuralgia, 5, 69
reflex tearing, 68
trigeminal neuralgia, 5, 69
Palinopsia, 275-276
achromatopsia and, 276
Capgrass syndrome and, 276
causes of, 276t
hallucinogens, 278
hyperglycemia and, 276
prosopagnosia and, 276
topographagnosia, 276
Palsies. *See specific nerve*
Panic attack
dizziness and, 643

imipramine for, 643
Papilla, usage of term, 77
Papilledema, 138, 139–142, 139t
conditions associated with, 143t
pseudotumor cerebri syndrome, 142
idiopathic intracranial hypertension, 143–145, 143t
pediatric, 479
secondary, 145
oral contraceptives, 145
venous sinus thrombosis, 145
Papillitis, 147, *148,* 151
Papillophlebitis, 110
Paraflocculi, ventral, of brain, eye movement control and, 353
Paranasal sinus disease
anatomy. *See* Orbit, anatomy
and optic neuropathy, 176
Paraneoplastic syndromes
ocular flutter, 394
optic chiasm, 225
retina (CAR), 112
Parasellar syndrome, 420, 430–436
and retina (CAR), 112
Parinaud syndrome (Dorsal midbrain), 60, 53, 351, 452, *453,* 548
Paralytic strabismus, 57
Paramedian pontine reticular formation (PPRF), 348, 357, 359, *347*
Parkinson's disease, 319, 362–363
blepharospasm, 318
gaze palsy, 352
motion sensitivity and, 47
square-wave jerk/oscillations, 392
visual hallucinations with, 277
Paroxysmal positional vertigo, benign, 640
Parry-Romberg syndrome, 315
Parvocellular layer, lateral geniculate nucleus, 84
Pattern ERG. *See* ERG
Pattern visual evoked potential. *See* Visual evoked potential
Pediatrics, 461–487
accommodative effort syndrome, 483
achromatopsia, 464
acquired visual loss in childhood, 467
adrenoleukodystrophy, neonatal, 464
Aicardi's syndrome, 467
gliomas, 467
blind infant, 464–467
cerebral blindness, 259
convergence insufficiencies, 482–483
delayed maturation of vision, 467
dyslexia, 478
esotropia
acquired, 482

Pediatrics, esotropia (contd.)
  acute comitant, 482
  cyclic, 482
  progressive, with myopia, 482
exotropic deviation, 479
fusional mechanisms, failure of,
      480–482
  acquired central defects, 480–481
  congenital anomalies, 481
  convergence insufficiency, 481
  microtropia, 481
gliomas, 172, 218–222, 467
headache, 479
  migraine, 479
  pseudotumor cerebri, 479
Heimann-Bielschowsky phenomenon,
      477
hypertropia deviation, 479
Jeune syndrome, 464
Joubert syndrome, 464
Leber's congenital amaurosis, 464
Leber's hereditary optic neuropathy, 467
migraine, 572–573
motor anomalies, congenital, 468–476
  innervation, 468–475
    Duane retraction syndrome,
        468–471
    Duane syndrome, 474
    elevator deficiencies, 472–474
    Marcus Gunn jaw-winking
        synkineses, 474–475
    Mobius syndrome, 471–472, 472
    synergistic divergence, 474
    synkinesis, defined, 474
    vertical retraction syndrome, 474
  restrictive syndromes, 475–476
    Brown tendon sheath syndrome,
        475–476
    familial fibrosis syndrome, 476
  vertical eye movement anomalies,
      472
neurodevelopmental milestones, 462t
neuronal ceroid lipofuscinosis, 464
night-blindness, stationary, congenital,
      464
nystagmus, 476–478
  congenital, 464, 476–477
  latent, 477
  periodic alternating, 477
  spasmus mutans, 219, 381, 478
ocular flutter, 478
ocular motor apraxia, congenital,
      477–478
ocular motor cranial neuropathies, 479
opsoclonus, 478
optic neuritis, 467

osteopetrosis, 464
patient encounter, 461–463
precocious puberty, 219
Refsum's disease, 464
sensory, strabismic abnormalities,
      479–483
sensory correspondence, 480
spasmus nutans, 219, 381, 478
strabismic amblyopia, 480
torticollis, 483
vision testing in children, 29, 29t, 30,
      53, 53, 463t
visual development, 463–464
  magnocellular pathways, 463
  parvicellular, 463
visual developmental, milestones, 463t
Peduncular hallucinations, 280–281
Pelli-Robinson chart, to measure visual
      acuity, 11, 19
Pendular nystagmus, acquired, 381
Penicillamine, myasthenia-like symptoms
      with, 442
Perilymphatic fistula, dizziness and,
      643–644
Perimetry, 23–42
  automated static threshold, 37–40
  static threshold, automated, 37–40
  visual field testing, 36
Perineuritis, 154
Periodic alternating nystagmus (PAN),
      385–386
Perseveration, visual, 274–276
Phakomatoses, 113
Phenothiazine, nystagmus induced by, 390
Phenytoin, dizziness from, 636
Phlebitis (Papillophlebitis)
  multiple sclerosis with, retina, 110
  retinal vasculitis and, 110
Phonologic dyslexia, 270
Phosphenes, 2
Photoreceptor cells, in retina, 8
Photostress test, 21–23
Phycomycoses. See Mucormycosis
Pick's sign, lid nystagmus, 63
Pickwickian syndrome, pseudotumor
      cerebri and, 145
Pigmentary retinopathies, 97–99, 98, 99.
      See also Leber's congenital
      amaurosis
Pinealomas, Parinaud syndrome, 453
Pits, of optic disc, 121–123, 122
Pituitary apoplexy, 210–211, 213
Pituitary metastases, and optic chiasm,
      227
Pituitary tumors, 205–209
Plant (plant dynamics), defined, 403

Plasticity, eye movement, 332–333
Polio, facial nerve, 311, 315–316
Polyarteritis nodosa
  retinal vasculitis and, 110
Polycythemia, with papilledema,
      intracranial pressure, 143
Polymyalgia rheumatica, cranial arteritis
      and, 163
Polymyositis
  retinal vasculitis and, 110
Polyneuropathy (polyneuritis), infectious,
      424–425
  acute, 423–425
  bulbar polyneuritis, 424
  facial palsy, 308
  Fisher syndrome, 424, 427
  Guillain-Barré syndrome, 424
Polyopia, 55, 276
Polypeptides, myasthenia-like symptoms
      with, 442
Polyradiculopathy. See Polyneuropathy
Pontine paramedian reticular formation
      (PPRF). See Eye movement,
      supranuclear disorders
Porphyria
  facial nerve, 314, 315, 316
Port-wine angioma, with Sturge-Weber
      syndrome, 617, 617
Position error, defined, 403
Positional nystagmus, 388–389, 389t
Posturography, dizziness, 638
Precocious sexual development,
      hypothalamic glioma and, 219
Pregnancy
  lymphocytic adenohypophysitis, 232
  optic chiasm, 232–233
Prochlorperazine, transient myopia from,
      549
Progressive external ophthalmoplegia,
      446–450
Progressive supranuclear palsy, 351, 392
Prolactinomes, 205
Promethazine (phenergan), transient
      myopia from, 549
Prophylactic treatment, migraine, 581–583
Proptosis. See Exophthalmos
Prosopagnosia, 276
Prosopagnosia, anterograde 267
Prozosine, dizziness and, 636
Pseudo-isochromatic plates, 20
Pseudoglaucoma, 169
Pseudoneuritis, optic disc, 124
Pseudopapilledema, 124–127
Pseudotumor cerebri. See Papilledema
Pseudotumor orbit. See Orbit,
      inflammations

Psychic paralysis of gaze, 270
Ptosis, 61–63, 61t. *See also* Eyelid
  with Grave's disease, 493
Pulfrich's phenomenon, 147
Pulse, defined, 403
Pulse-step, defined, 403
Pulseless disease
  disc swelling and, 169
  retinal arterial occlusion, 107
Pupil, 527–552
  abnormal, 532–548, 533t
  accommodation, disorders of, 548–549
  afferent pupillary defect, relative, 17,
    21, 533–536, *534, 535*
  in Alzheimer's disease, 542
  anatomy, 528–532
    accommodation, 532
    light reflex pathway, 528–531, *528*
    near reflex, 532
    ocular sympathetic pathways,
      531–532, *531*
  anisocoria, essential, 538–539, *538, 539*
  Argyll Robertson pupil, *536,* 536–537,
    536t
    characteristics of, 536t
  episodic dysfunction, 547–548
  hippus, 527
  Horner syndrome. *See*
    Oculosympathetic defects
  light-near dissociation syndromes, 537,
    537
  mydriasis, swinging flashlight test, *535*
  near reflex, 532
  oculosympathetic defects, 542–546
    abducens palsy and, 544, *545*
    carotid artery dissection and, 544
  pharmacologic accidents, 546–547,
    547
  springing, 547
  swinging flashlight test, afferent pupil
    defect, *534*
  tadpole, 547
  tonic pupil syndrome, 539–541, 538t,
    540, 541
Pupillary light response, 21
  Marcus Gunn pupil, 21
  neural density filter, 21
  photostress test, 22
  relative afferent pupillary defect, 21
  strabismus, 21
  swinging flashlight test, 21
Pursuit, eye movement, 333

Q

Quadrantanopia, 245, *251, 29*
  and Kestenbaum vertex sign, 102

Quinidine therapy, ocular symptoms of,
  112
Quinine, dizziness from, 636

R

Racemose hemangiomas of retina,
    thalamus, and midbrain, 619–620
Radiation therapy (radionecrosis)
  complications, optic chiasm, 229–232
  optic nerve and, 188
Ramp, defined, 403
Ramsay Hunt syndrome, 70, 307–308
RAPD. *See* Relative afferent pupillary
    defect
Rathke's cleft cyst, 226
Rathke's pouch, cyst of, 225
Reading. *See also* Acuity
  in alexia, 278
  assessment of, 270
  attention and, 269
  eye movements and, 269
  visual loss and, 269
Rebound nystagmus, 387
  Creutzfeldt-Jakob disease, 387
Recording techniques, eye movement,
    340–343
  afterimages, 340–341
  contact lens, 342
  corneal reflection, 341
  electro-oculography, 342
  electromagnetic search coil, 342
  mechanical transducers, 341
  ocular electromyography, 343
  photoelectric oculography, 342
  photography, 341
  video, 342–343
Recovery nystagmus, 382
Rectilinear, defined, 403
Reflex tearing, 68
Refsum's disease 99, 464
Regan, Neima charts, 19
Relative afferent pupillary defect (RAPD).
    See Pupil, afferent pupillary defect,
    relative
Release hallucinations, 278
  Charles Bonnet syndrome, 277–278
Restrictive syndromes, pediatric, 475–476
  Brown tendon sheath syndrome,
    475–476
  familial fibrosis syndrome, 476
Retina, 8–10
  abiotrophies, 97–99
  acute zonal occult outer retinopathy, 96
  anatomy, 76–77
  cone-rod dystrophy, 97–99
  diagnoses 95–17

diagnosis, 95–117
  acquired immunodeficiency
    syndrome, 111
  arterial occlusion, 102–109
    amaurosis fugar, 102, 103
    Barlow's syndrome, 107
    carotid atheromatous disease,
      102–107, 104t
    chronic ocular hypoxia, 105
    Ehler-Danlos syndrome, 107
    factor V Leiden, 108
    fibromuscular dysplasia, 107
    Marfan's syndrome, 107
    pulseless disease, 107
    transient obscuration of vision,
      104t
    venous stasis retinopathy, 105
  cardiac glycosides, 112
  chorio-retinal inflammation, 99–100
  cone-rod dystrophies, 97–99
  congenital hamartoma syndromes,
    112–114
    neurofibromatosis, 114
    tuberous sclerosis, 113–114
  constricted field, with retained acuity,
    97t
  heredodegenerations, 97–99
  human immunodeficiency virus
    infection, 111
  Leber's congenital amaurosis, 97
  macular changes, storage diseases
    with, 101t
  metabolic storage disorders, 100–102
  migraine, 108–109
  monocular visual deficit, temporal
    profile, 96
  pigmentary retinopathies, 97
  rod, monochromatism, 99
  toxic retinopathies, 111–112
  uveo-meningeal syndromes, 110–111,
    111t
  vasculitis, 109–110
    autoimmune vasculitis without
      systemic disease, 110
    Behçet's disease, 110
    dermatomyositis, 110
    Goodpasture syndrome, 110
    lupus erythematosus, 110
    multiple sclerosis with phlebitis, 110
    polyarteritis nodosa, 110
    polymyositis, 110
    sarcoidosis, 110
    ulcerative colitis, 110
    Wegener's syndrome, 110
    Whipple's disease, 110
  vein occlusion, 108

Jeune syndrome, 464
Joubert syndrome, 464
macropsia, 281
metamorphopsia, 282
micropsia, 281
migraine, 108–109, 566–569
    clinical features, 568–569
multifocal retinitis, 100
osteopetrosis, 464
photoreceptor cells, 8
receptive fields, 8
Refsum's disease, 464
retino-cortical visual pathway, 9
Retinal arterial occlusion. See Retina,
        diagnoses, arterial occlusion
Retinal-slip velocity, defined, 403
Retinal vein occlusion, 108
Retinal venous sheathing, with optic
        neuritis, 150
Retinitis pigmentosa, 97
    motion sensitivity and, 47
    nystagmus with, 384
Retinocerebellar angiomatosis (von
        Hippel-Lindau disease), 615–617
Retinol therapy, ocular symptoms of, 112
Retinopathies, toxic, 111–112
Retinotopic organization, sensory system,
        89–91
Retro-bulbar arachnoid cysts, 123
Retro-bulbar infarction, disc swelling and,
        168
Retro-bulbar neuritis, 137
Retrochiasmal visual pathways, 239–290
Rheumatoid arthritis
    disc swelling and, 169
    juvenile, Brown's syndrome and, 416
Riley-Day syndrome, pupillotonia with,
        541
Romberg test, dizziness, 637, 638
Rotary chair, dizziness, 638
Rotary nystagmus, 384
Rotational nystagmus, 388
Rubella, neuritis and, 151
Rubeola, neuritis and, 151
Russell's diencephalic syndrome
    glioma and, 219
    optic chiasm, 219

S
Saccade, 329–333
    defined, 403
Saccadic intrusions, oscillations, 391–396
    bobbing, 396
    characteristics of, 393t
    dipping, 396
    double saccadic pulses, 394

dysmetria, 394
    flutter, 394
    macro-saccadic oscillations, 393
    myoclonus, 395
    myokymia, superior, oblique, 395–396
    opsoclonus, 394–395
    saccadic pulses/pulse trains, 393–394
    square-wave jerk/oscillations, 392
    square-wave pulses, 392–393
    voluntary "nystagmus," 396
Saccadic oscillations, 391–396
Saccadic palsy, congenital, 361
Saccadic pulses/pulse trains, 393–394
Saccular aneurysm, 591–596
Sampled data, defined, 403
Sandlfy fever, with papilledema, 143
Sarcoidosis, 154
    facial nerve, 314, 315
    facial nerve paresis and, 316
    optic neuritis and, 154
    optic chiasm, 224
    retina, 110
Schilder's disease, with papilledema, 143
Schizophrinia, square-wave
        jerk/oscillations, 392
Scintillating scotoma, migraine, 279
Scopolamine, dizziness and, 636
Scorpion toxin, myasthenia-like symptoms
        with, 442
Scotoma, 16, 23, 32
    syndromes, central, 185–187
    Uhthoff's phenomenon, 3
See-saw nystagmus, 384–385
Seizures
    dizziness, 644
    visual, 278–279
Semicircular canals, 631, 632
    dizziness, 632–633
    vestibular system, 632–633
Sensory correspondence, usage of term,
        480
Septo-optic dysplasia, 121, 464, 121
    nystagmus, 384
Serotonin antagonists, migraine, 582–583
Sheridan-Gardner acuity test, 18
Sickle cell disease, disc swelling and, 169
Signal, defined, 403
Simultagnosia
Sine wave grating, 13, 19
Sinusoidal, defined, 403
Sixth nerve palsy. See Adducens palsy
Sjogren's syndrome, optic neuropathy and,
        169
Slow eye movement, 333–336
Smooth pursuit vestibulo-ocular reflex
        cancellation, dizziness, 635

Snellen chart, to measure visual acuity,
        11–12
Snellen letter visual acuity testing, 17
Sonography. See Ultrasonography
Spasm, hemifacial, 319–320
Spasmus nutans, 381
    glioma and, 219
    pediatric, 478
Spasticity of conjugate gaze, 58–59
Sphenoidal mucocele, optic chiasm,
        227–228
Spider toxin, myasthenia-like symptoms
        with, 442
Spinning inside of head, as symptom, 634
Spinocerebellar degenerations, 97
    downbeat nystagmus and, 386
Spread of comitance, diplopia and, 57
Springing pupil, 547
Square-wave jerk/oscillations, 392
    Parkinson's disease, 392
    progressive supranuclear palsy, 392
    schizophrinia, 392
Square-wave pulses, 392–393
Stabilization, ocular, 51–52
Stance, dizziness and, 637–638
Startle myoclonus, 395
Static threshold perimetry, automated,
        37–40
Stationary night-blindness, congenital, 464
Step, defined, 403
Step-ramp, defined, 403
Stereopsis, 23
Sternocleidomastoid muscle, and ocular
        torticollis, 483
Strabismic abnormalities, pediatric,
        479–483
Strabismic amblyopia, 480
Strabismus, pupillary light response, 21
Strabismus, surgery for nystagmus, 477
Streptomycin
Superior colliculus, build-up neurons, 358
    disequilibrium from, 635
    dizziness from, 636
Striate cortex, 244
Stroke
    with clinical features of migraine, 563
    with features of migraine, 563
    with migraine, 563
    migraine-induced, 563
    migraine-related, classification of, 563t
Sturge-Weber syndrome. See
        Encephalotrigeminal angiomatosis
Subnucleus magnocellularis, 66
Subsystem synergism, eye movement, 337
Sulfa-derived drugs, transient myopia
        from, 549

Sumatriptan, migraine, 580–581
Superior oblique paresis. *See* Trochlear palsies
Supranuclear disorders, eye movement and, 345–368
  brain stem, saccade circuits, cortical projections, 357–358
  candate nucleus, saccade, 358
  cerebellum
    influences, 353–355
    lesions
      effects of, 354
      ocular motor disorders caused by, 353t
    vascular syndromes of, 354–355
  cerebral control, eye movements, 355–363
  collicular-burst neurons, 358
  colliculus, superior, 358–359
  frontal eye fields, saccade generation, 357
  frontoparietal lesions, acute, bilateral, ocular motor apraxia, 361–362
  gaze
    functional disturbances of, 363
    holding, 360
  hemispheric lesions, unilateral, disturbances of gaze with, 360–361
  horizontal gaze, brain stem control, 346–349
    internuclear ophthalmoplegia, causes of, 347t
    motor commands, conjugate horizontal movements, 346
    pons, lesions, horizontal gaze and, 346–349
    saccades, slow, causes of, 347t
  Huntington disease, 363
  oculomotor apraxia, congenital, 361
  parietal eye fields, saccade generation, 356
  Parkinson disease, 362–363
  prefrontal cortex, dorsolateral, saccade generation, 357
  pursuit system, 359–360
  saccade
    generation, cortical areas, 355–357
    roles, 355
  saccadic palsy, congenital, 361
  saccadic system, 355–357
  substantia nigra pars reticulata, 358
  supplemental eye fields, saccade generation, 357
  vergence eye movements, brain stem control, 352–353
    disorders, 353

divergence paresis, paralysis, 353
motor commands, 352–353
spasm of near reflex, 353
vertical movements, brain stem connections, 349–352
  dorsal midbrain syndrome, 351
  midbrain lesions, 350
  skew deviation, 351
  supranuclear palsy, progressive, 351–352
  sustained vertical deviations, 350–351
  vestibulo-ocular system, 360
  Wallenberg syndrome, 354
Supranuclear palsy, progressive 450, *450*
  square-wave jerk/oscillations, 392
  Whipple disease, differentiated, 352
Suprasellar aneurysm, and optic chiasm, 222
Surface dyslexia, 270
Susac syndrome, 110
Sweating, gustatory, 321
Swimming inside of head, as symptom, 634
Swinging flashlight test, 21
  afferent pupil defect, *534*
Swollen disc
  diagnosis, 138–139
  etiology, 138t
Sympathetic pathways, pupil, 531–532
Symptoms, visual, 16–17
  blurring, 16
  color
    faded, 16
    shades of, darker, 16
  elucidation of, 1–6
  "ghost image," 16
  hemianopsia, *17*
  macropsia, 16
  macular sparing, 17
  metamorphopsia, 16
  micropsia, 16
Synergistic divergence, pediatric, 474
Synkinesis
  defined, 474
  facial, 305–306, 320–321
  oculomotor, 422–423
Syphilis, 152
  cross-reactivity with Lyme disease, 310
  facial palsy and, 307, 311
  perineuritis, 152
  and ureomeningeal syndrome, 111
Syringomyelia, with papilledema, 143
Systemic lupus erythematosus, Brown's syndrome and, 416
  optic neuropathy and, 151, 169, *170*

T
Takayasu's disease, 107. *See also* Pulseless disease
Tamoxifen therapy, ocular symptoms of, 112
Tangent screen
  chiasmal syndrome, 35
  homonymous hemianopsia, 35
  ischemic optic neuropathy, 35
  optic neuritis, 35
  visual field testing, 32–36
Tapetoretinal degeneration, 97–99, 467
Target, defined, 403
Taste, evaluation in facial palsy, 304
Tay-Sachs disease, 100, *100,* 101t
Tears, tearing, defects, 68–69
  crocodile. *See* Gustatory tearing
  function, and facial nerve, 304
Teller acuity card testing, 452
Temporal arteritis. *See* Cranial arteritis
Tensilon test, 62, *438, 440*
Tension headache, 574
Terminal, video, effect on vision, 2
Terosine, dizziness and, 636
Terson syndrome, 590, *591*
Tetanus, facial nerve and, 311
Tetracycline
  with papilledema, 143
  transient myopia from, 549
Tetrahydrocannabinol, and hallucinations, 27
Thalamus, disturbances of eye movements, 357
Thermal burns, and optic neuropathy, 188
Thiamine, deficiency, and optic neuropathy, 183. *See also* B-complex vitamins
Thymoma, myasthenia with, 437
Thyroid-gland
  autonomous, 445
  myopathy, 442–446. *See also* Graves' disease
Thyroid myopathy, 429
Thyrotoxicosis, with papilledema, 143
Thyrotropin-releasing hormone, 445–446
TIA. *See* Transient ischemic attacks
Tiapride, hallucinations with, 278
Tic douloureux, 573
Tick toxin, myasthenia-like symptoms with, 442
Time constant, defined, 403
Tobacco, nystagmus induced by, 390
Tobacco-alcohol amblyopia, 183–185
Tobramycin
  disequilibrium from, 635
  dizziness and, 636

Todd's paralysis, 319
Tolosa-Hunt syndrome, 429–430
   Hashimoto's thyroiditis, 430
   headache with, 576
   Wegener granulomatosis and, 430
Tonic pupil syndrome. *See* Pupil
Topographagnosia, 276
Torsional eye movements, brain stem
   connections, 349–352
Torsional nystagmus, 384
Torticollis, pediatric, 483
Toxacara canis, and optic neuropathy 154
Toxic optic neuropathy, 25
Toxins, 185
   nystagmus from, 390
   optic neuropathies, 181
   retinopathies, 111–112
Toxoplasmosis
   central nervous system infection with,
      436
   ophthalmyoplegia with, 427
Tracts, optic. *See* Optic tracts
Trajectory, defined, 403
Tranquilizers, nystagmus induced by,
   390
Tranquillizers, dizziness and, 636
Transfer function, defined, 403
Transient cerebral blindness, 259
   post-traumatic, 259
Transient ischemic attacks. *See also*
   Amaurosis fugax
   dizziness and, 644
Transient obscuration of vision, 104t
Traquair, island of vision model, 24,
   26–27
Trauma
   aneurysm, 597
   facial nerve, 311
   head, dizziness and, 642
   optic chiasm, 228–229
   optic neuropathy, 187–188, 523–524
   orbit, diagnosis, 504–505
Treacher Collins syndrome, 62
TRH. *See* Thyrotropin-releasing hormone
Triazolam, dizziness and, 636
Trichromacy, anomalous, 14
Trichromatic color, 14
Tricyclic antidepressants, migraine, 582
Trigeminal nerve, 64–67, *64, 68*
   afferents, peripheral, 66
   ascending pathways, 66–67
   function, clinical evaluation, 67
   neuralgia, 5, 573
   neuropathy, 70
   sensory complex, 64–66
Trigeminovascular system, migraine, 556

Tritan color defect, 15, dominant optic
   atrophy and, 130, *131*
Trochlear palsy, 413–416
   Graves' disease, 413
   myasthenia and, 413
Tuberculosis
   facial nerve, 311
   meningitis and, 225
   optic chiasm, 225
Tuberous sclerosis, retina, 112–114, *113*
Tubular field defects, 97, 97t
Tumor. *See under specific type*

U

Uhthoff's phenomenon, 3, 147
Ulcerative colitis
   retinal vasculitis and, 110
Ultrasonography
   and arterio-venous list, 504
   and Graves' disease, 444, *445*
   and optic nerve disease, 138, 139,
   142,
   and orbital disease, 429, 506, 507
Upbeat nystagmus, 387
   meningitis and, 387
   organophosphate poisoning, 387
   Wernicke's encephalopathy and, 387
Uveo-meningeal syndromes, 110–111
   retina, 110–111, 111t

V

Valsalva maneuver. *See* Orbit
Vascular compression, 179–181
Vascular anatomy. *See specific structure*
Vascular lesions. *See specific structure*
Vascular system, visual pathways, 91–92
Vasculitis
   autoimmune vasculitis without systemic
      disease, 110
   Behçet's disease, 110
   dermatomyositis, 110
   Goodpasture's syndrome, 110
   lupus erythematosus, 110
   multiple sclerosis with phlebitis, 110
   optic neuropathy, 151, *170*
   polymyositis, 110
   retina, 109–110
   sarcoidosis, 110
   ulcerative, colitis, 110
   Wegener's syndrome, 110
   Whipple's disease, 110
Vein occlusion, retina, 108
Velocity, retinal-slip, defined, 403
Velocity error, defined, 403
Venous sheathing, with optic neuritis,
   demyelination and, 150

Venous sinus thrombosis, and
   pseudotumor cerebri, 145
Venous stasis retinopathy, 105
Venous varix, lymphangioma. *See* Orbit,
   vascular anomalies
Verapamil, and migraine therapy, 581
   dizziness and, 636
Vergence eye movements, 337, 352–355
Vernier alignment, 12
Vertical eye movement. *See also* Parinaud
   syndrome
   disorders, 349–352, 472
Vertical retraction syndrome, 474
Vertigo, 634. *See also* Dizziness
   paroxysmal positional, benign, 640
Vestibular dynamic visual acuity test, 635
Vestibular neuritis, dizziness and, 639–640
Vestibular nystagmus, 383t
Vestibular suppressants, dizziness and, 636
Vestibular system, 629–645
   disorder. *See* Dizziness
   otoliths, 633
   semicircular canals, 632–633
Vestibular tone imbalance, nystagmus,
   370–371
Vestibulo-ocular reflex, 334–335, *352,* 360
   dizziness, 635
Video display terminal, effect on vision, 2
Vidian neuralgia, migraine and, 572
Vincristine, visual hallucinations with, 277
Vistech wall chart, 20
Visual acuity, 10–12, 17–19
   optical abberation, 10
   Pelli-Robson chart, 11
   Snellen chart, 11–12
Visual acuity testing
   central scotoma, 18
   fractional notation, 18
   Sheridan-Gardner test, 18
Visual agnosia, 264–267
   face perception, disorders of, 267
   prosopagnosia, 266–267
Visual association areas, anatomy, 86–88
Visual cortex. *See* Cortex, occipital,
   anatomy
Visual development, 463–464
   magnocellular pathways, 463
   milestones, 463t
   parvicellular, 463
Visual evoked potential, 15, 45, *46*
Visual field, 23–42
   anatomy, 23–26
   automated interpretation, 40–42
      reliability index, 40–42
         blue-on-yellow stimulus, 42
         color perimetry, 42

corrected loss variance, 41
deviation, empiric probability and, 41
false-positive response, 41
fixation losses, 40–41
global visual field index, 41
loss variance, 41
mean defect, 41
mean sensitivity, 41
clinical testing, 27–42
automated static threshold perimetry, 37–40
automated visual field interpretation, 40–42
cartography, 40
clinical perimetry, 36
color comparison, 31–32
confrontation methods, 27–28
corrected loss variance, 41
deviation, 41
factitious fields, 36
false-negative responses, 41
false-positive responses, 41
finger counting, 29
finger mimicking, 29
fixation losses, 40
global visual field indices, 41
Goldmann kinetic perimetry, 36–37
graphic display, 40
gray-scale symbols, 40
hand comparison, 29–31
loss variance, 41
mean defect, 41
mean sensitivity, 41
numeric display, 40
probability maps, 40
reliability indices, 40
short-term fluctuation, 41
tangent screen, 32–36
visually elicited eye movements, 29
defects, 248–254
defined, 23
empiric probability maps, 41
interpretation, automated, 40–42
physiology, 26–27
differential light sensitivity, 26
suprathreshold static perimetry, 27
Visual function, neuro-ophthalmic evaluation, 15–23
binocular function, 23
color vision, 20–21
contrast sensitivity, 19–20
graphs, 19
foveal function, tests of, 17–21

macular function, tests of, 17–21
metamorphopsia, 19
optotypes, 17
photostress test, 21–23, 22
pupillary light response, 21, 528, 533
in coma, 72t
swinging flashlight test, 21
stereopsis, 23
symptoms, 16–17
blurring, 16
color
darker, 16
faded, 16
"ghost image," 16
hemianopsia, 17
macropsia, 16
macular sparing, 17
metamorphopsia, 16
micropsia, 16
visual acuity, 17–19
Visual hallucinations, 276–281
Visual pathways. See specific structures
Visual pathways, sensory physiology of, 8–15
color vision, 14–15
anomaloscope, 14
color vision, trichromacy, 14
trichromacy, anomalous, 14
contrast sensitivity, 12–13
function, 13
retina, 8–10
ganglion cells, 8–9
on/off dichotomy, 8–9
parallel visual pathways, 9–10
magnocellular parallel pathways, 9–10
on-, off-pathways, 9
parvicellular parallel pathways, 9–10
receptive fields, 8
retino-cortical visual pathway, 9
visual acuity, 10–12
visual cortex, magnification factor, 10
Visual radiations. See Optic (Genizulo-calcarine) radiations
Visual sensory system examination, 7–49, 3
Visual-vestibulo-ocular response, 336
Visually elicited eye movement
foveation reflex, 29
visual field testing, 29
Vitamin A intoxication, pseudotumor cerebri and, 145
Vitamin A therapy, ocular symptoms of, 112

Vitamin B deficiency, optic neuropathy and, 183
Vitamin deficiency, 183–185
thiamine, 183
Vogt-Koyanagi-Harada syndrome, 110
Vogt Spielmeyer syndrome, 101
Voluntary "nystagmus," 396
von Hippel-Lindau disease (retinocerebellar angiomatosis), 112, 615, 616
von Recklinghausen's disease. See Neurofibromatosis

W

Wallenberg syndrome, 354
medullary plate infarction syndrome, 542
midbrain lesion and, 350
Warfarin, dizziness and, 644
Wasp toxin, myasthenia-like symptoms with, 442
Weber syndrome, fascicular lesions, 417–418
WEBINO, 347
Wegener granulomatosis, 110, 177
arteritis and, 166
optic neuropathy and, 154
paranasal sinus disease and, 177
retinal vasculitis and, 110
and Tolosa-Hunt syndrome, 430
Wernicke's
alcohol ophthalmoplegia, 4
encephalopathy, upbeat nystagmus and, 386
hemianopic pupil, cerebrovisual loss and, 242
Whipple disease
progressive supranuclear palsy, differentiated, 352
retina, 110
retinal vasculitis and, 110
vertical gaze, 352
Wildervanck cervico-oculoacoustic symptoms, in child, 471
Wilson's disease, ophthalmoplegia and, 454
Wolfram's syndrome, 128, 129
Wyburn-Mason syndrome (racemose hemangiomas of retina and brain), 172, 600, 619, 621, 620, 621

Y

Yoke muscles, eye movement and, 55–56